AF672599

Operative Techniques and Recent Advances in Acute Care and Emergency Surgery

Paolo Aseni • Luciano De Carlis
Alessandro Mazzola • Antonino M. Grande
Editors

Operative Techniques and Recent Advances in Acute Care and Emergency Surgery

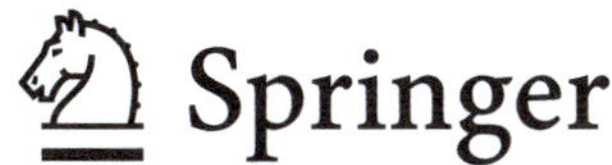

Editors
Paolo Aseni
Dipartimento di Emergenza Urgenza
ASST Grande Ospedale Metropolitano Niguarda
Milan, Milano
Italy

Luciano De Carlis
School of Medicine
University of Milano-Bicocca, Niguarda Hospital
Milan, Milano
Italy

Alessandro Mazzola
Department of Cardiac Surgery
IRCCS MultiMedica
Milan, Milano
Italy

Antonino M. Grande
Department of Cardiac Surgery
IRCCS Fondazione Policlinico San Matteo
Pavia
Italy

ISBN 978-3-319-95113-3 ISBN 978-3-319-95114-0 (eBook)
https://doi.org/10.1007/978-3-319-95114-0

Library of Congress Control Number: 2018966517

This Springer imprint is published by the registered company Springer Nature Switzerland AG
The registered company address is: Gewerbestrasse 11, 6330 Cham, Switzerland

"Ancora imparo" I'm still learning.
(Michelangelo at 87)

Foreword

Across the globe, trauma systems and approaches to the care of critically injured patients vary widely. The emerging paradigm of "acute care surgery" has provided grounds for discussion and debate in the surgical community. First, there appears to exist some confusion related to the underlying terminology. In essence, acute care surgery is defined as a service line that encompasses trauma surgery, emergency general surgery, and surgical critical care. Based on this pragmatic definition, many US surgeons argue that their European colleagues do *not* truly practice acute care surgery, as the component of surgical critical care has been largely outsourced to intensivists and anesthesiologists in European institutions. There is also an argument that many trauma centers in the United States have indeed been practicing the acute care surgery paradigm for decades, dating back to the pioneering work by John Border in the 1970s. Similarly, European countries have historically endorsed the analogy of the "combat surgeon" model which evolved in the aftermath of the Franco-Prussian War in 1870. In the twentieth century, Germany took a leadership position as a driver of integrated trauma care. This "European model" is reflective of the notion that trauma represents a disease of its own, rather than just the sum of specific injuries, and should therefore be managed by one single specialist—the trauma surgeon. The "Hannover school" founded by Harald Tscherne in the 1970s was further refined under Otmar Trentz in the 1990s who established trauma as a true scientific research-based discipline with an impressive measurable impact on the quality of trauma care and on patient outcomes. Academic institutions in Italy have recently taken a leading position in Europe by driving best practice guidelines in trauma and acute care surgery. In support of this statement, this first-edition textbook is preeminently written by Italian authors and edited by four distinguished experts from renowned institutions in Italy. The groundbreaking work provides a compelling testimonial on the current state of research and innovation in the field. This essential textbook will hopefully contribute to the prioritization and optimization of multi-disciplinary protocols and standardized processes for managing the vulnerable population of critically ill and severely injured patients. The editors have to be commended for mastering the gargantuan task of providing a compelling overview on all pertinent disciplines in trauma, acute care surgery, and emergency general surgery, by integrating these distinct entities in an elegant fashion into a new and invaluable "bible" for clinicians.

Philip F. Stahel
Rocky Vista University, College of Osteopathic Medicine
Parker, CO, USA

Ernest E. Moore
Department of Surgery
University of Colorado, School of Medicine, Denver Health Medical Center
Denver, CO, USA

Contents

Part I

General Principles

1 Surgical Education and Training for Emergency Surgery and Surgical Specialties

Antonello Forgione and Salman Y. Guraya

Key Points

- The aim of a standard surgical training program is to provide a competent surgeon, trained and assessed by an effective curriculum, who is ready for unsupervised practice.
- Several assessment tools are available in the workplace-based assessment strategy such as direct observation of procedural skills, mini-CEX, case-based discussions, and objective structured clinical examination (OSCE).
- A myriad of state-of-the-art surgical training tools is available for the trainees and senior surgeons that can serve the purpose of complementing the accredited surgical residency programs outside the OR.
- Simulation carries the promise to promote experiential learning, to secure patient safety, and to recreate scenarios that are rarely encountered and can assess the trainees' skills and competence in diverse situations.
- The mechanical box simulators are designed as boxes with objects or organs that are accessed using surgical instruments. The quality of the tactile feedback is perceived to be the same as in the OR, and the surgical performance can be monitored by trained surgeons.
- Telemedicine sweeps away distance barriers and can provide sufficient expertise to novices in remote rural areas. This innovative technology provides a high-definition profile of operative field, allows verbal communication between the mentor and mentee, and allows the trainer to point on the screen for further operative steps.

1.1 Introduction

Training and education of the surgical trainees is a dedicated, expensive, and demanding exercise that needs continuous supervision and transfer of surgical expertise in a structured fashion. This phenomenon envisages a myriad of learning tools, technologies, opportunities, and stakeholders [1]. The aim of a standard surgical training program is to provide a competent surgeon, trained and assessed by an effective curriculum, who is ready for unsupervised practice. This produce of an accredited surgical training program shall be able to function independently through an effective collaborative interprofessional practice that is known to have a positive impact on the delivery of health-care system, enhances patient satisfaction, reduces medical errors, and promotes efficiency and appropriate use of health services [2]. Such training programs must also ensure that the trainee surgeons develop the right personality, attitudes, and skills who can deliver with exceptional leadership capabilities in the high-tech operating rooms equipped with cutting-edge technologies [3, 4].

The orthodox apprenticeship approach of surgical training, where trainees would learn incidentally from their supervisors while essentially delivering service, is no longer sustainable due to major flaws such as unstructured training in a noneducational environment. Furthermore, the absence of a robust workplace-based assessment model leads to inadequate supervision of the trainees with insufficient feedback and ineffec-

A. Forgione (✉)
Niguarda Cà Granda Hospital, Milan, Italy

AIMS Academy, Milan, Italy
e-mail: antonello.forgione@ospedaleniguarda.it

S. Y. Guraya
Clinical Sciences Department, College of Medicine, University of Sharjah, Sharjah, United Arab Emirates
e-mail: sguraya@sharjah.ac.ae

P. Aseni et al. (eds.), *Operative Techniques and Recent Advances in Acute Care and Emergency Surgery*,
https://doi.org/10.1007/978-3-319-95114-0_1

tive assessment [5, 6]. Several assessment tools are available in the workplace-based assessment strategy such as direct observation of procedural skills [7], mini-CEX [8], case-based discussions [9], and objective structured clinical examination (OSCE) [10]. Of these, DOPS and OSCE carry a great potential for assessing the surgical competencies in a supervised learning environment with the possibility of immediate feedback. Traditionally, operating room has been the center-point of surgical training and has been considered as a stand-alone trusted platform for surgical education. However, in the recent past, the landscape of surgical training environment within which surgical education takes place has significantly changed due to the incorporation of ambulatory care, day-care surgery, computer-integrated surgery, concerns about patient safety, operating time, quality control, and ethical issues [11, 12].

The surgical rotations in accredited residency programs do not essentially articulate well with the career goals of the learners, ending up with less satisfied learners and suboptimal placements. In view of these shortcomings, parallel surgical training programs and modalities are needed that can bridge educational gaps within the context of skills [13]. In addition to the overarching need for adjuvant training conventions for the surgical trainees, there is also pressing need to provide surgical training opportunities to the trained and established surgeons. This urge to update the skills of surgical trainees will allow them to synchronize and modernize their skills with the evolving surgical technologies and emerging protocols. Unfortunately, there is dearth of evidence that can shed light on such surgical educational programs. In addition, the literature fails to provide a stand-alone comprehensive platform that can help the surgical trainers and trainees to fulfill their professional desire to accomplish surgical competence and to update their surgical skills. This book chapter explicitly sheds light on the current state-of-the-art modern surgical educational tools and programs with the aim to provide a precise note on merits and demerits of each modality.

1.2 Surgical Education and Training for Emergency Surgery

The sensitivity and presentation of patients in emergency room [14] necessitate instant lifesaving action plans by physicians that not only require clinical competence but also depend upon the physician's personality and character [15]. Periodic and systematic examinations have the potential to enhance the quality of patients' care and satisfaction and tend to reduce patients' stress in the ER [16]. Such unique approaches demand a multidimensional set of competencies that should be inculcated in ER physicians for developing their core skills in professional domains. These opportunities should be provided to them during the preclinical and clinical years.

The International Federation for Emergency Medicine (IFEM) has developed a 4-year structured universal standard curriculum for emergency medicine that can be conveniently embedded in the medical curricula [17]. This curriculum has been designed by an international consortium of specialists, health-care experts, and physicians and includes core domains of teaching emergency medicine to medical students. The key focus remains on improving the fundamental knowledge of clinical sciences employed in emergency medicine such as acquiring basic life-support cardiopulmonary resuscitation skills, to institute therapy of first aid for airway obstruction, to manage all types of shocks in all age groups, to administer cerebral resuscitation in brain illness and injury, to initiate basic principles of stabilization in life-threatening illness or injury, and to help the students to develop professional behavior, probity, and communication skills. The surgical components of IFEM curriculum emphasize on emergency management of trauma to all regions of the body including head and neck, chest, abdomen, musculoskeletal, vascular, urological, and dental trauma. Another body with a more precise focus on surgery, recognized as the European Society for Trauma and Emergency Surgery (ESTES), aims to advance the professional practice of emergency and trauma surgery right from the prehospital care through diagnosis, intervention, and intensive care to rehabilitation [18]. The core contents of the ESTES teaching model envisages to enable students to be competent in disaster and military surgery, emergency surgery, polytrauma and visceral surgery, and sports and skeletal trauma. In partnership with the German Society for Orthopedics and Trauma Surgery, ESTES offers a DGOU fellowship program that endeavors to provide the clinical and scientific training, medical education, and clinical exchange among the European nations.

The American College of Surgeons (ACS) offers an accredited certification as the Fellow of the American College of Surgeons (FACS) to all surgical specialties including emergency and trauma surgery [19]. The fellowship program entails submission of application and evaluation of the applicant's professional career. The grant of fellowship is based on the evaluation reports about the candidate's professional competence, ethical conduct, and surgical judgment. Since the eligibility to apply demands that the applicant should have a postgraduate certificate and should be a practicing surgeon, the FACS per se does not directly evaluate the surgical competence of the candidate; rather it relies on the feedback from supervisors and licensing bodies. It is commonly perceived that the working climate between the surgeon and his technical staff in the operating room performs optimally when this hierarchy is diligently followed by all stakeholders [20]. The Advanced Trauma Operative Management (ATOM) by ACS is an effective educational tool for enhancing surgical competence of trainees in the operative management of penetrating injuries to the abdomen and chest [21]. The ATOM course consists of six 30-min lectures followed by a 3-h lab session. The lectures entail penetrating trauma management by trauma laparotomy for injuries of the spleen and diaphragm;

liver, pancreas, and duodenum; and genitourinary and cardiovascular systems. The lab sessions consolidate the knowledge gained by theoretical sessions in the form of hands-on surgical management of the aforementioned injuries.

1.2.1 The Pitfalls and Challenges in Harmonizing a Universally Accredited Curriculum for Emergency Surgery

In the wake of scattered and non-integrated curricula and programs for emergency surgical training, there is pressing need to understand the value and place of such courses that can be embedded into MBBS curricula. On the basis of the community needs, resources, and faculty expertise, the medical educators would be able to incorporate a horizontal or, preferably, a vertical integration. For the postgraduate accredited residency programs, there is a dearth of a standard emergency surgery curriculum. The absence of an internationally acceptable program eventually deters the migration of international graduates across regions and countries due to varying contents, credit hours, and the level and depth of training they attain. A universally acknowledged curriculum for emergency surgery can be produced by an int'l consortium of field experts that can address the core contents and learning objectives across the globe.

1.3 Surgical Education and Training Tools

A myriad of state-of-the-art surgical training tools is available for the trainees and senior surgeons that can serve the purpose of complementing the accredited surgical residency programs outside the OR. The following section elaborates some of the surgical education tools and models using modern, cutting-edge technologies being used across the world.

1.3.1 Simulation-Based Surgical Tools

Literature has shown that as much as 10% of the admitted patients encounter various forms of unwanted surgical complications due to human error [22]. Unfortunately, the orthodox surgical practice of "see one, do one, teach one" approach exposes patients to inexperienced trainees that endanger patients' health and safety [23]. Henceforth, the surgical trainees can no longer rely only on human beings to attain their skills with the potential of trial and error. This necessitates the urge to explore, define, and implement versatile surgical educational models that do not jeopardize patient safety [14]. One such model implies simulation that refers to "a technique to replace or amplify real patient experiences with guided experiences, artificially contrived, that evokes or replicates substantial aspects of the real world in a fully interactive manner" [24]. Simulation carries the promise to promote experiential learning, to secure patient safety, and to recreate scenarios that are rarely encountered [25] and can assess the trainees' skills and competence in diverse situations [26].

The two most commonly used simulation-based surgical training models are described hereunder in detail.

1.3.1.1 Mechanical Simulators

The mechanical box simulators are designed as boxes with objects or organs that are accessed using surgical instruments [27]. The novice surgeons, starting to learn laparoscopic skills, can practice on synthetic materials as well as animal organs or tissues [28]. The quality of the tactile feedback is perceived to be the same as in the OR, and the surgical performance can be monitored by trained surgeons. A more refined version of commercially available mechanical box simulators is LapSim virtual reality simulator that is perceived to carry high fidelity with more precision [29].

1.3.1.2 Virtual Reality Simulators (VRS)

The VRSs facilitate the surgical trainees in developing their psychomotor skills and manual dexterity and in recreating the OR environment without supervision or time constraints. These modern surgical tools permit the learners to acquire the required skills with confidence at their own learning pace [30]. Modern VRSs such as the well-recognized MIST-VR and the newer LapSim (Surgical Science, Gothenburg Sweden) have built-in abstract graphics than can provide a high-fidelity simulation for trainees and assessors [31]. The commercially available laparoscopic VRS software replicate tasks such as grasping, cutting, and suturing, which help the trainees to acquire psychomotor skills essential to perform real-time procedures [32].

1.3.2 Video Games

There is growing evidence that video games have a positive effect on sharpening the basic laparoscopic surgical skills [33]. Apart from the numerous negative impacts of excessive game playing [34], several studies have argued that video gaming promotes spatial attention and hand-to-eye coordination [35]. The trainees invariably encounter technical challenges during laparoscopic surgery such as loss of depth perception, haptic feedback, and fulcrum effect [36]. Video games have the potential to overcome these barriers by providing a cost-effective and widely available surgical training tool for developing cognitive skills [37]. Despite these promising signals, there is currently, however, no standardized method to assess that video games are effective in transferring the desired surgical skills that are comparable to the OR experience.

1.3.3 Animal Lab Simulation

Labs using animal models provide substantial support in surgical training, education, and research. At the same time, animal labs offer a useful platform for the initial applications of innovative technique [38]. Live animal surgery remains the best training model, offering high fidelity that is unmatched by other kinds of simulation models [39]. From the medicolegal perspective, the use of animal labs is considered where no reliable alternative for surgical training and education is available. Nevertheless, in such situations, implementation of the legislative framework about 3 Rs, "Refine the procedure to limit suffering, Reduce the number of animals to a minimum, Replace the use of animals with non-animal alternatives when appropriate," should be closely adhered to [40].

1.3.4 Cadaveric Lab Simulation

Training of surgical skills on cadavers offers the best anatomy realism that can effectively prepare the trainee before working on living human beings [41]. Research has shown that surgical training on human cadaver model significantly augments reality simulation for the acquisition of laparoscopic colorectal skills. Thus, although difficult, the human cadaver model is perceived to be better acknowledged than simulators for laparoscopic sigmoid colectomy [42]. There is abundance of evidence that the simulator-based training followed by cadaver training can be conveniently integrated into surgical learning curve [43].

1.4 Mini-fellowship Surgical Training Programs

Well-crafted structured mini-fellowship surgical training programs, tailored to the needs of practicing surgeons, containing hands-on operative and clinical sessions have shown strong potential in transferring the desired laparoscopic surgical competence [44, 45]. A mini-fellowship surgical training program was successfully employed at the AIMS Academy that included telementoring sessions in the remote area of Russia [46]. The key highlights of this program reflect that, for being a competent surgeon, the acquisition of technical competence is as important as the attainment of clinical knowledge. Exploring the effectiveness of another surgical training program, Jenkins et al. studied a proficiency-based structured task-specific training model for laparoscopic colorectal surgery, and the authors have proposed that multimodality training with a modular operative approach substantially shortened the time to gain proficiency with low morbidity with an error rate of 25% [47]. Nevertheless, Simpson and Scheer have argued that all such mini-fellowship programs should have a standard set of program evaluation that can constantly evaluate its impact on trainers and trainees [48].

1.5 Preceptoring and Proctoring for Surgical Training

Preceptoring refers to the situation when an experienced surgeon scrubs with the learner to supervise the surgical procedure or is ready to intervene. In contrast, a proctor is a supervisor who monitors surgery, shares advice, and intervenes when necessary. Preceptoring is often employed before the trainee has attained the intended surgical skills for a given surgical procedure. Because of the growing concerns about the ethical and medicolegal issues, preceptoring permits training on patients while adhering to the standards set forth for patient safety [49].

1.6 Telementoring for Surgical Training

Telementoring refers to "the process of remote guidance and technical assistance to surgical procedures, utilizing telecommunication techniques" [50]. Telemedicine sweeps away distance barriers and can provide sufficient expertise to novices in remote rural areas. This innovative technology provides a high-definition profile of operative field, allows verbal communication between the mentor and mentee, and allows the trainer to point on the screen for further operative steps [51]. Since the mentoring process is not restricted by distance, the costs of formal mentoring programs may be reduced, and remote assistance can be incorporated into formal training schedule [52]. Forgione et al. developed a comprehensive theoretical and practical min-fellowship program that incorporated telementoring mode of training at the Advanced International Mini-invasive Surgery Academy at Milan, Italy [46]. A Russian surgeon, after successfully passing the required theoretical and practical sessions at AIMS, was telementored at the Northern Medical Clinical Centre Arkhangelsk Russia, about 2868 km from Milan, by experts from AIMS Academy Milan. Several other successful telementoring training events have been reported from across the world [53–55].

1.7 Telerobotic Manipulation and Assistance

By using Zeus TS micro joint system (Computer Motion Inc., Santa Barbara, CA), an expert robotic surgeon can provide telepresence for trainee surgeons in rural and

Table 1.1 Advantages and disadvantages of the commercially available surgical training models

No.	Surgical training model	Advantages	Disadvantages
1	Mechanical simulator	• Reproducible • Standardized • Training of isolated skills • Cheap	• No high fidelity • No tissue rendering
2	Virtual reality simulator	• Performance of real operations • Evaluation of isolated skills • Instant objective feedback	• Expensive • Questionable software and interface reliability
3	Animal lab	• Easy availability • Good tissue handling	• Ethical issues • Expensive
4	Cadaver lab	• High fidelity • Same anatomy (included individual variation) • No time pressure	• Ethical issues • Limited availability • Non-compliant bloodless tissues
5	Telementoring	• Exact anatomy • Realistic bleeding • Real OR setting • Independence of first operator	• Requires another surgeon throughout surgery • Expert surgeon cannot operate directly
6	Telerobotic assistance	• Exact anatomy • Realistic bleeding • Real OR setting	• Expensive • Requires another surgeon throughout surgery • Pressure of training

remote areas across the world. The telerobotic expert can guide intraoperatively at a remote site, looking at the same images as the primary surgeons, as both are located outside the surgical field [56]. Following the principles of telerobotic assistance for surgical training, Anvari et al. established the world's first remote telerobotic surgical service by connecting St Joseph's Hospital in Hamilton and North Bay General Hospital, situated about 400 km north of Hamilton. Twenty-one telerobotic laparoscopic operations were performed without any intraoperative complication. The investigators have argued that refinements in the robotic and telecommunication technology can offer a platform for routine use of the state-of-the-art laparoscopic surgical practice in rural communities that can be run by a close collaboration between surgeons in high-volume tertiary and rural hospitals.

The key features of all described surgical educational modalities along with the advantages and disadvantages are elaborated in Table 1.1.

1.8 Objective Assessment of Technical and Nontechnical Surgical Skills

1.8.1 Objective Structured Assessment of Technical Skills (OSATS)

A fundamental element of the accredited surgical training is an objective and meticulous assessment of the surgical trainee. Unfortunately, owing to variations in understanding and diverging parameters used by assessors, there has always been low validity and reliability by subjective assessment of any skill or competence. On the contrary, objective assessment follows a precise and explicit track with no room for personal judgment by the assessors. OSATS is a valuable objective assessment tool that can provide both a holistic and in-depth evaluation of open surgical skills [57]. This modality contains standard assessment forms with pre-defined criteria indicating how to score performance in the technical domain.

1.8.2 Fundamentals of Laparoscopic Surgery [58]

FLS, a joint consortium developed by SAGES and the American College of Surgeons, aims to teach and assess the knowledge, judgment, and skills inherently required for laparoscopic surgery, independent of the surgical specialty [58]. During the assessment, a physical endotrainer box simulator is used. "The optical system shows a monocular view of a series of objects that must be manipulated to perform five tasks of increasing complexity; peg transfer, cutting/dissecting, placement of a ligating loop to secure a tubular structure, and intra-corporeal or extra-corporeal knot tying" [59]. A trained proctor supervises this process and awards marks to each task. FLS offers a convenient and feasible tool for teaching laparoscopic surgery with an added advantage of being a validated assessment modality [60].

1.8.3 Fundamentals of Endoscopic Surgery [2]

Flexible endoscopy is a key component of surgical practice as surgeons perform upper and lower GI endoscopy during the preoperative work-up, intraoperative evaluation, and postoperative to identify the anatomic changes induced by surgical intervention [61]. The Society of American Gastrointestinal and Endoscopic Surgeons (SAGES) and the American Board of Surgery have jointly developed FES curriculum, a comprehensive educational tool very similar to FLS that includes Web-based didactic component of flexible endoscopy containing 12 units of teaching domains, written multiple choice exam (cognitive component), and a 5-module virtual reality skills exam (hands-on component).

1.8.4 Fundamental Skills for Robotic Surgery (FSRS)

FSRS has been validated as an effective, feasible, and structured curriculum that verifies its effectiveness by remarkable advancements in basic robotic surgery skills [62]. The system involves a simulation-based robotic curriculum that can be conveniently embedded in surgical training and educational programs.

1.8.5 Measuring Nonsurgical Skills: The Nontechnical Skills for Surgeons

Surgical educators have agreed that critical, cognitive, and interpersonal skills of surgeons significantly complement surgeons' technical abilities [63]. The Surgical Team Assessment Record (STAR) is one of the instruments that is designed to evaluate the human behaviors in the OR [64]. This scale attempts to determine the organizational, situational, team, and personal factors that might influence the surgical performance in the OR. A surgeon's intraoperative nontechnical skills are strongly correlated with the surgical outcomes, and breakdowns in surgeon's behavior in the OR negatively affect nontechnical characteristics such as teamwork, leadership, communication, confidence, and decision [65]. This emphasizes the need to embed fundamental domains of NOTSS such as communication, decision-making, situation awareness, leadership, teamwork, professionalism, and task management into the existing surgical training curricula [3, 66, 67]. Education and assessment of nontechnical skills in surgery lead to enhanced surgeons' performance in the OR that will improve quality as well as patient safety [4, 68].

Policymakers and surgical educators are increasingly incorporating virtual and e-Learning tools into the surgical training, and the distance learning arm of these modalities makes e-Learning more attractive and feasible. However, the fidelity and effectiveness of surgical educational platforms and training centers in delivering the desired skills by online video libraries and e-Learning platforms needs to be tested and validated by accrediting bodies.

1.9 Trainees' Perceptions of Surgical Education Tools and Strategies

While training the surgical residents and practicing surgeons, its customary to deeply understand the preferred resources of surgical education as desired by the learners. This understanding is driven by the fact that each learner has a distinct learning style and identification of these unique learning preferences can help trainers in improving the delivery of surgical education [69]. Guraya et al. explored the preferred learning resources of the participants attending surgical courses at the AIMS Academy during 2010 to 2013 and noted that the majority of participants (467/636; 73%) preferred "direct experience in the OR" as their favorite learning strategy, followed by "tutoring by skilled trainer" proposed by 426/636 respondents [13]. The study had concluded that surgical trainees preferred hands-on training and mini-fellowship courses for enhancement of their surgical skills.

In the later section of this article, we have described few popular surgical training centers.

1.10 State-of-the-Art Surgical Training and Education Centers

Some of the most popular surgical education and training centers, worldwide, that offer training services both in "dry and wet labs" using world-class laparoscopic instruments using theoretical as well as practical learning sessions are shown in Table 1.2. The l'Institut de Recherche contre les Cancers de l'Appareil Digestif (IRCAD) offers the opportunity to train with animals, while the UK centers use cadavers, as animal surgical training is forbidden. The AIMS Academy is a state-of-the-art training venue for hands-on surgical training along with the opportunity for in-campus and telementoring laparoscopic surgery courses and fellowship programs.

The commonly accessed online resources for surgical education and training are provided by WebSurg, SAGES Online, European Association for Endoscopic Surgery (EAES), and American Society for Gastrointestinal Endoscopy (ASGE). A host of recorded videos by field

Table 1.2 World's most popular surgical training and education centers

No.	Training center	Country
1	IRCAD[a]	Strasbourg, France Taichung, Taiwan Barretos, Brasil
2	AIMS[b]	Milan, Italy
3	Minimal Access Therapy Training Unit (MATTU) Centre	Guilford, UK
4	Cuschieri Skills Centre	Dundee, UK
5	Methodist Institute for Technology, Innovation and Education (MITIE)	Houston, USA
6	Center for the Future of Surgery	San Diego, USA
7	European Surgical Institute	Norderstedt, Germany

[a] l'Institut de Recherche contre les Cancers de l'Appareil Digestif
[b] Academy for International Minimally Invasive Surgery

experts with insightful remarks at key surgical steps along with a range of theoretical knowledge-based material make these portals extremely useful for the surgical trainees and practicing surgeons.

Conclusion

Financial constraints, quality control, and patient safety have urged the surgical educators to explore and develop more cost-effective, state-of-the-art surgical educational platforms that can be employed outside the OR. Simultaneously, the practicing senior surgeons are desired to periodically refresh and update their surgical skills that will allow them to get acquaintance with the modern surgical technologies. A myriad of cutting-edge technical innovations are now commercially available such as the simulation-based mechanical and virtual reality simulators, animal and cadaveric labs, telementoring, telerobotic-assisted surgery, and video games. The existing world-renowned surgical training centers employ various clusters of training tools that aim to embed the acquisition of surgical knowledge and technical skills. This research demands the initiation of concerted efforts in developing a blended and unified structured surgical training program that can be employed across the world.

References

1. Collins JP, Gough IR, Civil ID, Stitz RW. A new surgical education and training program. ANZ J Surg. 2007;77(7):497–501.
2. Al-Qahtani MF, Guraya SY. Measuring the attitudes of healthcare faculty members towards interprofessional education in KSA. J Taibah Univ Med Sci. 2016;11(6):586–93.
3. Khoshhal KI, Guraya SY. Leaders produce leaders and managers produce followers: a systematic review of the desired competencies and standard settings for physicians' leadership. Saudi Med J. 2016;37(10):1061.
4. Cuschieri A. Lest we forget the surgeon. Surg Innov. 2003; 10(3):141–8.
5. Guraya SY. Workplace-based assessment; applications and educational impact. Malays J Med Sci. 2015;22(6):5–10.
6. Barrett A, Galvin R, Steinert Y, Scherpbier A, O'Shaughnessy A, Horgan M, et al. A BEME (Best Evidence in Medical Education) review of the use of workplace-based assessment in identifying and remediating underperformance among postgraduate medical trainees: BEME Guide No. 43. Med Teach. 2016;38(12):1188–98.
7. Chuan A, Thillainathan S, Graham PL, Jolly B, Wong DM, Smith N, Barrington MJ. Reliability of the Direct Observation of Procedural Skills assessment tool for ultrasound-guided regional anaesthesia. Anaesth Intensive Care. 2016;44(2):201.
8. Lee V, Martin J. Factors impacting on Mini-CEX assessor judgments in Australian and New Zealand emergency departments: a mixed methods exploratory study. Emerg Med Australas. 2016;28:34.
9. Nurudeen SM, Kwakye G, Berry WR, Chaikof EL, Lillemoe KD, Millham F, et al. Can 360-degree reviews help surgeons? Evaluation of multisource feedback for surgeons in a multi-institutional quality improvement project. J Am Coll Surg. 2015;221(4):837–44.
10. Guraya S, Alzobydi A, Salman S. Objective structured clinical examination: examiners' bias and recommendations to improve its reliability. J Med Med Sci. 2010;1(7):269–72.
11. Taylor RH, Menciassi A, Fichtinger G, Dario P. Medical robotics and computer-integrated surgery. In: Springer handbook of robotics. Springer; 2008. p. 1199–222.
12. Guraya SY, London N, Guraya SS. Ethics in medical research. J Microsc Ultrastruct. 2014;2(3):121–6.
13. Guraya SY, Forgione A, Sampogna G, Pugliese R. The mapping of preferred resources for surgical education: perceptions of surgical trainees at the Advanced International Minimally Invasive Surgery Academy (AIMS), Milan, Italy. J Taibah Univ Med Sci. 2015;10(4):396–404.
14. Aggarwal R, Mytton OT, Derbrew M, Hananel D, Heydenburg M, Issenberg B, et al. Training and simulation for patient safety. Qual Saf Health Care. 2010;19(Suppl 2):i34–43.
15. Hobgood C, Anantharaman V, Bandiera G, Cameron P, Halperin P, Holliman J, et al. International Federation for Emergency Medicine model curriculum for medical student education in emergency medicine. Emerg Med Australas. 2009;21(5):367–72.
16. Schull MJ, Ferris LE, Tu JV, Hux JE, Redelmeier DA. Problems for clinical judgment: 3. Thinking clearly in an emergency. Can Med Assoc J. 2001;164(8):1170–5.
17. Hobgood C, Anantharaman V, Bandiera G, Cameron P, Halperin P, Holliman J, et al. International Federation for Emergency Medicine Model curriculum for medical student education in emergency medicine. Afr J Emerg Med. 2011;1(3):139–44.
18. Ruchholtz S. [The Trauma Registry of the German Society of Trauma Surgery as a basis for interclinical quality management. A multicenter study of the German Society of Trauma Surgery]. Unfallchirurg. 2000;103(1):30–7.
19. Debas HT, Bass BL, Brennan MF, Flynn TC, Folse JR, Freischlag JA, et al. American surgical association blue ribbon committee report on surgical education: 2004. Ann Surg. 2005;241(1):1–8.
20. Jacobs LM, Burns KJ, Kaban JM, Gross RI, Cortes V, Brautigam RT, et al. Development and evaluation of the advanced trauma operative management course. J Trauma Acute Care Surg. 2003;55(3):471–9.
21. Jacobs LM, Burns KJ, Luk SS, Marshall WT III. Follow-up survey of participants attending the Advanced Trauma Operative Management (ATOM) Course. J Trauma Acute Care Surg. 2005;58(6):1140–3.
22. Fabri PJ, Zayas-Castro JL. Human error, not communication and systems, underlies surgical complications. Surgery. 2008;144(4):557–65.
23. Gorrindo T, Beresin EV. Is "see one, do one, teach one" dead? Implications for the professionalization of medical educators in the twenty-first century. Acad Psychiatry. 2015;39(6):613–4.
24. Jakimowicz J, Fingerhut A. Simulation in surgery. Br J Surg. 2009;96(6):563–4.
25. Arriaga AF, Bader AM, Wong JM, Lipsitz SR, Berry WR, Ziewacz JE, et al. Simulation-based trial of surgical-crisis checklists. N Engl J Med. 2013;368(3):246–53.
26. Thomsen ASS, Subhi Y, Kiilgaard JF, la Cour M, Konge L. Update on simulation-based surgical training and assessment in ophthalmology: a systematic review. Ophthalmology. 2015;122(6):1111–30.e1.
27. Torkington J, Smith S, Rees B, Darzi A. The role of simulation in surgical training. Ann R Coll Surg Engl. 2000;82(2):88.
28. Villegas L, Schneider B, Callery M, Jones D. Laparoscopic skills training. Surg Endos Other Intervent Tech. 2003;17(12):1879–88.
29. Munz Y, Kumar B, Moorthy K, Bann S, Darzi A. Laparoscopic virtual reality and box trainers: is one superior to the other? Surg Endos Other Intervent Tech. 2004;18(3):485–94.
30. Susmitha WK, Mathew G, Devasahayam SR, Perakath B, Velusamy SK. Factors influencing forces during laparoscopic pinching: towards the design of virtual simulator. Int J Surg. 2015;18:211–5.

31. Cannon WD, Garrett WE, Hunter RE, Sweeney HJ, Eckhoff DG, Nicandri GT, et al. Improving residency training in arthroscopic knee surgery with use of a virtual-reality simulator. J Bone Joint Surg Am. 2014;96(21):1798–806.
32. Lamata F, Antolin M, Rodriguez S, Oltra A. Study of laparoscopic forces perception for defining simulation fidelity. Medicine meets virtual reality 14: accelerating change in healthcare: next medical toolkit. Stud Health Technol Inform. 2006;119:288.
33. Jalink MB, Goris J, Heineman E, Pierie J-PE, Henk O. The effects of video games on laparoscopic simulator skills. Am J Surg. 2014;208(1):151–6.
34. Giannotti D, Patrizi G, Di Rocco G, Vestri AR, Semproni CP, Fiengo L, et al. Play to become a surgeon: impact of Nintendo Wii training on laparoscopic skills. PLoS One. 2013;8(2):e57372.
35. Rosser JC, Lynch PJ, Cuddihy L, Gentile DA, Klonsky J, Merrell R. The impact of video games on training surgeons in the 21st century. Arch Surg. 2007;142(2):181–6.
36. Hafford ML, Van Sickle KR, Willis RE, Wilson TD, Gugliuzza K, Brown KM, et al. Ensuring competency: are fundamentals of laparoscopic surgery training and certification necessary for practicing surgeons and operating room personnel? Surg Endosc. 2013;27(1):118–26.
37. Kennedy A, Boyle E, Traynor O, Walsh T, Hill A. Video gaming enhances psychomotor skills but not visuospatial and perceptual abilities in surgical trainees. J Surg Educ. 2011;68(5):414–20.
38. Sun YH, Wu Z, Yang B. The laparoscopic animal lab training module. The training courses of urological laparoscopy. Springer; 2012. p. 45–59.
39. Swindle MM, Smith AC, Hepburn BJ. Swine as models in experimental surgery. J Invest Surg. 1988;1(1):65–79.
40. Mutter D, Dallemagne B, Perretta S, Vix M, Leroy J, Pessaux P, et al. Innovations in minimally invasive surgery: lessons learned from translational animal models. Langenbecks Arch Surg. 2013;398(7):919–23.
41. Jacobson S, Epstein SK, Albright S, Ochieng J, Griffiths J, Coppersmith V, et al. Creation of virtual patients from CT images of cadavers to enhance integration of clinical and basic science student learning in anatomy. Med Teach. 2009;31(8):749–51.
42. Leblanc F, Champagne BJ, Augestad KM, Neary PC, Senagore AJ, Ellis CN, et al. A comparison of human cadaver and augmented reality simulator models for straight laparoscopic colorectal skills acquisition training. J Am Coll Surg. 2010;211(2):250–5.
43. Porzionato A, Polese L, Lezoche E, Macchi V, Lezoche G, Da Dalt G, et al. On the suitability of Thiel cadavers for natural orifice transluminal endoscopic surgery (NOTES): surgical training, feasibility studies, and anatomical education. Surg Endosc. 2015;29(3):737–46.
44. Cottam D, Holover S, Mattar SG, Sharma SK, Medlin W, Ramanathan R, et al. The mini-fellowship concept: a six-week focused training program for minimally invasive bariatric surgery. Surg Endosc. 2007;21(12):2237–9.
45. Agrawal S. Post-CCT national surgical fellowship in bariatric and upper GI surgery. Bull R Coll Surg Engl. 2010;92(10):354–7.
46. Forgione A, Kislov V, Guraya SY, Kasakevich E, Pugliese R. Safe introduction of laparoscopic colorectal surgery even in remote areas of the world: the value of a comprehensive telementoring training program. J Laparoendosc Adv Surg Tech. 2015;25(1):37–42.
47. Jenkins JT, Currie A, Sala S, Kennedy RH. A multi-modal approach to training in laparoscopic colorectal surgery accelerates proficiency gain. Surg Endosc. 2015;30(7):3007–13.
48. Simpson JS, Scheer A. A review of the effectiveness of breast surgical oncology fellowship programs utilizing Kirkpatrick's evaluation model. J Cancer Educ. 2016;31(3):466–71.
49. Sachdeva AK. Acquiring skills in new procedures and technology: the challenge and the opportunity. Arch Surg. 2005;140(4):387–9.
50. Antoniou SA, Antoniou GA, Franzen J, Bollmann S, Koch OO, Pointner R, et al. A comprehensive review of telementoring applications in laparoscopic general surgery. Surg Endosc. 2012;26(8):2111–6.
51. Sebajang H, Trudeau P, Dougall A, Hegge S, McKinley C, Anvari M. The role of telementoring and telerobotic assistance in the provision of laparoscopic colorectal surgery in rural areas. Surg Endosc Other Intervent Tech. 2006;20(9):1389–93.
52. Sebajang H, Trudeau P, Dougall A, Hegge S, McKinley C, Anvari M. Telementoring: an important enabling tool for the community surgeon. Surg Innov. 2005;12(4):327–31.
53. Lee B, Png D, Liew L, Fabrizio M, Li M, Jarrett J, et al. Laparoscopic telesurgery between the United States and Singapore. Ann Acad Med Singap. 2000;29(5):665–8.
54. Bogen EM, Augestad KM, Patel HR, Lindsetmo R-O. Telementoring in education of laparoscopic surgeons: an emerging technology. World J Gastrointest Endosc. 2014;6(5):148.
55. Shin DH, Dalag L, Azhar RA, Santomauro M, Satkunasivam R, Metcalfe C, et al. A novel interface for the telementoring of robotic surgery. BJU Int. 2015;116(2):302–8.
56. Yu W, Alqasemi R, Dubey R, Pernalete N, editors. Telemanipulation assistance based on motion intention recognition. In: Proceedings of the 2005 IEEE International Conference on Robotics and Automation. IEEE; 2005.
57. Hatala R, Cook DA, Brydges R, Hawkins R. Constructing a validity argument for the Objective Structured Assessment of Technical Skills (OSATS): a systematic review of validity evidence. Adv Health Sci Educ. 2015;20(5):1149–75.
58. Fried GM. FLS assessment of competency using simulated laparoscopic tasks. J Gastrointest Surg. 2008;12(2):210–2.
59. Xeroulis G, Dubrowski A, Leslie K. Simulation in laparoscopic surgery: a concurrent validity study for FLS. Surg Endosc. 2009;23(1):161–5.
60. Okrainec A, Soper NJ, Swanstrom LL, Fried GM. Trends and results of the first 5 years of Fundamentals of Laparoscopic Surgery (FLS) certification testing. Surg Endosc. 2011;25(4):1192–8.
61. Hazey JW, Marks JM, Mellinger JD, Trus TL, Chand B, Delaney CP, et al. Why fundamentals of endoscopic surgery (FES)? Surg Endosc. 2014;28(3):701–3.
62. Stegemann AP, Ahmed K, Syed JR, Rehman S, Ghani K, Autorino R, et al. Fundamental skills of robotic surgery: a multi-institutional randomized controlled trial for validation of a simulation-based curriculum. Urology. 2013;81(4):767–74.
63. Yule S, Flin R, Maran N, Rowley D, Youngson G, Paterson-Brown S. Surgeons' non-technical skills in the operating room: reliability testing of the NOTSS behavior rating system. World J Surg. 2008;32(4):548–56.
64. de Leval MR, Carthey J, Wright DJ, Farewell VT, Reason JT. Human factors and cardiac surgery: a multicenter study. J Thorac Cardiovasc Surg. 2000;119(4):661–72.
65. Yule S, Flin R, Paterson-Brown S, Maran N. Non-technical skills for surgeons in the operating room: a review of the literature. Surgery. 2006;139(2):140–9.
66. Guraya SY, Norman RI, Roff S. Exploring the climates of undergraduate professionalism in a Saudi and a UK medical school. Med Teach. 2016;38(6):630–2.
67. Davidson PM. The surgeon for the future and implications for training. ANZ J Surg. 2002;72(11):822–8.
68. Pena G, Altree M, Field J, Thomas M, Hewett P, Babidge W, et al. Surgeons' and trainees' perceived self-efficacy in operating theatre non-technical skills. Br J Surg. 2015;102(6):708–15.
69. Guraya SS, Guraya SY, Habib FA, Khoshhal KI. Learning styles of medical students at Taibah University: trends and implications. J Res Med Sci. 2014;19(12):1155.

Pathophysiology of Acute Illness and Injury

2

Sergio Arlati

Key Points

- The inflammatory reaction is a highly adaptive, integrated response with a global protective effect against microbial pathogens or tissue damage. It provides for the elimination of pathogens, removal of cellular debris, and promotes tissue repair and healing.
- Multiple trauma or severe infection causes a widespread inflammatory reaction that causes diffuse endothelial activation (chemotaxis), damage (permeability edema), and vasodilation (hypotension-shock).
- Inflammation and coagulation are strictly coupled. As a general rule hyperinflammation means hypercoagulability. Coagulation has beneficial effects when inflammation is localized, but it becomes catastrophic when disseminated intravascular coagulation ensues.
- Humoral inflammatory mediators include cytokines, complement, thrombin, acute phase proteins, kinins, and PAF. Endothelial cells, monocytes, antigen-presenting cells (macrophages and dendritic cells), and neutrophils are the main effector cells.
- Neutrophils are responsible for tissue damage. Their widespread activation accounts for the noxious effects to innocent tissues with multiple organ damage.
- A counter-inflammatory response mounts immediately after the hyperinflammatory reaction. Such response is proportionate to inflammation along the whole course of disease.
- An immediate decrease of the acquired (lymphocytic) immune response occurs in parallel with inflammation leading to dysfunction and progressive immunoparalysis.
- Apoptosis of the cells of the immune system is the main responsible of immunoparalysis. This exposes to increased risks for opportunistic infections and sepsis/septic shock.

S. Arlati (✉)
Anesthesia and Intensive Care 1 (1st Dept),
ASST Grande Ospedale Metropolitano Niguarda, Milan, Italy
e-mail: sergio.arlati@ospedaleniguarda.it

2.1 Basic Concepts

The pathophysiology of acute care illnesses is a generalized, multi-systemic process that invariably activates the immune-inflammatory and coagulation systems with production of diffuse tissue and organ damage. The temporal development of acute care illnesses is quite variable although it usually evolves as a multiphasic process or more rarely as a single acute event that the body can't cope with. For example, multiple trauma causes the activation of the immune-inflammatory, coagulation, and neuroendocrine systems. Thus ischemia-reperfusion that follows severe post-traumatic hemorrhage with hypotension and tissue hypoperfusion activates the immune-inflammatory system with adhesion of polymorphonuclear leukocytes (PMNs) to the endothelium and increased capillary permeability, plasma fluid leakage, and tissue edema. The widespread activation of the coagulation creates a prothrombotic milieu with deposition of microthrombi, diffuse capillary obstruction, and further ischemic damage. Similarly, severe pneumonia challenges the circulating monocytes and resident tissue macrophages with a broad spectrum of microbial molecules. The subsequent activation of the inflammatory and coagulation systems causes the widespread activation of the endothelium with production of either local (e.g., ARDS) or distant organ damage (multiple organ dysfunction syndrome, MODS). However, the immune system provides a counter-regulatory response that limits the deleterious effects of the generalized inflammatory activation

P. Aseni et al. (eds.), *Operative Techniques and Recent Advances in Acute Care and Emergency Surgery*,
https://doi.org/10.1007/978-3-319-95114-0_2

(compensatory anti-inflammatory response syndrome, CARS) [1]. Although CARS opposes to the systemic inflammatory response syndrome (SIRS) [2], this is a double-edged sword because the risk of septic complications is increased. If unresolved, SIRS and CARS become the underlying players of a catabolic syndrome that leads to MODS and ultimately death [3]. In the past SIRS was viewed as an exaggerated response to inflammatory stimuli, but the latest experimental and observational data indicate that it is a rather predictable side effect of especially severe morbid events. In practice, SIRS and CARS result from the growing sophistication of ICU care that keeps patients alive during the early (acute) phase of traumatic and septic diseases. The protracted survival of formerly rapid lethal conditions makes now appreciable their natural evolution. Recent acquisitions also suggest that SIRS and CARS develop simultaneously rather than in sequence as previously believed. As a result a mixed antagonist response syndrome (MARS) was coined to reflect the balance between SIRS and CARS [4] (Fig. 2.1).

However, the phenotypic predominance of the hyperinflammatory state is the rule in early sepsis, hypoxia, or trauma as influenced by antigenic load, microbial virulence, host genetic factors, age, nutritional status, and comorbidities [5]. In the past CARS was believed to develop after SIRS exhaustion by repeated noxious stimuli (second hit theory) [5, 6]. According to this theory, recurrent morbid insults augment the inflammatory response by repeated stimulation of the inflammatory cascade. In this sense, SIRS would no longer depend by the initial insult but rather by the intensity and frequency of subsequent hits. However, the continuous challenge of the inflammatory system mounts an anti-inflammatory response that ultimately becomes predominant. So CARS does not develop simultaneously with SIRS, but only a minimal overlap would exist between the two phenomena. This pathophysiological view is derived from the observation that CARS prevails in the later stages of disease when the increased susceptibility to infections is associated with a weakened pro-inflammatory response (SIRS exhaustion). This concept translated into the linear transition from acute (early) SIRS to chronic (late) CARS with possible alternating recurrence of the two phases (MARS), (Fig. 2.2).

However, this view is no longer accepted as the historical belief of the "cytokine storm" after a catastrophic acute illness (e.g., meningococcal sepsis) giving the spectacular inflammatory reaction is not the rule [7]. Instead, the most common picture is by far a patient over 65 years of age with sepsis or recovering from multiple trauma/surgery and evidence of immunosuppression without the typical exaggerated acute phase inflammatory response [7]. In the past "cytokine storm" was synonymous of SIRS that is hyperinflammation defined by excessive release of classical pro-inflammatory cytokines including IL1, IL6, IL8, and TNFα. However, this concept is too narrow as it was quickly noted that "cytokine storm" is not the typical occurrence in late (chronic) sepsis or even in acutely septic patients with a weakened immune system [8, 9]. Similarly, it seems incorrect to define CARS on the basis of elevated release of anti-inflammatory cytokines in the blood. The current concept is rather that the magnitude of cytokine release depends on the premorbid immune-inflammatory status of the patient [10]. Otherwise stated the healthier the patient, the stronger will be the release of cytokines after stimulus. As a corollary, the more protracted is the disease, the more faded will be the inflammatory response over time (e.g., recurrent sepsis in postsurgical or trauma patient). However, an acute inflammatory response although typical of the acute phase may occur at any time of the disease profile if the host is sufficiently immunologically responsive. This view holds for

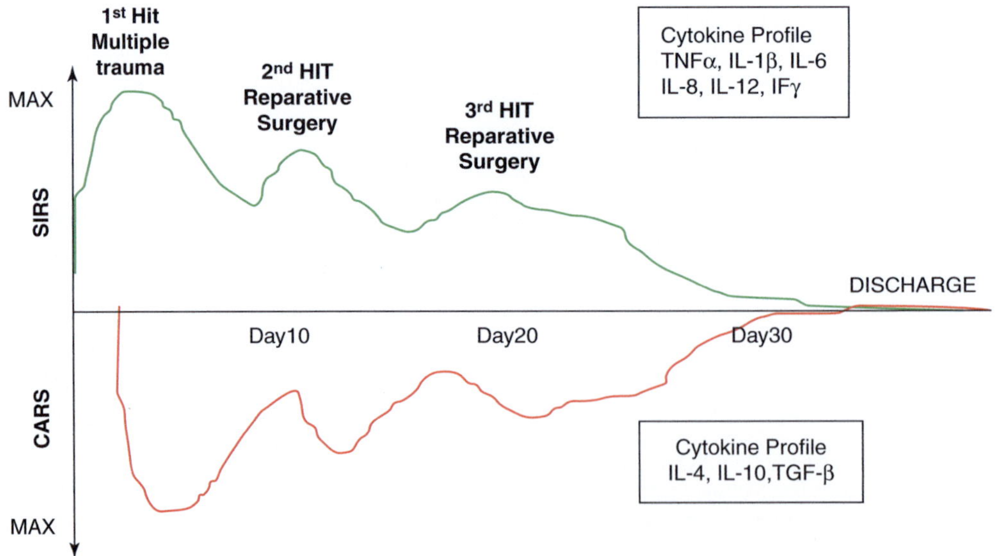

Fig. 2.1 Temporal profile of pro-inflammatory and anti-inflammatory cytokines according to the most recent hypothesis of simultaneous development of SIRS and CARS. So MARS is always ongoing

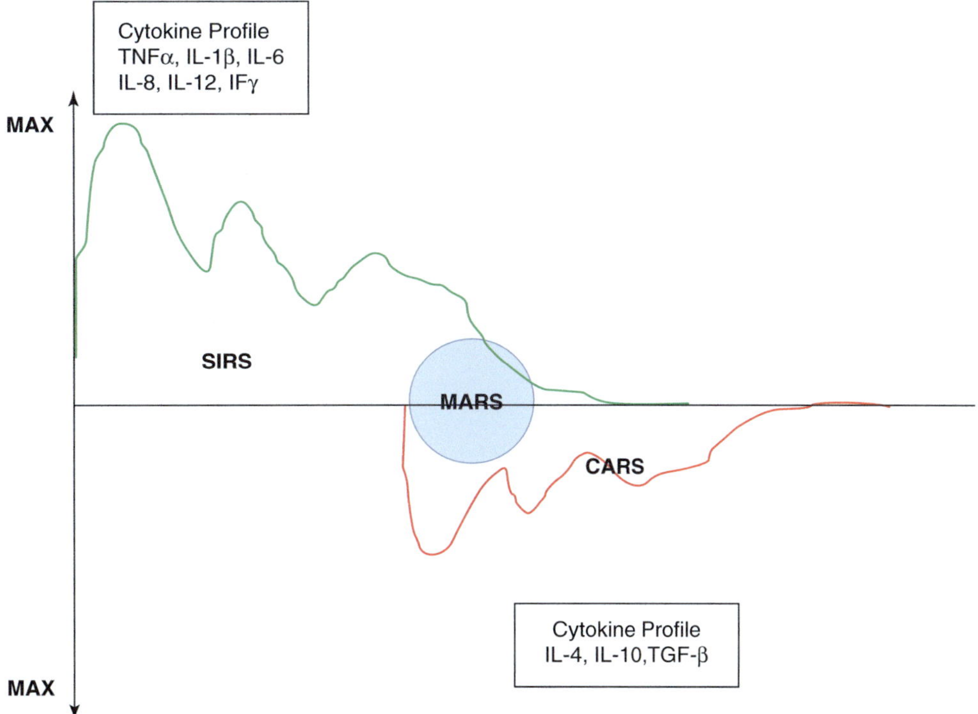

Fig. 2.2 Temporal profile of pro-inflammatory and anti-inflammatory cytokines according to the hypothesis of sequential development of SIRS and CARS. MARS is a transitional state in-between them

both the pro-inflammatory and anti-inflammatory cytokines, so it is incorrect to define the patient's inflammatory status on the basis of his/her cytokine profile [10]. Therefore, the mixed cytokine response pattern better represents the patient's inflammatory status leading to the paradigm "Sepsis: Always in MARS" [11]. Thus a hyperinflammatory status at the onset of sepsis or multiple trauma reflects the ability of the host to release a great amount of pro-inflammatory and anti-inflammatory mediators. Such ability is destined to fade over time with progression to a late (chronic) inflammatory status. In recent years, the immunocompetent cells have emerged as a new relevant player for the appearance of immunosuppression or immunoparalysis that often characterizes the host's response during the more chronic disease stages. At present, the process of immunosuppression (decreased T-cell proliferation and production of IL2, decreased monocyte and macrophage function) is believed to occur in parallel with the hyperinflammatory status of early sepsis of traumatic or surgical origin [12, 13]. Animal studies indicate that in non-survivors, the immune cell suppression progresses indefinitely up to anergy from the very beginning to the more chronic stages in a time-independent manner [10]. As a result, the phenotype of immunosuppression does not often correspond to the cytokine pattern of peripheral blood.

Prior to early deaths, cellular immunosuppression develops rapidly together with high pro-inflammatory and anti-inflammatory cytokine release (MARS-like) [14]. Conversely, the chronic state is preceded by a progressive (subacute or chronic) impairment of immune cells function with robust pre-lethal signs of anergy and a deteriorating but MARS-like cytokine profile (simultaneous presence of both pro-inflammatory and anti-inflammatory mediators in the blood) [10]. The spread of the inflammatory process starting from a single organ or tissue is by far the most frequent event in the pathophysiology of acute diseases. The inflammatory response is a highly coordinated process, which has evolved to limit the spread of noxious stimuli, eliminates pathogens and necrotic cellular debris, and promotes the healing of damaged tissues. It is subjected to multiple activations and control mechanisms and whose efficiency is largely dependent on genetic predisposition, age, and neurovegetative and hormonal milieu derived from the stress response. Finally, inflammation and immunity are tightly related in a complex network of multiple interconnections and reverberating loops. However, extremely intense or repeated stimulations may disturb their tuned response so that the inflammatory mediators spill over the anatomical barriers and multiple organs dysfunction syndrome ensues. Cardinal inflammation phenomena are local vasodilation, increased endothelial permeability, and chemotactic cells activation from the natural (granulocytes and monocytes) and acquired immune system (lymphocytes). The vascular mechanisms that lead to the four cardinal signs of inflammation are resumed in Fig. 2.3.

Neutrophils and monocytes are activated to infiltrate the site of infection with subsequent phagocytosis and lysis of bacterial products or cellular debris. In the meanwhile, the activated coagulation system seals the site of inflammation and provides a meshwork of fibrin that helps in the reparation process. Therefore, increased membrane permeability,

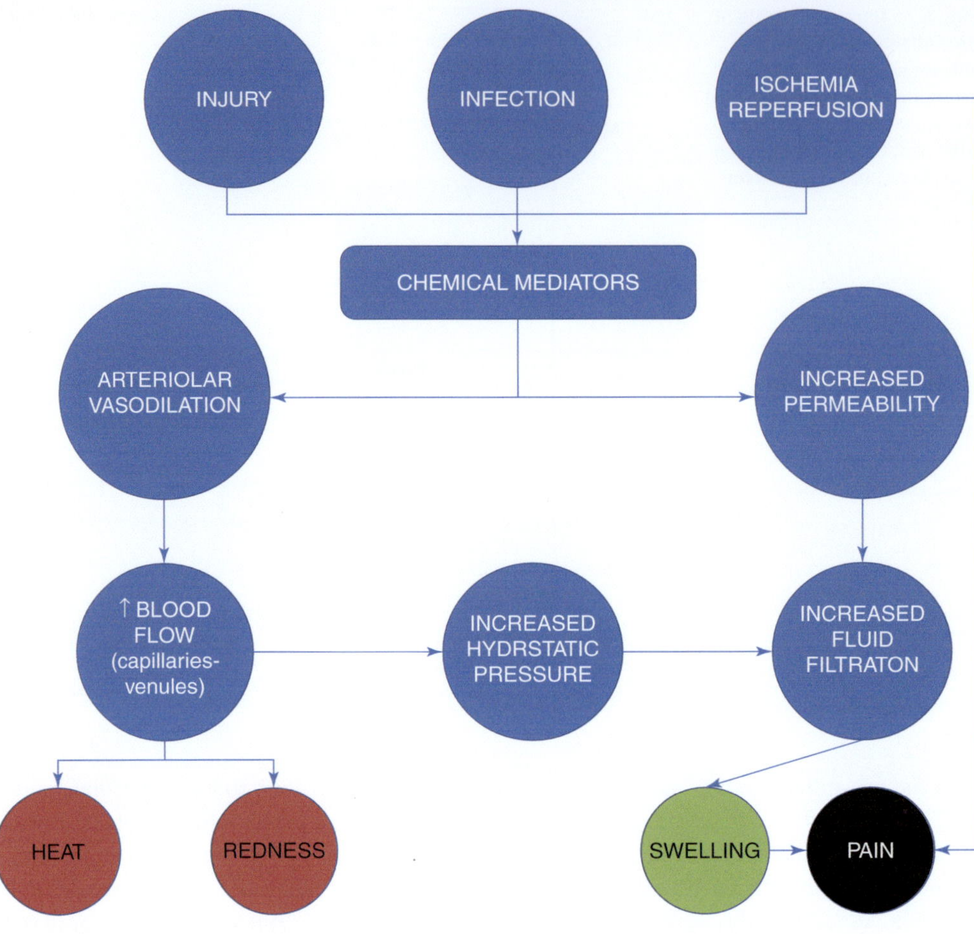

Fig. 2.3 Vascular mechanisms at the origin of the cardinal signs of inflammation. Arteriolar vasodilation and increased permeability are responsible for augmentation of blood flow (redness and heat) and fluids accumulation in tissue (swelling and pain)

capillary vasodilation, chemotaxis, and phagocytosis are defensive mechanisms that act in concert to ensure the maximum of protection against any threat or danger. A multiplicity of cell types (e.g., endothelium, monocytes, platelets) as well as humoral factors (complement, leukotrienes, kinins) acts following a synergistic and often redundant logic to activate, propagate, and maintain the inflammation so that the host defense is guaranteed. Nevertheless, the uncontrolled diffusion of inflammatory mediators causes hypotension and tissue edema by generalized vasodilation and increased endothelial permeability. Furthermore, the diffuse deposition of microthrombi by disseminated intravascular coagulation worsens the oxygen supply to tissues this, in turn, contributing to ischemic cells damage, further inflammation (ischemia/reperfusion injury), and MODS. The local action of the inflammatory system is similar to a well-refined military strategy. After an enemy attack (e.g., trauma) that engages the local garrison (resident macrophages and glial cells), the combat zone is rapidly enclosed and sealed by reinforcement troops (chemotactic activation of PMNs and intravascular coagulation). Thereafter, the soldiers get into the battlefield (increased membrane permeability and leukocytes migration) and shoot at the enemy destroying him (phagocytosis, proteases, and toxic oxygen products). However, after a massive attack, the hurried and often disorganized mobilization of the reserve troops makes difficult or even impossible to implement an effective defense. The recruitment of soldiers is often chaotic and uncoordinated (widespread chemotactic activation), the effective concentration of troops is impossible (generalized increase of endothelial permeability), and military patrols often shoot at innocent people (organ damage). Thus, pneumococcal pneumonia can transform into severe sepsis or septic shock if a generalized inflammatory reaction develops by either cellular (neutrophils, monocytes, macrophages, endothelium) or humoral effectors (complement, contact phase proteins, leukotrienes, cytokines, chemokines) resulting into increased capillary permeability (tissue edema), vasodilation (hypotension), and coagulation activation (ischemic organ damage). Generally, the pathophysiological mechanisms that lead to a systemic inflammatory reaction are infections, trauma, and ischemia-reperfusion damage. Each of them can act by itself or in combination with the other two. For example, multiple trauma causes the activation of immune-inflammatory mechanisms by itself (tissue necrosis), or as a consequence of ischemia-reperfusion damage (e.g., gut ischemia by post-traumatic mesenteric hematoma or post-ischemic muscular tissue reperfusion after hemorrhagic shock). Apart from the abovementioned mechanisms, the uncontrolled activation of the immune system (autoimmune diseases), massive cytokines production (metastatic cancer, leukemia, or lymphoma), and the unrestrained activation of serum proteases (acute pancreatitis) are less frequent causes of generalized inflammatory activation.

2.2 How the Systemic Inflammatory Reaction Develops

The widespread activation of the inflammatory system (systemic inflammatory reaction syndrome, SIRS) originates from the site of trauma, infection, or hypoxic cell damage (ischemia/reperfusion). Infection, traumatic or hypoxic injury, causes the release of a heterogeneous pattern of endogenous and exogenous molecules that trigger the innate immune system as chemoattractants and activators of antigen-presenting cells.

2.2.1 Alarmins

Infection from bacterial, viral, and fungal agents releases signaling substances that are recognized by the innate immune system due to their characteristic molecular pattern (pathogen-associated molecular patterns, PAMPs) [15]. Conversely, traumatic or hypoxic cell injury releases the so-called damage-associated molecular patterns (DAMPs) [16, 17] which represent the correlate of PAMP for danger signals of endogenous origin. PAMPs and DAMPs are grouped into the larger family of "alarmins" in assignment to the term danger signals [15]. Otherwise stated PAMPs and DAMPs constitute a physiologic signaling system that alerts the body to the presence of foreign invaders or noxious stimuli. "Alarmins" activate specific receptors of the superfamily of the Toll-like receptors (TLRs) [18, 19], expressed on endothelial and innate immune cells like macrophages, dendritic cells (antigen-presenting cells, APCs), monocytes, and PMNs [20]. APCs act as an intermediate between innate and acquired immune system. Their main function is to process antigen material and to present it to effector T cells of the immune system. TLR receptors recognize a variety of peptides that are important signaling molecules for activation and production of a multiplicity of inflammatory mediators. In addition, DAMPs are potent activators of the complement system [21–23] whose anaphylatoxins attract monocytes and PMNs on the endothelium. The high mobility group box protein (HMGB) is one of the most studied "alarmin." HMBG is a protein molecule derived from the nucleus of damaged cells [15, 24]. It is released by activated myeloid cells (e.g., neutrophils) [20], macrophages, dendritic cells [25–27], or necrotic cells [26] and acts as a chemoattractant for monocytes, macrophages, dendritic cells, neutrophils, and ϒδ cells [3]. It also participates to the secretion of pro-inflammatory cytokines [28] and mediates the monocyte-endothelial interaction by increasing vascular leakage [24, 29]. Fragments of DNA and histones are other well-known potent "alarmins." They originate from damaged tissues and microbial digestion by resident tissue macrophages or activated neutrophils. Peptides and mitochondrial DNA are vigorous alert molecules probably because of their vestigial origin from intracellular bacteria [3].

2.2.2 Pro-inflammatory Phospholipase Pathway

In addition to "alarmins," the release of phospholipids by damaged cell membranes (cellular hypoxia and trauma) or exogenous lipopolysaccharides (e.g., LPS-endotoxin) and polymers (lipoteichoic acid and peptidoglycans) alert the innate immune system by activating the complement and the contact phase proteins system (FXII, kallikrein, and kininogen). Phospholipids activate the phospholipases A_2 and C [30] with the production of arachidonic acid metabolites as leukotriene B_4, prostaglandin E_2, and thromboxane A_2 [31]. The activation pathway of phospholipase A_2 and C is detailed in Fig. 2.4.

In addition, mast cells release histamine and bradykinin with resulting vasodilation and increased capillary permeability and edema [32]. Just 20–30 min after trauma or microbial invasion, the innate immune cells become activated, Fig. 2.5.

2.2.3 Innate Cellular Immune Defense

The first line of the innate immune defense is represented by PMNs, mostly neutrophils, and monocytes. PMNs are chemoattracted by locally produced cytokines (e.g., TNF-α), leukotrienes, platelet-activating factor (PAF), and complement fragments (c5a) [33–36]. These inflammatory mediators also activate PMNs to express adhesion surface molecules for appropriate ligands on the activated endothelium [37]. This receptor-ligand interaction allows for adhesion of leukocytes to the capillary wall. Thereafter PMNs migrate through the endothelial barrier into the tissues by opportune signaling receptors on the inner surface of the endothelium. In the meanwhile, resident macrophages secrete cytokines (TNFα and IL-1) and chemokines (IL-8) which help the immune and inflammatory cells in self-regulating and crosstalking each other.

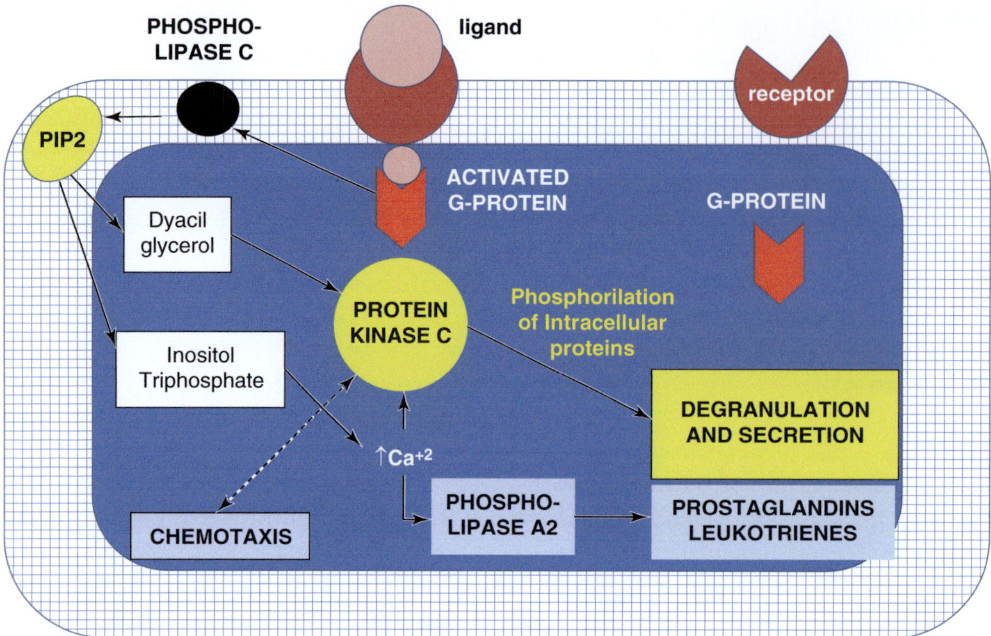

Fig. 2.4 Metabolic pathways of phospholipase A_2 and C. After ligand binding to the appropriate receptor, G protein is activated, this in turn activating the membrane phospholipase C to cleave phosphatidylinositol (PIP2) into diacylglycerol (DAG) and inositol triphosphate. DAG subsequently activates protein kinase C to promote phosphorylation of intracellular proteins that in turn leads leukocytes to degranulate and secrete proteases and other toxic substances. Conversely inositol triphosphate induces the mobilization of calcium ions from storage pools with subsequent activation of phospholipase A_2 by a Ca^{2+}-dependent mechanism. Phospholipase A_2 catalyzes the synthesis of prostaglandins and leukotrienes by arachidonic acid

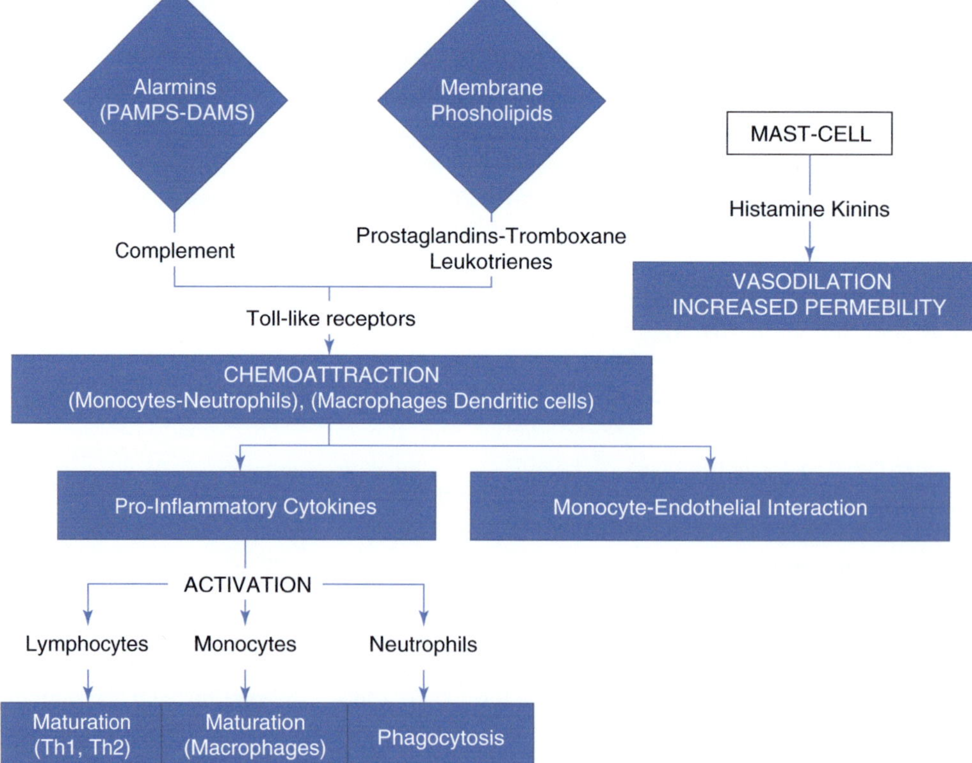

Fig. 2.5 Main humoral and cellular steps of the hyperinflammatory immune response

2.2.4 Pro-inflammatory Cytokines

Cytokines and chemokines are pleiotropic molecules with a great variety of effects that act in a paracrine and autocrine fashion. Among the most important cytokines secreted in the hyper-acute phase, TNF-α and IL-1β act within 1–2 h after trauma or sepsis, while IL-6, IL-10, and the chemokine IL-8 are subacute mediators [38]. Among the most relevant properties of cytokines, there is the ability to activate monocytes (innate immune system) and lymphocytes (acquired immune system) [39]. Under the appropriate cytokine pattern, the circulating monocytes differentiate into resident macrophages, while lymphocytes mature into different cell lines having immune-stimulatory (Th-1), immune-depressant (Th-2), and immune-modulatory (Treg) action [40]. Pro-inflammatory cytokines trigger both the recruitment and the phagocytic activity of leukocytes [41]. They also stimulate the release of proteases and increase the production of free oxygen radicals from activated neutrophils [41].

1. One of the best characterized cytokines is TNF which can produce SIRS when injected experimentally in high doses [39]. Its actions include the stimulation of many cell types and survival or apoptosis [42], cytokine secretion (IL-6, IL-8, IFϒ, IL-10), activation of the arachidonic acid pathways (thromboxane A2 and prostaglandin E2) and nitric oxide, induction of fever and production of selectins, and PAF (see below). TNF secretion is stimulated by many physiological stresses (hemorrhage, hypoxemia) as well as ischemia-reperfusion, endotoxin, and complement system. Macrophages and monocytes are the main TNF producers, although activated T cells are also implicated. Tumor necrosis factor acts via its receptors TNFR1 and TNFR2 with effects that depend on the specific receptor binding and environmental factors influence. Binding of TNF-α to TNFR1 leads to transcription of pro-inflammatory genes via the NF-Kb transcription factor. However, TNFR1 possesses a death domain at the cytoplasmic tail so that its stimulation also induces apoptosis via the caspase enzymes cascade (see below). Although these two effects seem contradictory, they might represent an adaptive mechanism that has evolved to protect cells against excessive stimulation (see below: Kidney Dysfunction). In contrast to the almost ubiquitous TNF1R, TNFR2 is expressed on immune and endothelial cells only and becomes activated by membrane-bound TNF-α [42, 43]. Binding to TNFR2 leads to activation and proliferation of neutrophils and many immune cells as NK cells, B cells, and peripheral T cells [44].
2. Interleukin-1-beta is the other well-studied cytokine that acts synergistically with TNF-α. Its actions include fever induction, cytokine and chemokine secretion [45], T cell and macrophage stimulation and various inflammatory mediators (including adhesion molecules), acute phase proteins, and NO synthesis. It also induces the release of neutrophils from the bone marrow and stimulates the expression of proteases and metalloproteases by tissues. IL-1β is secreted by macrophages, monocytes, and endothelial cells. Stimuli for IL-1β include TNF, complement, endotoxin, hemorrhage, and ischemia. The effects of IL-1β are mediated by the type IL-1 receptor (IL-1RI) which belongs to the IL-1 receptor superfamily. Besides IL-1β, another molecule that binds IL-1RI is the so-called soluble IL-1 receptor antagonist (IL1-RA) suggesting a controlling role in IL-1-mediated immune response.
3. The third important cytokine in the early inflammatory response is IL-6. Its secretion is induced by TNF and IL-1 [46]. Although it does not induce SIRS when injected into experimental animals, IL-6 has vasodilatory properties as it induces the production of nitric oxide by the endothelial cells. IL-6 is a subacute cytokine with marked regulatory properties on immune cell growth and differentiation. It inhibits apoptosis of neutrophils and stimulates the hepatic acute phase protein synthesis but also exhibits an anti-inflammatory action [47] by inducing the release of soluble TNFR and IL-1RA [48]. It seems, therefore, to play a dual role in the inflammatory response by acting both as a pro-inflammatory and anti-inflammatory mediator [49, 50]. Clinical studies demonstrated increased plasma levels in non-survivor septic patients so that IL-6 has been proposed as a prognostic marker [51–53].
4. The chemokine IL-8 is the most powerful chemoattractant for PMNs and monocytes [54]. Chemokines control the traffic of the immune cells, which are the main effectors of the immune system. Their binding to G-protein-coupled receptors leads to dose-dependent effects including chemotaxis and activation of immune cells. After stimulation by IL-1, TNF-α, complement, microbial products (e.g., LPS), hypoxia, and reperfusion, IL-8 increases neutrophils degranulation, adherence, and chemotaxis. Interestingly, chemokines act as chemoattractants in lower doses and potent activators of immune cells function in higher doses. Recently a group of so-called silent chemokine receptors has been described suggesting a role as decoy or scavenger receptors. The Duffy antigen receptors for chemokines (DARC), first described as blood group antigen, have been shown to bind IL-8 and other chemokines thus suggesting a regulatory action against excessive leukocyte activation in the systemic circulation [39].

Table 2.1 Main cellular source and effects of pro-inflammatory cytokines

Name	Main source	Immune cells activation	Immune-inflammatory mediators	Apoptosis
TNF-α	Macrophages Monocytes T cells (T_H1)	Macrophages, monocytes, NK cells	Cytokines, NO, arachidonic acid metabolites, PAF, selectins, adhesion molecules	Yes
IL-1	Macrophages Monocytes Endothelial cells	Macrophages, T cells	Cytokines, chemokines, acute phase proteins, tissue proteases, adhesion molecules	–
IL-6	Macrophages Monocytes Endothelial cells T-cells	Growth and differentiation of T and B cells, NK cells	Release of TNFR and IL-1RA, acute phase proteins	Inhibited
IL-8	Macrophages Monocytes Any somatic cell	Activation and chemotaxis of immune cells	Leukotrienes, PAF	–

The cellular source and the main effects of pro-inflammatory cytokines are resumed in Table 2.1.

2.2.5 Local and Systemic Inflammatory Mediators

Apart from cytokines, other important mediators of the hyper-acute phase are the arachidonic acid metabolites (leukotrienes, prostaglandins, and thromboxane). They are responsible for the activation of PMNs and endothelium and platelet aggregation. These substances are generated by activation of the phospholipases A2 and C (PLA_2 and PLC) which follows the entry of Ca^{2+} ions into damaged cells. PLA_2 also induces the release of PAF from the endothelium. PAF is an important inflammatory mediator with marked effects on macrophages, endothelial cells, and platelets aggregation. The inflammatory response is promptly propagated and amplified by important circulating mediators as the complement system, the contact phase proteins (kallikrein-kinins), and the coagulation cascade.

1. The complement cascade is a series of enzymatic cleavage reactions that are activated via the classical route by antigen-antibody complexes (IgM and IgG) or alternatively by bacterial degradation products (e.g., LPS, endotoxin) [32, 55, 56]. The latter pathway does not require prior immunization and thus represents an immediate defense mechanism against microbes. Conversely, the "natural antibodies" activate the complement by forming antigen-antibody complexes with different molecular species from exogenous (microbial) or endogenous (necrotic cells) origin [57–59]. "Natural antibodies" are physiologically circulating antibodies that arise in serum independently from prior host immunization [60]. They are mainly produced by a subpopulation of $CD5^+$ B cells and are poly-reactive with different antigens as peptides, phospholipids, and polysaccharides [60–62]. In musculoskeletal trauma and ischemia-reperfusion injury, the intense antigenic stimulation leads to binding of natural IgM antibodies and development of post-traumatic "innate autoimmunity" [63]. Complement activation leads to the formation of opsonins, anaphylatoxins, and the membrane attack complex, a multiprotein complex responsible for the increased capillary permeability [32]. Anaphylatoxins and opsonins are involved in important inflammatory processes such as opsonization, chemotaxis, and neutrophils degranulation. Complement also promotes the synthesis of acute phase proteins by the liver and stimulates the degranulation of mast cells with histamine release (vasodilation) [32, 64]. In practice, the activated complement is involved in all the most relevant inflammatory processes as immune cells attraction to the site of trauma or infection, microbial phagocytosis and lysis, antigens opsonization, platelets activation, and histamine release. The complement cascade is, therefore, a fundamental component of the innate host defense as it can be rapidly activated in a non-specific manner after injury or infection. It is phylogenetically ancient due to its basic role in the host response to bacterial pathogens. However, the systemic activation of the complement leads to severely deleterious effects such as shock and tissue edema due to massive vasodilation and increased membrane permeability.
2. Coagulation factor XII and kallikrein, together with kininogen, represent the contact phase system. These proteins activate each other by forming an integrated, highly amplified system for activation of the coagulation cascade. Kallikrein also stimulates the formation of the vasodilator bradykinin from kininogen. Kinins are potent vasodilators and vigorous effectors of increased vascular permeability [65]. A close interconnection exists between hemostasis and the inflammatory system. For example, the activated platelets aggregate with circulating leuko-

cytes to stimulate the immune cells system with production of endothelial damage [66]. Platelets also release pro-inflammatory mediators that excite the immune system [67] thus creating a vicious circle that produces more and more SIRS. The activated coagulation cascade after trauma or infection is primarily intended to stop the loss of blood and to seal the lesion. Thereafter, phagocytic and immune cells eliminate necrotic cells and invading microbes. However, the uncontrolled activation of the coagulation cascade causes the widespread deposition of microthrombi, this in turn causing hypoxic cellular damage and increased risk for hemorrhagic complications due to consumption of platelets and coagulation factors [68–71]. Disseminated intravascular coagulation (DIC) is a pathophysiological mechanism that frequently occurs after multiple trauma [68, 70, 71] and severe infections [68, 70]. DIC is responsible for diffuse microthrombi deposition, capillary blockade with heterogeneous microcirculatory perfusion, tissue ischemia, and production of hypoxic cellular damage [68, 72].

3. Acute phase proteins are synthesized in the liver by induction of the locally (Kupffer cells) produced cytokines (TNF-α, IL1-β, and IL6). This process is amplified by circulating cytokines that spillover from injured or infected tissue (overflow theory). Acute phase proteins include C-reactive protein (CRP), α-1-antitrypsin, α-2-macroglobulin, ceruloplasmin, lipopolysaccharide-binding protein (LPB), fibrinogen, and prothrombin [73]. These proteins have several inflammatory and anti-inflammatory properties. For example, CRP increases the surface expression of tissue factor (TF) [74], a procoagulant membrane-bound 4.5 kD protein on PMNs, monocytes, and tissue macrophages (see below). Conversely, α-1-antitrypsin neutralizes leukocyte proteases and free oxygen radicals, while α-2-macroglobulin and ceruloplasmin are inhibitory cofactors for the synthesis of cytokines [74]. Finally, high concentrations of LPB suppress LPS activity [75].

2.2.6 Phagocytosis

At this step of the inflammatory process, the injured or infected tissue is invaded by activated PMNs, mainly neutrophils that release proteases (elastase), exert their phagocytic and digestive properties (phagolysosomes), and produce free oxygen radicals (e.g., hydrogen peroxide) [76] and reactive NO species (e.g., peroxynitrite) [77]. Both neutrophils and macrophages kill bacteria. The first step involves phagocytosis of opsonized microbes. Opsonization means that bacteria are covered with host proteins (e.g., antibodies and complement fragments) and appropriately recognized by cell surface receptors such as TLR and receptors for the Fc portion of the immunoglobulins. The phagocytosed bacteria are typically inserted into a vacuole, the phagosome, which fuses with primary (azurophilic) or secondary granules to form phagolysosomes. Azurophilic granules contain antimicrobial proteases such as elastase and bactericidal/permeability increasing proteins, while secondary granules contain antiseptic peptides as lysozyme, lactoferrin, and metalloproteases. Fusion of granules with phagosomes creates a hostile environment that kills the pathogen (Fig. 2.6).

At the same time, the resident macrophages and circulating monocytes begin to phagocyte cellular and microbial

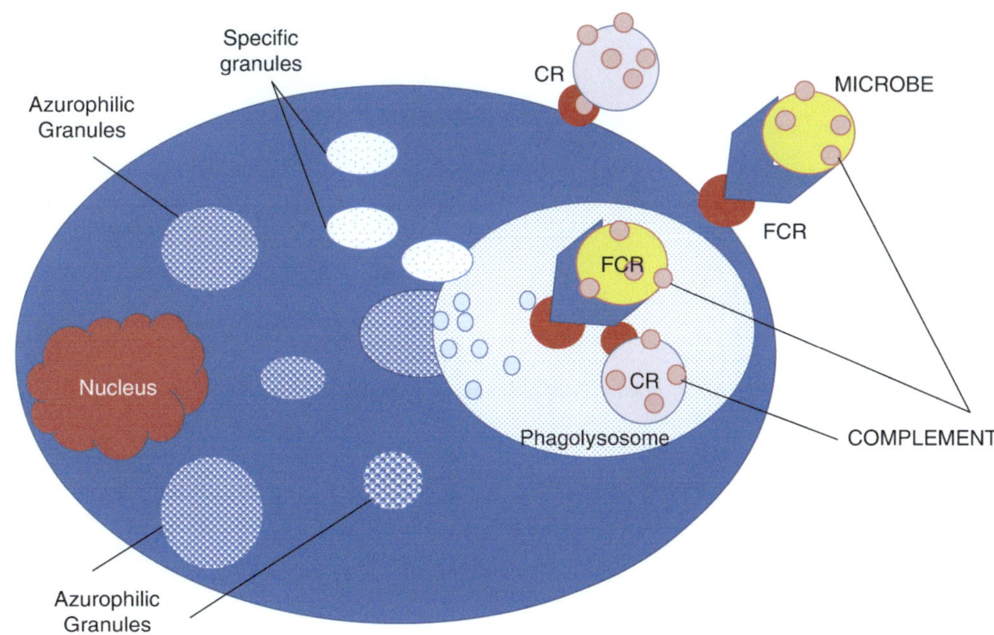

Fig. 2.6 Mechanism of phagocytic-cell destruction of bacteria. Opsonized bacteria bind to complement receptors (CRs) and FC receptors (FCRs) on the surface of phagocytic cells. Thereafter the bacterium is taken into the cytoplasm and included into a phagosome. The fusion of phagosome with specific and azurophilic granules gives a phagolysosome that destroys the bacterium by toxic and enzymatic digestion

debris. These cells produce cytokines and express membrane surface antigens that originate from the digestion process (see Fig. 2.7 for details).

Such molecules activate the endothelium to express adhesion molecules for further neutrophils chemoattraction. In the meanwhile, macrophages interact with T helper cells ($CD4^+$) that secrete interferon ϒ (IFϒ) and other cytokines for phagocytic cells activation. Finally, their interaction with B lymphocytes produces antimicrobial antibodies. This is a highly coordinated process, able to eliminate foreign bodies or cellular debris so ensuring the most effective protection against any insult of whatever origin.

2.3 The Anti-inflammatory Response

Besides the plethora of pro-inflammatory mediators, many anti-inflammatory substances play a counter-regulatory role in the development of CARS. IL-4, IL-10, IL-13, and transforming-growth-factor β (TGF-β) are among the most important anti-inflammatory and immunosuppressant mediators. The main actions of anti-inflammatory cytokines are shown in Table 2.2.

Besides these anti-inflammatory cytokines, several immune effector cells develop their actions immediately after the onset of the acute inflammatory response. The nature of their response is largely determined by the expressed membrane antigenic pattern as it determines their subsequent cellular interactions and biochemical reactions. From the native, multipotent $CD4^+$ T helper 0 cell (Th0), two main cell lines differentiate depending on cytokine environment, either into Th1 helper cell by IL-12 or Th2 helper cell by IL-4 [78].

1. The Th1 helper lymphocytes initiate and augment the delayed immune response by macrophage and neutrophil activation, promoting the production of opsonizing antibodies and stimulating the development of cytotoxic T cells. Their cytokines secretion includes IL-2, IFϒ, and TNFα. IFϒ activates macrophages and iNOS to produce

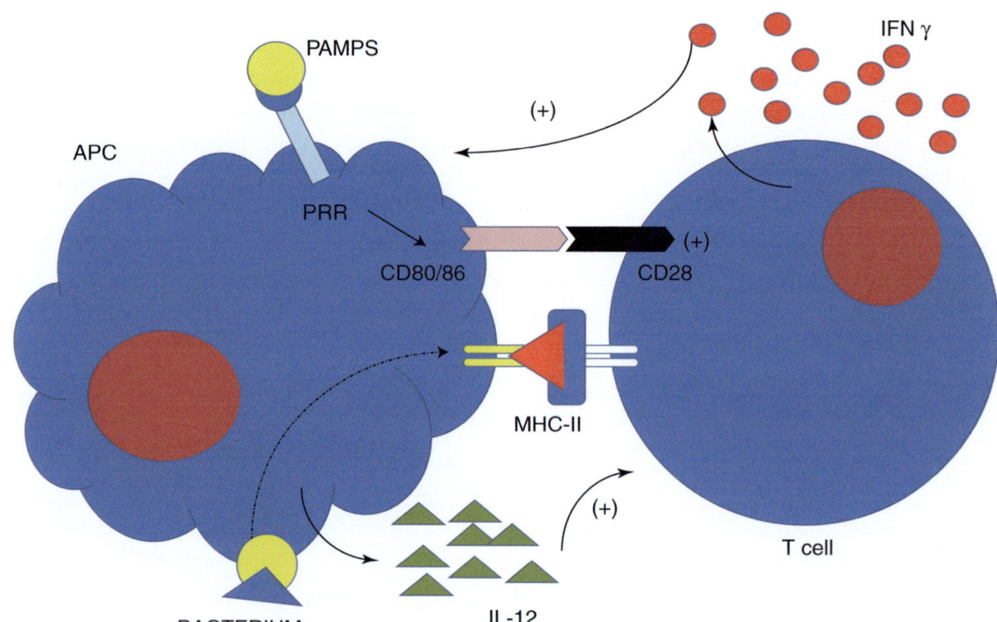

Fig. 2.7 Antigen presenting cells recognize microbial infection by binding of pathogen-associated molecular patterns (PAMPs) to pattern recognition receptors (PRRs) as well as by phagocytosis of bacteria. Thereafter IL-12 is produced, and opportune co-stimulatory molecules (CD80/86) are expressed together with MHCII antigens that bind to corresponding T-cell ligands. This binding results into T-cell activation and proliferation. The production of interferon γ stimulates the macrophages to kill intracellular bacteria

Table 2.2 Main cellular source and effects of anti-inflammatory cytokines

Cytokine	Source	Actions
IL-4	T cells (T_H2), basophils, mast cells	T and B cells
IL-10	Monocytes/macrophages, T cells (T_H2, T_{reg})	Inhibits monocyte/macrophage activation
IL-13	T cells (T_H2)	Inhibits monocyte/macrophage cytokine production
TGF-β	Monocytes, T cells (T_H2, T_{reg})	Inhibits monocyte/macrophage proliferation and activation
IL-1RA	Hepatocytes, monocytes/macrophages, PMNs	Inhibits IL-1 action by blocking the IL-1 receptor

NO free radicals [79]. Th1 helper cells are therefore involved in the classical inflammatory response. Overactivation of Th1-type cells produces type 4 delayed hypersensitivity.
2. Conversely, Th2-type lymphocytes show marked anti-inflammatory properties by producing anti-inflammatory cytokines as IL-4, IL-5, IL-10, and IL-13 [80]. Overactivation causes type 1 IgE-mediated allergy and hypersensitivity.

    Other important players of the cell-mediated immune response in trauma and sepsis are the regulatory T (Treg-type) cells and T17-type cells.
3. Treg-type cells formerly known as suppressor T cells are modulator and deactivator of the immune response. They are immunosuppressive and generally downregulate the activation and proliferation of effector T cells (T cells that responds to a stimulus including helper and killer lymphocytes). Treg-type cells produce IL-10 and TGFβ a potent anti-inflammatory cytokine. Elevated levels of circulating Treg cells have been observed in the blood of immune-paralyzed infected patients [81, 82].
4. The Th17-type cells are a subset of T helper cells so named because of production of the cytokine IL-17. They exert protective effects on the gastrointestinal mucosal barrier function [83]. There is general agreement that Th17-type lymphocytes are protective against extracellular bacterial and fungal infections [84, 85]. The decrease of Th17 cells population contributes to immunoparalysis [86].

It is widely accepted that the development of a successful immune response requires the balance between Th1 and Th2 helper cells. In the early stage of sepsis and trauma, a phenotypic Th1-type cells profile predominates with IFϒ production which activates the bactericidal action of macrophages and induces B cell production of opsonizing and complement-fixing antibodies. Conversely, later (chronic) stages are characterized by a shift from the Th1-type profile into a predominantly Th2-type response leading to immunoparalysis, reduced antigen recognition and cellular anergy (see below) [87]. Other more complex anti-inflammatory actions include the decreased production of monocyte-derived cytokines by reduced transcriptional factors (NF-kB) for the encoding genes [88]. Also, the reduced expression of membrane surface receptor CD14 on monocytes (LPS-receptor) blunts their pro-inflammatory activity. Also the expression of MHC (major histocompatibility complex) class II molecules HLA-DR (human leukocyte antigen) is downregulated [89] with interference in the elimination of infected cells and maturation of several immune cell lines. These anti-inflammatory effects play an important compensatory role in the development of the counter anti-inflammatory response syndrome (CARS). Ideally CARS is

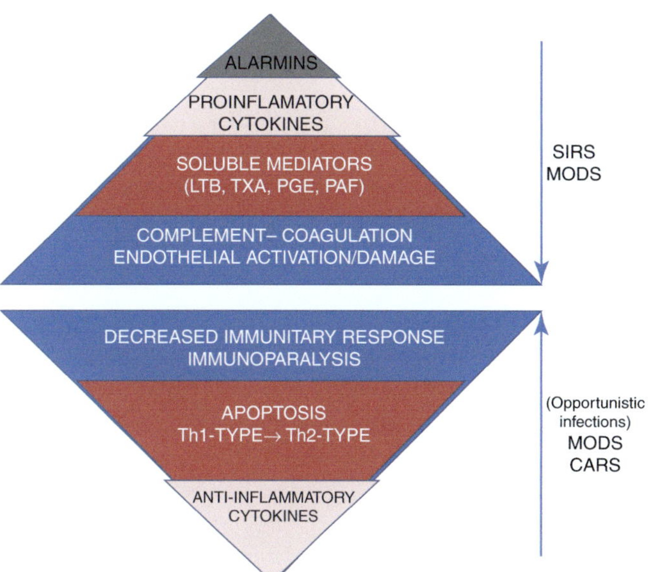

Fig. 2.8 Main steps of SIRS and CARS development with subsequent production of multiple organs dysfunction (MODS)

the physiological response to the risks of tissue damage by uncontrolled inflammation. The main SIRS and CARS events are summarized in Fig. 2.8.

The highly integrated, redundant, and coordinated immune-inflammatory system makes easy its comparison with a great classical orchestra. As a classical orchestra, there are players (neutrophils), soloists (monocytes and macrophages), and the musical score (humoral mediators). This score may be harmoniously classical (locally coordinated inflammatory response) or dissonantly dodecaphonic (SIRS). But who is the conductor?

2.4 The Endothelium

This fundamental role is covered by the endothelium. The acquisition that the endothelium orchestrates a complex, often redundant network of the immune-inflammatory players is quite recent. The endothelium is the interface between coagulation and inflammation in sepsis and trauma. Endothelial cells line the vessels in every organ by forming a barrier with organ-specific properties. So the vascular permeability is virtually null in capillaries of the brain and almost complete in the kidney with intermediate levels in the liver, muscle, and lung. The main properties of the endothelium are:

1. Lining the vascular system thus separating the blood from the cells and interstitium
2. Regulating the vascular tone with a net vasodilatory effect

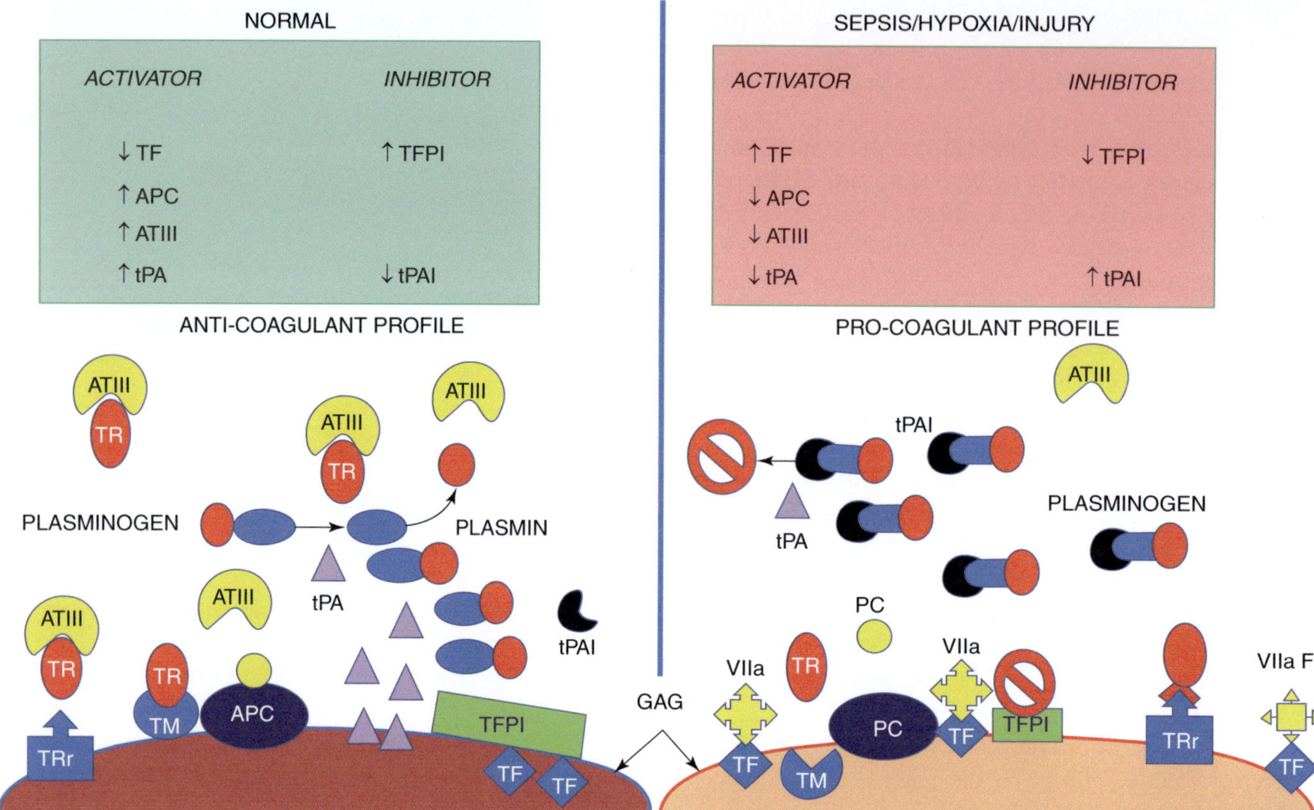

Fig. 2.9 Coagulation profile of endothelial surface during normal (left panel) and activated state (right panel). The anticoagulant profile is normally obtained by inhibition of thrombin (TR) activation of factor X by thrombomodulin (TM) expression on endothelial surface with formation of the activated protein C complex (APC). Antithrombin III (ATIII) further inhibits Thrombin activity by preventing its binding with receptor (TRr). Also tissue factor (TF) is not expressed on the endothelium, while its main physiological inhibitor, tissue factor pathway inhibitor (TFPI), is normally released by the intact endothelium. Finally the tissue plasminogen activator (tPA) catalyzes the zymogen plasminogen into plasmin, while tissue plasminogen activator inhibitor type-1 (tPAI-1) is reduced. After hypoxia, injury, or sepsis, the damaged endothelium expresses large amounts of TF, while TFPI release is inhibited. Also thrombomodulin receptor is internalized thus reducing APC formation, while decreased ATIII synthesis and degradation by serine protease increases the activity of thrombin. Finally tPAI-1 synthesis and release are increased thus reducing the formation of plasmin

3. Promoting anticoagulation by anti-thrombotic and profibrinolytic effects
4. Inhibiting the endothelial adhesion of platelets and leukocytes thus keeping the vessel clear

After trauma, hypoxic damage, or sepsis, the injured endothelium becomes prothrombotic and anti-fibrinolytic (Fig. 2.9).

2.4.1 Endothelial-Mediated Procoagulant State

The endothelium is involved in all the three major pathogenic pathways of septic and traumatic coagulopathy: tissue factor-mediated thrombin generation, dysfunctional anticoagulation, and fibrinolysis impairment [90]. Moreover, its activation by inflammatory stimulus leads to platelet and leukocyte adhesion and inhibition of vasodilation. Endothelial injury can be documented microscopically by a visible change of cell shape or damage and defects of endothelial lining. Indirect evidence of the damaged endothelium is the finding of elevated soluble markers of cell injury notably thrombomodulin, intercellular adhesion molecule, and E-selectin and von Willebrand factor [91, 92]. After endothelial damage, inflammatory fluids and cells can shift from the blood into the interstitial space. Endothelial injury is sustained over time so that its property loss is long-standing [93, 94]. Experimental animal and human studies demonstrated that after injury, the full recovery of endothelial lining occurs within 21 days [93]. The denudation of the vessel wall exposes tissue factor (TF), the principal activator of the extrinsic coagulation pathway with the risk of intravascular coagulation [93, 94]. Normally the outer endothelium expresses various membrane-bound molecules with anticoagulants properties among which are cell surface heparin-like molecules [95] and thrombin-binding protein thrombomodulin (TM). Heparin-like molecules are supported by glycosaminoglycans which cover the endothelial surface [90]. They act as cofactors for the antithrombin-mediated inhibition of thrombin and activate factor X (Stuart-Power factor) [95]. TM is the major responsible for thrombin inactivation as when bound to thrombin, forms a potent protein C (PC) activator complex that equips the endothelium with anticoagulant properties. However, the inflammatory or septic stimuli decrease the anticoagulant properties of the endothelial cells by loss or internalization of TM [96], while the contemporaneous stimulation of the thrombin receptor increases the inflammatory pathways. Finally, the action of neutrophil proteases also contributes to reduced TM expression. Moreover, the release of tissue plasminogen activator (TPa) is decreased, while its main physiological inhibitor, the plasminogen activator inhibitor-1 (PAI-1), increases so that the profibrinolytic properties of the endothelium are diminished. TF is increasingly expressed on both monocyte and macrophage membranes as well as on other cell types, while the function of its main physiological inhibitor, the tissue factor pathway inhibitor (TFPI), is decreased by reduced synthesis of glycosaminoglycans on endothelial surface [97]. In practice, any single procoagulant or profibrinolytic has its physiological inhibitor. Thus, TF is inhibited by TFPI [98], the coagulation system is counteracted by the activated protein C system [99], and tissue plasminogen activator (TPA) is coupled with tissue plasminogen activator inhibitor (TPAi) [100]. The imbalance between these systems results in a net procoagulant state with increased fibrin deposition, microvascular thrombotic occlusion, and risk for tissue ischemia [101]. Direct endothelial damage as occurs after trauma or ischemia-reperfusion injury contributes to activation of coagulation by decreased production of endothelial-derived substances as PGI and NO. The anti-adhesive properties of such molecules reduce leukocytes and platelets aggregation and counteract the procoagulant effectors. Localized coagulation has protective effects in discrete traumatic injuries, but its widespread activation is deleterious to the host with risk for multiple organ dysfunction and death [102, 103].

2.4.2 Endothelial Pro-adhesive Activation

Endothelial activation refers to the increased expression of adhesion molecules on endothelium surface. Complementary molecules are also expressed on the outer membrane of neutrophil and monocyte cells [104]. The surface expression, modulation, and activity of these molecules are highly regulated by locally produced cytokines (endothelial and monocyte cells) as the chemokine IL8 or PAF, IL1-β, and TNFα. The first step of the adhesion process consists of a "rolling" of leukocytes on the endothelial surface. This process involves selectins which are molecules expressed on leukocytes (L-selectin), endothelial cells (E-selectin), and platelets (P-selectin). Selectins act as receptors that permit a loose binding with the endothelial surface thus allowing for leukocyte rolling in proximity of opportune signaling molecules expressed on the endothelium. The second step involves the linkage of integrins with receptors of the immunoglobulins superfamily expressed on the endothelium surface. Integrins are a group of three heterodimer proteins expressed on the outer surface of activated leukocytes and collectively termed the CD11/CD18 complex. Adhesion molecules include ICAMs, E-selectins, PECAM (platelet endothelial cell adhesion molecules), and VECAM (vascular endothelial cell adhesion molecules). The final step consists of migration of activated leukocytes to the borders of endothelial cells and interaction with the endothelial-expressed adhesion molecules ICAM, PECAM, E-selectin, and VECAM [105]. Adhesion can occur without intervention of adhesion molecules in the lung and liver. It has been suggested that actin-containing stress fibers increase at the leukocyte periphery, this, in turn, causing decreased PMNs deformability and sequestration into the pulmonary and hepatic capillary beds [106]. The main effects of endothelial cells activation are summarized in Fig. 2.10.

2.4.3 Dysfunctional Endothelial Permeability

Thrombin is the main effector of increased endothelial permeability thus reaffirming the bidirectional interplay between the coagulation and the inflammatory cascade (Fig. 2.11). Thrombin can cleave a set of protease-activated receptors (PAR1-4) expressed on the endothelium [90, 107] that induces Rho-dependent cytoskeletal derangement in endothelial cells [108, 109].

PAR1 receptor activates Rho kinase which inhibits the dephosphorylation of myosin light chains (MLC) [110]. Phosphorylated MLC causes the actin-myosin interaction at the cell-to-cell contacts with contraction and rounding of endothelial cells and increased of vascular permeability.

This facilitates the passage of protein molecules and leukocytes from the blood into the interstitial space (Fig. 2.12).

Furthermore, the formation of gaps in the endothelial barrier exposes the proteins of the external coagulation pathway to the abundant TF amount expressed by the basement membrane and vessel adventitia. Clot formation is thus initiated, while collagen fibers from the extracellular matrix prompt vWf to polymerize and platelets to adhere.

Endothelial dysfunction refers to decreased NO release and reduced expression or synthesis of the constitutive NO synthase enzyme (eNOS). Abnormality of endothelial relaxation properties lasts for many days after the acute insult (endothe-

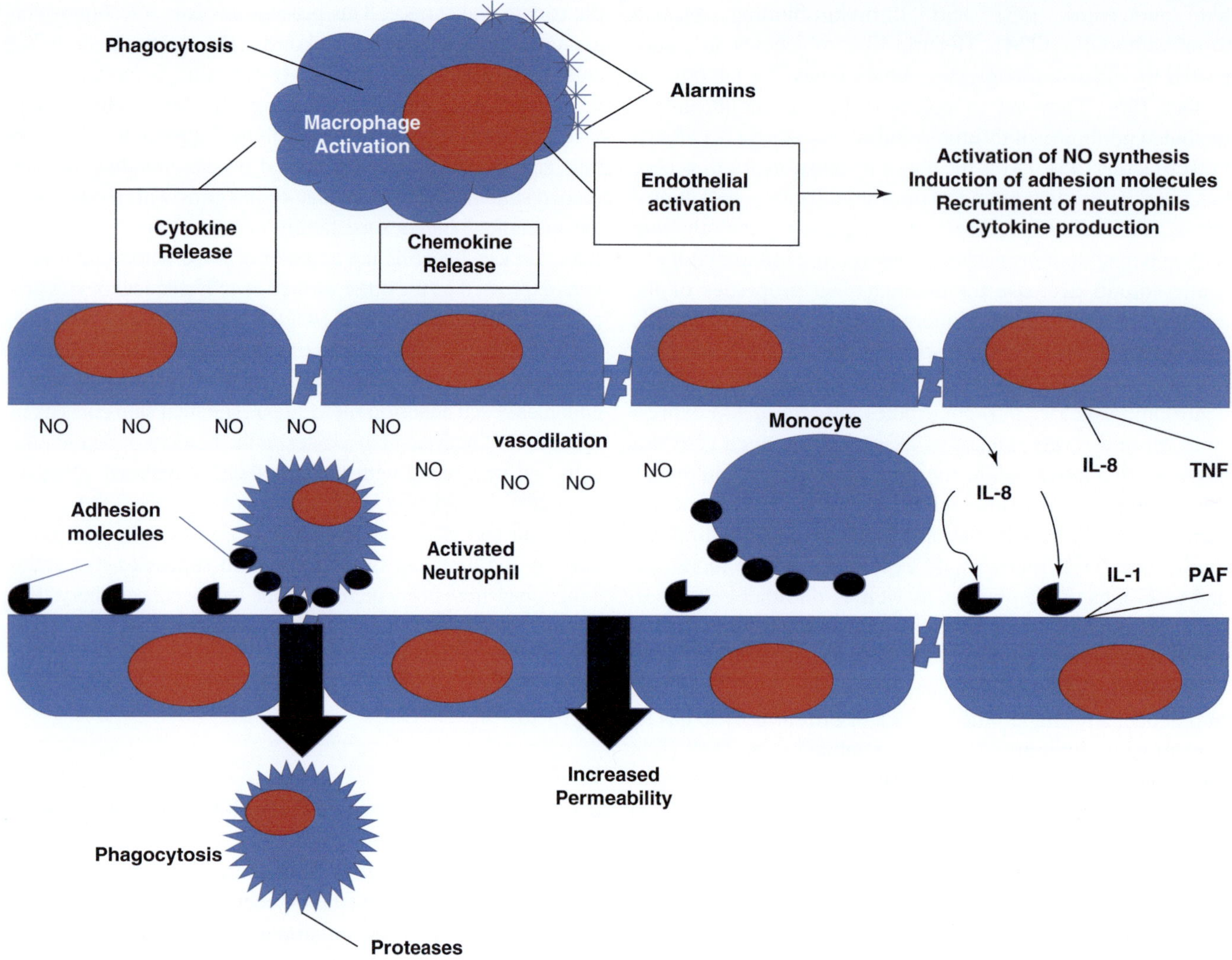

Fig. 2.10 Macrophage secretion of chemokines and cytokines stimulates the synthesis of adhesion molecules on the surface of endothelial cells. Neutrophils are recruited through the vascular wall to the site of inflammation. Monocytes are also stimulated to produce chemokines (mainly IL-8). The activated endothelium maintains inflammation by producing cytokines and other pro-inflammatory mediators. Finally nitric oxide synthesis is induced with vasodilation and loss of autoregulation of microcirculatory blood flow

lial stunning) [111]. The impairment of NO and PGI release by endothelial dysfunction have a profound impact upon cellular oxygenation with direct effects on tissues and organs well-being (Fig. 2.10). According to the concept of intrinsic metabolic regulation, oxygen supply and demand are constantly matched. Local vascular relaxation is therefore in dynamic equilibrium with the nervous-mediated vasoconstriction so that capillary blood flow is finely tuned to peripheral requirements. The endothelium plays a crucial role as a sensor of the local blood flow because of functional and structural coupling with the smooth muscle of arterioles and arteries.

Sensing is realized by depolarization/hyperpolarization of the endothelial cells, while communication involves electronic spread via endothelium/muscle cell-cell gap junctions [112]. Therefore, the hyperpolarization of the capillary endothelium induces the upstream vasodilation of the feeding arterioles and arteries [113, 114]. When inflammation impairs this finely tuned cell-cell communication, a "malignant intravascular inflammation" ensues [115]. The abnormal vascular reactivity, increased fibrin deposition, and cells adhesion may well account for heterogeneity of intra-organ perfusion and impaired oxygen delivery. The relationship between organ perfusion heterogeneity, impaired organ oxygen supply, and development of metabolic acidosis has been demonstrated in an animal model of endotoxic shock [116]. In an in vivo model of septic shock, a 36% reduction of perfused capillary density with increased perfusion heterogeneity and mean intercapillaries distance contributed to functional shunting [117] with impaired oxygen extraction after endotoxin challenge or fecal peritonitis [118, 119].

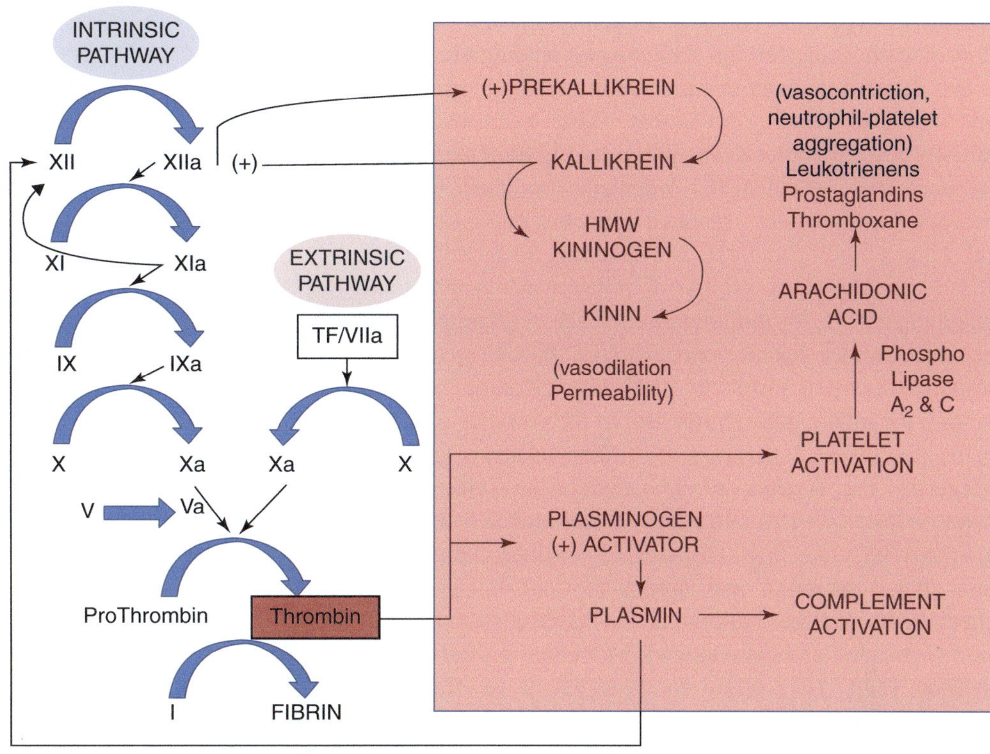

Fig. 2.11 Crosstalk between coagulation, fibrinolysis, and inflammation. (1) After its activation, thrombin stimulates tissue plasminogen activator (tPA) to catalyze the activation of plasmin that in turn stimulates the complement cascade. Thrombin also activates platelets to form arachidonic acid metabolites by membrane-bound phospholipases. (2) Also the Hageman factor (factor XII) stimulates the cleavage of prekallikrein into kallirein and subsequent kinins formation. This effect is potentiated by the positive feedback of plasmin and kallirein with the Hageman factor

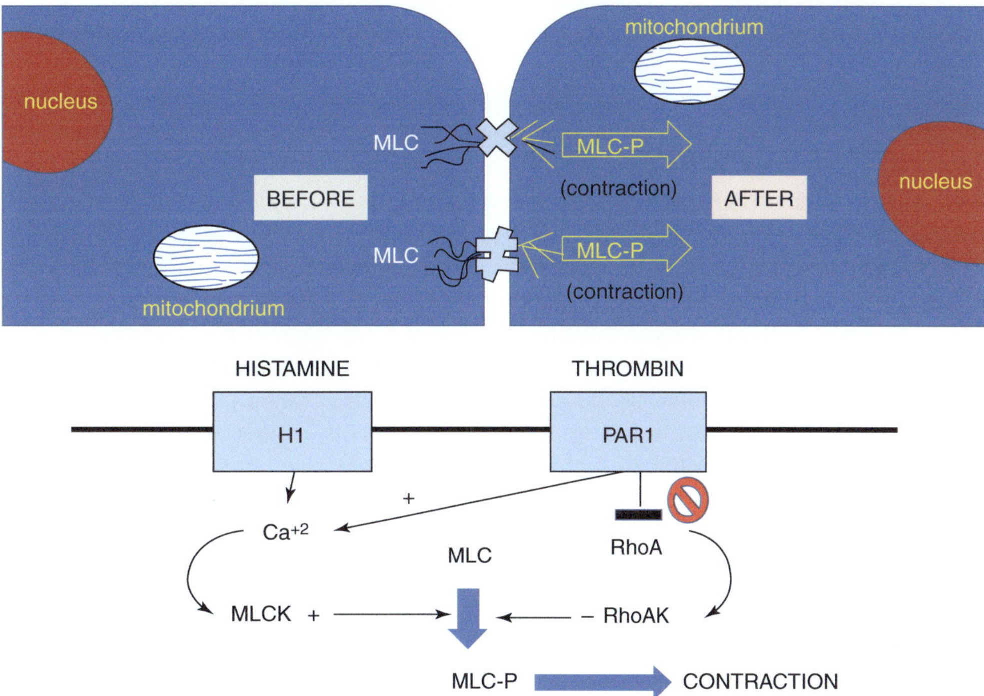

Fig. 2.12 Main pathways of increased vascular permeability. Myosin light-chain phosphorylation induces the reorganization of the actin cytoskeleton with acton-non-muscle-myosin interaction and subsequent loss of tight junctions and adherence junction stability

2.5 The Monocyte and Macrophage Cell

The other fundamental player of the systemic immune-inflammatory activation after trauma and ischemia-reperfusion or sepsis is the monocyte/macrophage cell. Monocytes are the circulating form of resident macrophages and dendritic cells. Resident macrophages can be found in the liver (Kupffer cells), lung (alveolar macrophages), lymphoid tissue (spleen and lymph nodes), and kidney (intra-glomerular mesangial macrophages). All these cells are very active in the synthesis of cytokines and removal of particulate antigens. In addition, they play a central role in antigen presentation to the innate Th1-type cells. APCs are fundamental for the eradication of pathogens, foreign antigens, or autologous cellular debris. Their key functions include the recognition, uptake, and killing of invading organisms. Tissue macrophages are initially activated after tissue injury by ischemic necrosis of mesenchymal cells in an IL1-α-dependent process. After the necrotic insult IL1-α is released from the dying cells with subsequent binding to the IL-1 macrophage surface receptors. IL1-α activates the assembly of inflammasome within the macrophage cytosol. Inflammasomes are multiprotein cytoplasmic complex that cooperate with the Toll-like receptors to respond to various insults by processing cytokines and promoting the inflammatory response. In the presence of pathogenic stimuli (e.g., alarmins), the inflammasome opens up so triggering the conversion of immature pro-inflammatory cytokines (e.g., IL1-β) into mature forms and activating pro-apoptotic enzymes (e.g., caspases). Thereafter, the extracellular IL1-β secretion and upregulation of IL1-β-induced chemokines, together with the increased expression of adhesion molecules, and cytokines secretion on the nearby endothelium [120, 121] allow for recruitment of circulating neutrophils and monocyte. NO synthesis is activated with resulting vasodilation, opening of endothelial gaps, and loosening of endothelial barrier properties [122] (Fig. 2.8). Monocytes and macrophages are also pivotal cells for the interaction between myeloid and endothelial cells. After the expression of chemoattractant molecules (IL8, monocyte chemoattractant protein-1 MCP-1, or macrophage inhibitory protein-1 MIP-1), the endothelium attracts monocytes to the inflammatory focus where they migrate into the tissue and become macrophages. Finally, the activated monocytes express large amounts of TF to propagate the procoagulant activity. After major uncomplicated trauma, the ability of APCs to express MHCII surface antigens is reduced [122] and returns to normal within a week [123]. After severe injuries, the APCs show a continuously decreased function. This deactivation leads to reduced expression of MHCII surface antigens and decreased ability to secrete cytokines which result into the increased susceptibility to infections [124].

2.6 Apoptosis

Many research findings have focused on the existence of premature programmed cell death (apoptosis) after injury, ischemia-reperfusion, and sepsis [125, 126]. Although apoptosis is an adaptive mechanism in several tissue and organs, namely, the lymphoid tissue and gut, its role seems deleterious in acute inflammatory states. Several studies suggest that the programmed cell death contributes to the derangement of cellular homeostasis in parenchymal (lung endothelial cells, kidney tubular cells, and skeletal muscle cells) and lymphoid organs with increased risk for sepsis and development of

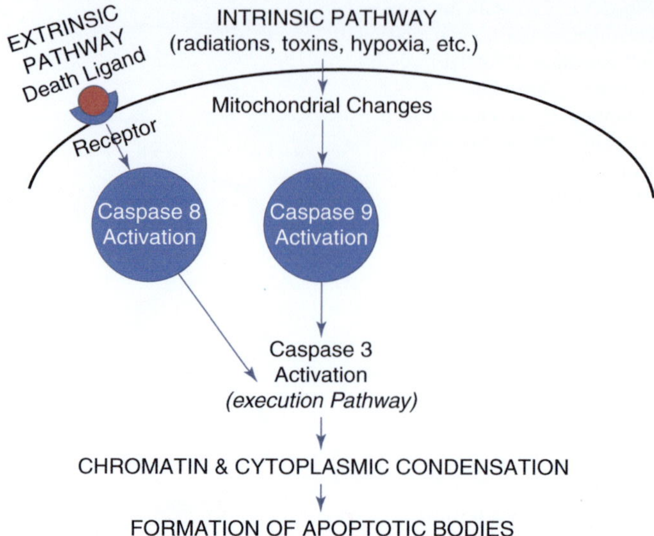

Fig. 2.13 The two main pathways of apoptosis are extrinsic and intrinsic pathway. Each requires specific triggering signals and activates its own initiator caspase which in turn activate the executioner caspase-3. The execution pathway includes cell shrinkage, chromatin condensation, cytoplasmic blebbing, and formation of apoptotic bodies. Finally phagocytosis of apoptotic bodies is performed by adjacent parenchymal cells or macrophages

multiple organ dysfunction [87]. Accelerated apoptosis induces lymphocytopenia [127] and decreased monocyte survival as reflected by loss of monocyte CD14 expression (co-receptor for the detection of bacterial lipopolysaccharide-LPS) [82]. Autoactivation of cytosolic and mitochondrial caspases are the two major pathways involved in apoptosis [128] (Fig. 2.13). Briefly, the extrinsic pathways activate caspases via binding to members of the TNF-receptor superfamily, while the mitochondrial induced pathway requires the emission of cytochrome c, otherwise essential for mitochondrial survival, into the cytosol with subsequent caspases activation [129]. Caspases are a family of proteolytic enzymes synthesized as inactive zymogens and activated by appropriate stimuli to express a death effector domain [130]. Apoptosis is a series of coordinated processes [131] that lead to DNA fragmentation, chromatin condensation, and blebs formation in the plasma membranes. Most important this controlled form of cellular degradation carries out with minimal effects on surrounding tissues. Therefore, apoptosis in a crucial physiological process during fetal development and throughout life as it maintains the normal development and regulation of cellular proliferation.

For example, during organ development apoptosis eliminates those cells that are no longer necessary. It has been estimated that without apoptosis, about 2 tons of bone marrow and lymphoid tissue would accumulate in the body [132]! Conversely accelerated apoptosis of lymphocytes is as detrimental as delayed apoptosis in neutrophils. Neutrophil cells are constitutively apoptotic as this ensures a tight control of the inflammatory response, but upon delayed apoptotic stimuli (cytokines), neutrophils become persistently activated and contributes to extensive organ damage by continuous release of toxic products (protease enzymes and reactive oxygen species) [133].

2.7 Immunoparalysis and Chronic Inflammatory States

Apoptosis causes a profound depression of immune functions with immunoparalysis and depletion of several immune cells including helper (CD4$^+$) and suppressor (CD8$^+$) T cells, B lymphocytes, and APCs (antigen presenting cells) [134]. Postmortem studies have confirmed immune cells apoptosis in all age groups [134, 135]. It can be speculated that apoptosis of gut-associated lymphoid tissue (GALT) [136] may be involved in bacterial translocation (see below). Several findings support the current view of immunoparalysis as a dominant feature of patients surviving the early hyperinflammatory phase. Although focal regions of inflammation ischemia and necrosis undoubtedly occur and contribute to the development of multiple organ dysfunction, death is the consequence of failure to control the primary infection or the development of new hospital-acquired infections often with opportunistic pathogens. This does not necessarily mean that infection is the main responsible for the patient's death and in fact many postmortem results are inconclusive. However, the severe decrease of innate immune function and the widespread hibernation of nonimmune cell type (cellular hibernation response) [137, 138] make apoptosis a primary mechanism for multiple organ dysfunction and ultimately death. Interestingly cancer and sepsis show similar immune defects [139], and increased survival after improving host immunity in cancer patients is encouraging to the field of sepsis. The most frequent manifestations of immunoparalysis include profound and persistent lymphopenia, loss of delayed type 4 hypersensitivity reaction [140], reactivation of latent viruses infections (herpes simplex virus and cytomegalovirus) [141, 142], and infection by low-virulent pathogens (e.g., *Stenotrophomonas* spp., *Candida* spp., *Acinetobacter* spp.) [143, 144]. Decreased pro-inflammatory cytokines production including IFϒ, TNF, and IL-2, increased IL-10 and other anti-inflammatory cytokines, decreased monocyte/macrophage and dendritic cells function with increased expression of apoptotic surface markers, and decreased cell survival are the hallmarks of immunoparalysis. Dendritic cells and monocytes play a pivotal role in the development of decreased immune function. Their reduced survival (apoptosis susceptibility) and function abnormalities (reduced HLA-DR expression and increased production of IL-10) induces T helper cell anergy and Treg cell proliferation. The reduced capacity of monocytes to release pro-inflammatory cytokines (e.g., TNF, IL-1, IL-6, IL-12), whereas the release of anti-inflammatory mediators (e.g., IL-10, IL-1RA) is not impaired or even enhanced [145] suggest for cellular reprogramming toward the anti-inflammatory pathway [146]. Monocyte dysfunction is known as endotoxin tolerance that is reduced cellular response to an endotoxin challenge. The main consequence of endotoxin tolerance is the increased susceptibility to nosocomial infections and death. Decreased immune T-cell function and T-cell exhaustion are the other leading causes of immunoparalysis.

1. The high antigenic load and the elevated pro- and anti-inflammatory cytokine profile of the early phase of trauma and sepsis are ideal for the development T-cell exhaustion. Phenotypic features of exhausted T cells are a decreased production of pro-inflammatory cytokines, mainly IFϒ and TNF, decreased cellular proliferation and cytotoxic function by excessive expression of PD-1 inducible co-stimulatory molecule and programmed cell death ligand PDL-1, and decreased expression of the IL-7 receptor [148]. IL-7 is a multipotential cytokine that acts to reverse immunosuppression by multiple mechanisms. It has shown to induce the two- to threefold increase of both naïve (Th0-type) and CD4/CD8 cells in cancer [149] and HIV patients [150] so reversing their major pathological abnormality, i.e., profound lymphopenia. Other effects include blockade of apoptosis [151], reversal of T-cell exhaustion [152], increased IFϒ [152] production leading to macrophage activation, and increased adhesion molecules expression on activated T lymphocytes [153].

   The decrease of Th1-type, Th2-type [86, 154–156], and Th17-type cells [86, 157] with maintenance of the number of Treg cells leads to the relative increase of regulatory functions and downregulation of effector T-cell response [86, 157]. The reduction of Th17-type cells contributes to the increased susceptibility to fungal infection due to their important role in protecting against extracellular bacterial and fungal invasion [158]. The relative increase of Treg cells is deleterious as being is associated with decreased effector T-cell proliferation and function. Their increased resistance to apoptosis with respect to the other T-cell type is probably responsible for their increased proportion [159, 160]. Treg cells can also suppress innate immune cells thus inhibiting myeloid-derived cell function [161]. Therefore, increased Treg cells impair the immune function by acting both on innate and adaptive immunity. Neutrophils, NK cells, and ϒδ T cells are other effectors whose function is decreased or impaired during immunoparalysis.
2. Briefly circulating neutrophils are markedly increased during the hyperinflammatory phase due to delayed apoptosis and release of immature cellular forms [162, 163]. Loss of chemotactic activity is their most frequently encountered dysfunction [164, 165]. A subset of

neutrophils with suppressive properties similar to the myeloid-derived suppressor cells (MDSCs) contributes to the development of immunoparalysis by production of large amounts of IL-10 [166] and interference in proliferation and function of effector T cells [167]. MDSCs are a heterogeneous group of myeloid cells that expand during chronic inflammatory states and cancer as a result of altered hematopoiesis. MDSCs possess strong immunosuppressive properties of both humoral and cellular type [168].

3. NK cells are markedly reduced both in peripheral blood and tissues where they are most abundant [169]. Impaired IFϒ by NK cells increases the host susceptibility to viral infections and reactivation of latent viruses, notably herpes simplex and cytomegalovirus [141, 142].
4. ϒδ T cells are a subset of lymphocytes that possess functions common to the innate and adaptive immune systems. They are particularly abundant in the intestinal mucosa with innate-like defense mechanism (IFϒ and IL-17 cytokines production). Intestinal ϒδ T cells are a first-line defense against infections [170], and their decreased number exposes to the risk of microbial invasion of the blood and peritoneal cavity.

The main effects of chronic inflammation upon innate and acquired immune cells are shown in Figs. 2.14 and 2.15.

2.8 How Multiple Organ Dysfunction (MODS) Develops

Multiple organ dysfunction syndrome (MODS) is defined as "the presence of altered organ function in an acutely ill patient such that homeostasis cannot be maintained without intervention" [2]. The mechanisms implicated in the development of MODS include:

1. Induction of cellular apoptosis
2. Translocation of microbes or microbial cellular debris from the gastrointestinal tract

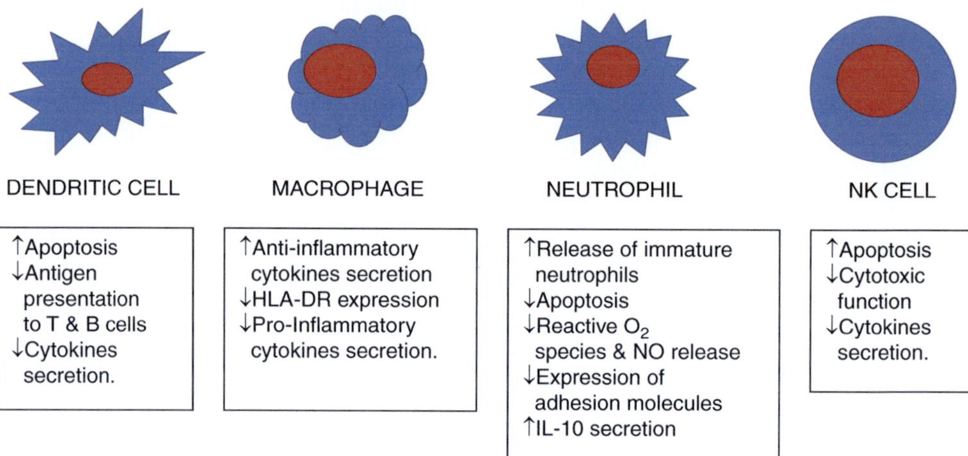

Fig. 2.14 Main effects of chronic sepsis (inflammation) on innate immune cells. Sepsis rapidly triggers extensive apoptosis in dendritic cells, monocytes, and natural killer (NK) cells, while neutrophils apoptosis is contemporarily delayed. Large amount of immunosuppressive IL-10 are released (neutrophils), while the decreased HLA-DR expression (monocytes and dendritic cells) impairs the optimal killing of bacteria

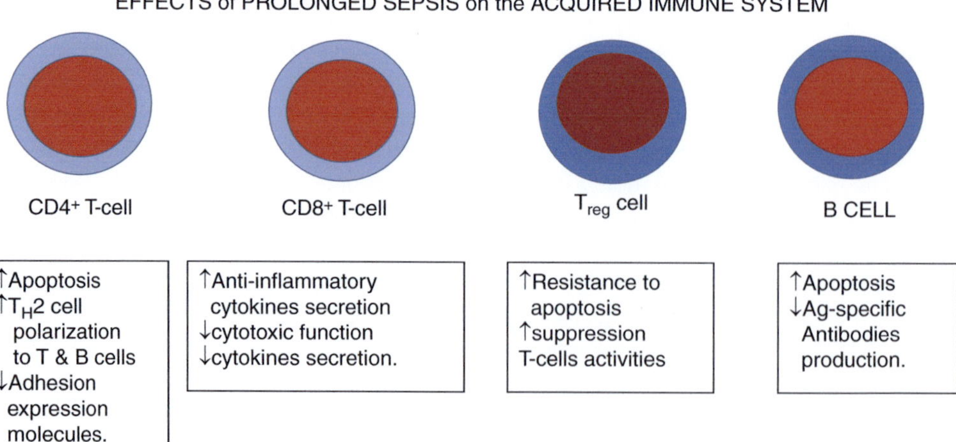

Fig. 2.15 Main effects of chronic sepsis (inflammation) on acquired immune cells. Lymphocytopenia results from massive loss of T helper and T suppressor lymphocytes. T regulatory cells are more resistant to apoptosis so that an immunosuppressive phenotype results. Surviving T cells shift from a pro-inflammatory Th-1 cell-type to an anti-inflammatory Th-2 cell-type profile

3. Immune system dysregulation
4. Mitochondrial dysfunction

Although the above mechanisms can interact in a variety of ways and combinations, immune system dysregulation and mitochondrial dysfunction seem to play a prevalent role. As detailed above, the immune system dysregulation is the imbalance between pro-inflammatory and anti-inflammatory mechanisms. CARS is a coordinated anti-inflammatory response to severe inflammatory stimuli that allows for the maintenance of immune system homeostasis. The "purpose" of CARS is to limit the noxious effects of SIRS while not interfering with pathogen elimination or healing of the injured tissue. However, CARS may be dangerous when its effects lead to a condition known as "immunoparalysis" with an increased risk of nosocomial sepsis and septic shock. Mitochondrial dysfunction with its hypoxic cellular implications is also important in the pathogenesis of MODS. PMNs production of reactive oxygen species (superoxide and peroxynitrite) and inflammatory cytokines induces oxidative stress that leads to uncoupling of oxidative phosphorylation. The derangement in cellular energy metabolism is known as cytophathic hypoxia, a functional concept that points out the imbalance between adequate oxygen delivery and poor oxygen utilization at the mitochondrial level. When cytophathic hypoxia develops, the result is cellular dysfunction and death. Although "bad" from a clinical point of view, cytophathic hypoxia may be a cellular adaptive response [171] as it can be viewed as a cellular hibernation-like state. However, if this phenomenon occurs for too long, irreversible cellular damage may result [172].

Bacterial translocation is another proposed mechanism for sustained inflammation and development of multiple organ dysfunctions. Although the "sustained-hit model" [173] predicts that the persistent stimulation of natural and acquired immune system by noxious stimuli is responsible for the maintenance of the inflammatory status, recent acquisitions implicate the apoptotic loss of δϒ T cells in the intestinal mucosa [170]. There is good evidence that ischemia-reperfusion injury is the main mechanism for loss of gut barrier function [174]. As oxygenation of the villi is dependent on a counter-current mechanism such that O_2 tension at the tip of the villi is lower than that of arterial blood, any decrease in splanchnic blood flow may be associated with bacterial translocation. At this point endotoxin, bacteria, or gut ischemia can stimulate the gut-associated lymphoid tissue to generate an immune-inflammatory response that affects distant organs. Otherwise stated the gut becomes a pro-inflammatory organ, releasing cytokines and other inflammatory mediators which give origin to sepsis and MODS.

According to the point of view of the intensive care medicine, the whole body is constituted by seven physiologically interdependent organ systems: nervous, respiratory, cardiovascular, hepatic biliary, renal, digestive, and coagulation system. Although many of them can be involved, the respiratory and cardiovascular systems are most frequently damaged with acute lung injury (ALI)/acute respiratory distress syndrome (ARDS) and sepsis-induced hypotension being the commonest clinical presentations. It is well established that the number or dysfunctional organs affects the prognosis. Thus the probability to die with only one single dysfunctional organ is fairly less than half with respect to two or more organ dysfunction [175]. Moreover, a multicenter study established that the mortality increases almost linearly from 21.2 to 76.2% when organ dysfunction increases from 1 to ≥4 organ systems [176]. Mortality is also influenced by comorbidities notably chronic renal failure, diabetes, and cancer [176, 177]. Cumulative comorbidities also increase the risk for the development of MODS with the highest mortality rate [178]. By converse, survivors suffer from a persistent chronic illness that may last for months or even years. This illness is characterized by prolonged ICU stay, slow recovery from organs dysfunction, recurrent infections, progressive or permanent cognitive deficit, and loss of overall sense of well-being and function [179, 180]. So the duration of healthy life expectancy is reduced although the patient's overall life span is intact.

The common pathophysiological denominator of MODS is the loss of cell membrane barrier function. This finding is strikingly evident from the autopsies of patients who die as a result of multiple organs dysfunction syndrome. Despite the clinical evidence of acute myocardial dysfunction, progressive cholestatic jaundice, continuing impairment of renal function, and similar dysfunction of other organ systems, the histopathological findings are remarkably normal or limited to mild tissue edema. Therefore, the preserved organ morphology is strikingly in contrast with the impairment of organ function. The loss of cellular and tissue (endothelial) barrier function seems the cornerstone for this sort of hibernation that prevents the multiplicity of organ expression, variability, and communication. The commonest clinical presentations of single organ system dysfunctions are shown below.

2.8.1 Nervous System

Recent acquisitions indicate that the brain is often involved in sepsis and MODS as it is one target of SIRS either by direct activation of resident pro-inflammatory cells (neuroglia) or by mediators generated elsewhere (complement, cytokines). Although the CNS is considered an immune-protected organ due to the blood-brain barrier, the abundance of glial cells with their signaling receptors makes the brain one of the preferred target for organ system dysfunction.

Therefore, the local inflammatory reaction that follows traumatic or hypoxic (e.g., post-cardiac arrest) brain damage can spread outside the CNS thus exacerbating SIRS. Conversely, the circulating cytokines and other inflammatory mediators may increase the permeability of the blood-brain barrier thus causing brain damage [181]. Cytokines activate monocytes to transform into glial cells (equivalent to resident macrophages in extra-cerebral tissues) so that inflammation continues in the nervous tissue [182]. Circulating cytokines also can stimulate the afferent fibers of the vagus nerve that activate the central nervous system. After stimulation of vagus nerve endings, cerebral endothelial cells are activated resulting in the breakdown of the blood-brain barrier [183, 184]. The activation of cerebral endothelium also induces microvascular dysfunction, loss of cerebral vascular tone (autoregulation), and coagulopathy (microthrombi deposition) [185]. Receptors for the commonest cytokines have been found in the hippocampus, one of the most involved regions for mnemonic elaboration and neuroplasticity [181]. Chronic inflammation of the hippocampus can lead to irreversible cognitive decline, especially in the elderly. Histopathologic lesions of the brain in sepsis include cerebral edema, infarct and ischemic lesions, and microabscesses [185]. Sepsis-associated encephalopathy has been reported in 23% of people in the ICU [186]. However, the true incidence is difficult to estimate because of lack of clear definition and subjective nature of its assessment. Moreover, sedative drugs may blunt the symptoms thus making the diagnosis difficult. Symptoms include changes in consciousness, awareness, cognition, and behavior. Symptoms seem correlated with the global severity of illness as assessed by the Acute Physiology and Chronic Health Evaluation II score (APACHE II score).

2.8.2 Respiratory System

It is by far the commonest organ system involved. ALI and ARDS are the two clinical manifestations of respiratory dysfunction. ALI is defined as the presence of bilateral pulmonary infiltrates on chest radiograph and arterial hypoxemia ($PaO_2/FiO_2 < 300$). If the PaO_2/FiO_2 drops below 200, the condition is classified as ARDS [187]. ARDS can originate from two distinct pathways:

1. Direct pulmonary damage as occurs after trauma, infection, aspiration, or inhalation injury
2. Indirect damage as occurs with sepsis, pancreatitis, extra-pulmonary trauma and burns, blood transfusions, and fat embolism [188, 189]

Respiratory dysfunction span from extremely severe forms requiring immediate tracheal intubation, mechanical ventilation, and paralysis to milder forms with mild hypoxia and tachypnea. The lung is the most frequent organ involved in sepsis and trauma probably because it is the single organ with the largest vascular bed and it harbors one of the largest populations of resident macrophages. ARDS is characterized by neutrophil infiltration, alveolar-capillary barrier disruption, pulmonary vascular leakage, and edema. In most severe forms the alveoli contain eosinophilic protein-rich exudate with presence of hyaline membrane [190]. Electron microscopic examination reveals extensive damage to type I alveolar pneumocytes with cellular swelling and blebbing of the plasma membranes [190]. Pulmonary edema and absorption atelectasis decrease the pulmonary volume with the occurrence of refractory hypoxia by increased pulmonary shunt. Moreover, the widespread deposition of microthrombi and hypoxic pulmonary vasoconstriction impose a pressure overload upon the right ventricle with myocardial dysfunction and failure. The initial clinical presentation is often subtle with tachypnea, dyspnea, dry cough, and agitation. Hypoxia with hypocapnia is the most prominent laboratory feature. The magnitude of hypoxia is often unexplained by the mild or absent roentgenographic signs. CT scan reveals diffuse but nonuniform ground-glass consolidations often with a non-conformal gravitational distribution [191]. In more severe forms, multiple patchy areas of lung consolidation coalesce in massive airspace consolidation [191]. Characteristically the distribution is uniform and affects all lung zones extending to the extreme periphery of the lung fields. Hypoxia and interstitial/alveolar edema stimulate the carotid body chemoreceptors and intraparenchymal lung mechanoreceptors to hyperventilate with decreased arterial carbon dioxide tension. In the latest phases, normocapnia ensues mainly as result of increased respiratory work due to alveolar collapse, decreased pulmonary volume, and respiratory compliance. The mechanical disadvantage of decreased pulmonary compliance causes the abnormal increase of trans-pulmonary pressure (the pressure across the alveoli) that is the driving force for pulmonary expansion. The shear stress upon the delicate alveolar and interstitial structure causes further inflammation as a vicious cycle ensue with endothelial activation and worsening of pulmonary function that influences each other. Mortality from ARDS ranges from 15 to 80% [189, 192] with average values of about 30% according to most recent ventilatory strategies [193].

2.8.3 Cardiovascular Dysfunction

It is one of the commonest organ dysfunction of septic and/or traumatic origin. Some studies report an incidence of up to 66% [194, 195] with a mortality rate as high as 70% [195, 196]. The cardiovascular dysfunction has long been recognized as a consequence of the generalized inflammatory reaction [197]. Its most prominent clinical features are (1) myocardial dysfunction with biventricular dilation and reduced ejection fraction [198] and (2) arterial hypotension despite fluid volume infusion and decreased response to vasoactive drugs. It generally accepted that the decreased cardiac function is the product of circulating myocardial depressant factors (endotoxin, IL1β, TNFα, IL6, PAF, and others) and mitochondrial damage [199–201]. Some experimental evidence indicates that endotoxin acts by inducing an inflammatory response through heart tissue macrophage, mast cells, and infiltrating blood leukocytes. The clinical picture includes the following: arterial hypotension, mental impairment, warm and dry skin, oliguria, elevated arterial blood lactates, and higher than normal mixed or central venous saturation. The hemodynamic pattern shows a high cardiac output and decreased peripheral vascular resistance [202, 203]. The picture of low cardiac output state (pale and wet skin, oliguria, and hypotension) is rarely seen and indicates a more severe form of cardiac depression [202, 203]. When examined in detail, the cardiac function appears depressed as, despite the high output state, the ejected volume is lower than normal (reduced stroke volume), the ventricle is dilated (increased diastolic volume), and its contractile state is impaired with reduced ejection fraction (increased end-systolic volume). These changes are often masked by the decreased peripheral vascular resistance. The reduced afterload allows for the maintenance of a high output state as the dysfunctional ventricle pump blood against a dilated arterial system. When the ventricular dysfunction is severe, the clinical picture resembles that of cardiogenic shock with low cardiac output, high arterial lactates, and intense peripheral vasoconstriction. Several studies have shown that cardiac dysfunction is biventricular in origin and that is potentially reversible by 7–10 days [204].

The other essential feature of cardiovascular dysfunction is arterial hypotension by decreased peripheral arterial resistance. Because a major fraction of peripheral vascular resistance is located in peripheral arteries, this segment is designated as the resistance vessels. Resistance vessels control the blood flow to organs, and it is under the control of either intrinsic (e.g., metabolic) or extrinsic (e.g., neural and humoral) factors. Intrinsic regulation plays a fundamental role in pressure-flow autoregulation (ability of an organ to keep constant the blood flow despite fluctuations in arterial pressure), reactive hyperemia (ability to increase the blood flow after relief of a vascular obstruction), and functional hyperemia (ability to cope the organ blood flow in accordance with local metabolic needs) [205, 206]. In sepsis, intrinsic regulation is compromised in all the vascular beds with the exception of the cerebral vasculature [207, 208]. This can explain the mismatch between whole oxygen supply and metabolic demands of septic shock. The increased cardiac output does not cope with the cellular energy requirements so that hypoxia and increased acid production develop. By converse, the extrinsic regulation of resistance vessels is responsible for maintenance of arterial pressure and blood flow to the whole organs. During sepsis and after trauma or ischemia-reperfusion injury, a marked hypo-responsiveness to vasopressor agents is a frequent finding with development of arterial hypotension and tissue hypoperfusion. It is generally accepted that the decreased responsiveness to vasoconstrictor stimuli is consequent to increased production of endothelial nitric oxide (NO) by the induced nitric oxide synthase (iNOS) [209]. In normal arterioles, a small amount of NO is produced by endothelial NOS (eNOS) as maintenance of cardiovascular homeostasis [209]. However, cytokines and endotoxins induce iNOS to produce large quantities of NO [209, 210]. Although iNOS induction can be viewed as an adaptive response to noxious stimuli, the resulting hypotension by massive NO production is deleterious for organs and tissues. Also, there is some evidence that vascular smooth muscle can be another relevant source of NO production. In smooth muscle, neural NOS (nNOS) is upregulated thus contributing to NO generation in septic animals [211]. Another factor implicated in arteriolar hypo-responsiveness may be the complex of morphological alterations of the endothelial lining of the arterioles. Experimental studies show that the endotoxin challenge results into endothelium disruption with cell swelling, pseudopod formation, and frank denudation of the endothelial lining [212, 213]. Finally, the loss of capillary to arteriolar signaling may induce the hypo-responsiveness of arterioles to vasopressor stimuli. In normal conditions, capillaries may regulate the arteriolar tone by the upstream spread of electronic signaling along the endothelium. In sepsis, the cell-to-cell communication is impaired so that the modulation of blood flow delivery to capillaries is severely compromised [214]. Taken all together the above mechanisms may lead to the inappropriate redistribution of blood flow to tissues and organs [215, 216]. Because the arterial control of blood flow is responsible for the convective flux of oxygen to capillaries, the alteration of arterial tone may cause regional hypoxia [215] and ultimately multiple organ dysfunction. Treatment principles of hyperdynamic shock are briefly outlined in Chap. 3.

2.8.4 Coagulation Dysfunction

The coagulation system is designed:

1. To stop active blood loss
2. To seal the site of lesion, thus allowing for pathogens destruction and removal of debris
3. To initiate the healing process

The most severe form of coagulation disorder is the disseminated intravascular coagulation (DIC). This pathophysiologic mechanism results from the imbalance between coagulation and fibrinolysis with upregulation of the procoagulant pathway, downregulation of anticoagulant pathway (namely, ATIII, protein C, and S system), and decreased fibrinolysis. Coagulation is regulated by three main anticoagulant mechanisms: antithrombin, the protein C system, and the tissue factor pathway inhibitor (TFPI). The loss of physiologic anticoagulation in sepsis results from the action of several humoral (IL1-β, TNF-α, and IL6, C-reactive protein) and cellular (vascular endothelial cells, monocytes, macrophages, and platelet) pro-inflammatory mediators. Furthermore, monocytes and macrophages are the main source of tissue factor (TF) a potent thrombin generator via the VII (extrinsic) pathway. The widespread fibrin deposition causes the formation of microthrombi with diffuse microcirculatory flow disturbance. TF is a membrane-bound protein that possesses the most important procoagulant activity [217]. After its expression on the cellular membranes, it forms complexes with the circulating factor VII of the coagulation cascade (extrinsic pathway) thus activating the formation of thrombin [218]. TF is abundant in the subcutaneous tissue and virtually in all blood-tissue barrier [219]. As seen above, TF is also inducible on monocyte and macrophage surfaces. In meningococcal septicemia, large quantities of TF have been localized in microparticles (MPs) shed from platelets and leukocyte aggregates [220]. After trauma or infection, large amount of TF can be expressed by the denuded endothelium, damaged subcutaneous, and muscular tissues with priming of the coagulation cascade. Similarly, sepsis can induce disseminated intravascular coagulation by cytokines production and monocyte adhesion to the activated endothelium with further TF expression. After thrombin formation, the von Willebrand factor (vWf) is released from the Weibel-Palade bodies of endothelial cells. vWf binds to platelet glycoprotein IIb to stabilize the adhesion of platelets and entrapped white blood cells aggregates to the injured endothelium [221]. Normally vWf multimers are cleaved by the protein complex ADAMTS13, and this process is stimulated under conditions of shear stress. Sepsis is associated with decreased circulating ADAMTS13 levels resulting in increased levels of ultra-large vWf multimers [221]. After adhesion to the endothelium (white thrombus formation), platelets enhances the inflammatory and coagulation cascade by expression of TF on activated monocytes and endothelial cells [222]. Clinical conditions associated with overt DIC are summarized in Table 2.3.

The role of DIC in the pathogenesis of MODS is widely supported by experimental and postmortem findings. Firstly, the demonstration of intravascular thrombi at autopsy appears related to the clinical dysfunction of the organ [223]. Secondly, experimental studies demonstrated the deposition of intravascular and extravascular fibrin in the kidneys, lung, liver, and brain [223]. Finally, clinical studies demonstrated the prognostic importance of DIC as being an independent predictor of death [224].

Table 2.3 Clinical pictures often associated with overt DIC

• Sepsis/severe infection (any microorganism)
• Trauma
• Serine protease activation (e.g., pancreatitis)
• Malignancy (solid or myeloproliferative/lymphoproliferative tumors)
• Obstetrical catastrophes (amniotic fluid embolism, abruptio placentae)
• Vascular abnormalities (aneurysms, giant hematomas)
• Severe hepatic failure
• Toxic reactions (snake venoms, drugs)
• Immunological reactions (transplant rejection and transfusion reactions)

The clinical diagnosis of DIC relies upon the simultaneous presence of:

1. Consumption of coagulation factors (prolonged clotting times)
2. Consumption of coagulation inhibitors (e.g., decreased ATIII activity)
3. Platelets consumption or count of less than 100,000/mm^3
4. Presence of fibrin degradation products (increased D-dimer)
5. Presence of a condition known to be associated with DIC

In the past decade, clinical simple scoring systems for DIC were introduced (Table 2.4).

They have individual strengths (JAAM has the highest sensitivity, while ISTH is the most specific) and collective weaknesses (poor diagnostic sensitivity for late-onset DIC) [228]. Fibrinogen levels are not sensitive indicators of DIC as fibrinogen synthesis is increased during SIRS as occurs in the acute phase protein reaction. Finally, the diagnosis of DIC can be difficult in the presence of hepatic dysfunction or portal vein thrombosis as many of diagnostic clues of DIC are present in these pathologic conditions. Coagulation dysfunction affects up to 30% of patients with sepsis [229], while thrombocytopenia ($<10^5$ platelets/mm^3) occurs in up to 60% with an inverse relationship between platelet count and severity of disease [230, 231].

2.8.5 Renal Dysfunction

Acute kidney injury (AKI) is defined as an absolute increase in serum creatinine of 1.5-fold from baseline or a urine output <0.5 mL/Kg/h for 6 h [232]. Overall AKI frequency was reported over 20% in a large cohort study of 325,395 patients admitted to ICU with odds of death increasing in parallel with increased severity of acute kidney injury [233]. Crude mortality has been found ranging between 28 and 82% [234, 235].

Table 2.4 Most popular DIC scoring systems

	JMHW		ISTH		JAAM	
Underlying disease	Absent Present	0 1	Required		Required	
Clinical presentation No Bleeding Bleeding No MODS MODS	0 1[a] 0 1			No SIRS SIRS	0 1	
Platelet count	>120 80–120 50–80 ≤50	0 1[a] 2[a] 3[a]	>100 50–100 <50	0 1 2	≥120 80–120 or −30% reduction in 24 h <80 or −50% reduction in 24 h	0 1 2
FDP	<10 10–20 20–40 >40	0 1 2 3			<10 10–25 >25	0 1 2
Fibrin-related marker (e.g., *soluble fibrin monomer, FDP)*			Normal Moderate Strong	0 2 3		
Fibrinogen	>1.5 1.0–1.5 ≤1	0 1 2	>1.0 <1.0	0 1		
PT ratio	<1.25 1.25–1.67 ≥1.67	0 1 2			<1.2 ≥1.2	0 1
Prolonged prothrombin time			<3.0 s 3.0–6.0 s >6.0 s	0 1 2		
Diagnosis		**≥7**		**≥5**		**≥4**

JMHW Japanese Ministry of Health and Welfare [225], *ISTH* International Society of Thrombosis and Haemostasis [226], *JAAM* Japanese Association of Acute Medicine [227]

[a]If hematologic malignancy, 0 pts for bleeding and platelets and add 3 pts to the total score

Table 2.5 Criteria for acute kidney injury

Risk (R)	Serum creatinine increased ≥1.5 over baseline
Injury (I)	Serum creatinine increased ≥2 over baseline
Failure (F)	Serum creatinine increased ≥3 over baseline
Loss (L)	Loss of renal function >4 weeks
End-stage renal disease (E)	Loss of renal function >3 months

Modified from [236]

The severity of AKI is classified using the risk, injury, failure, loss and end-stage renal disease (RIFLE) criteria listed in Table 2.5, [236].

Two main pathways are responsible for AKI: one is characterized by acute tubular necrosis, renal hypoperfusion, and ischemia—despite common belief, this form accounts for only 22% of sepsis-induced AKI [237]—and the second form is specific to MODS, and its predominant mechanism is apoptosis induced by inflammatory cytokines [238]. This pathogenic mechanism is more adherent to the hyperdynamic circulatory state that follows post-traumatic SIRS and sepsis [239]. Experimental studies suggest that the decrease in glomerular filtration rate in AKI is the result of a disproportionate vasodilation of the efferent than the afferent glomerular arterioles [240]. In normal condition, the vascular tone of afferent and efferent vessels is regulated by humoral intra-glomerular factors (mainly angiotensin, thromboxane A2, and PGI2). The interplay between vasoconstrictor (angiotensin and thromboxane A2) and vasodilator (PGI2) factors causes the tone of efferent vessels to increase with respect to the afferent arterioles. This allows for the glomerular capillary pressure to ensure normal filtration. During SIRS or sepsis, the dilation of the efferent arterioles decreases the glomerular pressure and hence the filtration rate [241]. This pathophysiologic mechanism can explain the positive effects of norepinephrine or vasopressin infusion in patients with SIRS and oliguria. Despite the common belief, norepinephrine and vasopressin have been reported to increase the urinary output in patients with hyperdynamic shock. Their vasoconstrictor effect is probably helpful in restoring the tone of the efferent arteriole with resulting increase of capillary perfusion pressure. In addition to glomerular hemodynamic changes, circulating or locally (mesangial cells) produced TNFα induces tubular cell apoptosis with imbalance in water and electrolytes homeostasis [242]. AKI is an important form of organ dysfunction because of its association with high mortality rates. In a multinational, multicenter study, the prevalence of AKI has been estimated to be 5–6% of people with only 40% of them discharged alive [243]. Septic shock is the most common cause of AKI with a prevalence of 65% [244]. Trauma patients who developed AKI showed 29% of mortality rate as compared with 9% of the overall mortality rate [245].

2.8.6 Hepatic and Gut Dysfunction

The gut has long been recognized as the "motor" of MODS due to its capability of amplifying the SIRS response during shock and gut hypoperfusion. The incidence of gastrointestinal dysfunction is difficult to estimate due to the subjective nature of diagnosis and the lack of a clear diagnostic definition. Symptoms and signs of intestinal dysfunction include hyporexia, anorexia, inability to tolerate enteral feeding, decreased intestinal motility, and diarrhea often of hemorrhagic type [246, 247]. After a catastrophic hypoperfusion of the gut as occurs with cardiac arrest or severe multiple trauma, the normal intestinal flora is destroyed and substituted by an increasing number of pathogens [248]. This phenomenon is detrimental because the normal flora protects against the colonization of microbial pathogens thus preventing bacterial translocation (see above) [249]. However, the change of normal flora together with reduced intestinal motility and disruption of normal gut mucosal barrier increase the risk for bacterial translocation and development of MODS. The loss of mucosal barrier function is the result of endotoxin, inflammatory cytokines, and decreased production of tight junction proteins [250].

Hepatic dysfunction is schematically divided into two clinical forms: hypoxic hepatitis (HH) and jaundice-induced cholestasis (JIC). HH can result from absolute (e.g., cardiogenic) or relative decrease in cardiac output with reduced oxygen supply to the liver. During septic shock, cardiac output and oxygen delivery are increased albeit not enough to cope with the high oxygen requirement of the liver and the inability of cells to extract oxygen [45]. Moreover, the hepatic arterial buffer response and other vascular mechanisms of defense against portal blood flow reduction are impaired [251]. HH is also the product of oxidative stress after ischemia/reperfusion injury and the action of endotoxin and other inflammatory mediators which lead to activation of Kupffer cells and activation and recruitment of leukocytes. The diagnosis of HH requires:

1. A clinical setting of impaired oxygen delivery (usually due to cardiac and/or respiratory failure)
2. A greater than 20-fold increase in serum aminotransferase activity
3. The exclusion of other causes of liver cell necrosis [252, 253]

Another landmark of HH is the acute drop of prothrombin levels which gives origin to a hemorrhagic syndrome [254]. These acute biochemical changes, especially those reflecting acute liver cells necrosis, decrease rapidly within 2 or 3 days and normalize within approximately 2 weeks. The delayed elevation of serum bilirubin is often seen but without apparent jaundice. Jaundice-induced cholestasis is a more subtle form of hepatic jaundice usually associated with severe infections [255, 256]. The increase of bilirubin is a late event in these septic patients [257], and histological studies reveal the intrahepatic origin of the cholestasis [258]. The reduction of bile salt excretion in the gut is responsible for the atrophy of the mucosal gut barrier [259] with loss of integrity and increased risk of bacterial translocation. Moreover, the gut is deprived by the bacteriostatic action of bile salts with proliferation of pathogens and increased production of endotoxin [260, 261]. This creates a vicious circle that perpetuates the infection and hence further cholestatic liver damage. The production and transport of bile salts are a complex, highly coordinated, and energy-dependent mechanism. During sepsis many of these mechanisms are impaired because of a lack of energy due to hypoxia or hypoperfusion or both [262]. The major limiting factor for the bile flow at the canalicular level is the ATP-dependent bile salt export pump that is severely impaired in the septic liver [262]. The severity of hyperbilirubinemia appears directly related to the severity of impairment in the various steps of bile formation. No specific therapies can be recommended for acute liver dysfunction. The most recommended measures are merely supportive including the normalization of perfusion pressure and restoration of oxygen delivery [263], the maintenance of normal oxygen tension, and serum glucose levels. The early use of enteral nutrition is also helpful in counteracting the atrophy of gut mucosal barrier and reducing the intestinal pathogens [264].

Case Scenario

A high-impact trauma victim was admitted to ED with head trauma and severe hemorrhagic shock by ruptured spleen and multiple bone fractures. The patient was unconscious; his blood pressure was 85/55 mmHg with 135 bpm pulse rate. Metabolic acidosis (pH 7.27, PaCO2 32 mmHg) and hyperlactacidemia (7.5 mmol/L) were also present. Splenectomy and external fixation of bone fractures were quickly performed. During surgery, the blood pressure remained at about 100/60 with an average 120 bpm pulse rate. Despite several liters of crystalloids and transfusion of blood products (4 PRC and 4 FFP), an infusion of norepinephrine up to 0.15 μg/Kg/min was started. At ICU admission, the patient had stable vital signs (AP 115/50 mmHg) a mild tachicardia (HR 115 bpm), and compensated metabolic acidosis (pH 7.37, PaCO2 30 mmHg) with elevated arterial blood lactates (7 mmol/L). After 12 h from ICU admission, the resuscitation phase appeared complete. At 24 h, fever of 38.8 °C, leukocytosis 21,000 cells/mm^3, respiratory alkalosis, and tachycardia prompted the execution of a total body CT scan.

1. ***What is the most probable diagnosis?***
   A. ***Sepsis***
   B. ***SIRS***
   C. ***Intra-abdominal abscess***
   D. ***Fever of CNS origin***

2. ***Which are the cytokines involved in the onset of fever and leukocytosis?***
   A. ***IL-4 and IL-10***
   B. ***IL-1 and TNF***
   C. ***IL-6 and IL-7***
   D. ***None of the above answers***

The CT scan excluded intra-abdominal abscesses and revealed large bilateral psoas muscle and pelvic hematomas. Microbiological cultures from urine, bronchial tube drainage fluids were negative. Within 5 days fever and tachycardia disappeared so that the definitive fixation of bone fractures was scheduled for the following week.

At day 10, a new appearance of fever and leukocytosis occurred.

3. ***What is the most probable origin of fever in this patient?***
   A. ***Infection***
   B. ***SIRS***
   C. ***Drugs-induced fever***
   D. ***Fever of unknown origin***

The chest roentgenogram showed a right perihilar infiltrate and purulent bronchial secretions. Broad spectrum antibiotics were started, but 24 h thereafter the patient develops hypotension, oliguria, metabolic acidosis, altered mental status, and decreased platelet count.

4. ***What is the most probable cytokines profile?***
   A. ***Increased pro-inflammatory and decreased anti-inflammatory cytokines (SIRS)***
   B. ***Predominance of anti-inflammatory upon pro-inflammatory cytokine profile (CARS)***
   C. ***Balanced pro- and anti-inflammatory cytokines profile (MARS)***
   D. ***None of the above answers***

A multi-sensitive *Klebsiella pneumoniae* was isolated from blood cultures, and antimicrobial therapy allows for rapid control of the septic source and resolution of the clinical picture. The patient was discharged from intensive care after 15 days and returned at home within 60 days from the hospital admission.

Please see Chap. 58 for the correct answer.

References

1. Bone RC. Sir Isaac Newton, sepsis, SIRS and CARS. Crit Care Med. 1996;24:1125–8.
2. American College of Chest Physicians/Society of Critical Care Medicine Consensus Conference: definitions for sepsis and organ failure and guidelines for the use of innovative therapies in sepsis. Crit Care Med. 1992;20:864–74.
3. Lord JM, Midwinter MJ, Chen Y, Belli A, Brohi K, Kovacs EJ, Koenderman L, Kubes P, Lilford RJ. The systemic immune response to trauma: an overview of pathophysiology and treatment. Lancet. 2014;384:1455–65.
4. Osuchowski MF, Craciun F, Weixelbaumer KM, Duffy ER, Remick DG. Sepsis chronically in MARS: systemic cytokine responses are always mixed regardless of the outcome, magnitude, or phase of sepsis. J Immunol. 2012;189(9):4648–56.
5. Hotchkiss RS, Karl IE. The pathophysiology and treatment of sepsis. N Engl J Med. 2003;348:138–50.
6. Oberholzer A, Oberholzer C, Moldawer LL. Sepsis syndromes: understanding the role of innate and acquired immunity. Shock. 2001;16:83–96.
7. Hotchkiss RS, Monneret G, Payen D. Immunosuppression in sepsis: a novel understanding of the disorder and new therapeutic approach. Lancet Infect Dis. 2013;13:260–8.
8. Riche FC, Cholley BP, Panis YH, Laisne MJ, Briard CG, Grauler AM, Gueris JL, Valleur PD. Inflammatory cytokine response in patients with septic shock secondary to generalized peritonitis. Crit Care Med. 2000;28:433–7.
9. Brunialti MK, Martins PS, de Carvalho B, Machado FR, Barbosa LM, Salomao R. TLR2, TLR4, CD14, CD11B, and CD11C expressions on monocytes surface and cytokine production in patients with sepsis, severe sepsis and septic shock. Shock. 2006;25:351–7.
10. Iskander KN, Osuchowski MF, Stearns-Kurosawa DJ, Kurosawa S, Stepien D, Valentine C, Remick DG. Sepsis: multiple abnormalities, heterogeneous responses, and evolving understanding. Physiol Rev. 2013;93:1247–88.
11. Osuchowski MF, Welch K, Yang H, Siddiqui J, Remick D. Sepsis: always in MARS. Shock. 2006;25:5.
12. Heidecke CD, Hensler T, Weighardt H, Zantl N, Wagner H, Siewert JR, Holzmann B. Selective defects on T lymphocytes function in patients with lethal intraabdominal infection. Am J Surg. 1999;178:288–92.
13. Ploder M, Pelinka L, Schmuckenschlager C, Wessner B, Ankersmit HJ, Fuerst W, Redl H, Roth E, Spittler A. Lipopolysaccharide-induced tumor necrosis factor alpha production and not monocyte human leukocyte antigen-DR expression is correlated with survival in septic trauma patients. Shock. 2006;25:129–34.
14. Cavaillon JM, Adib-Conquy M, Cloez-Tayarani I, Fitting C. Immunodepression in sepsis and SIRS assessed by ex-vivo cytokine production is not a generalized phenomenon: a review. J Endotoxin Res. 2001;7:85–93.
15. Bianchi ME. DAMPs, PAMPs and alarmins: all we need to know about danger. J Leukoc Biol. 2007;81:1–5.
16. Pugin J. How tissue injury alarms the immune system and causes a systemic inflammatory response. Ann Intensive Care. 2012;2:22.
17. Zhang Q, Raoof M, Chen Y, Sumi Y, Sursal T, Junger W, Brohi K, Itagaki K, Hauser CJ. Circulating mitochondrial DAMPSs cause inflammatory response to injury. Nature. 2010;464:104–7.
18. Chen G, Li J, Ochani M, Rendon-Mitchell B, Qiang X, Susarla S, Ulloa L, Yang H, Fan S, Goyert SM, Wang P, Tracey KJ, Sama AE, Wang H. Bacterial endotoxin stimulates macrophages to release HMGB1 partly through CD14- and TNF-dependent mechanisms. J Leukoc Biol. 2004;76:994–1001.
19. Zedler S, Faist E. The impact of endogenous triggers on trauma-associated inflammation. Curr Opin Crit Care. 2006;12:595–601.
20. Manson J, Thiemermann C, Brohi K. Trauma alarmins as activators of damage-induced inflammation. Br J Surg. 2012;99(Suppl 1):12–20.
21. Burk AM, Martin M, Flierl MA, Rittirsch D, Helm M, Lampl L, Bruckner U, Stahl GL, Blom AM, Perl M, Gebhard F, Huber-Lang MS. Early complementopathy after multiple injuries in humans. Shock. 2012;37(4):348–54.
22. Neher MD, Weckbach S, Flierl MA, Huber-Lang MS, Stahel PF. Molecular mechanisms of inflammatory and tissue injury after major trauma-is complement the "bad guy"? J Biomed Sci. 2011;18(1):90.
23. Huber-Lang MS, Kotvun A, Ignatius A. The role of complement in trauma and fracture healing. Semin Immunol. 2013;25:73–8.
24. Harris HE, Raucci A. Alarmin(s) news about danger: workshop on innate danger signals and HMGB1. EMBO Rep. 2006;7:774–8.

25. Wang H, Vishunabhakat JM, Bloom O, Zhang M, Ombrellino M, Sama A, tracey KJ. Proinflammatory cytokines (tumor necrosis factor and interleukin 1) stimulate release of high mobility group protein-1 by pituicytes. Surgery. 1999;126:389–92.
26. Scaffidi P, Misteli T, Bianchi ME. Release of chromatin protein HMGB1 by necrotic cells triggers inflammation. Nature. 2002;418:191–5.
27. Gardella S, Andrei C, Ferrera D, Lotti LV, Torrisi MR, Bianchi ME, Rubartelli A. The nuclear protein HMGB1 is secreted by monocytes via a non-classical, vesicle-mediated secretory pathway. EMBO Rep. 2002;3:995–1001.
28. Andersson U, Wang H, Palmblad K, Aveberger AC, Bloom O, Erlandsson-Harris H, Janson A, Kokkola R, Zhang M, Yang H, Tracey KJ. High mobility group 1 protein (HMG-1) stimulates proinflammatory cytokine synthesis in human monocytes. J Exp Med. 2000;192:565–70.
29. Rouhianen A, Kuja-Panula J, Wilkman E, Pakkanen J, Stenfors J, Touminen RK, Leptanlo M, Carpén O, Parkkinen J, Rauvala H. Regulation of monocyte migration by amphoterin (HMGB1). Blood. 2004;104:1174–82.
30. Roumen RM, Redl H, Schlag G. Inflammatory mediators in relation to the development of multiple organ failure in patients after severe blunt trauma. Crit Care Med. 1995;23:474–80.
31. Rose S, Marzi L. Pathophysiology of polytrauma. Zentralbl Chir. 1996;121(11):896–913.
32. Mollnes TE, Fosse E. The complement system in trauma-related and ischemic tissue damage: a brief review. Shock. 1994;2:301–10.
33. Biffl WL, Moore EE, Moore FA, Carl VS, Kim FJ, Franciose RJ. Interleukin-6 potentiates neutrophil priming with platelet-activating factor. Arch Surg. 1994;129:1131–6.
34. Friese RS, Rehring TF, Wollmering M, Moore EE, Ketch LL, Banerjee A, Harken AH. Trauma primes cells. Shock. 1994;1:388–94.
35. Hietbrink F, Koenderman L, Rijkers G, Leenen L. Trauma: the role of the innate immune system. World J Emerg Surg. 2006;1:15.
36. Partrick DA, Moore FA, Moore EE, Barnett CC Jr, Silliman CC. Neutrophil priming and activation in the pathogenesis of postinjury multiple organ failure. New Horiz. 1996;4:196–210.
37. Alcaide P, Auerbach S, Luscinskas FW. Neutrophil recruitment under shear flow: it's all about endothelial rings and gaps. Microcirculation. 2009;16:43–57.
38. Giannoudis PV, Hildebrand F, Pape HC. Inflammatory serum markers in patients with multiple trauma. Can they predict outcome. J Bone Joint Surg Br. 2004;86(3):313–23.
39. Lenz A, Franklin GA, Cheadle WG. Systemic inflammation after trauma. Injury. 2007;38:1336–45.
40. Zhu J, Yamane H, Paul WE. Differentiation of effector C4 T cell populations. Annu Rev Immunol. 2010;28:445–89.
41. Botha AJ, Moore FA, Moore EE. Postinjury neutrophil priming and activation: an early vulnerable window. Surgery. 1995;118:358–65.
42. DeLong WG Jr, Born CT. Cytokines in patients with polytrauma. Clin Orthop Relat Res. 2004;422:57–65.
43. Grell M, Becke FM, Wajant H, Mannel DN, Scheurich P. TNF receptor type 2 mediates thymocyte proliferation independently of TNF receptor type 1. Eur J Immunol. 1998;28:257–63.
44. Carpentier I, Coonaert B, Beyaert R. Function and regulation of tumor necrosis factor type 2. Curr Med Chem. 2004;11:2205–12.
45. Dinarello CA. Interleukin-1 beta. Crit Care Med. 2005;33:S460–2.
46. Shalaby MR, Waage A, Espevik T. Cytokine regulation of interleukin 6 production by human endothelial cells. Cell Immunol. 1989;121:372–82.
47. Opal SM, DePalo VA. Anti-inflammatory cytokines. Chest. 2000;117:1162–72.
48. Tilg H, Trehu E, Atkins MB, Dinarello CA, Mier JW. Interleukin-6 (IL-6) as an anti-inflammatory cytokine. Induction of circulating IL-1 receptor antagonist and soluble tumor necrosis factor receptor p55. Blood. 1994;83:113–8.
49. Lin E, Calvano SE, Lowry SF. Inflammatory cytokines and cell response in surgery. Surgery. 2000;127:117–26.
50. Xing Z, Gauldie J. Cox G IL6 is an anti-inflammatory cytokine required for controlling local or systemic acute inflammatory responses. J Clin Invest. 1998;101:311–20.
51. Jekarl DW, Lee SY, Park YJ, Kim Y, Park JH, Wee JH, Choi SP. Procalcitonin as a diagnostic marker and IL-6 as a prognostic marker for sepsis. Diagn Microbiol Infect Dis. 2013;75(4):342–7.
52. Takahashi W, Nakada TA, Yazaki M, Oda S. Interleukin-6 levels act as a diagnostic marker for infection and a prognostic marker in patients with organ dysfunction in the intensive care unit. Shock. 2016;46(3):254–60.
53. Inagaki T, Hoshino M, Hayakawa T, Ohara H, Yamada T, Yamada H, Lida M, Nakazawa T, Ogasawara T, Uchida A, Hasegawa C, Miyaji M, Takeuchi T. Interleukin 6 is a useful marker for early prediction of the severity of acute pancreatitis. Pancreas. 1997;14(1):1–8.
54. Keane MP, Strieter RM. Chemokine signaling in inflammation. Crit Care Med. 2000;28:N13–26.
55. Fosse E, Pillgram-Larsen J, Svennevig JL, Nordby C, Skulberg A, Mollnes TE, Abdelnoor M. Complement activation in injured patients occurs immediately and is dependent on the severity of the trauma. Injury. 1998;29(7):509–14.
56. Stahel PF, Morganti-Kossman MC, Kossmann T. The role of the complement system in traumatic brain injury. Brain Res Rev. 1998;27:243–56.
57. Buzdon MM, Napolitano LM, Shi HJ, Ceresoli DM, Rauniya R, Bass BL. Femur fracture induces site-specific changes in T-cells immunity. J Surg Res. 1999;82(2):201–8.
58. Weiser MR, William JP, Moore FD Jr, Kobzik L, Ma M, Hechtman HB, Carroll MC. Reperfusion injury of ischemic skeletal muscle is mediated by natural antibody and complement. J Exp Med. 1996;183(5):2343–8.
59. Zhang M, Alicot EM, Chiu I, Li J, Verna N, Vorup-Jensen T, Kessler B, Shimaoka M, Chan R, Friend D, Mahmood U, Weissleder R, Moore RD, Carrol MC. J Exp Med. 2006;203(1):141–52.
60. Bouvet Zouali M. Silent antibodies. Arch Inst Pasteur Tunis. 2005;83:3–8.
61. Carrol MC, Holers VM. Innate autoimmunity. Adv Immunol. 2005;86:137–57.
62. Fleming SD. Natural antibodies, autoantibodies and complement activation in tissue injury. Autoimmunity. 2006;39:379–86.
63. Stahel PF, Smith WR, Moore EE. Role of biological modifiers regulating the immune response after trauma. Injury. 2007;38:1409–22.
64. Schmidt OI, Infanger M, Heyde CE, Ertel W, Stahel PF. The role of neuroinflammation in traumatic brain injury. Eur J Trauma. 2004;30:135–49.
65. Sugimoto K, Hirata M, Majima M, Katori M, Ohwada T. Evidence for a role of kallikrein-kinin system in patients with shock after blunt trauma. Am J Physiol. 1998;274:1556–60.
66. Van Gils JM, Zwaginga JJ, Hordijk PL. Molecular and functional interactions among monocytes, platelets, and endothelial cells and their relevance for cardiovascular diseases. J Leukoc Biol. 2009;85:195–204.
67. Jenne CN, Urrutia R, Kubes P. Platelets: bridging hemostasis, inflammation and immunity. Int J Lab Hematol. 2013;35:254–61.
68. Abraham E. Coagulation abnormalities in acute lung injury and sepsis. Am J Respir Cell Mol Biol. 2000;22:401–4.
69. Fan J, Kapus A, Li YH, Rizoli S, Marshall JC, Rotstein OD. Priming for enhanced alveolar fibrin deposition after hemorrhagic shock: role for tumor necrosis factor. Am J Respir Cell Mol Biol. 2000;22(4):412–21.

70. Levi M, de Jonge E, Van der Poll T. New treatment strategies for disseminated intravascular coagulation based on current understanding of the pathophysiology. Ann Med. 2004;36:41–9.
71. Gando S, Kameue T, Matsuda N, Sawamura A, Hayakawa M, Kato H. Systemic inflammation and disseminated intravascular coagulation in early stage of ALI and ARDS: role of neutrophil and endothelial activation. Inflammation. 2004;28(4): 237–44.
72. Lo EH, Wang X, Cuzner ML. Extracellular proteolysis in brain injury and inflammation: role for plasminogen activators and matrix metalloproteinases. J Neurosci Res. 2002;69:1–9.
73. Whicher JT, Westacott CI. The acute phase response. In: Whicher JT, Evans SW, editors. Biochemistry of inflammation. London: Kluwer Academic; 1992. p. 243–71.
74. Du Clos TW. Function of C-reactive protein. Ann Med. 2000;32:274–8.
75. Zweigner J, Gramm HJ, Singer OC, Wegscheider K, Schumann RR. High concentrations of lipopolysaccharide-binding protein in serum of patients with severe sepsis or septic shock inhibit the lipopolysaccharide response in human monocytes. Blood. 2001;98(13):3800–8.
76. Fujishima S, Aikawa N. Neutrophil-mediated tissue injury and its modulation. Intensive Care Med. 1995;21:277–85.
77. Laroux FS, Pavlick KP, Hines IN, Kawachi S, Harada H, Bharwani S, Hoffman JM, Grisham MB. Role of nitric oxide in inflammation. Acta Physiol Scand. 2001;173(1):113–8.
78. Mosmann TR, Sad S. The expanding universe of T-cell subsets: Th1 and Th2 and more. Immunol Today. 1996;17:138–46.
79. Blanchette J, Jaramillo M, Olivier M. Signalling events involved in interferon-gamma-inducible macrophage nitric oxide generation. Immunology. 2003;108(4):513–22.
80. Kelso A. Th1 and Th2 subsets: paradigms lost? Immunol Today. 1995;16:374–9.
81. Monneret G, Debard AL, Venet F, Bohe J, Hequet O, Bienvenu J, Lepape A. Marked elevation of human circulating $CD4^+CD25^+$ regulatory T cells in sepsis induced immunoparalysis. Crit Care Med. 2006;34:2561–6.
82. Venet F, Pachot A, Debard AL, Bienvenu J, Lepape A, Powell WS, Monneret G. Human $CD4^+CD25^+$ regulatory T lymphocytes inhibit lipopolysaccharide-induced monocyte survival through a Fas/Fas ligand-dependent mechanism. J Immunol. 2006;177(9): 6540–7.
83. Romani L. Immunity to fungal infections. Nat Rev Immunol. 2011;11:275–88.
84. Blaschitz C, Raffatellu M. Th17 cytokines and the gut mucosal barrier. J Clin Immunol. 2010;30(2):196–203.
85. Van de Veerdonk FL, Mouktaroudi M, Ramakers BP, Pistiki A, Pickkers P, van der Meer JWM, Netea MG, Giammarellos-Bourboulis EJG. Deficient candida-specific T-helper 17 response during sepsis. J Infect Dis. 2012;206:1798–802.
86. Pachot A, Monneret G, Voirin N, Leissner P, Venet F, Bohé J, Payen D, Bienvenu J, Mougin B, Lepape A. Longitudinal study of cytokine and immune transcription factor mRNA expression in septic shock. Clin Immunol. 2005;114(1):61–9.
87. Tschoeke SK, Ertel W. Immunoparalysis after multiple trauma. Injury. 2007;38:1346–57.
88. Rossato M, Curtale G, Tamassia N, Castellucci M, Mori L, Gasperini S, Mariotti B, De Luca MC, Mirolo M, Cassatella MA, Locati M, Bazzoni F. IL-10-induced micro-RNA-187 negatively regulates TNF-alpha, IL-6 and IL-12p40 production in TLR4-stimulated monocytes. Proc Natl Acad Sci U S A. 2012;109:E3101–10.
89. Monneret G, Lepape A, Voirin N, Bohé G, Venet F, Debard AL, Thizy H, Bienvenu J, Gueyffier F, Vanhems P. Persisting low monocyte human leukocyte antigen-DR expression predicts mortality in septic shock. Intensive Care Med. 2006;32:1175–83.
90. Schouten M, Wiersinga WJ, Levi M, van der Poll T. Inflammation endothelium and coagulation in sepsis. J Leukoc Biol. 2008;83(3):536–45.
91. Bajaj MS, Tricomi SM. Plasma levels of the three endothelial-specific proteins von Willebrand factor, tissue factor pathway inhibitor, and thrombomodulin do not predict the development of acute respiratory distress syndrome. Intensive Care Med. 1999;25:1259–66.
92. Kayal S, Jais JP, Aguini N, Chaudiere J, Labrousse J. Elevated circulating E-selectin, intercellular adhesion molecule 1, and von Willebrand factor in patients with severe infection. Am J Respir Crit Care Med. 1998;157:776–84.
93. Leclerc J, Pu Q, Corseaux D, Haddad E, Decoene C, Bordet R, Six I, Jude B, Vallet B. A single endotoxin injection in the rabbit causes prolonged blood vessel dysfunction and a procoagulant state. Crit Care Med. 2000;28:3672–8.
94. Wiel E, Vallet B. Vascular endothelial cell dysfunction in septic shock. Crit Care Med. 2001;29(Suppl):S36–41.
95. Bombeli T, Mueller M, Haeberli A. Anticoagulant properties of the vascular endothelium. Thromb Haemost. 1997;77:408–23.
96. Rapaport S, Rao L. Initiation and regulation of tissue factor-dependent blood coagulation. Arterioscler Thromb. 1992;12:1111–21.
97. Ott I, Miyagi Y, Miyazaki K, Heeb MJ, Mueller BM, Rao LV, Ruf W. Reversible regulation of tissue factor-induced coagulation by glycosyl phosphatidylinositol-anchored tissue factor pathway inhibitor. Arterioscler Thromb Vasc Biol. 2000;20(3):874–82.
98. Monroe DM, Key NS. The tissue factor-factor VIIa complex: procoagulant activity, regulation, and multitasking. J Thromb Haemost. 2007;5:1097–105.
99. Esmon CT. Protein C anticoagulant pathway and its role in controlling microvascular thrombosis and inflammation. Crit Care Med. 2001;29:S48–51.
100. Binder BR, Christ G, Gruber F, Grubic N, Hufnagl P, Krebs M, Mihaly J, Prager GW. Plasminogen activator inhibitor 1: physiological and pathophysiological roles. News Physiol Sci. 2002;17(2):56–61.
101. Regoeczi E, Brain MC. Organ distribution of fibrin in disseminated intravascular coagulation. Br J Haematol. 1969;17:73–81.
102. Carr C, Bild GS, Chang AC. Recombinant E. coli-derived tissue factor pathway inhibitor reduces coagulopathic and lethal effects in the baboon gram-negative model of septic shock. Circ Shock. 1994;44:126–37.
103. Camerota AJ, Creasey AA, Patla V, Larkin VA, Fink MP. Delayed treatment with recombinant human tissue factor pathway inhibitor improves survival in rabbit gram-negative peritonitis. J Infect Dis. 1998;177:668–76.
104. Springer T. Traffic signals on endothelium for lymphocyte recirculation and leukocyte emigration. Annu Rev Physiol. 1995;57:827–72.
105. Varani J, Ward P. Mechanisms of endothelial cell injury in acute inflammation. Shock. 1994;2:311–9.
106. Doerschuk CM. Leukocyte trafficking in alveoli and airway passage. Respir Res. 2000;1:136–40.
107. Levi M, van der Poll T. Endothelial injury in sepsis. Intensive Care Med. 2013;39:1839–42.
108. Riewald M, Ruf W. Mechanistic coupling of protease signaling and initiation of coagulation by tissue factor. Proc Natl Acad Sci U S A. 2001;98:7742–7.
109. Riewald M, Petrovan RJ, Donner A, Mueller BM, Ruf W. Activation of endothelial cell protease activated receptor 1 by the protein C pathway. Science. 2002;296:1880–2.
110. Kimura K, Ito M, Amano M, Chihara K, Fukata Y, Nakafuku M, Yamamori B, Feng J, Nakano T, Okawa K, Iwamatsu A, Kaibucki K. Regulation of myosin phosphatase by Rho and Rho-associated kinase (Rho-kinase). Science. 1996;273:245–8.

111. Bhagat K, Moss R, Collier J, Vallance P. Endothelial "stunning" following a brief exposure to endotoxin: a mechanism to link infection and infarction? Cardiovasc Res. 1996;32:822–9.
112. Sandow SL, Hill CE. Incidence of myoendothelial gap junctions in the proximal and distal mesenteric arteries of the rat is suggestive of a role in endothelium-derived hyperpolarizing factor-mediated response. Circ Res. 2000;86:341–6.
113. Emerson GG, Segal SS. Endothelial cell pathway for conduction of hyperpolarization and vasodilation along hamster feed artery. Circ Res. 2000;86:94–100.
114. Segal SS. Microvascular recruitment in hamster striated muscle: role for conducted vasodilation. Am J Physiol. 1991;261:H180–9.
115. Pinsky MR. Regional blood flow distribution. In: Pinsky MR, Dhainaut JF, Artigas A, editors. The splanchnic circulation: no longer a silent partner. Berlin: Springer; 1995. p. 1–13.
116. Nelson DP, Samsel RW, Wood LDH, Schumacker PT. Pathological supply dependence of systemic and intestinal O2 uptake and endotoxemia. J Appl Physiol. 1988;64:2410–9.
117. Lam C, Tyml K, Martin C, Sibbald W. Microvascular perfusion is impaired in a rat model of normotensive sepsis. J Clin Invest. 1994;94(5):2077–83.
118. Humer MF, Phang PT, Friesen BP, Allard MF, Goddard CM, Walley KR. Heterogeneity of gut capillary transit times and impaired gut oxygen extraction in endotoxemic pigs. J Appl Physiol. 1996;81:895–904.
119. Elis CG, Bateman RM, sharpe MD, Sibbald WJ, Gill R. Effect of a maldistribution of microvascular blood flow on capillary O2 extraction in sepsis. Am J Physiol Heart Circ Physiol. 2002;282:H156–64.
120. Eigenbrod T, Park JH, Harder J, Iwakura Y, Nunez G. Cutting edge: critical role of mesothelial cells in necrosis-induced inflammation through the recognition of IL-1 alpha released from dying cells. J Immunol. 2008;181:8194–8.
121. Dinarello CA. Interleukin-1 in the pathogenesis and treatment of inflammatory diseases. Blood. 2011;117:3720–32.
122. Koppelman B, Neefjes JJ, de Vries JE, de Waal Malefyt R. Interleukin-10 down regulates MHC class II alphabeta peptide complexes at the plasma membrane of monocytes by affecting arrival and recycling. Immunity. 1997;7:861–71.
123. Giannoudis PV, Smith RM, Perry SL, Windsor AJ, Dickson RA, Bellamy MC. Immediate IL-10 expression following major orthopaedic trauma. Relationship to anti-inflammatory response and subsequent development of sepsis. Intensive Care Med. 2000;26:1076–81.
124. Galbraith N, Walker S, Galandiuk S, Gardner S, Polk HC Jr. The significance and challenges of monocyte impairment: for the patient and the surgeon. Surg Infect. 2016;17:303–12.
125. Hotchkiss RS, Tinsley KW, Swanson PE, Grayson MH, Osborne D, Wagner TH, Cobb JP, Coppersmith C, Karl IE. Depletion of dendritic cells, but not macrophages, in patients with sepsis. J Immunol. 2002;168:2493–500.
126. Wesche DE, Lomas-Neira JL, Perl M, Chung CS, Ayala A. Leukocyte apoptosis and its significance in sepsis and septic shock. J Leukoc Biol. 2005;78:325–37.
127. Delogu G, Moretti S, Antonucci A. Apoptosis and surgical trauma: dysregulated expression of death and survival factors on peripheral lymphocytes. Arch Surg. 2000;135:1141–7.
128. Danial NN, Korsmeyer SJ. Cell death: critical control points. Cell. 2004;116:205–19.
129. Zimmermann KC, Green DR. How cells die: apoptosis pathways. J Allergy Clin Immunol. 2001;108:S99–S103.
130. Pop C, Salvesen GS. Human caspases: activation, specificity, and regulation. J Biol Chem. 2009;284:21777–81.
131. Pinheiro da Silva F, Nizet V. Cell death during sepsis: integration of disintegration in the inflammatory response to overwhelming infection. Apoptosis. 2009;14:509–21.
132. Melino G. The sirens' song. Nature. 2001;412:23.
133. Jimenez MF, Watson RW, Parodo J, Evans D, Foster D, Steinberg M, Rotstein OD, Marshall JC. Dysregulated expression of neutrophil apoptosis in the systemic inflammatory response syndrome. Arch Surg. 1997;132:1263–70.
134. Hotchkiss RS, Swanson PE, Freeman BD, Tinsley KW, Cobb JP, Matischak GM, Buchman TG, Karl IE. Apoptotic cell death in patients with sepsis, shock and multiple organ dysfunction. Crit Care Med. 1999;27:1230–51.
135. Felmet KA, Hall MW, Clark RS, Jaffe R, Carcillo J. Prolonged lymphopenia, lymphoid depletion and hypoprolactinemia in children with nosocomial sepsis and multiple organ failure. J Immunol. 2005;174:3765–72.
136. Hotchkiss RS, Schmieg RE Jr, Swanson PE, Freeman BD, Tinsley KW, Cobb JP, Karl IE, Buchman TG. Rapid onset of intestinal epithelial and lymphocyte apoptotic cell death in patient with trauma and shock. Crit Care Med. 2000;28:3207–17.
137. Fink MP, Evans TW. Mechanisms of organ dysfunction in critical illness: report from a round table conference held in Brussels. Intensive Care Med. 2002;28:369–75.
138. Abraham E, Singer M. Mechanisms of sepsis-induced organ dysfunction. Crit Care Med. 2007;35:2408–16.
139. Hotchkiss RS, Monneret G, Payen D. Sepsis-induced immunosuppression: from cellular dysfunctions to immunotherapy. Nat Rev Immunol. 2013;13:862–74.
140. Meakins JL, Pietsch JB, Bubenick O, Kelly R, Rode H, Gordon J, MacLean LD. Delayed hypersensitivity: indicator of acquired failure of host defenses in sepsis and trauma. Ann Surg. 1977;186:241–50.
141. Luyt CE, Combes A, Deback C, Aubriot-Lorton MH, Nieszkkowska A, Trouillet JL, Capron F, Agut H, Gilbert C, Chastre J. Herpes simplex virus lung infection in patients undergoing prolonged mechanical ventilation. Am J Respir Crit Care Med. 2007;175(9):935–42.
142. Limaye AP, Kirby KA, Rubenfeld GD, Leisenring WM, Bulger EM, Neff MJ, Gibran NS, Huang ML, Santo Hayes TK, Corey L, Boeckh M. Cytomegalovirus reactivation in critically immunocompetent patients. JAMA. 2008;300:413–22.
143. Otto GP, Sossdorf M, Claus RA, Rodel J, Menge K, Reinhardt K, Bauer M, Riedemann NC. The late phase of sepsis is characterized by an increased microbiological burden and death rate. Crit Care. 2011;15(4):R183.
144. Kollef KE, Schramm GE, Wills AR, Reichley RM, Micek ST, Kollef MH. Predictors of 30-day mortality and hospital costs in patients with ventilator-associated pneumonia attributed to potentially antibiotic-resistant gram-negative bacteria. Chest. 2008;134:281–7.
145. Cavaillon M, Adib-Conquy M. Bench to bedside review: endotoxin tolerance as a model of leukocyte reprogramming in sepsis. Crit Care. 2006;10:233. https://doi.org/10.1186/cc5055.
146. Biswas SK, Lopez-Collazo E. Endotoxin tolerance: new mechanisms, molecules and clinical significance. Trends Immunol. 2009;30:475–87.
147. Zhang X, Morrison DC. Lipopolysaccharide structure-function relationship in activation versus reprogramming of mouse peritoneal macrophages. J Leukoc Biol. 1993;54:444–50.
148. Boomer JS, To K, Chang KC, Takasu O, Osborne DF, Walton AH, Bricker TL, Jarman SD II, Kreisel D, Krupnick AS, Srivastava A, Swanson PE, Green JM, Hotchkiss RS. Immunosuppression in patients who die of sepsis and multiple organ failure. JAMA. 2011;306:2594–605.
149. Morre M, Beq S. Interleukin-7 and immune reconstitution in cancer patients: a new paradigm for dramatically increasing overall survival. Target Oncol. 2012;7:55–68.
150. Levy Y, Sereti I, Tambussi G, Routy JP, Leliévre JD, Delfraissy JF, Molina JM, Fischl M, Goujard C, Rodriguez B, Rouzioux C,

Avettand-Fenoel V, Croughs T, Beq S, Morre M, Poulin JF, Sekaly RP, Thiebaut R, Lederman MM. Effects of recombinant human interleukin-7 on T-cell recovery and thymic output in HIV-infected patients receiving antiretroviral therapy: result of a phase I/IIa randomized, placebo-controlled, multicenter study. Clin Infect Dis. 2012;55:291–300.

151. Hotchkiss RS, Swanson PE, Knudson CM, Chang KC, Cobb JP, Osborne DF, Zollner KM, Buchman TG, Korsemeyer SJ, Karl IE. Overexpression of Bcl-2 in transgenic mice decreases apoptosis and improves survival in sepsis. J Immunol. 1999;162:4148–56.
152. Venet F, Foray AP, Villars-Mechin A, Malcus C, Poitevin-Later F, Lepape A, Monneret G. IL-7 restores lymphocyte function in septic patients. J Immunol. 2012;189:5073–81.
153. Usinger J, McGlynn M, Kasten KR, Hoekzema AS, Watanabe E, Muenzer JT, McDonough JS, Tschoep J, Ferguson TA, McDunn JE, Morre M, Hildeman DA, Caldwell CC, Hotchkiss RS. IL-7 promotes T cell viability, trafficking, and functionality and improves survival in sepsis. J Immunol. 2010;184:3768–79.
154. Cheadle WG, Pemberton RM, Robinson D, Livingstone DH, Rodriguez JL, Polk HC Jr. Lymphocyte subset responses to trauma and sepsis. J Trauma. 1993;35:844–9.
155. Gouel-Cheron A, Venet F, Allaouchiche B, Monneret G. CD4+ T-lymphocyte alterations in trauma patients. Crit Care. 2012;16:432.
156. Le Tulzo Y, Pangault C, Gacouin A, Guilloux V, Tribut O, Amiot L, Tattevin P, Thomas R, Fauchet R, Drenou B. Early circulating lymphocyte apoptosis in human septic shock is associated with poor outcome. Shock. 2002;18:487–94.
157. Venet F, Davin F, Guignant C, Larue A, Cazalis MA, Darbon R, Allombert C, Mougin B, Malcus C, Poitevin-Later F, Lepape A. Early assessment of leukocyte alterations at diagnosis of septic shock. Shock. 2010;34(4):358–63.
158. Monneret G, Venet F, Kullberg BJ, Netea MG. ICU-acquired immunosuppression and the risk for secondary fungal infections. Med Mycol. 2011;49(Suppl 1):S17–23.
159. Venet F, Chung CS, Monneret G, Huang X, Horner B, Garber M, Ayala A. Regulatory T cell populations in sepsis and trauma. J Leukoc Biol. 2008;83(3):523–35.
160. Leng FY, Liu JL, Liu ZJ, Qu HP. Increased proportion of CD4(+) CD25(+)Foxp3(+) regulatory T cells during the early-stage sepsis in ICU patients. J Microbiol Immunol Infect. 2013;46(5):338–44.
161. Delano MJ, Scumpia PO, Weinstein JS, Coco, Nagaraj S, Kelly-Scumpia KM, O'Malley KA, Wynn JL, Antonenko S, Al-Quran SZ, Swan R, Chung CS, Atkinson MA, Ramphal R, Gabrilovich DJ, Reeves W, Ayala A, Phillips J, Laface D, Heyworth PG, Clare-Salzler M, Moldawer LL. J Exp Med. 2007;204(6):1463–74.
162. Drifte G, Dunn-Siegrist I, Tissieres P, Pugin J. Innate immune functions of immature neutrophils in patients with sepsis and severe systemic inflammatory response syndrome. Crit Care Med. 2013;41:820–32.
163. Alves-Filho JC, Spiller F, Cunha FQ. Neutrophil paralysis in sepsis. Shock. 2010;34(Suppl 1):15–21.
164. Kovach MA, Standiford TJ. The function of neutrophils in sepsis. Curr Opin Infect Dis. 2012;25:321–7.
165. Cummings CJ, Martin TR, Frevert CW, Quan JM, Wong VA, Mongovin SM, Hagen TR, Steinberg KP, Goodman RB. Expression and function of the chemokine receptor CXCR1 and CXCR2 in sepsis. J Immunol. 1999;162(4):2341–6.
166. Kasten KR, Muenzer JT, Caldwell CC. Neutrophils are significant producers of IL-10 during sepsis. Biochem Biophys Res Commun. 2010;393:28–31.
167. Pillay J, Kamp VM, van Hoffen E, Visser T, Tak T, Lammers JW, Ulfman LH, Leenen LP, Pickkers P, Koenderman L. A subset of neutrophils in human systemic inflammation inhibits T cell responses through Mac-1. J Clin Invest. 2012;122:327–36.
168. Makarenkova VP, Bansal V, Matta BM, Perez LA, Ochoa JB. CD11+/Gr-1+ myeloid suppressor cells cause T cell dysfunction after traumatic stress. J Immunol. 2006;176(4):2085–94.
169. Souza-Fonseca-Guimaraes F, Parlato M, Phillipart F, Misset B, Cavaillon JM, Adib-Conquy M. Captain study group. Toll-like receptors expression and interferon-gamma production by NK cells in human sepsis. Crit Care. 2012;16:R206.
170. Andreu-Ballester JC, Tormo-Calandin C, Garcia-Ballestreros C, Perez-Griera J, Amigò V, Almela-Quilis A, Ruiz del Castillo J, Penarroja-Otero C, Ballester. Association of ϒδ Tcells with disease severity and mortality in septic patients. Clin Vaccine Immunol. 2013;20(5):738–46.
171. Singer PM, De Santis V, Vitale D, Jeffcoate W. Multiorgan failure is an adaptive, endocrine-mediated, metabolic response to overwhelming systemic inflammation. Lancet. 2004;364:545–8.
172. Mizock BA. The multiple organ dysfunction syndrome. Dis Mon. 2009;55:476–526.
173. Moore FA, Moore EE. Evolving concepts in the pathogenesis of postinjury multiple organ failure. Surg Clin North Am. 1995;75:257–77.
174. MacFie J. Current status of bacterial translocation as a cause of surgical sepsis. Br Med Bull. 2004;71:1–11.
175. Umegaki T, Ikai H, Imanaka Y. The impact of acute organ dysfunction on patients' mortality with severe sepsis. J Anaesthesiol Clin Pharmacol. 2011;27:180–4.
176. Angus DC, Linde-Zwirble WT, Lidicker J, Clermont G, Carcillo J, Pinsky MR. Epidemiology of severe sepsis in the United States: analysis of incidence, outcome and associated costs of care. Crit Care Med. 2001;29:1303–10.
177. Danai PA, Moss M, Mannino DM, Martin GS. The epidemiology of sepsis in patients with malignancy. Chest. 2006;129(6):1432–40.
178. Esper AM, Moss M, Lewis CA, Nisbet R, Mannino DM, Martin GS. The role of infections and comorbidity. Factors that influence disparities in sepsis. Crit Care Med. 2006;34(10):2576–82.
179. Angus DC. The lingering consequences of sepsis: the hidden public health disaster? JAMA. 2010;304:1833–4.
180. Chavan SS, Huerta PT, Robbiati S, Valdes-Ferrer SI, Ochani M, Dancho M, Frankfurt M, Volpe BT, Tracey KJ, Diamond B. HMGB1 mediates cognitive impairment in sepsis survivors. Mol Med. 2012;18:930–7.
181. Rothwell NJ, Hopkins SJ. Cytokines and the nervous system II: actions and mechanisms of action. Trends Neurosci. 1995;18:130–6.
182. Terrando N, Eriksson LI, Ryu JK, Yang T, Monaco C, Felmann M, Jonssson Fagerlund M, Charo IF, Akassoglou K, Maze M. Resolving postoperative neuroinflammation and cognitive decline. Ann Neurol. 2011;70:986–95.
183. Sonneville R, Verdonk F, Rauturier C, Klein IF, Wolff M, Annane D, Chretien F, Sharshar T. Understanding brain dysfunction in sepsis. Ann Intensive Care. 2013;3:1–11.
184. Lamar CD, Hurley RA, Taber KH. Sepsis-associated encephalopathy: review of neuropsychiatric manifestations and cognitive outcome. J Neuropsychiatry Clin Neurosci. 2011;23:237–41.
185. Sharshar T, Annane D, de la Grandmaison GL, Brouland GP, Hopkinson NS, Francoise G. The neuropathology of septic shock. Brain Pathol. 2004;14:21–33.
186. Sprung CL, Peduzzi PN, Shatney CH, Schein RM, Wilson ME, Sheagren JN, Hinshaw LB. Impact of encephalopathy on mortality in the sepsis syndrome. The veterans Administration Systemic Sepsis Cooperative Study Groups. Crit Care Med. 1990;18(8):801–6.
187. ARDS Definition Task Force, Ranieri VM, Rubenfeld GD, Thompson BT, Ferguson ND, Caldwell E, Fan E, Camporota L, Slutsky AS. Acute respiratory distress syndrome: the Berlin definition. JAMA. 2012;307(23):2526–33.

188. Pelosi P, Caironi P, Gattinoni L. Pulmonary and extrapulmonary forms of acute respiratory distress syndrome. Semin Respir Crit Care Med. 2001;22:259–68.
189. Blank M, Napolitano LM. Epidemiology of ARDS and ALI. Crit Care Clin. 2011;27:439–58.
190. Woolf N. Chapter 33: Pulmonary edema (including respiratory distress syndrome). In: Pathology: basic and systemic. London: WB Saunders Ed; 1998. p. 446–51.
191. Muller NL, Frase RS, Colman NC, Paré PD. Chapter 14: Pulmonary edema. In: Radiologic diagnosis of diseases of the chest. London: WB Saunders Ed; 2001. p. 432–51.
192. Agarwal R, Srinivas R, Nath A. Is the mortality higher in the pulmonary vs the extrapulmonary ARDS? A meta-analysis. Chest. 2008;133:1463–73.
193. The Acute Respiratory Distress Syndrome Network, Brower RG, Matthay MA, Morris A, Schoenfeld D, Thompson BT, Wheeler A. Ventilation with lower tidal volumes as compared with traditional tidal volumes for acute lung injury and the acute respiratory distress syndrome. N Engl J Med. 2000;342:1301–8.
194. Rohde JM, Odden AJ, Bonham C, Kuhn L, Malani P, Flanders S, Iwashyna TJ, Chen LM. The epidemiology of acute organ system dysfunction from severe sepsis outside the intensive care unit. J Hosp Med. 2013;8:243–7.
195. Ogura H, Gando S, Saitoh D, Takeyama N, Kushimoto S, Fujishima S, Mayumi T, Araki T, Ikeda H, Kotani J, Miki Y, Shiraishi S, Suzuki K, Suzuki Y, Takuma K, Tsuruta R, Yamaguchi Y, Yamashita N, Aikawa N. Epidemiology of severe sepsis in Japanese intensive care units: a prospective multicenter study. J Infect Chemother. 2014;20(3):157–62.
196. Guidet B, Aegerter P, Gauzit R, Meshaka P, Dreyfuss D, CUB-Réa Study Group. Incidence and impact of organ dysfunctions associated with sepsis. Chest. 2005;127:942–51.
197. Kumar A, Haery C, Parrillo JE. Myocardial dysfunction in septic shock: part 1. Clinical manifestation of cardiovascular dysfunction. J Cardiothorac Vasc Anesth. 2001;15(3):364–76.
198. Parker MM, Shelhamer JH, Bacharach SL, Green MV, Natanson C, Frederick TM, Damske BA, Parrillo JE. Profound but reversible myocardial depression in patients with septic shock. Ann Intern Med. 1984;100(4):483–90.
199. Hassoun SM, Marechal X, Montaigne D, Bouazza Y, Decoster B, Lancel S, Neviere R. Prevention of endotoxin-induced sarcoplasmic reticulum calcium leak improves mitochondrial and myocardial dysfunction. Crit Care Med. 2008;36:2590–6.
200. Kao YH, Chen YC, Cheng CC, Lee TI, Chen YJ, Chen SA. Tumor necrosis factor-alpha decreases sarcoplasmic reticulum Ca2+-ATPase expressions via the promoter methylation in cardiomyocytes. Crit Care Med. 2009;38(1):217–22.
201. Stein B, Frank P, Schmitz W, Scholz H, Thoenes M. Endotoxin and cytokines induce direct cardiodepressive effects in mammalian cardiomyocytes via induction of nitric oxide synthase. J Mol Cell Cardiol. 1996;28(8):1631–9.
202. MacLean LD, Mulligan WG, McLean APH, Duff JH. Patterns of septic shock in man: a detailed study of 56 patients. Ann Surg. 1967;166:543–62.
203. Waisbren BA. Bacteremia due to gram-negative bacilli other than the Salmonella: a clinical and therapeutic study. Arch Intern Med. 1951;88(4):467–88.
204. Parker MM, McCarthy KE, Ognibene FP. Right ventricular dysfunction and dilatation, similar to left ventricular changes, characterize the cardiac depression of septic shock in humans. Chest. 1990;97:126–31.
205. Granger DN, Kvietys PR, Korthuis RJ. Microcirculation of the intestinal mucosa. In: Wood JD, editor. Handbook of physiology section 6. The gastrointestinal system vol. 1: motility and circulation. Part II. American Physiological Society; 1989. p. 1405–74.
206. Granger HJ. Autoregulation of tissue perfusion and oxygenation. In: Kamada T, Shiga T, McCuskey RS, editors. Tissue perfusion and organ function: ischemia/reperfusion injury. Amsterdam: Elsevier-Science; 1996. p. 29–45.
207. Matta BF, Stow PJ. Sepsis-induced vasoparalysis does not involve the cerebral vasculature: indirect evidence from autoregulation and carbon dioxide reactivity studies. Br J Anaesth. 1996;76:790–4.
208. Parker JL, Emerson TE Jr. Cerebral hemodynamics vascular reactivity and metabolism during canine endotoxin shock. Circ Shock. 1977;4:41–53.
209. McCormack DG. Control of vascular reactivity. New Horiz. 1995;3:248–56.
210. Scott JA, Machoun M, McCormack DG. Inducible nitric oxide synthase and vascular reactivity in rat thoracic aorta: effect of aminoguanidine. J Appl Physiol. 1996;80:271–7.
211. el-Dwairi Q, Comtois A, Guo Y, Hussain SN. Endotoxin induced skeletal muscle contractile dysfunction: contribution of nitric oxide synthases. Am J Physiol. 1998;274:C770–9.
212. Goddard CM, Poon BY, Khu ME, Wiggs BR, VanEden SF, Hogg JC. KR. Leukocyte activation does not mediate myocardial leukocyte retention during endotoxemia in rabbits. Am J Physiol. 1998;275:H1548–57.
213. Sutton ET, Norman JC, Newton CA, Hellermann GR, Richard IS. Endothelial structural integrity is maintained during endotoxic shock in an interleukin-1 type 1 receptor knockout mouse. Shock. 1997;7:105–10.
214. Tyml K, Yu J, McCormack DG. Capillary and arteriolar responses to local vasodilators are impaired in a rat model of sepsis. J Appl Physiol. 1998;84:837–44.
215. Vallet B. Vascular reactivity and tissue oxygenation. Intensive Care Med. 1998;24:3–11.
216. Lang CH, Bagby GJ, Ferguson JL, Spitzer JJ. Cardiac output and redistribution of organ blood flow in hypermetabolic sepsis. Am J Physiol. 1984;246:R331–7.
217. Mann KG, Van't Veer C, Cawthern K, Butenas S. The role of the tissue factor pathway in initiation of coagulation. Blood Coagul Fibrinolysis. 1998;9(Suppl):S3–7.
218. Ruf W, Edgington TS. Structural biology of tissue factor, the initiator of thrombogenesis in vivo. FASEB J. 1994;8:385–90.
219. Camerer E, Kolsto AB, Prydz H. Cell biology of tissue factor, the principal initiator of blood coagulation. Thromb Res. 1996;81:1–41.
220. Nieuwland R, Berckmans RJ, McGregor S, Boing AN, Romijn FP, Westendorp RG, Hack CE, Sturk A. Cellular origin and procoagulant properties of microparticles in meningococcal sepsis. Blood. 2000;83:861–7.
221. Bockmeyer CL, Claus RA, Budde U. Inflammation-associated ADAMTS13 deficiency promotes formation of ultra-large von Willebrand factor. Hematologica. 2008;93:137–40.
222. Osterud B. Tissue factor expression by monocytes: regulation and pathophysiological roles. Blood Coagul Fibrinolysis. 1998;9(Suppl):S9–S14.
223. Gando S. Microvascular thrombosis and multiple organ dysfunction syndrome. Crit Care Med. 2010;38(2 Suppl):S35–42.
224. Dhainault JF, Jan SB, Joyce DE, Pettila V, Basson BR, Brandt JT, Sundin D, Levi M. Treatment effects of drotrecogin alfa (activated) in patients with severe sepsis with or without overt disseminated intravascular coagulation. J Thromb Haemost. 2004;2:1924–33.
225. Kobayashi N, Maekawa T, Takada M, Tanaka H, Gonmori H. Criteria for diagnosis of DIC based on the analysis of clinical and laboratory findings in 345 DIC patients collected by the Research Committee on DIC in Japan. Bibl Haematol. 1983;49:265–75.

226. Taylor FB, Toh CH, Hoots WK, Wada H, Levi M. Towards definition, clinical and laboratory criteria, and a scoring system for disseminated intravascular coagulation. On behalf of the Scientific Subcommittee on Disseminated Intravascular Coagulation (DIC) of the International Society of Thrombosis and Haemostasis (ISTH). Thromb Haemost. 2001;86:1327–30.
227. Gando S, Iba T, Eguchi Y, Ohtomo Y, Okamoto K, Koseki K, Mayumi T, Murata A, Ikeda T, Ishikura H, Ueyama M, Ogura H, Kushimoto S, Saitoh D, Endo S, Shimazaki A. A multicenter, prospective validation of disseminated intravascular coagulation diagnostic criteria for critically ill patients: comparing current criteria. Crit Care Med. 2006;34:625–31.
228. Takemitsu T, Wada H, Hatada T, Ohmori Y, Ishikura K, Takeda T, Sugiyama T, Yamada N, Maruyama K, Katayama N, Isaji S, Shimpo H, Kusunoki M, Nobori T. Prospective evaluation of three different diagnostic criteria for disseminated intravascular coagulation. Thromb Haemost. 2011;105:40–4.
229. Aird WC. The hematologic system as a marker of organ dysfunction in sepsis. Mayo Clin Proc. 2003;78:869–81.
230. Brun-Buisson C, Doyon F, Carlet J, Dellamonica P, Gouin F, Lepoutre A, Mercier JC, Offenstadt G, Régnier B. Incidence, risk factors, and outcome of severe sepsis and septic shock in adults: a multicenter prospective study in intensive care unit. French ICU group for Severe Sepsis. JAMA. 1995;274:968–74.
231. Mavrommatis AC, Theodoridis T, Orfanidou A, Roussos C, Christopolou-Kokkinou V, Zakynthinos S. Coagulation system and platelets are fully activated in uncomplicated sepsis. Crit Care Med. 2000;28(2):451–7.
232. Parmar A, Langerberg C, Wan L, May CN, Bellomo R, Bagshaw SM. Epidemiology of sepsis acute kidney injury. Curr Drug Targets. 2009;10:1169–78.
233. Thakar CV, Christianson A, Freyberg R, Almenoff P, Render ML. Incidence and outcomes of acute kidney injury in intensive care units: a Veterans Administration Study. Crit Care Med. 2009;37(9):2252–8.
234. Hoste EA, Kellum JA. Incidence classification and outcomes of acute kidney injury. Contrib Nephrol. 2007;156:32–8.
235. Kellum JA, Levin N, Bouman C, Lameire N. Developing a consensus classification system for acute renal failure. Curr Opin Crit Care. 2002;8:509–14.
236. Bellomo R, Ronco C, Kellum JA, Metha RL, Palevsky P. Acute Dialysis Quality Initiative workgroup: acute renal failure-definition, outcome measures, animal models, fluid therapy and information technology needs: the Second International Consensus Conference of the Acute Dialysis Quality Initiative (ADQI) Group. Crit Care. 2004;8:R204–12.
237. Langenberg C, Bagshaw SM, May CM, Bellomo R. The histopathology of septic acute kidney injury: a systematic review. Crit Care. 2008;12(2):R38.
238. Messmer UK, Winkel G, Briner VA, Pfeilschifter J. Glucocorticoids potently block tumor necrosis factor-alpha and lipopolysaccharide-induced apoptotic cell death in bovine glomerular endothelial cells upstream of caspase 3 activation. Br J Pharmacol. 1999;127:1633–40.
239. Langenberg C, Wan L, Egi M, May CN, Bellomo R. Renal blood flow distribution in experimental septic acute renal failure. Kidney Int. 2006;69:1996–2002.
240. Wan L, Bagshaw SM, Langenberg C, Saotome T, May C, Bellomo R. Pathophysiology of septic acute kidney injury: what do we really know? Crit Care Med. 2008;36(4 Suppl):S198–203.
241. Wan L, Langenberg C, Bellomo R, May CN. Angiotensin II in experimental hyperdynamic sepsis. Crit Care. 2009;13:R190.
242. Baud L, Oudinet JP, Bens M, Noe L, Peraldi MN, Rondeau E, Etienne J, Ardaillou R. Production of tumor necrosis factor by rat mesangial cells in response to bacterial lipopolysaccharide. Kidney Int. 1989;35(5):1111–8.
243. Uchino S, Kellum JA, Bellomo R, Doig GS, Morimatsu H, Morgera S, Schetz M, Tan I, Bouman C, Macedo E, Gibney N, Tolwani A, Ronco C. Beginning and Ending Supportive Therapy for the kidney (BEST Kidney). Acute renal failure in critically ill patients: a multinational multicenter study. JAMA. 2005;294:813–8.
244. Bagshaw SM, Lapinsky S, Dial S, Arabi Y, Dodek P, Wood G, Ellis P, Guzman J, Marshall J, Parrillo JE, Skrobik Y, Kumar A. Cooperative Antimicrobial Therapy of Septic Shock (CATSS) Database Research Group. Acute kidney injury in septic shock: clinical outcomes and impact of duration of hypotension prior to initiation of antimicrobial therapy. Intensive Care Med. 2009;35:871–81.
245. Podoll AS, Kozar R, Holcomb JB, Finkel KW. Incidence and outcome of early acute kidney injury in critically ill trauma patients. PLoS One. 2013;8:1–5.
246. Ulkeja A. Altered gastrointestinal motility in critically ill patients: current understanding of pathophysiology, clinical impact, and diagnostic approach. Nutr Clin Pract. 2010;25:16–25.
247. Chapman MJ, Nguyen NQ, Deane AM. Gastrointestinal dysmotility: clinical consequences and management of the critically ill patient. Gastroenterol Clin North Am. 2011;40:725–39.
248. Hayakawa M, Asahara T, Henzan N, et al. Dramatic changes of the gut flora immediately after severe and sudden insults. Dig Dis Sci. 2011;56:2361–5.
249. Guarner F, Malagelada JR. Gut flora in health and disease. Lancet. 2003;361:512–9.
250. Farrell CP, Barr M, Mullin JM, Mullin JM, Lande L, Zitin M. Epithelial barrier leak in gastrointestinal disease and multiorgan failure. J Epithel Biol Pharmacol. 2012;5:13–8.
251. Lautt WW. Mechanism and role of intrinsic regulation of hepatic arterial blood flow: hepatic arterial buffer response. Am J Physiol. 1985;249:G549–56.
252. Furhmann V, Kneidinger H, Herkner H, Heinz G, Nikfardjam M, Bojic A, Schellongowski P, Angermayr B, Kitzberger R, Warszawska J, Holzinger U, Schenk P, Madi C. Hypoxic hepatitis: underlying conditions and risk factors for mortality in cirtically ill patients. Intensive Care Med. 2009;35:1397–405.
253. Henrion J, Schapira M, Luwaert R, Colin L, Delanoy A, Heller FR. Hypoxic hepatitis: clinical and hemodynamic studies in 142 consecutive cases. Medicine (Baltimore). 2003;82:392–406.
254. Henrion J. Hypoxic hepatitis. Liver Int. 2012;32(7):1039–52.
255. Gimson AE. Hepatic dysfunction during bacterial sepsis. Intensive Care Med. 1987;13:162–6.
256. Banks JG, Foulis AK, Ledingham IM, MacSween RN. Liver function in septic shock. J Clin Pathol. 1982;35:1249–52.
257. Moreno R, Vincent JL, Matos R, Mendoca A, Cantraine F, Thijs L, Takala J, Sprung C, Antonelli M, Bruining H, Willats S. The use of maximum SOFA score to quantify organ dysfunction/failure in intensive care. Results of a prospective, multicenter study. Working Group on Sepsis relate Problems of the ESICM. Intensive Care Med. 1999;25:686–96.
258. Moseley RH. Sepsis and cholestasis. Clin Liver Dis. 2004;8:83–94.
259. Assimakopoulos SF, Scopa CD, Vagianos CE. Pathophysiology of increased intestinal permeability in obstructive jaundice. World J Gastroenterol. 2007;13:6458–64.
260. Kamiya S, Nagino M, Kanazawa H, Komatsu S, Mayumi T, Takagi K, Asahara T, Nomoto K, Tanaka R, Nimura Y. The value of bile replacement during external biliary drainage: an analysis of intestinal permeability, integrity, and microflora. Ann Surg. 2004;239:510–7.
261. Padillo FJ, Muntane J, Montero JL, Briceno J, Mino G, Solorzano G, Stiges-Serra A, Pera-Madrazo C. Effect of internal biliary drainage on plasma levels of endotoxin, cytokines, and C-reactive protein in patients with obstructive jaundice. World J Surg. 2002;26:1328–32.

262. Fuchs M, Sanyal AJ. Sepsis and cholestasis. Clin Liver Dis. 2008;12:151–72.
263. Dellinger RP, Levy MM, Carlet JM, Bion J, Parker MM, Jaeschke R, Reinhart K, Angus DC, Brun-Buisson C, Beale R, Calandra T, Dhainaut JF, Gerlach H, Harvey M, Marini JJ, Marshall J, Ranieri M, Ramsay G, Sevransky J, Thompson BT, Townsend S, Vender JS, Zimmerman JL, Vincent JL. Surviving Sepsis Campaign: international guidelines for management of severe sepsis and septic shock: 2008. Crit Care Med. 2008;36:296–327.
264. McClave SA, Martindale RG, Vanek WW, McCarthy M, Roberts P, Taylor B, Ochoa JB, Napolitano L, Cresci G. Guidelines for the provision and assessment of nutrition support therapy in the adult critically ill patient: Society of Critical Care Medicine (SCCM) and American Society for Parenteral and Enteral Nutrition (A.S.P.E.N.). JPEN J Parenter Enteral Nutr. 2009;33:277–316.

Shock States in Acute Care Surgery

3

Sergio Arlati

Key Points

- Shock is defined as a condition of reduced oxygen delivery to tissues in relation to metabolic demands. Shock is not synonymous with hypotension although hypotension is very often associated with shock states.
- Hypovolemic (haemorrhagic) shock is the most frequent form of shock in the acute surgical setting. Its main pathophysiological feature is reduced venous return by a decrease of the stressed volume. For any given volume deficit, the oxygen debt is more severe with haemorrhage than pure hypovolemia due to haemoglobin loss.
- Prolonged hypovolemic shock accumulates a severe oxygen debt with global ischaemia-reperfusion injury, subsequent inflammatory response and generalized organ dysfunction and damage.
- Irreversible shock is characterized by diffuse vasodilation, unresponsiveness to vasopressors, severely depressed myocardial function, cellular energy depletion with metabolic acidosis that culminate in cardiovascular collapse and ultimately death.
- The absolute priority during hypovolemic shock is the rapid restoration of circulating volume. Red blood cells are the first therapeutic options, but any fluid can temporary be used to restore the intravascular volume.

3.1 Introduction

Shock is defined as a condition of reduced oxygen delivery to tissues with respect to metabolic demands [1]. The reduction of oxygen supply is by far the most frequent mechanism of tissue hypoxia. This causes the shift from aerobic to anaerobic metabolism, the depletion of intracellular ATP stores and the production of metabolic acidosis. The reduction of oxygen flow to tissues may be due to low cardiac output states as occurs in hypovolemic, cardiogenic and obstructive shock or to the combination of elevated tissue oxygen requirements, high cardiac output state and microcirculatory perfusion mismatch as occurs in septic shock. This chapter will deal with the pathophysiology of haemorrhagic shock and the role of compensatory mechanisms acting to ensure O_2 flow to vital organs. The consequences of tissue and organ hypoxia together with the effect of ischaemia-reperfusion injury after the resumption of adequate oxygen supply will also be considered. Clinical features and treatment principles will be derived from physiological principles. Finally, the haemodynamic profile and pathophysiology of cardiogenic and septic shock will be summarized. The haemodynamic effects of positive pressure ventilation will be briefly outlined as CPAP, and non-invasive pressure ventilation is increasingly used in surgical patients.

3.1.1 Haemorrhagic Shock

It is estimated that five million people per year die as a result of trauma and that in 50% of cases, death is a result of haemorrhagic shock [2]. Haemorrhagic shock is by far the main manifestation of post-traumatic and surgical shock, the other causes being obstructive shock (tension pneumothorax, pericardial tamponade), cardiogenic shock (myocardial contusion or infarction) and spinal shock (trauma of the spinal column).

Shock is defined as inadequate oxygen supply to tissues regardless of systemic arterial pressure. Otherwise stated arterial hypotension is not synonymous with shock although they are frequently associated. The inadequate oxygen supply causes a shift of cellular metabolism from aerobic (36 moles of ATP produced per 1 mole of oxygen consumed) to

S. Arlati (✉)
Anesthesia and Intensive Care (1st Department), ASST Grande Ospedale Metropolitano Niguarda, Milan, Italy
e-mail: sergio.arlati@ospedaleniguarda.it

P. Aseni et al. (eds.), *Operative Techniques and Recent Advances in Acute Care and Emergency Surgery*,
https://doi.org/10.1007/978-3-319-95114-0_3

anaerobic (2 moles of ATP per 1 mole of oxygen) with intracellular ATP depletion and production of metabolic acidosis (lactic acid). This causes progressive mitochondrial dysfunction (uncoupling of the oxidative phosphorylation), further ATP depletion with increased membrane permeability, cellular swelling and rupture thus leading to irreversible organ damage. The normalization of blood pressure does not guarantee the adequacy of resuscitation as oxygen flow depends on tissue perfusion rather than arterial blood pressure. Hence the primary goal of resuscitation is the rapid correction of hypovolemia and hypoperfusion. When resuscitation is incomplete, prolonged hypoperfusion leads to progressive shock with accumulation of further oxygen debt and extensive cells and tissues damage. Moreover the more prolonged is hypoperfusion, the worse will be the resulting ischaemia-reperfusion injury with activation of the systemic inflammatory response syndrome (SIRS) and multiple organ dysfunction (MODS) and failure occurrence. If unresolved the hypoperfusion may progress into irreversible shock characterized by loss of vasomotor tone, progressive hypotension unresponsive to both fluids and vasoactive drugs, severe metabolic acidosis, irreversible cardiac failure and ultimately death. For details about the inflammatory mechanisms triggered by ischaemia-reperfusion injury, refer to Chap. 2.

A typical case of haemorrhagic shock is described here:

A 42-year-old man is admitted to the ED following a high-energy trauma. Clinical examination and CT scan reveal an incomplete splenic rupture, a femur shaft fracture and an unstable fracture of the pelvic ring. He is hypotensive (90/60 mmHg) and tachycardic (pulse rate 120 bpm) on admission. Arterial blood gas analysis reveals a compensated metabolic acidosis (pH 7.36, PaCO2 29 mmHg) with elevated arterial blood lactates (8.5 mmol/L). The initial haemoglobin level is 10 g/dL. An emergency laparotomy is performed due to ongoing intra-abdominal bleeding. Thereafter the orthopaedist provides for the external fixation of femur and pelvis. In OR the patient receives three packed red blood cell transfusion and 2500 mL crystalloids. After surgery, he is transferred to the ICU where he appears restless and anxious. His blood pressure on admission is 125/65 mmHg, and the pulse rate is 110 bpm. The neurological status is attributed to anxiety and incomplete pain control for which the patient receives low doses of i.v. opioids and benzodiazepine with improvement of the symptoms. Twelve hours later, the vital signs are normalized, but arterial blood lactates remain elevated (4.0 mmol/L), and oliguria is present despite 1000 mL of crystalloids infusion. In the following 12 h, arterial hypotension and metabolic acidosis (pH 7.29, PaCO2 31) develop. An infusion of low-dose norepinephrine is started with normalization of arterial blood pressure. An invasive haemodynamic monitoring is implemented by the transpulmonary thermodilution technique that allows the estimation of cardiac preload by measurement of global end-diastolic volume (GEDV). The first haemodynamic measurement reveals a normal cardiac output but a decreased stroke volume. The GEDV measurement is normal. Arterial blood lactates increase to 11.2 mmol/L reflecting a severe global perfusion deficit. The central venous oxygen saturation (Sc_vO_2) is lower than normal. Low values of Sc_vO_2 indicate inadequate oxygen supply either due to high oxygen consumption (e.g. shivers) or inadequate delivery (low-output states). The combination of a lower than normal Sc_vO_2 value, metabolic acidosis and elevated arterial lactates suggests the presence of inadequate oxygen delivery, accumulation of an oxygen debt and increased anaerobic metabolism. A mild to moderate arterial hypoxia develops requiring endotracheal intubation and mechanical ventilation. The persistence of oliguria with elevated serum BUN and creatinine levels prompts the institution of continuous renal replacement therapy. A decreased platelet count and increased serum bilirubin also develop. The patient is discharged from the ICU 12 days later and will return home after 3 months of hospitalization.

The following key points can be drawn:

1. Blood pressure is not a reliable index of circulating volume and adequate perfusion to tissue. In our patient, a normal blood pressure coexists with abnormal global perfusion indexes as reflecting tissue hypoperfusion.
2. The adequacy of volume resuscitation cannot be based upon vital signs but on the evaluation of global perfusion indexes. The presence of oliguria and elevated arterial blood lactates in the context of hypovolemic shock reflects an incomplete resuscitation. In addition, elevated lactate levels in association with metabolic acidosis are suggestive for the presence of anaerobic metabolism. In this context, the patient's restlessness was mistakenly attributed to pain and anxiety, and the apparent improvement after small doses of opioids and anxiolytic drugs delays the correct interpretation of the neurological status. Restlessness and anxiety are probably the results of diffuse co-activation of the hypothalamic-pituitary axis and noradrenergic networks during the response to stress [3]. This closely recalls the inexperienced physician who slows down the diagnostic process of the acute abdomen after morphine administration. The relief of pain is thus confused with the healing of the disease!
3. The persistence of hypovolemic shock leads to the progressive decrease of peripheral vascular resistances with requirement of vasopressor drugs. This is in contrast with the early hypovolemic shock when blood pressure is kept normal by high sympathetic neural output, increased blood levels of circulating epinephrine and norepinephrine and activation of the renin-angiotensin-aldosterone system. The accumulation of an elevated oxygen debt leads to diffuse endothelial and smooth muscle cell dys-

function with arteriolar vasodilation and hypotension. If the oxygen debt becomes massive, refractory hypotension and cardiovascular collapse ensue.

4. After prolonged shock, there is a myocardial dysfunction as evidenced by the decrease in stroke volume. Note that this occurs in spite of a normal cardiac preload (GEDV) and decreased afterload (arterial vasodilation). In the presence of normal cardiac function, the combination of normal preload and decreased afterload would increase the stroke volume thus keeping the blood pressure normal. In our patient, the decreased stroke volume reflects the presence of a mild to moderate myocardial dysfunction. Therefore arterial hypotension and tachycardia ensue.
5. Hypotension worsens both cellular hypoxia and anaerobic metabolism thus leading to decompensated metabolic acidosis (low pH despite compensatory $PaCO_2$ decrease).
6. The partial correction of ischaemia in our patient leads to ischaemia-reperfusion injury thus, in turn, causing a systemic inflammatory syndrome (SIRS) with activation of the coagulation and platelet consumption (decreased platelet count). Multiple end-organ damage ensues with renal, respiratory and hepatic dysfunction.

Let us now look at the physiopathology of the haemorrhagic shock in its early stage. The main problem of haemorrhagic shock is hypovolemia or more precisely the decrease of stressed volume [4]. Stressed volume is a somewhat complex physiological concept described by Guyton, who defined it as the volume that actively stretches the vein wall beyond its elastic point of equilibrium [5]. In practice, the stressed volume is the volume that generates a positive filling pressure (Fig. 3.1, left). It is this 7–8 mmHg pressure as estimated from animal studies that return the blood to the hearts [6]. If the stressed volume changes, the mean filling pressure changes as well, and so it does the venous return provided that the vascular resistances remain constant. During hypovolemic shock, the decrease in stressed volume decreases the mean filling pressure and, consequently, venous return (Fig. 3.1, middle). The stressed volume represents only about 30% of the total volume that is 1.5 L of the estimated 5 L in a 70 kg man [4]. This volume represents just under half of the blood volume contained in the venous reservoir which is about 3200 mL. The difference between total venous volume and the stressed volume (3200–1500 mL) is the unstressed volume or the volume that remains in the venous system when the mean filling pressure is zero [4]. This occurs when no active (muscular) or passive (elastic) forces operate on the vein wall. As a consequence, the vein does not need this volume to remain open. From a physiological standpoint, a null intravascular filling pressure occurs when the smooth muscular fibres are relaxed and the intramural elastic fibres are at their resting length so that no tension can be generated across the vein wall. The unstressed volume represents a reservoir volume that can be mobilized in numerous pathophysiological conditions, firstly of all if hypovolemia occurs [4, 7]. Its mobilization requires the active contraction of the venous muscular fibres by increased orthosympathetic stimulation so increasing the intravascular pressure and hence venous return (Fig. 3.2,

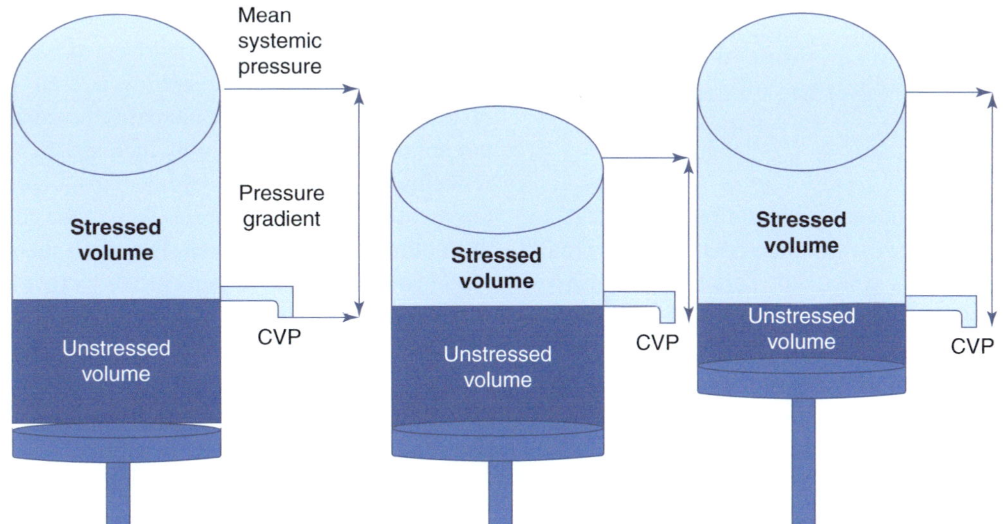

Fig. 3.1 Left: schematic representation of the venous compartment. The upper part is the stressed volume that generates the intravascular pressure for venous return. The unstressed volume is placed underneath the outflow so that it does not contribute generating a pressure gradient. Middle: venous compartment after acute hypovolemia. The stressed volume is reduced so that the venous return decreases by a diminution of the pressure gradient. Right: unstressed volume is squeezed into the stressed volume so that the venous pressure gradient is restored and the venous return returns normal

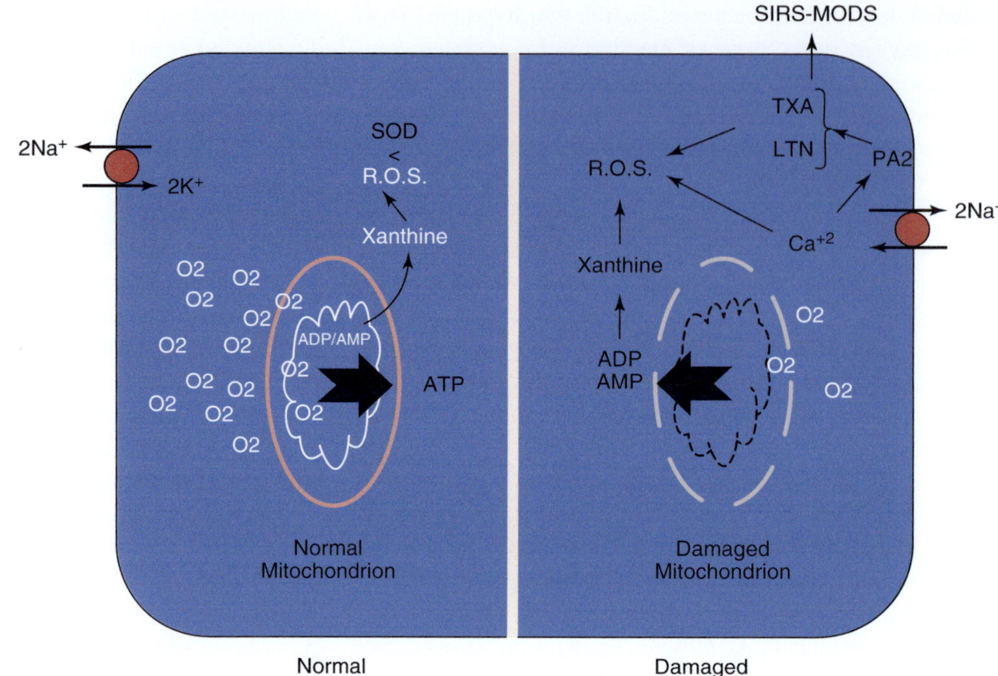

Fig. 3.2 Schematic representation of normal (left side) and pathological (right side) cellular events during normoxia and hypoxia. Decreased oxygen supply causes the production of ROS (reactive oxygen species) and increased Ca^{+2} entry with cytoskeleton and mitochondrial damage (broken line). Abbreviations: *TXA* thromboxane, *LTN* leukotrienes, *PA2* phospholipase A2

Table 3.1 Clinical presentation based upon estimated blood losses[a]

	Class I	Class II	Class III	Class IV
Blood loss (mL)	Up to 750	750–1500	1500–2000	>2000
Blood loss (%)	Up to 15%	15–30%	30–40%	>40%
Pulse rate	<100	>100	>120	>140
Blood pressure	Normal	Normal	Decreased	Decreased
Resp. rate	Normal	20–30	30–40	>35
Urine output mL/h	>30	20–30	5–15	Negligible
Mental status	Slightly anxious	Mildly anxious	Anxious, confused	Confused, lethargic

[a]Modified from American College of Surgeons Committee on Trauma 2004

right). The active smooth muscular contraction operates a squeezing of the smaller veins into the greater ones so that a sort of autotransfusion is generated. This mechanism is so efficient that keeps the venous return normal for blood loss up to 750 mL. The compensatory mechanism is so efficient that blood pressure can remain normal for blood loss up to 30% of the total blood volume (Table 3.1). This classification is purely indicative because it does not take into account the rate of blood loss. For example, a penetrating wound at the groin with lesion of the femoral artery causes the immediate loss of more than 1000 mL of blood with sudden hypotension and tachycardia that would be classified as class III or IV haemorrhage. However, it clearly shows that arterial blood pressure is not related to circulating blood volume and hence to flow. As a consequence, if the goal of volume resuscitation is normalization of the blood pressure instead of restoration of adequate whole-body perfusion, the patient is at high risk for prolonged shock.

The mobilization of the unstressed volume is the only compensatory mechanism that allows for the maintenance of normal blood pressure and heart rate [4, 7, 8]. Other mechanisms can compensate for the reduction of blood pressure, but they cannot compensate for the increased pulse rate (Table 3.1, class II shock). Thus, the isolated increase of arterial vascular resistances can normalize blood pressure, but it has no effects on venous return which relies upon the volume that fills the veins above the unstressed volume. As a consequence, the isolated increase of arterial pressure cannot restore flow. Similarly, the increase of cardiac contractility is not helpful because it can only increase the venous return by reducing the right atrial pressure. This, in turn, will increase the pressure gradient between the veins and the atrium thus promoting the venous return. However, the right atrial pressure is already close to zero in the hypovolemic patient so that the gradient cannot be increased. Moreover, the reduction of intravascular pressure below zero causes the collapse of the intrathoracic veins during expiration. This limits the possibility of increasing the total venous return as the effective time of venous drainage is shortened. For the same reason, vasoactive and inotropic drugs increase blood pressure by augmenting the cardiac inotropic state or the peripheral vascular resistances. They are of little help in hypovolemic shock as their effect on venous return is negligible.

However, the hypoperfusion consequent to hypovolemic shock stimulates a variety of neurohormonal compensating mechanisms that produce an efficient, highly integrated response so that blood pressure and pulse rate are maintained normal up to 30% of blood volume losses.

1. Firstly, stimulation of carotid and aortic baroreceptors stimulates the vasopressor centres in the brain medulla. This activation produces immediate peripheral vasoconstriction by increased norepinephrine spillover from the orthosympathetic nerve endings. The contraction of the smooth muscle layers in the small venous and arterial vessels improves both the cardiac filling volume by increasing venous return and rising of arterial blood pressure by peripheral arterial vasoconstriction. These compensatory measures allow for maintenance of cerebral and coronary perfusion pressure.
2. Secondly, the decrease in ventricular filling pressure inhibits the production of natriuretic peptide, thus reducing natriuresis and its vasodilator effect upon the small arterial vessels.
3. Chemoreceptors on the juxtaglomerular apparatus react to the reduced sodium concentration in the distal tubule by stimulating the renin-angiotensin-aldosterone system with production of intense peripheral vasoconstriction (angiotensin II), renal reabsorption of sodium and water (aldosterone).
4. Pain also has intense neuroendocrine effects as it stimulates the norepinephrine, serotonin and endorphins networks in the central nervous system. The activation of the hypothalamus and brain stem further stimulates the orthosympathetic nervous system.
5. The adrenal gland is activated by sympathomimetic vegetative fibres. The increased release of epinephrine and norepinephrine stimulates β1-adrenergic receptors with tachycardia (chronotropic effect) and increased myocardial contraction (inotropic effect). Tachycardia is an extremely effective way for to maintenance of the cardiac output. The increased pulse rate compensates for the decreased stroke volume due to preload reduction. Tachycardia also contributes to rising the diastolic blood pressure, thus keeping pulse pressure (P_{syst}-P_{dia}) normal or even increased when stroke volume reduction is mild (class I shock). Stimulation of α1-adrenergic receptors by norepinephrine produces vasoconstriction especially of renal, cutaneous and splenic vascular beds. This causes redistribution of blood to heart and brain thus preserving vital organ perfusion. The sympathomimetic stimulation of the α1-adrenergic receptors contributes to keep blood pressure near to normal, mainly by increasing the diastolic blood pressure (increased peripheral vascular resistance). By progression of the haemorrhage, the systolic pressure decreases due to decreased stroke volume. The pulse pressure also decreases, but the diastolic pressure remains near to normal thus maintaining normal the mean arterial pressure too. Please note that mean arterial pressure is the main determinant of cerebral and coronary perfusion. Peripheral vasoconstriction also acts on the microcirculation by promoting the intravascular absorption of fluids from the interstitium [9]. As arteriolar vasoconstriction drops the hydrostatic pressure into the capillaries, the filtration of fluids into the interstitial space may cease. The further drop in pressure causes a reverse flow phenomenon with absorption of water and electrolytes from the interstitium into the capillary. This compensatory mechanism helps in the maintenance of intravascular volume when hypovolemic shock is prolonged. However, it may be responsible for the shifts of large amounts of water from the interstitial to the vascular space.
6. The hypothalamic stimulation by peripheral and central afferents produces ADH that is an effective vasopressor and contributes to the maintenance of extracellular volume by reabsorption of free water from the collecting tubule.
7. Finally, the stimulation of the hypothalamus-pituitary axis releases ACTH and growth hormone with resulting hyperglycaemia by activation of glycogenolysis and gluconeogenesis (in cooperation with increased blood levels of glucagon and circulating catecholamine). The hyperglycaemia pulls water out of the cells and contributes to the maintenance of circulating volume by cellular shrinkage.

All these mechanisms make complex the estimation of resuscitative volume that is needed to recover from hypovolemic shock. As a result, the total infused volume is often in excess with respect to that predicted by simple blood loss estimation.

A major problem with haemorrhagic shock concerns the type of fluid losses. Unlike hypovolemic shock where only plasma (e.g. burns) or water (e.g. bowel obstruction) is lost, the decrease of haemoglobin levels in haemorrhagic acts synergistically with hypovolemia to the further reduction of oxygen delivery. The following example is useful as explanation. In a 70 kg man, having an estimated blood volume of 5 L, a resting cardiac output of 5.5 L/min and a haemoglobin level of 15 g/dL (haematocrit 45%), the oxygen delivery to tissues is about 1000 mL/min. This calculation is as follows:

O_2 delivery = [(1.34 × Hb × SaO_2) × Cardiac Output × 10] (neglecting the contribution of dissolved O_2 in arterial blood). After 1/3 of plasma losses (−900 mL), the circulating volume decreases from 5 to about 4 L, but the haemoglobin level increases to 18.5 g/dL. If the cardiac output decreases to about 3.5 L/min as due to hypovolemia, the O_2 delivery to tissues is now 830 mL/min (−17% reduction). However when 900 mL of blood are lost by haemorrhage, the O_2 delivery reduces to 680 mL/min only with −32% reduction. The restoration of circulating volume by rapid crystalloid infusion allows for the cardiac output to return normal or even supranormal thus compensating for the decrease of haemoglobin. So, after 2 L of intravenous crystalloids, the cardiac output rises to 6 L/min, the haemoglobin level falls to 12 g/dL and the oxygen delivery returns near to normal (950 mL/min). Therefore the timely restoration of circulating volume is fundamental to minimize the accumulation of the oxygen debt that ensues during acute haemorrhage.

Theoretical considerations suggest that a haemoglobin level of 7 g/dL is adequate for sufficient O_2 delivery provided that circulating volume is restored and/or that metabolic demands are normal Whenever an imbalance occurs between oxygen delivery and extraction, an oxygen debt ensues. The larger is the discrepancy between O_2 supply and requirement, the larger will be the debt to be paid. The oxygen debt is relatively independent on the time needed to gather it. Several studies have shown that the accumulation of an oxygen debt greater than 140 mL/kg is invariably lethal in a dog model of haemorrhagic shock [9]. These studies also offer the possibility of estimating the specific probability of death in relation to the lethal dose of oxygen debt (LDO_{2debt}). Thus an exponential relationship has been found between the LDO_{2debt} and the probability of death [10]. A 50% probability of death corresponds to a LD_{50} of 113.5 mL/kg of oxygen debt in dogs and 95 mL/kg in pigs [10, 11]. Such interspecies difference seems related to the higher percentage of body fat in the pig. The determination of the oxygen debt is not easy to obtain in humans, but a good correlation can be found with common indicators of metabolic acidosis such as arterial blood lactates and the base deficit (BD) value. BD is defined as the amount of bases to be added to 1 L of fully oxygenated blood to bring back the pH value to 7.40 at a temperature of 37 °C and a PCO2 of 40 mmHg. Both arterial blood lactates and BD correlate with the amount of tissue hypoxia. BD seems to perform better than arterial lactates as suggested by several experimental and human studies [12]. It has been shown that a BD lower (more negative) than −6 mmol/L reflects accurately the trend of shock towards a potentially lethal condition [13]. As a rough approximation, an oxygen debt of 30 mL/kg corresponds to 4.5 mmol/L of arterial blood lactates and −6.0 mmol/L of BD. When the oxygen debt reaches 150 mL/kg, the average arterial blood lactates and BD value are, respectively, 22.5 mmol/L and −25 mmol/L. This corresponds to about +1.3 mmol/L of arterial blood lactates, and −1.5 mmol/L of BD occur for any 10 mL/kg increase of oxygen debt.

In the emergency department, the patient with traumatic shock is usually monitored by serial measurements of vital parameters and common clinical signs of hypoperfusion (capillary refill, skin temperature and colour, mental status and urine output). In adjunct, serial determinations of arterial blood lactates or base deficit is usually performed. Repeated determination of haemoglobin levels is also useful to detect occult or active bleeding, especially if clinical deterioration occurs.

Other common monitoring parameters are central venous pressure (CVP) and haemoglobin saturation of central (right atrial) venous blood (Sc_vO_2).

The purpose of the monitoring is:

1. To assess the haemodynamic status
2. To assess the severity of tissue hypoperfusion
3. To evaluate the effectiveness of resuscitative efforts in restoring tissue perfusion

Although CVP is not a reliable index of cardiac preload, it is widely used to assess fluid responsiveness of the cardiovascular system. The CVP value cannot reflect preload mainly because the ventricular compliance and volume are not linearly related each other. This means that the stretch of the ventricular wall for any given increase in volume is not constant but a curvilinear pressure-volume relationship exists. Therefore, the initial CVP value cannot infer about the adequacy of the cardiac preload, but its changes are useful to assess the adequacy of the right ventricle to manage a volume load. This approach can also be used to evaluate the efficacy of the resuscitative efforts during hypovolemic shock. If the rapid infusion of crystalloids increases the CVP value by more than 5 mmHg, the infusion is stopped and resumed if 10 min thereafter the CVP has decreased by 2 mmHg [14]. Although not verified experimentally, this 5 to 2 rule is widely used in clinical practice to estimate whether the right ventricle can handle the infused volume. However, remember that the amount of volume to be infused in a single patient cannot be predicted by this approach. It only answers the question if the right ventricle can handle such volume load. However, the combination of CVP changes, clinical evaluation and serial measurements of BD and lactates is probably the best way to assess the effectiveness of resuscitative efforts in a patient with shock at the bedside. So, if the rapid infusion of crystalloids increases the CVP value (increased preload) with improvement of arterial pressure and subsequent increase of urine output and decreased arterial blood lactates, this means that the infused volume has been effective. Please also note that if after a volume bolus the cardiac output increases with no CVP changes, the responsible mechanism is the improvement of myocardial contractility by increased coronary perfusion pressure.

In this discussion, I have emphasized the use of CVP instead of pulmonary artery occlusion pressure (PAOP). Although PAOP is informative about the function of the left ventricle and its increase alerts the physician against the occurrence of pulmonary oedema, CVP is by far more widely used in clinical practice. Moreover, any increase in the right atrial pressure (CVP) reflects the increase of cardiac output provided that the ventricle is normal and that is working on the rising portion of the Frank-Starling curve. Physiologically the stretching of the ventricle by increased preload increases its force of contraction with augmentation of the stroke volume. As the initial CVP value does not predict the amount of volume to be infused, this value does not even predict whether and how much the patient will be a volume responder [15]. Otherwise stated the only way to test the patient's fluid responsiveness is to test it by a volume bolus. This is because the pressure value at which the ventricular function curve reaches its plateau is largely individual. Therefore, the right atrial pressure will be high in the presence of pulmonary hypertension (low ventricular compliance), moderate in the patient with left ventricular dilatation that limits the pericardial stretch by impinging on the right ventricle and low in normal individuals. In the last decade, the bedside use of ultrasound (US) in the patient with hypovolemia and shock has gained popularity. US examination allows for rapid, non-invasive and repeatable estimation of cardiac preload and function in many acute care settings [16]. Moreover, it has been demonstrated a valuable tool in guiding the resuscitation of patients with shock [17]. For a detailed description of US examination in the acute care setting, see Chap. 6.

The above physiological analysis predicts the efficacy and role of vasoactive drugs in hypovolemic shock. Although any pharmacological intervention is by far less effective than volume infusion, norepinephrine infusion may have a role in the emergency treatment of hypovolemic shock. Its stimulation of α1-receptors reduces the capacitance of the venous system (venous squeezing), thus allowing for increasing the stressed volume [18]. This sort of autotransfusion contributes to venous return until the unstressed volume is available. In addition, the arterial vasoconstriction increases the perfusion pressure to vital organs. Nevertheless, remember that pressure is not synonymous with perfusion so that norepinephrine must be used with caution in the hypovolemic patient as it may worsen tissue perfusion albeit blood pressure returns normal.

3.1.2 Cardiogenic Shock

The primary problem in cardiogenic shock is the reduction of cardiac function with consequent decrease of stroke volume, increased ventricular end-diastolic volume and pressure. This raises the right atrial pressure (CVP) with reduction of the venous return to the heart and distension of peripheral veins. However, this increases the mean systemic pressure thus allowing for venous return to come back to the previous level, albeit at higher intravascular pressure. This is only a temporary measure as the progressive decline of myocardial contractility produces a low-output state with venous congestion and peripheral oedema due to increased filtration at the capillary level. The same pattern occurs when pulmonary artery occlusion pressure increases with reduced left ventricular function, but here the decreased cardiac output is associated with pulmonary oedema. The most important therapeutic aspects of cardiogenic shock are the increase of ventricular performance and the decrease of afterload. Any increase in heart rate is of little help firstly because tachycardia is already present as a compensatory measure of the low-output state and secondly because it may worsen the perfusion of the coronary bed due to reduction of the diastolic time. Therefore, the only option is to administer an inotrope as dobutamine (usually 5–8 microg/kg/min up to 20 microg/kg/min). This drug has both inotropic and vasodilator effects. Caution must be used if the myocardium cannot increase its inotropic state as the vasodilator effect of dobutamine reduces the systemic vascular resistances with drop of systemic and coronary perfusion pressure. The intra-aortic balloon pump represents the best ideal choice in cardiogenic shock when inotropes fail to increase the cardiac output. It provides a decrease of left ventricular load while ensuring coronary perfusion at the same time. However, this device can be used as a temporary measure to buy time in the stunned myocardium or to allow for surgical interventions such as revascularization, cardiac transplantation and repair of a ruptured valve. The right-side heart failure as imposed by pulmonary embolism poses additional problems. When the right heart fails, especially if the rising of right ventricular pressures impinges on the filling of the left chambers, there is a fall in systemic arterial pressure that reduces the coronary perfusion [19]. At this point, a negative feedback ensues as the reduced coronary perfusion pressure causes ischaemic ventricular dysfunction with further drop of contractility, decrease of arterial blood pressure that ultimately leads to death. In this situation dobutamine is potentially dangerous as the fixed pulmonary obstruction may not allow for the increase of cardiac output despite the augmented inotropism. The result is worsening of arterial hypotension due to its vasodilatory effect with rapidly fatal consequences. Therefore, dobutamine is not indicated in patients with fixed low-output states, including those with end-stage cardiac disease [20]. In this situation, epinephrine (0.08–0.15 microg/kg/min) or low-dose norepinephrine (less than 0.1 microg/kg/min) is more useful as their α1 effect preserves coronary perfusion by increasing systemic vascular resistance and maintenance of arterial pressure. Nevertheless, this is only a temporary measure, as if the patient remains dependent on norepinephrine, the prognosis is poor.

3.1.3 Septic Shock

The haemodynamic features of early septic shock are complex and include low peripheral vascular resistances, increased cardiac output with decreased blood pressure, decrease in stressed vascular volume and mild decrease in cardiac function [21–23]. In the later stage, the cardiac function worsens, and peripheral resistances increase thus in turn causing the drop in cardiac output [23]. The increased cardiac output in early septic shock must be associated with increased venous return. Once again the venous return can increase by diminution of right atrial pressure or changes in the stressed volume, vascular resistances, vascular compliance and venous distribution of flow. Right atrial pressure is higher than normal in septic shock due to decreased ventricular function so that it cannot be responsible for the increase in cardiac output [24]. The total vascular volume is also decreased due to increased capillary leak, but it is unknown if the unstressed volume can compensate for this reduction. Some evidence indicates that the redistribution of flow from the splanchnic to the muscle reduces the time constant for venous drainage so increasing the return of blood to the heart [25]. Initially, the reduction of peripheral arterial resistance is compensated by the increased cardiac output so that arterial blood pressure remains normal. However, when venous return cannot be furtherly increased, arterial blood pressure decreases and hypotension ensues. This certainly contributes to the inadequate oxygen supply in septic shock, but abnormal regulation of microcirculatory flow and increased oxygen demands also play a role as blood flow seems to pass through the equivalent arteriovenous fistulas.

Which are the therapeutic options? As mean arterial pressure is given by the product of cardiac output by peripheral vascular resistance, the main therapeutic options are the increase of venous return by fluid administration or the use of vasopressors that increase peripheral vascular resistance. The increase in venous return certainly rises the cardiac output by increasing the stressed volume. However, the decreased vascular resistance and increased capillary leak make volume replacement quite ineffective as several litres of crystalloids are required to increase the filling pressure of the heart so rising the cardiac output. The intravenous volume in fact raises the mean systemic venous pressure, but this also increases the leak of plasma water from the injured capillaries. A more convenient approach is to raise the systemic vascular resistances with norepinephrine. It acts by squeezing the venous compartment, thus realizing a sort of autotransfusion that increases the stressed volume [17]. Moreover, the increased arteriolar resistance causes the capillary pressure to drop thus reducing the leak of fluids into the interstitium. This approach has the advantage that it can be quickly turned off, while the infused fluids can only be excreted by the kidney over time. In the past some concerns were raised about the use of norepinephrine in septic shock as it was thought that its vasopressor effect could decrease the renal blood flow with worsening of the renal function. Nevertheless, the clinical experience has shown that it increases the urine output probably by increased glomerular filtration. In fact, the combined increase of venous return and peripheral vascular resistance by norepinephrine augment the arteriolar pressure in the glomerulus thus increasing the urine output [26]. Therefore, the vasoconstrictor effect of norepinephrine has a detrimental effect under conditions of high peripheral resistances as hypovolemic or cardiogenic shock, but it seems advantageous if peripheral resistances are abnormally low.

The lowering in peripheral arterial resistances is invariably associated with the decrease of blood pressure unless the cardiac output increases so compensating for it. However cardiac output is tightly coupled with peripheral oxygen requirements, and if metabolic demands do not change, cardiac output will not change too. As a consequence, when decreased peripheral resistances are the primary mechanism of arterial hypotension, tissue perfusion remains adequate provided that cardiac output does not change. The main example of this condition is traumatic spinal shock and the use of sedative drugs. Tissue hypoperfusion only occurs if the venous return decreases with increased venous capacitance. This is a good example of hypotension without shock, and the usual clinical picture is the hypotensive patient with normal mental status and urine output and no arterial blood lactate elevation. Usually, there is no tachycardia as this would reflect the need for a compensatory mechanism that comes into play when hypotension is associated with decreased cardiac output. However, these patients have lowered cardiovascular reserves to compensate for further cardiovascular challenges. Moreover, the possibility for cerebral vascular autoregulation is potentially lost. Arterial pressure can be raised in two ways. Firstly, intravenous volume can be given to increase the stressed vascular volume. This would increase the venous return so that cardiac output could raise blood pressure in spite of decreased peripheral resistances. However, it should be remembered that the blood volume is not decreased and that undue volume infusion will be easily excreted by the kidney provided that the renal perfusion is normal. Otherwise stated, the infusion of crystalloids is only a temporary measure for raising blood pressure. Another way is to start a low-dose vasopressor as norepinephrine that increases the stressed volume by operating small veins squeezing.

Hypotension frequently occurs in the postoperative period when positive pressure ventilation or CPAP is applied to restore the decreased functional residual capacity after surgery. The reduction of blood pressure is essentially dependent on decreased venous return [27]. The increase of intrathoracic pressure causes the CVP to raise so that the pressure gradient for venous return is reduced [28, 29]. The net effect of positive pressure relies upon the possibility of the unstressed volume to compensate for the reduction of venous return. If the total blood volume is severely decreased, the application of a positive intrathoracic pressure causes a reduction in the stressed volume that cannot be furtherly compensated by the formerly decrease of unstressed volume. On the contrary, if the positive pressure is applied to a patient without volume depletion, PEEP shows only a transitory effect on venous return as the increased CVP causes the upstream mean systemic pressure to increase so normalizing the pressure gradient once again [30]. The therapeutic implication of the above analysis is obvious as the most important step is to restore blood volume so that the positive intrathoracic pressure has a minimal impact on venous return.

Whatever is its origin, shock can be viewed as a whole-body ischaemia-reperfusion injury. Ischaemia leads sequentially to intracellular anaerobic metabolism, reduced ATP stores, cellular damage and cell necrosis. Reperfusion also causes further cellular damage either locally and diffusely by widespread activation of inflammatory mediators. Briefly, ischaemia reduces the oxygen supply to the cells with consequent ATP depletion and accumulation of its degradation products as AMP and ADP. These metabolites are converted to hypoxanthine by the hypoxia-induced O-form of xanthine oxidase and then furtherly degraded to reactive oxygen species (ROS), namely, superoxide O_2^-, hydrogen peroxide H_2O_2 and hydroxyl radical OH^- [31]. Reperfusion increases dramatically the production of ROS molecules as new oxygen is supplied to the enzymes of the intra-mitochondrial respiratory chain [32]. Hypoxia also produces mitochondria dysfunction with swelling and further decrease of ATP production. This generates a vicious cycle with further energy depletion and ROS species production which causes direct damage to membrane proteins and lipids [33]. Finally, the ATP depletion activates the caspase enzymes with subsequent cellular apoptosis [34]. Lipid peroxidation and ROS species cause damage to the endothelium with disruption of the endothelial membrane barrier. The increased permeability causes the leakage of plasma into the interstitium with oedema formation and decreased circulating volume. Another important feature of hypoxic cellular damage is the cytosol increase of Ca^{2+} ion. The entry of calcium into the cells activates several proteases and endonucleases with further cell damage [35]. The membrane Ca^{+2}-dependent phospholipase A2 is also activated with production of arachidonic acid metabolites (thromboxane, leukotrienes) which are potent inflammatory mediators [36]. The entry of ionized calcium in the cells is the consequence of cellular energy depletion [37]. Under normal circumstances, intracellular H^+ ions are exchanged with extracellular sodium by the Na^+-H^+ exchanger (NHE), in an electroneutral process. Na^+ cations are then pumped out of the cells by the Na^+/K^+-ATPase-dependent exchanger. However, the depletion of ATP stores inactivates the Na^+/K^+-ATPase pump so that Na^+ is pumped out the cells by the $2Na^+/Ca^{2+}$ exchanger that does not require ATP. The influx of Ca^{2+} triggers a vicious circle as new ROS are generated with further cellular damage and entry of Ca^{2+} into the cells.

A schematic overview of the cellular mechanisms during hypoxia is shown in Fig. 3.2. Besides the tissue damage, the ischaemia-reperfusion mechanism activates a generalized immune-inflammatory response that causes endothelial dysfunction and damage. Increased membrane permeability occurs with cellular swelling and cytoskeletal derangement. Moreover, the increased permeability of the endothelial barrier allows for increased filtration of plasma water in the interstitium and accumulation of oedema fluid. Finally the activation of endothelial cells by several cytokines, chemokines, platelet aggregating factor (PAF) and complement factors is responsible for activation and recruitment of polymorphonucleates (PMNs) and monocytes which causes further inflammation and damage [38, 39]. PMNs are responsible for direct ROS production and release of proteolytic enzymes, while the monocytes amplify the immune-inflammatory response by regulating the cross-talking between innate and acquired immune system. Finally, the damaged endothelium reduces the synthesis of the vasodilator nitric oxide (NO), while potent vasoconstrictors as endothelin and thromboxane are released. Therefore, the loss of autoregulation results in capillary vasoconstriction [40]. This adds to endothelial cell swelling and interstitial oedema in worsening the perfusion tissues with further ischaemic damage [41, 42]. Finally the systemic release of cytotoxic mediators propagates the damage to distant organs with multiple organ dysfunction and failure (MODS).

Conclusions

Shock states in acute care settings are very frequent. Haemorrhagic shock is by far the most frequent type of surgical and traumatic shock. Prompt recognition of shock is essential for rapid institution of resuscitative manoeuvers designed to minimize the accumulation of oxygen debt. Prolonged shock results from incomplete resuscitation. It is associated with global ischaemia-reperfusion injury that triggers a generalized inflammatory state and development of multiple organ dysfunction and failure.

Clinical Scenario

A 72-year-old man is admitted to the emergency surgical ward with a diagnosis of intestinal obstruction by a large metastatic cancer of the prostate. At clinical examination, he appears confused and lethargic with a rapid pulse rate (120 bpm), hypotension (85/40 mmHg) and oliguria. The skin is warm and pale, and rectal temperature is 38.7 °C. The haemoglobin level is 9 g/dL, serum proteins are 7.5 g/dL, serum creatinine is 1.89 mg/dL and BUN is 98 mg/dL. The coagulation profile and platelet count are normal. After placement of arterial and venous lines, the CVP value is 6 mmHg. Arterial blood gas analysis reveals a compensated metabolic acidosis (pH 7.38 and PaCO2 31 mmHg) with increased arterial blood lactates (3 mmol/L).

1. What is the main pathophysiological diagnosis of the shock state?
   A. Hypovolemic shock
   B. Haemorrhagic shock
   C. Septic shock
   D. Cardiogenic shock

Comment: This patient probably has a mixed shock. He is hypovolemic due to bowel sequestration of water and electrolytes. The serum protein level appears normal, a very unusual finding in a patient with disseminated cancer. However, the value is falsely increased by the reduction of plasma volume. For the same reason, the decreased haemoglobin level is even lower than it would seem. The patient is febrile, and sepsis might well be associated with bowel obstruction due to bacterial translocation. A more careful observation at his blood pressure values reveals that both diastolic and systolic pressure are decreased. This is unusual in pure hypovolemic shock as peripheral vascular resistances rise the diastolic pressure value, thus reducing the pulse pressure. In our patient, the pulse pressure is near to normal (45 mmHg), as both systolic and diastolic pressure are reduced. This probably reflects peripheral vascular dilation, a well-known cardiovascular marker of sepsis. Finally the CVP value is higher than expected if hypovolemia is associated with a normal cardiac function. The higher than normal CVP value is consistent with a mild impairment of ventricular function, a frequent finding in sepsis. In conclusion this patient suffers from hypovolemic shock although sepsis cannot be excluded.

2. What is the main mechanism responsible for the decreased blood pressure?
   A. Decreased peripheral resistances
   B. Decreased cardiac contractility
   C. Decreased venous return
   D. None of these

Comment: The primary mechanism of hypovolemic shock is the reduction of venous return due to decreased stressed vascular volume. Normally the unstressed volume is the physiological reserve for stressed volume reduction as small vessels are squeezed into large veins to restore the venous return. However severe volume depletion reduces the effectiveness of this compensatory mechanism so that venous return reduces and blood pressure falls. This mechanism is emphasized by reduction of peripheral resistances as occurs during sepsis. In our patient, both mechanisms might operate to reduce arterial blood pressure.

3. What is the first therapeutic manoeuver to increase blood pressure?
   A. Fluids
   B. Inotropes
   C. Vasopressors
   D. Packed red cells

Comment: The first therapeutic measure in our patient is to give fluids as this will restore venous return. This is the most effective therapeutic approach in hypovolemic shock. However, a very large amount of fluids may be needed before the ventricle could fill enough to increase its output. This is even more difficult to achieve when hypovolemia is associated with arterial vasodilation. Our patient's mental status suggests that blood pressure is no more adequate to ensure vital organ perfusion. This is a true emergency as if prolonged, hypotension may worsen coronary perfusion with impairment of cardiac function, further drop of cerebral perfusion pressure, loss of brain control of peripheral vascular tone, sudden cardiovascular collapse and ultimately death. The use of norepinephrine in this context seems justified as the increase of peripheral vascular resistances allow for the rapid restoration of safer blood pressure values. A convenient approach may be as follows: after 1 L of crystalloids, a low dose of norepinephrine infusion is started simultaneously with another fluid bolus if hypotension persists. Norepinephrine is titrated to achieve at least 55–60 mmHg of mean blood pressure.

Remember that fluids remain the cornerstone of therapy and norepinephrine is only a temporary measure to ensure adequate perfusion pressure to vital organs!

The use of inotropes has no rationale in these hypovolemic patients. These drugs often increase blood pressure by increasing the heart rate. However the concomitant decrease of peripheral vascular resistance reduced the compensatory effect of tachycardia. Finally, the use of inotropic drugs in severely hypovolemic patients exposes to the risk of arrhythmias as atrial fibrillation and supraventricular tachycardia.

Although red packed cells are not indicated in pure hypovolemic shock, blood transfusion in our patient needs a brief comment. The repletion of circulating volume by crystalloids or colloids decreases the haemoglobin level by dilution of the erythrocyte mass volume. In our patient, the slightly reduced haemoglobin level coexists with severe hypovolemia. By consequence, any fluid that replaces the circulating volume leads to a severe decrease in the erythrocyte mass. This is potentially dangerous as oxygen delivery might be decreased in spite of restoration of cardiac output. Remember that oxygen delivery is as follows:

$$[\text{Hb}] \times 13.4 \times \text{SaO}_2 / 100 \times \text{cardiac output}.$$

Therefore, if severe, the decrease of [Hb] cannot be adequately matched by the even greatest increase of cardiac output. Attention must be paid to avoid the excessive reduction of haemoglobin level in our patient as insufficient oxygen supply might occur if severe anaemia develops.

4. What is the less appropriate vasoactive agent?
   A. Epinephrine
   B. Norepinephrine
   C. Dobutamine

Comment: Certainly the less appropriate agent in this patient is dobutamine. This drug has marked inotropic and vasodilatory effects so that tachycardia would be the main effect in this hypovolemic patient. Conversely norepinephrine allows for internal autotransfusion (see text for details) thus increasing the venous return. Moreover, its vasoconstrictor effect helps in raising arterial blood pressure by increasing of peripheral vascular resistance.

Please see Chap. 58 for the correct answer.

References

1. Baron BJ, Scalea TM. Acute blood loss. Emerg Med Clin North Am. 1996;14:35–55.
2. World Health Organization. Injury chart book. A graphical overview of the global burden of injuries. Department of injuries and violence prevention. Noncommunicable diseases and Mental Health Cluster. Geneva: World Health Organization; 2002. http://www.who.int/violence _injury_prevention/pubblication/other_injury/chart/en/.
3. Chrousos GP. The hypothalamic-pituitary-adrenal-axis and immune mediated inflammation. N Engl J Med. 1995;332:1351–62.
4. Rothe CF. Reflex control of veins and vascular capacitance. Physiol Rev. 1983;63(4):1281–95.
5. Guyton AC, Jones CE, Coleman TG. Circulatory physiology: cardiac output and its regulation. In: Guyton AC, editor. Philadelphia: WB Saunders; 1973.
6. Guyton AC, Lindsey AW, Kaufman BN. Effect of mean circulatory filling pressure and other peripheral circulatory factors on cardiac output. Am J Physiol. 1955;180:659–77.
7. Rothe CF, Drees JA. Vascular capacitance and fluid shifts in dogs during prolonged hemorrhagic hypotension. Circ Res. 1976;38(5):347–56.
8. Rothe CF, Johns BL, Bennett TD. Vascular capacitance of dog intestine using mean transit time of indicator. Am J Physiol. 1978;234(1):H7–H13.
9. Crowell JW, Smith EE. Oxygen deficit and irreversible hemorrhagic shock. Am J Physiol. 1984;206:313–6.
10. Dunham CM, Siegel JH, Weireter L, Fabian M, Goodarzi S, Guadalupi P, Gettings L, Linberg SE, Vary TC. Oxygen debt and metabolic academia as quantitative predictors of mortality and the severity of the ischemic insult in hemorrhagic shock. Crit Care Med. 1991;19:231–43.
11. Rixen D, Raum M, Holzgraefe B, Sauerland S, Nagelshmidt M, Neugebauer EA. Shock and trauma study group. A pig hemorrhagic shock model: oxygen debt and metabolic academia as indicators of severity. Shock. 2001;16:239–44.
12. Rixen D, Siegel JH. Bench-to-bedside review: oxygen debt and its metabolic correlates as quantifiers of the severity of hemorrhagic and post-traumatic shock. Crit Care. 2005;9:441–53.
13. Rixen D, Raum M, Bouillon B, Lefering R, Neugebauer E. Arbeitsgemeinschaft 'Polytrauma' of the Deutschen Gesellschaft Fur Unhallchirurgie: base deficit development and its prognostic significance in posttrauma critical illness: an analysis by trauma registry of the Deutsche Gesellschaft fur Unfallechirurgie. Shock. 2001;15:83–9.
14. Weil MH, Henning RJ. New concepts in the diagnosis and fluid treatment of circulatory shock. Thirteenth annual Becton, Dickinson and Company Oscar Schwidetsky Memorial Lecture. Anesth Analg. 1979;58(2):124–31.
15. Magder SA, Georgiadis G, Cheong T. Respiratory variations in right atrial pressure predict the response to fluid challenge. J Crit Care. 1992;7(2):76–85.
16. Feissel M, Michard F, Faller JP, Teboul JL. The respiratory variations in inferior vena cava diameter as a guide to fluid therapy. Intensive Care Med. 2004;30(9):1834–7.
17. Barbier C, Loubiere Y, Schmit C, Hayon J, Ricome JL, Jardin F, Veillard-Baron A. Respiratory changes in inferior vena cava diameter are helpful in predicting fluid responsiveness in ventilated septic patients. Intensive Care Med. 2004;30(9):1740–6.
18. Appleton C, Olajos M, Morkin E, Goldman S. Alpha-1 adrenergic control of the venous circulation in intact dogs. J Pharmacol Exp Ther. 1985;233(3):729–34.
19. Calvin JE, Quinn B. Right ventricular pressure overload during acute lung injury: cardiac mechanics in the pathophysiology of right ventricular systolic dysfunction. J Crit Care. 1989;4(4):251–65.
20. Calvin JE. Right ventricular afterload mismatch during acute pulmonary hypertension and its treatment with dobutamine: a pressure segment length analysis in a canine model. J Crit Care. 1989;4(4):239–50.
21. Chien S, Dellenback RJ, Usami S, Treitel K, Chang C, Gregersen MI. Blood volume and its distribution in endotoxin shock. Am J Physiol. 1966;210(6):1411–8.
22. Lang CH, Bagby GJ, Ferguson JL, Spitzer JJ. Cardiac output and redistribution of organ blood flow in hypermetabolic sepsis. Am J Physiol. 1984;246:R331–7.
23. MacLean MR, Mulligan WG, MacLean APH, Duff JH. Patterns of septic shock in man-a detailed study of 56 patients. Ann Surg. 1967;166:543–62.
24. Parker MM, Parrillo JE. Septic shock: hemodynamic and pathogenesis. JAMA. 1983;250(24):3324–7.
25. Magder SA, Quinn R. Endotoxin and the mechanical properties of the canine peripheral circulation. J Crit Care. 1991;6(2):81–8.

26. Desjars P, Pinaud M, Bugnon D, Tasseau F. Norepinephrine therapy has no deleterious renal effects in human septic shock. Crit Care Med. 1989;17(5):426–9.
27. Cournard A, Motley HL, Werko L. Physiological studies of the effect of intermittent positive pressure breathing on cardiac output in man. Am J Physiol. 1948;152:169–74.
28. Scharf SM, Brown R, Tow DE, Parisi AF. Cardiac effects of increasing lung volume and decreasing pleural pressure. J Appl Physiol Respir Environ Exerc Physiol. 1979;47:253–62.
29. Scharf SM, Caldini P, Ingram RH. Cardiovascular effects of increasing airway pressure in the dog. Am J Physiol. 1977;232(1):H35–43.
30. Fessler HE, Brower RG, Wise RA, Permutt S. Effects of positive end-expiratory pressure on the gradient for venous return. Am Rev Respir Dis. 1991;143:19–24.
31. Chambers DE, Parks DA, Patterson G, Roy R, McCord JM, Yoshida S, Parmley LF, Downey JM. Xanthine-Oxidase as a source of free radical damage in myocardial ischemia. J Mol Cell Cardiol. 1985;17:145–52.
32. Becker LB. New concepts in reactive oxygen species and cardiovascular reperfusion physiology. Cardiovasc Res. 2004;61:461–70.
33. Maxwell SR, Lip GY. Reperfusion injury: a review of the pathophysiology, clinical manifestation and therapeutic optioins. Int J Cardiol. 1997;58:95–117.
34. McCully JD, Wakiyama H, Hsieh YJ, Jones M, Levitsky S. Differential contribution of necrosis and apoptosis in myocardial ischemia-reperfusion injury. Am J Physiol Heart Circ Physiol. 2004;286:1923–35.
35. Seal JB, Gewertz BL. Vascular dysfunction in ischemia reperfusion injury. Ann Vasc Surg. 2005;19:572–84.
36. Ernster L. Biochemistry of reoxygenation injury. Crit Care Med. 1988;16:947–53.
37. Mentzer RM, Lasley RD, Jessel A, Karmazyn M. Intracellular sodium hydrogen exchange inhibition and clinical myocardial protection. Ann Thorac Surg. 2003;75:S700–8.
38. Barry MC, Wang JH, Kelly CJ, Sheenan SJ, Redmond HP, Bouchier-Hayes DJ. Plasma factors augment neutrophil and endothelial activation during aortic surgery. Eur J Vasc Endovasc Surg. 1997;13:381–7.
39. Barry MC, Kelly C, Burke P, Sheehan S, Redmond HP, Bouchier-Hayes D. Immunological and physiological responses to aortic surgery: effect of reperfusion on neutrophil and monocyte activation and pulmonary function. Br J Surg. 1997;84:513–9.
40. Hill JH, Ward PA. The phlogistic role of C3 leukotactic fragment in myocardial infarct in rats. J Exp Med. 1971;133:855–900.
41. Boyle EM, Pohlman TH, Cornejo CJ, Verrier ED. Ischemia-reperfusion injury. Ann Thorac Surg. 1997;64:S24–30.
42. Menger MD, Rucker M, Vollmar B. Capillary dysfunction in striated muscle ischemia/reperfusion on the mechanisms of capillary “no-reflow”. Shock. 1997;8:2–7.

Preoperative Assessment of the Acute Critically Ill Trauma Patient in the Emergency Department

4

Bianca M. Wahlen and Andrea De Gasperi

Key Points

- In the acutely ill trauma patient, a rational, sequential, and rapid approach is mandatory: time is critical but rationality should always be used.
- To secure the airway is a "class one priority": a delay in securing the airway may lead to rapidly progressing hypoxemia and risk of life-threatening complications.
- A comprehensive approach to manage hemodynamic instability is warranted, including management of hemorrhagic hypovolemic shock, hemodilution, hypothermia, coagulopathy, electrolyte abnormalities, and acid-base derangements and alternative etiologies (if present) of shock after trauma.
- The role of ultrasound (US) in the acute care of trauma is rapidly evolving and gaining a pivotal role: it should be implemented and expanded according to the most recent guidelines.
- Acute coagulopathy of trauma (ACT) is receiving an ever-increasing attention due to the relevant impact researches on the outcome: viscoelastic tests (TEG/ROTEM) seem to have a relevant impact on the management of the bleeding trauma patients. Antifibrinolytics are becoming a mainstay in the trauma management.

B. M. Wahlen
Department of Trauma Surgery, Hamad General Hospital, Doha, Qatar

A. De Gasperi (✉)
2 Servizio Anestesia e Rianimazione, Ospedale Niguarda CaGranda, Milan, Italy
e-mail: andrea.degasperi@ospedaleniguarda.it; andrea.degasperi@mpcnet.it

4.1 Introduction

Trauma, defined as a "serious bodily injury or shock caused by an external source," is nowadays a leading cause of morbidity and mortality worldwide, and it is predicted to become the third largest contributor to the global burden of disease by 2020. The initial evaluation of an acute critically ill trauma patient is a challenging task, particularly in the bleeding, unstable patient. Time is of utmost importance (Grade 1A in the last release of the European guideline on management of major bleeding and coagulopathy following trauma) [1]: in some cases, seconds make the difference between life and death [2, 3]. A great number of traumatized patients require emergent resuscitation, surgical management for temporary stabilization (or definitive treatment) of injuries, and perioperative critical care management [1, 2]. Accordingly, the time available for preassessment varies, and a multidisciplinary approach is warranted to care for individuals who have suffered a severe traumatic injury: anesthesiologists, as perioperative care physicians, should have, when present, a leading role in managing trauma patients, enabling early airway management, appropriate and timely resuscitation, basic (or advanced) neurologic evaluation, hypothermia prevention, analgesia and sedation as needed, and transfer of the patient to the operating room without delay [2, 3].

The main goals of preoperative assessment in the trauma setting are:

1. To evaluate the patient's conditions
2. To determine if lab or instrumental tests are needed (testing should be performed based on clinical suspicion and limited to those able to change the management)
3. To estimate the risks
4. To consider any intervention able to reduce or impact on the perioperative surgical and medical risks

Depending on the urgency, the interventions are categorized since 2004 in lifesaving, urgent, expedited, and elective

P. Aseni et al. (eds.), *Operative Techniques and Recent Advances in Acute Care and Emergency Surgery*,
https://doi.org/10.1007/978-3-319-95114-0_4

[4]. Among interventions able to reduce injuries from the environmental exposure, hypothermia (defined as a core temperature below 35 °C, mild hypothermia being classified as a core temperature between 32 and 35 °C) should be addressed and treated immediately or, if possible, prevented. As a matter of fact, hypothermia may heavily impact on both coagulopathy and the development of multiple organ dysfunction [3]. Whenever possible, a medications list, particularly of drugs able to impact on hemostasis (antiplatelet, anticoagulant drugs and particularly the new direct anticoagulants) and the cardiovascular system (antihypertensives, particularly ACE inhibitors and beta-blockers), should be obtained.

4.2 Pulmonary Assessment

In case of emergency, surgical or interventional procedures, postoperative pulmonary complications, (reported in up to 6% of the cases after major abdominal surgery), along with cardiac, thromboembolic, and infectious complications, are among the major postoperative medical sequelae: they contribute significantly to overall perioperative morbidity and mortality in the acute trauma setting [4, 5] and are almost always associated with longer hospital stay, higher treatment costs, and worst outcome [6].

4.2.1 Airway Assessment

Following the ABC algorithm, to secure the airway is the priority. This is especially true in acute critically ill patients who are at risk for respiratory distress or aspiration. In specific trauma patients (e.g., patient with head and midface trauma or neck injuries), a fast and accurate evaluation of the airway might be lifesaving. Every patient should be assessed for mask ventilation, tracheal intubation, and / or surgical airway access. As most of these patients are at increased risk for aspiration, the supraglottic airway devices play a minor role in the airway management. Since the LEMON score has been included in the 8th edition of the *Advanced Trauma Life Support* (ATLS) Manual in 2009, it should be incorporated as a standard in the assessment of the airway of every trauma patient (or at least an effort has to be done) [3, 7] (Table 4.1).

Commonly used criteria for endotracheal intubation (ETI) include:

1. Inability to maintain airway or oxygenation
2. Respiratory distress (also without hypoxia or hypoventilation)
3. Moderate cognitive impairment
4. Glasgow Coma Scale < 9
5. Inability to protect the airway against aspiration
6. Unstable midface trauma and/or airway injuries

Table 4.1 LEMON score

L	Look externally (Facial trauma, large incisors, beard or mustache, large tongue)
E	Evaluate the 3-3-2 rule – Incisor distance: 3 FB – Hyoid-mental distance: 3 FB – Thyroid-to-mouth distance: 2 FB
M	Mallampati score ≥ 3
O	Obstruction Presence of any condition like epiglottitis, peritonsillar abscess, trauma
N	Neck mobility (limited neck mobility)

Furthermore, early ETI may be indicated in cervical spine injury with any evidence of respiratory failure. Complete cervical spinal cord injury or incomplete injury above C6 will lead, due to a decreased innervation of the respiratory muscles (especially intercostal muscles), to breathing difficulties. Instead, lesions above C3 determine complete and immediate respiratory arrest. Eligible patients undergo an immediate rapid sequence intubation and/or surgical airway access, depending on the underlying trauma [8]. Any form of cervical spine pathology should be excluded if to secure the airway is not time-critical and an emergent priority: even if rare, intubation-related cervical spine injuries have been described [3, 9, 10]. If cervical spine injuries cannot be excluded, manual in-line stabilization (MILS) is the gold standard, as direct laryngoscopy might become more difficult if not impossible. Videolaryngoscopes are well-recognized alternatives, often offering, compared to conventional direct laryngoscopy, a better view. However, a possible longer intubation time has to be considered [8]. Other devices for a backup plan might include flexible fiberscope or optical stylets such as Bonfils or Bullard: all are mentioned in international guidelines [8, 11, 12]. However, all those alternatives imply an experienced user and a laryngeal view not compromised by blood or other secretions [3]. More important, indirect optical devices may be useless in ongoing bleeding, as to be expected, for example, in midface or neck injuries. According to ASA (American Society of Anesthesiologists) recommendations [2, 12], in case of problematic intubations, alternatives include (but are not limited to) combinations of solutions or techniques: among them, laryngeal mask airway as an intubation conduit (with or without flexible scope guidance), flexible scope intubation, intubating stylet or tube changer, and light wand. In patients with maxillofacial, laryngeal or tracheal trauma, oral or nasal blind intubation is discouraged, and surgical airway facilities should be immediately available [3]. For the most updated algorithms, see those endorsed by ASA [2, 8, 12].

4.3 Assessment of Breathing

4.3.1 Physical Examination

The primary tool for diagnosis and differential diagnosis is still the physical examination. Auscultation may display normal bronchial bilateral breath sounds, crackles, pleural rubs, wheezing, or silent chest. Respiratory depth and rate have to be determined, chest wall asymmetry and paradoxical chest wall motion are to be evaluated, and the patient has to be examined for penetrating wounds, seat belt, or steering wheel marks. Chest wall tenderness or other signs indicating rib fractures have to be excluded; subcutaneous emphysema or tracheal deviation has to be ruled out. Hyperresonance or dullness to chest percussion may indicate tension pneumothorax or hemothorax. Studies give evidence that experienced users in lung ultrasound (LUS) will be able to rule out in a fast, safe, and radiation-free way life-threatening conditions like hemothorax and tension pneumothorax, large pleural effusions, or misplaced tubes [13–15]. Furthermore, lung ultrasound in some situations (e.g., identification of pneumothorax after blunt trauma, misplacement of endotracheal tubes or pleural effusion) might be even superior to conventional imaging techniques [13–16].

4.3.2 Imaging: From Chest X-Ray to Chest Ultrasonography and CT Scan

One of the first routine examinations in trauma patients is still a standard chest radiograph [3]. In the further clinical course, or according to the clinical scenario, plain radiographs may be foregone in favor of immediate chest CT scanning [15]. Although both methods are still important and necessary, chest ultrasonography (US) plays more and more a role in trauma patients, especially in time-critical situations. Among major advantages of US are lack of radiations and immediate availability. Studies give evidence that the quality of radiography and ultrasonography, when US is used by experienced and/or specifically trained examiners, is similar [13–16].

One of the risks in trauma patients is a post-intubation tension pneumothorax, to be immediately ruled out by all means for the dramatic and life-threatening hemodynamic and respiratory effects. The fastest and therefore safest method in the operating theater will be the ultrasonography. For pneumothorax, the sensitivity is 91% and the specificity 98%. In an expert review done by Wilkerson et Stone and quoted by Blanco et al. [14] and Volpicelli et al. [16], the AAs concluded that bedside thoracic US is an even more sensitive screening test than supine AP chest radiography for the detection of pneumothorax in adult patients with blunt chest trauma. Since 2012, the lung US for pneumothorax has been incorporated in the international evidence-based recommendations for point-of-care lung ultrasound [16]. With a *level A* evidence, the signs of pneumothorax include the presence of lung point(s), the absence of lung sliding, the absence of B-lines, and the absence of lung pulse. In the OR, another application for ultrasonography is the confirmation of a correct endotracheal intubation. Particularly in trauma patients, when intubation under direct vision could be difficult, and the help of capnography is lacking, US seems to be a useful tool to confirm correct intubation, as proved in a very recent experience [17].

4.3.3 Gas Exchange

Patients with aspiration, hemo- or pneumothorax, and lung contusion are at extreme risk of developing rapidly progressing hypoxemia and/or acute lung injury [18, 19]. Additional risks may arise from massive transfusion (by transfusion of packed red blood cells, fresh frozen plasma, and/or platelets), volume overload, and fluid shift. These conditions may result in ventilation/perfusion mismatch, increased intrapulmonary shunt, increased extravascular lung water, segmental lung damage, and/or loss of compliance, further aggravating pulmonary gas exchange [18–20]. Protective ventilation is warranted in this scenario.

4.3.3.1 Monitoring Gas Exchange and Acid-Base Equilibrium (ABE)

(a) **Arterial Oxygen Saturation (SaO_2)**—Continuous oxygen saturation monitoring should be standard in all trauma patients. In case of mechanical ventilation, $SaO_2 > 92$ is the target [8].
(b) **End-tidal Carbon dioxide ($EtCO_2$)**—$EtCO_2$ monitoring should be used in all intubated patients. In non-intubated patients the micro-stream, nasal capnographic monitoring as a semi-quantitative measurement should be considered both during spontaneous and, when indicated, during noninvasive ventilation (NIV).
(c) **Blood Gas Analysis (BGA)**—As in the acute critically ill patients, arterial line placement should be standard. An experienced provider, guided by US in problematic or difficult cases, should insert the arterial line within few minutes (often less than one). Intermittent blood gas analysis immediately reveals changes in oxygenation and acid-base balance. Base excess (BE) and lactate blood level provide a way to assess the severity of shock. Blood gas analysis and acid-base equilibrium allow within seconds decisions concerning ventilation, replacement of volume, administration of electrolytes, and/or packed red blood cells (PRBCs). Metabolic acidosis is not infrequent in the

hyperacute setting: adequate fluid resuscitation and, when needed, pressor or inotropes (and not bicarbonate!) are the mainstays to restore blood pressure and to maintain tissue perfusion [8, 15].

4.3.4 Lung Protective Ventilation

Patients intubated in the prehospital triage have to be assessed for adequate ventilation. Most of the trauma patients, particularly those with accompanying blunt chest trauma due to fall from height or motor vehicle accident, suffer from single or multiple, uni- or bilateral rib fractures, flail chest, hemothorax or tension pneumothorax, as well as lung contusion: they require immediate intubation and lung protective ventilation, to be continued both in the OR and in the ICU [8, 21]. Ventilation parameters have to be assessed and, if necessary, appropriately adjusted. Typically, the ventilator settings would require tidal volume of 6–8 mL/kg (predicted body weight) and a respiratory rate (RR) of 12–16 breaths/min using a volume- or pressure-limited ventilation. RR at 8–10 breaths/min, with adequate expiratory time to reduce air trapping (i.e., inspiratory-to-expiratory [I:E] ratio of 1:3), might also be considered, allowing a permissive hypercapnia ($PaCO_2$ 40–45 mmHg) if not otherwise contraindicated (e.g., evidence of brain injury or metabolic acidosis) [8]. Mean airway pressure should be kept as low as possible and ideally below 25–30 mmHg. An individualized "open-lung PEEP" (OL-PEEP, the level resulting in maximal dynamic compliance during a decremental PEEP trial) should be applied [21, 22]. According to some Authorities [8], in the specific setting of trauma, no PEEP has to be used until having achieved a hemodynamic stability after adequate resuscitation. After stabilization, PEEP could be increased to 5–10 cm H_2O, main being the balance between minimization of lung injury and hemodynamic optimization. FiO_2 should be titrated aiming at SaO2 > 92% [8, 21, 22].

4.3.4.1 ECMO: The Case for Very Selected Indications

Evaluation of patients who are "critical" concerning the pulmonary gas exchange should be immediately performed, and their referral to extracorporeal membrane oxygenation (ECMO) team might be considered [23, 24]. As a matter of fact, its use in ARF after trauma is controversial and seldom reported [24]: the decision to activate the ECMO team differs from center to center. Nevertheless, accepted criteria refer commonly to the Murray score (see Table 4.2) [18]. Usually patients with potentially reversible causes and a Murray score ≥ 3.5 might benefit from ECMO and should be discussed with the ECMO team [23, 24]. According to the most recent experience, mortality was higher in patients with high injury severity score and lower arterial pH on arrival. Ability to tolerate systemic anticoagulation was associated with improved survival [24].

Table 4.2 Murray score

Point(s)	0	1	2	3	4
PaO2/FiO2 FiO2 100% For 20 min	≥300	225–299	175–224	100–174	≤100
PEEP	≤5	6–8	9–11	12–14	≥15
CRX, number of quadrants infiltrate	0	1	2	3	4
Compliance (cm H_2O)	80	60–79	40–59	20–39	≤19

4.3.5 Previous History

Underlying injuries, especially neck or midface injuries, may comprise the airway and/or breathing capacity of a trauma patient. Besides that, additional preexisting patient-related factors can aggravate this condition. Therefore, if possible, the past and present history of the patient should be taken, to be aware of other comorbidities able to complicate perioperative ventilation and/or oxygenation further. Age >50 years [3, 4], chronic obstructive pulmonary disease [25], congestive heart failure, poor general health status (American Society of Anesthesiologists [ASA] class >2), obstructive sleep apnea, smoking [26], pulmonary hypertension [27–29], low oxygen saturation, and serum albumin < 3.5 g/dL are patient-related risk factors able to heavily impact on postoperative pulmonary complications [5]. As in every kind of risk assessment in surgery, the patient's comorbidities and the type surgery are the two main drivers able to qualify the patient at "high risk." Emergency surgery increases the risk for pulmonary complications above average [5, 30]. The incidence of complications is inversely related to the distance of the surgical incision from the diaphragm [5]. Thus, the complication rate is significantly higher for thoracic and upper abdominal surgery than for lower abdominal and all other procedures [31].

Therefore close communication between anesthesia, surgery, radiology, and operating room staff should be continuous, concise, clear, and guaranteed: a dedicated communication training is suggested by some authors [3, 8].

4.4 Circulation (Cardiac) Assessment

Among the causes of shock (classically defined as the acute imbalance between oxygen supply and demand but practically defined in the trauma setting as an acute, critical hypotension) in the critically ill acute trauma patient, hemorrhage is reported as the most common [1]. Classified in four classes, hemorrhage becomes critical when blood losses involve ≥30% of the blood volume (class III), with critical fall of systolic blood pressure [15]. Chest, abdomen, retroperitoneum, and thighs are reported to be the most frequent sites of (massive) hemorrhage [3]. In case of urgent surgical intervention, anesthesia and the surgical procedure can influence cardiac performance in several ways. Decreased cardiac preload due to blood loss, fluid shifts, and compressed venous blood flow and afterload changes due to anesthetic agents, bowel manipulation, pulmonary emboli, as well as stress on cardiac compensation caused, for example, by stress, pain, tachycardia, and/or anemia can adversely impact on intraoperative hemodynamics. Other potential causes of hemodynamic impairment to be considered (and possibly ruled out) are cardiac tamponade, tension pneumothorax, hemothorax, spinal cord injury, and fat or air emboli [15]. Initially, detailed patient history (including drugs taken by the patient), skin temperature, and capillary refill (press centrally for 5 s and release: normal color should return within 2 s) and, if possible, auscultation and electrocardiogram (ECG) should be the first steps in evaluating a trauma patient [8, 15].

4.4.1 Auscultation

Besides all types of heart murmurs, which might be present in any patients, special attention has to be paid to patients with blunt chest trauma. Patients with suspected myocardial contusion might display, besides usually very unspecific signs, *pulsus paradoxus*, muffled heart sounds, and pericardial friction rub. This is the setting where US, the real new millennium stethoscope, could make the difference.

4.4.2 EKG

When possible, a 12-lead EKG should be recorded in every trauma patients: on the one hand to exclude acute conditions (pulmonary embolism, myocardial infarction, cardiac contusion, electrolyte imbalances), on the other hand as a baseline for future comparison. In suspected cardiac contusion, EKG is a class I recommended test in the initial treatment of a patient with significant chest trauma. One might get a hint if the probability of a traumatic contusion is high [31–34]: as a matter of fact, 40–83% of the patients will have an abnormal EKG. There is no correlation between the severity of contusion and any kind of arrhythmia. Most likely contusion of the left ventricle will present as an abnormality of ST-T and pathological Q waves. Also common is a right bundle branch block, whereas AV-Block I°, left bundle branch block, hemiblocks, and AV-Block III° are less common.

4.4.3 Biomarkers

In general serum lactate, arterial blood gas analysis, and renal and liver function tests are included in an emergency routine [8]. Measuring biomarkers (troponin I and troponin T, N terminal pro BNP) initially and after a 4–6-h interval, particularly in patients with blunt chest trauma, belongs to the tests with negative predictive value of class II and should be assessed [35–38].

4.4.4 Echocardiography

If ECG and the results of biomarkers are not within normal limits, further investigations (mainly echocardiography) are recommended as a class II recommendation and should be considered [39]. In *time-critical cases,* the bedside cardiac ultrasound is a useful tool in the emergency environment [14]. The subxiphoid four-chamber view is an excellent cross-longitudinal section of the heart. The size of the right ventricle can easily be compared to the left ventricle size. Contractility of each chamber, mitral valves, and the descending thoracic aorta in cross section next to the left atrium can be evaluated. Simple question concerning the overall activity of the heart as well as a possible pericardial effusion/tamponade can be ruled out or confirmed quickly and precisely. Adequate image quality on transthoracic echocardiography (TTE) may be technically challenging in the acute trauma patients. Consequently, TTE might be required in some of the more acutely ill patients and have relevant information also of the aortic pathology (i.e., dissection). In *less time-critical cases,* and if and when possible, transesophageal echocardiography (TEE) could find its strength in the emergency department for the evaluation of hemodynamically unstable patients, providing selective functional and anatomic information to differentiate the underlying disturbance, being perhaps superior to other invasive monitors. As a semi-invasive method to assess the left ventricular (LV) volumes and ejection fraction, TEE provides fast information about heart pump function, acute myocardial infarction (MI) or pulmonary embolism (PE), heart and systemic volume status (hypovolemia), obstructive flow patterns (dynamic LV flow obstruction, cardiac tamponade), and unexplained hypoxemia. Because the management of MI, PE, hypovolemia, or obstruction is different, the early placement of TEE can significantly assist in forming and optimizing the treatment plan. TEE has already been well established for patient monitoring during cardiac surgery. In 2010 the American Society of Anesthesiologists updated their practice guidelines for perioperative TEE use [40]. Recommendations for TEE use for non-cardiac surgery were established. The American Society of Anesthesiologists (ASA) practice guidelines recommend the use of TEE when the nature of surgery or the patient's known or suspected cardiovascular pathology might result in severe hemodynamic, pulmonary, or neurologic compromise. TEE should be used when unexplained life-threatening hemodynamic instability persists despite corrective therapy if equipment and expertise are available. According to the ASA, patients with potential benefit of TEE monitoring might include those with known or suspected cardiovascular compromise, patients with unexplained persistent hypotension, or unexplained persistent hypoxemia, as well as patients with major thoracic or abdominal trauma. However, depending on comorbidities, clinical condition and surgical invasiveness, intraoperative TEE can help to optimize perioperative care, assessing LV function and volume load, recognizing early regional wall motion abnormalities, and guiding fluid, vasopressor or inotropic therapy [41].

4.4.5 Evaluation of Volume Status and the Impact of Renal Function

Assessment of the volume status is of the utmost importance and one of the most challenging tasks in the acute critically ill trauma patient. Fluid resuscitation with respect to optimal volume and type of fluids is under constant debate [15]. Strategies which include delayed fluid resuscitation and/or controlled hypotension are relevant in some trauma scenarios but, according to very recent reviews, are to be taken and applied wisely (cum grano salis!) [42]. On the contrary, volume overload might have a devastating impact not only on kidney function but also on the overall mortality. It is known that acute kidney injury (AKI) develops in 55–66% of critically ill patients with a mortality rate ranging 15–80%, depending on the severity of renal dysfunction [43, 44]. Recent reports highlight that fluid overload is an independent risk factor for AKI in the critically ill patients. It is biologically plausible that volume overloading leads to organ congestions thus resulting in decreased renal blood flow [45–50]. Furthermore, it has been shown that fluid overload is related to an increase in overall mortality with critical illness. If both factors are combined, fluid overload in an already established AKI has been correlated with lower renal functional recovery and lower survival [51, 52]. Patients with chronic kidney disease (CKD) are at increased risk of perioperative morbidity and mortality. Preexisting chronic kidney diseases can be ruled out reviewing serum creatinine, glomerular filtration rate, and blood urea nitrogen (BUN). Acute trauma and urgent/emergent trauma surgery increase the risk of acute kidney injury (AKI). In trauma patients, an indwelling urinary catheter is the rule, allowing, on the one hand, an immediate detection of urinary tract injuries and, on the other hand, continuous measurement of urine output (UO). In a large ICU population, intensive UO monitoring was associated with improved detection of AKI and reduced 30-day mortality in patients developing AKI; less fluid overload was also reported for all monitored patients [53].

Among the methods used to assess volume status, measurement of central venous pressure (CVP), equivalent to right atrial pressure (RAP) when the vena cava is continuous with the right atrium, is still considered a standard of monitoring [54, 55]. This is confirmed by studies, which give evidence that large part of the anesthesiologists uses the CVP to assess volume status and to guide volume therapy and fluid management decisions [54, 55]. This in spite of some relevant studies clearly shows limitations of this use of CVP in this setting [56]. Other concerns expressed by experts are the risk of complications (among them, infection, catheter-induced thrombosis, and arrhythmias). Furthermore, occasionally, in time-critical situations or in very peculiar conditions when central venous catheterization is not possible, the use of noninvasive or dynamic techniques to assess the volume status is crucial to rule out (or in..!) hypovolemia [57]. As a matter of fact, preload static parameters such as CVP or wedge pressure may not predict volume status and/or fluid responsiveness. RAP is related to venous return, which in turn depends on venous capacitance gradient. Cyclic changes of ventricular filling induced by increased intrathoracic pressure variations and heart-lung interaction during mechanical ventilation lead to delta-up and delta-down variations of stroke volume and inferior vena cava (IVC) size. Fluid responder is usually defined the patient whose stroke volume increases by 10–15% following a 3 mL/kg (usually 250 mL) crystalloid or colloid fluid bolus. Dynamic parameters (systolic pressure variation, SPV; stroke volume variation, SVV; pulse pressure variation, PPV), instead of the time-honored “static” parameters (CVP is an example), are in the last few years on the rise both in anesthesia and ICU settings [58]. An alternative and quick method to assess the volume status is the sonographic assessment of the venous collapsibility index (VCI) using respiratory variation of IVC (inferior vena cava) diameter. VCI measures the fractional change in major venous diameters through the respiratory cycle rather than relying on a single measurement of venous diameter. Results of a recent review article confirm that sonographic measurement of IVC diameter and collapsibility is under certain circumstances a valid method of estimating CVP and RAP (right atrial pressure) [59]. Technically, the measurement of the IVC diameter can be performed in the subxiphoid, lateral, and even supra-iliac position. However, ICV diameter can be affected by high intra-abdominal pressure and is therefore limited in patients with blunt abdominal trauma or patients scheduled for emergency re-laparotomy. In case of problematic conditions, superior vena cava (SVC) collapsibility index might be an alternative: SVC needs of course of a TTE monitoring, neither always possible in the trauma setting not everywhere available. Vignon et al. in a very recent experience tried to identify responders to volume expansion using 10 mL/kg of colloid solution among septic shock patients under mechanical ventilation. Using for SVC a threshold of 36%, collapsibility had sensitivity of 90% and specificity of 100% in detecting an 11% rise in cardiac index after volume expansion [60].

4.5 Neurologic Assessment

Once addressed and, if possible, solved the problems associated with the safety of the airway, breathing, and circulation, a focused neurologic examination is needed. Neurologic assessment should be performed according to the Glasgow Coma Scale (Table 4.3), able also to grade the severity of neurological impairment. Also to be addressed any lateralizing signs and the level of sensation if a spinal cord injury is present (Table 4.4).

Further assessment should include pupillary size and responsiveness. In less time-critical cases, assessment of gross motor and sensory function in all four limbs should be carried out. If a spinal cord injury is present, a full neurological assessment is vital at the earliest opportunity—an example is the check for priapism, loss of anal sphincter tone, and the bulbocavernosus reflex.

For the experienced physician, most of the cranial nerves can be easily assessed as reported below (Table 4.5).

In conscious trauma patients, motor function can also be easily assessed using the "American Spinal Injury Association (ASIA) Motor Key" (Tables 4.6 and 4.7).

Table 4.3 Glasgow Coma Scale (GCS)

Behavior	Response	Score
Eye opening response	Spontaneously	4
	To speech	3
	To pain	2
	No response	1
Best verbal response	Oriented to time, place, and person	5
	Confused	4
	Inappropriate words	3
	Incomprehensible sounds	2
	No response	1
Best motor response	Obeys commands	6
	Moves to localized pain	5
	Flexion withdrawal from pain	4
	Abnormal flection (decorticate)	3
	Abnormal extension (decerebrate)	2
	No response	1
Total score	Best response	15
	Comatose patient	8 or less
	Totally unresponsive	3

Table 4.4 Level of consciousness according to GCS

GCS 13–15, mild	Normal to lethargic, mildly disoriented
GCS 9–13, moderate	Lethargic to obtunded, follows commands with arousal, confused
CGS 3–8, severe	(Comatose, no eye opening or verbalization, does not follow commands with arousal)

Table 4.5 Cranial nerve assessment

Cranial nerves (CN)	
CN I	Olfactory Nerve
	Non-noxious stimulus (e.g., coffee) testing each nostril separately
CN II	Optic nerve (visual fields, pupillary reaction to light)
CN III, IV, VI	Oculomotor, trochlear, abducens
CN V	Trigeminal nerve (motor and sensory divisions to be tested)
CN VII	Facial nerve (facial expression and taste sensation)
	Muscles for facial expression (smile and wrinkle the brow)
CN VIII	Vestibular-auditory nerve (snapping the fingers together to compare the two sides)
CN IX, X	Glossopharyngeal and vagus nerves IX, mainly sensory; X, mainly motor
Gag reflex:	Test the posterior third of the tongue and oropharynx
Hoarseness:	CN X or lesion nucleus ambiguous
Unilateral lesion CN X:	Uvula deviation
Bilateral lesions CN X:	Palate elevates poorly when saying "Ah" but rapidly when gag reflex elicited
CN XI	Spinal accessory (ipsilateral SCM and trapezius muscle)
	(weakness of turning the head to the opposite side)
CN XII	Hypoglossal nerve
	Tongue protrudes toward the side of lesion

Table 4.6 Function and muscles involved in movements

Root	Function	Muscle
C5	Elbow flexors	Biceps
C6	Wrist extensors	Extensor carpi radialis longus and brevis
C7	Elbow extensors	Triceps
C8	Finger flexors	Flexor digitorum profundus
T1	Finger abductors	Abductor digiti minimi
L2	Hip flexors	Iliopsoas
L3	Knee extensors	Quadriceps
L4	Ankle dorsiflexors	Tibialis anterior

Table 4.7 Muscle grading

Grade	Strength
0	Total paralysis
1	Palpable or visible contraction
2	Active movement, full range of motion, gravity eliminated
3	Active movement, full range of motion, against gravity
4	Active movement, full range of motion, against gravity, and provides some resistance
5	Active movement, full range of motion, against gravity, and provides normal resistance
NT	Not tested

Patients with neurotrauma are at extreme risk. Hypotension (one single systolic blood pressure measurement <90 mmHg) doubles mortality. Hypoxia, defined as apnea or cyanosis, or PaO_2 < 60 mmHg on the arterial blood gas analysis, is also known to increase mortality. Combination of both usually triples mortality in patients with neurotrauma. Patients have to be assessed for neurogenic shock and basal skull fracture. Neurogenic shock refers to a hemodynamic condition characterized by hypotension, bradycardia, and hypothermia: usually occurs in spinal cord injuries above T1. Below the level of injury, loss of vasoconstrictive effect might be lost. Its incidence increases in injuries above T6. As parasympathetic effects are relatively unopposed, this condition usually results in bradycardia, lower systemic vascular resistance, and venous pooling. Basal skull fractures are usually heralded by some characteristic signs and symptoms. Among them (the list is not complete) are Raccoon's eyes, Battle's sign, cerebrospinal fluid rhinorrhea (patients usually describe salty or metallic taste)/otorrhea, hemotympanum, or laceration of external auditory canal.

4.5.1 Coagulation and the Trauma-Associated Coagulopathy

Close to one third of the severely injured trauma patients develop an "evident" coagulopathy with relevant hemorrhage [61–63]. Hypothermia, acidosis, and hemodilution ("the lethal triad") are among the physiologic derangements often present in the acute phase of trauma. Bleeding after major trauma has been associated with hemostatic alterations associated with the "lethal triad": (1) acidosis (due to inadequate tissue perfusion and able to impact in part on coagulation process), (2) hypothermia (due to conduction/convection mainly associated with physical exposure and cold fluids), and (3) hemodilution (multiple hemostatic defects due to large volumes of unbalanced fluids and/or unbalanced administration of blood components). Disseminated intravascular coagulation (DIC) occurs early after the injury and is mainly associated with consumption coagulopathy (increased consumption vs. inadequate repletion) together with diffuse microvascular thrombosis [61]. However, together with DIC, there is an early "biological" response to trauma and shock, the acute traumatic coagulopathy (ATC), not associated with the "triad", and possibly overlapping to DIC. As a matter of fact, trauma-induced coagulopathy (TIC) is defined as the acute traumatic coagulopathy (ATC, a sort of "innate" component) together with "coagulopathies" which further develop, frequently iatrogenic and related to unbalanced fluid resuscitation, suboptimal temperature control, or delayed hemorrhage control [63].

As a matter of fact, according to the most recent theories [61–63], the so-called ATC is evident prior to and independent from the "lethal triad," worsens with hypotension and head injury, and differs from the hemostatic alterations observed in other potentially problematic settings (e.g., liver surgery, cardiac surgery, or obstetrics). When compared with trauma patients without ATC, individuals with ATC show to three- to fourfold greater mortality, particularly in the first 24 h following the trauma [61–63]. ATC should be defined an early and endogenous hemostatic alteration triggered by endothelial hypoperfusion associated with massive tissue injury and characterized by hypocoagulation, hyperfibrinolysis, early and enhanced fibrinogen depletion, and platelet dysfunction [62–65]. Interestingly enough, minor prolongations of clotting times and preserved thrombin generation are associated with reduced clot generation and clot strength, as if an endogenous process could be responsible for the hemostatic derangements. The exact mechanism of ATC is still a matter of debate [61–63, 66, 67]. It is postulated a "switch" of thrombin from the "usual" procoagulant action toward an anticoagulant effect: the switch is sustained by an increase in soluble thrombomodulin levels secondary to endothelial hypoperfusion and glycocalyx disruption [62, 63, 66]. Thrombomodulin-bound thrombin gives rise to an "excess" activation of protein C (activated protein C, aPC), able to cleave FV and FVIII [62, 63]. Fibrinolytic state is enhanced by (1) increase in tissue plasminogen activator (tPA)-mediated conversion of plasminogen to plasmin, (2) decreased plasminogen activator inhibitor-1 (PAI-1), and (3) decreased thrombin-activatable fibrinolysis inhibitor (TAFI). The hyperfibrinolytic state observed in trauma patients with ATC is associated with increased D-dimer level and reduced level of native PC [61].The PC depletion could suggest a potential mechanism to explain, after the early hypocoagulable phase lasting up to 24 h, the second, hypercoagulable phase observed up to 48–72 h. Hypofibrinogenemia and enhanced fibrinolysis are associated with elevated D-dimer and reduced fibrinogen, usually documented with conventional lab tests (D-dimer, Clauss fibrinogen). As abovementioned, increasing severity of injuries correlates with elevated markers of endothelial cell and glycocalyx damage, protein C activation, clotting factor consumption, and fibrinolysis. In spite of that, as reported by Johansson et al., [67] INR and aPTT values (everywhere available and then always to be considered in first-line diagnostics) were within the normal range. Interestingly enough, when prolonged (in 10–30% of the traumatized patients), aPTT was more specific than PT-INR to define the severity of coagulopathy [61, 67].

Nowadays, the viscoelastic approach (more dynamic than conventional lab tests) is increasingly used, due to the relevant advances in thromboelastography/thromboelastometry made possible by the newest release of both TEG (Haemonetics, USA) and ROTEM (TEM International, Germany). Thromboelastography is an "holistic approach," able to provide simultaneously on a small sample of whole or citrated fresh blood and in a short timespan (15 min), information usually obtained from multiple time-consuming tests (PT, PTT, thrombin time, fibrinogen level, and platelet count) regarding clot initiation/formation, clot strength, and (hyper) fibrinolysis [1, 68, 69] (Fig. 4.1) (table of reference values for TEG and ROTEM).

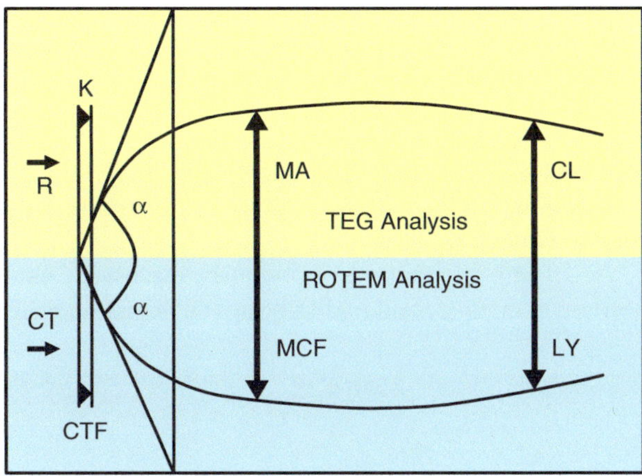

Reference values for TEG					
	r- time reaction time (min)	*K* time (min)	*α*-angle	MA maximum amplitude (mm)	LY lysis (%)
Whole blood	4–8 min	1–4 min	47–74°	55–73 mm	
Citrated blood+ kaolin	3–8 min	1–3 min	55–78°	51–69 mm	
r-TEG	0–1 min	1–2 min	66–82°	54–72	0.0–7.5
Citrated blood+ kaolin and heparinase	Comparison with kaolin test: a shortening in CT in kaolin and heparinase indicates the presence of heparin or heparin-like substances				
ROTEM	EXTEM (tissue factor)		Extrinsic activator (tissue factor); not affected by aprotinin, sensitive to heparin; fast assessment of clot formation		
	INTEM (contact activator)		Intrinsic activator: sensitive to heparin: assessment of clot formation and fibrin polymerisation		
	HEPTEM (contact activator + heparinase)		Neutralises heparin effects; specific detection of heparin		
	FIBTEM (tissue factor+ platelet antagonist cytochalasin D)		Pharmacologic inactivation of platelet cytoskeleton by cytochalasin D; FIBTEM represents the strength of the clot under platelet inhibition		
	APTEM (tissue factor + aprotinin)		Inhibition of premature lysis by the addition of aprotinin: fast detection of fibrinolysis when compared at the same time to EXTEM		
	ECATEM (ecarin)		Used in the management of direct thrombin inhibitors		

Reference ranges for ROTEM					
	CT Clotting time (s)	CFT Clot formation time (s)	A 10 Amplitude 10 min after CT (mm)	MCF Maximum clot firmness (mm)	ML Maximum lysis (% of MCF)
INTEM	100–240 s	30–110 s	44–66	50–72 mm	<15 %
EXTEM	38–79 s	34–159 s	43–65	50–72 mm	<15 %
FIBTEM			8–24	9–25 mm	
APTEM	Comparison with EXTEM: a stable MCF confirms hyperfibrinolysis				
HEPTEM	Comparison with INTEM: a shortening in HEPTEM CT indicates the presence of heparin or heparin-like substances				

Fig. 4.1 Nomenclature, reference values, and "signatures" of TEG and ROTEM [69]

In trauma patients, early traces show a reduction in clot amplitude (reduced MA) and reduced alfa angle. Low fibrinogen (fibrinogen monitoring is available on both TEG and ROTEM) in turn can also influence the platelet function thus contributing to the reduced MA (Fig. 4.2).

Thromboelastography/elastometry is the only way to clearly demonstrate hyperfibrinolysis (both primary or secondary) (see Figs. 4.3 and 4.4) for TEG and ROTEM hyperfibrinolysis traces.

Also possible is the demonstration of a "laboratory detectable autoheparinization" (heparin-like effect) due to liberation of endothelial components (glycosaminoglycans): this condition could be documented in vitro and reversed with heparinase. The clinical meaning and the correction of heparin effect in specific surgical or medical settings is under discussion (Fig. 4.5).

According to what was previously discussed, increased fibrinolytic activity and rapid fibrinogen depletion character-

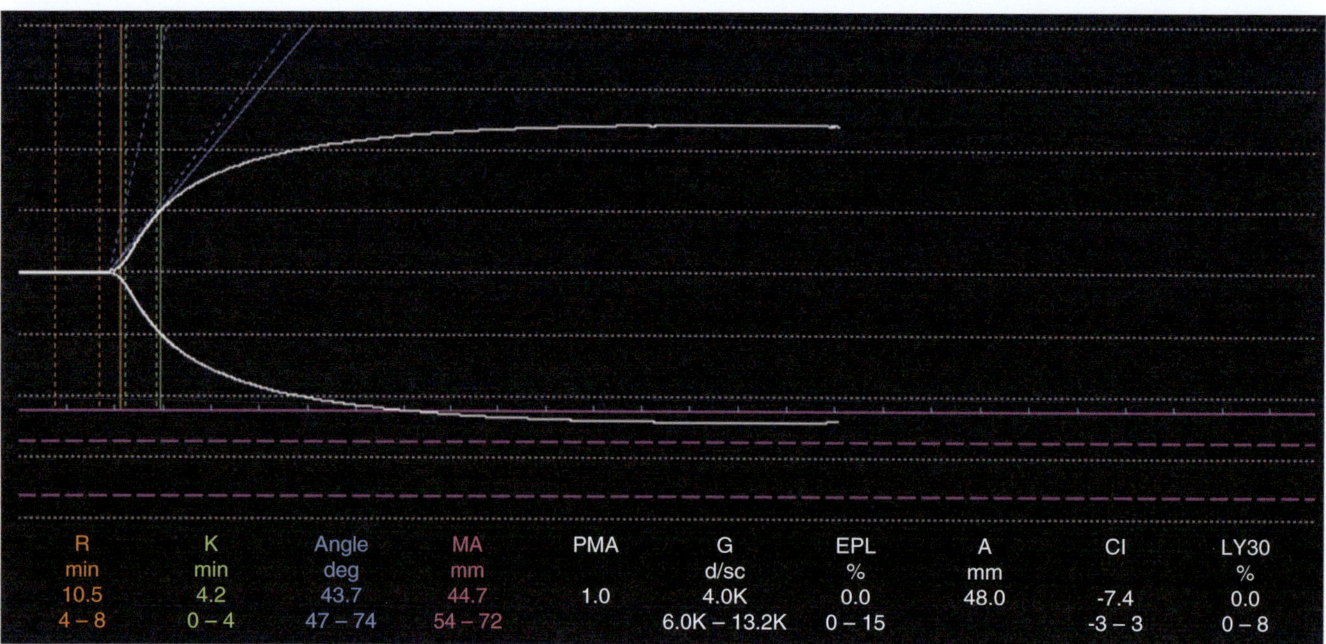

Fig. 4.2 TEG in a trauma patient (upon ED arrival)

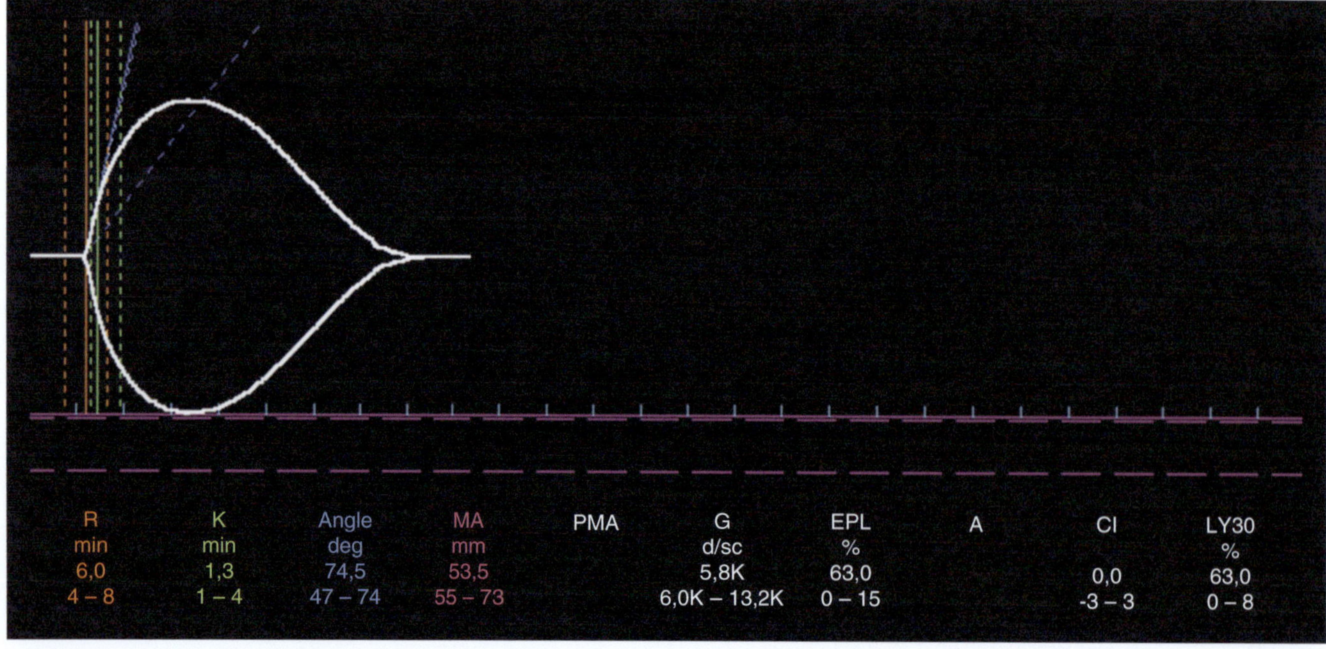

Fig. 4.3 Hyperfibrinolysis on TEG

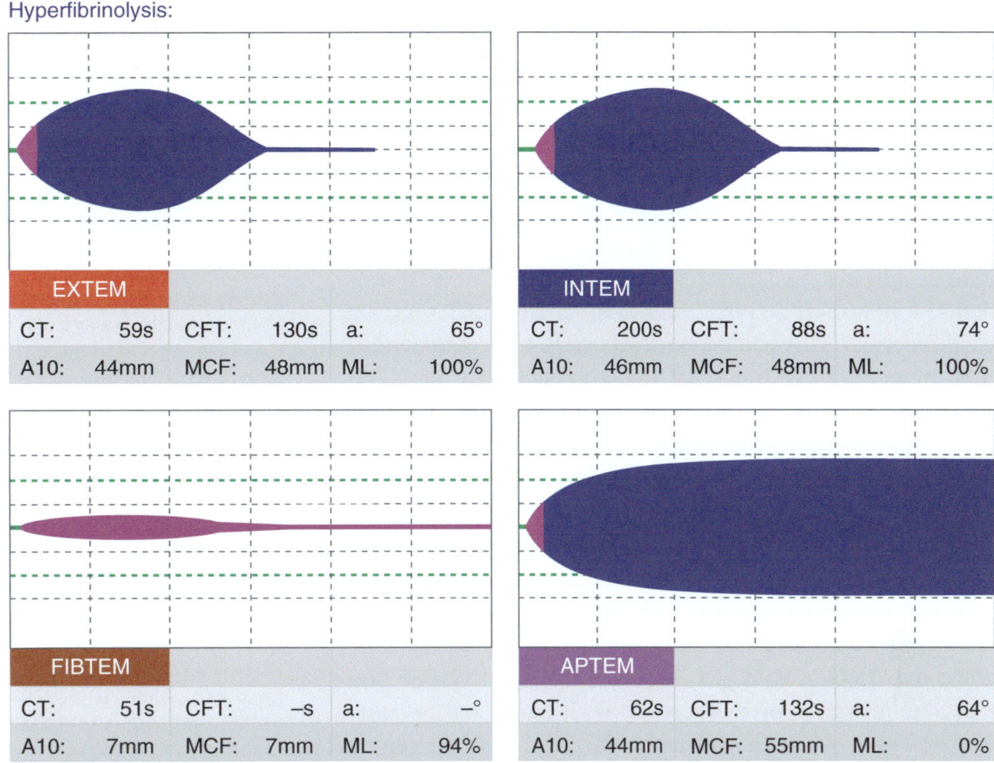

Fig. 4.4 Hyperfibrinolysis on ROTEM

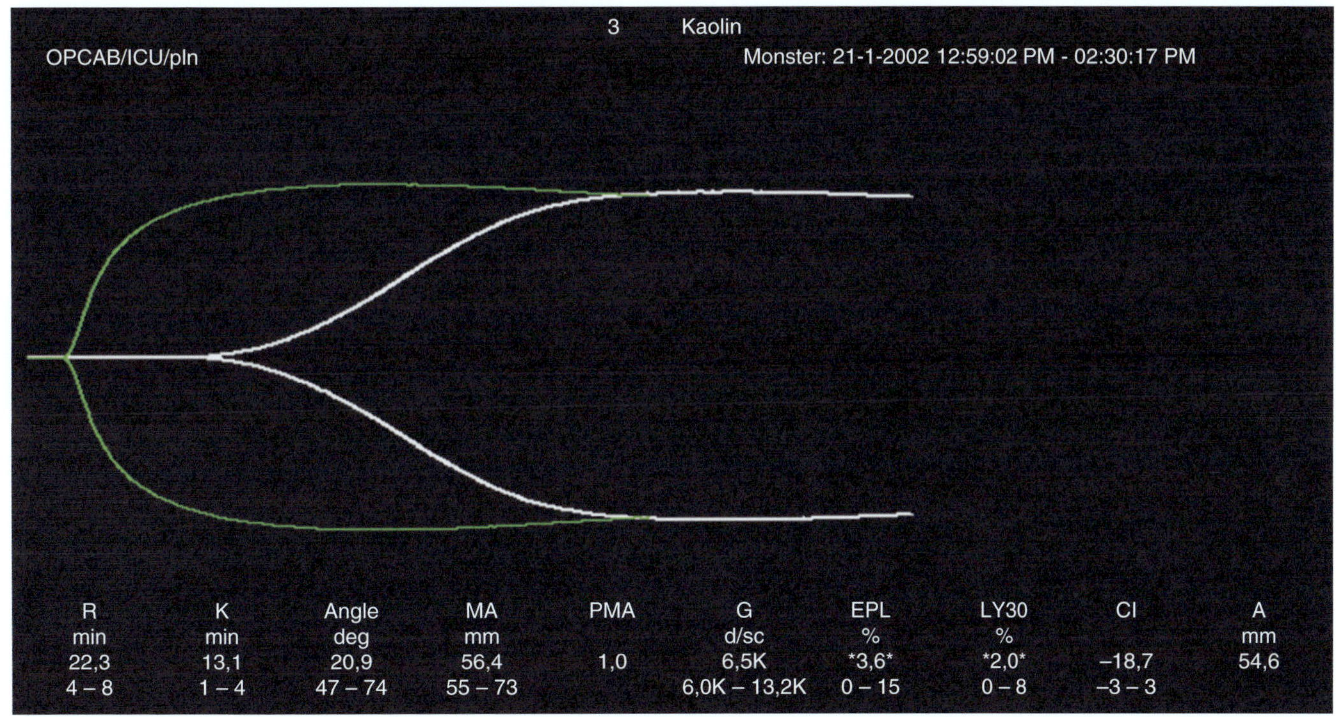

Fig. 4.5 Heparin-like effect (white line) and correction with heparinase (green line)

ize the ATC: as very recently demonstrated by Davenport et al. [62, 63], PC pathway should provide a "mechanistic link between the two main theories of early trauma coagulopathy", (1) DIC with fibrinolytic phenotype and (2) primary aPC-driven fibrinolysis (and possible fibrinogenolysis) [62, 63]. As stated by Davenport et al. [62], a unifying hypothesis defined by aPC generation and widespread fibrinolytic activation provides support to the improved outcomes in trauma patients (both in cohort studies and in randomized controlled trial) when the early empiric administration of an antifibrinolytic drugs was used [69]. Since long time antifibrinolytic drugs were available to minimize blood loss in various surgical setting (orthopedic, cardiac, liver transplant surgeries, obstetrics). Since the publication of the CRASH-2 trial (the first randomized, placebo-controlled, multicenter trial of tranexamic acid in trauma patients) [68, 70], it is standard to infuse 1 g of tranexamic acid (TXA) over a 10-min period followed by an infusion of another gram of TXA over an 8-h period. This has been incorporated as recommendation number 25 (Grade 1A recommendation) in "The European Guideline on the management of major bleeding and coagulopathy following trauma: fourth edition" [1]. This, as well as the infusion of fibrinogen, is standard of care in most of the centers dealing with trauma patients. However, once the main source of bleeding is controlled by damage control surgery (DCS) and additional factors like hypothermia and acidosis (together with hypotension, the already mentioned components of the "lethal triad") are excluded or corrected, TEG or ROTEM are excellent tools to guide further administration of blood products. It turned out to be of extraordinary value in patients with massive crush injury (e.g., caused by rollover), where one or more extremities are without blood supply for several hours. Once the supplying vessels are reanastomosed, the reperfusion may severely compromise the coagulation within minutes, leading to significantly prolonged R-times (reperfusion syndrome or ischemia-reperfusion injury).

References

1. Rossaint R, Bouillon B, Cerny V, Coats TJ, Duranteau J, Fernandez-Modejar E, et al. The European guideline on management of major bleeding and coagulopathy following trauma: fourth edition. Crit Care. 2016;20:100. https://doi.org/10.1186/s13054-016-1265-x.
2. Statements of principles: trauma anesthesiology, ASAHQ 16.10. 2013 (as accessed on 20 Aug 2017). www.asahq.org.
3. Raja A Zane RD. Initial management of the trauma in adults. UPTODATE Section Editor: Maria E Moreira, MD; Deputy Editor: Jonathan Grayzel, MD, FAAEM. Last update August 2017.
4. National confidential enquiry into patient outcome and death. London: the NCEPOD classification of interventions [Online]; 2004. http://www.ncepod.org.uk/pdf/NCEPODClassification.pdf.
5. Yang CK, Teng A, Lee DY, Rose K. Pulmonary complications after major abdominal surgery: National Surgical Quality Improvement Program analysis. J Surg Res. 2015;198:441.
6. Dimick JB, Chen SL, Taheri PA, et al. Hospital costs associated with surgical complications: a report from the private-sector National Surgical Quality Improvement Program. J Am Coll Surg. 2004;199:531.
7. Kortbeek JB, Al Turki SA, Ali J, Antoine JA, Bouillon B, Brasel K, et al. Advanced trauma life support, 8th edition, the evidence for change. J Trauma. 2008;64:1638–50.
8. Galvano S, McCunn M. Anesthesia for adult trauma patients. UPTODATE 2017. Deputy Editor Nussmeier N. Literature review current through Jul 2017. | This topic last updated: 7 Aug 2017.
9. McLeod AD, Calder I. Spinal cord injury and direct laryngoscopy—the legend lives on. Br J Anaesth. 2000;84:705–9.
10. Hindman BJ, Palecek JP, Posner KL, Traynelis VC, Lee LA, Sawin PD, et al. Cervical spinal cord, root, and bony spine injuries: a closed claims analysis. Anesthesiology. 2011;114:782–95.
11. Frerk C, Mitchell VS, McNarry AF, Mendonca C, Bhagrath R, Patel A, et al. Difficult Airway Society 2015 guidelines for management of unanticipated difficult intubation in adults. DAS intubation guidelines working group. Br J Anaesth. 2015;115:827–48.
12. Hagberg CA, Kaslow O. Difficult airway management algorithm in trauma: updated by COTEP. ASA Monitor. 2014;78:56. American Society of Anesthesiologists. Excerpted from ASA Monitor 2014 of the American Society of Anesthesiologists.
13. Zanobetti M, Poggioni C, Pini R. Can chest ultrasonography replace standard chest radiography for evaluation of acute dyspnea in the ED? Chest. 2011;139:1140–7.
14. Blanco P, Volpicelli G. Common pitfalls in point-of-care ultrasound: a practical guide for emergency and critical care physicians. Crit Ultrasound J. 2016;8:15. https://doi.org/10.1186/s13089-016-0052-x.
15. Colwell C. Initial evaluation and management of shock in adult trauma. UPTODATE 2017. Deputy Editor Grayzel J. Literature review current through Jul 2017.
16. Volpicelli G, Elbarbary M, Blaivas M, Lichtenstein DA, Mathis G, Kirkpatrick AW, et al. International Liaison Committee on Lung Ultrasound (ILC-LUS) for International Consensus Conference on Lung Ultrasound (ICC-LUS). Intensive Care Med. 2012;38:577–91. https://doi.org/10.1007/s00134-012-2513-4.
17. Ramsingh D, Frank E, Haughton R, Schilling J, Gimenez KM, Banh E, Rinehar J, Cannesson M. Auscultation versus Point-of-care Ultrasound to determine endotracheal versus bronchial intubation. A diagnostic accuracy study. Anesthesiology. 2016;124:1012–20.
18. Murray JF, Matthay MA, Luce JM, Flick MR. An expanded definition of the adult respiratory distress syndrome. Am Rev Respir Dis. 1988;138:720–3. [PubMed].
19. Ranieri VM, Rubenfeld GD, Thompson BT, Ferguson ND, Caldwell E, Fan E, et al. Acute respiratory distress syndrome: the Berlin Definition. JAMA. 2012;307:2526–33.
20. Pfeifer R, Heussen N, Michalewicz E, Hilgers RD, Pape HC. Incidence of Adult Respiratory Distress Syndrome (ARDS) in trauma patients: a systematic review and meta-analysis over a period of three decades. J Trauma Acute Care Surg. 2017;83(3):496–506. PubMed id: 28590348.
21. Ferrando C, Suarez-Sipmann F, Tusman G, León I, Romero E, Gracia E, et al. Open lung approach versus standard protective strategies: effects on driving pressure and ventilatory efficiency during anesthesia—a pilot, randomized controlled trial. PLoS One. 2017;12:e0177399.
22. Stueber T, Karsten J, Voigt N, Wilhelmi M. Influence of intra-operative positive end-expiratory pressure level on pulmonary complications in emergency major trauma surgery. Arch Med Sci. 2017;13:396–403.
23. Ried M, Bein T, Philipp A, Müller T, Graf B, Schmid C, et al. Extracorporeal lung support in trauma patients with severe chest injury and acute lung failure: a 10-year institutional experience. Crit Care. 2013;17:R110. https://doi.org/10.1186/cc12782.
24. Ahmad SB, Menaker J, Kufera J, O'Connor J, Scalea TM, Stein DM. Extracorporeal membrane oxygenation after traumatic injury. J Trauma Acute Care Surg. 2017;82:587–91.
25. Gupta H, Ramanan B, Gupta PK, et al. Impact of COPD on postoperative outcomes: results from a national database. Chest. 2013;143:1599.
26. Grønkjær M, Eliasen M, Skov-Ettrup LS, et al. Preoperative smoking status and postoperative complications: a systematic review and meta-analysis. Ann Surg. 2014;259:52.

27. Meyer S, McLaughlin VV, Seyfarth HJ, et al. Outcomes of noncardiac, nonobstetric surgery in patients with PAH: an international prospective survey. Eur Respir J. 2013;41:1302.
28. Lai HC, Lai HC, Wang KY, et al. Severe pulmonary hypertension complicates postoperative outcome of non-cardiac surgery. Br J Anaesth. 2007;99:184.
29. Memtsoudis SG, Ma Y, Chiu YL, et al. Perioperative mortality in patients with pulmonary hypertension undergoing major joint replacement. Anesth Analg. 2010;111:1110.
30. Qaseem A, Snow V, Fitterman N, et al. Risk assessment for and strategies to reduce perioperative pulmonary complications for patients undergoing noncardiothoracic surgery: a guideline from the American College of Physicians. Ann Intern Med. 2006;144:575.
31. Clancy K, Velopulos C, Bilaniuk JW, Collier B, Crowley W, Kurek S, et al. Eastern Association for the Surgery of Trauma Screening for blunt cardiac injury: an Eastern Association for the Surgery of Trauma practice management guideline. J Trauma Acute Care Surg. 2012;73:S301–6.
32. Alborzi Z, Zangouri V, Khodaei S. Diagnosing myocardial contusion after blunt chest trauma. J Tehran Heart Cent. 2016;13(11):49–54.
33. Bansal MK, Maraj S, Chewaproug D, Amanullah A. Myocardial contusion injury: redefining the diagnostic algorithm. Emerg Med J. 2005;22:465–9.
34. Holanda MS, Domínguez MJ, López-Espadas F, López M, Díaz-Regañón J, Rodríguez-Borregán JC. Cardiac contusion following blunt chest trauma. Eur J Emerg Med. 2006;13:373–6.
35. Dogan H, Sarikaya S, Neijmann ST, Uysal E, Yucel N, Ozucelik DN, et al. N-terminal pro-B-type natriuretic peptide as a marker of blunt cardiac contusion in trauma. Int J Clin Exp Pathol. 2015;8:6786–9.
36. Kelley WE, Januzzi JL, Christenson RH. Increases of cardiac troponin in conditions other than acute coronary syndrome and heart failure. Clin Chem. 2009;55:2098–112.
37. Swaanenburg JC, Klaase JM, DeJongste MJ, Zimmerman KW, ten Duis HJ. Troponin I, troponin T, CKMB-activity and CKMB-mass as markers for the detection of myocardial contusion in patients who experienced blunt trauma. Clin Chim Acta. 1998;272:171–81.
38. St Louis P, Gandhi S. Cardiac contusion and creatine kinase-MB: a pertinent case history and brief review of the utility of CK-MB. Clin Biochem. 1994;27:105–11.
39. ASA statement: Statement on Transesophageal Echocardiography: last amended on October 28, 2015. ASA guidelines. www.asahq.org.
40. Practice guidelines for perioperative transesophageal echocardiography. An updated report by the American Society of Anesthesiologists and the Society of Cardiovascular Anesthesiologists Task Force on Transesophageal Echocardiography. Anesthesiology. 2010;112:1–13.
41. Hahn RT, Abraham T, Adams MS, Bruce CJ, Glas KE, Lang RM, et al. Guidelines for performing a comprehensive transesophageal echocardiographic examination: recommendations from the American Society of Echocardiography and the Society of Cardiovascular Anesthesiologists. J Am Soc Echocardiogr. 2013;26:921–64.
42. Kwan I, Bunn F, Chinnock P, Roberts I. Timing and volume of fluid administration for patients with bleeding. Cochrane Database Syst Rev. 2014. PMID 24599652.
43. Wong F, O'Leary JG, Reddy KR, Patton H, Kamath PS, Fallon MB, et al. New consensus definition of acute kidney injury accurately predicts 30-day mortality in patients with cirrhosis and infection. Gastroenterology. 2013;145:1280–8.e1.
44. Salahuddin N, Sammani M, Hamdan A, Joseph M, Al-Nemary Y, Alquaiz R, et al. Fluid overload is an independent risk factor for acute kidney injury in critically ill patients: results of a cohort study. BMC Nephrol. 2017;18:45. https://doi.org/10.1186/s12882-017-0460-6.
45. Liu KD, Thompson BT, Ancukiewicz M, Steingrub JS, Douglas IS, Matthay MA, et al. Acute kidney injury in patients with acute lung injury: impact of fluid accumulation on classification of acute kidney injury and associated outcomes. Crit Care Med. 2011;39:2665–71.
46. Prowle JR, Echeverri JE, Ligabo EV, Ronco C, Bellomo R. Fluid balance and acute kidney injury. Nat Rev Nephrol. 2010;6:107–15.
47. de Almeida JP, Palomba H, Galas FR, Fukushima JT, Duarte FA, Nagaoka D, Torres V, Yu L, Vincent JL, Auler O Jr, et al. Positive fluid balance is associated with reduced survival in critically ill patients with cancer. Acta Anaesthesiol Scand. 2012;56:712–7.
48. Salahuddin, Bouchard J, Soroko SB, Chertow GM, Himmerlfarb J, Ikizler TA. Fluid accumulation, survival and recovery of kidney function in critically ill patients with acute kidney injury. Kidney Int. 2009;76:422–7.
49. Payen D, de Pont AC, Sakr Y, Spies C, Reinhart K, Vincent JL. A positive fluid balance is associated with a worse outcome in patients with acute renal failure. Crit Care. 2008;12:R74.
50. Teixeira C, Garzotto F, Piccinni P, Brienza N, Iannizzi M, Gramaticopolo S, Forfori F, Pelaia P, Rocco M, Ronco C, et al. Fluid balance and urine volume are independent predictors of mortality in acute kidney injury. Crit Care. 2013;17:R14.
51. Bellomo R, Cass A, Cole L, Finfer S, Gallagher M, Lee J, et al. An observational study fluid balance and patient outcomes in the randomized evaluation of normal vs. augmented level of replacement therapy trial. Crit Care Med. 2012;40:1753–60.
52. Heung M, Wolfgram DF, Kommareddi M, Hu Y, Song PX, Ojo AO. Fluid overload at initiation of renal replacement therapy is associated with lack of renal recovery in patients with acute kidney injury. Nephrol Dial Transplant. 2012;27:956–61.
53. Jin K, Murugan R, Sileanu FE, Folde E, Priyanka P, Clermont G, Kellum JA. Intensive Monitoring of urine output is associated with increased detection of acute kidney injury and improve outcomes. Chest. 2017;152(5):972–9. https://doi.org/10.1016/j.chest.2017.05.011.
54. Cannesson M, Pestel G, Ricks C, Hoeft A, Perel A. Hemodynamic monitoring and management in patients undergoing high risk surgery: a survey among North American and European anesthesiologists. Crit Care. 2011;15:R197.
55. Biancofiore G, Cecconi M, Della Rocca G. A web-based Italian survey of current trends, habits and beliefs in hemodynamic monitoring and management. J Clin Monit Comput. 2015;29:635–42.
56. Marik PE, Cavallazzi R. Does the central venous pressure predict fluid responsiveness? An updated meta-analysis and a plea for some common sense. Crit Care Med. 2013;41:1774–81.
57. Beigel R, Cercek B, Luo H, Siegel RJ. Noninvasive evaluation of right atrial pressure. J Am Soc Echocardiogr. 2013;26:1033–42.
58. Vincent JL, Rhodes A, Perel A, Martin GS, Della Rocca G, Vallet B, et al. Clinical review: update on hemodynamic monitoring—a consensus of 16. Crit Care. 2011;15:229.
59. Ciozda W, Kedan I, Kehl DW, Zimmer R, Khandwalla R, Kimchi A. The efficacy of sonographic measurement of inferior vena cava diameter as an estimate of central venous pressure. Cardiovasc Ultrasound. 2016;14:33. https://doi.org/10.1186/s12947-016-0076-1.
60. Vignon P, Repessé X, Bégot E, Léger J, Jacob C, Bouferrache K, Slama M, Prat G. Comparison of echocardiographic indices used to predict fluid responsiveness in ventilated patients. Am J Respir Crit Care Med. 2017;195:1022–32. https://doi.org/10.1164/rccm.201604-0844OC.
61. Cohen MJ, Kutcher ME. Coagulopathy associated with trauma. UPTODATE 2017. Deputy Ed Collins KA, Literature review current through: Jul 2017. | Last updated: 29 Aug 2016.
62. Davenport RA, Guerreiro M, Frith D, Rourke C, Platton S, Cohen M, Pearse R, et al. Activated protein C drives the hyperfibrinolysis of acute traumatic coagulopathy. Anesthesiology. 2017;126:115–27.

63. Gall LS, Brohi K, Davenport R. Diagnosis and treatment of hyperfibrinolysis in trauma. Semin Thromb Hemost. 2017;43:224–34.
64. Castellino FJ, Chapman MP, Donahue DL, Thomas S, Moore EE, Wohlauer MV, et al. Traumatic brain injury causes platelet adenosine diphosphate and arachidonic acid receptor inhibition independent of hemorrhagic shock in humans and rats. J Trauma Acute Care Surg. 2014;76:1169–76.
65. Lee TH, Hampton DA, Diggs BS, McCully SP, Kutcher M, Redick BJ, et al. Traumatic brain injury is not associated with coagulopathy out of proportion to injury in other body regions. J Trauma Acute Care Surg. 2014;77:67–72.
66. Cohen MJ, Call M, Nelson M, Calfee CS, Esmon CT, Brohi K, Pittet JF. Critical role of activated protein C in early coagulopathy and later organ failure, infection and death in trauma patients. Ann Surg. 2012;255:379.
67. Johansson PI, Sørensen AM, Perner A, Welling KL, Wanscher M, Larsen CF, Ostrowski SR. Disseminated intravascular coagulation or acute coagulopathy of trauma shock early after trauma? An observational study. Crit Care. 2011;15:R272.
68. Ganter MF, Huber C. Coagulation monitoring: current techniques and clinical use of viscoelastic point of care devices. Anesth Analg. 2008;106:1366.
69. Grassetto A, Paniccia R, Biancofiore G. Chap. 2: General aspects of viscoelastic tests. In: Ranucci M, Simioni P, editors. Point of care tests in severe hemorrhage. Cham: Springer. p. 19–34. https://doi.org/10.1007/978-3-319-24795-3.
70. Shakur H, Roberts I, Bautista R, et al. Effects of tranexamic acid on death, vascular occlusive events, and blood transfusion in trauma patients with significant hemorrhage (CRASH-2): a randomized, placebo-controlled trial. Lancet. 2010;376:23–32.

Invasive and Noninvasive Hemodynamic Monitoring

5

Stefano Orsenigo and Marco Pulici

Key Points

- Patient hemodynamic status should be early understood, in order to improve patient outcome.
- A single hemodynamic index is often insufficient in establishing patient perfusion status.
- Tissue perfusion depends on oxygenation and cardiac output, which depends on preload, afterload, cardiac contractility, and heart rate.
- Preoperative fluid deficit should be assessed and preemptively compensated.
- Central venous pressure and pulmonary arterial wedge pressure are not reliable in assessing fluid responsiveness.
- Noninvasive hemodynamic monitoring systems include physical examination, peripheral oxygen saturation, blood pressure and heart rate measurement, electrocardiogram, vena cava assessment, and transthoracic echocardiography.
- Invasive hemodynamic indexes include central venous oxygenation, central venous to arterial carbon dioxide gap, lactates, pulse contour-derived CO, transesophageal echocardiography, gastric tonometry, and thermodilution CO.

5.1 Background

Hemodynamic monitoring is the main diagnostic and therapeutic approach to the instable critical patient: hypoperfusion can be prevented, leading to better outcomes and avoiding shock. That is especially true in surgical patients who have, by definition, increased hypoperfusion risks: vena cava compression by positive-pressure ventilation, reduction in muscle tone, and some drugs used during surgery may redistribute blood flow and therefore normal perfusion; moreover, the maintenance of normothermia, starvation, and inflammatory response may increase oxygen consumption [1]. A correct optimization of cardiac output (CO) in patients undergoing major surgery may decrease postoperative complications and length of stay [2].

In a setting of decreased oxygen delivery and increased oxygen consumption, especially in a patient with pre-existing organ failure, hypoperfusion and thus tissue damage may develop [1]. According to L.M. Bigatello and E. George, hypotension is the most common cause of hemodynamic instability in surgical patients [3]: bleeding, inadequate fluid replacement, and vasodilation must be considered [4]. Hypotension can result in myocardial infarction, stroke, renal failure, and bowel ischemia [4].

Hypertension (arbitrarily defined as systolic blood pressure (BP) > 190 mmHg and/or diastolic BP > 100 mmHg [5]) is most commonly seen in patient who does not receive their usual medications before surgery and whether fluid therapy has been excessive or pain has been undertreated [4]. Pain often begins 10–20 min after surgery, lasting up to 4 h. If left untreated, it may increase the risk of bleeding, cerebrovascular events, and myocardial infarction [5].

Since no single value is sufficient to estimate patient hemodynamic condition, over the years, various monitoring strategies have been proposed (over the years): beginning with physical examination to more complex monitoring systems.

5.2 Hemodynamic Status Monitoring

Box 5.1 Cardiac Output

$$CO = SV \times hr$$

where
SV = stroke volume
hr = heart rate

S. Orsenigo (✉) · M. Pulici
Department of Anesthesia and Intensive Care, Niguarda Ca' Granda Hospital, Milan, Italy
e-mail: marco.pulici@ospedaleniguarda.it

P. Aseni et al. (eds.), *Operative Techniques and Recent Advances in Acute Care and Emergency Surgery*,
https://doi.org/10.1007/978-3-319-95114-0_5

Hemodynamic status monitoring measures the organism's ability to deliver oxygen to its tissues.

Tissue oxygenation is consequently determined by oxygen delivery (DO_2), which is in turn determined by the product of arterial blood oxygen content (i.e., oxyhemoglobin concentration) and CO [6].

CO can consequently be considered as a good index of tissue oxygenation, given a sufficient blood oxygen content. CO is entirely determined by cardiac preload, afterload, contractility, and heart rate [7].

Preload is defined as myocardial distension before systole. As stated by Frank-Starling relationship, myocardial contraction force depends on muscle fiber stretch: an increase in preload in a healthy patient should trigger an increase in CO (within certain ranges). In this case, the patient is considered as fluid responder (see below).

Afterload is the resistance against which the ventricles must push the blood. Hence, afterload is inversely proportional to CO [8].

Each of these element functions may be measured via different monitoring systems, which are reviewed below.

5.2.1 Physical Examination

According to *European Journal of Anaesthesiology* (EJA) intravascular volume therapy guidelines, each patient suspected with hypovolemia should receive a careful physical examination, looking for signs of hemorrhage, dehydration, or other causes of volume loss. Tongue appearance, jugular vein filling, and capillary refill (tested using nail blanch test) should be evaluated; search for pleural effusion (auscultation and percussion), ascites or distended intestinal loops (abdominal palpation), and edema or skin turgidity (inspection of lower limbs) should be performed. Previous medical history should also be taken into account [9].

However, some authors demonstrated poor agreement between examiners, poor positive predictive value, and poor diagnostic accuracy of physical examination in assessing fluid responsiveness [10].

EJA guidelines concludes that even if physical examination alone is not reliable, it should be used together with other indexes, hence improving clinical accuracy [9].

5.2.2 Peripheral Oxygen Saturation

Peripheral oxygen saturation (SpO_2) is an easy and noninvasive estimation of arterial oxygen saturation (fraction of oxygen-saturated hemoglobin relative to total) and can give some initial yet important information about tissue oxygenation.

It is calculated using a sensor placed on the fingertip, which measures light absorbance changes and provides SpO_2 and heart rate.

Many are its limitations: patient movements, vasoconstriction, hypoperfusion, hypothermia, shock, unskilled clinician, probe misplacement, use of nail polish, severe anemia, high-intensity ambient light, and abnormal pulses (such as venous pulse and large dicrotic notch) may result in SpO_2 inaccurate measurement. Furthermore, pulse oximetry is not able to discern functional hemoglobin from nonfunctional ones (carboxyhemoglobin and methemoglobin [4, 11]).

SpO_2 of 92% (95% in black patients) reliably predict an arterial oxygen partial pressure of at least 60 mmHg (lower level that does not produce hypoxemia [4]).

Recently plethysmography analyses have been reviewed, and some system can give some information about CO and fluid responsiveness, though limitation has been reported [12].

5.2.3 Blood Pressure

Blood arterial pressure can be measured via sphygmomanometer or via arterial catheter. The pros are to be noninvasive for the first one and to be continuous and more accurate for the latter: edema, swelling, and very high or very low BP can impair sphygmomanometer values.

Manual pressure measurement is based on Korotkoff sound detection (at the pressure at which it is heard, the first sound is considered the systolic blood pressure; at the pressure at which it disappears, it is considered the diastolic pressure), while automated sphygmomanometer measurement relies on oscillometry: small changes in cuff pressure during its deflation are used to estimate mean arterial pressure (MAP). Proprietary algorithms are then used to calculate systolic and diastolic blood pressure, which are respectively underestimated and overestimated and are thereby, in this case, less reliable than MAP [13].

MAP > 70 mmHg is generally considered to be an index of good tissue perfusion [3]. However, blood pressure is physiologically autoregulated, and its measure can't predict whether the patient is hemodynamically stable or he or she is compensating an instable situation. Hypotension is a late sign of low tissue perfusion, and it reflects a failure in compensatory mechanism which usually avoids BP falls.

Although rare, noninvasive blood pressure measurement has also some complications: compartment syndromes may develop in the setting of frequent cuff inflations [13]. Despite these limitations, blood pressure should be measured, as low blood pressure is a negative prognostic indicator [14].

5.2.4 Electrocardiogram

Normal lead II electrocardiogram (ECG) is used in every hospital ward, and moreover in ICUs, in order to gather important information about ischemic heart diseases [14] as well as heart rate.

ST alterations and arrhythmias may impair normal myocardial contractility and, hence, CO. Multi-lead ECG monitor is advised for special coronary conditions.

5.2.5 Heart Rate Assessment

As stated above, heart rate may be assessed both via pulse oximetry and ECG. The main difference is that the first one measures pulse rate (arterial pulsation), while the latter measures heart rate (electrical stimulation of the heart). Some conditions, such as atrial fibrillation and pulseless electrical activity, may impair pulse rate, while the ECG keeps showing heart rate [13].

Tachycardia is a non-specific sign of hypovolemia (in order to keep a normal BP, during hypovolemia, sympathetic tone is increased and, consequently, also heart rate).

In athletes and in the elderly and with some medication, however, tachycardia may not develop [14].

5.2.6 Vena Cava Assessment

Box 5.2 Distensibility Index

$$DI_{IVC} = \frac{d_{max} - d_{min}}{d_{min}}$$

where
DI_{IVC} is distensibility index
d_{max} is maximum cava diameter
d_{min} is minimum cava diameter

Central venous pressure (CVP) can be measured invasively via central venous catheter (CVC) as a measure of cardiac preload. Inferior vena cava (IVC) diameter can also be used as a noninvasive volemic measure via ultrasonographic techniques.

CVC can be inserted in internal or external jugular, subclavian, femoral, or axillary veins. Furthermore, central catheters can be placed peripherally, for example, from the basilic vein (peripherally inserted central venous catheters or PICC).

If placed correctly, CVC should be able to measure central venous pressure. Ideally, the CVC tip should lie within the superior vena cava, below the clavicles and above the third rib. CVC placement successfulness should be assessed by X-ray imaging [13].

In clinical practice, CVP measurement is often considered as a good index of volemic status; however, there is strong evidence of poor correlation [2, 9, 15–18] between CVP tracing and patient volemia or fluid responsiveness: CVP may be influenced by many other factors such as peripheral vascular tone, right ventricular compliance, pulmonary vascular resistance, and, in ventilated patients, intrathoracic pressure [9].

CVP can be useful as an upper threshold at which stopping fluid therapy, a positive trend reaching high values (CVP > 8 mmHg), may inform the clinician that there is no more need of fluid replacement, but it should not be considered an absolute target [19] of fluid therapy.

Distensibility index of IVC in mechanical ventilated patients, however, can be used to accurately predict fluid responsiveness [20]. This technique is less reliable in spontaneously breathing or with high intra-abdominal pressure patients and may be difficult to obtain in the obese ones [2].

In mechanical ventilated patients, a threshold of 18% has demonstrated high sensitivity and specificity (90%) [9].

Although distensibility index appeared to be more accurate than IVC diameter, it can be stated that IVC diameter less than 10 mm may be suggestive of hypovolemia and IVC diameter more than 22 mm may be suggestive of hypervolemia [9].

5.2.7 Pulmonary Artery Catheter

A pulmonary artery catheter (PAC), or Swan-Ganz catheter, is a 110-cm-long, 7–9 Fr in circumference catheter, equipped with a balloon at the tip. It is also provided with two ports, one at the tip and the other 30 cm proximally, and a temperature thermistor, also at the tip.

PAC may be inserted in the same sites by which CVC are inserted (see above). The balloon should then be inflated with air and the catheter advanced through right atrium, tricuspid valve, right ventricle, pulmonic valve, and finally pulmonary artery. Here, the PAC wedge on pulmonary artery, and the balloon is then deflated.

Once successfully placed, Swan-Ganz catheter gathers continuously CVP and pulmonary artery pressure, as well as pulmonary artery wedge pressure (PAWP) when the balloon is inflated.

PAWP is an indirect measure of pulmonary venous pressure and left atrium pressure, and thus left ventricle telediastolic pressure, which can be considered as left cardiac chamber preload. However, tip position can alter reliability of PAWP measurement decreasing its accuracy.

Furthermore, PAWP can't be continuously monitored; nevertheless, when pulmonary venous resistance is low, pulmonary artery diastolic pressure (PADP) approximates wedge pressure, allowing continuous assessment.

PADP can thereby be theoretically used to guide fluid therapy, as it should be directly proportional to patient's volemia. This is true when both juxtacardiac and ventricle compliance are normal. In a setting of increased juxtacardiac pressure (e.g., in cardiac tamponade, pericardial constriction, or positive-pressure ventilation) or altered ventricle compliance (e.g., in diastolic dysfunction), PADP is unable to assess patient fluid responsiveness at any given preload.

Thus, PADP poorly correlates with blood volume and cannot predict preload or patient fluid responsiveness.

Swan-Ganz catheter and CVC can also be used to assess hemodynamic variables such as systemic (SVR) and pulmonary vascular resistance (PVR).

Considering human cardiovascular system as a hydraulic fluid model, and hence assuming it has a continuous and laminar flow through rigid pipes, it can be stated that:

$$\mathrm{SVR} = \frac{\mathrm{MAP} - \mathrm{CVP}}{\mathrm{CO}}$$

and that

$$\mathrm{PVR} = \frac{\mathrm{MPAP} - \mathrm{PAWP}}{\mathrm{CO}}$$

where MPAP is mean pulmonary arterial pressure.

However, these formulas excessively oversimplify cardiovascular system behavior, and some authors advocate that it should not be used in clinical practice [13].

5.2.8 Central Venous Pressure

Central venous oxygenation is measured by sampling pulmonary artery blood (SvO_2) via Swan-Ganz catheter. However, $ScvO_2$ is obtained from vena cava blood sampling. It is less invasive and it fairly correlates with SvO_2 [21].

$ScvO_2$ value is then subtracted from arterial oxygenation (SaO_2) to calculate oxygen consumption. In a healthy patient, oxygen extraction is approximately 25% [21] of the total amount of oxygen delivered to peripheral tissue by a completely oxygenated arterial blood. This results in a 75% oxygen-saturated central venous hemoglobin.

$ScvO_2$ shows early patient hemodynamic imbalance, prior to other hemodynamic or lab value changes; it's considered a valid endpoint for shock resuscitation [22].

Oxygen saturation less than 60–65% has been shown to predict adverse outcome after surgery [4].

Many factors may alter oxygen saturation: with normal oxygen arterial content, decreased $ScvO_2$ can estimate decreased CO, although decreased $ScvO_2$ is also an index of imbalance between oxygen supply and consumption, even in the presence of normal or increased CO.

Hence, used alone, it shows low accuracy in the determination of hemodynamic status. Other parameters are still needed to better understand $ScvO_2$ measure [21].

5.2.9 Central Venous to Arterial Carbon Dioxide Gap

Carbon dioxide in blood is mainly present in the form of bicarbonate. Relationship between total blood CO_2 and CO_2 partial pressure (pCO_2) is influenced by oxygen saturation (Haldane effect), hematocrit, temperature, and blood pH, and it's hence a curvilinear relationship.

By applying the Fick equation (normally used to calculate oxygen consumption) to CO_2, it can be stated that CO_2 production (VCO_2) is proportional to CO and venous ($CvCO_2$) to arterial ($CaCO_2$) carbon dioxide gap:

$$\mathrm{VCO_2} = \mathrm{CO} \times \left(\mathrm{CvCO_2} - \mathrm{CaCO_2}\right)$$

However, the relationship between total blood carbon dioxide and pCO_2, over CO_2 physiological ranges, may be considered rather linear, and difference in concentration between venous and arterial carbon dioxide (dCO_2) may be used instead:

$$\mathrm{VCO_2} = \mathrm{CO} \times \mathrm{dCO_2}$$

Thus, dCO_2 is directly proportional to CO_2 production and inversely to CO [23].

dCO_2 has been proven to be a good and early index of tissue perfusion imbalance in critical ill patient [24, 25]. Furthermore, if impairment is confirmed with low $ScVO_2$, there is an improvement in its specificity and positive and negative predictive values [24].

In a setting of constant ventilation, a dCO_2 greater than 6 mmHg is considered an index of low tissue perfusion.

5.2.9.1 Partial CO_2 Rebreathing

Based on the same principle as dCO_2, partial rebreathing CO_2 technique is accomplished using a specially designed breathing system that allows brief (50 s) increase of dead space. In this manner, CO_2 is rebreathed, allowing the use of the Fick equation on its minimum and maximum values.

This technique allows a safe and noninvasive measurement of CO, but it is applicable only in intubated patients. Changing ventilation patterns and pulmonary shunts may impair its diagnostic accuracy, and increased intracranial pressure represents a relative contraindication. Moreover, clinical trials were small and mainly focused on specific patient groups [13].

5.2.10 Lactates

Lactate is the metabolic end product of anaerobic glycolysis. Lactate clearance can be used to monitor tissue perfusion [26]; however, it can be elevated in other scenarios: some drugs, seizures, malignancy, thiamine deficiency, and hepatic failure are associated with higher lactate levels [27].

Normalization of lactate level is considered a valid endpoint for shock resuscitation [22], especially if a trend is used [24] rather than its static value. Persistent elevated lactate levels are associated with poor clinical outcome and death.

5.2.11 Fluid Responsiveness

Fluid responders are defined as those patients that increase stroke volume more than 10% after a fluid bolus (e.g., fluid challenge) [18]. Stroke volume is not easily measured at bedside even with advanced monitoring systems.

It is important to discriminate fluid responder and non-fluid responder patients: studies showed that half of ICU patients are non-responders [19].

Aya et al. demonstrated that the minimal volume that should be administered is 4 mL/kg in 5 min [28], even if there is evidence that the protocol may be liberalized [26].

Passive leg raise (PLR) is a maneuver that mimics fluid challenge without actually giving any fluids. PLR should be started with the patient in semi-recumbent position: it is performed lowering the trunk while raising the legs [29]. Positive prediction of fluid responsiveness should be assessed with CO or stroke volume measurement (threshold, a raise between 8 and 15%) or, if unavailable, radial pulse pressure (threshold, a raise between 9 and 12%) [9]; other CO measurement techniques validated with PLR include pulse contour CO, echocardiography, and esophageal Doppler [29]. CVP, PAWP, and PADP should not be used as poor correlation has been shown [13] (Fig. 5.1).

As it has no side effects, PLR should be considered as a replacement of standard bolus for the fluid challenge [29] when feasible: patient condition (e.g., intra-abdominal hypertension, leg or pelvic injuries) may contraindicate PLR.

5.2.12 Fluid Balance

Fluid balance is the sum of fluid parenterally or enterally administered to the patient and fluid loss (urine output, gastrointestinal drainage tubes and respiratory water loss, and diaphoresis) [30].

It's monitored in clinical practice to estimate fluid status in critically ill patients.

Patient weight, a more accurate fluid balance indicator, can be difficult to obtain at bedside with sufficient precision.

Hourly urine output is commonly used to judge hemodynamic adequacy. It is noninvasive but yields little information about the causes of hemodynamic imbalance.

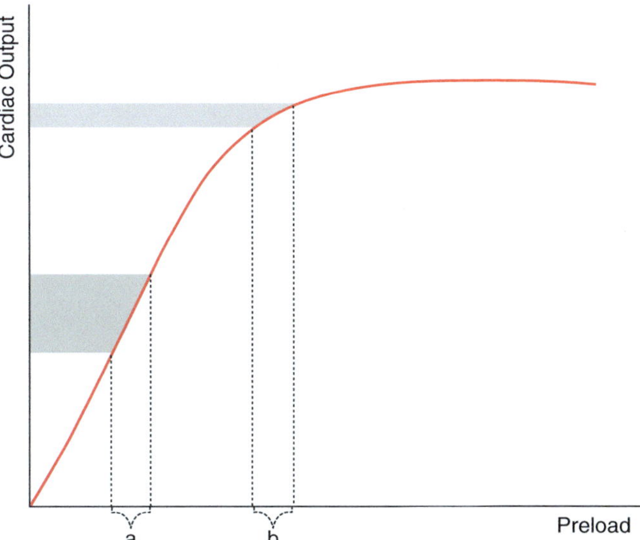

Fig. 5.1 Frank-Starling relationship. In order to understand if the patient will benefit from fluid infusion, it is important to understand where he or she is on the curve. If he is on the steep part (patient a in the picture), fluid therapy would increase preload and therefore cardiac output. Otherwise, if he is on the flat part, fluid infusion would increase preload without increasing cardiac output (patient b)

A treatment goal of at least 0.5 mL/kg/h is often used in clinical practice, even if it has not been validated [31]: sure enough, oliguria may be a signal of decreased renal perfusion [26] as a consequence of impaired hemodynamics.

5.2.13 Pulse Contour-Derived CO

Pulse contour CO systems are based on the principle that pulse pressure strictly reflects left ventricular stroke volume [19].

The area described by pulse pressure tracing is proportional to CO, once vascular compliance is known or estimated.

These systems, often used in postoperative care units, also calculate fluid responsiveness dynamic indexes such as pulse pressure variation (PPV) and stroke volume variation (SVV) [19].

These indexes are derived from heart-lung interaction during positive-pressure ventilation: by compressing vena cava, preload may decrease in fluid-responding patients, resulting in decreased stroke volume and pulse pressure during inspiration (Fig. 5.2). Therefore, wide changes on stroke volume and/or pulse pressure are strong predictors of fluid responsiveness.

Changes in pulse pressure can also be evaluated at a glance, with an estimated failure ratio in detecting fluid responsiveness of 4.4% [13].

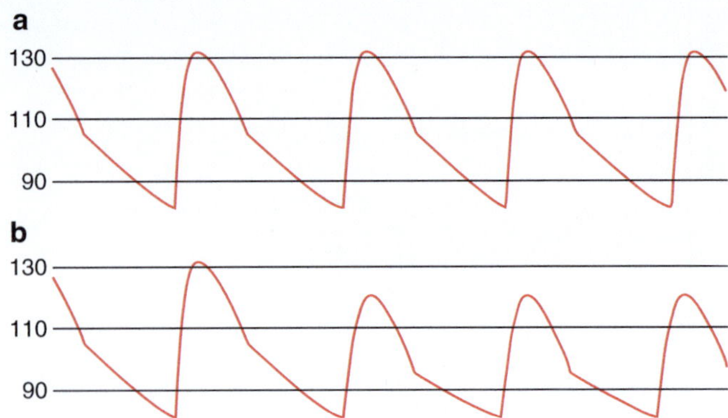

Fig. 5.2 (**a**) Pulse pressure in a (probably) *non*-fluid-responding patient. As you can notice, there is no difference between peaks at each pulse. (**b**) Pulse pressure in a (probably) fluid-responding patient. During inspiration, vena cava collapses and preload decreases and also pulse pressure

By using these systems, a patient is defined as not fluid responder with a SVV less than 10% and PPV less than 9% and responders with SVV major than 14% and PPV major than 13%. The areas between these values are considered gray areas, in which these systems are not able to provide reliable information [13].

Pulse contour analysis flaws are invasiveness, as they require a proper arterial line, with good tracing, and need of frequent recalibration with an independent measure of CO [19], in order to measure vascular compliance variations. Furthermore, their accuracy is very low in non-mechanically ventilated patients or in patients receiving a tidal volume less than 8 mL/kg and positive-end expiratory pressure less than 5 mmHg [9] or in patients with irregular cardiac rhythm, abnormal abdominal pressure, or open chest. Also, changes while assuming lateral position or steep Trendelenburg position are still not clear [13].

5.2.14 Ultrasonographic Techniques

Ultrasonographic techniques include transthoracic echocardiography, IVC diameter evaluation (described above), and esophageal Doppler determination of CO.

Transthoracic echocardiography is a reliable procedure if performed by expert investigators: volume status can be estimated by left and right ventricle filling state. However, unskilled practitioners may reduce its accuracy; volume deficit is considered safely assumed only in the event of ventricle kissing (US image of ventricle wall touching each other) [9].

Esophageal Doppler may provide continuous estimation of aorta blood flow by ultrasound Doppler determination of blood velocity and echographic evaluation aortic diameter.

Since only the descending thoracic aorta is measured, and CO may vary through arterial system, bias may be present, especially in patients with shock and/or receiving vasoactive drugs [19]. An empirically determined correction of 1.4 is often used, but, even if highly accurate, it cannot be considered universally applicable [13].

Furthermore, the patient needs to be well sedated to prevent probe movements, which would interfere with measurement reliability.

5.2.15 Gastric Tonometry

Box 5.3 Henderson-Hasselbalch Equation

$$\mathrm{pH} = \mathrm{pK_a} + \log_{10}\left(\frac{\left[\mathrm{HCO_3^-}\right]}{0.0307 \times \mathrm{pCO_2}}\right)$$

where pK_a is acid dissociation constant

Since splanchnic perfusion is early impaired in a setting of tissue hypoperfusion, by knowing the values of organ pH and CO_2, it may be possible to early detect hemodynamic impairment.

By deploying a modified nasogastric tube into the stomach, equipped with a balloon filled with an indicator (e.g., saline or air), it is possible to measure gastric intramucosal pCO_2 and, then, calculate by using Henderson-Hasselbalch equation, intramucosal pH (pHi).

The indicator must be sampled using a blood gas analyzer or air tonometry after at least 90 min in the stomach.

Since CO_2 removal decreases with hypoperfusion, by knowing pHi and arterial-gastric intramucosal pCO_2 gradient, it is possible to detect low organ perfusion states: high CO_2 levels mean low pHi and, hence, low perfusion.

Even if a large meta-analysis showed how the use of gastric tonometry could decrease patient's mortality, this system is not very commonly used in ICUs worldwide [32, 33].

5.2.16 Transpulmonary Thermodilution CO

Box 5.4 Modified Stewart-Hamilton Equation

$$\mathrm{CO} = \frac{V_i \times (T_b - T_i) \times K}{\int \Delta T_b(t)\,dt}$$

where
V_i = injected volume
T_b = body temperature
T_i = injectate temperature
K = computation constant

Generally considered the gold standard of CO measurement, thermodilution techniques are based on temperature difference of an indicator in different circulation sites.

Thermodilution technique was originally performed via a pulmonary artery catheter (Swan-Ganz catheter, see above). This technique measured temperature difference in pulmonary artery blood. CO was then calculated with the modified Stewart-Hamilton equation. CO changes during respiration could impair measurement [7].

Transpulmonary thermodilution CO is a newer and less invasive technique which measures temperature either at femoral or axillary artery, via an arterial line. A bolus of cold solution is injected through a CVC. Since the measurement is made over a longer period, it is unaffected by CO respiratory changes.

Temperature falls between injection site and measurement site is proportional to CO.

These systems also permit indirect calculation of other variables such as extravascular lung water index (ELWI), as a measure of pulmonary edema, useful in guiding fluid administration, and global end-diastolic volume (GEDV), as a more reliable measure of preload than CVP or PADP [13].

Severe right-sided valvular regurgitation or intracardiac shunts and concomitant fluid infusion may impair CO measurement [7].

The major flaw of transpulmonary thermodilution system is invasiveness: an artery central line and a CVC are still needed, leading to increased infection risks [19].

5.3 Drugs

5.3.1 Crystalloids

Fluids represent the cornerstone of hemodynamic management. Their judicious use has been shown to improve patient outcome [34].

However, as any other drugs, adverse effects may show up: excessive fluid administration may lead to tissue edema and pulmonary edema [26]. A large work from Brandstrup et al. showed that perioperative fluid restriction reduces incidencc of anastomotic leakage, pulmonary edema, pneumonia, and wound infection [35].

Recent reviews indicated fluid overload as a negative prognostic factor in many critical ill patients [19, 36].

Fluids are especially needed in postoperative patients, as it's been estimated that major surgery can cause a deficit of 3–6 L persisting up to 72 h after surgery. This delay is usually explained by the shift in the third space [35].

Even if some studies reported that preoperative compensation of possible fluid deficit is associated with less postoperative nausea and vomiting and improved postoperative hemodynamic profile, none has succeeded in showing decreased mortality. However, as stated by EJA guidelines, preemptive compensation seems reasonable, and it's considered prudent in any preoperative fluid deficit [9].

Literature suggests the use of balanced salt solutions (Hartmann's or Ringer's) over NaCl 0.9% saline: the use of the first is associated with lesser incidence of postoperative infections and acute kidney injury; furthermore, overloads with normal saline may cause hyperchloremic metabolic acidosis [37].

Intravenous fluids should be evaluated as any other drug, with the aim of maximizing efficacy and minimizing iatrogenic toxicity [37].

5.3.2 Colloids

Albumin is considered to be the reference colloidal solution. Its safety is still questioned: in 1998 the Cochrane Injuries Group Albumin Reviewers published a meta-analysis which showed a significant increase in the rate of death in patient receiving albumin instead of crystalloids [38], while Australian and New Zealand investigators published the Saline versus Albumin Fluid Evaluation (SAFE) study, comparing saline and albumin in randomized clinical trial. The latter study showed, in patients receiving albumin, an increased rate of death in those with head injury and decreased rate of death in those with sepsis [39].

A more recent study by Italian investigators (ALBIOS, Albumin Italian Outcome Sepsis) showed a clinically relevant improvement in hemodynamic, without any change in mortality in patients with severe sepsis receiving 20% albumin and crystalloids or crystalloids alone [40]. Anyway, albumin infusion has little or no other clinical risk or major complications.

Thus, the efficacy of albumin in fluid resuscitation, and its possible improved outcome in certain population, still needs to be determined [37].

Other colloid solutions available include 6% hydroxyethyl starch (HES) and gelatin [9].

5.3.3 Red Cell Transfusion

Each blood donation (about 470 mL) is filtered in order to remove white cells, platelets, and plasma. Red cell units are then resuspended in saline, adenine, glucose, and mannitol and stored.

Red cells can be administered as a therapy to both acute and chronic anemia [41].

Anemia is quite common in postoperative patient and has to be treated as it impairs oxygen delivery causing tissue hypoperfusion and myocardial ischemia [42].

In the last years, many studies had shown that a more conservative approach (7 g/dL as threshold in healthy patients, even if some authors advice that it should be used for every kind of patient) decreases pulmonary edema, organ failure rates, and patient mortality, compared with a liberal transfusion strategy [42].

ABO-incompatible red cell transfusion is the primary hazard of transfusions; other transfusion-related adverse effects include acute lung injury, volume overload, virus-infected units (hepatitis C virus and human immunodeficiency virus), bacterial infected units (which are very rare), and other less clinically relevant conditions such as non-hemolytic fever transfusion reactions and urticaria [41].

5.3.4 Inotropes and Vasopressors

The most used inotropes and vasopressors are epinephrine, norepinephrine, dopamine, dobutamine, and levosimendan. They are usually administered in order to increase myocardial contractility and/or vascular tone in critical ill patient with marked hemodynamic impairment [43]. During the use of such medications, CO measurement is highly recommended.

Epinephrine is both a β and α agonist, having thereby important effects on CO. It rapidly increases heart rate, ventricular contraction strength, and vasoconstriction, raising blood pressure. Clinical indications are emergency situations such as anaphylaxis and cardiac arrest. Adverse reactions include cerebral hemorrhage, ventricular arrhythmias, and splanchnic ischemia.

Norepinephrine is equipotent to epinephrine in stimulating β1 receptors but has little action on β2 and a potent action on α. This means that norepinephrine raises peripheral resistance, increasing blood pressure, but has little chronotropic effect, overcome by vagal compensatory reflex. Clinical indication for norepinephrine is the treatment of hypotension and hypoperfusion in non-fluid responder patients, especially in order to maintain cerebral perfusion pressure [43]. Adverse reactions include severe hypertension and reduced blood flow to the kidneys and intestines.

Dopamine is the metabolic precursor of norepinephrine and epinephrine. It stimulates DA1, DA2, β, and α receptors in a dose-depending fashion. It was known to have protective renal effects at low doses in oliguric states. In the last years, many studies have proven that low-dose dopamine is not clinically effective and may instead induce harm [44].

Adverse effects include nausea, vomiting, tachycardia, anginal pain, arrhythmias, and hypertension [45].

Dobutamine is a β-adrenergic drug with also some α-adrenergic effects which limits the increase in heart rate compared with pure β stimulation. Dobutamine is the medication of choice in low cardiac output patients who already received proper fluid administration. Even if it has been used by Rivers et al. in septic shock patients in order to improve $ScvO_2$, its value should not be used as a target, since it has been associated with worse outcomes [7].

Levosimendan is a relative new drug which increases calcium sensitization of troponin C in myocardiocytes. It also has effects on ATP-dependent potassium channels on the sarcolemma, leading to peripheral and coronary dilation, and on mitochondrial potassium channels, granting cardioprotection. Shortly following a bolus infusion, levosimendan has been shown to improve cardiac output, stroke volume, and heart rate and to decrease pulmonary wedge pressure and total peripheral resistance and therefore arterial blood pressure. It also affects renal circulation, causing preglomerular vasodilation and so improving renal flow.

Levosimendan produces an active metabolite, named OR-1896, which prolongs drug effects up to 7–9 days after stopping infusion.

Many studies have compared levosimendan with dobutamine: levosimendan produced greater increase in cardiac output, decreased mortality, improved renal function, reduced hospital length of stay, but showed higher atrial fibrillation incidence [46].

However, a recent randomized placebo-controlled study proved no mortality reduction in patients undergoing cardiac surgery after low-dose levosimendan administration [47].

Adverse effects mainly include hypotension, headache, atrial fibrillation, and tachycardia. Even after prolonged infusion (up to 48 h), no tolerance has been observed [46].

No randomized controlled trials have shown the superiority of any inotropic drugs, if compared in terms of major clinical outcomes [47].

5.3.5 Vasodilators

Vasodilators, together with β-blockers, are the mainstay of pharmacological approach to postoperative hypertension [5].

The main vasodilators are angiotensin-converting enzyme inhibitors (ACEi), angiotensin II receptor blockers (ARBs), calcium channel antagonists, urapidil, nitrates, and sodium nitroprusside.

ACEi inhibit the conversion from angiotensin I to angiotensin II, resulting in reduced vasoconstriction and increased bradykinin concentration, leading to vasodilation [48]. Their adverse reactions include cough, hypotension, skin rash, angioedema, acute renal failure, and hyperkalemia. Since surgical patients are at increased risk for circulatory decompensation, ACEi should not be considered as first-line agents for perioperative hypertension [5].

ARBs inhibit angiotensin I receptors reducing biological effects of angiotensin II, reducing AP. Although it is still an issue whether ARBs are equivalent to ACEi in therapeutic effects, adverse reactions with ARBs are comparable with that of placebo [48].

Ca2+ channel antagonists inhibit calcium channel function, leading to relaxation of arterial smooth muscles and inotropic and chronotropic effect on the heart, compensated by baroreflex increase in sympathetic tone. Adverse reactions include hypotension, pulmonary edema, dizziness, headache, and nausea [48].

Sodium nitroprusside acts by releasing NO, which is usually produced by endothelial cells to promote vasodilation. Thus, sodium nitroprusside causes vasodilation in both arterioles and venules, modest increase in heart rate, and overall reduction of myocardial O_2 consumption. Adverse effects include excessive vasodilation and, less commonly, accumulation of cyanide leading to lactic acidosis [48].

Urapidil is an α1-receptor blocker but also has a central hypotensive effect. It is used for hypertensive crises, severe or treatment-resistant, and perioperative and postoperative hypertension. Adverse effects include dizziness, nausea, headaches, fatigue, and orthostatic hypotension [49].

5.3.6 Diuretics

Diuretics are used to reduce preload, pulmonary edema, fluid overload, duration of oliguria, and need for dialysis [50]. The most used diuretics in the postoperative period are loop diuretics, especially furosemide, due to their increased potency. Furosemide inhibits the sodium-potassium-chloride channel, consequently inhibiting Na+ reabsorption and promoting diuresis [51].

Adverse effects of furosemide include hypovolemia, electrolyte imbalance (e.g., hypokalemia, hypomagnesemia, hypocalcemia, hyponatremia, hyperuricemia), hypersensitivity, and ototoxicity [51].

5.3.7 Beta-Adrenergic Blockers

β-adrenergic blocking agents lower CO by decreasing myocardial contractility, heart rate, and consequently oxygen consumption. They are mainly used in hypertension management and to reduce morbidity and mortality in myocardial infarctions survivors.

They also have significant side effects, such as bronchospasm, impotence, depression, and psychosis. Furthermore, multiple interactions with other medications have been reported [7].

Even if beta-blockers were initially discontinued before surgery, evidence showed that sudden withdrawal can actually worsen hypertension [7]: both European Society of Cardiology and American College of Cardiology Foundation/American Heart Association guidelines agree that patients on chronic treatment with such medications should be maintained throughout perioperative period with fairly good evidence [52–54].

Worth of notice, among β-adrenergic blocking agents, esmolol is the one with shortest half-life (distribution half-life of 2 min and elimination half-life of 9 min), making it the drug of choice in perioperative patients [4].

Conclusion

Even though many monitoring techniques have been developed, correctly assessing patient hemodynamic status and fluid responsiveness is still a challenge.

No index is sufficient by itself and often more than a single index is needed.

Moreover its value should be analyzed in terms of dynamic changes during patient observation, rather than its static measurement.

Therapy aimed to improve patient hemodynamic status should be properly thought, as different conditions need different approaches.

So, what kind of monitor for which patient?

As we have seen previously in this chapter, there is no such thing as the perfect monitoring system. Every patient has different needs, and hemodynamic monitoring should be tailored with respect to patient clinical condition, monitoring invasiveness, and, of course, expensiveness. After surgery, it is important to identify where the patient should be transferred. Classically, the choice is between the ward and the ICU (Fig. 5.3).

Patient hemodynamic status should play a large role in this decision, as ICUs are equipped with systems unavailable in the wards.

Clinicians should remember that ICUs are considered appropriate for every patient who requires vasoactive drugs, support for circulatory instability due to hypovolemia from any cause and which is unresponsive to modest volume replacement, or patients resuscitated following cardiac arrest where intensive care is considered appropriate [55].

Type of surgery (i.e., major versus minor) and American Society of Anesthesiologists (ASA) score may guide clinician decision.

Clinicians should always bear in mind that choosing not to monitor hemodynamic status (i.e., not choosing the best possible monitoring technique available) *always* means to be unaware of the actual patient hemodynamic status and therefore what the best therapeutic option is.

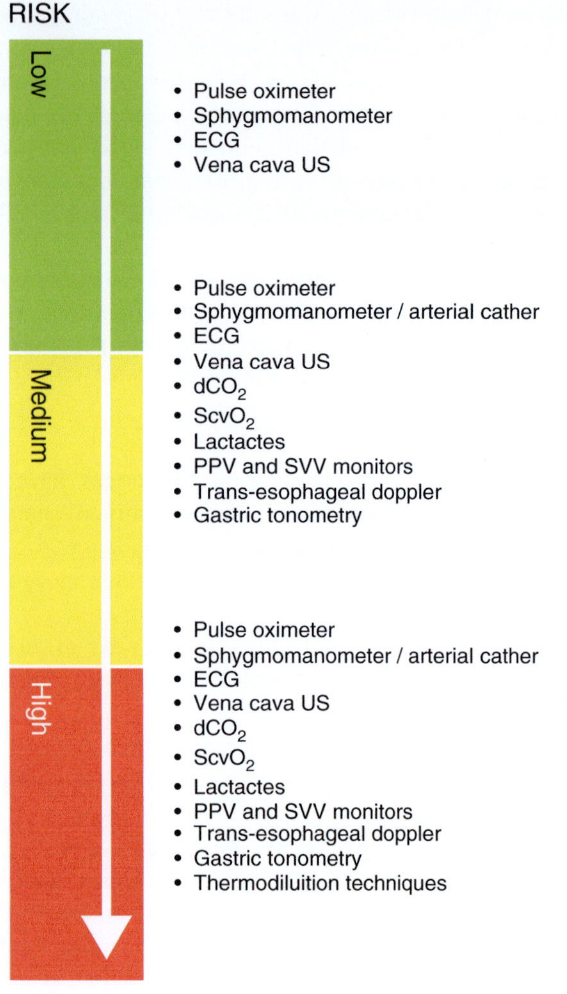

Fig. 5.3 Which monitor for which patient? Hemodynamic risk should guide your decision about monitoring strategies

Case Scenario

Male, 56 years old, ASA 2

Medical history includes chronic obstructive pulmonary disease (COPD) and post-ischemic dilatative cardiomyopathy.

He was scheduled for ileal and sigmoid resection and colostomy, classified as ASA 2.

Surgery was uncomplicated and it lasted about 4 h.

A CVC has been placed and BP has been measured with automatic sphygmomanometer. Intraoperative diuresis has been estimated to 100 mL.

During surgery, fluid replacement has been performed, drove by PA 70/40 mmHg, CVP 3 mmHg, and oliguria. After Ringer lactate 9000 mL, CVP increased to 7 mmHg and BP to 110/60 mmHg.

On his arrival in the ward, he has been extubated. He looks painless.

He is oliguric and has a BP of 140/60 mmHg, heart rate 67, SpO_2 94%, and respiratory rate 24.

1. Does this patient need more fluids?
   A. No: CVP is greater than 6 mmHg.
   B. No: BP is sufficient.
   C. Yes: he is oliguric.
   D. We should gather more indexes to assess his volemic status.

2. Which of the following monitoring techniques would you use postoperatively?
   A. Lactate levels
   B. Thermodilution
   C. PLR or fluid challenge
   D. Vena cava US evaluation

3. How would you change this patient management?
   A. I would have gathered some preoperative information about patient's hemodynamic status.
   B. I would have gathered other intraoperative information about patient's hemodynamic status, rather than only diuresis, BP, and CVP.
   C. I would have done as the anesthetist did.
   D. I would have administered the same fluid volume, but, instead of Ringer lactate, I would have used saline 0.9%.

4. What are the determinants of cardiac output?
   A. Preload and afterload
   B. Heart contractility and heart rate
   C. Arterial blood oxygen content
   D. Blood pressure value

Please see Chap. 58 for the correct answer.

References

1. Webb AR, Shapiro MJ, Singer M, Suter P. Oxford textbook of critical care. Oxford: Oxford University Press; 1999. p. 907.
2. Marik PE, Monnet X, Teboul JL. Hemodynamic parameters to guide fluid therapy. Ann Intensive Care. 2011;1:1.
3. Bigatello LM, George E. Hemodynamic monitoring. Minerva Anestesiol. 2002;68:219–25.
4. Longnecker DE, Brown DL, Newman MF, Zapol WM. Anesthesiology. 2012:1280–9.
5. Varon J, Marik PE. Perioperative hypertension management. Vasc Health Risk Manag. 2008;4(3):615–27.
6. McLellan SA, Walsh TS. Oxygen delivery and haemoglobin. Contin Educ Anaesth Crit Care Pain. 2004;4:123–6.
7. Longnecker DE, Brown DL, Newman MF, Zapol WM. Anesthesiology. 2012;418

8. Vincent JL. Understanding cardiac output. Crit Care. 2008;12(4):174.
9. Marx G, Schindler AW, Mosch C, Albers J, Bauer M, Gnass I, Hobohm C, Janssens U, Kluge S, Kranke P, Maurer T, Merz W, Neugebauer E, Quintel M, Senninger N, Trampisch HJ, Waydhas C, Wildenauer R, Zacharowski K, Eikermann M. Intravascular volume therapy in adults: guidelines from the Association of the Scientific Medical Societies in Germany. Eur J Anesthesiol. 2016;33(7):488–521.
10. Saugel B, Kirsche SV, Hapfelmeier A, Phillip V, Schultheiss C, Schmid RM, Huber W. Prediction of fluid responsiveness in patients admitted to the medical intensive care unit. J Crit Care. 2013;28(4):537.e1–9.
11. Ortega R, Hansen CJ, Elterman K, Woo A. Pulse oximetry. N Engl J Med. 2011;364:e33.
12. Moore LJ, Wade CE, Vincent L, Podbielski J, Camp E, Junco DD, Radhakrishnan H, McCarthy J, Gill B, Holcomb JB. Evaluation of noninvasive hemoglobin measurements in trauma patients. Am J Surg. 2013;206(6):1041–7.
13. Miller RD, Cohen NH, Eriksson LI, Fleisher LA, Wiener-Kronish JP, Young WL. Miller's anesthesia. 8th ed. Philadelphia, PA: Saunders; 2015. p. 1362–48.
14. Pinsky MR. Functional hemodynamic monitoring. Crit Care Clin. 2015;31(1):89–111.
15. Marik PE, Lemson J. Fluid responsiveness: an evolution of our understanding. Br J Anaesth. 2014;112(4):617–20.
16. Marik PE, Cavallazzi R. Does the central venous pressure predict fluid responsiveness? An updated meta-analysis and a plea for some common sense. Crit Care Med. 2013;41(7):1774–81.
17. Cherpanath TGV, Geerts BF, Lagrand WK, Schultz MJ, Groeneveld ABJ. Basic concepts of fluid responsiveness. Neth Heart J. 2013;21:530–6.
18. Lobo SM, de Oliveira NE. Clinical review: what are the best hemodynamic targets for noncardiac surgical patients? Crit Care. 2013;17(2):210.
19. Teboul JL, Saugel B, Cecconi M, De Backer D, Hofer CK, Monnet X, Perel A, Pinsky MR, Reuter DA, Rhodes A, Squara P, Vincent JL, Scheeren TM. Less invasive hemodynamic monitoring in critically ill patients. Intensive Care Med. 2016;42(9):1350–9.
20. Feissel M, Michard F, Faller JP, Teboul JL. The respiratory variation in inferior vena cava diameter as a guide to fluid therapy. Intensive Care Med. 2004;30:1834–7.
21. Reyer E. The hemodynamic and physiological relevance of continuous central venous oxygenation monitoring: it's not just for sepsis. ICU Medical Inc; 2013. p. 1–8.
22. Mesquida J, Saludes P, Gruartmoner G, Espinal C, Torrents E, Baigorriand F, Artigas A. Central venous-to-arterial carbon dioxide difference combined with arterial-to-venous oxygen content difference is associated with lactate evolution in the hemodynamic resuscitation process in early septic shock. Crit Care. 2015;19:126.
23. Mallat J, Lemyze M, Tronchon L, Vallet B, Thevenin D. Use of venous-to-arterial carbon dioxide tension difference to guide resuscitation therapy in septic shock. World J Crit Care Med. 2016;5(1):47–56.
24. Tánczos K, Németh M, Molnár Z. The multimodal concept of hemodynamic stabilization. Front Public Health. 2014;2:34.
25. Mallat J, Salaun P, Gasan G, Tronchon L, Thevenin D. Venoarterial carbon dioxide gradient at the early stage of septic shock. Crit Care. 2010;14(Suppl 1):P156.
26. Vincent JL, Weil MH. Fluid challenge revisited. Crit Care Med. 2006:1333–7.
27. Andersen LW, Mackenhauer J, Roberts JC, Berg KM, Cocchi MN, Donnino MW. Etiology and therapeutic approach to elevated lactate. Mayo Clin Proc. 2013;88(10):1127–40.
28. Aya H, Rhodes A, Grounds RM, Cecconi M. Minimal volume for a fluid challenge in postoperative patients. Crit Care. 2015;19(Suppl 1):P189.
29. Monnet X, Teboul JL. Passive leg raising: five rules, not a drop of fluid! Crit Care. 2015;19(1):18.
30. Perren A, Markmann M, Merlani G, Marone C, Merlani P. Fluid balance in critically ill patients. Should we really rely on it? Minerva Anestesiol. 2011;77:802–11.
31. Sevransky J. Clinical assessment of hemodynamically unstable patients. Curr Opin Crit Care. 2009;15(3):234–8.
32. Mythen MG. Does gastric tonometry-guided therapy reduce total mortality in critically ill patients? Crit Care. 2015;19:172.
33. Zhang X, Zuan W, Yin P, Wang L, Wu X, Wu Q. Gastric tonometry guided therapy in critical care patients: a systematic review and meta-analysis. Crit Care. 2015;19:22.
34. Cecconi M, Hofer C, Teboul JL, Pettila V, Wilkman E, Molnar Z, Della Rocca G, Aldecoa C, Artigas A, Jog S, Sander M, Spies C, Lefrant JY, De Backer D. Fluid challenges in intensive care: the FENICE study. Intensive Care Med. 2015;41:1529–37.
35. Strunden MS, Heckel K, Goetz AE, Reuter DA. Perioperative fluid and volume management: physiological basis, tools and strategies. Ann Intensive Care. 2011;1:2.
36. Cordemans C, De Laet I, Van Regenmortel N, Schoonheydt K, Dits H, Huber W, Malbrain MLNG. Fluid management in critically ill patients: the role of extravascular lung water, abdominal hypertension, capillary leak, and fluid balance. Ann Intensive Care. 2012;2(Suppl 1):S1.
37. Myburgh JA, Mythen MG. Resuscitation fluids. N Engl J Med. 2013;369:1243–51.
38. Abi B. Cochrane injuries group albumin reviewers Why albumin may not work. Br Med J. 1998;317:235.
39. The SAFE Study Investigators. A comparison of albumin and saline for fluid resuscitation in the intensive care unit. N Engl J Med. 2004;350:2247–56.
40. Caironi P, Tognoni G, Masson S, Fumagalli R, Pesenti A, Romero M, Fanizza C, Caspani L, Faenza S, Grasselli G, Iapichino G, Antonelli M, Parrini V, Fiore G, Latini R, Gattinoni L. Albumin replacement in patients with severe sepsis or septic shock. N Engl J Med. 2014;370(15):1412–21.
41. Contreras M. ABC of transfusion. New York, NY: John Wiley & Sons; 2009.
42. Hébert PC, Carson JL. Transfusion threshold of 7g per deciliter—the new normal. N Engl J Med. 2014;371(15):1459–61.
43. Bangash MN, Kong M, Pearse RM. Use of inotropes and vasopressor agents in critically ill patients. Br J Pharmacol. 2010;165(7):2015–33.
44. Holmes CL, Walley KR. Bad medicine: low-dose dopamine in the ICU. Chest. 2003;123(4):1266–75.
45. Brunton L, Parker K, Blumenthal D, Buxton I. Goodman & Gilman's manual of pharmacology and therapeutics. New York: McGraw-Hill; 2008. p. 149–58.
46. Nieminen MS, Fruhwald S, Heunks LMA, Suominem PK, Gordon AC, Kivikko M, Pollesello P. Levosimendan: current data, clinical use and future development. Heart Lung Vessel. 2013;5(4):227–45.
47. Landoni G, Lomivorotov VV, Alvaro G, Lobreglio R, Pisano A, Guarracino F, Calabrò MG, Grigoryev EV, Likhvantsev VV, Salgado-Filho MF, Bianchi A, Pasyuga VV, Baiocchi M, Pappalardo F, Monaco F, Boboshko VA, Abubakirov MN, Amantea B, Lembo R, Brazzi L, Verniero L, Bertini P, Scandroglio AM, Bove T, Belletti A, Michienzi MG, Shukevich DL, Zabelina TS, Bellomo R, Zangrillo A. Levosimendan for hemodynamic support after cardiac surgery. N Engl J Med. 2017;376:2021–31.

48. Brunton L, Parker K, Blumenthal D, Buxton I. The Goodman & Gilman's manual of pharmacology and therapeutics. New York: McGraw-Hill; 2008. p. 519–36.
49. Buch J. Urapidil, a dual-acting antihypertensive agent: current usage considerations. Adv Ther. 2010;27(7):426–43.
50. Sear JW. Br J Anesth. 2005;95(1):20–32.
51. Oh SW, Han SY. Loop diuretics in clinical practice. Electrolyte Blood Press. 2015;13(1):17–21.
52. Sear JW, Foex P. Recommendations on perioperative beta-blockers: differing guidelines: so what should the clinician do? Br J Anaesth. 2010;104(3):273–5.
53. Poldermans D, Bax JJ, Boersma E, et al. Guidelines for pre-operative cardiac risk assessment and perioperative cardiac management in non-cardiac surgery: the Task Force for Preoperative Cardiac Risk Assessment and Perioperative Cardiac Management in Non-cardiac Surgery of the European Society of Cardiology (ESC) and endorsed by the European Society of Anaesthesiology (ESA). Eur Heart J. 2009;30:2769–812.
54. Fleischmann KE, Beckman JA, Buller CE, et al. CCF/AHA focused update on perioperative beta blockade. J Am Coll Cardiol. 2009;54:2102–28.
55. Intensive Care Society. Standards for intensive care units. 1996.

6 Point-of-Care Ultrasound Management and Monitoring in Critical Care

E. Storti and S. Rossi

Key Points

- Point-of-care clinical ultrasound (PoCUS) is an ultrasonography brought to the patients in multiple settings and performed by the provider in real time; it is a multi-goal, dynamic, problem-based, and time-effective evaluation that allows the assessment of multiple districts and integration in the clinical evaluation granting the recognition, through the images, of specific patterns of disease.
- PoCUS can be used for airway and lungs assessment; it allows the evaluation of airway patency and effective breathing in emergency conditions. In the daily practice, it can help in the evaluation of patients in spontaneous and artificial ventilation guiding the intubation maneuvers and granting dynamic lung assessment.
- Using a combined ultrasonographic evaluation of multiple districts (inferior vena cava, heart chambers, and lung parenchyma), it is possible to determine the hemodynamic status of the patient and to assess its changes in relation to the treatment performed.
- FAST, being an easily replicable exam, is suitable for those patients with blunt abdominal trauma in whom a nonoperative management was chosen and in which repeated reevaluations will be necessary.
- PoCUS, for its intrinsic characteristic of being fast, reliable, and easily replicable, is particularly useful for the periodic assessment of relevant clinical variables; it can be used as a valid instrument to constantly monitor the patient's status, anticipating potential detrimental evolutions, thereby configuring itself as a precious tool guiding in the correct management of critical patients.

E. Storti (✉)
General Intensive Care Unit and Intermediate Care Unit, Ospedale Maggiore, Lodi, Italy
e-mail: enrico.storti@asst-lodi.it

S. Rossi
Pediatric Unit, Department of Molecular and Developmental Medicine, University of Siena, Siena, Italy
e-mail: serena.rossi02@universitadipavia.it

6.1 Introduction

Healthcare technology is becoming more and more advanced and portable.

The process of advancement has also been applied to imaging techniques and especially to ultrasound. This constant development affected the field of ultrasound very deeply because, throughout the years, machines have undergone a "miniaturization" process in terms of dimensions with a concomitant boosting/improvement in relation to their technical effectiveness.

Nowadays ultrasound machines are highly performant, portable, and light instruments, equipped with advanced settings (i.e., store and forward wireless capabilities) and long-lasting batteries that allow their use in various settings; the new maneuverable ultrasound machines can, therefore, be easily transported and used throughout the emergency rooms, in intensive care units (ICU), operating rooms (OR), and hospital wards.

The technological evolution of point-of-care ultrasound has determined its rapid diffusion in different medical fields, allowing its use by a growing number of physicians like anesthesiologists, surgeons, and emergency medicine doctors that previously relied only on ultrasonographic diagnosis performed by radiologists or other specialists (cardiologists, gynecologists, urologists) [1–5].

P. Aseni et al. (eds.), *Operative Techniques and Recent Advances in Acute Care and Emergency Surgery*,
https://doi.org/10.1007/978-3-319-95114-0_6

6.2 Point-of-Care Ultrasound in Critical Care Medicine

The many applications, extensive diagnostic possibilities, and comprehensive view of problems that ultrasound has in the experienced hands of the radiologists are well known, but a paradigmatic shift is necessary when dealing with a patient in a critical care setting.

During the evaluation of a patient in an emergency situation, there are a number of factors that can profoundly condition the treatment and the subsequent course of action. Those factors should be promptly recognized and handled with the right set of priorities in order to define a fast, proper diagnostic and therapeutic strategy.

Surely, one of the most relevant elements when dealing with a critical patient is "time." The clinical presentation of this type of patients is often dramatic and rapidly evolving with nonspecific and non-univocal signs and symptoms.

While the diagnostic definition and treatment of acute pathologies are radically different, the time span between the identification of the problem and its treatment is directly related to the patient's survival.

In light of these considerations, the cost/benefit ratio between the definition of the most effective diagnostic modality and the time needed to put that in place should be accurately considered.

In relation to this, the use of ultrasound in a critical, time-dependent, and undifferentiated setting cannot be intended as the traditional "vertical" screening and evaluation of a single organ.

The traditional "organ-based" ultrasound evaluation should be replaced, in a critical setting, by a "problem-based," comprehensive examination directly performed by the clinician that allows a rapid integration of the images with the clinical picture of the patient.

Point-of-care ultrasound (PoCUS) is defined as ultrasonography brought to the patients in multiple settings and performed by the provider in real time, allowing findings to be directly correlated with the patients presenting signs and symptoms; it's an extension of the classical physical examination that allows the recognition, from the images, of specific patterns of disease that will help to tackle the presenting problems in a faster and effective way.

It is a rapid examination (<10 min) that allows the assessment of multiple districts (head, neck, thorax, abdomen, vessels, and even bones) and that can be performed without interrupting the clinical evaluation and the resuscitation maneuvers.

It is a multi-goal, patient-centered, dynamic, problem-based, and time-effective technology that can enable doctors (or different providers) to have a peculiar vision of patients' care.

PoCUS is performed directly by the physicians that treat the patient with the primary goal of rapidly defining (or excluding) pathologies that can be the cause of complex and rapidly evolving clinical pictures.

The images have to be of rapid interpretation allowing the recognition of specific patterns of disease through simple scans and have to grant the answer to bimodal questions (yes/no questions) like: Is there intrathoracic fluid? Is there a pneumothorax? Is there a cardiac tamponade? Is there intra-abdominal fluid?

Even expert sonologists have difficulties obtaining complex images and measurements in critical patients that are often poorly compliant, with life-threatening vital parameters or extensive bleeding; the help provided by PoCUS approach allows the clinicians to interpret the clinical condition rapidly and to best direct subsequent care.

6.3 "Ultrasound-Enhanced ABCDE Management"

Everybody is now familiar with the conceptual revolution that FAST (Focused Assessment with Sonography in Trauma) brought to the medical and surgical community. The trauma patients' evaluation changed radically when ultrasound (US) was introduced in the picture.

FAST is a safe, effective, and replicable technique to detect intraperitoneal free fluid accumulations in the peritoneal recesses and pouches [6].

An extended version of the standard FAST examination (E-FAST) has been developed and offers further information; in addition to the abdominal images, the E-FAST examination includes views of bilateral hemithoraces to assess for hemothorax and views of bilateral upper anterior chest walls to assess for PNX [7, 8].

In recent years a further notable step has been taken, and it has been proven that the integration of a comprehensive PoCUS approach in the critical care setting evaluation is surely beneficial; parallel to the ABCDE clinical approach, originally proposed for the assessment of the critically ill patients, a consolidated stepwise method can be used to integrate the US in the clinical evaluation, thus empowering the physician even more in the diagnostic process (Table 6.1).

In the first few minutes of the primary and secondary assessments of the patient, a trained critical care physician looking for very basic ultrasound findings like abnormal movements and air and fluid collections could quickly go through airway, respiratory, cardiovascular, and neurologic systems (or through the skull, chest, abdomen, and limbs); this will grant a critical, real-time insight to refine and dramatically improve diagnosis, treatments, and procedures [9].

PoCUS constitutes a relevant added value regarding the definitions of airway problems, lung pathologies (breathing), hemodynamically unstable situations (circulation), neurological damages (disability), and the complete definition of other lesions (exposure) related to the clinical picture of the patients.

Keeping in mind the correspondence with the ABCDE sequence used for life support, we will describe the impact of

Table 6.1 The table shows the integration of ultrasound in the ABCDE clinical evaluation of critical patients

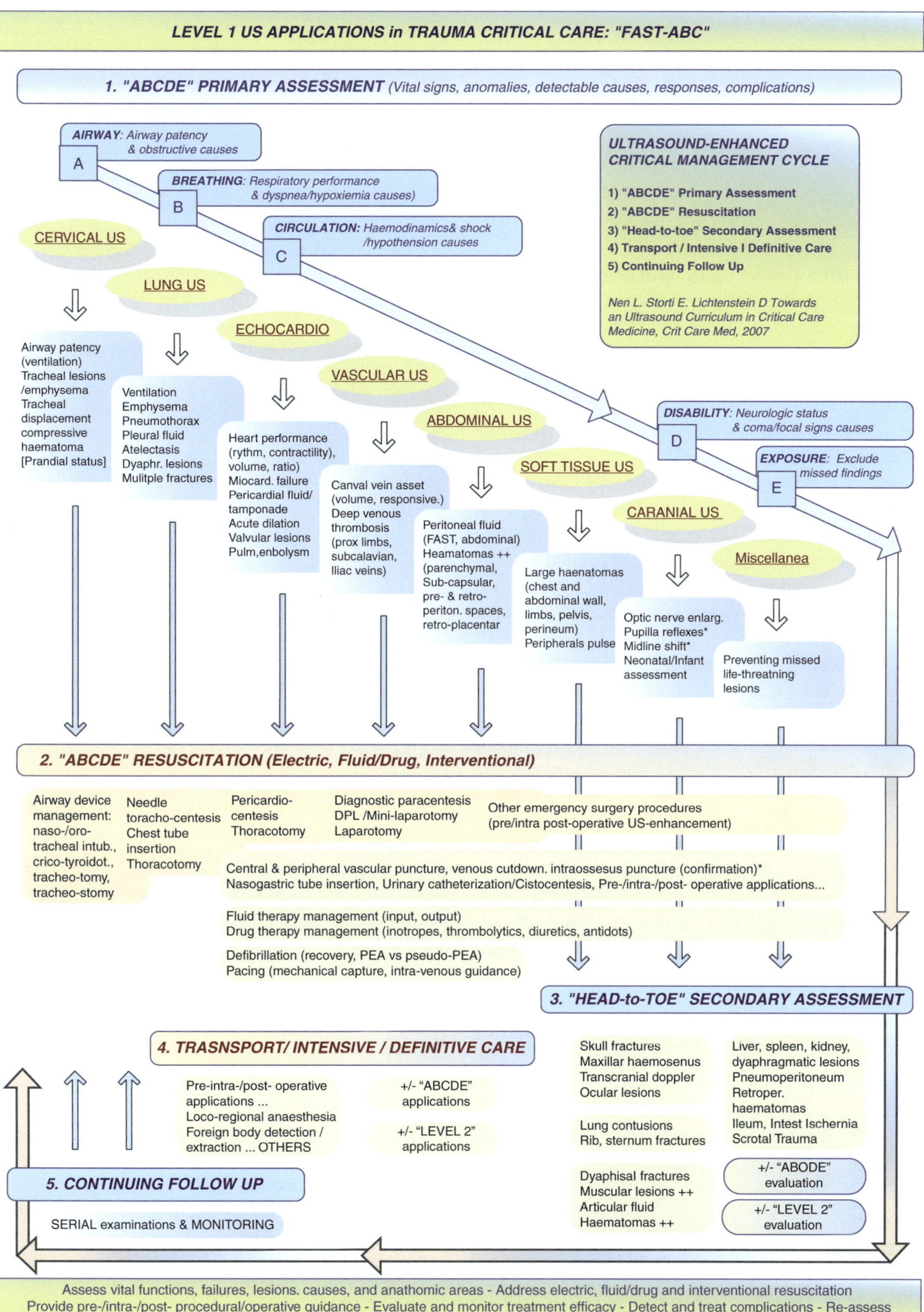

Adapted from *Neri L, Storti E, Lichtenstein D. Toward an ultrasound curriculum for critical care medicine. Crit Care Med. 2007 May;35(5 Suppl):S290–304*

the most recent PoCUS applications in the assessment and treatment of critically ill patients.

6.3.1 Airways

Airway management constitutes one of the most critical steps in the care of unstable patients. The patency of the airways is the fundamental prerequisite in order to obtain and maintain proper tissue oxygenation and to avoid hypoxic cardiac arrest.

The sonographic assessment of the airway may be easily performed before, during, and after securing the airway.

With a high-frequency linear probe, it is possible to obtain, rapidly and accurately, the exact position of the patient's trachea and to evaluate any deviation from the neck midline. Those deviations can be associated with rapidly evolving conditions that could threaten patient's life like tension PNX or hematomas of the neck.

Using a transverse scan of the neck (distally from the thyroid cartilage), it is possible to align the midpoint of the ultrasound probe with the longitudinal axis of the trachea; once the exact position of the trachea with respect to the midline of the neck is defined, it is possible to obtain the longitudinal scan by simply rotating the US probe 90° clockwise (Fig. 6.1).

With a longitudinal scan (Fig. 6.2), it is possible to localize the cricothyroid cartilage in about 10 s (the timing is similar to manual palpation/localization), and it's also possible to precisely evaluate the anatomy of the trachea even in subjects with complex neck anatomy (short neck, obese people, burn victims, etc.) or with abnormal vessels crossing in front of the tracheal tube, giving a clear advantage in gaining tracheal access both in emergency and elective conditions (cricothyrotomy and tracheotomy) [10–12].

Failure in identifying the trachea with the US is essentially due to the presence of air in the subcutaneous tissue that will impede the passage of ultrasounds and that will generate comet-tail artifacts known as "E-lines" (Fig. 6.3). This pattern appears even for small air collections that won't generate the classical snow-crunching crepitations felt with palpation; in this way, it is possible to rapidly and accurately diagnose lesions of the tracheobronchial tree, quickly confirming decisions and priorities to the evolving patient condition [8].

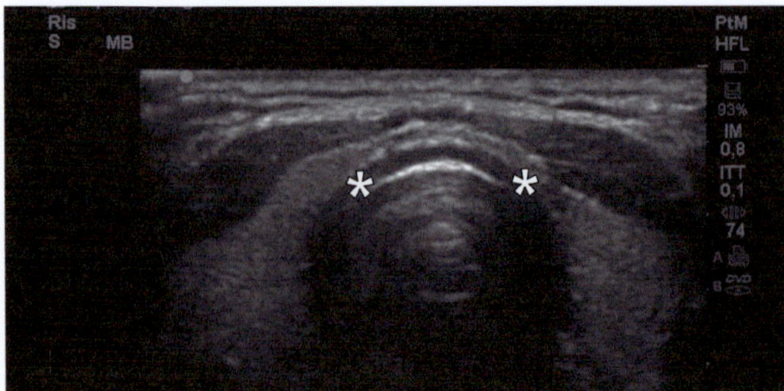

Fig. 6.1 Transverse scan of the anterior part of the neck. It allows the visualization of tracheal rings (white asterisks), evaluating their distance from the skin level

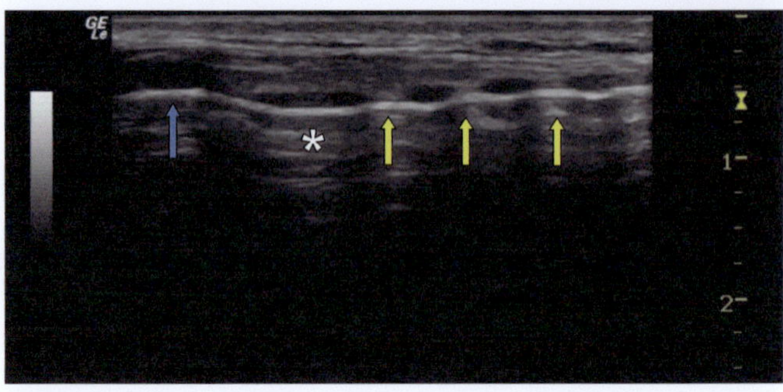

Fig. 6.2 Longitudinal scan of the trachea. It allows the precise detection of the cricoid cartilage (blue arrow), the first tracheal ring (asterisk), and the spaces between the proximal tracheal rings (yellow arrows)

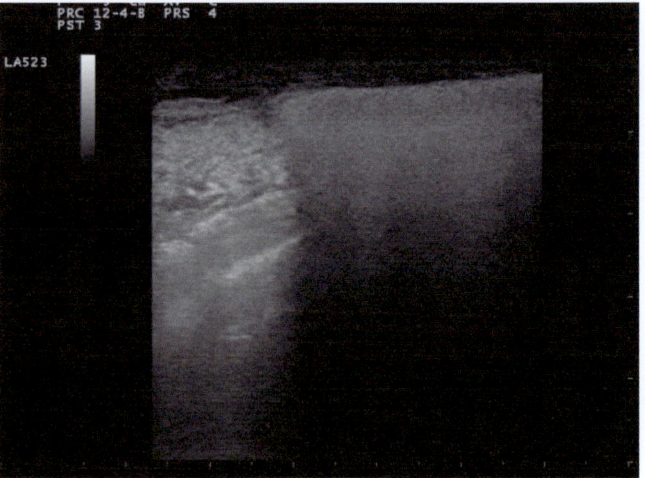

Fig. 6.3 Transverse scan of the neck with a linear probe. The visualization of the trachea is impaired due to the presence of air in the subcutaneous tissue (right portion of the image). There is a clear demarcation between the right side filled with air and the left side where air is not present, thus allowing the visualization of neck structures

One of the most important uses of PoCUS in the field of airway management in the critically ill patients is the possibility to accurately check the position of the endotracheal tube (ETT) and the possibility to provide guidance during the intubation maneuvers [13].

This technique is called TRUE (tracheal rapid ultrasound exam) and was found to have a pooled sensitivity of 98.9% and specificity of 94.1% in the detection of proper tracheal intubation with a median operating time of 9 s.

Airway US for ETT position confirmation is best used when auscultation is unreliable, the end-tidal CO2 monitor is not accurate, radiology is unavailable, or the patient does not respond as expected after intubation [14–16].

Confirmation of the correct tracheal tube placement is performed indirectly by visualizing the esophagus during advancement of an endotracheal tube. Due to the sonographic presence of air filling the trachea, it is virtually impossible to identify a correctly placed endotracheal tube searching only for the precise position of its tip. In contrast, recognition of an endotracheal tube as it passes through the esophagus, left and posterolateral to the trachea, is easier and indicative of an esophageal intubation; it will be definitively demonstrated by a well-defined, round-shaped, hyperechoic (white) artifact caused by ETT surface with a shadow (black) stating immediately beneath (Fig. 6.4a, b).

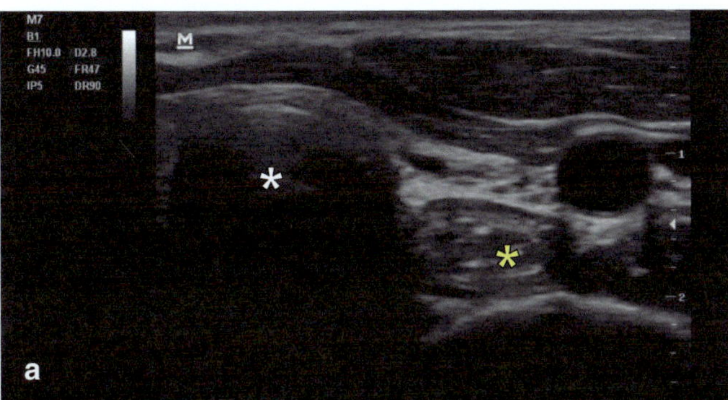

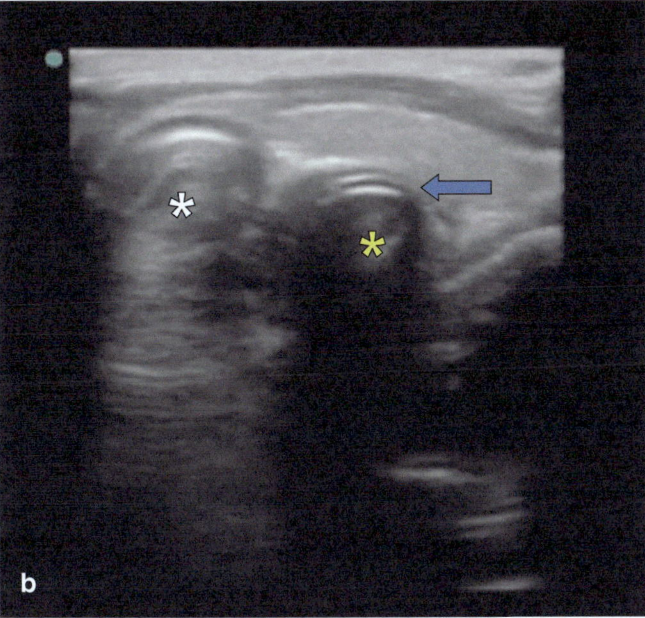

Fig. 6.4 (**a**) Left transverse anterolateral scan of the neck. The anatomical relations between the trachea (white asterisk) and esophagus (yellow asterisk) are shown. Right to the esophagus, the left common carotid artery is visible. (**b**) Using the same scan as in (**a**), it is possible to visualize the trachea (white asterisk) and the tram-track hyperechoic profile of the endotracheal tube (blue arrow) incorrectly placed in the esophagus (esophageal intubation). The yellow asterisk shows the posterior shadowing generated by the tube, impairing correct esophageal visualization

If a tube is not visualized in the esophagus, correct endotracheal placement is thereby confirmed indirectly [17].

Another way of indirectly confirming the proper positioning of the tip of the ETT above the carina is by visualizing the pleural sliding, scanning both lungs, meaning that the tidal volume is uniformly delivered in both hemithoraces.

Selective intubation can be easily and immediately detected by visualizing the so-called lung pulse in the excluded lung (most commonly the left lung). Lung pulse is indicative of an expanded but non-inflated lung and is defined as minimal pleural pulsations, synchronous with cardiac contractions and not with breathing acts [18, 19].

It has been demonstrated that the use of PoCUS to determine the correct ETT position has a much higher sensitivity and specificity than auscultation alone allowing the physicians to correctly identify the location of the ETT in 95% of cases [20]. Moreover, all these evaluations can be performed at the patient's bedside in less than 60 s allowing the operator to omit emergency chest X-ray imaging that will take a much longer time to be obtained.

6.3.2 Breathing

For many years "the dogma" that lung parenchyma couldn't be visualized with ultrasound dominated the minds of sonographers in the world that were aware that air would act as an obstacle to ultrasound wave propagation.

In the 1990s, the revolutionary idea that the artifacts generated by air could be interpreted and used to indirectly assess the status of the lung tissue was postulated by *D. Lichtenstein* [21].

From that initial statement, there was an exceptional evolution that brought lung ultrasound to be the rigorous standard of care [22].

The linear artifacts mentioned above were classified as horizontal and vertical ones; using these lines it is possible to evaluate rapidly the most important alterations of pleura and lung parenchyma.

All artifacts originate from the pleural line that appears as a hyperechoic (white) line that moves horizontally with every breathing act (lung sliding).

The basic ultrasound scan is the so-called bat sign; it is given by a longitudinal scan of the thorax in which the hyperechoic pleural line is comprised between and position about 5 mm lower than two anechoic shadow images generated by two consecutive ribs that stop the passage of ultrasounds by their total reflection (Fig. 6.5).

"A lines" are hyperechoic horizontal linear artifacts that appear in a repetitive pattern on the screen under the pleural line and are associated with a normal lung pattern.

"B lines" are vertical artifacts (Fig. 6.6) that originate from the pleural line and look like comet tails; these lines

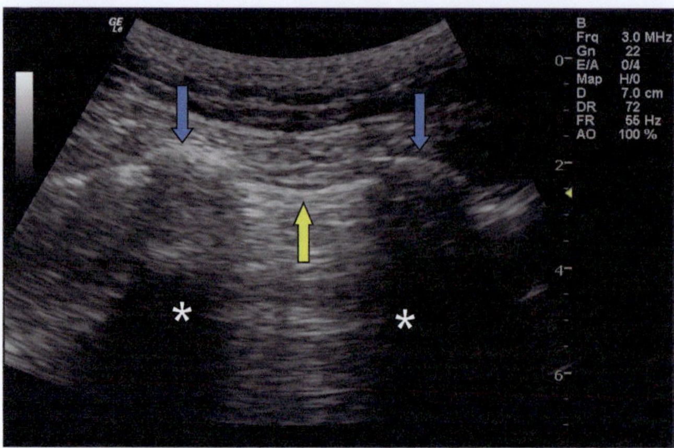

Fig. 6.5 The "bat sign" obtained with a longitudinal scan of the thorax. Two contiguous ribs (blue arrows) with their anechoic shadowing and the pleural line (yellow arrow) are shown. An "A line" is visible as a linear hyperechoic artifact (between the two white asterisks)

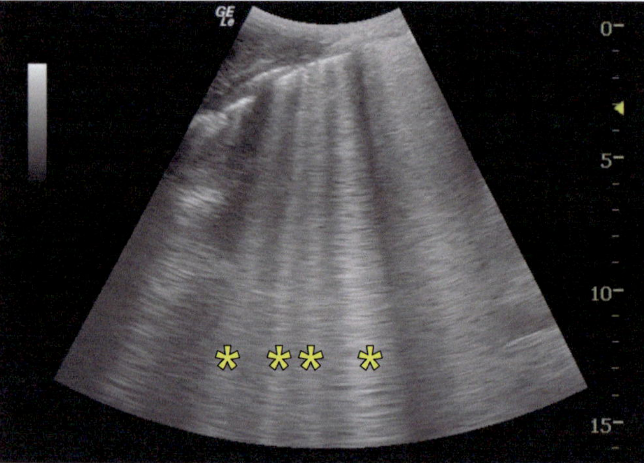

Fig. 6.6 Longitudinal scan of the thorax at the level of the midaxillary line obtained using a convex probe. It shows multiple vertical artifacts, "B lines" (yellow asterisks), originating from the pleural line

appear because of the coexisting presence of two media with different acoustic impedance (e.g., air/water) in conditions like the wet lung.

The diffuse, bilateral appearance of B lines will represent the presence of water within the lungs and will allow the clinician to make a rapid diagnosis of pulmonary edema (cardiogenic or lesional) [23].

Facing a dyspnoic patient, lung ultrasound will help the physician in the definition of the genesis of that respiratory failure, making an accurate and quick discrimination between pulmonary edema (B lines present) and COPD exacerbation (B lines absent) possible.

The presence of B lines allows the rapid discrimination between pulmonary edema and asthma/COPD recurrence with very high sensitivity and specificity (sens 100%, spec 92%) [24, 25].

In adjunct to the evaluation of these artifacts that will help the clinician to rapidly differentiate between normal and pathologic lungs, many other applications of the technique have been studied.

Pleural effusions can be rapidly and effectively identified and quantified using PoCUS; it has been proven that the thickness (expressed in mm) of the pleural effusion correlates positively with the volume of the fluid collection (expressed in mL) [26]. Moreover, having the visual support of US, the physician can accurately and safely evaluate the possibility of positioning a drainage in the best possible location without venturing in risky procedure guided only by semeiotics and chest X-rays [27].

Another useful application of lung ultrasound in emergency settings is the possibility to effectively rule in or rule out (in a few seconds) pneumothorax (PNX). The presence of pleural sliding, B lines, and consolidation allows to rule out PNX; in order to rule in the diagnosis, the so-called lung point sign has to be demonstrated. Lung point is defined as the exact point in which the detached visceral pleura, during inspiration, touches again the parietal pleura; lung point also allows to map the extension of the PNX and to monitor the evolution of the clinical picture. The specificity of lung point is nearly 100% [28].

Among the many applications of lung US, one of the most useful is undoubtedly the possibility of detecting lung consolidations (pneumonia, atelectasis, contusions) directly at the patients' bedside [29].

Consolidations appear as areas of tissue-like echo texture with shred, inferior margins. The differentiation between pneumonia and atelectasis relies on the evaluation of the air bronchogram (hyperechoic lines or dots within a hypoechoic area, representing air trapped in small airways) and on the clinical/lab findings: the visualization of a dynamic air bronchogram (that moves with breathing) has a PPV for pneumonia of 97%, while a static air bronchogram is more suggestive of atelectasis [30] (Fig. 6.7).

It has been proven that PoCUS has a high sensitivity and specificity also in diagnosing ARDS through the recognition of a typical pattern characterized by B lines, spared areas, pleural line thickening, and subpleural consolidations (Fig. 6.8). Although CT-scan quantitative analysis represents the gold standard to assess lung aeration and recruitment in ARDS patients, ultrasound changes can be assessed (at a given location on the chest) using the following four sonographic findings, often in progression: normal pattern, multiple spaced B lines, coalescent B lines, and consolidation.

This method has been proposed as a non-irradiating alternative to identify patients that might benefit from higher PEEP levels [31–33].

All these applications can be performed both during the initial evaluation of the patient in the emergency room and

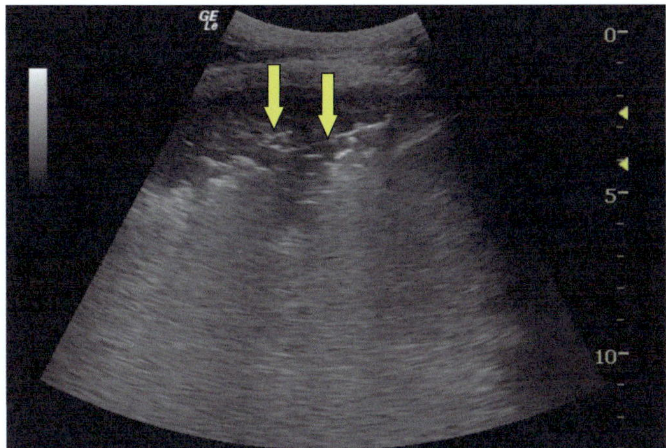

Fig. 6.7 Longitudinal scan of the thorax at the level of the midaxillary line, obtained with a convex probe, showing an extensive area of lung consolidation. Note the tissue-like echographic appearance of the consolidation with its irregular inferior profile (shred sign). Two yellow arrows point to the air bronchogram visible as two linear hyperechoic findings

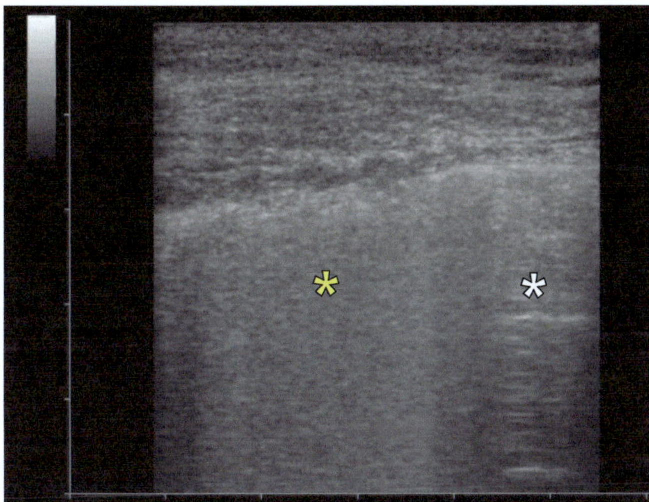

Fig. 6.8 Transverse thoracic scan at the level of anterior axillary line showing a spared area in a patient with ARDS. Spared areas are areas of normal lung pattern (white asterisk) in at least one intercostal space surrounded by areas of coalescent B lines or "white lung" (yellow asterisk) appearance for each examined area. Also note pleural line abnormalities defined as thickenings greater than 2 mm, evidence of small subpleural consolidations, or coarse appearance on the left side, whereas on the right side, the pleural line has a normal appearance

any other hospital setting (e.g., ICU or other hospital wards) configuring a versatile option that will aid in the definition of an often problematic clinical picture.

Familiarizing with lung ultrasound is important for the evaluation of critically ill patients because it allows the diagnostic definition and subsequent noninvasive monitoring of many conditions that present during the hospital stay in ICU. Moreover, it helps in monitoring the efficacy of the therapeutic strategies put in place (drainages, lung recruitment maneuvers, diuretic therapy, etc.) giving the physician a comprehensive view of the patient's condition.

6.3.3 Circulation

The application of PoCUS concept allows simplifying the management of cardiological emergencies.

It's possible to evaluate, through easily teachable scans, the morphology of cardiac chambers and the position of the interventricular septum or to rapidly estimate the ejection fraction [34].

Moreover, the presence/absence of pericardial fluid can be rapidly and effectively evaluated allowing the physician to assess the cardiac function in emergency conditions [35].

One of the most interesting aspects of point-of-care ultrasound is the possibility to make a comprehensive differential diagnosis of the many causes of pulseless electrical activity (PEA), namely, cardiac tamponade, tension pneumothorax, pulmonary embolism, and hypovolemia.

All these conditions can be quickly identified using US even during CRP maneuvers, and US scans can guide the operator in positioning the therapeutic cardiac or thoracic drainages in safe conditions [36].

Moreover, the acquisition of scans of the neck and thoracic inlet regions (internal jugular vein, subclavian vein, axillary vein), arms, and legs (superficial and deep femoral vein, saphenous vein) helps in the direct visualization of thrombi inside the vessel lumen or in the indirect hypothesis of a venous thrombosis secondary to a non-compressibility of the vessel itself (Fig. 6.9).

Compression ultrasonography (CUS) is now a well-established bedside technique to assess for deep vein throm-

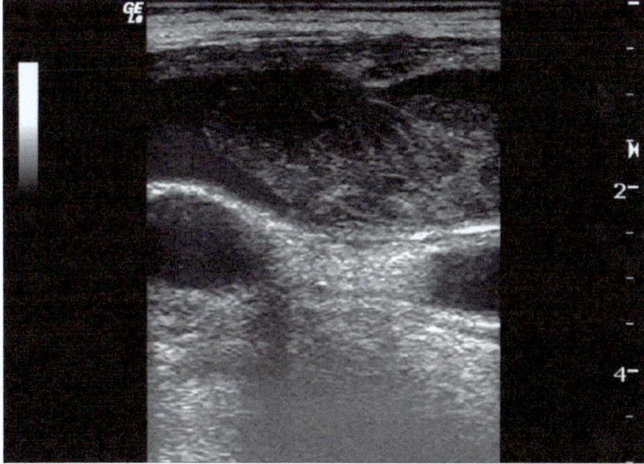

Fig. 6.9 Longitudinal scan performed with a linear probe at the level of right internal jugular vein (RIJV) showing massive occlusive thrombosis with compression/distortion at the level of the carotid, located inferiorly

bosis (DVT). By performing a two-point compression technique (at femoral and popliteal vein level), it is possible to rapidly detect a DVT with high sensitivity and specificity. Complete compression of the vein rules out a DVT, whereas the inability to completely compress the vein rules in a DVT [37–39].

One of the most dreadful causes of severe hemodynamic instability is represented by massive hemorrhages.

Internal bleeding is one of the predominant causes of preventable death in patients with major trauma. It is well known that there is a strict correlation between the delay in providing care to patients with major trauma and mortality rate; there is an increase in mortality rate of 1% every 3 min.

This rationale guided the evolution, at the beginning of the 1990s, of the first clinical-ultrasonographic protocol called FAST [6]. FAST ultrasound is considered the prototype of point-of-care ultrasound and allowed to start the process of integration of US in the clinical evaluation.

FAST is a focused ultrasound investigation centered in the detection of free fluid inside the peritoneum (hepatorenal, splenorenal, pelvic spaces), the pleura, and the pericardium using easily acquired and highly replicable scans (Fig. 6.10).

FAST US has now become a fundamental part of the emergency protocols in all trauma centers allowing a rapid evaluation of the hemodynamically unstable patient.

Using the FAST approach has many advantages: it is rapid (2–3 min) and noninvasive, and it's able to reduce the rate of explorative laparotomies (13 vs. 36%) and CT exams (26 vs. 56%). From an organizational point of view, it allows reducing the risk connected with the transfer of critical patients around the hospital, because the exam can be done at the bedside and, in the end, it can take part in the reduction of the costs of the patient's hospital stay [40].

It is important to notice how FAST US had an impact on the evaluation of trauma also in the pediatric population, thereby greatly reducing exposure to radiation, a concerning event in this type of population [41].

It is important to make a consideration when using this technique in critical patients; the diagnostic impact of ultrasound in trauma patients with hemodynamically stable conditions, with absent hemoperitoneum, with retroperitoneal lesions, or with lesions of a hollow organ is lower. However, it has been widely demonstrated that the impact of this diagnostic technique in blunt and unstable abdominal trauma is substantial, leading to a significant improvement in patients' care [42, 43].

6.3.4 Disability

For the evaluation of the neurological damages in a critical patient, CT scan is undoubtedly the gold standard, but, in conditions in which the CT confirmation cannot be obtained, the US use, especially when integrated with the clinical picture, constitutes a valuable diagnostic alternative that permits a resourceful modulation of the subsequent patients' management.

Point-of-care ultrasound in the evaluation of neurological damage is a relatively new and advanced concept that is still not diffusely known nor used; it provides real-time information about possible gross anomalies of the CNS structures helping in the definition of the neurological state of a patient in the emergency room or prehospital settings.

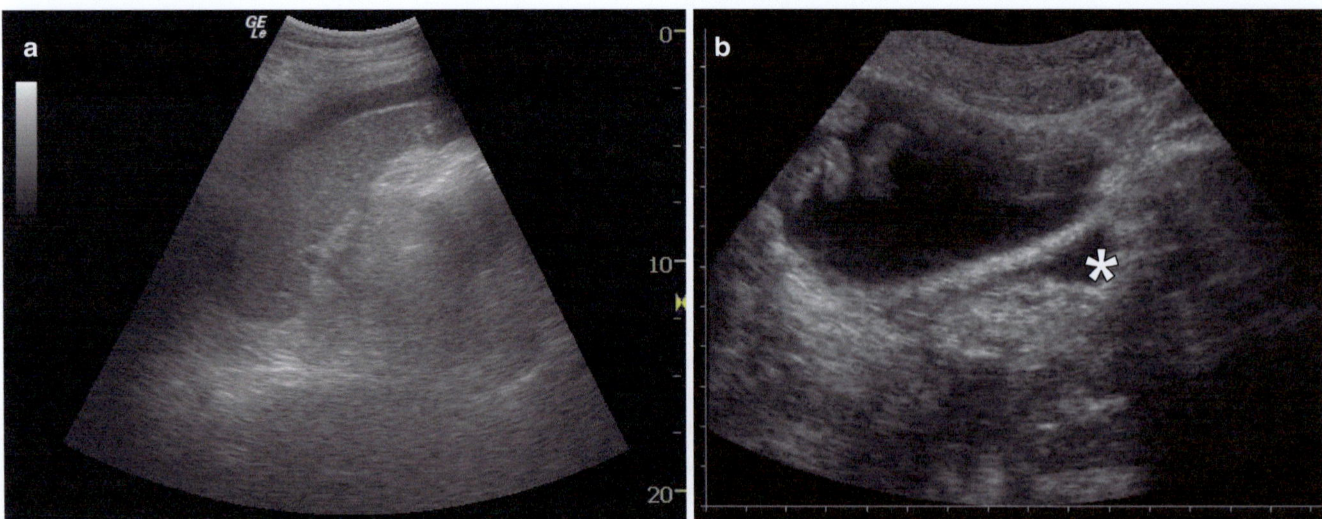

Fig. 6.10 (**a**) Left upper quadrant abdominal scan showing subdiaphragmatic/perisplenic fluid (anechoic). (**b**) Pelvic scan with a large fluid collection; bowel loops can be seen floating inside the free fluid collection (floating gut sign). The asterisk marks an almost empty urinary bladder

The eye scan with a linear or microconvex probe constitutes a valid screening tool able to confirm an increase in ICP through the measurement of the proximal optic nerve.

The optic nerve head belongs anatomically to the central nervous system, and it is invested by the three meningeal sheaths in which the cerebrospinal fluid flows; therefore any increase in intracranial pressure (ICP) will be transmitted at the optic nerve level, determining an increase in the diameter of the optic disc (papilledema).

In order to perform this type of ultrasound, trans-palpebral scans should be acquired paying attention to exert the lowest possible pressure as not to cause reflex bradycardia.

Generally, diameters >5 mm (depending on scan technique) are pathological in adults and children older than 4 years with an accuracy of 95% [44, 45] (Fig. 6.11).

Of course, this echographic evaluation of the optic nerve as an indirect, qualitative index of increased ICP should be confirmed as soon as possible with a brain CT scan that is still the gold standard in this field.

Another relatively new application is the use of ultrasound in the determination of pupillary diameter in patients with massive head trauma and with periorbital edema or blood collections that impede the palpebral movements preventing the direct eye visualization and the exclusion of possible pupillary asymmetry [46] (Fig. 6.12).

Using the same scan, it is possible to see the anterior eye chamber, the lens, and the posterior chamber. In the event of facial trauma, it's feasible to rapidly demonstrate anterior chamber collapse, dislocation of the lens, vitreous bleeding, or the presence of retrobulbar air. It generates comet-tail artifacts similar to those seen in the lungs, which will impede and complicate the optic nerve visualization. This finding orients toward an orbital bone fracture that must be carefully evaluated (Fig. 6.13).

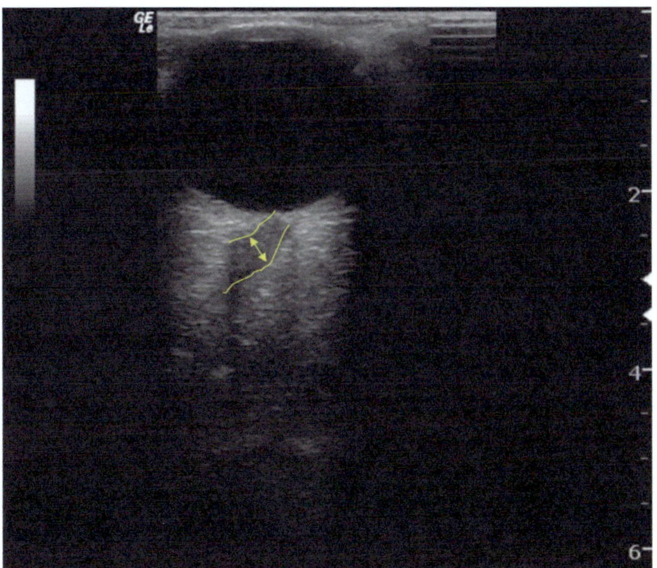

Fig. 6.11 Transverse scan, tangential to the eyeball (linear probe), allows optic nerve localization (yellow lines) and the evaluation of its diameter (yellow arrow)

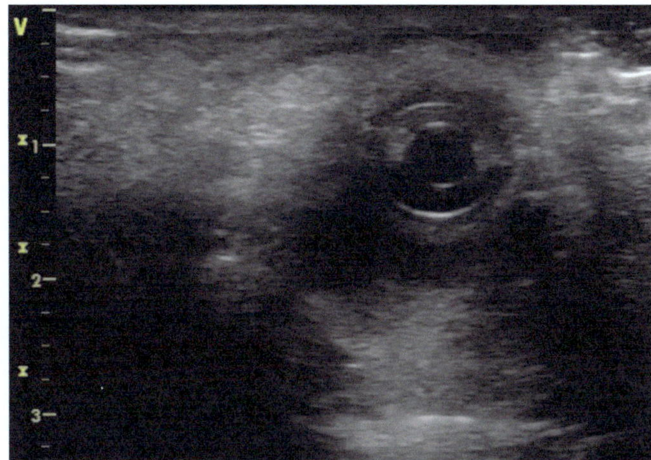

Fig. 6.12 Transverse scan of the eyeball using a linear probe; it helps in determining pupillary diameter and reactivity with the eyes closed (bilateral periorbital hematomas)

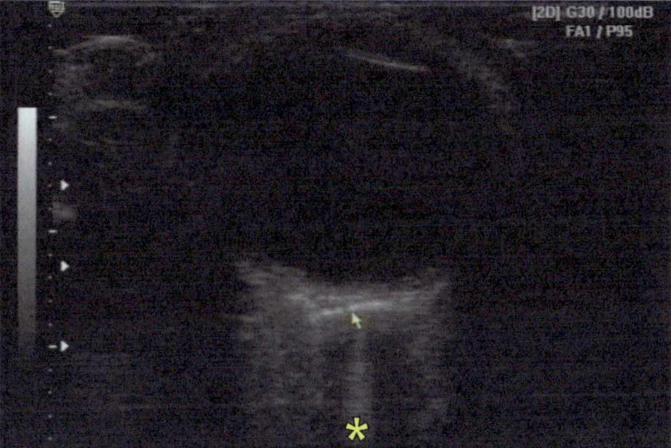

Fig. 6.13 Transverse ocular scan performed with a linear probe. The retrobulbar area (arrow) is hyperechoic due to the presence of air that generates a comet-tail artifact (yellow asterisk). Courtesy of M. Blaivas

The managerial and diagnostic impact of this technique on emergency services will be the avoidance of "over-" and "under-triage" of eye problems, possibly generated by the sole external eye evaluation; the aid given by ultrasound allows to appropriately direct the timing of the ophthalmologic evaluation (urgent or deferred) [47].

6.3.5 Exposure

In this phase, after the lifesaving stabilization of vital parameters, it is possible to reassess, using the ABCDE steps, all the findings that emerged during the primary evaluation, combining the clinical evaluation with a longer and more accurate PoCUS exam. The goal is to perform a complete assessment, to integrate anamnestic and clinical data with a more precise echographic evaluation of every district of the body, searching for new elements not diagnosed during the primary evaluation and timely recognizing emerging complications.

It is important to specify that, in front a stable and transportable patient, it is mandatory to always refer to the diagnostic gold-standard exam (e.g., CT, MRI, angiography, etc.) and to consult the appropriate specialists in relation to the ongoing clinical problem.

We report a couple of examples that clearly point to the importance of "exposure" phase.

In the exposure phase after a trauma, lesions at the level of limbs or joints become more evident; using a linear probe, integrating longitudinal and transverse scans, it is possible to demonstrate bone fractures. A fracture appears as an abrupt interruption of the hyperechoic cortical portion of the bone; a gap between the two residual bone fragments is visible, and usually, a hypoechoic collection of the surrounding muscles is present (hematoma) [48] (Fig. 6.14).

This approach allows diagnosing fractures of the long bones without transporting the patient, preventing a delayed discovery that might cause a potential "C problem" (hemorrhage), granting, therefore, a more specific and accurate management of a patient in the "exposure phase," such as the presence of air in the peritoneal cavity which, in the absence of a penetrating injury, points to perforation of a hollow viscus.

In the supine position, air tends to localize in ventral and cranial areas of the body and has to be searched in the contact zones between the diaphragm and the liver or spleen. In the event of a perforation, hyperechoic comet-tail artifacts will be present preventing the visualization of the underlying parenchyma of the liver and spleen.

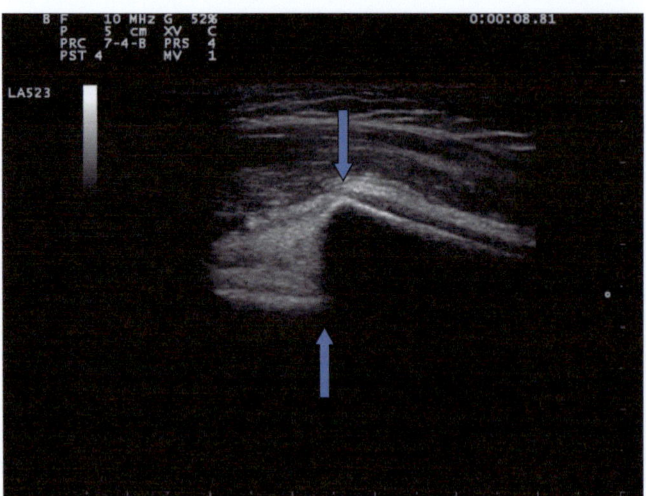

Fig. 6.14 Longitudinal scan performed with a linear probe at the level of the right humeral diaphysis. The gap between the two linear hyperechoic structures representing the bone fragments (blue arrows) is clearly visible

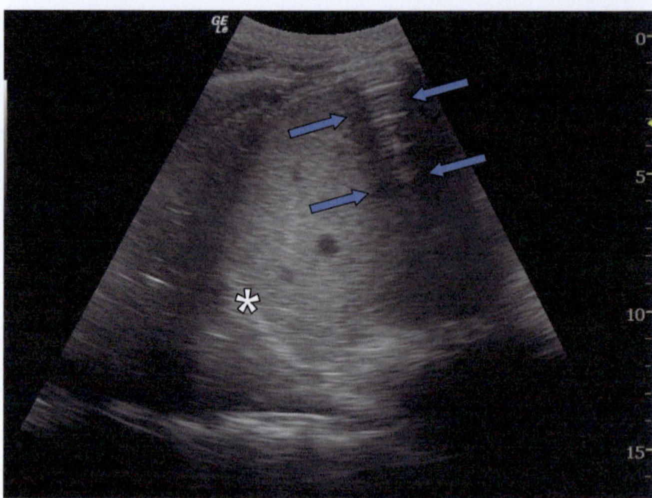

Fig. 6.15 Longitudinal scan (convex probe) of the thoracoabdominal area at the level of the anterior axillary line. The diaphragm is indicated by the white asterisk; blue arrows point to the comet-tail artifact generated by the presence of intraperitoneal air that prevents the visualization of the hepatic parenchyma

By changing the patient's decubitus (when not contraindicated) to a lateral position, air will move up to the opposite side, with a consensual shift of the artifact location [49] (Fig. 6.15).

6.4 PoCUS Use in Invasive Procedures

In the last few years, one of the applications in which real-time bedside ultrasound established its supremacy, is the field of invasive procedures.

As mentioned before, the concept of PoCUS is based on multiple-organ evaluation in order to simplify complex diagnoses in time-dependent situations.

In these circumstances, the necessity to rapidly perform invasive procedures on patients with many comorbidities and taking many medications, even when performed by expert physicians, determines an elevated rate of failure or complication, potentially causing iatrogenic damage [50].

The use of ultrasound as a guide before and during an invasive maneuver has given the physician a higher level of confidence in many applications like the positioning of central venous catheters, tracheotomy, pericardiocentesis, paracentesis, abscess drainage, etc.

An extensive discussion on all the possible ultrasound-guided procedures is beyond the purpose of this chapter; however, a brief explanation of the potential benefits of two of the most commonly performed procedures (chest drainage and vascular access) will be made.

During the primary assessment of a trauma patient, PNX and massive hemothorax with active bleeding might be a potential cause of death, if not promptly identified.

Regarding hemothorax, it is possible to use an approach similar to the one utilized for PNX: real-time rule-in and rule-out together with bedside monitoring of its progression or regression can be performed.

Once the effusion is identified as a hypoechoic space and is quantified using as a parameter its cranio-caudal and dorsal extension, it is possible to precisely determine the distance between the two pleural sheets using a transverse thoracic scan [51].

The intrapleural distance allows to easily evaluate the effusion's size and progression, unequivocally quantifying the distance between the lung and the thoracic wall (Fig. 6.16).

This measure, together with the detection of the diaphragm position, allows to better define the indication for the insertion of a chest drainage, the proper insertion site, and the best procedure timing according to the diagnostic and therapeutic strategy in place.

Another growing field of interest is the ultrasound-guided positioning of central venous catheters (CVC). Percutaneous insertion of CVC is a routinely, rapid, and minimally invasive procedure; unfortunately, when performed without a "visual guidance," this procedure still bears some alarming complications (e.g., carotid puncture, PNX) that can endanger the life of the patient and that can, in the end, prolong the hospital stay.

Ultrasound-guided CVC insertion shows numerous advantages with respect to the old "blind" technique based only on anatomical criteria.

Using US during the procedure allows the precise localization of the vessel in relation to the skin and surrounding structures (e.g., the lung or other vessels), the estimation of its diameter, and the confirmation of the patency of the lumen, and, moreover, it allows to directly visualize the needle during insertion and to follow the progression of the guide wire in longitudinal scans (Fig. 6.17).

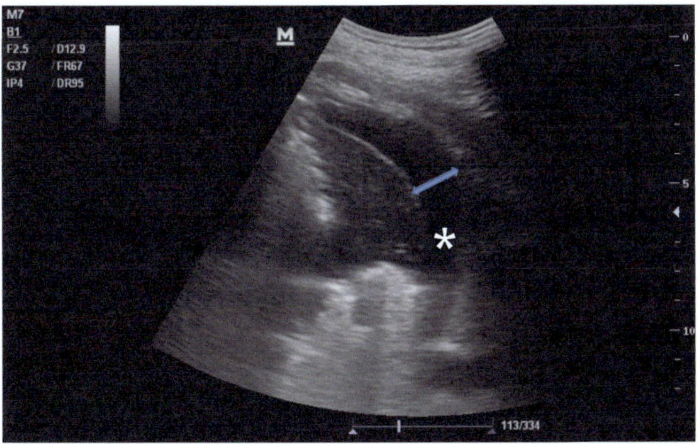

Fig. 6.16 Transverse right supradiaphragmatic scan at the level of the midaxillary line. White asterisk shows the pleural effusion. Blue arrow identifies the intrapleural distance that, by referring to the graduated scale on the right part of the image, can be estimated to be 2 cm wide

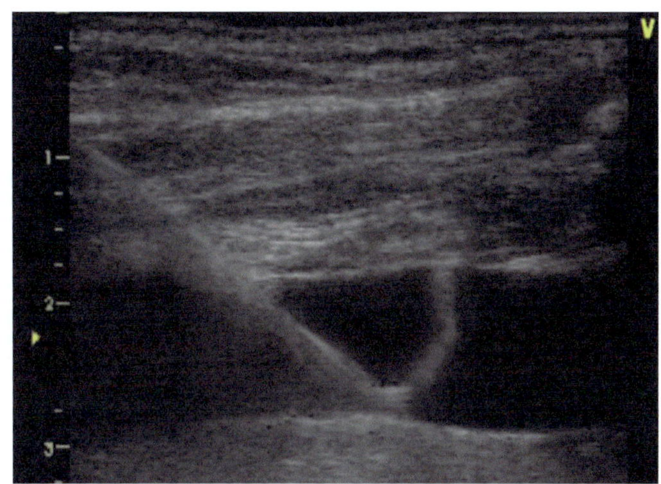

Fig. 6.17 Longitudinal scan (linear probe) of the right internal jugular vein. It is possible to appreciate, inside the vessel lumen, the presence of the guide wire during US-guided incannulation (Seldinger technique)

After an adequate training, the use of US-guided insertion both for the internal jugular vein and the subclavian vein allows to reduce the failure rate (up to 60% reduction), to reduce the mean time needed for a correct cannulation (up to 80% reduction), and to reduce the number of attempts to puncture (by a half).

With this visual approach, the procedure-related complications drop (PNX decreased by 80%), and, if those happen, they can be easily recognized and promptly treated.

The advantages of this method are best demonstrated in those complicated cases in which the blind technique alone could have a very high rate of failures like anatomical variants, obesity, burns, radiotherapy sequelae, venous thrombosis, or limited experience of the operator [52–56].

Considerable advantages have also been shown in the pediatric/neonatal field where the procedure appears to be safer because it rapidly allows confirming, with precise measurement, the compatibility between the catheter caliber and the vessel diameter [57–59].

By adding a brief training in the use of US to the on-field experience, the physicians will gain a level of confidence and safety that could not be achievable with the blind technique only.

It's possible to conclude that PoCUS use during primary and secondary critical patients' evaluation allows to rapidly indicate to perform an invasive procedure, to assess the difficulty level, to guide or assist during the procedure, to verify its effectiveness, and to demonstrate in real time the possible intra- and post-procedural complications.

6.5 Patients' Monitoring

We have illustrated the many useful applications of PoCUS in emergency situations; in the emergency setting of the ER, PoCUS has the purpose of better evaluating unstable patients allowing a fast definition of the patient's clinical picture and related diagnostic pathway. The emergency ultrasonographic ABCDE approach is fundamental in order to obtain control over a life-threatening situation, but, in the context of critical care medicine, it is also of prominent importance to perform regular reevaluations of the patients' condition in order to better direct the subsequent management.

After the stabilization of critical patients in the context of the ER, PoCUS is undoubtedly suitable also for the continuous reassessment and seriate evaluation of critical and potentially unstable patients, like the ones admitted in ICU. Having learned the basic applications of US in emergency situations, it is possible to transfer, with even more feasibility because of the absence of a specific time constraint, the stepwise US approach in the repeated monitoring of the patients' in ICU.

As a matter of fact, "good monitoring should assess relevant variables, provide interpretable data, be easy to implement, and not cause harm. The ideal monitoring should be reliable, continuous, noninvasive, operator-independent and cost-effective, and should have a fast response time" [60].

PoCUS, integrated with the clinical signs and symptoms and with laboratory studies, can, therefore, be used as an instrument to keep track of the changes in the patient's clinical picture and can be used as a valid instrument to monitor the patient's status.

Doctors working in ICU will, therefore, benefit from the dynamic, flexible, and bedside purpose that PoCUS will provide, gaining a full and integrated view of the problems that they will have to face.

As anticipated before, the fundamental premise to ultrasound use as a monitoring tool in the ICU is a specific training that has to ensure the right set of skills and the proper minimal requirements in order to grant a comprehensive and multi-organ echographic evaluation.

An analytical description of the many validated applications for ultrasound monitoring could not be thoroughly performed in this chapter.

To better perceive the added value that PoCUS could have in ICU as an integrated part of the patients' clinical evaluation and monitoring, the most common situations that could benefit from this innovative approach will be presented.

Intubation maneuvers and rapid checking of the ETT position are among the most common ICU necessities.

Through simple scans of the neck and thorax using a linear probe, it is possible to assess the correct position of the ETT above the carina, excluding an esophageal intubation. The visualization of the virtual lumen of the esophagus, not occupied by the tube, allows to confirm indirectly the correct tracheal intubation concomitantly with the presence of bilateral pleural sliding (symmetrical ventilation with the tip of the ETT above the carina) or the presence of lung pulse in one hemithorax (selective homolateral lung intubation).

The use of lung US has radically changed the approach to diagnostic imaging in ICU with particular advantage for those patients that present highly complex pictures that could prevent intrahospital transfer to a radiology department.

Ultrasound also allows a bedside dynamic lung assessment, a decisive part in the evaluation of the resistive characteristics of the tissue and its interaction with the ventilator.

The use of ultrasound grants a bedside dynamic vision of the state of the lungs allowing the physician to follow the evolution in time of a particular lung condition; with a peculiar focus on the densitometric lung tissue characteristics, the operator can clearly identify a dry lung (A pattern), a wet lung (B pattern), or a consolidated/non-ventilated lung (C pattern).

The seriate ultrasound monitoring of consolidated areas, regardless of blood gas analysis that can sometimes be of non-univocal interpretation, grants the possibility to effectively document and quantify the degree of lung reopening; this process is represented by the transition from a C pattern to an A or B pattern (Fig. 6.18) [61].

The evolution of consolidated areas generated by infectious pathologies (i.e., pneumonia) could be equally observed in relation to the real effectiveness of antibiotic therapy performed adding a consistent bedside indicator to be evaluated in order to maintain or modify antibiotic therapy (Table 6.2).

All the applications explained above converge into the ultimate goal to measure lung aeration, which allows to follow the evolution of various lung pathologies and to adjust mechanical ventilation (Fig. 6.19).

Until recently, the quantitative analysis of thoracic CT scans has been the only way to assess lung aeration; in recent years, ultrasound was used to dynamically monitor the changes in lung aeration using ultrasonographic aeration scores. It has been found that those scores are correlated with CT-measured fractional pulmonary tissue volume [62, 63] (Fig. 6.20).

Among the many possible applications, one of the most useful in the ICU setting, as described above, is the possibility to observe in real time how the lungs will respond to a change in the settings of a mechanical ventilator (plateau pressure, tidal volume, peep level, etc.) and recruiting maneuvers (i.e., prono-supination).

With lung US, the clinicians, for example, can evaluate the hemodynamic impact of the recruiting maneuvers assessing the effects exerted by the progressive increase of insufflation pressures on the venous return by simply monitoring the dimensions of IVC and cardiac chambers.

Lung US can also be used to evaluate the likelihood of a successful weaning from the mechanical ventilator.

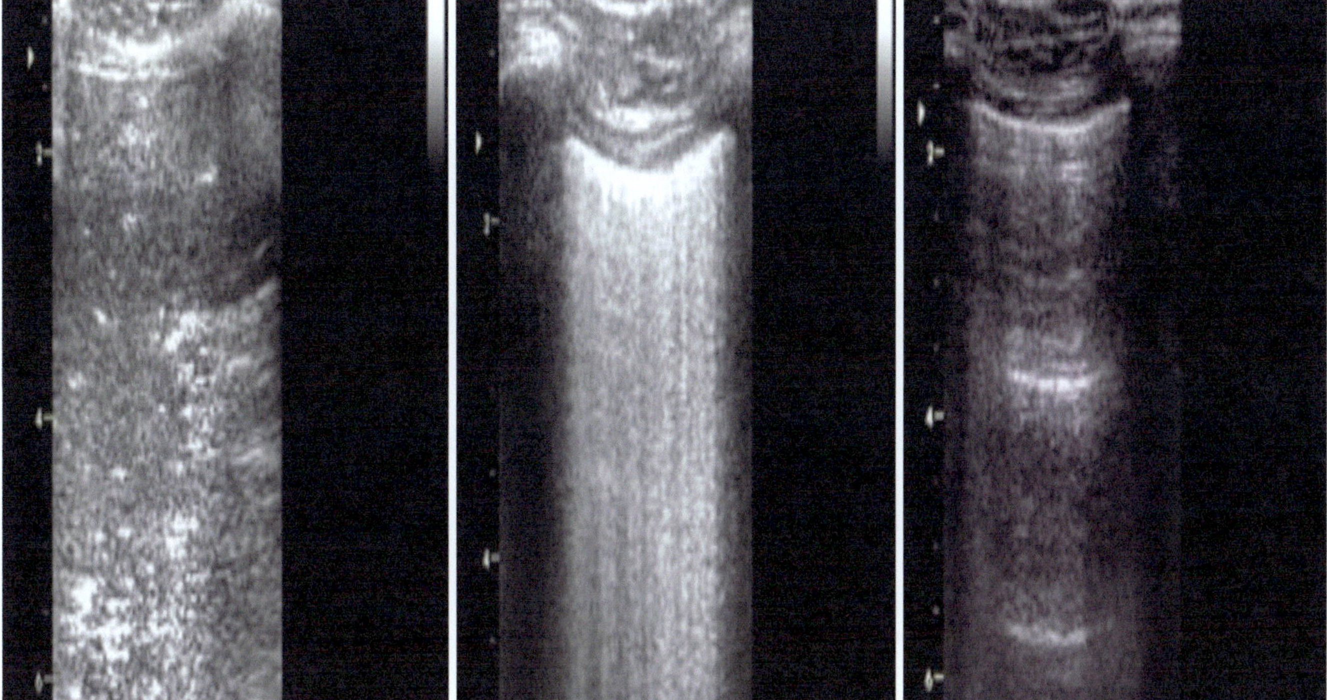

Fig. 6.18 Longitudinal thoracic scans (linear probe) of the same lung area of a single patient. The picture shows the progressive lung reaeration demonstrated by a gradual evolution from a consolidation pattern to a normal pattern with A lines, indicating the effective reaeration of the explored area

Table 6.2 Lung ultrasound reaeration score aimed at evaluating the effects of antibiotics on lung aeration

Quantification of reaeration			Quantification of loss of aeration		
1 point	3 points	5 points	−5 points	−3 points	−1 point
B1 → N	B2 → N	C → N	N → C	N → B2	N → B1
B2 → B1	C → B1			B1 → C	B1 → B2
C → B2					B2 → C

With the lung aeration score, it is possible to objectively quantify the degree of lung aeration based on ultrasound findings

N, normal pattern, *B1* well-defined and irregularly spaced B lines, *B2* coalescent B lines, *C* alveolar consolidation

This score can be used as a dynamic monitoring tool suitable for periodic reevaluations and for assessing the efficacy of the therapeutic actions put in place (e.g., antibiotic therapy)

Adapted from Bouhemad B, Brisson H, Le-Guen M, Arbelot C, Lu Q, Rouby J-J. Ultrasound assessment of antibiotic-induced pulmonary reaeration in ventilator-associated pneumonia. Crit Care Med. 2010 Jan;38(1):84–92

Predicting post-extubation distress is a major issue in critically ill patients. The possibility to observe in real time the tendency to lung deflation and toward the development of a wet lung (B pattern), during the progressive reduction of ventilatory support, from CPAP to spontaneous breathing trials, orients consistently toward a safe extubation, thereby reducing premature reintubations [64].

Furthermore, ultrasonographic assessment of the diaphragm thickening fraction is a noninvasive method that may prove useful in evaluating the diaphragmatic function and its contribution to respiratory workload in intensive care unit patients.

Ultrasound can be used to determine diaphragm excursion, which may help to identify patients with diaphragm dysfunction. Ultrasonographic examination can also allow for the direct visualization of the diaphragm thickness in its zone of apposition. Thickening of the diaphragm has been proposed to reflect the magnitude of diaphragmatic effort, similarly to an ejection fraction of the heart.

Diaphragm thickness may be measured in the zone of apposition during tidal ventilation, and the thickening fraction (TF) can be calculated as (thickness at inspiration − thickness at expiration)/thickness at expiration.

Diaphragmatic thickening fraction can be used as an index of diaphragmatic efficiency as a pressure generator.

One useful application of diaphragm US is to help in predicting a failure of the weaning from the mechanical ventilator; it has been shown that patients that present diaphragmatic dysfunction at US showed frequent early and delayed weaning failures [65–67].

Even with these brief exemplifications of some lung PoCUS uses, it is possible to understand how this rapid, bedside, replicable, and noninvasive evaluation is useful to follow the evolution of a parenchymal consolidation, pneumonia, or atelectasis, monitoring the response to therapy or the progression toward a more complicated picture.

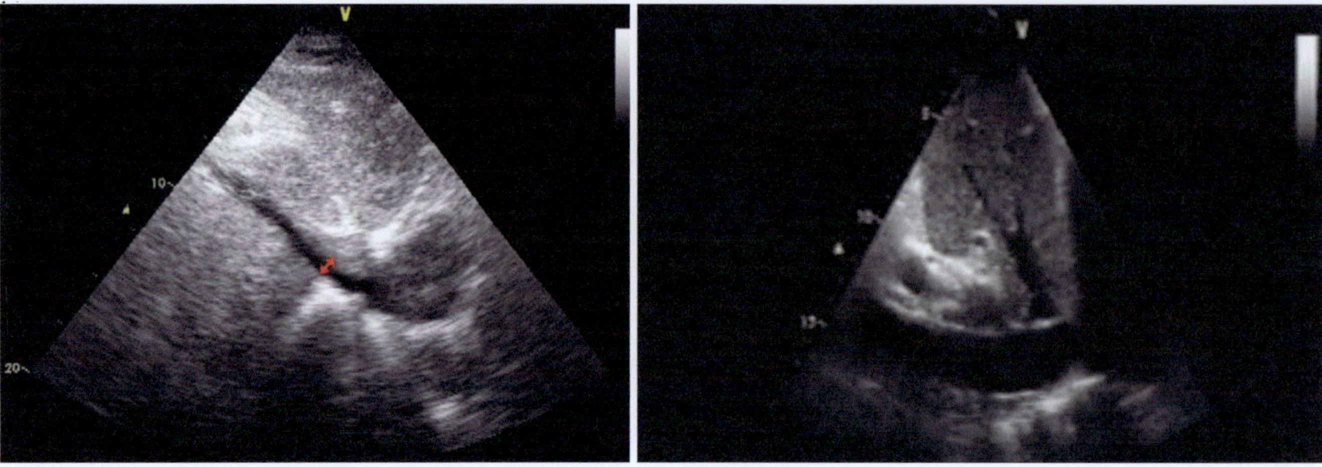

Fig. 6.19 Subxiphoid longitudinal window. It allows to easily visualize IVC. On the left the IVC in a hypovolemic patient is totally collapsed; on the right is shown IVC in a hypervolemic condition

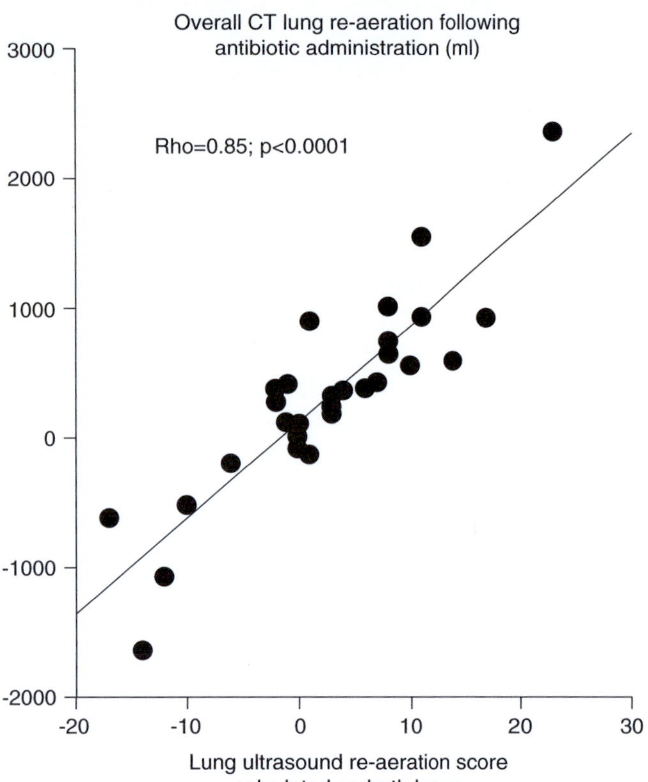

Fig. 6.20 The table shows the positive correlation between ultrasound lung aeration score and the CT-measured lung aeration. Adapted from Bouhemad B, Brisson H, Le-Guen M, Arbelot C, Lu Q, Rouby J-J. Ultrasound assessment of antibiotic-induced pulmonary reaeration in ventilator-associated pneumonia. Crit Care Med. 2010 Jan;38(1):84–92

It is also possible to assess, through simple scans, the hemodynamic status of the patient in relation to the treatment performed.

After having controlled and stabilized a massive hemorrhage, it is important to keep track of the volemic state of the patient and to check, with seriate evaluations, the presence of residual bleeding allowing a rapid intervention in case of recurrence. This approach will be particularly useful in those patients with blunt abdominal trauma in which a nonoperative management (NOM) was chosen and in which repeated reassessment would be necessary.

Having a constant awareness of the hemodynamic status of a patient is especially important in the context of ICU where fluid administration has to be carefully evaluated and titrated.

An integrated use of bedside US is relevant in this circumstance because, through the visualization of the IVC diameters and collapsibility and through the assessment of the heart kinetics and the visualization of the lung water content, it assists the clinicians in performing safe corrections of the patient's volemia.

Of particular interest is the possibility to integrate the vital parameters of spontaneously breathing patients with an indirect estimate of the central venous pressure; with the evaluation of the diameter and collapsibility of the inferior vena cava during inspiration, it is possible to evaluate the CVP and to correlate this finding with the volemic status of the patient and with the diuretic or rehydrating therapy.

For example, an IVC < 15 mm (in spontaneous ventilation) with an evident inspiratory collapse, especially if associated with a small and hyperkinetic right ventricle, is unequivocally sign of hypovolemia (low CVP); an IVC > 20 mm, which shows no collapse during inspiration, with diffuse B lines identified with a lung ultrasound, points clearly to a condition of hypervolemia (high CVP).

When indicated and purely as guidance, it is possible to calculate the caval index (CI), which allows to quantitatively indicate the need for fluid therapy [CI = (IVC-exp diameter − IVC insp diameter)/(IVC-exp diameter) * 100]. A CI >50% strongly suggests fluid responsiveness (Table 6.3).

Table 6.3 Correlation between RA pressure (CVP) and IVC appearance

CVP (cm H2O)	Inspiratory IVC collapse (%)	IVC diameter (cm)
0–5	100	<1.5
5–10	>50	1.5–2.5
11–15	<50	1.5–2.5
16–20	<50	>2.5
>20	0	>2.5

The table shows the correlation between right atrial pressure and the inferior vena cava diameter and collapsibility assessed with ultrasound *Feissel M, Michard F, Faller JP, Teboul JL. The respiratory variation in inferior vena cava diameter as a guide to fluid therapy. Intensive Care Med 2004;30:1834–7*
Harshitha Sridhar, Pavan Mangalore, V. P. Chandrasekaran, and Rishya Manikam, "Caval Aorta Index and Central Venous Pressure Correlation in Assessing Fluid Status! "Ultrasound Bridging the Gap"," *ISRN Emergency Medicine, vol. 2012, Article ID 828626, 5 pages, 2012.* doi:https://doi.org/10.5402/2012/828626

In mechanically ventilated patients, the effect exerted by the positive pressure on venous return has to be considered; during inspiration there will be an increase in intrathoracic pressure that will be transmitted to the right atrium, thereby squeezing blood from the thorax to the abdomen. Therefore, the dynamic variation of the IVC diameter will be reversed, showing an increased diameter during inspiratory phase and a decreased one in expiratory. As in spontaneous breathing, these variations tend to disappear in hypervolemic conditions [68].

Similarly, to the aforementioned description of the IVC evaluation in spontaneously breathing patients, in mechanically ventilated patients, given the reversed thoracic pressure dynamic, it is possible to calculate the distensibility index (DI) of the vena cava. [DI = (maxIVC − minIVC)/minIVC] where a DI <18% indicates that the patient is unlikely to benefit from fluid bolus.

In emergency situations, the evaluation of these indexes can be performed using the same qualitative approach applied for the evaluation of the global heart function; these parameters can be estimated through a rapid visual assessment rather than a precise calculation, leaving the quantitative rigorous evaluations for hemodynamically stable patients in order to keep an effective management in time-dependent patients.

In the ICU setting, both an excessive use of inotropic and/or vasoconstrictor drugs and the maintenance of a long-lasting hemodynamic supportive therapy are frequent events.

The revaluation of the patients' hemodynamic status after the beginning and adjustments of therapy with amines (i.e., noradrenaline, dobutamine) allows to directly evaluate both the desired and undesired effects.

Moreover, whenever it is essential to infuse high doses of vasoactive and/or inotropic drugs, it is essential to constantly consider the effects of drug doses on the mechanical heart function in order to administer the lower effective dose, thereby reducing undesired complications.

One practical example occurs in the septic, hypotensive patients. After a primary emergency evaluation, usually performed in the emergency department, an excellent systolic heart function is frequently observed, with an ejection fraction >60–65%. Lower peripheral resistances, a consequence of the vasodilation induced by sepsis, cause an overestimation of the systolic heart function. After the beginning of the treatment with noradrenaline, a sudden worsening of heart function that requires treatment with an inotropic drug like dobutamine is frequently observed; this is due to a normalization of the afterload revealing a contractile dysfunction that was usually present from the beginning but was masked by peripheral vasodilation.

A simple global evaluation of the kinetic properties of the heart chambers obtained during amine dose titrations, together with the evaluation on the IVC diameters and with the appearance/reduction of cardiogenic pulmonary edema (bilateral diffused B pattern), allows to choose the best possible drug and to obtain a dose optimization without an invasive hemodynamic monitoring that is usually not easy to timely put in place especially in the first and most delicate phases of septic shock [69–71].

It has been demonstrated that the integration of US in a stepwise approach to the patient's status is capable of reducing the number of differential diagnoses in the physician's head and of simplifying the decisional process and the therapeutic strategy [72].

In this way the physician can promptly adjust the management in relation to the evolving clinical conditions, being able to anticipate potential detrimental evolution of the clinical picture.

Following the precise PoCUS rules, the clinicians will gain confidence with a valuable tool to perform periodical reevaluations, thereby identifying the variations of the clinical picture, keeping a constant surveillance on the evolution of the patient's status toward a positive or negative outcome.

At the end of this description of the prominent aspects and more recent uses of PoCUS, it is possible to conclude that the introduction of a rigorous algorithm, which is able to identify potentially lethal conditions through a rapid, simple, intuitive, and systematic sequence, constitutes the prerogative for a correct management of unstable patients.

Given the spread of the PoCUS use, guidelines regarding the use of US by non-radiologists were created, and many educational programs were successfully developed in order to effectively teach the use of this technique to different specialists [73–75].

Only through an internationally shared definition of the minimal requirements needed by physicians and through constant updating and research on modern and growing applications of US it will be possible to promote and guarantee a higher level and comprehensive development of PoCUS in critical care medicine [9].

References

1. Spevack DM, Spevack DM, Tunick PA, Kronzon I. Hand carried echocardiography in the critical care setting. Echocardiography. 2003;20(5):455–61.
2. Martin LD, Howell EE, Ziegelstein RC, Martire C, Whiting-O'Keefe QE, Shapiro EP, et al. Hand-carried ultrasound performed by hospitalists: does it improve the cardiac physical examination? Am J Med. 2009;122(1):35–41.
3. Vignon P, Chastagner C, François B, Martaillé J-F, Normand S, Bonnivard M, et al. Diagnostic ability of hand-held echocardiography in ventilated critically ill patients. Crit Care. 2003;7(5):R84–91.
4. Gillman L, Kirkpatrick A. Portable bedside ultrasound: the visual stethoscope of the 21st century. Scand J Trauma Resusc Emerg Med. 2012;20:18.
5. Wittenberg M. Will ultrasound scanners replace the stethoscope? BMJ. 2014;3463:1–3.
6. Scalea T, Rodriguez A, Chiu W. Focused Assessment with Sonography for Trauma (FAST): results from an international consensus conference. J Trauma. 1999;46(3):466–72.
7. Kirkpatrick W, Sirois M, Laupland K, Liu D, Rowan K, Ball C, et al. Hand-held thoracic sonography for detecting post-traumatic pneumothoraces: the extended focused assessment with sonography for trauma (EFAST). J Trauma. 2004;57(2):288–95.
8. Lichtenstein DA. Lung ultrasound in the critically ill. Ann Intensive Care. 2014;4(1):1.
9. Neri L, Storti E, Lichtenstein D. Toward an ultrasound curriculum for critical care medicine. Crit Care Med. 2007;35(5 Suppl):S290–304.
10. Frerk C, Mitchell VS, McNarry AF, Mendonca C, Bhagrath R, Patel A, et al. Difficult Airway Society 2015 guidelines for management of unanticipated difficult intubation in adults. Br J Anaesth. 2015;115(6):827–48. Oxford University Press.
11. Kristensen MS, Teoh WH, Rudolph SS, Tvede MF, Hesselfeldt R, Børglum J, et al. Structured approach to ultrasound-guided identification of the cricothyroid membrane: a randomized comparison with the palpation method in the morbidly obese. Br J Anaesth. 2015;114(6):1003–4.
12. Dinsmore J, Heard AM, Green RJ. The use of ultrasound to guide time-critical cannula tracheotomy when anterior neck airway anatomy is unidentifiable. Eur J Anaesthesiol. 2011;28(7):506–10.
13. Das SK, Choupoo NS, Haldar R, Lahkar A. Transtracheal ultrasound for verification of endotracheal tube placement: a systematic review and meta-analysis. Can J Anesth. 2015;62(4):413–23.
14. Chou H-C, Tseng W-P, Wang C-H, Ma MH-M, Wang H-P, Huang P-C, et al. Tracheal rapid ultrasound exam (T.R.U.E.) for confirming endotracheal tube placement during emergency intubation. Resuscitation. 2011;82(10):1279–84.
15. Chou EH, Dickman E, Tsou P-Y, Tessaro M, Tsai Y-M, Ma MH-M, et al. Ultrasonography for confirmation of endotracheal tube placement: a systematic review and meta-analysis. Resuscitation. 2015;90:97–103.
16. Gottlieb M, Bailitz J. Can transtracheal ultrasonography be used to verify endotracheal tube placement? Ann Emerg Med. 2015;66(4):394–5.
17. Chun R, Kirkpatrick AW, Sirois M, Sargasyn AE, Melton S, Hamilton DR, et al. Where's the tube? Evaluation of hand-held ultrasound in confirming endotracheal tube placement. Prehosp Disaster Med. 2004;19(4):366–9.
18. Lichtenstein DA, Lascols N, Prin S, Mezire G. The "lung pulse": an early ultrasound sign of complete atelectasis. Intensive Care Med. 2003;29(12):2187–92.
19. Saporito A, Lo Piccolo A, Franceschini D, Tomasetti R, Anselmi L. Thoracic ultrasound confirmation of correct lung exclusion before one-lung ventilation during thoracic surgery. J Ultrasound. 2013;16(4):195–9.
20. Ramsingh D, Frank E, Haughton R, Schilling J, Gimenez KM, Banh E, et al. Auscultation versus point-of-care ultrasound to determine endotracheal versus bronchial intubation. Anesthesiology. 2016;124(5):1012–20.
21. Lichtenstein D. General ultrasound in the critically ill. Springer; 2005. 199 p.
22. Volpicelli G, Elbarbary M, Blaivas M, Lichtenstein DA, Mathis G, Kirkpatrick AW, et al. International evidence-based recommendations for point-of-care lung ultrasound. Intensive Care Med. 2012;38(4):577–91.
23. Picano E, Pellikka PA. Ultrasound of extravascular lung water: a new standard for pulmonary congestion. Eur Heart J. 2016;37(27):2097–104.
24. Lichtenstein D, Mezière G. A lung ultrasound sign allowing bedside distinction between pulmonary edema and COPD: the comet-tail artifact. Intensive Care Med. 1998;24(12):1331–4.
25. Dietrich CF, Mathis G, Blaivas M, Volpicelli G, Seibel A, Wastl D, et al. Lung B-line artefacts and their use. J Thorac Dis. 2016;8(6):1356–65.
26. Balik M, Plasil P, Waldauf P, Pazout J, Fric M, Otahal M, et al. Ultrasound estimation of volume of pleural fluid in mechanically ventilated patients. Intensive Care Med. 2006;32(2):318–21.
27. Cao W, Wang Y, Zhou N, Xu B. Efficacy of ultrasound-guided thoracentesis catheter drainage for pleural effusion. Oncol Lett. 2016;12(6):4445–8.
28. Moore C, Copel J. Point-of-care ultrasonography. N Engl J Med. 2011;364:749–58.
29. Alzahrani SA, Al-Salamah MA, Al-Madani WH, Elbarbary MA. Systematic review and meta-analysis for the use of ultrasound versus radiology in diagnosing of pneumonia. Crit Ultrasound J. 2017;9:6.
30. Lichtenstein D, Mezière G, Seitz J. The dynamic air bronchogram. Chest. 2009;135(6):1421–5. American College of Chest Physicians.
31. Lichtenstein D, Goldstein I, Mourgeon E, Cluzel P, Grenier P, Rouby J-J. Comparative diagnostic performances of auscultation, chest radiography, and lung ultrasonography in acute respiratory distress syndrome. Anesthesiology. 2004;100(1):9–15.
32. Copetti R, Soldati G, Copetti P. Chest sonography: a useful tool to differentiate acute cardiogenic pulmonary edema from acute respiratory distress syndrome. Cardiovasc Ultrasound. 2008;6(1):16.
33. Algieri I, Mongodi S, Chiumello D, Mojoli F, Cressoni M, Via G, et al. CT scan and ultrasound comparative assessment of PEEP-induced lung aeration changes in ARDS. Crit Care. 2014;18(Suppl 1):285.
34. Kimura BJ. Point-of-care cardiac ultrasound techniques in the physical examination: better at the bedside. Heart. 2017;103(13):987–94.
35. Ceriani E, Cogliati C. Update on bedside ultrasound diagnosis of pericardial effusion. Intern Emerg Med. 2016;11(3):477–80.
36. Connolly JA, Dean AJ, Hoffmann B, Jarman RD. Emergency point of care ultrasound. 2017. 488 p.
37. Blaivas M. Ultrasound in the detection of venous thromboembolism. Crit Care Med. 2007;35(5 Suppl):S224–34.
38. Jang T, Crisp J, Lovato L. Compression ultrasonography of the lower extremity with portable vascular ultrasonography can accurately detect deep venous thrombosis in the emergency department. Ann Emerg Med. 2010;56(6):601–10.
39. Pomero F, Dentali F, Borretta V, Bonzini M, Melchio R, Douketis JD, et al. Accuracy of emergency physician–performed ultrasonography in the diagnosis of deep-vein thrombosis. Thromb Haemost. 2012;109(1):137–45.
40. Branney SW, Moore EE, Cantrill SV, Burch JM, Terry SJ. Ultrasound based key clinical pathway reduces the use of hospital resources for the evaluation of blunt abdominal trauma. J Trauma. 1997;42(6):1086–90.
41. Coley BD, Mutabagani KH, Martin LC, Zumberge N, Cooney DR, Caniano DA, et al. Focused abdominal sonography for trauma

(FAST) in children with blunt abdominal trauma. J Trauma. 2000;48(5):902–6.
42. Holmes JF, Kelley KM, Wootton-Gorges SL, Utter GH, Abramson LP, Rose JS, et al. Effect of abdominal ultrasound on clinical care, outcomes, and resource use among children with blunt torso trauma. JAMA. 2017;317(22):2290. American Medical Association.
43. Natarajan B, Gupta PK, Cemaj S, Sorensen M, Hatzoudis GI, Forse RA. FAST scan: is it worth doing in hemodynamically stable blunt trauma patients? Surgery. 2010;148(4):695–701.
44. Raffiz M, Abdullah JM. Optic nerve sheath diameter measurement: a means of detecting raised ICP in adult traumatic and non-traumatic neurosurgical patients. Am J Emerg Med. 2017;35(1): 150–3.
45. Dubourg J, Javouhey E, Geeraerts T, Messerer M, Kassai B. Ultrasonography of optic nerve sheath diameter for detection of raised intracranial pressure: a systematic review and meta-analysis. Intensive Care Med. 2011;37(7):1059–68.
46. Chiao L, Sharipov S, Sargsyan AE, Melton S, Hamilton DR, Mcfarlin K, et al. Ocular examination for trauma; clinical ultrasound aboard the International Space Station. J Trauma. 2005;58: 885–9.
47. Blaivas M, Theodoro D, Sierzenski PR. A study of bedside ocular ultrasonography in the emergency department. Acad Emerg Med. 2002;9(8):791–9.
48. Weinberg ER, Tunik MG, Tsung JW. Accuracy of clinician-performed point-of-care ultrasound for the diagnosis of fractures in children and young adults. Injury. 2010;41(8):862–8.
49. Hoffmann B, Nürnberg D, Westergaard MC. Focus on abnormal air: diagnostic ultrasonography for the acute abdomen. Eur J Emerg Med. 2012;19(5):284–91.
50. Farcy DA, Chiu W, Marshall JP, Osborn TM. Critical care emergency medicine. 2nd ed. 688 p.
51. Krackov R, Rizzolo D. Real-time ultrasound-guided thoracentesis. J Am Acad Phys Assist. 2017;30(4):32–7.
52. Brass P, Hellmich M, Kolodziej L, Schick G, Smith AF. Ultrasound guidance versus anatomical landmarks for internal jugular vein catheterization. In: Brass P, editor. Cochrane Database of Systematic Reviews, vol. 1. Chichester: Wiley; 2015. p. CD006962.
53. Hind D, Calvert N, McWilliams R, Davidson A, Paisley S, Beverley C, et al. Ultrasonic locating devices for central venous cannulation: meta-analysis. BMJ. 2003;327(7411):361–0.
54. Stolz LA, Stolz U, Howe C, Farrell IJ, Adhikari S. Ultrasound-guided peripheral venous access: a meta-analysis and systematic review. J Vasc Access. 2015;16(4):321–6.
55. Reusz G, Csomos A. The role of ultrasound guidance for vascular access. Curr Opin Anaesthesiol. 2015;28(6):1.
56. Egan G, Healy D, O'Neill H, Clarke-Moloney M, Grace PA, Walsh SR. Ultrasound guidance for difficult peripheral venous access: systematic review and meta-analysis. Emerg Med J. 2013;30(7): 521–6.
57. Benkhadra M, Collignon M, Fournel I, Oeuvrard C, Rollin P, Perrin M, et al. Ultrasound guidance allows faster peripheral IV cannulation in children under 3 years of age with difficult venous access: a prospective randomized study. Pediatr Anesth. 2012;22(5): 449–54.
58. Aouad-Maroun M, Raphael CK, Sayyid SK, Farah F, Akl EA. Ultrasound-guided arterial cannulation for paediatrics. In: Aouad-Maroun M, editor. Cochrane Database of Systematic Reviews, vol. 9. Chichester: Wiley; 2016. p. CD011364.
59. Shime N, Hosokawa K, MacLaren G. Ultrasound imaging reduces failure rates of percutaneous central venous catheterization in children. Pediatr Crit Care Med. 2015;16(8):718–25.
60. Tobin M. Post graduate course on ICU monitoring. ATS Conference, San Diego; 2006.
61. Via G, Storti E, Gulati G, Neri L, Mojoli F, Braschi A, et al. Lung ultrasound in the ICU: from diagnostic instrument to respiratory monitoring tool. Minerva Anestesiol. 2012;78(11):1282–96. Agosto.
62. Bouhemad B, Brisson H, Le-Guen M, Arbelot C, Lu Q, Rouby J-J. Ultrasound assessment of antibiotic-induced pulmonary reaeration in ventilator-associated pneumonia. Crit Care Med. 2010;38(1):84–92.
63. Grondin Beaudoin B, Chartrand-Lefebvre C, Girard M. Comparison of four scores for ultrasound assessment of pulmonary aeration. Am J Respir Crit Care Med. 2016;193:A5156.
64. Mongodi S, Via G, Bouhemad B, Storti E, Mojoli F, Branchi A. Usefulness of combined bedside lung ultrasound and echocardiography to assess weaning failure from mechanical ventilation: a suggestive case. Crit Care Med. 2013;41(8):e182–5.
65. Mongodi S, Via G, Bouhemad B, Storti E, Mojoli F, Braschi A. Usefulness of combined bedside lung ultrasound and echocardiography to assess weaning failure from mechanical ventilation: A suggestive case. Crit Care Med. 2013;41(8):e182–5.
66. Umbrello M, Formenti P, Longhi D, Galimberti A, Piva I, Pezzi A, et al. Diaphragm ultrasound as indicator of respiratory effort in critically ill patients undergoing assisted mechanical ventilation: a pilot clinical study. Crit Care. 2015;19(1):161. BioMed Central.
67. Matamis D, Soilemezi E, Tsagourias M, Akoumianaki E, Dimassi S, Boroli F, et al. Sonographic evaluation of the diaphragm in critically ill patients. Technique and clinical applications. Intensive Care Med. 2013;39(5):801–10.
68. Kim WY, Suh HJ, Hong S-B, Koh Y, Lim C-M. Diaphragm dysfunction assessed by ultrasonography: influence on weaning from mechanical ventilation. Crit Care Med. 2011;39(12):2627–30.
69. Boyd JH, Sirounis D, Maizel J, Slama M. Echocardiography as a guide for fluid management. Crit Care. 2016;20(1):274. BioMed Central.
70. Barbier C, Loubires Y, Schmit C, Hayon J, Ricme J-L, Jardin F, et al. Respiratory changes in inferior vena cava diameter are helpful in predicting fluid responsiveness in ventilated septic patients. Intensive Care Med. 2004;30(9):1740–6.
71. Durairaj L, Schmidt GA. Fluid therapy in resuscitated sepsis. Chest. 2008;133(1):252–63.
72. Jones A, Tayal V, Sullivan M, Kline J. Randomized, controlled trial of immediate versus delayed goal-directed ultrasound to identify the cause of nontraumatic hypotension in emergency department patients. Crit Care Med. 2004;32:1703–8.
73. Cinel I, Nanda R, Dellinger RP. Cardiac dysfunction in septic shock. Berlin, Heidelberg: Springer; 2008. p. 43–54.
74. Kotagal M, Quiroga E, Ruffatto BJ, Adedipe AA, Backlund BH, Nathan R, et al. Impact of point-of-care ultrasound training on surgical residents' confidence. J Surg Educ. 2015;72(4):e82–7. NIH Public Access.
75. Killu K, Coba V, Mendez M, Reddy S, Adrzejewski T, Huang Y, et al. Model point-of-care ultrasound curriculum in an intensive care unit fellowship program and its impact on patient management. Crit Care Res Pract. 2014;2014:934796.

Part II

Trauma

Critical Care Resuscitation in Trauma Patients: Basic Principles and Evolving Frontiers

7

Cherisse Berry, Ronald Tesoriero, and Thomas Scalea

Key Points

- Hypovolemia secondary to uncontrolled hemorrhage is the most common cause of shock after injury.
- Endpoints of resuscitation including lactate, base deficit, and central venous oxygen saturation are key to developing an optimal resuscitation strategy.
- The primary objectives in the clinical management of shock are to stop hemorrhage, establish vascular access, restore circulating volume, and improve tissue oxygen delivery.
- The patient's response to initial fluid resuscitation is the key to determining subsequent therapy.
- The concept of permissive hypotension was developed to limit the volume of resuscitation administered to the bleeding trauma patient by targeting a lower than normal blood pressure to avoid exacerbating hemorrhage by hydrostatic clot disruption while maintaining adequate end-organ perfusion.
- Damage control surgery (DCS) involves rapid emergency department evaluation, followed by abbreviated laparotomy or thoracotomy.
- Damage control resuscitation (DCR) involves minimization of crystalloids, permissive hypotension, early use of plasma with transfusion of balanced ratio of blood products, and goal-directed correction of coagulopathy.
- Point-of-care functional tests such as thromboelastography (TEG) and rotational thromboelastometry (ROTEM) are being used more often for the diagnosis and management of patients with trauma-induced coagulopathy (TIC).
- Resuscitative endovascular balloon occlusion of the aorta (REBOA) has been pioneered as an alternative to ED thoracotomy when the indication is simply to cross-clamp the aorta with more favorable outcomes.

7.1 Introduction

Shock is the failure of the circulatory system to provide adequate tissue oxygenation and organ perfusion required to meet cellular metabolic demands [1]. The etiologies of shock include hypovolemic, obstructive, neurogenic, or distributive. In the trauma patient, shock is most commonly from bleeding. However, shock can be nonhemorrhagic such as blunt cardiac injury causing cardiogenic shock, cardiac tamponade and tension pneumothorax causing obstructive shock, delayed presentation of penetrating injury to the abdominal viscera with feculent peritonitis causing septic shock, and acute spinal cord injury causing neurogenic shock [1, 2].

Uncontrolled hemorrhage results in a decrease in cardiac output leading to inadequate oxygen delivery. At the level of the microcirculation, the cells compensate for a decrease in oxygen delivery by increasing oxygen extraction. However, when oxygen extraction can no longer meet cellular demand, a critical oxygen delivery point is met. This point reflects the transition from aerobic metabolism to anaerobic metabolism, resulting in the formation of lactic acid, metabolic acidosis, and cellular dysfunction leading to cellular dysfunction and ultimately cell death.

C. Berry · R. Tesoriero · T. Scalea (✉)
R Adams Cowley Shock Trauma Center, University of Maryland School of Medicine, Baltimore, MD, USA
e-mail: Cherisse.Berry@nyumc.org; rtesoriero@umm.edu; tscalea@umm.edu

P. Aseni et al. (eds.), *Operative Techniques and Recent Advances in Acute Care and Emergency Surgery*,
https://doi.org/10.1007/978-3-319-95114-0_7

Table 7.1 Estimated blood loss

	Class I	Class II	Class III	Class IV
Blood loss (mL)	Up to 750	750–1500	1500–2000	>2000
Blood loss (% blood volume)	Up to 15%	15–30%	30–40%	>40%
Pulse rate (BPM)	<100	100–120	120–140	>140
Systolic blood pressure	Normal	Normal	Decreased	Decreased
Pulse pressure (mmHg)	Normal or increased	Decreased	Decreased	Decreased
Respiratory rate	14–20	20–30	30–40	>35
Urine output (mL/h)	>30	20–30	5–15	Negligible
CNS/mental status	Slightly anxious	Mildly anxious	Anxious, confused	Confused, lethargic
Initial fluid replacement	Crystalloid	Crystalloid	Crystalloid and blood	Crystalloid and blood

Reproduced from ATLS [2], 9th Edition

7.2 Identifying Blood Loss

Hypovolemia secondary to uncontrolled hemorrhage is the most common cause of shock after injury [2]. As described by ATLS, hemorrhage is classified into four classes based on clinical signs at the patient's initial presentation (Table 7.1). This classification system allows for the estimation of acute blood loss, which can help guide intravenous fluid replacement or the administration of blood products [1]. Developing an optimal resuscitation strategy including type, quantity, and timing of fluid therapy is key to the resuscitation of the severely injured trauma patient [3].

While Table 7.1 can serve as a useful guide, it is important to remember that not every patient behaves according to these classes of hemorrhagic shock. Even if these were accurate, they are relatively nonspecific. Class I shock is almost completely undetectable. Measured vital signs are normal. While patients may be slightly anxious, many patients are anxious following injury. Thus, patients may lose 1.5 units of blood over a relatively short period of time, and this will be clinically undetectable.

Even patients with class II shock may be difficult to identify in the resuscitation bay. Again, vital signs are relatively normal. There may be some mild tachycardia, but heart rate like mental status is also nonspecific. Heart rate can be increased from anxiety as well as blood loss. Thus, patients may lose up to 3 units of blood and not exhibit obvious deterioration in their clinical status. By the time patients are obviously hemodynamically unstable, the blood loss is often close to 40% of the total circulating blood volume, a significant amount.

Other factors may impact the patients on presenting vital signs. Young patients have an extraordinary ability to compensate for acute blood loss. Their blood vessels are highly reactive, and they can develop profound vasoconstriction, preserving blood flow to the central organs and the brain. It is estimated that young people can lose in excess of 50% of their circulating blood volume before developing clinical signs. Unfortunately, these young patients often develop sudden and profound hemodynamic collapse when blood loss becomes symptomatic.

Conversely, older patients tolerate blood loss poorly and may develop signs of shock with a relatively small-volume blood loss. The use of beta-blockers may limit the older patients' ability to compensate for blood loss, as heart rate cannot increase. In addition, IV fluids given in the prehospital phase of care may allow patients to partially compensate for blood loss, even if it is of high volume. Thus, clinicians must be vigilant, repeatedly assess patients with high-risk mechanisms for blood loss, and not trust vital signs which may underestimate the volume of hemorrhage.

7.3 Estimating the Depth of Shock and Adequacy of Resuscitation

As normally measured vital signs often underestimate the depth of shock, other measures must be used to reliably estimate the degree of shock a patient may be in at the time of presentation. In order to be clinically useful, these parameters must be easy to measure and rapidly available and, ideally, may be measured in serial fashion to gauge response to stabilization efforts.

Base deficit (BD) is defined as the amount of base required to raise 1 L of whole blood to a normal pH. The degree of acidosis should estimate the degree of tissue hypoperfusion. Mutschler [4] evaluated 16,305 patients and stratified BD into four classes: class I (BD < 2 mmol/L), class I (BD > 2–6 mmol/L), class III (BD > 6–10 mmol/L), and class IV (BD > 10 mmol/L). They found that mortality, transfusion, and coagulopathy correlated in a linear way with increasing BD classification. In addition, Davis et al. [5] have demonstrated that BD correlates with 24-h transfusion requirements, total transfusion requirements, ICU length of stay, and mortality. An arterial blood gas is easy to obtain and rapid to run and can be repeated as needed. Thus, obtaining a blood gas at the time of admission in all patients with high-risk mechanisms of injury is a useful way to estimate shock.

The BD is likely a surrogate measure of serum lactate. However, in some patients, there may be other reasons for acidosis other than shock. Thus, directly measuring a serum lactate level would be a more direct measure of inadequate cellular perfusion. Lactate can be obtained as a point-of-care test, making it available almost immediately. If point-of-care testing is not available, sending blood to the laboratory for a lactate measurement likely means it will take 30–40 min before the result is available. This obviously makes the test less useful.

Some questioned the utility of either BD or lactate in trauma patients, as drug and/or alcohol intoxication which is common in trauma patients may make the tests less useful. However, Dunne et al. [6] clearly demonstrated that the measurements are useful even in the face of intoxication. While the absolute measurements may be slightly different, the utility remains the same.

When cellular perfusion is inadequate, cells extract additional oxygen at the tissue level in order to support aerobic metabolism. Thus, measuring venous oxygen saturation, ideally when venous blood is fully mixed in the pulmonary artery, might be a useful measure of shock. Accessing the pulmonary artery in the resuscitation bay is virtually impossible. However, Scalea et al. [7] clearly demonstrated that central venous oxygen saturation is an early and reliable measure of loss of circulating blood volume starting to fall after a blood loss of 3%. The same group also demonstrated that the measurement was clinically useful in trauma patients [8]. Central venous oxygen saturation can be obtained from a central line, which is often placed to aid in resuscitation.

Either mixed or central venous oxygen saturation represents blood from a variety of vascular distributions. However, venous extraction happens in some vascular beds before others. Measuring perfusion in a vascular bed in which changes occur early would be more useful than a global measurement. The splanchnic bed extracts oxygen early. Several investigators have demonstrated that measurement of sublingual pCO2, an indirect measurement of cellular pH in the splanchnic bed, correlates with degree of shock [9–12]. Unfortunately, devices to measure this are no longer available. However, alternate transcutaneous measurements of peripheral oxygen saturation, such as in the thenar eminence, are easy to obtain and have shown some promise in quantifying blood loss [13].

It would be attractive if the same measures that estimate depth of shock could be used to estimate adequacy of resuscitation. Unfortunately, this does not appear to be the case. Of all measures available, serum lactate is the most accurate measure of resuscitation. Abramson et al. [14] demonstrated the time to clear lactate to normal was the most accurate predictor of survival. Dezman et al. [15] more recently found that failure to clear lactate to normal had a nearly sevenfold increase in 24-h mortality when compared to those in which lactate normalized.

The relationship between BD and anion gap lactate, which seems tightly correlated initially, becomes more variable as resuscitation continues. In the ICU, utilizing BD or anion gap as a surrogate for serum lactate results in a nearly 50% rate of poor decision-making [16]. The relationship seems to recouple at 48 h. While the reason for this is not completely clear, it is likely that shock induces changes in the distal tubular cells of the kidney, and they are no longer able to maintain accurate acid-base homeostasis. This seems to recover as the patient recovers from the initial shock insult.

7.4 Focused Rapid Echocardiographic Evaluation (FREE)

Both depth of shock and adequacy of resuscitation can also be evaluated by a bedside central ultrasound. We developed a focused rapid echocardiographic evaluation (FREE). FREE is a comprehensive, transthoracic examination, designed for the ICU, which measures left ventricular ejection fraction (EF), stroke volume (SV), cardiac output (CO), and cardiac index (CI). These measurements allow examination of cardiac function using EF, CO, and CI [17]. By incorporating hemodynamic information from the echocardiographic evaluation with the patient's clinical scenario, treatment recommendations about the use of fluid, inotropic agents, and vasopressors can be made. A variation of this exam has been found to be useful in the resuscitation bay to estimate volume status even after trauma [18]. It can be performed reliably by emergency physicians and surgeons.

7.5 Initial Management

The primary objectives in the clinical management of shock are to stop hemorrhage, establish vascular access, restore circulating volume, and improve tissue oxygen delivery [1]. Early control of hemorrhage is first accomplished by direct compression of external wounds, limb tourniquets, immobilization of long bone fractures, and/or the use of pelvic binders for unstable pelvic fractures. Once bleeding is controlled early, current strategies for definitive hemorrhage control include an abbreviated initial surgery (damage control surgery), planned definitive surgery after resuscitation has been completed, angioembolization and other endovascular techniques, and topical hemostatic agents such as collagen, gelatin- and cellulose-based products, fibrin, and synthetic glues [19].

In the hypotensive trauma patient, ATLS recommends giving an initial 1–2 L bolus of warm isotonic fluid to adults and 20 mL/kg for pediatric trauma patients and then observing the patient's response [2]. The patient's response to initial fluid resuscitation is the key to determining subsequent therapy. Patients who respond rapidly to the initial fluid bolus and maintain hemodynamic stability are known as "rapid responders." No further volume resuscitation is recommended. "Transient responders" are patients who respond to the initial fluid bolus and achieve hemodynamic stability but then begin to deteriorate and become hemodynamically unstable. Volume resuscitation with blood and other blood products is recommended. Patients who fail to respond to initial fluid administration and have persistent hemodynamic instability are known as "nonresponders" [2].

Historically, restoring circulating volume involved aggressive fluid resuscitation with large volumes of isotonic fluids such as lactated ringers or normal saline followed by blood, plasma, and then platelets. However, more modern resuscitation strategies suggest that aggressive fluid resuscitation with crystalloids is associated with tissue edema, an increased incidence of abdominal compartment syndrome, and hyperchloremic metabolic acidosis, thus worsening outcomes [19, 20]. Ley et al. [21] retrospectively evaluated nearly 3000 trauma patients and found that while volume of crystalloid up to 1 L did not negatively affect patients, infusion of 1.5 L or greater of crystalloid was independently associated with increased mortality.

Large-volume fluid resuscitation with crystalloids depletes clotting factors and worsens trauma-induced coagulopathy. Additionally, in patients with penetrating injury with hemorrhage, aggressive fluid resuscitation can cause disruption of preformed clot, leading to rebleeding or further blood loss [1]. Thus, the concept of permissive hypotension was developed to limit the volume of resuscitation administered to the bleeding trauma patient by targeting a lower than normal blood pressure to avoid exacerbating hemorrhage by hydrostatic clot disruption while maintaining adequate end-organ perfusion [22, 23]. Current recommendations advocate for the administration of small boluses of fluid (250 mL) to obtain a palpable radial pulse (equating to approximately 80–90 mmHg or a mean arterial pressure of 50 mmHg) in trauma patients without head injury [1].

There are two randomized prospective trials that compare aggressive fluid resuscitation to limited fluid resuscitation. In the first, Bickell et al. [24] randomized nearly 700 patients with penetrating trauma in the field to IV fluids with the goal to raise BP to 100 mmHg against no fluid regardless of hemodynamics until OR arrival. There was a statistically significant survival advantage to withholding fluid.

Dutton et al. [25] randomized patients with both blunt and penetrating injuries to fluid to attain a BP of 100 mmHg versus fluid to achieve a BP of 70 mmHg. The protocol was continued until hemostasis was achieved. Survival was the same, and the authors concluded there was no advantage to aggressive fluid therapy.

7.6 Direct Peritoneal Resuscitation (DPR)

Traditional resuscitation in patients with hemorrhagic shock using intravenous fluid and blood has been shown to restore central hemodynamics; however, splanchnic and end-organ perfusion remains inadequate with increased risk of hypoperfusion [26]. When local metabolic demands are not achieved, tissue hypoxia, endothelial cell dysfunction, cytokine release, oxygen radicals, and multi-organ failure result. By exposing the viscera and solid organs to a hyperosmolar dialysis solution, vasodilation, increased blood flow, and hyperperfusion occur [27, 28]. In addition to these protective effects on the microcirculation, DPR has the ability to decrease tissue edema. Tissue edema results when fluid shifts from the intravascular to the extravascular space during large-volume resuscitation often delaying abdominal closure in DCS patients [29].

In a recently published randomized control trial, Smith et al. [30] found that when compared with DCS patient receiving conventional resuscitation, DCS patients receiving DPR had decreased time to definitive abdominal closure (4.1 days vs 5.9 days; $p \leq 0.002$), had lower rates of intra-abdominal complications (8% vs 18%) with lower rates of abscess formation (3% vs 14%; $p < 0.05$), and had a trend toward lower 30-day mortality rates (13% vs 28%; $p = 0.06$) [30].

7.7 Damage Control Surgery (DCS) and Damage Control Resuscitation (DCR)

In the late 1980s and early 1990s, there was a huge increase in the incidence of penetrating trauma on the streets in the United States. High-velocity weapons became common, as did multiple trajectories. Patients required long operative procedures and virtually always arrived in the ICU in profound shock, hypothermic, acidotic, and coagulopathic. Many failed to resuscitate and died early. Those that lived often succumbed to multiple organ failure days or weeks later.

Trauma surgeons realized that a different strategy was needed. The concept of damage control was born to deal with the subset of patients with exsanguinating hemorrhage. DCS involves rapid ED evaluation, followed by abbreviated laparotomy or thoracotomy. Only immediately life-threatening injuries are repaired. Other injuries, such as those to the G.I. tract, are temporized. Nonsurgical bleeding was controlled by packing, and the patient was brought to the ICU. After normalization of temperature, correction of coagulation, and resuscitation, the patient returns to the OR for definitive care of all injuries.

As trauma care evolved, we realized that resuscitation techniques must be part of this new paradigm of care. Thus, patients with hypotension at the time of ED presentation now receive minimal crystalloid. The target blood pressure is 80 mmHg. We realized that early blood use was wise. Finally plasma is now used much earlier than previously thought prudent. In essence, we strive to prevent coagulopathy, not treat it.

7.8 Massive Transfusion (MT)

Trauma patients in severe hemorrhagic shock often require the activation of a massive transfusion protocol (MTP). Massive transfusion (MT) is defined as transfusion of at least 10 units of packed red blood cells within 24 h. The early identification of patients who will require MT is critical to developing an optimal resuscitation strategy. Cotton et al. [31] published a multicenter validation study of the assessment of blood consumption (ABC) score in 2010 which gives 1 point for each of the following: penetrating mechanism, systolic blood pressure (SBP) less than 90 mmHg, heart rate greater than 120 beats per minute, and positive focused abdominal sonography in trauma (FAST) examination. An ABC score of 2 or more points predicted the need for massive transfusion within 24 h with a sensitivity of 75–90%, specificity of 67–86%, and overall accuracy 84–86%.

The American College of Surgeons (ACS) Trauma Quality Improvement Program (TQIP) Massive Transfusion in Trauma Guidelines [32] recommends the initiation of a MTP if one or more of the following criteria are met: ABC score of 2 or more, persistent hemodynamic instability, active bleeding requiring operation or angioembolization, or blood transfusion in the trauma bay. If MTP criteria are met, the guidelines recommend initiating DCR by starting universal blood product infusion rather than crystalloid or colloid solutions, transfusing universal red blood cells (RBCs) and plasma in a ratio between 1:1 and 1:2 (plasma/platelets/packed red blood cells), transfusing 1 single donor apheresis or random donor platelet pool for each 6 units of RBC, automatically sending for blood products by the transfusion service in established ratios, delivering subsequent coolers at 15-min intervals until the MTP has been completed, and keeping the goal at least 1 MTP cooler ahead for the duration of the MTP activation.

Transfusion of a balanced ratio of blood products is an essential component of DCR. The PROPPR randomized clinical trial [33] sought to determine the effectiveness and safety of transfusing patients with severe trauma and major bleeding using plasma, platelets, and red blood cells in a 1:1:1 ratio compared with a 1:1:2 ratio. After randomizing 680 severely injured trauma patients from 12 level I trauma centers to 1:1:1 blood product ratios (plasma/platelets/packed red blood cells) vs 1:1:2 blood product ratios (plasma/platelets/packed red blood cells) during active resuscitation, no significant difference in mortality was found at 24 h or 30 h, and there was no difference in complications including acute respiratory distress syndrome, multiple organ failure, venous thromboembolism, sepsis, and transfusion-related complications. However, in the 1:1:1 group, exsanguination was significantly decreased (9.2% vs 14.6%, $p = 0.03$), and more patients achieved hemostasis (86% vs 78%, $p = 0.006$).

The timing of transfusions during active resuscitation was evaluated in the PROMITT study [34], a prospective cohort study that sought to relate in-hospital mortality to early transfusion of plasma and/or platelets. One thousand two hundred forty-five severely injured adult trauma patients from ten level I trauma centers, who survived 30 min of trauma after admission, received a transfusion of at least 1 unit of RBCs within 6 h of admission, and received at least 3 units of RBCs, plasma, or platelets within 24 h, were included. In the first 6 h, patients with ratios less than 1:2 were three to four times more likely to die than patients with ratios of 1:1 or higher. Thus, higher plasma and platelet ratios early in resuscitation were associated with decreased mortality in patients who received transfusions of at least 3 units of blood products during the first 24 h after admission.

7.9 The Coagulopathy of Trauma

Acute traumatic coagulopathy is another potential complication of severe injury and MT. Together with acidosis and hypothermia, coagulopathy after trauma has been recognized for several decades as part of a lethal triad of death. This classic description of trauma-induced coagulopathy (TIC) occurs late after injury, as a result of ongoing hemorrhage and subsequent dilution from fluid administration and massive transfusion [35].

However, over the past 10 years, studies have shown that some trauma patients arrive to the emergency department with an established coagulopathy [35]. Acute traumatic coagulopathy (ATC) impairs clot formation, promotes fibrinolysis, and occurs soon after injury [36]. ATC is an endogenous hypocoagulable state that occurs in the setting of tissue hypoperfusion and is primarily mediated by the activation of protein C [37].

Many prospective trials have shown an association between ATC and activated protein C resulting in increased risk of acute lung injury, ventilator-associated pneumonia, multi-system organ failure, and death [37–40]. A diagnosis of ATC on admission is associated with increased mortality rates, increased transfusions, greater risks of complications, and longer hospital length of stays [41]. While the etiology of ATC has yet to be completely elucidated, evidence suggests that factors such as tissue injury, tissue hypoperfusion, clotting factor dilution, hypocalcemia, hypothermia, acidosis, inflammation, and fibrinolysis may contribute to its development [42]. Thus, ATC should be considered where inflammation and coagulation abnormalities collide, producing a complex cascade that, if unchecked, is highly morbid.

7.10 Point-of-Care Testing to Assess Coagulopathy

Recognition of ATC and subsequent treatment early is key to optimal care. Traditional plasma-based conventional coagulation tests (CCTs) including prothrombin time (PT) and its standardized international normalized ratio (INR), activated partial thromboplastin time, and fibrinogen are based on isolated, static endpoints [42, 43]. Some evidence has suggested that rapid, real-time functional assessment of coagulation function is imperative in guiding goal-directed therapy for specifically identified coagulation abnormalities [42].

Point-of-care functional tests such as thromboelastography (TEG) and rotational thromboelastometry (ROTEM) are being used more often for the diagnosis and management of patients with TIC [38]. Unlike traditional coagulation tests, TEG is a dynamic test and continuously assesses real-time viscoelastic properties of coagulation including time to clot initiation (*R* time), time to achieve clot strength (*K* time), rate of clot formation (α angle), clot strength (MA), and clot breakdown or fibrinolysis (LY30) [44] (Fig. 7.1) [45]. Da Luz and colleagues [46] performed a meta-analysis of 55 studies involving 12,489 patients and found limited observational data showing both TEG and ROTEM may be useful for diagnosis of early trauma coagulopathies, specifically hypocoagulability, hypercoagulability, hyperfibrinolysis, and platelet dysfunction. In addition, they may also be used to direct blood and blood product transfusion (Fig. 7.2) [45]. A recent randomized trial by Gonzalez et al. [47] demonstrated a highly significant survival advantage to TEG-based resuscitation compared to resuscitation based on routine lab tests.

Hyperfibrinolysis is the most lethal phenotype of ATC resulting in a mortality rate of 50–100% [48–50]. The association between increased mortality and hyperfibrinolysis was the foundation for the Clinical Randomization of an Antifibrinolytic in Significant Hemorrhage (CRASH-2) trial [51] which sought to determine the benefit of early empiric antifibrinolytic therapy with tranexamic acid (TXA) on mortality, vascular occlusive events, and blood transfusions in 20,211 trauma patients from 40 countries.

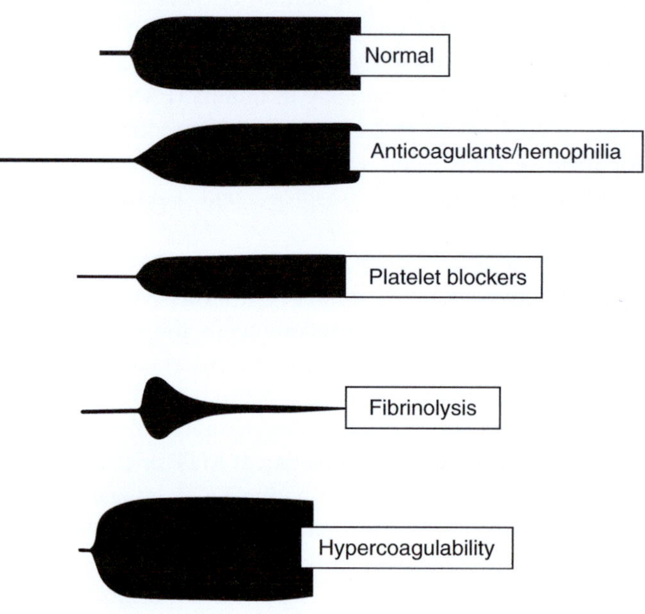

Fig. 7.2 Examples of normal and abnormal tracings on TEG. Reproduced from da Luz [45]

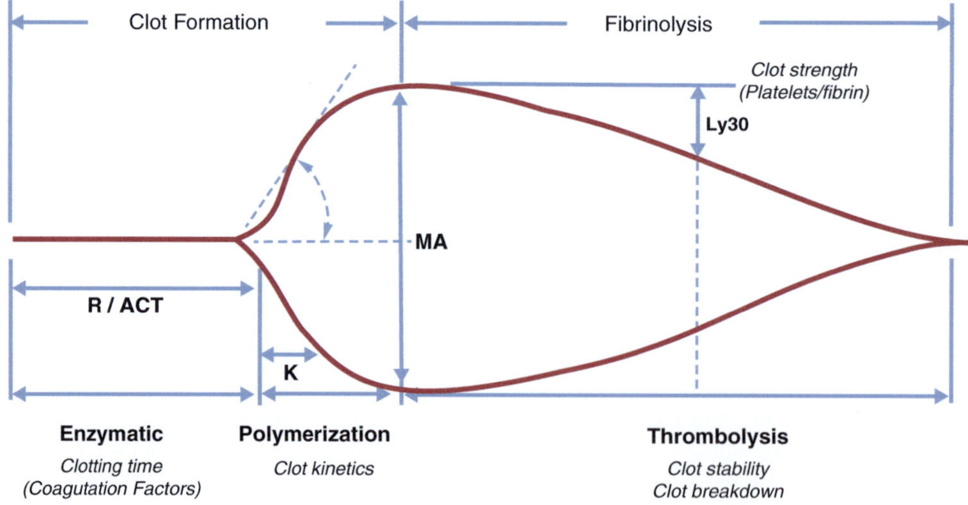

Fig. 7.1 Example of TEG findings. The typical presentation of measurement data obtained by TEG® is shown. The data are displayed in a graph in which the horizontal axis is time (min) and the vertical axis is clot firmness, similar to the ROTEM® system. Parameters are the duration from the start of the measurement to the beginning of clotting (R-time), duration from the beginning of clotting to the time when the amplitude of clot firmness reaches 20 mm (K-time), clot firmness (MA) and the fibrinolytic index (LY30) (with permission of Springer Nature; from: Sakamoto Y, Koami H, and Miike T. Monitoring the coagulation status of trauma patients with viscoelastic devices. Journal of Intensive Care; 2017; 5:7-11)

TXA inhibits fibrinolysis by preventing the binding of plasminogen to fibrin. This landmark study found that early treatment (<1 h from injury) with TXA (1 g loading dose over 10 min followed by an infusion of 1 g over 8 h) significantly reduced the risk of death due to bleeding (5.3% vs 7.7%, $p < 0.0001$) when compared to placebo. Treatment with TXA given between 1 and 3 h after injury also reduced the risk of death due to bleeding (4.8% vs 6.1%, $p = 0.03$) when compared to placebo. However, treatment with TXA given after 3h from injury significantly increased the risk of death due to bleeding (4.4% vs 3.1%, $p = 0.004$) when compared to placebo [51].

However, two large retrospective studies challenged the results of the CRASH-2 trial by showing no survival benefit in using TXA in trauma patients [52, 53]. These findings support the theory that trauma patients may develop coagulopathy or hypercoagulopathy after early injury [54]. The spectrum of post-injury fibrinolysis involves three unique phenotypes: hyperfibrinolysis (LY30 > 3%), physiologic fibrinolysis (LY 30 between 0.8 and 3%), and physiologic shutdown (LY30 < 0.8%). The key to optimizing early trauma resuscitation is to understand the mechanism for each one [49].

Systemic hyperfibrinolysis as diagnosed by TEG is driven by hypoperfusion and has been found to be associated with increased levels of tissue plasminogen activator (tPA) [49]. Hypofibrinolysis or fibrinolysis shutdown is the most prevalent phenotype and is associated with delayed mortality from multi-organ failure, involving direct tissue injury [55]. Meizoso [54] recently performed TEG on 181 adult trauma patients on admission to the ICU and at 1 week in 78 adult trauma patients. Followed by physiologic fibrinolysis (38%) and hyperfibrinolysis (4%), fibrinolysis shutdown was found to not only be the most prevalent phenotype (58%) but it was also found to be an independent predictor of mortality (OR 8.48; 95% CI 1.35–53.18; $p < 0.022$).

7.11 Endovascular Hemostasis for Trauma

The traditional therapy for hemostasis is operative exploration followed by repair, ligation, or resection of a damaged nonessential organ. However, this requires open surgery, which itself is morbid, and causes blood loss and heat loss. In some cases, a different approach may be preferable. This would be particularly true in cases where the cause of hemorrhage is not surgically accessible.

Endovascular therapy has the potential to arrest hemorrhage by occluding damaged blood vessels from the inside. Since 1976, endovascular care has been used to treat pelvic fracture hemorrhage with great success. Bleeding from pelvic fractures is often located deep in the pelvis in the hypogastric arterial distribution. These vessels are not easily approached via laparotomy so arterial embolization is far more affective in achieving hemostasis. Similar techniques have been used to treat bleeding in the spleen, kidney, and the liver.

Injuries to the thoracic aorta had been traditionally repaired via left thoracotomy. However, for almost 20 years, endovascular care has been possible [56–59]. TEVAR is now the standard of care for management in many trauma centers. In a large multi-institutional AAST series, TEVAR use was associated with a statistically significant improvement in mortality [60].

ED thoracotomy is a potentially lifesaving maneuver to treat patients with cardiac or proximal pulmonary injuries when they present in extremis. The same technique has been used to treat non-compressible torso hemorrhage such as intra-abdominal or pelvic bleeding. Thoracotomy and aortic cross-clamping just above the diaphragm control inflow to the area of injury and preserve cerebral and coronary perfusion during profound hemorrhagic shock. However, survival from this approach has traditionally been reported at less than 10%. Seamon et al. [61] reported an 8.5% overall survival in patients in 10,238 patients treated with ED thoracotomy.

More recently, use of a transfemoral aortic balloon has been pioneered as an alternative to ED thoracotomy when the indication is simply to cross-clamp the aorta. Resuscitative endovascular balloon occlusion of the aorta (REBOA) has shown more favorable outcomes as a bridge to the finish of hemostasis by cheating temporary inflow occlusion leading to hemodynamic stability [62].

Moore et al. [63] compared patients undergoing ED thoracotomy versus REBOA at level I trauma centers over an 18-month period. Patient treated with REBOA had fewer early deaths and overall improved survival. The Aortic Occlusion for Resuscitation in Trauma and Acute Care Surgery (AORTA) registry collected by the American Association for the Surgery of Trauma prospectively identifies trauma patients requiring aortic occlusion at eight level I trauma centers found no difference in mortality between REBOA and ED thoracotomy [64]. However, overall survival for aortic occlusion was 21%, a significant improvement when compared to historical controls.

In the past, REBOA was placed via a 12-French sheath, requiring open repair of the femoral artery when the sheets was removed. However, the newer ER REBOA catheters (Prytime) are placed via a 7-French sheath which does not mandate open femoral artery repair. It is likely that will increase. Hopefully insertion site complications will be small.

Extracorporeal therapies are another type of endovascular care that is used in injured patients. While the need is rare, when needed, immediate availability of these resources is necessary in order to save lives.

Extracorporeal warming is the most rapid way to reverse hypothermia. This can be accomplished with a number of circuits. In essence, blood is removed from the patient, warmed in the circuit, and then returned to the patient. In patients with severe hypothermia, little else is effective. We recently cared for a young man with profound hypothermia from exposure who presented with a cardiac arrest. He had 90 min of closed chest CPR during which we warmed him with an extracorporeal circuit. When his temperature became approximately 88 °F, he had a ventricular fibrillation. He responded to a single shock, had sustained sinus rhythm, and ultimately recovered.

Venovenous bypass can be used as part of resuscitation in selected patients with severe liver injuries. Cannulae are placed in the jugular vein and the vena cava just below the liver. Decompressing the hepatic venous circulation decreases bleeding from the retrohepatic vena cava and/or hepatic veins. This facilitates operative care in patients with complex posterior liver injuries.

7.12 ECMO

Complications from MT in trauma patient include transfusion-related lung injury (TRALI), transfusion-associated circulatory overload (TACO), and acute respiratory distress syndrome (ARDS) which may require the use of venovenous extracorporeal membrane oxygenation (ECMO) due to refractory hypoxemia (PaO2 < 65 mmHg) despite maximal ventilatory support and adjunct therapies such as inhaled nitric oxide, prostacyclins, and proning [65]. Because the ECMO circuit is optimized with systemic heparinization, its use in trauma patients is controversial. However, Ahmed et al. [65] recently published a single-center experience using ECMO in 39 trauma patients and found that 44% survived to discharge and, of those who survived, 94% were anticoagulated with heparin suggesting that the ability to tolerate heparin is associated with improved survival.

Case Scenario

A 21-year-old male presents after a high-speed motor vehicle crash. He is hypotensive in the field but is rapidly transported to the trauma center. Upon arrival, his blood pressure is 90/50, and his heart rate is 135 beats/min. On exam, his breath sounds are clear, his abdomen is soft, but his pelvis is unstable. In addition, he has obvious bilateral femur fractures.

The patient has a large bore IV access obtained, and a massive transfusion event is declared. He is initially resuscitated with a balanced transfusion strategy using 1 unit of red blood cells for every unit of plasma. Further resuscitation is guided by serial TEGs.

Initial FAST is negative and radiographs demonstrate an APC III fracture. He is placed in a pelvic binder but remains hypotensive. Right femoral arterial access is obtained, and a Zone III REBOA deployed when he fails to resuscitate. He is brought to the hybrid operating room where he undergoes internal iliac artery embolization. He then stabilizes.

Postoperatively, the patient has a whole-body CT scan which reveals no additional injuries. He is stabilized and then goes for early long bone fracture fixation. He recovers well and is discharged to rehabilitation 2 weeks later.

1. Resuscitation for profound hemorrhagic shock should involve:
   A. 4 L of crystalloid followed by blood
   B. Early blood and plasma with 1 unit of plasma for every unit of blood
   C. Hypertonic saline followed by crystalloid
   D. 1 unit of plasma for every 10 units of blood
2. Elements of damage control resuscitation include:
   A. Balanced blood and plasma use
   B. Allowing blood pressure to remain low until hemostasis is obtained
   C. Use of a massive transfusion protocol
   D. All of the above
3. REBOA use is most appropriate for:
   A. Patients with blunt aortic injury in the chest
   B. Patients with mild blood loss
   C. Non-compressible torso bleeding
   D. Extremity bleeding
4. Thromboelastography (TEG) measures:
   A. Clot strength
   B. Clot breakdown
   C. Rate of (fibrinolysis) clot
   D. All of the above
5. Direct peritoneal resuscitation uses which solution:
   A. Hyperosmolar dialysis solutions
   B. Normal saline
   C. High glucose fluids
   D. Sterile water

Please see Chap. 58 for the correct answer.

References

1. Pearson JD, Round JA, Ingram M. Management of shock in trauma. Anaesth Intensive Care Med. 2011;12(9):387–9.
2. American College of Surgeons Committee on Trauma. ATLS advanced trauma life support- student course manual, Chapter 3. 9th ed. Chicago, IL: American College of Surgeons; 2012. p. 66–88.

3. Chang R, Holcomb JB. Optimal fluid therapy for traumatic hemorrhagic shock. Crit Care Clin. 2017;33:15–36.
4. Mutschler M, Nienaber U, Brockamp T, et al. Renaissance of base deficit for the initial assessment of trauma patients: a base deficit based classification for hypovolemic shock developed on data from 16,305 patients derived from the TraumaRegister DGU®. Crit Care. 2013;17(2):R42.
5. Davis JW, Parks SN, Kaups KL, et al. Admission base deficit predicts transfusion requirements and risk of complications. J Trauma. 1996;41(5):769–74.
6. Dunne JR, Tracy JK, Scalea TM, Napolitano LM. Lactate and base deficit in trauma: does alcohol or drug use impair their predictive accuracy. J Trauma. 2005;58(5):959–66.
7. Scalea TM, Holman M, Fuortes M, et al. Central venous blood oxygen saturation: an early, accurate measurement of volume during hemorrhage. J Trauma. 1988;28(6):725–32.
8. Scalea TM, Hartnett RW, Duncan AO, et al. Central venous oxygen saturation: a useful clinical tool in trauma patients. J Trauma. 1990;30(12):1539–42.
9. Baron BJ, Dutton RP, Zehtabchi S, et al. Sublingual capnometry for rapid determination of the severity of hemorrhagic shock. J Trauma. 2007;62(1):120–4.
10. Baron BJ, Sinert R, Zehtabchi S, et al. Diagnostic utility of sublingual PCO2 for detecting hemorrhage in penetrating trauma patient. J Trauma. 2004;57(1):69–74.
11. Pellis T, Weil MH, Tang W, et al. Increases in both buccal and sublingual partial pressure of carbon dioxide reflect decreases of tissue blood flows in a porcine model during hemorrhagic shock. J Trauma. 2005;58(4):817–24.
12. Ristagno G, Tang W, Sun S, Weil MH. Role of buccal PCO2 in the management of fluid resuscitation during hemorrhagic shock. Crit Care Med. 2006;34(12):S442–6.
13. Crookes BA, Cohn SM, Bloch S, et al. Can near-infrared spectroscopy identify the severity of shock in trauma patients. J Trauma. 2005;58(4):813–6.
14. Abramson D, Scalea TM, Hitchcock R, et al. Lactate clearance and survival following injury. J Trauma. 1993;35(4):584–8.
15. Dezman ZDW, Comer AC, Smith GS, et al. Failure to clear lactate predicts 24-hour mortality in trauma patients. J Trauma Acute Care Surg. 2015;79:580–5.
16. Mikulaschek A, Henry S, Donovan R, Scalea TM. Serum lactate is not predicted by anion gap or base excess after trauma resuscitation. J Trauma. 1996;40:218–24.
17. Murthi SB, Hess JR, Hess A, et al. Focused rapid echocardiographic evaluation versus vascular catheter-based assessment of cardiac output and function in critically ill trauma patients. J Trauma. 2012;72(5):1158–64.
18. Ferrada P, Murthi SB, Anand RJ, et al. Transthoracic focused rapid echocardiographic examination: real-time evaluation of fluid status in critically ill trauma patients. J Trauma. 2011;70:56–64.
19. Madigan MC, Kemp CD, Johnson JC, Cotton BA. Secondary abdominal compartment syndrome after severe extremity injury: are early, aggressive fluid resuscitation strategies to blame? J Trauma. 2008;64:280–5.
20. Handy JM, Soni N. Physiological effects of hyperchloraemia and acidosis. Br J Anaesth. 2008;101:141–50.
21. Ley EJ, Clond MA, Srour MK, et al. Emergency department crystalloid resuscitation of 1.5 L or more is associated with increased mortality in elderly and nonelderly trauma patients. J Trauma. 2011;70(2):398–400.
22. Giannoudi M, Harwood P. Damage control resuscitation: lessons learned. Eur J Trauma Emerg Surg. 2016;42:273–82.
23. Kaafarani HMA, Velmahos GC. Damage control resuscitation in trauma. Scand J Surg. 2014;103(2):81–8.
24. Bickell WH, Wall MJ, Pepe PE, et al. Immediate versus delayed fluid resuscitation for hypotensive patients with penetrating torso injuries. NEJM. 1994;331:1105–9.
25. Dutton RP, Mackenzie CF, Scalea TM. Hypotensive resuscitation during active hemorrhage: impact on in-hospital mortality. J Trauma. 2002;52:1141–6.
26. Matheson PJ, Mays CJ, Hurt RT, Zakaria ER, et al. Modulation of mesenteric lymph flow and composition by direct peritoneal resuscitation from hemorrhagic shock. Arch Surg. 2009;44(7):625–34.
27. Garrison RN, Conn AA, Harris PD, Zakaria el R. Direct peritoneal resuscitation as adjunct to conventional resuscitation from hemorrhagic shock: a better outcome. Surgery. 2004;136(4):900–8.
28. Hurt RT, Zakaria el R, Matheson PJ, et al. Hemorrhage-induced hepatic injury and hypoperfusion can be prevented by direct peritoneal resuscitation. J Gastrointest Surg. 2009;13(4):587–94.
29. Smith JW, Garrison RN, Matheson PJ, et al. Direct peritoneal resuscitation accelerates primary abdominal wall closure after damage control surgery. J Am Coll Surg. 2010;210:658–64.
30. Smith JW, Matheson PJ, Franklin GA, et al. Randomized control trial evaluating the efficacy of peritoneal resuscitation in the management trauma patients undergoing damage control surgery. J Am Coll Surg. 2017;224(4):396–404.
31. Cotton BA, Dossett LA, Haut ER, et al. Multicenter validation of a simplified score to predict massive transfusion in trauma. J Trauma. 2010;69(Suppl 1):S33–9.
32. ACS TQIP. Massive transfusion in trauma guidelines. American College of Surgeons. https://www.facs.org/%7E/media/files/quality%20programs/trauma/tqip/massive%20transfusion%20in%20trauma%20guildelines.ashx.
33. Holcomb JB, Tilley BC, Baraniuk BC, et al. Transfusion of plasma, platelets, and red blood cells in a 1:1:1 vs a 1:1:2 ratio and mortality in patients with severe trauma: the PROPPR randomized clinical trial. JAMA. 2015;313(5):471–82.
34. Holcomb JB, del Junco DJ, Fox EE, et al. The prospective, observational, multicenter, major trauma transfusion (PROMMTT) study: comparative effectiveness of a time-varying treatment with competing risk. JAMA Surg. 2013;148(2):127–36.
35. Frith D, Brohl K. The pathophysiology of trauma-induced coagulopathy. Curr Opin Crit Care. 2012;18(6):631–6.
36. Brohi K, Cohen MJ, Ganter MT, et al. Acute coagulopathy of trauma: hypoperfusion induces systemic anticoagulation and hyperfibrinolysis. J Trauma. 2008;64:1211–7.
37. Cohen MJ, Call M, Nelson M, et al. Critical role of activated protein C in early coagulopathy and later organ failure, infection and death in trauma patients. Ann Surg. 2012;255(2):379–85.
38. Cohen MJ, Christie SA. Coagulopathy of trauma. Crit Care Clin. 2017;33:101–18.
39. Brohi K, Cohen MJ, Ganter MT, et al. Acute traumatic coagulopathy: initiated by hypoperfusion: modulated through the protein C pathway? Ann Surg. 2007;245(5):812–8.
40. Cohen MJ, Kutcher M, Redick B, et al. Clinical and mechanistic drivers of acute traumatic coagulopathy. J Trauma Acute Care Surg. 2013;75(1 Suppl 1):S40–7.
41. Hunt H, Stanworth S, Curry N. Thromboelastography (TEG) and rotational thromboelastometry (ROTEM) for trauma induced coagulopathy in adult trauma patients with bleeding. Cochrane Database Syst Rev. 2015;2:1–4.
42. Kashuk JL, Moore EE, Sawyer M. Goal directed resuscitation via POC thrombelastography. Ann Surg. 2010;251:604–14.
43. Goodman MD, Mackley AT, Hanseman DJ. All the bangs without the bucks: defining essential point-of-care testing for traumatic coagulopathy. J Trauma Acute Care Surg. 2015;79(1):117–24.
44. Thakur M, Ahmed AB. A review of thromboelastography. Int J Periop Ultrasound Appl Technol. 2012;1(1):25–9.
45. Da Luz LT, Nascimento B, Rizoli. Thrombelastography (TEG): practical considerations on its clinical use in trauma resuscitation. Scand J Trauma Resusc Emerg Med. 2013;21:29.
46. Da Luz LT, Nascimento B, Shankarakutty AK. Effect of thromboelastography (TEG®) and rotational thromboelastometry

(ROTEM®) on diagnosis of coagulopathy, transfusion guidance and mortality in trauma: descriptive systematic review. Crit Care. 2014;18:518.
47. Gonzalez E, Moore EE, Moore HB, et al. Goal-directed hemostatic resuscitation of trauma-induced coagulopathy: a pragmatic randomized clinical trial comparing a viscoelastic assay to conventional coagulation assays. Ann Surg. 2016;263(6):1051–9.
48. Moore HB, Moore EE, Gonzalez E, et al. Hyperfibrinolysis, physiologic fibrinolysis, and fibrinolysis shutdown: the spectrum of postinjury fibrinolysis and relevance to antifibrinolytic therapy. J Trauma Acute Care Surg. 2014;77(6):811–7; discussion 7.
49. Moore HB, Moore EE, Morton AP, et al. Shock-induced hyperfibrinolysis is attenuated by plasma first resuscitation. J Trauma Acute Care Surg. 2015;79:897–904.
50. Cotton BA, Harvin JA, Kostousouv V, et al. Hyperfibrinolysis at admission is an uncommon but highly lethal event associated with shock and prehospital fluid administration. J Trauma Acute Care Surg. 2012;73(2):365–70; discussion 70.
51. CRASH-2 Trial Collaborators, Shakur H, Roberts I, Bautista R, et al. Effects of tranexamic acid on death, vascular occlusive events, and blood transfusion in trauma patients with significant haemorrhage (CRASH-2): a randomised, placebo-controlled trial. Lancet. 2010;376(9734):23–32.
52. Valle EJ, Allen CJ, Van Haren RM, et al. Do all trauma patients benefit from tranexamic acid? J Trauma Acute Care Surg. 2014;76:1373–8.
53. Harvin JA, Peirce CA, Mims MM, et al. The impact of tranexamic acid on mortality in injured patients with hyperfibrinolysis. J Trauma Acute Care Surg. 2015;78:905–11.
54. Meizoso JP, Karcutsie CA, Ray JJ, et al. Persistent fibrinolysis shutdown is associated with increased mortality in severely injured trauma patients. J Am Coll Surg. 2017;224(4):575–82.
55. Moore HB, Moore EE, Liras IN, et al. Acute fibrinolysis shutdown after injury occurs frequently and increases mortality: a multicenter evaluation of 2,540 severely injured patients. J Am Coll Surg. 2016;222:347–55.
56. Neschis DG, Moainie S, Flinn WR, Scalea TM, Bartlett ST, Griffith BP. Endograft repair of traumatic aortic injury-a technique in evolution: a single institution's experience. Ann Surg. 2009;250:377–82.
57. Neschis DG, Scalea TM. Endovascular repair of traumatic aortic injuries. Adv Surg. 2010;44:281–92.
58. Garcia-Toca M, Naughton PA, Matsumura JS, et al. Endovascular repair of blunt traumatic thoracic aortic injuries: seven-year single-center experience. Arch Surg. 2010;145:679–83.
59. Willis M, Neschis D, Menaker J, et al. Stent grafting for a distal thoracic aortic injury. Vasc Endovasc Surg. 2011;45:187–90.
60. Demetriades D, Velmahos GC, Scalea TM, et al. Operative repair or endovascular stent graft in blunt traumatic thoracic aortic injuries: results of an American Association for the Surgery of Trauma Multicenter Study. J Trauma. 2009;66:967–73.
61. Seamon MJ, Haut ER, Van Arendonk K, et al. An evidence based approach to patient selection for emergency department thoracotomy: a practice management guideline from the Eastern Association for the Surgery of Trauma. J Trauma Acute Care Surg. 2015;79(1):159–273.
62. Qasim Z, Brenner M, Menaker J, Scalea TM. Resuscitative endovascular balloon occlusion of the aorta. Resuscitation. 2015;96: 275–9.
63. Moore LJ, Brenner M, Kozar RA. Implementation of resuscitative endovascular balloon occlusion of the aorta as an alternative to resuscitative thoracotomy for noncompressible truncal hemorrhage. J Trauma Acute Care Surg. 2015;79(4):523–32.
64. Dubose JJ, Scalea TM, Brenner M. The AAST prospective Aortic Occlusion for Resuscitation in Trauma and Acute Care Surgery (AORTA) registry: data on contemporary utilization and outcomes of aortic occlusion and resuscitative balloon occlusion of the aorta (REBOA). J Trauma Acute Care Surg. 2016;81(3):409–19.
65. Ahmed S, Menaker J, Kufera J, et al. Extracorporeal membrane oxygenation after traumatic injury. J Trauma Acute Care Surg. 2017;82(3):587–91.

Prehospital Care and In-Hospital Initial Trauma Management

8

Riccardo Pinciroli, Giacinto Pizzilli, Emanuele Vassena, Simone Checchi, Monica Ghinaglia, and Gabriele Bassi

Key Points

- More than half of trauma-related deaths occur within the first 24 h after the primary injury. Thus, the early phases are crucial in the management of the trauma patient.
- The timely delivery of a functioning prehospital emergency trauma care is a key challenge, potentially impacting the survival of trauma victims.
- The emergency medical service (EMS) can be divided into three broad categories: (1) basic life support (BLS) EMS system, (2) advanced life support (ALS) EMS system, and (3) physician-led ALS (MD-ALS) system.
- In the prehospital emergency assistance of traumatized patients, two main strategies can be pursued: "Stay & Play" and "Scoop & Run."
- A brief assessment of the surrounding trauma scene is conducted prior to evaluating an individual patient. Next, the "primary survey" is performed, to identify life-threatening conditions prompting immediate support therapy.
- Endotracheal intubation is the key intervention for securing the airway, thus preserving ventilation and oxygenation. It is an advanced technical skill, potentially lifesaving, but not free from risks.
- Controversy exists on the role of intravenous crystalloids to compensate shock in the out-of-hospital setting. A preliminary issue is the difficult evaluation of the shock entity and the subsequent determination of the potential benefit associated with an intravenous fluid bolus.
- The allocation of the right medical resource for each trauma patient is based on the limited information provided by first responders on the scene; for this reason prehospital trauma triage is a challenging task.
- The development of a quick, safe, and effective triage algorithm is of critical importance, contributing to both patients' outcome and optimal resource allocation.
- Major trauma management requires several different procedures, which must be performed in the shortest time possible, often concomitantly. A team-based approach is mandatory. Shared institutional protocols should be established, where any team member is assigned to specific tasks.
- The purpose of the primary evaluation is to recognize patients who need emergent endotracheal intubation, fluid resuscitation, and/or resuscitation maneuvers for treatment of imminent threats to life (e.g., decompression of a tension pneumothorax, relief of cardiac tamponade, drainage of massive hemothorax).

R. Pinciroli (✉)
University of Milan-Bicocca Medical School, Monza, MB, Italy

Anesthesia and Intensive Care 1, ASST Grande Ospedale Metropolitano Niguarda, Milan, MI, Italy

G. Pizzilli
Emergency Department, Anesthesia and Intensive Care Unit, M. Bufalini Hospital, Cesena, CE, Italy
e-mail: giacinto.pizzilli@ospedaleniguarda.it

E. Vassena · S. Checchi
University of Milan-Bicocca Medical School, Monza, MB, Italy

M. Ghinaglia
Emergency Department, ASST Grande Ospedale Metropolitano Niguarda, Milan, MI, Italy
e-mail: monica.ghinaglia@ospedaleniguarda.it

G. Bassi
Anesthesia and Intensive Care 1, ASST Grande Ospedale Metropolitano Niguarda, Milan, MI, Italy

Emergency Department, ASST Grande Ospedale Metropolitano Niguarda, Milan, MI, Italy
e-mail: gabriele.bassi@ospedaleniguarda.it

P. Aseni et al. (eds.), *Operative Techniques and Recent Advances in Acute Care and Emergency Surgery*,
https://doi.org/10.1007/978-3-319-95114-0_8

- Once the ABCDE and resuscitation algorithms have been carried out, a secondary survey is performed with the aim of obtaining the list of the patient's injuries and establishing therapeutic priorities.
- The principles of damage control resuscitation are avoiding/reversing hypothermia, delaying complete volume resuscitation until definitive hemostasis is achieved, minimizing crystalloid administration, applying massive transfusion protocols, minimizing delays in surgical or angiographic interventions, use of functional coagulation point-of-care tests to guide ongoing resuscitation, and administration of tranexamic acid to aid hemostasis.

8.1 The Trauma System

More than half of trauma-related deaths occur within the first 24 h after the primary injury. Thus, the early phases are crucial in the management of the trauma patient. Prehospital and in-hospital emergent care are the two necessary elements of a healthcare system whose aims include the treatment of major traumatic injuries.

Nevertheless, a true consensus about the overall standards in trauma care is far from being reached, due to the significant heterogeneity in terms of clinical approaches and logistics, typical of each country's emergency care system. The available high-quality evidence is, therefore, scarce, with several, still unresolved, controversies.

Overall, effective teamwork, the development of shared local guidelines, and multidisciplinary algorithms are recognized as the cornerstones of a functioning "trauma system."

The aim of this chapter is to outline the different phases of early trauma management, in both the pre- and in-hospital settings.

8.2 Prehospital Trauma Care

The timely delivery of a functioning prehospital emergency trauma care is a key challenge, potentially impacting the survival of trauma victims [1]. The main goals are to:

1. Ensure a prompt dispatch.
2. Detect and treat all life-threatening injuries (if possible).
3. Identify the most appropriate hospital for each patient, avoiding under-triage and over-triage.
4. Effectively communicate with the destination facility.
5. Minimize the delay of potentially definitive care.

However, due to clear logistic and ethical limitations, few randomized controlled trials have been carried out on prehospital trauma care. Moreover, several dissimilarities must be considered among the different countries, including cultural, geographical, and economical aspects, as well as the existing regional policies [1].

8.2.1 Prehospital Trauma Care: "Who?"

In general, a structured approach should be adopted in the treatment of acute trauma [2]. Among western countries, several different models of prehospital trauma care can be identified. At present, no system can be considered better performing in terms of clinical outcome [3]. Generally speaking, the emergency medical service (EMS) can be divided into three broad categories:

1. *Basic life support (BLS) EMS system*
   A BLS team provides noninvasive support care. Systems including this first-level rescue team provide trained volunteers or technicians. In the trauma scenario, their aim is to rapidly transport patients to a medical care facility.
2. *Advanced life support (ALS) EMS system*
   The team is staffed with paramedics, healthcare professionals working as emergency medical technicians in the out-of-hospital setting. They perform invasive procedures, such as tracheal intubation and intravenous fluid therapy.
3. *Physician-led ALS (MD-ALS) system*
   A medical doctor is part of the first-responder emergency team, which usually also include a technician and nurse with specific emergency care training. The dispatch of such a highly specialized team is generally considered according to a pre-specified protocol, based on the available information coming from the trauma scene.

In 2007, Roudsari et al. conducted an international study to compare these three main EMS staffing philosophies. The authors reported substantial heterogeneity in the performance according to the team composition, even within the same prehospital trauma care system. Particularly, the early trauma fatality rate was significantly lower in MD-ALS EMS systems compared with ALS EMS systems. Nevertheless, the incidence of shock in the emergency department did not vary significantly [4, 5]. There is no convincing evidence that, in the urban setting of western countries, compared to BLS, the use of prehospital ALS teams provides any benefit to injured patients in terms of either morbidity or mortality [6]. This is likely due to the proximity of the scene to an available trauma center and the prevalent role of time in the management of acute trauma. Recently, Garner et al. designed a randomized controlled trial to evaluate the impact of prehospital physician intervention in the setting of severe traumatic brain injury. Although, unfortunately, the study was discontinued early, intention-to-treat analysis showed no significant difference in 30-day mortality. The sensitivity analyses suggest a clinically significant mortality reduction in patients with GCS < 9 receiving physician prehospital care [7]. In a recent systematic review, Wilson et al. analyzed whether prehospital management by doctors affects outcomes in major trauma when compared to management by other advanced life support providers. Data shows insufficient evidence to conclude that prehospital management by doctors improves outcomes in patients with major trauma [8].

8.2.2 Prehospital Trauma Care: "How?"

In the prehospital emergency assistance of traumatized patients, two main strategies can be pursued:

1. *Stay & Play*: as much as possible, the patient is stabilized at the scene and then transported to the hospital.
2. *Scoop & Run*: the team reaches the closest available trauma center as soon as possible, without any medical intervention being performed to stabilize the patient.

The *Stay & Play* strategy is usually preferred in European countries, while North American systems favor a *Scoop & Run* approach.

In order to *Stay & Play*, the appropriate advanced equipment and trained personnel must timely reach the patient at the scene. Stabilization includes, after a systematic assessment, at least the capability to perform (a) endotracheal intubation, (b) tube thoracostomy, and (c) ensuring an intravenous line to start the fluid resuscitation therapy. Conversely, the *Scoop & Run* strategy involves the shortest possible arrival to the trauma center, while managing the immediately life-threatening injuries during transportation. A few emergency medical systems try to combine the two approaches. The principle of the fastest possible arrival to a trauma referral center is constantly preserved. However, limited therapeutic interventions are quickly performed at the scene, to allow for more secure transportation. Other necessary lifesaving maneuvers can also be carried out in the ambulance, on the way to the hospital.

The appropriateness of invasive maneuvers being performed on-site, relatively to their impact on patients' outcomes, is currently debated, thus questioning the validity of either approach. Clearly, there is a close relationship between the composition of the emergency team dispatched on site (BLS vs. ALS vs. MD-ALS), the choice to whether or not perform rescue interventions, and the time needed to complete them successfully.

8.2.3 Prehospital Trauma Care: "What?"

Unnecessary interventions performed at the scene of major traumatic injuries are inevitably associated with an increased mortality rate [9]. For this reason, the identification of recommended vs. potentially detrimental maneuvers to be performed out of the hospital is of capital importance.

First, regardless of the training and education of the first responder, a schematic evaluation should guide further management of the injured patient in the prehospital phase (Fig. 8.1). Generally speaking, the classic American College of Surgeons' Advance Trauma Life Support approach is always valid.

A brief assessment of the surrounding trauma scene is conducted prior to evaluating an individual patient. Next, the

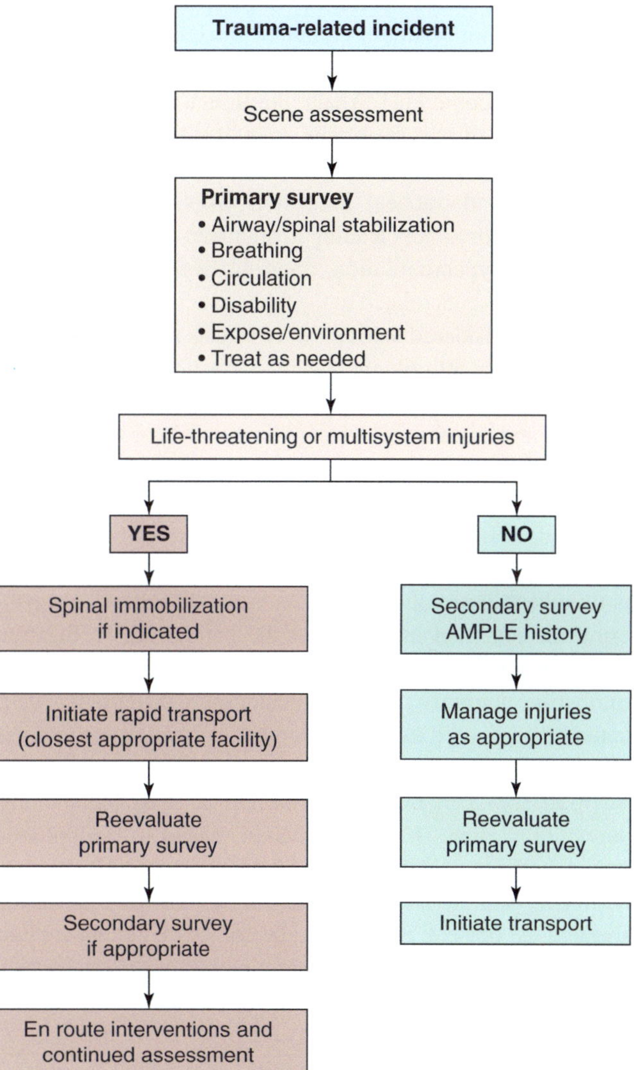

Fig. 8.1 Flowchart of the general on-scene approach to major trauma (Reproduced with permission from Salomone JP, Pons PT, McSwain NE, eds. PHTLS: Prehospital Trauma Life Support. 7th ed. St. Louis: Mosby; 2011:429. Copyright © Elsevier)

"primary survey" is performed, to identify life-threatening conditions prompting immediate support therapy, although uncertainty remains about which exact maneuver should be considered "lifesaving" in such setting. After the completion of the primary survey, the patient with identified life-threatening, or potentially life-threatening, injuries is rapidly prepared for transport to the closest available facility [10].

8.2.3.1 Endotracheal Intubation

Provided the integrity of the respiratory system, endotracheal intubation is the key intervention for securing the airway, thus preserving ventilation and oxygenation. It is an advanced technical skill, potentially lifesaving, but not free from risks (Fig. 8.2). The rationale for on-scene intubation is the maintenance of airway patency and oxygenation, both potentially altered, either primarily or secondarily, by the injury. Several studies report worse outcomes with out-of-hospital endotracheal intubation. While a common procedure in major traumas, only a few studies have actually demonstrated an improved outcome [11]. Again, the limitations of inadequate research design are important, with the literature currently mainly relying on observational studies with significant bias. Prehospital endotracheal intubation takes time and can be associated with factors leading to an adverse outcome such as inadvertent hyperventilation, transient hypoxia, bradycardia, and adverse events related to the maneuver itself [12]. Overall, it must be considered that untoward effects may counterweigh the potential benefit of emergent endotracheal intubation [11]. The literature is also inconclusive relatively to the optimal sedation and/or paralysis strategy to pursue in order to achieve optimal and safe conditions for laryngoscopy, with no clear advantage of a rapid sequence intubation (RSI) protocol, although, clinically, this is usually the preferred approach [13]. The placement of a tube within the trachea out of the hospital and in the trauma setting is particularly difficult. Also considering the potential instability of the patient due to the traumatic lesions, and the importance of time, unsuccessful intubation attempts pose significant risks. Alternative dedicated devices, such as the Combitube® double-lumen endotracheal tube, or laryngeal mask airway devices, can also be used. Such devices can be blindly introduced into the patient's supraglottic space. Concerns remain related to the potential adverse effects and limitations of these devices. To date, no definitive data are available regarding their safety and effectiveness. At present, they should be considered either second-tier alternatives, particularly if no member of the onsite team is adequately trained for the proper placement of an endotracheal tube, or rescue devices, in case of failed intubation.

Indications for endotracheal intubation include:

- Inability of the patient to maintain a patent airway due to altered (or rapidly decaying) neurological status (Glasgow Coma Scale score ≤ 8)
- At-risk airway (e.g., non-readily resolving airway obstruction, major burns, neck hematomas, etc.)

Once an endotracheal tube has been placed, confirmation of the exact positioning within the trachea must be sought. This is based, first, on clinical data. Particularly, first, at laryngoscopy, the operator should be able to directly see the tube passing through the vocal cords. Then, bilateral breath sounds must be heard at ventilation, with no gastric inflation. The chest rising and tube fogging complete the clinical assessment. Furthermore, the visualization of CO_2, either through capnography or rapid colorimetric detectors, further confirms the correct tube placement within the airway. Finally, the tube is appropriately secured.

8.2.3.2 Intravenous Fluid Therapy

The rationale for placing an intravenous line to start fluid infusion is based on the perceived aim of rapidly stabilizing the hemodynamics of the trauma patient. The purpose is maintaining adequate perfusion pressures, thus avoiding further tissue damage. Again, controversy exists on the role of intravenous crystalloids to compensate shock in the out-of-hospital setting.

A preliminary issue is the difficult evaluation of the shock entity and the subsequent determination of the potential benefit associated with an intravenous fluid bolus. Although clinically useful, the validity of standard ATLS classification of shock (Table 8.1) has been recently put under scrutiny [14, 15]. New classifications, based on a more pathophysiological approach, have been proposed [16]. However, at present, no globally accepted evidence-based method has been established as a reference for the estimation of blood loss and fluid requirements in trauma patients. As a result, ATLS classification is still widely used, both clinically, and as a literature benchmark.

The role of fluid resuscitation itself also remains controversial. Most authors agree on the detrimental effect of an excessive increase in intravascular volume through an aggressive fluid resuscitation strategy, before the source of bleeding is effectively controlled. Forced hemodilution, due to a disproportionate infusion of crystalloids in hypovolemic hemorrhagic trauma patients, would ultimately lead to a decrease in distal organ perfusion. The three natural physiological defense mechanisms of hemostasis (arterial retraction/spasm, hypotension, and clotting) would be compromised. An increased risk of bleeding may result, with decreased arterial pressure [16]. No published study has ever demonstrated an improvement in survival associated with the prehospital administration of fluids. The most recent Cochrane systematic review on this topic gathered data from six prospective interventional RCTs. The authors found no conclusive evidence for, or against, earlier, or

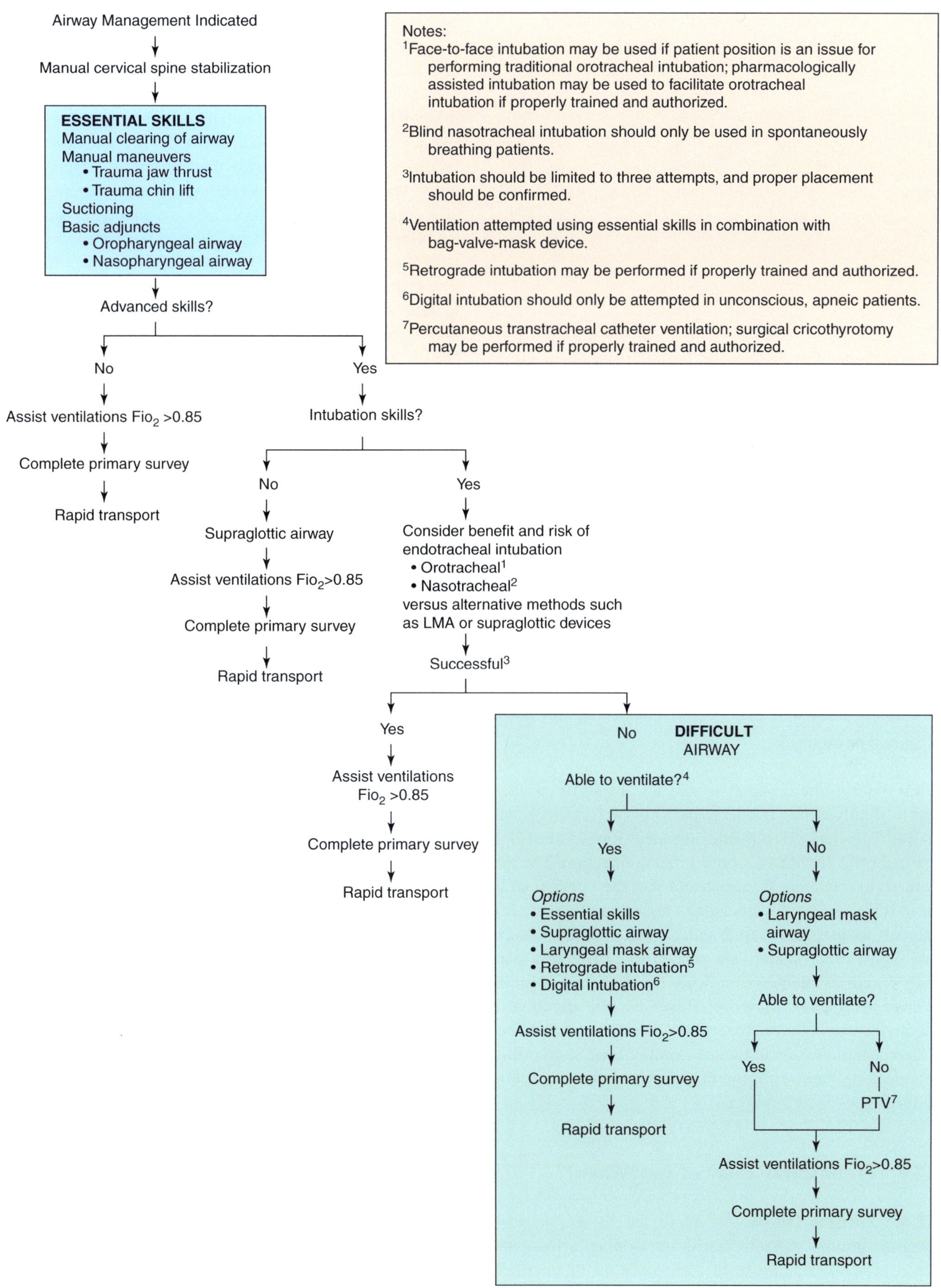

Fig. 8.2 Flowchart: prehospital airway management (Reproduced with permission from Salomone JP, Pons PT, McSwain NE, eds. PHTLS: Prehospital Trauma Life Support. 7th ed. St. Louis): Mosby; 2011:140. Copyright © Elsevier)

Table 8.1 Class of hemorrhagic shock—ATLS classification

	I	II	III	IV
Blood loss (mL)	Up to 750	750–1500	1500–2000	>2000
Blood loss (% of volume)	Up to 15	15–30	30–40	>40
Heart rate (bpm)	<100	100–120	120–140	>140
Respiratory rate (bpm)	14–20	20–30	30–40	>35
Urine output (mL/h)	>30	20–30	5–15	Negligible
Central nervous system/mental status	Slightly anxious	Mildly anxious	Anxious, confused	Confused, lethargic

larger-volume, intravenous fluid administration in uncontrolled hemorrhage [17].

In the absence of clear recommendations and lack of convincing evidence, in our opinion, trauma fluid resuscitation in the prehospital setting must be based on the available clinical data, collected after the on-scene primary assessment. Three general principles could be highlighted:

- If the patient shows signs of uncontrolled hemorrhage, with no evidence of traumatic brain injury (TBI), fluids can be infused, titrated to maintain systolic blood pressure (SBP) in the range of 80–90 mmHg.
- If TBI is suspected, in the context of multiple injuries, intravenous fluids should be administered at a rate sufficient to maintain a SBP of 90 mmHg.
- In case of isolated TBI, a SBP higher than 100 mmHg should be targeted.

En route to the destination hospital, the EMS providers should ideally obtain two large bore (14 or 16 gauge) intravenous catheters. If possible, lactated Ringer should be warmed (102 °F/38.8 °C) prior to administration. The time required to secure an IV access and start the infusion on the scene is also debated, with authors reporting minimum time intervals ranging between 2 and 12 min or more [18–20]. Although further studies are needed to clarify this issue, EMS providers should never delay transport just to initiate intravenous therapy. Moreover, fluids must be administered only to the extent they help reaching the SBP goal [1]. There is also uncertainty about the best kind of fluid to be infused in a bleeding trauma patient. Further randomized controlled trials are needed in this area.

8.2.4 Prehospital Trauma Care: "When?"

8.2.4.1 Trauma Triage

Triaging trauma patients means developing a pre-established method, leading to the prioritization of treatment, built on the baseline available information. Purpose of field triage is to select patients in order to appropriately allocate medical resources to those most likely to benefit. First and foremost, an effective triage should result in severely injured patients (even potential ones) being addressed to tertiary hospitals equipped with the staff, expertise, and facilities to adequately treat them, namely, "trauma centers." Statistically, only 7–15% of trauma patients actually require this higher level of assistance [1]. However, the allocation of the right medical resource for each trauma patient is based on the limited information provided by first responders on the scene. Prehospital trauma triage is, therefore, a true challenge. Several issues must be taken into account, such as (1) the time restraint of the situation; (2) the paucity of information available from the scene, whose reliability depends on the level of training of the first responder; (3) the unpredictable availability of hospitals to actually accept candidate patients; and (4) the variable geography of the area and its impact on the time needed for transport. Depending on the characteristics of the controlled area, emergency medical service dispatch centers continuously manage multiple trauma calls and perform triage on several, often concomitant, trauma cases. The development of a quick, safe, and effective triage algorithm is of critical importance, contributing to both patients' outcome and optimal resource allocation.

Once the patient has been directed to the selected treatment center, information about the patient's state is usually transmitted to the receiving facility. The availability of a clear and concise prehospital report allows the hospital team to anticipate emergent equipment and personnel needs.

Another issue is the definition of "major trauma victim." While easy to intellectualize, its exact quantification is complicated. The use of a precise classification is important, in order to standardize and compare triage systems, treatment protocols, and outcomes.

The Injury Severity Score (ISS) is an anatomical scoring system. An Abbreviated Injury Scale (AIS) score (1–6, "minor" to "unsurvivable") is assigned to the worst injury in each body system (head, face, chest, abdomen, extremities—including pelvis—external). The ISS is then computed as the sum of squares of the AIS scores in the three most injured regions. A maximum value of 75 is automatically assigned if an AIS 6 is present in any system [21].

The ISS is a useful tool to retrospectively classify major trauma victims, whereas an ISS > 15 usually is an accepted threshold.

The American College of Surgeons Committee on Trauma and the Centers for Disease Control and Prevention's 2011 Guidelines for Field Triage of Injured Patients outline anatomical, mechanical, and particular patient's conditions that raise suspicion of severe trauma.

Table 8.2 Markers of severe traumatic injury

Clinical indicators	Anatomical indicators	Mechanical indicators	Special considerations
GCS < 13	Penetrating injuries to the head, neck, torso, and extremities proximal to the elbow or knee	Falls >6 m (adults) >3 m (children)	Older adults (>55 years of age)
SBP < 90 mmHg	Chest wall instability or deformity	High-risk automobile crash	Pregnancy >20 weeks
RR >29 or <10 or altered respiratory mechanics or prehospital intubation	Two or more proximal long bone fractures	Car deformity with intrusion of the car body (including the roof) of >30 cm at the occupant site or >45 cm at any site	Anticoagulants
	Crushed, degloved, mangled, or pulseless extremity	Ejection (partial or complete) from automobile	Burns
	Amputation proximal to the wrist or ankle	Death in same passenger compartment	EMS team judgment
	Pelvic fractures	Vehicle telemetry data consistent with high risk of injury	
	Open or depressed skull fractures	Auto versus pedestrian (bicyclist thrown, run-over, or with significant (e.g 30 km/h) impact)	
	Paralysis	Motorcycle crash >30 km/h	

GCS Glasgow Coma Scale, *SBP* systolic blood pressure, *RR* respiratory rate, *EMS* emergency medical service

The ACS Field Triage System is a more complete, advanced triage scoring method. Indications are included for patient referral to a trauma center based on specific physiology and anatomy of the injury. The mechanism of injury and comorbid factors are considered as well. Interestingly, the EMS team judgment about the severity of the injury is also taken into consideration (Table 8.2 and Fig. 8.3) [1].

Conversely, several European countries do not have a national mandatory triage scale. Evidence is lacking about the usefulness of a trauma field triage system, nor comparisons about different systems, or the applicability of the same system within different nations, are currently available [22]. However, the absence of robust evidence on the effect of any particular prehospital triage algorithm, while a significant limitation, does not mean such systems should not be implemented. On the contrary, further research is needed in this critical aspect of the emergency and acute care medicine discipline.

A known indicator of the trauma center performance is the rate of under-triage and over-triage. Under-triage is defined as the misclassification of a patient as not in need of a higher level of care (mainly, the destination to a trauma center), when in fact he/she does. Under-triage is a medical problem that may easily result in a poor patient outcome, since the receiving medical facility may not be ready or adequate for the management of an unexpected major trauma victim.

On the other hand, over-triage is the incorrect classification of a patient as requiring admission to a trauma center, whenever such high-level resources were indeed not needed. An over-triaging system errs on the side of patient safety. However, it inevitably results in a poorer allocation of financial and human resources.

The American College of Surgeons Committee on Trauma (ACS-COT) recommends mature trauma systems to strive in order to achieve rates of <5% under-triage. Conversely, the ACS-COT defines as "acceptable" an over-triage rate of 25–50% [23].

8.2.4.2 Time vs. Outcome

The "golden hour" is a well-known key principle of trauma care, attributed to R. Adams Cowley, founder of Baltimore's renowned Shock Trauma Institute [9]. It is defined as the post-injury time interval when resuscitation and stabilization are expected to be the most beneficial for the trauma victim [6]. While a useful paradigm to stress the importance of time limitations in trauma care, the evidence supporting the "golden hour" concept is actually scarce. The 1-h cutoff has not been scientifically replicated, and its usefulness in the management of EMS systems has repeatedly been called into question [24]. Again, there is no large RCT conducted in the civilian population that either strongly supports or rejects the hypothesis that faster is universally better in trauma care [25]. A recent large systematic review conducted by Harmsen et al. showed a decreased mortality risk with shorter response time and transfer time. However, longer on-scene time and total prehospital time were associated with increased odds of survival [26]. Moreover, according to the authors, a swift transport does seem beneficial for patients suffering penetrating trauma, particularly if hemodynamically unstable and/or with associated TBI. According to other reports, longer prehospital time in patients with ISS > 15 was associated with an increased length of stay and complications, but not with increased mortality [27]. In conclusion, the "golden hour" seems to better apply to specific subgroups of patients, but there is no evidence favoring the

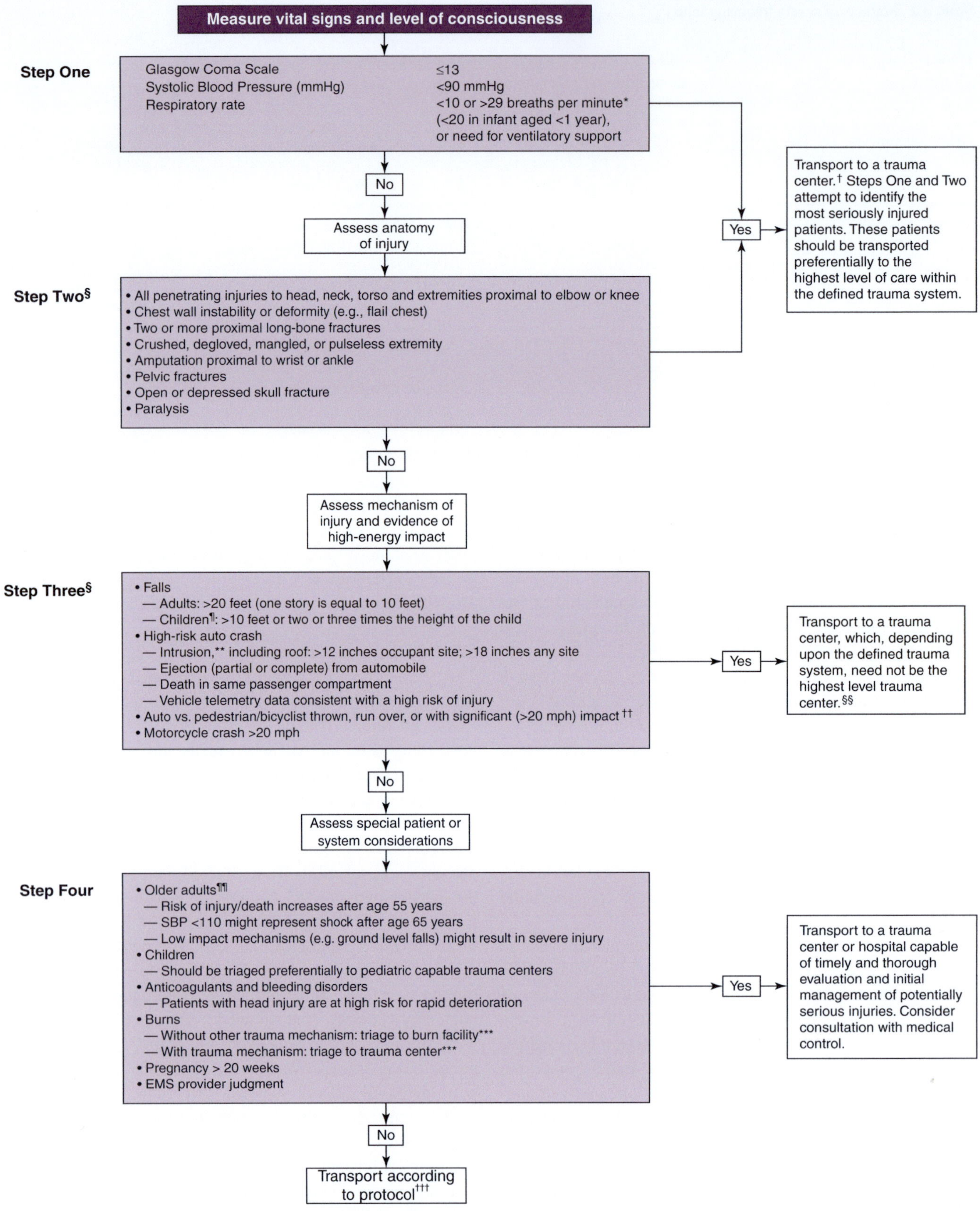

Fig. 8.3 2011 American College of Surgeons Guidelines for field triage of injured patients (reproduced with permission)

widespread application for every trauma. A much stronger factor favoring survival seems to be the referral of major trauma patients from the field directly to a specialized trauma center [28].

8.3 In-Hospital Initial Trauma Care

The emergency room is the place where, bypassing waiting rooms, the patient is rushed once arrived at the destination hospital. The availability, in modern emergency departments, of dedicated specialized rooms for the management of major traumas (e.g., "shock room," "trauma bay," Fig. 8.4) significantly facilitates the management of such cases. Patient's priorities are thereby established. In order to achieve this goal, similarly to the field approach, a strict protocol of evaluation and treatment should be observed. A primary and a secondary evaluation are planned. The aim of the primary evaluation is to recognize and treat immediately life-threatening conditions. The ATLS Airways, Breathing, Circulation, Deficit, and Exposure (ABCDE) systematic assessment is typically adopted. A secondary evaluation subsequently follows, including a head-to-toe physical examination, monitoring, imaging, and laboratory tests. Of note, the completion of the planned diagnostic and treatment course could be delayed in case of patient's instability. In that case, it is crucial to minimize the time elapsing from admission to operating room (OR) or interventional radiology (IR) transfer.

Early control of bleeding is mandatory for improving outcome. It is important to establish priorities and to identify patients who would benefit from early damage control surgery or IR. The patient's assessment should be coupled with a damage control resuscitation strategy whose aim is to prevent the lethal triad of (1) hypothermia, (2) acidosis, and (3) coagulopathy, as well as to identify patients for whom the activation of a massive blood transfusion protocol is needed.

Damage control resuscitation is currently the cornerstone of the management of major trauma patients. At the same time, damage control surgery aims at controlling early hemorrhage and minimizing operative time, by delaying definitive repair to the moment the patient will be stabilized.

8.3.1 The "Trauma Team"

Major trauma management requires several different procedures, which must be performed in the shortest time possible, often concomitantly. A team-based approach is mandatory. Shared institutional protocols should be established, where any team member is assigned to specific tasks.

The composition of the trauma team varies based on each institution's practice. However, the core of the team requires five to eight members.

The team leader is in charge, with direct responsibility on, mainly, (1) emergency room logistics, (2) the decision-making process about diagnostic and therapeutic priorities, and (3) communication, both within the team and with the

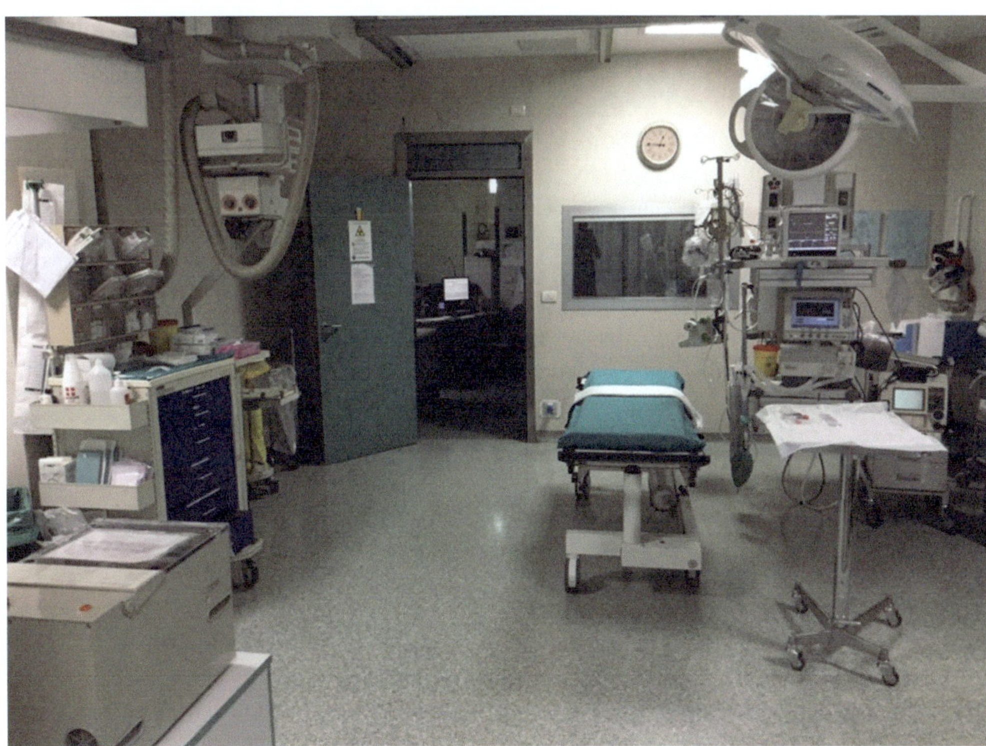

Fig. 8.4 Representative emergency department "shock room" for the comprehensive management of major trauma patients. The facility is a large space, fully equipped with all the necessary material for the emergency management and evaluation of traumatic injuries without the patient, nor the team, leaving the area (airway, IV access, ultrasound, X-ray tube, mechanical ventilation, monitoring, point-of-care testing, blood transfusion, body and fluids warming, spine and pelvis immobilization, etc.). If needed, emergent damage control surgical procedures (e.g., tube thoracostomy, extraperitoneal pelvic packing, emergency thoracotomy) can be performed

patient's relatives. The leader should be coordinating the team, without being involved in a specific clinical task. The role of team leader does not require specific training, but it is usually fulfilled by a physician, most often a surgeon. Intensivists, or emergency physician, can also act as team leaders, depending on the institutional setup.

An anesthesiologist/intensivist/emergency physician is the member of the team dedicated to airway management, central vascular accesses, volume resuscitation, and sedation/analgesia.

A surgeon is generally responsible for emergency chest decompression and chest tube placement, surgical management of bleeding, and head-to-toe physical examination of the victim.

At least two nurses should be part of the team, one assisting the airway expert, the other helping the surgeon. Peripheral vascular access, gastric tube placement, blood draw, and urethral catheter placement are usually performed by nurses, as well.

The presence of a radiologist, an orthopedic, and/or a neurosurgeon is often necessary in the emergency room for the first phases of severe trauma victim management.

Much emphasis should be put on communication and coordination among team members. It is well recognized that effective teamwork in severe trauma management can be lifesaving.

8.3.2 Primary Evaluation

During the primary evaluation, all immediately life-threatening conditions are detected, in a very short time frame (i.e., few minutes), and treated. The cornerstone of primary evaluation is the ABCDE assessment. ABCDE and resuscitation procedures should be carried out simultaneously, and the effect of any therapeutical intervention should be reassessed in a timely fashion. Complete primary evaluation and treatment must be carried out before proceeding with subsequent trauma protocol steps. The ABCDE should be reassessed periodically and/or whenever patient's conditions change.

The purpose of the primary evaluation is to recognize patients who need emergent endotracheal intubation, fluid resuscitation, and/or resuscitation maneuvers for treatment of imminent threats to life (e.g., decompression of a tension pneumothorax, relief of cardiac tamponade, drainage of massive hemothorax) [29].

8.3.2.1 Airway and Cervical Spine

Spine Protection

It is mandatory to minimize movement of the cervical spine during airway management. Neck immobilizing devices should be kept in place until cervical spine injury has been ruled out by imaging (CT scan being the gold standard technique, even though, in some cases, MRI is required). If immobilizing devices have to be removed, the head must be kept in neutral in-line position with manual immobilization by a member of the trauma team [29].

Endotracheal Intubation

Whenever the patient has already been intubated out-of-hospital, its correct placement should be checked by bilateral chest auscultation and capnography. If the tube is found in the esophagus, it should be kept in place until a definitive airway has been secured, as tube removal may elicit vomit.

In the trauma setting, several conditions may threaten airway integrity, such as foreign bodies, avulsed teeth or dentures, blood, vomit, expanding hematoma, edema, direct airway or circumferential neck burns, etc. Any such situation must be promptly detected. In general, a GCS < 8 is likely associated with loss of protective airway reflexes, increasing the risk of aspiration of gastric contents. Endotracheal intubation is generally indicated. Suction must always be in place and ready for use, being an essential device for safe airway management.

Ventilatory problems in the trauma patient include apnea/bradypnea due to unconsciousness or neuromuscular paralysis (e.g., spinal cord lesion above C5 level) or inadequate respiratory efforts. Hypoxia (defined as an SpO2 $< 90\%$ in reservoir bag mask) and acidosis (pH < 7.2) are commonly used parameters.

Combative patients may need sedation and intubation in order to carry out diagnostic and therapeutic procedures. Agitation could also be due to substance abuse, or even hypoxia.

The choice of the intubation technique is based upon the circumstances and the operator's skills. Intubation is often a challenging maneuver in the trauma victim. Equipment for the management of the difficult airway, including a surgical one, must be available and ready for use, in case conventional attemps fail. In the awake, spontaneously breathing patient, intubation with a "rapid sequence induction" is the most common approach. It allows to minimize the risk of aspiration by avoiding mask ventilation [29].

Advanced Airway Management

Videolaryngoscopy is an option, given the frequent limitation to neck hyperextension. Awake nasal or orotracheal intubation assisted by fiberoptic bronchoscopy also is a possibility, but it requires trained personnel and an awake, collaborative patient.

A supraglottic device (e.g., laryngeal mask) can be placed temporarily if intubation fails, in order to ensure ventilation. Notably, supraglottic devices do not protect from aspiration.

Cricothyroidotomy of tracheostomy may be the only way of securing the airway of patients with severe facial or laryngeal trauma.

8.3.2.2 Breathing

Prevention of hypoxemia is recommended in the severe trauma setting. Supplemental oxygen (at least 10 L/min with bag mask) should be provided to all spontaneously breathing patients with major trauma, in order to maintain an SpO_2 of 95% or higher.

Assessment

A focused physical examination can often lead to detect severe respiratory conditions requiring immediate intervention:

- A respiratory rate < 10/min indicates hypoventilation, likely associated with hypercapnia.
- A respiratory rate > 29/min suggests inadequate respiratory efforts.
- Symmetry of respiration should be assessed with both inspection and auscultation.
- Subcutaneous emphysema raises a high suspicion of pneumothorax, laryngeal, or tracheobronchial trauma.
- Central cyanosis is assessed by inspecting the color of lips or mucosae, keeping in mind that, in order to be observed, cyanosis requires at least 5 g/dL of unoxygenated hemoglobin (may not be evident with concomitant severe anemia).
- Diagnosis of tension pneumothorax should be clinical. The affected side is often elevated compared to the contralateral, its excursion is impaired, and the jugular tone can be increased. Reduced breath sounds and hyperresonance on percussion are characteristic features but may be difficult to assess in a noisy environment.
- In case of massive hemothorax, dyspnea is usually evident; limitation of excursion and reduced breath sounds also aid the diagnosis.
- Flail chest is detected by inspection and suggests underlying pulmonary contusion.

Treatment

Tension pneumothorax and massive hemothorax should be drained even before imaging is obtained, in case of a severe cardiovascular or respiratory derangement. Emergent treatment of tension pneumothorax is performed by needle decompression, placing a large bore IV cannula in the second intercostal space, just above the rib, on the midclavicular line. A chest drain tube should then be placed as soon as possible, possibly before positive-pressure mechanical ventilation is initiated. Treatment of massive hemothorax is by chest tube drainage. The amount of blood drained should be strictly monitored. Penetrating chest injuries may lead to open pneumothorax if the defect of the chest wall is wide enough. In this case, an occlusive dressing should be placed upon the wound, and a chest tube should be inserted in a different site. Invasive or noninvasive mechanical ventilation should be considered in case of flail chest.

Mechanical Ventilation

Mechanical ventilation in the trauma victim can be challenging. In the first phases of trauma management, positive-pressure ventilation can aggravate hypotension, decreasing venous return, especially in already hypovolemic patients. On the other hand, the risk of hypoxia due to alveolar derecruitment is concrete. Moreover, for the overall management of the trauma case, it is important to keep a SpO_2 of at least 95% for adequate oxygen delivery. A protective ventilation strategy should be early adopted to prevent ventilation-induced lung injury. Protective ventilation includes the use of low tidal volumes (6–8 mL/Kg predicted body weight) and moderate positive end-expiratory pressure (PEEP), targeting a plateau airway pressure below 30 cmH_2O. Respiratory rate should be titrated based on $PaCO_2$ levels, aiming at normocapnia (35–40 mmHg).

Hyperventilation, in order to keep moderate hypocapnia (30–35 mmHg), should be adopted, as a rescue therapy, only in case of imminent or ongoing cerebral herniation. The effect of PEEP on intracranial pressure has been shown to be negligible, as long as the $PaCO_2$ is controlled.

It is important to monitor respiratory mechanics and gas exchange with serial arterial blood gas analyses throughout the early phases of trauma management.

8.3.2.3 Circulation

Assessment

Circulation is first assessed by checking peripheral and central pulses, looking for signs of hypoperfusion and, most importantly, identifying potentially active sources of bleeding. The presence of a carotid pulse indicates a systolic blood pressure >40–50 mmHg, while a palpable radial pulse generally indicates a systolic pressure of at least 70 mmHg.

Heart rate, peripheral oxygen saturation (SpO_2), and noninvasive blood pressure should be assessed. Clinical signs of tissue hypoperfusion, such as augmented capillary refilling time (>3–4 s), cold extremities, and mottling, which is usually more evident around knee caps, may be present in spite of still normal blood pressure.

Jugular veins should always be inspected, as increased jugular filling and congestion of the head and neck suggest an obstructive cause of shock, such as tension pneumothorax or cardiac tamponade.

Cardiac arrest in the trauma setting is generally associated with a poor outcome, with extremely low survival rates.

Reversible causes of cardiac arrest (i.e., severe hypovolemia, or tension pneumothorax, cardiac tamponade) should immediately be detected and treated.

Cardiac tamponade diagnosis on clinical basis can be challenging. Beck's triad (jugular tension, severe hypotension, and dull heart sounds) raises the suspicion, but definitive diagnosis is made by point-of-care transthoracic echography. Needle pericardiotomy, or emergency thoracotomy, should be performed.

Treatment

At least two large bore peripheral venous catheters (best if 14 gauge) should be placed as soon as possible. If major vascular lesions are suspected, IV lines should be placed so that the potentially damaged vessel does not affect the continuity between the IV access and the right ventricle (i.e., place the IV above the diaphragm in case of abdominal injuries, below the diaphragm if superior vena cava affluent obstruction, or disruption, is suspected).

Intraosseous access is a valuable option for rapid fluid resuscitation in case an IV cannot be placed. It allows the infusion of crystalloids and blood components. The placement of central venous access and/or artery cannulation should not delay the initial trauma resuscitation. These procedures are usually carried out later on, during the secondary evaluation, or even after diagnostics have been completed.

Volume Resuscitation/Bleeding Control

Hemorrhagic shock resuscitation is based on prompt fluid replacement. Isotonic crystalloids are currently the first choice for early volume resuscitation. Despite their effectiveness in restoring intravascular volumes, synthetic colloids (starches) should be avoided, as they can impair platelet function and coagulation and increase the risk of kidney injury. Albumin is contraindicated in the presence of traumatic brain injury.

Balanced isotonic crystalloids are generally preferred, since the infusion of large volumes of normal saline may lead to hyperchloremic metabolic acidosis and impaired renal perfusion.

On the other hand, normal saline is the crystalloid of choice in patients with traumatic brain injury, in which hypotonic crystalloids must be avoided.

Controlling hemorrhage clearly is the crucial aspect of the vast majority of trauma cases.

Uncontrolled post-traumatic bleeding is the second leading cause of mortality after TBI. Trauma-related coagulopathy is a major issue in the trauma victim. Up to 30% of bleeding patients already show some degree of coagulation impairment at admission. Thus, the importance of the early recognition of active bleeding and coagulopathy is paramount for the improvement of trauma patients outcome. Hemostasis should be the first goal in the patient who is actively bleeding.

Aggressive crystalloid resuscitation in order to restore normal vital signs in the first phases of trauma care can lead to deleterious consequences, both primarily, like hypothermia and dilution coagulopathy, and secondarily, like fluid overload, abdominal compartmental syndrome, and ARDS. Moreover, a liberal fluid administration leading to an excessive elevation in arterial pressure might be detrimental, as it increases blood loss and prevents, or disrupts, the formation of clots at the bleeding site.

Mild, controlled hypotension (permissive hypotension) favors clot formation and slows bleeding rate from damaged vessels. Similarly to the prehospital setting, a SBP of 80–90 mmHg should be targeted in patients with ongoing hemorrhage, and no known TBI, until definitive bleeding control is achieved. Crystalloids should be titrated to achieve such target SPB, while overall crystalloids should be as minimized as possible, in favor of transfusing blood components whenever necessary.

For patients with active bleeding and concomitant traumatic brain or spinal cord injury, on the other hand, a higher blood pressure threshold should be observed (>100 mmHg of systolic or >80 mmHg mean arterial pressure), in order to assure adequate cerebral, or spinal cord, perfusion.

Vasopressors

Vasopressors should be considered only as a temporary measure to maintain tissue perfusion in case of severe hypotension unresponsive to volume therapy. Low-dosage norepinephrine is the most commonly used agent. Inotropes could be considered in case of suspected myocardial depression.

Patients with hemorrhagic shock and an identified source of bleeding should undergo immediate bleeding control procedures if they do not respond to the initial volume resuscitation.

Blood Transfusion

Massive transfusion protocols should be developed within each trauma center. Effective communication between the trauma team and the blood bank is extremely important in the management of the trauma victim requiring blood transfusion.

Transfusion goals should not be limited to ensure adequate oxygen delivery through hemoglobin supplementation, but should instead include adequate coagulation factors and platelet. A standard red blood cell (RBC)/fresh frozen plasma (FFP)/platelet (PLT) ratio of 1:1:1 is currently recommended.

Shock index (i.e., heart rate/systolic blood pressure ratio) is the most common trigger of massive transfusion protocol activation. Type 0 negative packed RBCs should be available as a temporary resource. A restrictive hemoglobin goal of 7 g/dL is recommended in trauma victims with no known cardiovascular disease.

Patient's hemodynamics and its responsiveness to volume resuscitation are crucial in defining further diagnostic and therapeutic paths. The stable patient can undergo accurate secondary evaluation, being addressed to CT scan, then possibly surgery or IR vs. conservative management and observation. On the other hand, the hemodynamically unstable (or the transiently responsive) patient should promptly undergo extended focus ultrasonography and bedside chest plus pelvis X-ray, in order to identify bleeding sources (usually thoracic, abdominal, or pelvic). The latter patient is likely to benefit from early damage control surgery, requiring a massive transfusion and strict coagulation monitoring.

Tranexamic Acid

The administration of tranexamic acid, an antifibrinolytic drug, is recommended within 3 h after injury (1 g should be administered in the prehospital setting, then an additional 1 g should be infused in 8 h) in order to avoid clot disruption.

Desmopressin (DDAVP) 0.3 mcg/kg could help hemostasis in patients with known von Willebrand disease or under antiplatelet drugs, together with platelets. Prothrombin complex concentrates are given to reverse the effect of vitamin K antagonist or factor Xa inhibitors. An antidote for direct thrombin inhibitor dabigatran is now available (idarucizumab) [30].

8.3.2.4 Disability

A first, rapid assessment of the level of consciousness can be obtained with the AVPU scale, which evaluates mental status defining the patient as:

- Alert
- Responsive to verbal stimuli
- Responsive to pain
- Completely unresponsive

The Glasgow Coma Scale (GCS) is the cornerstone of the assessment of the victim's state of consciousness. It evaluates three items (eye-opening, verbal, and motor response) resulting in a score from 3 to 15. In the intubated patients, always unable to speak, the motor response is crucial in defining mental status.

First neurological examination is completed assessing pupillary status: baseline diameter and response to light. Altered pupillary status is an early sign of cerebral herniation, which requires immediate treatment.

The GCS assessment should be systemically repeated, as well as the ABCDE, even after the first evaluation. Neuroworsening (defined as an impairment of two points of the GCS) should be promptly detected by periodic reassessment of GCS.

It must be noted that altered mentation in the severe trauma settings could be due not only to traumatic brain injury but also other factors like cerebral hypoxia due to shock hypoperfusion or hypoxemia, metabolics, and intoxication [10].

8.3.2.5 Exposure

Up to two-thirds of severe trauma victims presents some degree of hypothermia, which is an independent risk factor for mortality. Hypothermia has several detrimental effects on patients' outcome, mostly impairing platelets function and coagulation. Severe hypothermia (<32 °C) is associated with almost 100% mortality.

Risk factors of hypothermia include the severity of injury, CNS involvement, extremes of age, wet clothes, long extrication time, burns, large open wounds, blood loss, low environmental temperatures, and underlying medical conditions (e.g., hypothyroidism, adrenal failure, diabetes mellitus). A few iatrogenic factors may lead to increased heat loss as well, such as exposure, general anesthesia and muscle paralysis, large intravenous infusion of cold crystalloids or blood products, and lengthy (>3 h) surgery.

Since it is difficult to rewarm a patient in which considerable heat loss has occurred, any effort should be made in order to prevent hypothermia. The patient's body temperature should be periodically assessed. First-line strategies for keeping normothermia (i.e., a core temperature of 36–37 °C) should include removal of wet clothes, avoidance of cold surfaces, warm room environment, warm intravenous fluids, warm blankets, and forced-air blankets.

In case of hypothermia, active warming strategies should be implemented. Forced-air warming should be maximized, like other potentially available tools, like underbody heating pads, radiant warmer, humidified ventilation, or circulating water garment. Body cavity lavage with warm fluids during surgery is another option, although of uncertain efficacy. Of note, warming should be ceased in case the subject's temperature rose above 37 °C, as hyperthermia is associated with increased mortality as well.

Body temperature has a considerable impact on hemodynamics as well, especially in the trauma patients. Mild hypothermia stimulates sympathetic activity leading to increased heart rate and blood pressure, which can mask underlying hypovolemia. Attention should also be paid to avoid too rapid temperature shifts, particularly in patients with underlying cardiovascular disease [31].

TBI with associated intracranial hypertension could, on the other hand, benefit from mild hypothermia. As usual, pros and cons of hypothermia must be put on the balance.

8.3.3 Secondary Evaluation

Once the ABCDE and resuscitation algorithms have been carried out, a secondary survey is performed with the aim of obtaining the list of the patient's injuries and establishing therapeutic priorities.

During the secondary survey, vital signs must periodically be checked. It must be noted that this secondary evaluation is carried out only if the patient is stable or once stabilized by a successful resuscitation. In case of persisting instability, in spite of proper resuscitation maneuvers, the patient should be promptly transferred to the OR/IR for hemorrhage source control. In this case, the secondary survey is performed later on, as soon as the patient stabilizes.

The secondary assessment involves the collection of focused medical history (if feasible), a whole body physical exam, patient's monitoring, and imaging.

8.3.3.1 AMPLE

Interviewing the awake patient or, if not feasible, collecting information from the next of kin, a quick and focused past medical history can be obtained. The "AMPLE" mnemonic summarizes the most relevant medical issues to be evaluated in the trauma patient: allergies, medications, past illness, last meal, and events. Particularly, it is crucial to find out whether or not the patient is taking anticoagulant medications that might need immediate reversal.

8.3.3.2 Physical Examination

A systematic head-to-toe examination is performed, in order to detect all sites of possible injury:

- A rapid neurological exam of motor and sensory functions and cranial nerve assessment. Notably, scalp hemorrhage may lead to important blood loss, especially in children.
- Neck palpation, in order to recognize subcutaneous emphysema ("snowball crepitus"), swelling, or dislocation of structures.
- Inspection and palpation of the chest for the detection of chest wall fractures and flail chest.
- Inspection and palpation of the abdomen to exclude abdominal tenderness and/or wall tension.
- Evaluation of pelvic stability.
- Inspection of the perineum and digital rectal examination to detect bleeding and test sphincter tone.
- Evaluation of the urethral meatus.
- Examination of the extremities for fractures or misplacements; muscle palpation in order to rule out early compartment syndrome.
- Evaluation of the back with the log-roll maneuver: a group of operators rolls the patient on a side, keeping the long axis of the spine in-line, while inspection and palpation of the whole spine are performed, seeking for swelling, dislocation, or tenderness. Lifting up the scoop stretcher can be utilized in spite of log rolling for palpation of the spine in patients with suspected unstable pelvic fracture.

8.3.4 Laboratory Tests

Blood samples should be early drawn in the emergency department for point-of-care and a basic set of laboratory analyses.

An arterial blood gas analysis not only assesses pulmonary gas exchange but also the presence of metabolic acidosis, the level of hemoglobin, and the electrolytic balance. Lactate levels and base deficit are currently the standard markers of tissue perfusion. Their complete normalization within the first 24 h following injury should be the goal of resuscitation efforts. Thus, their trends should be monitored. Lactate clearance requiring more than 24 h is associated with the development of post-traumatic organ failure.

The analysis of venous blood gases, particularly from peripheral samples, cannot be considered a valid surrogate for the estimation of blood oxygenation, CO_2, and pH, but is reliable indicators of lactate levels.

Most importantly, a sample for the determination of blood type and cross-matching should always be drawn as soon as possible. A complete blood count is mandatory as well. Hemoglobin level at emergency department admission does not necessarily reflect the severity of blood loss. During hemorrhage, whole blood is lost; thus interstitial fluid shifts to restore intravascular volume, ultimately producing hemodilution, which, however, is not immediately measurable. As a consequence, normal hemoglobin levels do not rule out an ongoing bleeding. On the other hand, already low hemoglobin or hematocrit level at hospital admission must be considered an indicator of important bleeding, potentially associated with coagulopathy.

Standard coagulation tests, such as activated partial thromboplastin time (aPTT) and prothrombin time (PT), are mandatory minimum requirements for trauma care. An international normalized ratio (PT-INR) <1.5 should be sought. Nevertheless, standard coagulation tests are of limited help for the assessment of early trauma-induced coagulopathy. Thus, functional point-of-care whole blood viscoelastic coagulation tests, such as thromboelastography (TEG), should be obtained, in order to have a quicker and deeper understanding on the status of hemostasis (time of clot formation, strength of the clot, platelet aggregation, and fibrinolytic process). TEG-guided coagulation resuscitation is one of the key principles of the damage control approach. Fibrinogen levels must always be assessed together with platelet count and coagulation times, as fibrinogen is the first coagulation cascade factor to drop, due to consumption in the severe trauma bleeding patient.

Other basic laboratory studies aimed at assessing potential organ dysfunction include blood urea nitrogen, creatinine, liver enzymes, and glucose level. Baseline levels of blood muscle enzymes (creatine phosphokinase and myoglobin) should also be checked. Cardiac biomarkers can be required if cardiac contusion is suspected on the basis of dysrhythmias or echographic findings. Toxicology blood tests are often useful for both clinical and legal purposes. Finally, pregnancy status should be ruled out in all fertile-age females by testing urinary beta-hCG.

8.3.5 Monitoring

An arterial line can be placed before or after imaging, to obtain continuous invasive blood pressure and to draw blood samples for arterial blood gas analyses.

Establishing central venous access can be useful for monitoring and sampling purposes, as well as for the intraoperative and postoperative management of infusions, should surgery be needed.

A 12-lead electrocardiogram should be performed to evaluate possible cardiac injury. A nasogastric (orogastric, in case of basal skull fractures) tube is often placed.

All major trauma patients should receive urethral catheterization. If there's suspicion of perineal or pelvic injury involving the urethra or the bladder, urology consult should be sought.

8.3.6 Imaging

8.3.6.1 X-Ray and eFAST

Bedside chest and pelvis X-rays, and extended focused ultrasonography, are performed in all patients, regardless of the hemodynamic status, as they can be crucial in the prompt detection of bleeding or obstructive causes of shock. These exams are obtained directly in the emergency room.

Extended focused assessment with sonography for trauma has increasingly become an extension of physical examination. Moreover, in many protocols, emergency echocardiography for detection of cardiac tamponade or lung ultrasound for the diagnosis of pneumothorax has actually become part of ABCDE assessment itself.

Whenever an ultrasound (US) machine is available, the abdominal echographic examination has now replaced the diagnostic peritoneal lavage for the diagnosis of intra-abdominal bleeding. A positive US is very specific and accurate for detection of hemoperitoneum. On the other hand, a negative exam does not completely rule out intraperitoneal hemorrhage. In this case, further diagnostic (i.e., contrast-enhanced CT scan) might be considered.

8.3.6.2 CT Scan

Contrast medium-enhanced multislice CT assessment is the gold standard imaging exam for hemodynamically stable patients with a high-risk mechanism of injury. Ongoing bleeding with a minimum rate of 0.5 mL/min can be visualized. Trauma scan patterns often include the head, neck, chest, abdomen, and pelvis. If shock is present, CT is usually delayed, and sources of bleeding are first assessed by sonography or bedside X-ray of the chest and pelvis.

The availability, at some institutions, of CT-scan machines allowing the quick execution of the exam within the emergency room minimizes time, sometimes allowing the study to be completed even in the partially unstable patient, provided an at least initial response to resuscitation. However, the CT suite inevitably is an environment where the trauma victim is more vulnerable. Risks and benefits should be balanced by the team.

Today, emergent angiography has become an interventional, rather than diagnostic, procedure. The arterial bleeding is generally detected as a "blushing" on contrast-enhanced CT scan. If indicated, transfer to IR is prompted for the nonsurgical control of bleeding through the endovascular approach.

8.3.7 Damage Control Resuscitation and Surgery

The principles of damage control resuscitation are:

- Avoiding/reversing hypothermia
- Delaying complete volume resuscitation until definitive hemostasis is achieved
- Minimizing crystalloid administration
- Applying massive transfusion protocols
- Minimizing delays in surgical or angiographic interventions
- Use of functional coagulation point-of-care tests to guide ongoing resuscitation
- Administration of tranexamic acid to aid hemostasis

Damage control surgery essentially means a three-step approach to the severely injured patients:

1. First emergent intervention to control bleeding and contamination, which should last less than 90 min (e.g., abdominal or pelvic packing, exterior fixation of pelvis or fractured limbs)
2. Resuscitation and monitoring in the intensive care unit
3. Once resuscitation goals are achieved (usually within 12–48 h): definitive surgical repair

A damage control approach should not be used systematically in all severe trauma victims. Some of them could rather benefit from definitive surgery. Recommendations for damage control surgery include:

- Hypothermia
- Metabolic acidosis
- Presence of coagulopathy
- Hemodynamic instability
- Severe bleeding

all of which must be unresponsive to resuscitation [30, 32].

8.3.8 Pain Relief

Pain management is an often-overlooked issue in severe trauma. For patients with major trauma, intravenous morphine is a good first-line analgesic. Doses should be titrated based on the patient's response. The physician must be aware that, after the administration of opiates, the victim's adrenal response to pain is blunted, so systemic vascular resistances and cardiac output can rapidly decrease leading to sudden hypotension, due to a previously occulted hypovolemia.

Ketamine at analgesic doses is a valid option. Benzodiazepines like midazolam are often associated, in order to prevent hallucinations.

NSAIDs should be avoided in the early stages of severe trauma, due to their possible detrimental effects on platelet function and kidney perfusion.

8.3.9 Antibiotic Prophylaxis

The majority of severe trauma victims do not require any a priori antibiotic prophylaxis. Inappropriate use of antibiotics agent is responsible for selection of drug-resistant bacteria and fungi. The choice to administer antibiotic prophylaxis should be evaluated on individual basis. Specific conditions in which antibiotic prophylaxis is recommended include:

- Open traumatic brain injury
- Maxillary fractures
- Open limb fractures
- Hollow viscus injuries

Adjustment of antibiotics administration should be considered in patients undergoing massive transfusion.

Tetanus vaccination status of the patient should be assessed, and, if necessary, tetanus immunoglobulins, or vaccination refresh, should be administered.

8.4 Handover

Concisely passing thorough and correct information among healthcare professionals is particularly challenging in the trauma setting. This is due to the simultaneous involvement of several different operators, across multiple specialties and with different levels of training (technicians, nurses, physicians). Both in the prehospital and in-hospital settings, miscommunication may arise, associated with the emergency character of the situation, the multiple actions being undertaken at the same time, and the significant amount of information being passed along through the different phases of trauma care. A structured approach should be pursued in such circumstances, possibly with the aid of safety checklists.

References

1. Mattox K. Trauma. 7th ed. New York, NY: McGraw-Hill Companies; 2013.
2. Hofman M, Sellei R, Peralta R, Balogh Z, Wong T, Evans J, et al. Trauma systems: models of prehospital and inhospital care. Eur J Trauma Emerg Surg. 2012;38(3):253–60.
3. Oestern H-J, Trentz O, Uranues S. General trauma care and related aspects. Heidelberg: Springer; 2014.
4. Roudsari BS, Nathens AB, Arreola-Risa C, Cameron P, Civil I, Grigoriou G, et al. Emergency Medical Service (EMS) systems in developed and developing countries. Injury. 2007;38(9):1001–13.
5. Roudsari BS, Nathens AB, Cameron P, Civil I, Gruen RL, Koepsell TD, et al. International comparison of prehospital trauma care systems. Injury. 2007;38(9):993–1000.
6. Liberman M, Roudsari BS. Prehospital trauma care: what do we really know? Curr Opin Crit Care. 2007;13(6):691–6.
7. Garner AA, Mann KP, Fearnside M, Poynter E, Gebski V. The Head Injury Retrieval Trial (HIRT): a single-centre randomised controlled trial of physician prehospital management of severe blunt head injury compared with management by paramedics only. Emerg Med J. 2015. https://doi.org/10.1136/emermed-2014-204390.
8. Wilson SL, Gangathimmaiah V. Does prehospital management by doctors affect outcome in major trauma? A systematic review. J Trauma Acute Care Surg. 2017;83(5):965–74.
9. Cowley RA. A total emergency medical system for the State of Maryland. Md State Med J. 1975;24(7):37–45.
10. The ATLS Subcommittee, American College of Surgeons' Committee on Trauma, and the International ATLS Working Group. Advanced trauma life support (ATLS®): the ninth edition. J Trauma Acute Care Surg. 2013;74(5):1363.
11. Wang HE, Yealy DM. Out-of-hospital endotracheal intubation: where are we? Ann Emerg Med. 2006;47(6):532–41.
12. Dunford JV, Davis DP, Ochs M, Doney M, Hoyt DB. Incidence of transient hypoxia and pulse rate reactivity during paramedic rapid sequence intubation. Ann Emerg Med. 2003;42(6):721–8.
13. Davis DP, Fakhry SM, Wang HE, Bulger EM, Domeier RM, Trask AL, et al. Paramedic rapid sequence intubation for severe traumatic brain injury: perspectives from an expert panel. Prehosp Emerg Care. 2007;11(1):1–8.
14. Mutschler M, Nienaber U, Brockamp T, Wafaisade A, Wyen H, Peiniger S, et al. A critical reappraisal of the ATLS classification of hypovolaemic shock: does it really reflect clinical reality? Resuscitation. 2013;84(3):309–13.

15. Guly H, Bouamra O, Little R, Dark P, Coats T, Driscoll P, et al. Testing the validity of the ATLS classification of hypovolaemic shock. Resuscitation. 2010;81(9):1142–7.
16. Bonanno FG. Hemorrhagic shock: the "physiology approach". J Emerg Trauma Shock. 2012;5(4):285.
17. Kwan I, Bunn F, Roberts I. Timing and volume of fluid administration for patients with bleeding. Cochrane Database Syst Rev. 2003; https://doi.org/10.1002/14651858.CD002245.
18. Carr BG, Brachet T, David G, Duseja R, Branas CC. The time cost of prehospital intubation and intravenous access in trauma patients. Prehosp Emerg Care. 2008;12(3):327–32.
19. Zarate L, Mandleco B, Wilshaw R, Ravert P. Peripheral intravenous catheters started in prehospital and emergency department settings. J Trauma Nurs. 2008;15(2):47–52.
20. Seymour CW, Cooke CR, Hebert PL, Rea TD. Intravenous access during out-of-hospital emergency care of noninjured patients: a population-based outcome study. Ann Emerg Med. 2012;59(4):296–303.
21. Baker SP, O'Neill B, Haddon W Jr, Long WB. The injury severity score: a method for describing patients with multiple injuries and evaluating emergency care. J Trauma Acute Care Surg. 1974;14(3):187–96.
22. Lidal IB, Holte HH, Vist GE. Triage systems for pre-hospital emergency medical services—a systematic review. Scand J Trauma Resusc Emerg Med. 2013;21(1):28.
23. Sasser SM, Hunt RC, Faul M, Sugerman D, Pearson WS, Dulski T, et al. Guidelines for field triage of injured patients: recommendations of the National Expert Panel on Field Triage, 2011. Morb Mortal Wkly Rep Recomm Rep. 2012;61(1):1–20.
24. Newgard CD, Schmicker RH, Hedges JR, Trickett JP, Davis DP, Bulger EM, et al. Emergency medical services intervals and survival in trauma: assessment of the "golden hour" in a North American prospective cohort. Ann Emerg Med. 2010;55(3):235–46.e4.
25. Lerner EB, Moscati RM. The golden hour: scientific fact or medical "urban legend"? Acad Emerg Med. 2001;8(7):758–60.
26. Harmsen A, Giannakopoulos G, Moerbeek P, Jansma E, Bonjer H, Bloemers F. The influence of prehospital time on trauma patients outcome: a systematic review. Injury. 2015;46(4):602–9.
27. Báez AA, Lane PL, Sorondo B, Giráldez EM. Predictive effect of out-of-hospital time in outcomes of severely injured young adult and elderly patients. Prehosp Disaster Med. 2006;21(6): 427–30.
28. MacKenzie EJ, Rivara FP, Jurkovich GJ, Nathens AB, Frey KP, Egleston BL, et al. A national evaluation of the effect of trauma-center care on mortality. N Engl J Med. 2006;354(4): 366–78.
29. Mayglothling J, Duane TM, Gibbs M, McCunn M, Legome E, Eastman AL, et al. Emergency tracheal intubation immediately following traumatic injury: an Eastern Association for the Surgery of Trauma practice management guideline. J Trauma Acute Care Surg. 2012;73(5):S333–S40.
30. Rossaint R, Bouillon B, Cerny V, Coats TJ, Duranteau J, Fernández-Mondéjar E, et al. The European guideline on management of major bleeding and coagulopathy following trauma. Crit Care. 2016;20(1):100.
31. Perlman R, Callum J, Laflamme C, Tien H, Nascimento B, Beckett A, et al. A recommended early goal-directed management guideline for the prevention of hypothermia-related transfusion, morbidity, and mortality in severely injured trauma patients. Crit Care. 2016;20(1):107.
32. Cannon JW, Khan MA, Raja AS, Cohen MJ, Como JJ, Cotton BA, et al. Damage control resuscitation in patients with severe traumatic hemorrhage: a practice management guideline from the Eastern Association for the Surgery of Trauma. J Trauma Acute Care Surg. 2017;82(3):605–17.

From Trauma Scoring System to Early Appropriate Care

9

Anna Mariani, Gianpaolo Casella, and Paolo Aseni

Key Points

- Think of trauma as an illness, not as an organ injury.
- Think each patient has his/her own characteristic that you need to know as soon as possible.
- Do exactly what the patients need nothing more than that.
- Continue to study the patients to understand how he's managing the immune response to trauma.
- Consider the best option, damage control strategy vs. early definitive treatment, based on the information you can get (scores)

9.1 Introduction

Despite improvement traffic safety, emergency prehospital and in-hospital management, severe trauma still represents the most frequent cause of death in people below the age of 40 years in the Western world. Patients die as a direct consequence of their sustained injury or by the additional damage caused by subsequent immune reactions.

Mortality in trauma patients has been described as tri-modal type (Fig. 9.1):

A. Mariani (✉)
Department of General Surgery and Transplantation, ASST Grande Ospedale Metropolitano, Niguarda Ca' Granda Hospital, Milan, MI, Italy

G. Casella
Anesthesia and Intensive Care 1, ASST Grande Ospedale Metropolitano Niguarda, Milan, MI, Italy

P. Aseni
Dipartimento di Emergenza Urgenza, ASST Grande Ospedale Metropolitano Niguarda, Milan, Italy

- Immediately after trauma (injuries incompatible with life)
- After few hours (it depends in particular on primary brain injuries and haemorrhagic shock)
- Late mortality (after 7 days, it depends on secondary brain injuries and host-defense failure)

Medical trauma teams have to deal with the second and third type of mortality; the possibility to improve survival is depending on the ability to recognize patients with, or at higher risk of, haemorrhagic shock, severe brain injury and sepsis.

The amount of additional reactions to trauma is determined by both endogenous and exogenous factor [1].

Endogenous factors are determined in part by genetic predisposition and in part by physical conditions that form the basis of the patient's susceptibility to develop a multisystem organ dysfunction (MOD) [1, 2].

Two types of exogenous factors are usually recognized: the first hit (the injury itself) and second hit (a consequence of the injuries, resuscitation and surgical intervention) [2].

Medical team is largely involved in determining the second hit due to the different strategies of treatment for trauma patients. Even though trauma severity *scores* are not the key elements of *treatment*, proper application of these models may *help* in decision-making at the *right time* among the different trauma experts who can *choose* different variables and assign the weight for predicting the risk of mortality in surgical ICU.

9.2 Pathophysiology of Trauma

9.2.1 Theory: The *Two-Hit* Hyphothesis

When an injury occurs, the reactions of the body are due to endogenous factors and exogenous factors.

Endogenous factors, such as genetic predisposition and physical condition, form the basis of patient's susceptibility to

P. Aseni et al. (eds.), *Operative Techniques and Recent Advances in Acute Care and Emergency Surgery*,
https://doi.org/10.1007/978-3-319-95114-0_9

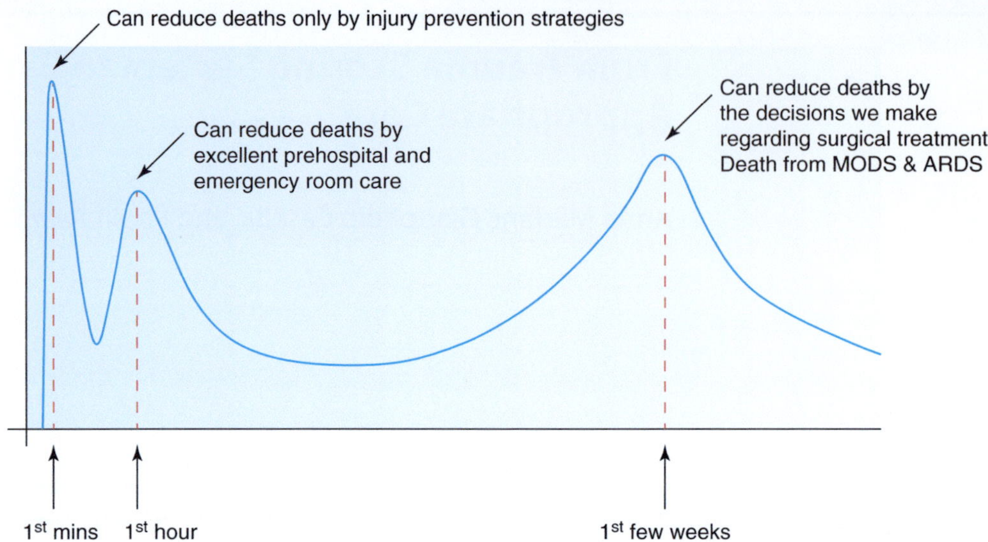

Fig. 9.1 Mortality trimodal type (Adapted from Trunkey DD. Trauma. Sci Am. 1983;249: 28–35)

develop organ failure [1]. Several studies have evidenced the strong correlation between some genetic variations and development of organ failure [1–5]. Exogenous factors, like the injury itself (the so-called first hit or trauma-load) and the resuscitation procedures or surgical interventions (the so-called second hit or intervention load), play a key role in the development and clinical presentation of organ failure [2, 6]. The complex of the host-defense response is stimulated by first and second hits [2]. "First hit" is represented by primary organ, or soft tissue, injuries and fractures with local tissue damage as well as by activation of the systemic inflammatory response.

"Second hit" is determined by hypoxia, repeated cardiovascular instability, hypothermia, metabolic acidosis, ischemic injury, dead tissue, contaminated catheters and tubes, respiratory distress, cerebral oedema, intracranial hypertension and infections [2, 4].

Moreover, surgical interventions with severe tissue damage, blood loss and consequent hypothermia, inadequate or delayed surgical care, after neglected or missed injury, as well as massive transfusions, represent the "second hit". Injury in each single anatomical area can induce a "second hit" due to the local and systemic inflammatory response. Neglected or missed injuries and delayed surgical or intensive care can amplify the "second hit" to potential irreversible phase of "second hit".

Thoracic injuries (multiple rib fractures, lung contusion, lung lacerations) are often complicated by local and systemic inflammation, with or without manifestation of pneumonia or acute respiratory distress syndrome.

Abdominal injuries are mainly represented by haemorrhagic events (liver, spleen, kidney, vascular injuries) and aseptic or septic peritonitis (pancreas or hollow viscus). All of these injuries can lead to acute abdominal compartment syndrome which reduces the blood flow to abdominal organs with consequent multiple organ dysfunction and death.

Soft tissue injuries or extremity injuries, especially in patients with haemorrhagic shock, are often complicated with hypoperfusion and hypoxia with a high risk of ischemia/reperfusion injuries and secondary infections [2].

9.2.2 SIRS, CARS, MARS and MODS

Endogenous factors and exogenous factors, with "first and second hits", play a key role in the development and clinical presentation of organ failure. Organ damage and subsequent organ failure are the result of a dysfunctional system [2, 3, 5]. A local inflammatory reaction is physiological and is explained by the "danger model" [7–9].

The "danger model" assumes that alarm signals, secreted by healthy cells or necrotic cells which are present after injury, can provoke an inflammatory reaction. The combination of the different type of tissue and the type of alarm signals are associated with the subsequent type of response.

Depending on the severity of trauma, different gene polymorphism and general condition of the host, both the local and systemic release of pro-inflammatory cytokines and phospholipids are present, assessing the complex of so-called systemic inflammatory response syndrome (**SIRS**) (Table 9.1).

SIRS was defined in 1991. *SIRS* was *defined* as fulfilling at *least two* of the *four* criteria summarized in Table 9.1 and is characterized by the local and systemic production and release of different mediators, such as pro-inflammatory cytokines, complement factors, proteins of the contact phase and coagulation systems, acute-phase proteins, neuroendocrine mediators and an accumulation of immunocompetent cells at the local site of tissue damage.

Depending on the severity of the injury and the post-traumatic course, anti-inflammatory mediators are also produced (Table 9.2). An overwhelming anti-inflammatory response seems to be responsible for post-traumatic immunosuppression with high susceptibility to infection and septic complication. This immunological status is called

Table 9.1 Clinical parameters of systemic inflammatory response syndrome (SIRS)

1	Heart rate > 90/min
2	Breathing rate > 20/min, respectively, hyperventilation with decrease of the arterial CO2 partial pressure (PaCO2) under 32 mmHg
3	Temperature >38° or <36°
4	Number of leukocytes >12,000/mm^3 or <4000 mm^3 or ≥10% juvenile neutrophil granulocytes

For the definition of SIRS, two or more parameters must be fulfilled

Table 9.2 *PMNL* polymorphonuclear leukocytes, *TNF-(* tumour necrosis factor (, *TNF-®* tumour necrosis factor ®, *IL-1®* interleukin 1 ®, *IL-6* interleukin 6, *IL-8 0* interleukin 8, *MMF* macrophage migratory factor, *HMG-1* high motility group protein, *IL-12* interleukin 12, *IL-18* interleukin 18, *IFN-©* interferon-© modulating cytokines, *Th 2 cells* T-helper lymphocytes

Pro-inflammatory mediators	Anti-inflammatory mediators
Activation of PMNL, monocytes, tissue macrophages, lymphocytes, natural killer cells and parenchymal cells	Few hours after trauma, Th2 cells and monocytes/macrophages release IL-4, IL-10, IL-13 and TGFβ.
1–2 h = TNF-α, IL-1	The readiness of blood monocytes from injured patients to release pro-inflammatory cytokines was decreased in in vitro studies after stimulation with Gram-negative (endotoxin, lipopolysaccharide, LPS) or Gram-positive (e.g. peptidoglycan, lipoteichoic acid), bacterial pro- ducts and correlated with the post-traumatic course
Subacute = IL-6, IL-8, MMF, HMG-1, IL-12, IL-18, IFN-©	

compensatory anti-inflammatory response syndrome (**CARS**) (Fig. 9.2).

Cellular/Molecular Elements

- Lymphocyte dysfunction (i.e. reduced proliferative and/or helper T cell (TH1) cytokine production in response-defined antigens or specific T cell stimuli)
- Lymphocyte apoptosis
- Downregulation of monocyte HLA receptors monocytes deactivation (i.e. reduced Th1/pro-inflammatory cytokine production in response stimuli)
- IL-10 production
- Transforming growth factors-beta production prostaglandin E2 production

Clinical Elements

- Cutaneous anergy
- Hypokalaemia
- Leukopenia

Table 9.3 Definition of MODS

Multiple organ dysfunction definition	
Cardiovascular system	– HR ≤ 54 – Medium blood pressure ≤ 49 mmHg – Fibrillation or ventricular tachycardia – Arterial pH ≤ 7.24 or PaCO2 < 40 mmHg
Respiratory system	– RR ≤5 or ≥49 – PaCO2 < 50 mmHg – Need of mechanical ventilation after the fourth day of recovery in ICU
Kidney	– Urine output ≤ 479 mL (die or ≤159 mL/8 h) – PaCO2 ≤ 50 mmHg – Serum creatinine > 3.5 mL/dL
Blood	– Leucocyte count ≤ 1000/μL – Platelets count ≤ 20,000/μL – Ht ≤ 20%
Liver	– Serum bilirubin > 3 mg/dL – SGOT > ×2 – INR > 1.5
Gastroenteric system	– Bleeding with need of transfusion or at least two units
Nervous system	– GCS < 6 without sedation

- Susceptibility to infection
- Failure to clear the infection

In the presence of an overreaction of the anti-inflammatory response, two clinical scenarios are possible: CARS or MARS [3, 10].

In both of these situations, the body is in a state of immune paralysis, and it is unable to produce an adequate reaction to a new threat (i.e. infection, surgical hit) (Fig. 9.3).

If the balance is achieved, the patient recovers, while if it fails, multiple organ dysfunction syndrome (**MODS**) may happen (Table 9.3).

The evolution of the physiological and reversible systemic inflammatory after trauma to a host-defense failure can be interpreted as an overload of primary and secondary hits and an imbalance of pro- and anti-inflammatory mechanism.

The elements involved in MODS are endothelial cell damage, dysfunction of vascular permeability with capillary leakage, microcirculatory disturbances with cellular hypoxia and finally apoptosis of parenchymal cells.

Dysfunctions of different systems are involved in MODS (respiratory, cardiovascular, renal, hepatic, gastrointestinal, haematological and central nervous system) [3, 9, 10].

9.3 Scoring Systems

A score in medicine is a one-dimensional value that describes a rather complex situation and is usually a combination of several aspects, each of which is expressed as a parametric value or categorical value [11].

All scores are intended to give supportive information for decision-making, especially in an emergency setting.

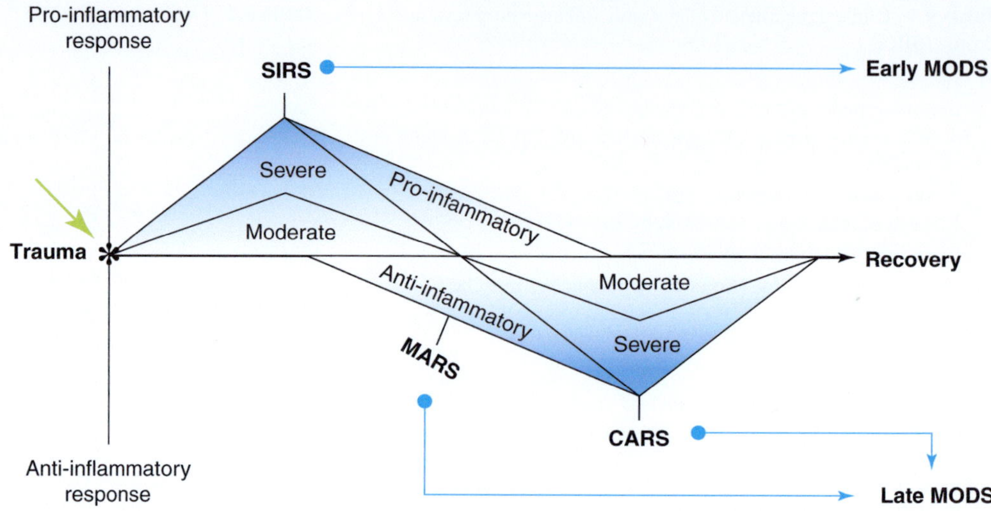

Fig. 9.2 The inflammatory response after trauma (adapted from F. Hietbrink, L. Koenderman, GT Rijkers and LPH Leenen. Trauma: the role of the innate immune system. World Journal of Emergency Surgery. 2006, 1:15–26)

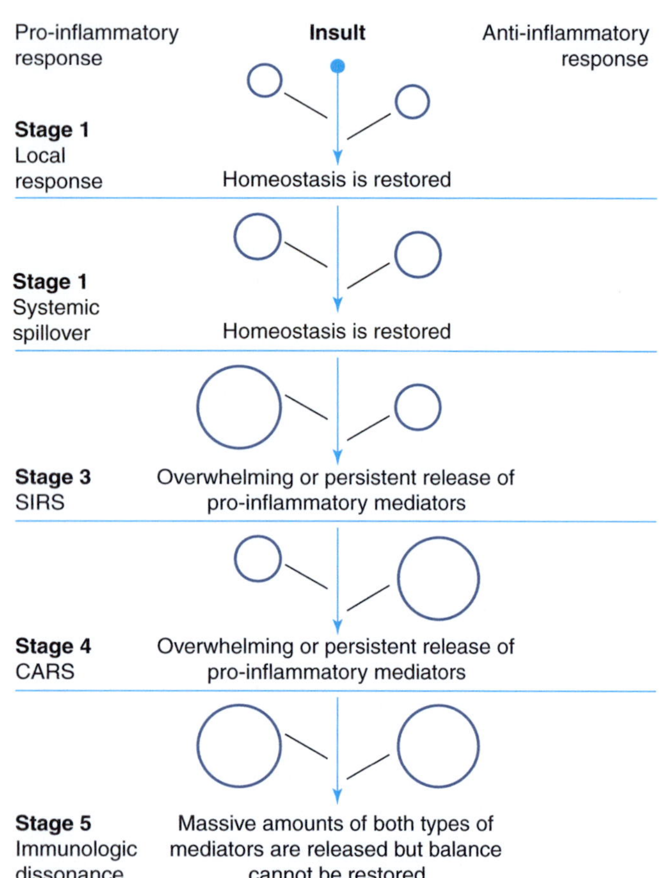

Fig. 9.3 Local and systemic inflammatory response. (Adapted from Aneta Malgorzata Binkowska, Grzegorz Michalak, Robert Slotwinski. Current views on the mechanisms of immune responses to trauma and infection. Central European Journal of Immunology. 2015; 40: 2)

There are four important characteristics of all scoring system: discrimination, precision, calibration and validation.

Discrimination describes the ability of a score to separate survivors from non-survivors.

Precision is the extent to which a prognostic score (i.e. a score that provides a risk of death estimate for each case) can closely predict the mortality rate observed.

Calibration is the extent to which the mentioned above precision is equally valid for low-risk and high-risk patients.

Validation refers to those properties of a scoring system (discrimination, precision, calibration) evaluated indifferent clinical setting.

Trauma setting scores are developed to describe the severity of injuries or the prognosis of a patient and correlate with severity. The triage scores are simply based on the patient observation and consider only a few items which are usually easy to calculate and are especially used in prehospital setting and at the admission to the emergency department. Prognostic scores describe a probability of survival from the score values.

Trauma severity score describes the injury pattern in a similar fashion, where injuries might affect different body systems and are divided into anatomical scores and physiological scores. Moreover, there is some score related to specific organ injuries.

9.3.1 Anatomical Scores

The principal anatomical scores used in trauma setting are abbreviated injury score (AIS), injury severity score (ISS) and new injury severity score (NISS).

The abbreviated injury scale (**AIS**) was introduced in 1969 [12]. Since that time it has been revised and updated (last time in 1998) against survival so that it now provides a reasonably accurate ranking of the severity of the injury. The AIS is monitored by a scaling committee of the Association for the Advancement of Automotive Medicine.

Injuries are ranked on a scale of 1–6, with 1 being minor, 5 severe and 6 a nonsurvivable injury (Table 9.4). Although

Table 9.4 AIS score [23]

	AIS
1	Minor
2	Moderate
3	Serious
4	Severe
5	Critical
6	Unsurvivable

AIS represents the degree of "threat to life" associated, it does not represent a comprehensive measure of severity. The AIS is not an injury scale, and the difference between AIS1 and AIS2 is not the same as that between AIS4 and AIS5. There are many similarities between the AIS scale and the organ injury scales of the AAST [13–17].

The injury severity score (**ISS**) provides an overall score for patients with multiple injuries. For each injury is assigned an AIS, and this is allocated to each of six body regions (head, face, chest, abdomen, extremities—including pelvis, external). Only the highest AIS score in each body region is used. The three most severely injured body regions have their score squared and added together to produce the ISS score.

The ISS score takes values from 0 to 75. If an injury is assigned an AIS of 6 (unsurvivable injury), the ISS score is automatically assigned to 75. A score more than 15 identifies a major trauma; this score includes patient with at least one injury with an AIS ≥ 4 or at least two injuries with AIS ≥ 3.

The ISS score is virtually the only anatomical scoring system in use and correlates linearly with mortality, morbidity and hospital stay.

As multiple injuries within the same body region are only assigned a single score, a proposed modification of the ISS, the "new injury severity score" (**NISS**), has been presented. This is calculated as the sum of the squares of the top three scores regardless of the body region. The NISS has been found to outperform the traditional ISS score statistically [18–20].

Even if all the anatomical scores correlate with mortality, all of them have a big limitation since they don't consider the risk related to each single patient as, for instance, the risk of an 80 years old man with cardiomyopathy who has the same score for similar injuries of a 20-year-old patient in previous health conditions.

9.3.2 Physiological Scores

The principal physiological scores in trauma setting used in the emergency department are Glasgow coma score (GCS) [17], revised trauma score (RTS), shock index (SI) [21–24], TRISS [25], TASH score [26]; APACHE, SAPS II, SOFA, and PIRO scores are usually emplyoied in ICU.

Table 9.5 GCS score

Best eye response (4)	Best verbal response (5)	Best motor response (6)
1. No eye opening	1. No verbal response	1. No motor response
2. Eye opening to pain	2. Incomprehensible sound	2. Extension to pain
3. Eye opening to verbal command	3. Inappropriate words	3. Flexion to pain
4. Eye open spontaneously	4. Confused	4. Withdrawal from pain
	5. Orientated	5. Localising pain
		6. Obeys commands

Table 9.6 Paediatric GCS score

Best eye response (4)	Best verbal response (5)	Best motor response (6)
1. No eye opening	1. No vocal response	1. No motor response
2. Eye opening to pain	2. Inconsolable agitated	2. Extension to pain
3. Eye opening to verbal command	3. Inconsistently consolable, moaning	3. Flexion to pain
4. Eye open spontaneously	4. Cries but is consolable, inappropriate interaction	4. Withdrawal from pain
	5. Smiles, oriented to sounds, follows objects, interacts	5. Localising pain
		6. Obeys commands

The Glasgow Coma Score (**GCS**) is scored between 3 and 15, 3 being the worst and 15 the best. It is composed of three parameters: best eye response, best verbal response and best motor response (choosing the best response if the response is different from the different side) [17] (Table 9.5).

Talking about GCS is important to break the total score down into its components (such as E3 V3 M5 = GCS 11), in which the "M" is the most important prognostic factor. A coma score of 13 or higher correlates with a mild brain injury; 9–12 is a moderate injury and 8 or less a severe brain injury [27].

In case of paediatric patients, the score has to be revised as below (Table 9.6):

The Revised Trauma Score (**RTS**) is a physiological scoring system, with high reliability and demonstrated accuracy in predicting death. It is scored from the first set of data obtained from the patient and consists of Glasgow Coma Scale, systolic blood pressure and respiratory rate.

Values for the RTS are in the range 0–7.8408 (Table 9.7). The RTS is heavily weighted towards the Glasgow Coma Scale to compensate for major head injury without multisys-

Table 9.7 RTS score calculation

Glasgow coma scale (GCS)	Systolic blood pressure (SBP)	Respiratory rate (RR)	Coded value
13–15	>89	10–26	4
9–12	76–89	>29	3
6–8	50–75	6–9	2
4–5	1–49	1–5	1
3	0	0	0
RTS = 0.9368 GCS + 0.7326 SBP + 0.2908 RR			

Table 9.8 *b* coefficients of TRISS calculation

	Blunt	Penetrating
*b*0	−0.4499	−2.5355
*b*1	0.8085	0.9934
*b*2	−0.8035	−0.0651
*b*3	1.7430	−1.1360

tem injury or major physiological changes. A threshold of RTS < 4 has been proposed to identify those patients who should be treated in a trauma centre, although this value may be somewhat low.

The trauma score—injury severity score (**TRISS**) determines the probability of survival (Ps) of a patient from the ISS and RTS using the following formulae: Ps = $1/(1 + e^{-b})$ [25].

Where "*b*" is calculated from (Table 9.8):

$$b = b0 + b1(\text{RTS}) + b2(\text{ISS}) + b3(\text{Age})$$

The coefficients *b*0, *b*3 are derived from multiple regression analysis of the major trauma outcome study database. Age index is 0 if the patient is below 54 years of age or 1 if 55 years and over. *b*0 to *b*3 are coefficients which are different for blunt and penetrating trauma. If the patient is less than 15, the blunt index for *b*3 (Age) is used regardless of mechanism.

The shock index (**SI**), defined by the ratio of heart rate to systolic blood pressure, has been advocated to better risk-stratify patients for increased transfusion requirements and early mortality.

SI upon emergency department arrival may be considered a clinical indicator of hypovolemic shock with respect to transfusion requirements, haemostatic resuscitation and mortality [23, 24].

There is a growing body of evidence that the ratio of HR to SBP, as reflected by the SI, is the most promising vital sign to detect acute hypovolaemia and circulatory failure.

Due to a negative relationship between SI and left ventricular stroke volume as well as cardiac output, the SI can be used clinically as the quickest non-invasive tool to assess cardiac function during acute hypovolaemia (Table 9.9).

The **trauma associated severe haemorrhage-score (TASH-Score)** is an easy-to-use scoring system that reliably predicts the probability for mass transfusion (MT) after multiple trauma. Taken as a surrogate for life-threatening bleeding calculation may focus attention on relevant variables indicative for risk and impact strategies to stop bleeding and stabilize coagulation in acute trauma care [11] (Table 9.10).

In the ICU setting is crucial to be able to identify those patients with a restored equilibrium from those who remain in unbalanced clinical status with an uncorrected immune response to decide the right timing for treatment.

Table 9.9 Classification of hypovolaemic shock based on SI

	Class I	Class II	Class III	Class IV
Shock	No shock	Mild shock	Moderate shock	Severe shock
SI at admission	<0.6	≥0.6 to <1	≥1 to <1.4	≥1.4
Need of blood products	Observe	Consider use of blood products	Prepare transfusion	Prepare massive transfusion

Table 9.10 TASH score: the TASH score of 18 equals a 50% risk of massive transfusion (MT) after severe multiple injuries

Variables	Variable	Points	Score
	<7	8	
	<9	6	
Haemoglobin (mg/dL)	<10	4	
	<11	3	
	<12	2	
	<−10	4	
Base excess (mmol/L)	<−6	3	
	<−2	1	
Systolic blood pressure (mmHg)	<100	4	
	<120	1	
Heart rate (beats/min)	>120	2	
Free intra-abdominal fluid (e.g. by FAST)		3	
Clinically instable pelvic fracture		6	
Open or dislocated femur fracture		3	
Male gender		1	
TASH (sum of score points) =			

Probability for mass transfusion	
TASH	*P*
1–8	<5%
9	6%
10	8%
11	11%
12	14%
13	18%
14	23%
15	29%
16	35%
17	43%
18	50%
19	57%
20	65%
21	71%
22	77%
23	82%
24+	>85%

Different scores, such as the MODS score (Goris score), MODS score (Marshall score), acute physiology and chronic health evaluation (APACHE) score or sequential organ failure assessment (SOFA) score, are available to describe dysfunctions of seven systems: respiratory, cardiovascular, renal, hepatic, gastrointestinal, haematological and central nervous systems. The MODS score published by Goris et al. in 1985 was one of the first attempts to quantify the severity of organ dysfunction and failure based on expert opinion about surgical patients admitted to ICU.

The attempt to define "early" and "late" MODS scores highlights another relevant issue about sequential organ failure monitoring. Lung failure and heart failure, if present, are often observed very early after admission to ICU. In contrast, the onset of liver failure is usually observed later. Patients with failure or dysfunction of all organs have a high rate of mortality. There is no threshold to define a rate of mortality or morbidity.

A lot of attempts to improve MODS score have been described. The scoring system (Table 9.11) was constructed using simple physiologic measures of organ dysfunction in six organ systems, and it is in strong relation with the ultimate risk of ICU and in hospital mortality. The modification of multiple organ dysfunction score reflects organ dysfunction developing during the ICU stay and therefore is potentially amenable to therapeutic prevention and manipulation.

APACHE II uses a point score based on initial values of 12 routine physiologic measurements, age and previous health status to provide a general measure of severity of disease. An increasing score (range 0–71) was closely correlated with the subsequent risk of hospital death. This relationship was also found for many common diseases. When APACHE II scores are combined with an accurate description of disease, they can prognostically stratify acutely ill patients and assist investigators comparing the success of new or differing forms of therapy. This scoring index can be used to evaluate the use of hospital resources and the treatment of patients (Tables 9.12 and 9.13).

SAPS II score (simplified physiology score) is one of the most used scores in ICU. It is used for ICU patients major than 15 years old. The final score is 0–163 points; it calculates 15 different topics; in this scoring system is indicated the worst value of the first 24 h after admission (Table 9.14).

Sepsis-related organ failure assessment score, also known as sequential organ failure assessment score (**SOFA score**), Table 9.15, is used to track a person's status during the stay in an intensive care unit to determine the extent of a person's organ function or rate of failure. The score is based on six different scores: respiratory, cardiovascular, hepatic, coagulation, renal, and neurological system.

Since sepsis is a common presenting illness to the emergency services and one of the leading causes of hospital mortality even in trauma patients, a lot of scoring systems has been created for defining sepsis. The predisposition, infection (or insult), response and organ dysfunction (**PIRO**) staging of sepsis might give better information (Table 9.16). PIRO system can classify patients by their predisposing conditions, the nature and extent of the infection, the nature and magnitude of the host response and the degree of concomitant organ dysfunction.

Table 9.11 MODS score. (PAR: Pressure adjusted hearth rate; HR heart rate; CVP central venous pressure; MAP mean arterial pressure)

	Score points				
Organ system	0	1	2	3	4
Respiratory (PaO2/FiO2)	>300	226–300	151–225	76–150	≤75
Renal (serum creatinine) mmol/L	≤100	101–200	201–350	351–500	<500
Hepatic (serum bilirubin) mmol/L	≤20	21–60	61–120	121–240	>240
Cardiovascular (PAR: HRx CVP/MAP)	≤10	10.1–15.0	15.1–20	20.1–30	>30
Hematologic (platelet count) mL/10q	>120	81–120	51–80	21–50	≤20
Neurologic (GCS)	15	13–14	10–12	7–9	≤6

Points	ICU mortality %	Hospitality mortality %	ICU stay days
0	0	0	2
1–4	1–2	7	3
5–8	3–5	16	6
9–12	25	50	10
13–16	50	70	17
17–20	75	82	21
21–24	100	100	

Table 9.12 APACHE II score

APACHE II score	
Age	Points
≤44 years	0
45–54 years	2
55–64 years	3
65–74 years	5
≥75 years	6
Chronic health points	
Nonoperative, or emergency post-op and any condition below[a]	5
Elective operation and any condition below[a]	2
[a]Cirrhosis w/portal hypertension or encephalopathy; class IV angina, chronic hypoxia, I CO2 or polycythemia; chronic dialysis immunocompromised	

Total APACHE score = APCHP + APS (sum age points (AP) + chronic health points (CHP) + acute physiologic score (APS) points)

[a]Sum all variables 1–12 for acute physiologic score (APS) (use one variable each for 5 and 9). Use the worst value from the preceding 24 h (Adapted from APACHE II: a severity of disease classification system. Crit care med 1985, 13:818–29)

Table 9.13 APS score

Acute physiologic score (APS)										
		Points								
Physiologic variable		4	3	2	1	0	1	2	3	4
1	Temp °F	≤85.9	86.0–89.5	89.6–93.1	93.2–96.7	96.8–101.2	101.3–102.1		102.2–105.7	≥105.8
	Temp °C	≤29.9	30–31.9	32–33.9	34–35.9	36–38.4	38.5–38.9		39–40.9	≥41
2	HR bpm	≤39	40–54	55–69		70–109		110–139	140–179	≥180
3	MAP, mmHg	≤49		50–69		70–109		110–129	130–159	≥160
4	RR, bpm	≤5		6–9	10–11	dic-24	25–34		35–49	≥50
5	Oxygenation: use A-a gradient (5a) if FiO2 ≥ 0.5 or use PaO2 (5b) if FiO2 > 0.5									
5a	A-a gradient					<200		200–349	350–499	≥500
5b	PaO2	≤54	55–60		61–70	>70				
6	Na+ (S, mmo/L)	≤110	111–119	120–129		130–139	150–154	155–159	160–179	≥180
7	K+ (S, mmo/L)	≤2.4		2.5–2.9	3.0–3.4	3.5–5.4	5.5–5.9		6.0–6.9	≥7.0
8	Cr (S, mg/dL)			<0.6		0.6–1.4		1.5–1.9	2.0–3.4	≥3.5
9	Arterial pH is preferred. Use venous HCO3 if no AGBs									
9a	pH (arterial)	≤7.14	7.15–7.24	7.25–7.32		7.33–7.49	7.5–7.59		7.6–7.69	≥7.7
9b	HCO3 (venous)	≤14	15–17.9	18–21.9		22–31.9	32–40.9		41–51.9	≥52
10	WBC, cells/μL	≤1		1.0–2.9		3.0–14.9	15–19.9	20–39.9		≥40
11	Hct, %	≤20		20–29.9		30–45.9	46–49.9	50–59.9		≥60
12	GCS coma	Score = 15 – GCL score (see below, record, e.g. "GCS 9 = E2 V4 M3 at 17:35 h")								

Score	Mortality (%)
0–4	4
5–9	4
10–14	15
15–19	25
20–24	40
25–29	55
30–34	75
>34	85

Table 9.14 SAPS score

Mortality (%)	SAPS II score
10	29 pts
25	40 pts
50	52 pts
75	64 pts
90	77 pts

SAPS score									
Variables	Score								
	+4	+3	+2	+1	0	+1	+2	+3	+4
Age					≤45	46–55	56–65	66–75	>75
HR	≥180	140–179	110–139		70–109		55–69	40–54	<40
SBP	≥190		150–189		80–149		55–79		<55
Temperature	≥41	39.0–40.9		38.5–38.9	36.0–38.4	34.0–35.9	32.0–33.9	30.0–31.9	<30
RR									
(Ventilation or CPAP)	≥50	35–49		25–34	12–24	10–11	6–9		<6
Urine output (L/24 h)			<5.00	3.50–4.99	0.70–3.49		0.50–0.69	Sì	>0.20
Urea	≥55.0	36.0–54.9	29.0–35.9	7.5–28.9	3.5–7.4	<3.5		0.20–0.49	
HT	≥60.0		50.0–59.9	46.0–49.9	30.0–45.9		20.0–29.9		<20.0
WBC	≥40.0		20.0–39.9	15.0–19.9	3.0–14.9		1.0–2.9		<1.0
Glu	≥44.5	27.8–44.4		14.0–27.7	3.9–13.9		2.8–3.8	1.6–2.7	<1.6
K	≥7.0	6.0–6.9		5.5–5.9	3.5–5.4	3.0–3.4	2.5–2.9		<2.5
Na	≥180	161–179	156–160	151–155	130–150		120–129	110–119	<110
HCO3		>40.0		30.0–39.9	20.0–29.9	10.0–19.9		5.0–9.9	<5.0
GCS					13–15	10–12	7–9	4–6	3

Table 9.15 The sequential organ failure assessment (SOFA)

	SOFA score				
Variables	0	1	2	3	4
Respiratory Pao2/FIO2, mmHg	>400	≤400	≤300	≤200[a]	≤100[a]
Coagulation Platelets × 103/UL[b]	>150	≥150	≤100	≤50	≤20
Liver Bilirubin, mg/dL[b]	<1.2	1.2–1.9	2.0–5.9	6.0–11.9	>12.0
Cardiovascular					
Hypotension	No hypotension	Mean arterial pressure < 70 mmHg	Dop ≤ 5 or Dob (any dose)[c]	Dop > 5, epi ≤ 0.1, or norepi ≤ 0.1[c]	Dop > 1 5, epi > 0.1, or norepi > 0.1[c]
Central nervous system Glasgow coma core scale	15	13–14	10–12	6–9	<6
Renal Creatinine, mg/dL or urine output, mL/24h	<1.2	1.2–1.9	2.0–3.4	3.5–4.9 or <500	>5.0 or <200

Norepi indicates norepinephrine, *Dob* dobutamine, *Dop* dopamine, *Epi* epinephrine, *FIO2* fraction of inspired oxygen
[a]Values are with respiratory support
[b]To convert bilirubin from ng/dL to mmol/L, multiply by 17.1
[c]Adrenergic agents, administered for at least 1 h (doses given are in µg/kg per minute)
[d]To convert creatinine from mg/dL to mmol/L, multiply by 88.4

Table 9.16 Classification on sepsis based on the PIRO system [31]

	P	I	R	O
Diagnostics	Predisposition	Infection	Response	Organ failure
Clinical	Age	Susceptibility to infection	SIRS	Organ failure according to the scale: MODS, SOFA, LODS, PEMOD, PELOD
	Comorbidity	Site of infection	Other clinical signs of sepsis	
	General condition	Pathogen identification		
	Cause of trauma/ infection (degree and severity)	Source of infection (hospital or nonhospital)	Shock CRP	
		Extent of the infection	Dysfunction	
Molecular	Genetics (Polymorphism TLR, TNF, IL-1, CD14)	Gene transcript profiles	Biomarkers	Monitoring of cell-mediated immunity (abnormal apoptosis, mitochondrial and endothelial damage and activation of adhesion molecules, cell hypoxia)
		Analysis of microbial products (LPS, mannan, bacterial DNA)	Nonspecific markers of inflammation (e.g. PCT, IL-6) or markers immune disorders (e.g. HLA-DR)	
		Assessment of virulence factors		

MODS multiple organ dysfunction syndrome, *SOFA* sequential organ failure assessment, *LODS* logistic organ dysfunction system, *PEMOD* paediatric multiple organ dysfunction, *PELOD* paediatric logistic organ dysfunction
Reference range
Risk of mortality
Mild = 0–1 point
High = 2 points
Very high = 3–4 points

9.3.3 Score Related to Specific Organ Injuries

Some specific injuries require a rapid treatment due to the possibility of worsening of the patient condition for the overwhelming immune response and the mediators that the injury itself can produce.

An example of this situation is the mangled extremity injuries [28]. Many mangled extremities are borderline cases, and the decision to amputate or to salvage a limb must be carefully evaluated. With advances in the medical field over the last 15 years, more mangled lower extremities are salvaged, especially in civilian injuries. The mangled extrem-

Table 9.17 MESS score

Mangled extremity severity score (MESS)
Skeletal/soft tissue injury
Low-energy injury (e.g. simple bone fracture)—1 point
Medium-energy injury (e.g. multiple bone fracture)—2 points
High-energy injury (e.g. car accidents)—3 points
Very-high-energy injury (e.g. high-speed trauma with severe contamination)—4 points
Limb ischemia
Normal perfusion with reduced or even absent pulse: 1[a] point
Absent pulse, paraesthesia, diminished capillary refill: 2 points
Cool, paralyzed, insensate limb: 3[a] points
Shock
Systolic blood pressure > 90 mmHg: 0 point
Hypotensive transiently: 1 point
Hypotensive persistent: 2 points
Age
<30 years: 0 point
30–50 years: 1 point
>50 years: 2 points

[a]The score is doubled for ischemia > 6 h

Table 9.18 Operational aortic injury risk score

Risk score criteria
Lactate > 4 mM
Mediastinal haematoma > 10 mm
Lesion/normal aortic ratio > 1.4
High risk for aortic rupture when any two factors are present

ity severity score, **MESS score,** helps physician to decide the correct treatment considering both anatomical and physiological conditions of the patients. A total score of six or less consistent with a salvageable limb, severe or greater amputation is generally the eventual result (Table 9.17).

The **aortic injury score** can be applied on admission using clinically relevant factors that incorporate patient physiology, the size of the aortic lesion and extent of the mediastinal haematoma [29]. The model reliably identifies and distinguishes patients with high-grade blunt traumatic aortic injuries (BTAI) who are at risk for early rupture from those with stable lesions (Table 9.18).

9.4 Using Score in Decision-Making for Trauma Patients

Time from admission to definitive care is very variable for each trauma patient; type of injury, physiological impact following trauma and immune response of the single patient are all factors interacting with each other [30, 31].

Few seconds after trauma, the immune system starts to react, and it continues till 3 weeks after trauma. A balance between SIRS and CARS have to be achieved by the patients, and a careful clinical monitoring can help to decide the right treatment in the right moment avoiding the second hit surgical procedure.

The current approach to the challenge of multivisceral high-energy trauma is based on a modified operative sequence, whereby rapid life-saving bail-out techniques are used to arrest haemorrhage and control spillage and fluid leakage avoiding resections and reconstructions. This is then followed by a period of secondary resuscitation and rewarming in the surgical intensive care unit (SICU), followed by a planned reoperation. This strategy is named damage control strategy and will be treated elsewhere in a dedicated chapter.

In the emergency, department trauma surgeons have to recognize all patients that need a damage control strategy [32]. This evaluation must be efficient and rapid. It is based on few parameters of patients and information derived from prehospital setting. Mortality in trauma is particularly related to haemorrhagic shock which in turn is related to avoidable mortality [33].

If signs of shock are present, clinicians have to consider a strategy to stop haemorrhage and rapidly treat the patients in ICU. A SI greater than 1.4, a TASH score greater than 18 and type of injury can suggest a damage control strategy.

The need for massive transfusion is related to the need for damage control surgery, and only the application of both damage control resuscitation and surgery can lead to improvement of the probability of patients' survival.

Sometimes the real challenge is to achieve control of bleeding and spillage in the shortest possible time to minimize the second hit. In these patients, the lethal triad (acidosis, coagulopathy and hypothermia) is going up, and the best option is to stop bleeding and spillage and to restore patient's resources in ICU.

9.4.1 Indications for Damage Control Strategy (DCS), Early Appropriate Care (EAC) and Definitive Care

ISS greater than 25, as well as an RTS greater than 4, can suggest DCS. Patients *in extremis* are easily candidate to DCS; however sometimes can be difficult to choose the right treatment in patients responders to the first load of fluids [30–32].

It is known that a temporary treatment of injuries such as long bone fracture can lead to respiratory problems or prolonged time to specific treatment due to infections. Recently a lot of research has been published to identify criteria to decide between DCS and EAC in patients with orthopaedic injuries.

When the probability of a complication has decreased to an acceptable level (below 20%), the EAC can be considered in a patient responding to resuscitation measures, which usually means a lactate <4.0 mmol/L, pH $\geq$ 7.25 or a base excess (BE) $\geq$ −5.5 mmol/L. The aim of an EAC with definitive management of mechanically unstable fractures of the axial skeleton and long bones within 36 h of injury can be an acceptable option as long as the patient has demonstrated response to resuscitation in consideration of the improvement of the acidotic state (lactate < 4.0 mmol/L, pH ≥ 7.25 or BE above 5.5 mmol/L) [31].

On the other side, DCS is recommended if a coagulopathy is already present at admission (INR > 1.2), lactate > 6 mmol/L, BD > 3 mmol/L or hypothermia with a body temperature less than 35 °C.

There is some particular evidence that brain trauma injuries (TBI) with AIS ≥ 3 who develop coagulopathy had a higher mortality rate than isolated severe TBI patients without coagulopathy.

A GCS which identifies a severe brain injury demands a damage control treatment to avoid the second hit due to blood loss and hypoperfusion in cerebral tissue even if in other patients without brain injury the same bleeding injury can be treated with a nonoperative management (NOM).

Patients can bleed from soft tissue without the possibility of a surgical control, e.g. obese subjects, in these setting DCS should be done by resuscitation with massive transfusion protocols.

Mangled injuries can lead to severe bleeding and contamination; it is important to treat the injury considering both the possibility of recovery of the limb and the second hit that a hypo-perfused district can provoke.

Damage control surgery includes abbreviated laparotomy with packing, control of bleeding and temporary closure of the abdomen; damage control thoracotomy may require emergency thoracotomy or sternotomy, temporary packing with vacuum, full control of the pericardium and temporary closure; damage control of pelvic fracture may require extraperitoneal pelvic packing, angiographic embolization or REBOA control.

Damage control resuscitation includes massive transfusion protocols, rewarming technique and coagulopathy control.

The possibility to choose correctly a DCS depends on the experience of the trauma surgeon, the presentation of the patients, the type of injuries due to trauma, available resources, and a correct interpretation of early scores [32, 33].

While a lot of literature can be found for DCS and decision-making in an emergency setting, it's hard to have a strict indication of how and when to perform a second look laparotomy or to definitively close the abdomen.

A correct decision should be taken considering both the recovery of the balance of the physiological parameters of the patients and the risk of overwhelming infection and organ failure (Fig. 9.4).

After 24 h of the DCS operation, adequate resuscitation is evidenced by a normalized lactate, base excess, pH and weaning from amines which could act as a guide to the timing for a second look laparotomy.

When surviving the first 72 h after injury, the risk of mortality in severely injured trauma patients managed with damage

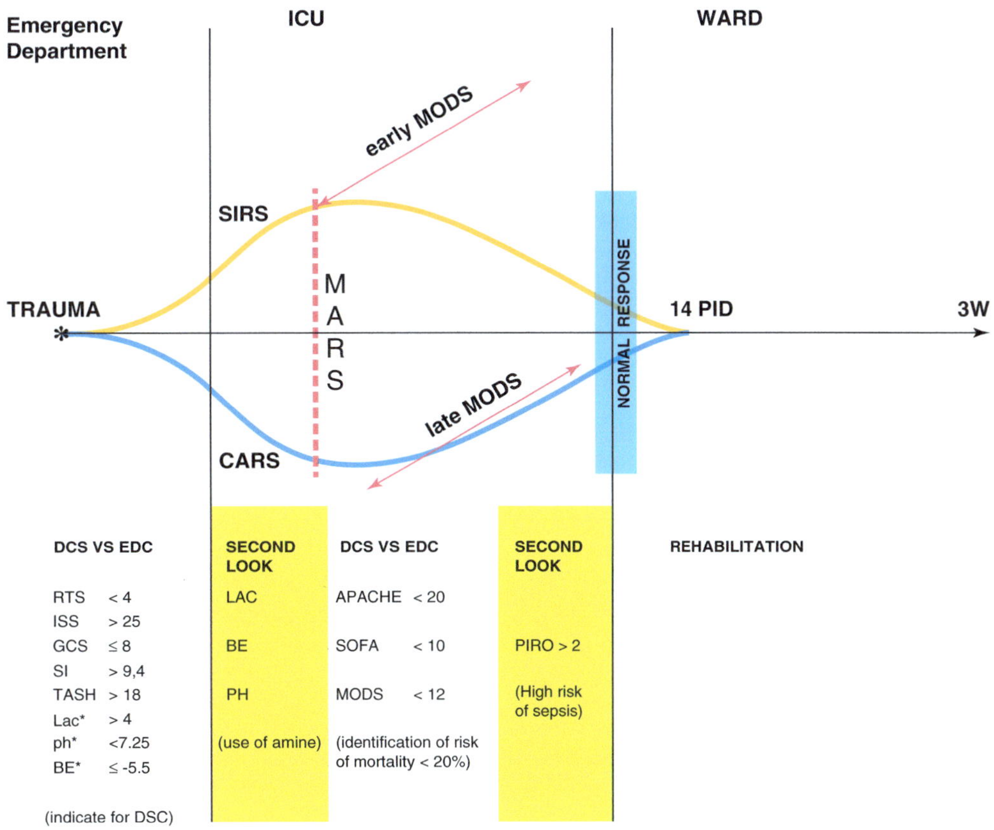

Emergency Department
ICU
WARD
early MODS
SIRS
M A R S
NORMAL RESPONSE
TRAUMA
14 PID
3W
late MODS
CARS
DCS VS EDC
RTS < 4
ISS > 25
GCS ≤ 8
SI > 9,4
TASH > 18
Lac* > 4
ph* <7.25
BE* ≤ -5.5
(indicate for DSC)
SECOND LOOK
LAC
BE
PH
(use of amine)
DCS VS EDC
APACHE < 20
SOFA < 10
MODS < 12
(identification of risk of mortality < 20%)
SECOND LOOK
PIRO > 2
(High risk of sepsis)
REHABILITATION

Fig. 9.4 *PID* post injury day, *DCS* damage control surgery, *EDC* early definite care, * after fluid challenge, *DSTC* definite surgical care control protocol is mainly related to sepsis, organ failure or severe brain injuries.

The patients may need a definite surgery even after 72 h from trauma, and choosing the correct timing can be paramount to improve patients' outcome.

The adoption of the principles of DCS has reduced post-traumatic complications in severly injured pateints. The development of better clinical monitoring by the wise use of scoring systems may help clinicians to improve the risk stratification and to select for each single patient the most appropriate time of treatment from DCS to definitive care.

References

1. Hietbrink F, Koenderman L, Rijkers GT, Leenen LPH. Trauma: the role of the innate immune system. World J Emerg Surg. 2006;1:15–26.
2. Keel M, Trentz O. Pathophysiology of polytrauma. Injury. 2005;36:691–709.
3. Gentile LF, Cuenca A, Efron PA, et al. Persistent inflammatory and immunosuppression: a common syndrome and new horizon for surgical intensive care. J Trauma Acute Care Surg. 2012;72:1491–501.
4. Hayakawa M. Pathophysiology of trauma-induced coagulopathy: disseminated intravascular coagulation with the fibrinolytic phenotype. J Intensive Care. 2017;5:14–20.
5. Gebhard F, Huber-Lang M. Polytrauma-pathophysiology and management principles. Langenbecks Arch Surg. 2008;393:825–31.
6. Saadia R, Shein M. Multiple organ failure. How valid is the "two-hit" model? J Accid Emerg Med. 1999;16:163–7.
7. Bone RC. Sir Isaac Newton, sepsis, SIRS, and CARS. Crit Care Med. 1996;24:1125–8.
8. Binkowska AM, Michalak G, Slotwinski R. Current views on the mechanisms of immune responses to trauma and infection. Cent Eur J Immunol. 2015;40:206–16.
9. Ward NS, Casserly B, Ayala A. The compensatory anti-inflammatory response syndrome (CARS) in critically ill patients. Clin Chest Med. 2008;29:617, viii.
10. Giannoudis PV, Hildebrand F, Pape HC, Gentile LF. Inflammatory serum markers in patients with multiple trauma. J Bone Joint Surg Br. 2004;86-B(3):313–23.
11. Lefering R. Trauma scoring. In: Oestern HJ, et al., editors. General trauma care and related aspects. European manual of medicine. Berlin: Springer; 2014. p. 25–9.
12. Baker SP, et al. The Injury Severity Score: a method for describing patients with multiple injuries and evaluating emergency care. J Trauma. 1974;14:187–96.
13. Moore EE, Shackford SR, Pachter HL, et al. Organ injury scaling: spleen, liver, and kidney. J Trauma. 1989;29:1664.
14. Moore EE, Cogbill TH, Malangoni MA, et al. Organ injury scaling II: pancreas, duodenum, small bowel, colon, and rectum. J Trauma. 1990;30:1427.
15. Moore EE, Cogbill TH, Jurkovich GJ, et al. Organ injury scaling III: chest wall, abdominal vascular, ureter, bladder, and urethra. J Trauma. 1992;33:337–9.
16. Moore EE, Malangoni MA, Cogbill TH, et al. Organ injury scaling IV: thoracic, vascular, lung, cardiac and diaphragm. J Trauma. 1994;36:299–300.
17. Moore EE, Cogbill TH, Jurkovich MD, et al. Organ injury scaling: spleen and liver (1994 revision). J Trauma. 1995;38:323–4.
18. Copes WS, Sacco WJ, Champion HR, Bain LW. Progress in characterising anatomic injury. In: Proceedings of the 33rd Annual Meeting of the Association for the Advancement of Automotive Medicine, Baltimore, MA. 1993. p. 205–18.
19. Champion HR, et al. Trauma score. Crit Care Med. 1981;9:672–6.
20. Champion HR, et al. A revision of the trauma score. J Trauma. 1989;29:623–9.
21. Fröhlich M, Driessen A, Böhmer A, et al. Is the shock index based classification of hypovolemic shock applicable in multiple injured patients with severe traumatic brain injury? Scand J Trauma Resusc Emerg Med. 2016;24:148.
22. Berger T, Green J, Horeczko T, et al. Shock index and early recognition of sepsis in the emergency department: pilot study. West J Emerg Med. 2013;14:168–74.
23. Haider AA, Azim A, Rhee P, et al. Substituting systolic blood pressure with shock index in the National Trauma Triage Protocol. J Trauma Acute Care Surg. 2016;81:1136–41.
24. Mutschler M, Nienaber U, Münzberg M, et al. The shock index revisited—a fast guide to transfusion requirement? A retrospective analysis on 21,853 patients derived from the Trauma Register DGU. Crit Care. 2013;17:R172.
25. Boyd CR, Tolson MA, Copes WS, et al. Evaluating trauma care: the TRISS method. J Trauma. 1987;27:370–8.
26. Yucel N, Lefering R, Maegele M, et al. Trauma associated Severe Hemorrhage (TASH)-score: probability of mass transfusion as surrogate for life threatening hemorrhage after multiple trauma. J Trauma. 2006;60:1228–36; discussion 1236–7.
27. Teasdale G, Jennett B. Assessment of coma and impaired consciousness. A practical scale. Lancet. 1974;2(7872):81–4.
28. Fodor L, Sobec R, Sita-Alb L, Fodor M, Ciuce C. Mangled lower extremity: can we trust the amputation scores? Int J Burns Trauma. 2012;2(1):51–8.
29. Harris DG, Rabin J, Kufera JA, et al. A new aortic injury score predicts early rupture more accurately than clinical assessment. J Vasc Surg. 2015;61:332–8.
30. Han G, Wang Z, Du Q, Xiong Y, et al. Damage-control orthopedics versus early total care in the treatment of borderline high-energy pelvic fractures. Orthopedics. 2014;37:1091–100.
31. Tasker A, Kelly MB. Managing trauma: the evolution from 'early total care'/'damage control' to 'early appropriate care'. J Trauma Orthop. 2014;2:66–70.
32. Voiglio EJ, Dubuisson V, Massalou D, et al. Abbreviated laparotomy or damage control laparotomy: why, when and how to do it? J Visc Surg. 2016;153:13–24.
33. Paffrath T, Lefering R, Flohè S, et al. How to define severely injured patients?—an Injury Severity score (ISS) based approach alone is not sufficient. Injury. 2014;45(Suppl 3):S64–9.

Airway Management in Trauma Patients

10

Michal Barak, Yoav Leiser, and Yoram Kluger

Key Points

- Airway control is the primary and principal task of the caregiver in trauma. Any flaw in airway management may lead to grave morbidity or mortality.
- Many factors may complicate airway management in trauma: patient's hemodynamic instability, C-spine injury, full stomach, emergency situation, and operator's lack of experience.
- A definitive airway is the superior method to secure the airway, which is a cuffed tube secured in the trachea. This includes orotracheal tube, nasotracheal tube, or surgical airway, meaning cricothyrotomy or tracheostomy.
- The physician may be challenged with a situation where it is difficult to intubate the patient. Being familiar with standard basic airway techniques and advanced airway devices may help in such situation. The assistance of colleagues, whose expertise includes the airways, is always recommended.
- In case of "cannot intubate, cannot ventilate" cricothyrotomy is a lifesaving procedure. It is superior to tracheostomy in emergency situations because the cricothyroid membrane is superficial and minimal dissection is required to get access to the airway. It is important that emergency department physicians are trained and practiced with this procedure.

10.1 Introduction

In compliance with the guidelines of advanced trauma life support (ATLS) for the management of patients who sustained life-threatening injuries, airway maintenance with cervical spine immobilization is a primary priority [1]. The loss of airway may be lethal and can happen faster than the loss of the ability to breathe or the onset of circulatory problems. Thus, lifesaving intervention should begin with airway management [1–3]. The main purpose is to ventilate the patient in order to facilitate tissue oxygenation, most importantly the brain and the heart. Timely, decisive, and skillful management of the airway may often make the difference between life and death or between ability and disability in such circumstances. One should be familiar with airway anatomy, the standard basic airway techniques and devices, situations that set airway difficulties, and advanced airway management in extreme situations. The assistance of colleagues, whose expertise includes the airways, is always recommended.

M. Barak (✉)
The Department of Anesthesiology, Rambam Health Care Campus, and the Ruth and Bruce Rappaport Faculty of Medicine, Technion-Israel Institute of Technology, Haifa, Israel
e-mail: m_barak@rambam.health.gov.il

Y. Leiser
The Department of Oral and Maxillofacial Surgery, Rambam Health Care Campus, and the Ruth and Bruce Rappaport Faculty of Medicine, Technion-Israel Institute of Technology, Haifa, Israel

Y. Kluger
Department of General Surgery, Pancreatic Surgery Service, Rambam Health Care Campus, and the Ruth and Bruce Rappaport Faculty of Medicine, Technion-Israel Institute of Technology, Haifa, Israel
e-mail: y_kluger@rambam.health.gov.il

10.2 Approach to the Airway of Trauma Patient

There are several aspects in managing the trauma patient's airway. The following are needed to be considered by the physician in charge:

P. Aseni et al. (eds.), *Operative Techniques and Recent Advances in Acute Care and Emergency Surgery*,
https://doi.org/10.1007/978-3-319-95114-0_10

(a) The primary caregiver has to determine whether the patient requires support in breathing and whether there is an indication to secure the airway and to ventilate the lungs.
(b) Airway assessment needs to be promptly executed within the limitation of time and the patient's cooperation.
(c) The physician has to determine whether there is likelihood for difficult mask ventilation or difficult endotracheal intubation, such as obesity or facial hair.
(d) What is the extent, the details, and the anatomy of the injury? Does it include the head and face and cervical (C) spine? Hemodynamic stability of the patient?
(e) What is the upcoming surgical procedure that the patient will need to have, and is prolonged mechanical ventilation predicted at this stage? [4]

10.2.1 Airway Assessment

The main purpose of airway evaluation is to determine whether difficulty in mask ventilation or endotracheal intubation is to be expected. In addition, while examining the patient's airway, the physician needs to decide which type and size of airway device is suitable for the patient and the situation. Airway assessment should be carried out as quickly as possible, and take into consideration the patient's ability to cooperate. Previous difficulty in intubation may be known to the patient or family [5, 6]. The condition of the face and neck, mouth, bony structure, and soft tissue is to be examined (Table 10.1). In addition, the inner view of the mouth is to be inspected, also known as Mallampati score (Fig. 10.1): poor vision of the hard and soft palate has a higher score and may indicate difficult intubation. Mallampati's oropharyngeal classification was first proposed as a hypothesis for prediction of difficult intubation [7, 8]; its efficacy in the prediction of difficulty at direct laryngoscopy was demonstrated later in clinical trials [8–11], and it became a part of pre-intubation airway examination.

10.2.2 Securing the Airways

In order to decide whether there is a need for airway management and for ventilation in a trauma patient, the following questions should be answered:

(a) Is the patient conscious?
(b) Is the patient breathing effectively?
(c) Is the patient hemodynamically stable?
(d) Does the patient require surgery or transporting to another facility?
(e) Does the trauma involve the maxillofacial region or the upper or lower airways?
(f) Is there a head trauma with increased ICP, which may necessitate hyperventilation?

Table 10.1 Airway assessment

• Medical history
– History of difficult intubation, including syndromes such as Down syndrome and Pierre-Robin syndrome
– Pathology of the oropharynx area or neck (e.g., maxillofacial trauma, cervical spine injury)
– Previous treatment to the oropharynx or neck (e.g., radiation to the neck, cervical neck fixation)
– Obstructive sleep apnea
• Physical examination
– Mouth opening (should be more than three fingerbreadths)
– Thyromental distance (should be more than three fingerbreadths)
– Condition of the mouth cavity and teeth (e.g., denture, bleeding)
– Temporomandibular joint and neck mobility
– Size of the tongue and mandible
– Mallampati score
– Facial hair

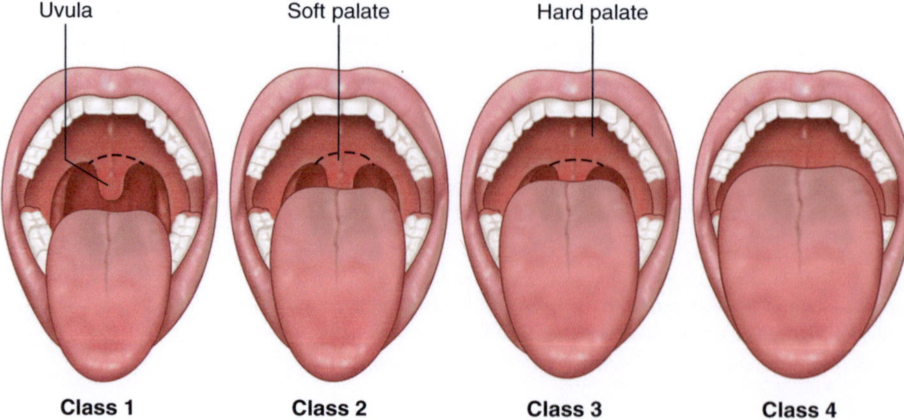

Fig. 10.1 The Mallampati score. Class 1: Complete visualization of the uvula, soft palate, and faucial pillars. Class 2: Visualization of the soft palate, major part of uvula, and faucial pillars. Class 3: Visualization of the soft palate and base of uvula. Class 4: Only hard palate visible

Table 10.2 Indications for definitive airway in trauma patient[a]

Need for airway protection	Need for ventilation or oxygenation
Severe maxillofacial trauma	Inadequate respiratory efforts • Tachypnea • Hypoxia • Hypercarbia • Cyanosis
Risk for obstruction • Neck hematoma • Laryngeal or tracheal injury • Stridor	Massive blood loss and need for volume resuscitation
Risk for aspiration • Bleeding • Vomiting	Severe closed head injury with need for brief hyperventilation and patients with GCS scores of 8 or less
Unconscious	Apnea

[a]Advanced Trauma Life Support Student Course Manual [12]

Trauma patients presenting with apnea or a gasping breathing pattern (respiratory rate < 6/min), hypoxia (oxygen saturation < 90% despite oxygen insufflation and after exclusion of tension pneumothorax), trauma-associated hemodynamic instability [systolic blood pressure (SBP) < 90 mmHg], severe chest trauma with respiratory insufficiency (respiratory rate > 29/min), or severe traumatic brain injury [Glasgow Coma Scale (GCS) < 9] require emergency airway assistance.

Ventilation and oxygenation can be achieved through several airway devices. However, the superior approach is to secure the airway with a definitive airway, which is a cuffed tube secured in the trachea. This includes orotracheal tube, nasotracheal tube, or surgical airway, meaning cricothyrotomy or tracheostomy [12, 13]. The definitive airway is advantageous since it enables ventilating directly and only the trachea; the cuff minimizes the risk for aspiration to the lungs, and fixation is superior to other means of ventilation, thus suitable for patient's transport.

The indications for achieving a definitive airway are specified in Table 10.2.

10.3 Techniques and Devices for Airway Management

There are many techniques and devices to manage the patient's airway; however, the basic and frequently practiced approaches are mask ventilation and endotracheal intubation. One should be familiar and experienced with these techniques before advancing to other airway techniques. The necessary equipment for mask ventilation and endotracheal intubation is to be prepared and checked: face mask, oral airway, reservoir bag, direct laryngoscope, endotracheal tube, oxygen supply, and suction catheter (Fig. 10.2).

10.3.1 Mask Ventilation

Ventilating the patient with a face mask is the primary and easiest method of ventilation and oxygenation. The physician should select the proper mask size that fits the patient's face in order to have effective ventilation. In some patients, an oral or nasal airway is required to ensure adequate air passage to the patient's larynx and lungs (Fig. 10.3).

The disadvantage of mask ventilation is that it is not a definitive airway; thus (a) it is difficult to continue managing the patient for a long time with mask ventilation, for transportation or for radiologic examination, and (b) there is a chance of inflating the stomach and increasing the risk of gastric content regurgitation followed by its aspiration into the lungs.

10.3.2 Tracheal Intubation

Orotracheal intubation with direct laryngoscopy is a simple and straightforward method for securing the airway in trauma patients. It is performed with a conventional laryngoscope, e.g., Macintosh blade, with a rapid sequence induction (RSI) in order to decrease the risk of pulmonary aspiration [14, 15]. However, the incidence of a difficult intubation in the emergency department is 3–5.3% for unanticipated difficult tracheal intubation and 0.5–1.2% for failed intubation [16]. Failure to achieve successful tracheal intubation to a maximum of three attempts is defined as failed tracheal intubation and indicates the need to change strategy [17, 18]. Multiple failed attempts at tracheal intubation injure the patient' larynx and may be harmful [19]. Every additional laryngoscopy causes soft tissue edema, bleeding, and secretions, thus worsening the airway condition and decreasing the likelihood of successful intubation. Analysis of failed cases identified gaps in care that included poor identification of at-risk patients, poor or incomplete planning, inadequate provision of skilled staff and equipment to manage these events successfully, delayed recognition of events, and failed rescue because of lack or failure of interpretation of capnography [16, 20]. Therefore, emergency airway management necessitates a firm concept of techniques of securing the airway and of dealing with the potential difficult intubation, whereby establishing a definite airway is not feasible with standard techniques [21].

10.3.3 The Difficult Airway

Difficulty in mask ventilation or tracheal intubation requires a quick response as to how to manage the patient's airway. Several professional societies, including the American Society of Anesthesiologists (ASA) and the Difficult Airway Society

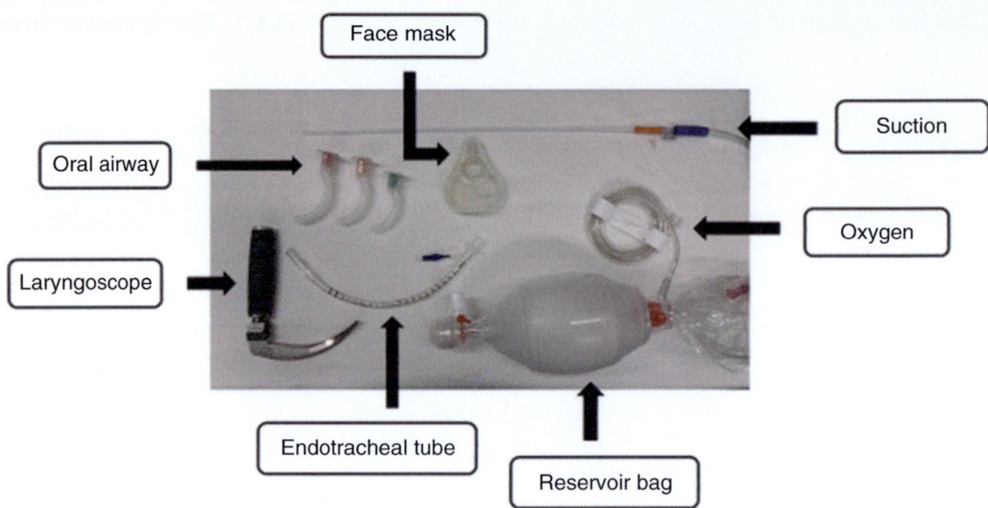

Fig. 10.2 Necessary equipment for basic airway management: face mask, oral airway, reservoir bag, direct laryngoscope, endotracheal tube, oxygen supply, and suction catheter

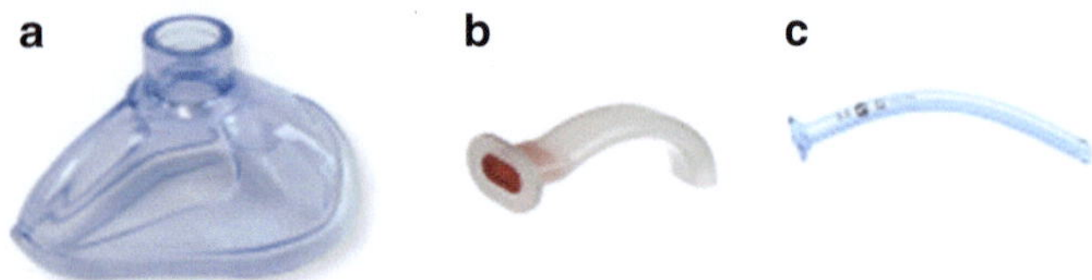

Fig. 10.3 (**a**) Face mask, (**b**) oral airway, (**c**) nasal airway

(DAS), have published guidelines to assist the physician in decision-making at that crucial point [18, 22]. The main issues are similar in all the guidelines, progressing from simple to more advanced airway devises, while maintaining the patient's safety.

Occasionally the difficult airway guidelines are not suitable in managing the trauma patient. Techniques of awake intubation are not always possible in a trauma patient, since these techniques are (a) time-consuming, (b) require special equipment, (c) necessitate operator's special expertise, and (d) require patient's cooperation, all of which are often absent in trauma. The hallmark of airway management of the difficult airway patient is maintaining the patient's spontaneous breathing as long as possible, which may be unfeasible in trauma patient. In addition, in a case of difficulty, the recommendations are either "cancel case" or "wake patient," neither of which is a realistic option with trauma patients. Thus, the physician in charge has to be prepared earlier than usual to proceed to the option of "invasive airway access," meaning surgical airway.

Figure 10.4 describes our suggested strategy for management of a difficult airway of trauma patient in emergency situation.

10.3.4 Alternative Airway Techniques and Devices

The main obstacle in performing successful endotracheal intubation is not having an unobstructed view of the vocal cords. Numerous airway devices and strategies have been developed to overcome this obstacle. Some devices, such as the flexible fiber-optic bronchoscope (FOB), enable an indirect view of the vocal cords. Other devices, such as the laryngeal mask airway (LMA) or the double lumen esophageal-tracheal Combitube, can be inserted blindly and do not require a view of the vocal cords by any means. Another option for endotracheal intubation of a patient with difficult intubation is to place an LMA and then pass an endotracheal tube through the LMA. The final option is the surgical one: to establish direct access to the trachea by performing a cricothyrotomy or a tracheotomy.

10.3.4.1 Fiber-Optic Bronchoscopy

Performing awake fiber-optic intubation under local anesthesia for achieving successful endotracheal intubation in the spontaneous breathing patient is one of the recommended methods in situations where airway management is difficult [18]. However, the use of a fiber-optic bronchoscope (FOB) is sometimes unfeasible in trauma patients. Blood, vomitus, and secretions in the patient's airway may preclude vision by fiber-optic instruments. Furthermore, the patient's cooperation is essential for such an approach, and this cooperation is not easy to obtain in the pain-suffering, anxious trauma patient.

10.3.4.2 The Video Laryngoscope

The video laryngoscope is a device that enables an indirect view of the epiglottis and the vocal cords, rather than a direct view as with conventional laryngoscopes. The images from the patient's larynx are displayed on a screen or a monitor in the operator's vicinity. There are many types of video laryngoscopes, such as GlideScope®, C-CAM, Truview PCD™, King Vision™, and others that are commonly used in difficult airway situations [23, 24].

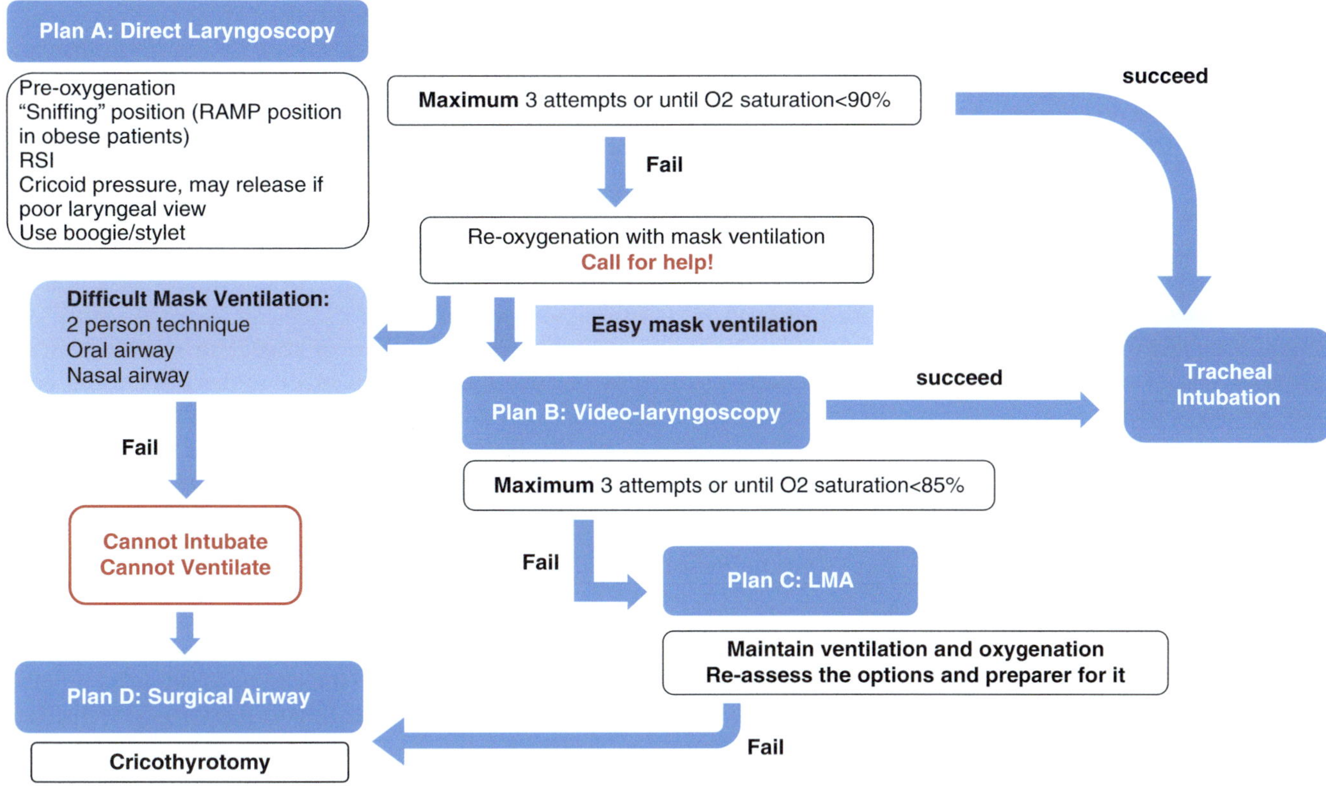

Fig. 10.4 Suggested strategy for difficult airway management of a trauma patient in an emergency situation. *RSI* rapid sequence induction

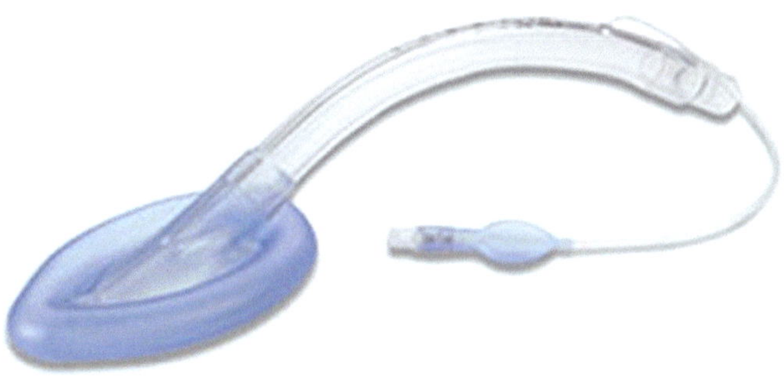

Fig. 10.5 Laryngeal mask airway (LMA)

Studies have shown that, when used for emergency intubations, video laryngoscopy was associated with better vocal cord visualization and a higher rate of first attempt successful intubations compared with a conventional direct laryngoscopy [25–27]. However, the successful use of a video laryngoscope relies on a good view of the inner airway, which may be precluded in the trauma patient by blood and secretions in the oral cavity.

10.3.4.3 Supraglottic Airway Devices

Supraglottic Airway Devices (SAD), such as the Laryngeal Mask Airway (LMA) (Fig. 10.5) and its several diverse variations, are very important devices for managing the difficult airway [18, 21]. The SAD is placed blindly in the oropharynx, and its successful placement requires minimal experience [28–30]. However, SADs do not provide a definitive airway and can be displaced when the patient is moved and transferred. Thus, it is not a final airway tool for managing trauma patients, especially for trauma patients who require maxillofacial surgery where the oral cavity is to be empty. However, a SAD is an ideal rescue device for ventilating the patient until the definitive airway is achieved, as has been repeatedly proven in combat casualties and many other trauma victims [31–33]. When definitive surgery is to be performed, the SAD may be a bridge until it is replaced by an endotracheal tube [34] or, alternatively, by a cricothyrotomy.

10.3.4.4 The Esophageal-Tracheal Combitube

The esophageal-tracheal double-lumen tube (Combitube) is an airway device that is inserted blindly into the oropharynx. It is a double lumen tube that facilitates ventilating the patient whether its distal tip is in the trachea or in the esophagus. The Combitube was presented for difficulty in airway management in trauma and resuscitation, since it is easy to use [35–37]. However, insertion of Combitube has been associated with serious injury to the upper airway and digestive tract, such as esophageal laceration and perforation, tongue edema, vocal cord injury, tracheal injury, aspiration pneumonitis, and pneumomediastinum [38].

10.3.4.5 Surgical Airway

Performing a cricothyrotomy is a lifesaving procedure in selected patients in the "cannot intubate, cannot ventilate" situation [13, 18, 22, 39, 40]. Surgical establishment of an airway is a safe method for securing the airway when the procedure is performed by an experienced surgeon. Factors that can make the cricothyrotomy particularly challenging are lack of familiarity with the procedure, poor anatomical landmark as in morbidly obese patient, previous radiation to the neck, hematoma, injury, or previous surgery to the laryngeal region. When a patient experiences acute respiratory distress and surgical airway access is performed under local anesthesia, the patient's movements may pose additional difficulty to the surgeon. Yet, patient's consciousness is required to maintain patent airway and preserve spontaneous breathing until secured airway is achieved. It is prudent to consider mild sedation (midazolam); however, it is better to have a restless alive patient with an open airway than a sedated or paralyzed patient with a complete airway obstruction.

Surgical Technique

The procedure is performed with the patient in a semirecumbent position. Neck overextension should be avoided since it further narrows the airway. Disinfection of the neck is important although time is limited. The use of a 2% lidocaine injection with epinephrine to facilitate local anesthesia and hemostasis in an awake patient is preferable. After standard preparation of the skin, a 2 cm vertical incision of the skin of the neck just below the laryngeal prominence (thyroid cartilage) is performed (Fig. 10.6). The next step is to make a transverse incision in the cricothyroid membrane which lies deep to this point. Then, a tracheostomy tube or endotracheal tube is inserted into the trachea, and its cuff inflated. Securing this precious airway is of utmost importance. The tube is to be fixated to the skin with a stich. There are several commercial supplies that are especially designed for this procedure and include all the equipment needed [41, 42]. It is recommended to have one of these in the emergency airway cart.

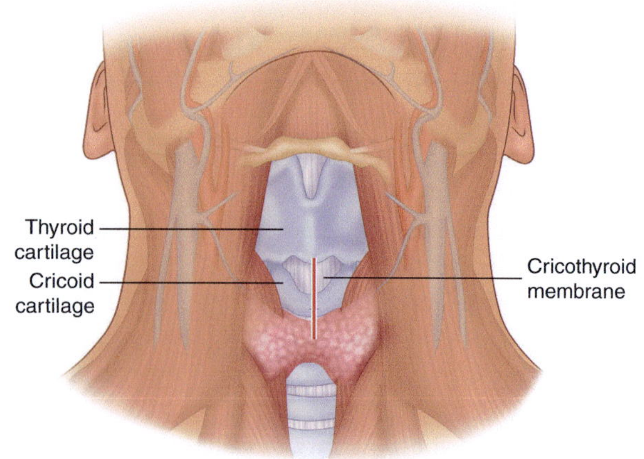

Fig. 10.6 Anatomical landmark for cricothyrotomy

Cricothyrotomy vs. Tracheostomy

The advantage of performing cricothyrotomy rather than tracheostomy is that the cricothyroid membrane is superficial and minimal dissection is required. The disadvantage of this approach is that the cricothyroid membrane's area is small and several adjacent structures may be injured, such as the cricothyroid muscles and the central cricothyroid artery. In case of cricoid cartilage damage due to pressure necrosis or unintentional scalpel damage, perichondritis may follow, with subsequent stenosis.

Although the procedure of choice in emergent situations is cricothyrotomy, in practice there seems to be a propensity for doing a tracheotomy rather than a cricothyrotomy. In their retrospective analysis of 4312 emergent airways, Dillon et al. found that 34 patients required emergency surgical access and, in these 34 patients, a tracheotomy was done in 24 and a cricothyrotomy in 10 patients [43]. This preference may be attributed to the higher failure risk of cricothyrotomy [44]. Emergency surgical access is not frequently used, yet the surgical airway may be the route of choice when the trauma is extensive and the patient requires prolonged postoperative mechanical ventilation.

The surgical airway procedure carries a 6% rate of complications, such as hemorrhage or pneumothorax, in an elective scenario [13] and higher complication rate when the procedure is performed in an urgent or emergent situation [45–47] and can, occasionally, be fatal [48].

When cricothyrotomy is carried out as a resuscitative effort during "cannot intubate, cannot ventilate" situation, it may be extremely stressful for the operator, especially the less experienced one [49, 50], and, as a rule, the procedure is best performed by the team's surgeon rather than the anesthesiologist. With that being said, it is important that emergency department physicians are trained and practiced with this procedure [51, 52].

10.4 General Consideration of a Trauma Patient's Airway Management

Apart from the possibility of facing difficult intubation, several other factors may worsen the scenario of managing the trauma patient's airway: hemodynamic instability, C-spine injury, full stomach, emergency situation, and operator's lack of experience.

10.4.1 Hemodynamic Instability

Airway management in the hemodynamic unstable patient is different than in the stable patient for several reasons. First and foremost, hemodynamic instability sets a very short time limit for airway control, since the physician has to aim the efforts in managing the cause for instability [53, 54]. Usually the patient is to be operated very soon and, in such circumstances, every minute counts. In cases where instability results from massive bleeding, the patient's peripheral perfusion is poor, and the extremities are cold, along with low arterial blood pressure and patient's movements. The pulse oximeter often fails to give accurate reading, and the patient's oxygenation is unknown to the caretaker [55, 56]. Perfusion is progressively decreasing to the lungs as well, and alveolar dead space is increased ("West zone 1"), causing tachypnea and worsening the tachycardia. For all these reasons, it is better to achieve a definitive airway as soon as possible.

10.4.2 C-Spine Injury

A patient with a supraclavicular injury or with blunt trauma is considered to have a C-spine injury, until proven otherwise by imaging [57]. Since a complete C-spine clearance may take several hours and sometimes days to achieve, the patient has to be fitted with a neck collar for cervical spine immobilization. At the time of intubation, the intubator's assistant performs "in-line stabilization" in order to support the head and neck in place and prevent neck movement throughout the procedure [58, 59]. However, several studies have indicated that direct laryngoscopy and intubation are unlikely to cause clinically significant neck movements. On the other hand, "in-line stabilization" may not always immobilize the injured segments effectively. In addition, "in-line stabilization" worsens the laryngoscopic view which may, in turn, worsen the outcome in traumatic brain injury by delaying endotracheal intubation and causing hypoxia [58, 59]. Using a video laryngoscope instead of a conventional laryngoscope with a Macintosh blade may be beneficial for intubating patients whose neck needs to be in a neutral position and whose cervical spine requires immobilization [60–62]. Neck movements during laryngoscopy using a conventional Macintosh laryngoscope have been compared to that using the Glidescope® video laryngoscope [61] and the Truview PCD™ laryngoscope [62]. Both these studies found that neck movements are reduced when using the video laryngoscopes for endotracheal intubation.

10.4.3 Full Stomach

All trauma patients must be assumed to have a "full stomach." Accordingly, the risk of regurgitation and aspiration is high. In order to diminish such risks, evacuating the contents of the stomach through the nasogastric tube before proceeding with airway management is recommended. However, insertion of a nasogastric tube in a confused, uncooperative, sometimes intoxicated patient who sustained a facial injury may, by itself, trigger vomiting. Another mean of reducing the risk of pulmonary aspiration of regurgitated gastric contents is to use Sellick's maneuver [63], a technique in which the esophagus is occluded by applying pressure on the cricoid cartilage, in order to compress the esophagus against the underlying vertebral body. Over the years Sellick's maneuver, which is also called cricoid pressure, has been incorporated into "rapid sequence induction" (RSI), a method intended to minimize the risk of gastric content aspiration during endotracheal intubation [14, 15]. Although Sellick's maneuver and RSI are widely used, the maneuver may significantly hamper endotracheal intubation because the laryngeal view is worsened [64–66]. Moreover, doing Sellick's maneuver forcefully may injure the esophagus or the laryngeal cartilages [67, 68].

10.4.4 Emergency Situations

Managing the airway in an emergent situation poses additional difficulties, resulting from the fact that the time to accomplish the task is short and the patient's condition may deteriorate quickly. Both decision-making and performance are impaired at such times. The performance of urgent or emergent intubation is associated with remarkably high complication rates, which may exceed 20% [19, 69]. This is the result of several factors, including repeated intubation attempts, performing direct laryngoscopy without muscle relaxation, and lack of operator experience.

10.4.5 Personnel Experience

In emergency situations, the care of acute trauma patients is provided by individuals who are often not experienced—the "inverse care law" [70]. The responsibility for acute airway management often falls into the hands of non-anesthesiologists [71, 72]. In their multicenter analysis of 8937 intubations in the emergency department, Walls et al. reported that anesthesiologists performed only 3% of the intubations, and the remaining 97% of the intubations were performed by emergency physicians (87%) and physicians from other specialties (10%) [72]. In order to improve the clinical outcome of trauma patients, skillful personnel should be tasked with their airway management. That indicates conducting a training program for teaching airway management to emergency department physicians and supplying the equipment and conditions that are suitable for performing endotracheal intubation.

10.5 Maxillofacial Trauma and Airway Injuries

The patient with maxillofacial trauma presents a special challenge in managing the airway. This is a situation that combines all the potential difficulties of airway management:

(a) We anticipate difficult mask ventilation and difficult intubation.
(b) The patient often swallows blood from the trauma site in the upper airways and is at a high risk for gastric content regurgitation.
(c) In many cases, the C-spine is injured, and securing the airway is to be done without moving the neck.
(d) Head injury is another component in many of these trauma patients.
(e) The patient who is starved for air and may already be hypoxemic could also be uncontrollable and combative.

In addition, the type of maxillofacial operation that is planned and the postoperative airway status of the patient are to be considered, since for some operations, the oral cavity needs to be empty for performing the procedure and closed with maxilla-mandibular fixation (MMF) at the end of surgery, and prolonged mechanical ventilation is sometimes expected.

10.5.1 Maxillofacial Trauma Anatomy

Safe and optimal airway management of the patient with maxillofacial trauma requires appreciation of the nature of the trauma. There are several maxillofacial injuries that require immediate treatment, especially in acute upper airway compromise and/or when profuse hemorrhage occurs. According to Hutchinson [73], there are six specific situations associated with maxillofacial trauma, which can adversely affect the airway:

1. Posteroinferior displacement of a fractured maxilla parallel to the inclined plane of the base of the skull may block the nasopharyngeal airway.
2. A bilateral fracture of the anterior mandible may cause the fractured symphysis and the tongue to slide posteriorly and block the oropharynx in the supine patient.
3. Fractured or exfoliated teeth, bone fragments, vomitus, blood, and secretions, as well as foreign bodies, such as dentures, debris, and shrapnel, may block the airway anywhere along the oropharynx and larynx.
4. Hemorrhage from distinct vessels in open wounds or severe nasal bleeding from the complex blood supply of the nose may also contribute to airway obstruction.
5. Soft tissue swelling and edema which result from trauma to the head and neck may cause delayed airway compromise.
6. Trauma to the larynx and trachea may cause swelling and displacement of structures, such as the epiglottis, arytenoid cartilages and vocal cords, thereby increasing the risk of cervical airway obstruction.

A high index of suspicion, a meticulous physical examination, and close observation of the patient may assist in the early detection of such situations. Once early airway management has been completed and hemorrhage is controlled at all sites, the patient should have a computerized tomography (CT) scan of the head and neck to provide more detailed information on the type and extent of the trauma for definitive management of bone and soft tissue injuries. The imaging and the definitive maxillofacial operation may be deferred until all life- and/or organ-threatening injuries have been properly managed.

10.5.2 Early Airway Management of Maxillofacial Trauma Patient

Endotracheal intubation is expected to be difficult in a maxillofacial trauma patient. The challenge in performing the intubation arises mainly from a difficulty in viewing the vocal cords using conventional direct laryngoscope. The oral cavity, pharynx, and larynx may be filled with blood, secretions, soft tissue, and bone fragments, all of which preclude a good view of the vocal cords. In patients where endotracheal intubation is expected to be feasible, it should be performed with RSI and a manual in-line stabilization maneuver, in order to decrease the risk of pulmonary aspiration and take into account a potential C-spine injury.

Regarding mask ventilation: mask ventilation is problematic in the patient with maxillofacial trauma because the anatomy of the oral cavity and/or oropharynx could be disarranged by the trauma and obscured by bleeding. Thus, the ventilation mask cannot be properly fitted to the face for effective mask ventilation. Furthermore, an injured airway may prevent efficient air transfer from the mask to the lungs.

10.5.3 Preparing the Patient for Maxillofacial Surgery

Maxillofacial surgery is done after stabilization of the patient and the radiographic tests have been performed and all the injuries identified. In some patients, maxillofacial surgery is performed at the same time as the surgery on other injured organs. Operating on patients with maxillofacial trauma, and especially those with severe complex comminuted panfacial fractures, is challenging for the surgeon. The surgeon has to perform fracture reduction, repair soft tissue injuries, and restore the occlusion. In order to facilitate optimal operating conditions and to achieve proper pre-traumatic figuration and function, the occlusion has to be maintained and checked at all times during the surgery. At the end of the surgery, the mouth is to be set closed with MMF. These surgical requirements preclude the use of an oral endotracheal tube. In cases when MMF is not required, an oral tube may be suitable. The choice of the airway device that will be used during the operation is to be agreed upon by the surgeon who is familiar with the planned procedure, including possible intraoperative change of plan and potential postoperative complications.

Some trauma patients reach the operating room conscious and spontaneously breathing and their maxillofacial trauma is not extensive. In selected patients, naso-endotracheal intubation can be used for airway control during surgery [74] (Fig. 10.7). However, naso-endotracheal intubation is relatively contraindicated in patients with midface fractures or fractures at the base of the skull [75].

Severely injured major trauma patients usually arrive at the operating room with one of the following airway control devices, namely, endotracheal tube, a SAD, a cricothyrotomy, or a tracheotomy, performed earlier in the field or emergency department. For these trauma patients where a tracheostomy or a cricothyrotomy was performed as the first line of securing the airway, it is useful subsequently for the

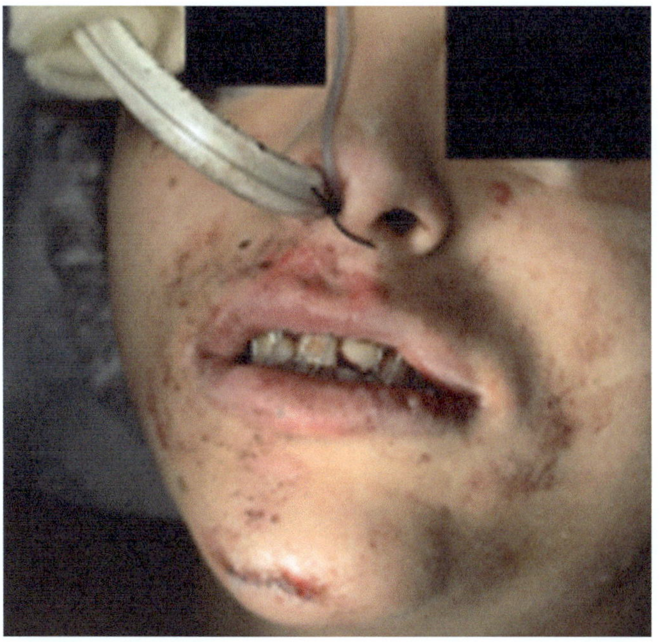

Fig. 10.7 Nasal endotracheal tube in a patient with maxillofacial trauma (From Barak M et al. [76] with permission)

surgery and postoperative recovery period. It is recommended, however, that cricothyrotomy be converted to tracheotomy at that time [76, 77]. If the patient arrives at the operating room with an oral endotracheal tube and prolonged ventilation is expected, the oral tube is to be changed to open tracheostomy. In a patient with no mandibular fracture, with a contraindication to nasal intubation, and there is no need for prolonged intubation, submental orotracheal intubation is to be used as the method for securing the airway during surgery [76, 78–80].

10.5.4 Submental Orotracheal Intubation

Submental orotracheal intubation was presented to avoid the need for tracheotomy and to permit unfettered access to the oral region. This type of intubation is done (a) in patients with comminuted fracture of the midface or the nose, where nasal intubation is contraindicated, (b) in patients who require restoration of the occlusion, and (c) in patients whose condition permits extubation at the end of surgery.

However, this type of intubation is contraindicated in patients with comminuted mandibular fractures.

10.5.4.1 Surgical Technique

Submental orotracheal intubation requires the use of a spiral reinforced armored endotracheal tube (Fig. 10.8) to prevent the tube from kinking during usage. Following an orotracheal intubation, a 2 cm incision is made halfway between the chin and the angle of the mandible, and blunt dissection is performed to the oral floor. A surgical access is made through the superficial fascia, platysma, and deep fascia. The opening is positioned in the floor of the mouth. After accomplishing the dissection, forceps are used to create a tunnel for passing the tube without interference. When creation of the surgical access is complete, the tube is pulled through the tunnel, using gentle rotational movements. Following this maneuver, sutures are used to fix the tube's position (Fig. 10.9). When indicated, extubation is done through the

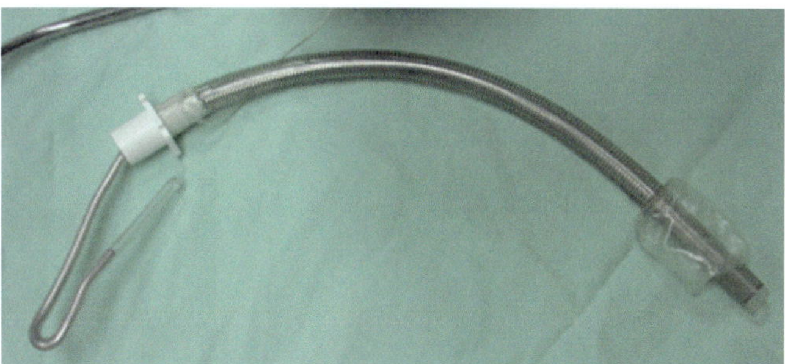

Fig. 10.8 Spiral reinforced armored tube, for the use in submental endotracheal intubation

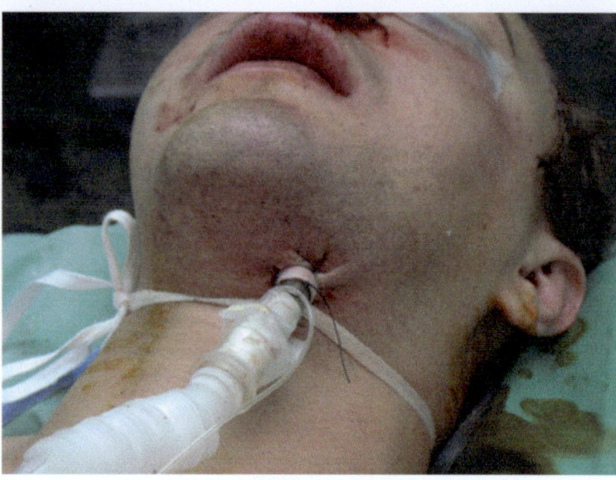

Fig. 10.9 Submental orotracheal tube in a patient with maxillofacial trauma (From Barak M et al. [76] with permission)

external skin incision. There is no need to suture the intraoral incision, and the skin incision is closed using the sutures that were placed at the time of intubation.

Complications from submental endotracheal intubation do occur and include bleeding, damage to the lingual nerve and the marginal mandibular branch of the facial nerve, damage to the duct of the submandibular gland, damage to the sublingual gland, salivary fistulae, and skin infections [81, 82].

10.6 Postoperative Airway Management of the Difficult Airway Patient

The patient with a difficult airway is also at high risk for post-extubation complications [83, 84]. Following surgery, the mucous membranes are edematous, the soft tissues are swollen, and the airway may be compressed. Neck expandability is relatively low, and even a small hemorrhage in the region could result in airway compromise. The risk of airway-related complications during the perioperative period was analyzed from the American Society of Anesthesiologists Closed Claims database in order to identify the patterns of liability associated with the management of the difficult airway. It was found that 12% of complications arose at extubation and 5% during recovery [85].

In intubated patients with maxillofacial trauma, extubation should be deferred until the edema subsides. During extubation, the patient should be monitored closely, and the care providers should be prepared for the possibility of re-intubation. It is important to prevent nausea and vomiting because of the risk of gastric content aspiration [86], especially in those patients with MMF because pulmonary aspiration is plausible. For those patients with a tracheotomy tube, the patient may be awakened and allowed to breathe spontaneously through the tracheostomy tube for a few days in order to ensure a safe recovery.

Case Scenario

A 30-year-old female patient sustained a superficial gunshot wound to the head, on her right temporal region. Emergency personnel found her conscious, breathing, and talking. Her blood pressure was 130/70, and her heart rate was 120/min.

1. At that point:
   A. The patient is to be intubated immediately.
   B. Emergency surgical airway (cricothyrotomy) is to be performed urgently.
   C. The patient is to be transferred to the hospital, breathing spontaneously with oxygen supplement.
   D. The patient is to be ventilated with LMA.
2. On arrival to the emergency department, the patient deteriorated rapidly, lost consciousness, and became hemodynamically unstable.
   A. The patient is to be intubated immediately.
   B. Emergency surgical airway (cricothyrotomy) is to be performed urgently.
   C. The patient can continue breathing spontaneously with oxygen supplement.
   D. It is better to use the Combitube to ventilate the patient.
3. The emergency department physician failed three times to intubate the patient. What is the best thing to do now?
   A. Try again, until success is achieved.
   B. Call for help.
   C. Mask ventilation with face mask and reservoir bag.
   D. B and C.
4. The patient further deteriorates during failed mask ventilation. Her O_2 saturation drops to 70%, followed by bradycardia of 40/min. Now is the time to:
   A. Try again to intubate the patient.
   B. Urgently perform an emergency surgical airway (cricothyrotomy).
   C. Get ready for resuscitation with drugs and chest compressions.
   D. B and C.
5. The emergency department surgeon performed cricothyrotomy on the patient. She was ventilated effectively, her O_2 saturation rose to 96%, and she was taken to the operating room for an urgent explorative laparotomy. At the end of the operation, it is planned to transfer the patient to the intensive care unit for prolonged mechanical ventilation. The best way to continue to ventilate her is:
   A. Continue to use the cricothyrotomy for ventilation.
   B. Change to a tracheostomy tube.
   C. Change to an endotracheal tube.
   D. Extubate the patient.

Please see Chap. 58 for the correct answer.

References

1. Committee on Trauma; American College of Surgeons. Advanced trauma life support for doctors ATLS. 8th ed. Chicago: American College of Surgeons; 2008.
2. Langeron O, Birenbaum A, Amour J. Airway management in trauma. Minerva Anestesiol. 2009;75:307–11.
3. Walls RM. Management of the difficult airway in the trauma patient. Emerg Med Clin North Am. 1998;16:45–61.
4. Mayglothling J, Duane TM, Gibbs M, McCunn M, Legome E, Eastman AL, Whelan J, Shah KH, Eastern Association for the Surgery of Trauma. Emergency tracheal intubation immediately following traumatic injury: an Eastern Association for the Surgery of Trauma practice management guideline. J Trauma Acute Care Surg. 2012;73:S333–40.
5. Lundstrøm LH, Møller AM, Rosenstock C, Astrup G, Gätke MR, Wetterslev J, Danish Anaesthesia Database. A documented previous difficult tracheal intubation as a prognostic test for a subsequent difficult tracheal intubation in adults. Anaesthesia. 2009;64:1081–8.
6. Vannucci A, Cavallone LF. Bedside predictors of difficult intubation: a systematic review. Minerva Anestesiol. 2016;82:69–83.
7. Mallampati SR. Clinical sign to predict difficult tracheal intubation (hypothesis). Can Anaesth Soc J. 1983;30:316–7.
8. Mallampati SR, Gatt SP, Gugino LD, Desai SP, Waraksa B, Freiberger D, Liu PL. A clinical sign to predict difficult tracheal intubation: a prospective study. Can Anaesth Soc J. 1985;32:429–34.
9. Rose DK, Cohen MM. The airway: problems and predictions in 18,500 patients. Can J Anaesth. 1994;41:372–83.
10. Shiga T, Wajima Z, Inoue T, Sakamoto A. Predicting difficult intubation in apparently normal patients: a meta-analysis of bedside screening test performance. Anesthesiology. 2005;103:429–37.
11. Healy DW, LaHart EJ, Peoples EE, Jewell ES, Bettendorf RJ Jr, Ramachandran SK. A Comparison of the Mallampati evaluation in neutral or extended cervical spine positions: a retrospective observational study of >80 000 patients. Br J Anaesth. 2016;116:690–8.
12. Advanced Trauma Life Support Student Course Manual, 9th ed, Chicago, IL; American College of Surgeons, 2012. Chapter 2 pp 31–49.
13. Hamaekers AE, Henderson JJ. Equipment and strategies for emergency tracheal access in the adult patient. Anaesthesia. 2011;66:65–80.
14. Mace SE. Challenges and advances in intubation: rapid sequence intubation. Emerg Med Clin North Am. 2008;26:1043–68.
15. Algie CM, Mahar RK, Tan HB, Wilson G, Mahar PD, Wasiak J. Effectiveness and risks of cricoid pressure during rapid sequence induction for endotracheal intubation. Cochrane Database Syst Rev. 2015;(11):CD011656.
16. Nemeth J, Maghraby N, Kazim S. Emergency airway management: the difficult airway. Emerg Med Clin North Am. 2012;30:401–20.
17. Law JA, Broemling N, Cooper RM, Drolet P, Duggan LV, Griesdale DE, Hung OR, Jones PM, Kovacs G, Massey S, Morris IR, Mullen T, Murphy MF, Preston R, Naik VN, Scott J, Stacey S, Turkstra TP, Wong DT. Canadian Airway Focus Group. The difficult airway with recommendations for management—part 1—difficult tracheal intubation encountered in an unconscious/induced patient. Can J Anaesth. 2013;60:1089–118.
18. Apfelbaum JL, Hagberg CA, Caplan RA, Blitt CD, Connis RT, Nickinovich DG, Hagberg CA, Caplan RA, Benumof JL, Berry FA, Blitt CD, Bode RH, Cheney FW, Connis RT, Guidry OF, Nickinovich DG, Ovassapian A, American Society of Anesthesiologists Task Force on Management of the Difficult Airway. Practice guidelines for management of the difficult airway: an updated report by the American Society of Anesthesiologists Task Force on Management of the Difficult Airway. Anesthesiology. 2013;118:251–70.
19. Mort TC. Emergency tracheal intubation: complications associated with repeated laryngoscopic attempts. Anesth Analg. 2004;99:607–13.
20. Stephens CT, Kahntroff S, Dutton RP. The success of emergency endotracheal intubation in trauma patients: a 10-year experience at a major adult trauma referral center. Anesth Analg. 2009;109:866–72.
21. Lockey DJ, Healey B, Crewdson K, Chalk G, Weaver AE, Davies GE. Advanced airway management is necessary in prehospital trauma patients. Br J Anaesth. 2015;114:657–62.
22. Frerk C, Mitchell VS, McNarry AF, Mendonca C, Bhagrath R, Patel A, O'Sullivan EP, Woodall NM, Ahmad I, Difficult Airway Society Intubation Guidelines Working Group. Difficult Airway Society 2015 guidelines for management of unanticipated difficult intubation in adults. Br J Anaesth. 2015;115:827–48.
23. Aziz MF, Healy D, Kheterpal S, Fu RF, Dillman D, Brambrink AM. Routine clinical practice effectiveness of the Glidescope in difficult airway management: an analysis of 2,004 Glidescope intubations, complications, and failures from two institutions. Anesthesiology. 2011;114:34–41.
24. Lewis SR, Butler AR, Parker J, Cook TM, Smith AF. Videolaryngoscopy versus direct laryngoscopy for adult patients requiring tracheal intubation. Cochrane Database Syst Rev. 2016;11:CD011136.
25. Jones BM, Agrawal A, Schulte TE. Assessing the efficacy of video versus direct laryngoscopy through retrospective comparison of 436 emergency intubation cases. J Anesth. 2013;27:927–30.
26. Sakles JC, Mosier J, Chiu S, Cosentino M, Kalin L. A comparison of the C-MAC video laryngoscope to the Macintosh direct laryngoscope for intubation in the emergency department. Ann Emerg Med. 2012;60:739–48.
27. Serocki G, Bein B, Scholz J, Dörges V. Management of the predicted difficult airway: a comparison of conventional blade laryngoscopy with video-assisted blade laryngoscopy and the GlideScope. Eur J Anaesthesiol. 2010;27:24–30.
28. Schalk R, Byhahn C, Fausel F, Egner A, Oberndörfer D, Walcher F, Latasch L. Out-of-hospital airway management by paramedics and emergency physicians using laryngeal tubes. Resuscitation. 2010;81:323–6.
29. Ruetzler K, Roessler B, Potura L, Priemayr A, Robak O, Schuster E, Frass M. Performance and skill retention of intubation by paramedics using seven different airway devices—a manikin study. Resuscitation. 2011;82:593–7.
30. Goliasch G, Ruetzler A, Fischer H, Frass M, Sessler DI, Ruetzler K. Evaluation of advanced airway management in absolutely inexperienced hands: a randomized manikin trial. Eur J Emerg Med. 2013;20:310–4.
31. Grier G, Bredmose P, Davies G, Lockey D. Introduction and use of the ProSeal laryngeal mask airway as a rescue device in a pre-hospital trauma anaesthesia algorithm. Resuscitation. 2009;80:138–41.
32. Mabry RL, Frankfurt A. Advanced airway management in combat casualties by medics at the point of injury: a sub-group analysis of the reach study. J Spec Oper Med. 2011;11:16–9.
33. Adams BD, Cuniowski PA, Muck A, De Lorenzo RA. Registry of emergency airways arriving at combat hospitals. J Trauma. 2008;64:1548–54.
34. Wong DT, Yang JJ, Mak HY, Jagannathan N. Use of intubation introducers through a supraglottic airway to facilitate tracheal intubation: a brief review. Can J Anaesth. 2012;59:704–15.
35. Idris AH, Gabrielli A. Advances in airway management. Emerg Med Clin North Am. 2002;20:843–57.
36. Rabitsch W, Schellongowski P, Staudinger T, Hofbauer R, Dufek V, Eder B, Raab H, Thell R, Schuster E, Frass M. Comparison of a conventional tracheal airway with the Combitube in an urban emergency medical services system run by physicians. Resuscitation. 2003;57:27–32.
37. Davis DP, Valentine C, Ochs M, Vilke GM, Hoyt DB. The Combitube as a salvage airway device for paramedic rapid sequence intubation. Ann Emerg Med. 2003;42:697–704.
38. Vézina MC, Trépanier CA, Nicole PC, Lessard MR. Complications associated with the Esophageal-Tracheal Combitube in the pre-hospital setting. Can J Anaesth. 2007;54:124–8.

39. Dob DP, McLure HA, Soni N. Failed intubation and emergency percutaneous tracheostomy. Anaesthesia. 1998;53:72–4.
40. Helm M, Gries A, Mutzbauer T. Surgical approach in difficult airway management. Best Pract Res Clin Anaesthesiol. 2005;19:623–40.
41. Benkhadra M, Lenfant F, Nemetz W, Anderhuber F, Feigl G, Fasel J. A comparison of two emergency cricothyroidotomy kits in human cadavers. Anesth Analg. 2008;106:182–5.
42. Murphy C, Rooney SJ, Maharaj CH, Laffey JG, Harte BH. Comparison of three cuffed emergency percutaneous cricothyroidotomy devices to conventional surgical cricothyroidotomy in a porcine model. Br J Anaesth. 2011;106:57–64.
43. Dillon JK, Christensen B, Fairbanks T, Jurkovich G, Moe KS. The emergent surgical airway: cricothyrotomy vs. tracheotomy. Int J Oral Maxillofac Surg. 2013;42:204–8.
44. Mabry RL. An analysis of battlefield cricothyrotomy in Iraq and Afghanistan. J Spec Oper Med. 2012;12:17–23.
45. Kearney PA, Griffen MM, Ochoa JB, Boulanger BR, Tseui BJ, Mentzer RM Jr. A single-center 8-year experience with percutaneous dilational tracheostomy. Ann Surg. 2000;231:701–9.
46. Yuen HW, Loy AH, Johari S. Urgent awake tracheotomy for impending airway obstruction. Otolaryngol Head Neck Surg. 2007;136:838–42.
47. Altman KW, Waltonen JD, Kern RC. Urgent surgical airway intervention: a 3 year county hospital experience. Laryngoscope. 2005;115:2101–4.
48. Gupta P, Modrykamien A. Fatal case of tension pneumothorax and subcutaneous emphysema after open surgical tracheostomy. J Intensive Care Med. 2014;29:298–301.
49. Cooper S. We need to cut the neck! Confronting psychological and moral distress during emergency cricothyrotomy. Narrat Inq Bioeth. 2013;3:E5–9.
50. Greenland KB, Acott C, Segal R, Goulding G, Riley RH, Merry AF. Emergency surgical airway in life-threatening acute airway emergencies—why are we so reluctant to do it? Anaesth Intensive Care. 2011;39:578–84.
51. King DR, Ogilvie MP, Velmahos G, Alam HB, Demoya MA, Wilcox SR, Mejaddam AY, Van Der Wilden GM, Birkhan OA, Fikry K. Emergent cricothyroidotomies for trauma: training considerations. Am J Emerg Med. 2012;30:1429–32.
52. King D, Ogilvie M, Michailidou M, Velmahos G, Alam H, deMoya M, Fikry K. Fifty-four emergent cricothyroidotomies: are surgeons reluctant teachers? Scand J Surg. 2012;101:13–5.
53. Kirkpatrick AW, Ball CG, D'Amours SK, Zygun D. Acute resuscitation of the unstable adult trauma patient: bedside diagnosis and therapy. Can J Surg. 2008;51:57–69.
54. Matthes G, Bernhard M, Kanz KG, Waydhas C, Fischbacher M, Fischer M, Böttiger BW. Emergency anesthesia, airway management and ventilation in major trauma. Background and key messages of the interdisciplinary S3 guidelines for major trauma patients. Unfallchirurg. 2012;115:251–64. In German.
55. Sinex JE. Pulse oximetry: principles and limitations. Am J Emerg Med. 1999;17:59–67.
56. Petterson MT, Begnoche VL, Graybeal JM. The effect of motion on pulse oximetry and its clinical significance. Anesth Analg. 2007;105:S78–84.
57. Crosby ET. Airway management in adults after cervical spine trauma. Anesthesiology. 2006;104:1293–318.
58. Manoach S, Paladino L. Manual in-line stabilization for acute airway management of suspected cervical spine injury: historical review and current questions. Ann Emerg Med. 2007;50:236–45.
59. Santoni BG, Hindman BJ, Puttlitz CM, Weeks JB, Johnson N, Maktabi MA, Todd MM. Manual in-line stabilization increases pressures applied by the laryngoscope blade during direct laryngoscopy and orotracheal intubation. Anesthesiology. 2009;110:24–31.
60. Kill C, Risse J, Wallot P, Seidl P, Steinfeldt T, Wulf H. Videolaryngoscopy with glidescope reduces cervical spine movement in patients with unsecured cervical spine. J Emerg Med. 2013;44:750–6.
61. Robitaille A, Williams SR, Tremblay MH, Guilbert F, Thériault M, Drolet P. Cervical spine motion during tracheal intubation with manual in-line stabilization: direct laryngoscopy versus GlideScope videolaryngoscopy. Anesth Analg. 2008;106:935–41.
62. Bhardwaj N, Jain K, Rao M, Mandal AK. Assessment of cervical spine movement during laryngoscopy with Macintosh and Truview laryngoscopes. J Anaesthesiol Clin Pharmacol. 2013;29:308–12.
63. Sellick BA. Cricoid pressure to control regurgitation of stomach contents during induction of anaesthesia. Lancet. 1961;2:404–6.
64. Haslam N, Parker L, Duggan JE. Effect of cricoid pressure on the view at laryngoscopy. Anaesthesia. 2005;60:41–7.
65. Ellis DY, Harris T, Zideman D. Cricoid pressure in emergency department rapid sequence tracheal intubations: a risk-benefit analysis. Ann Emerg Med. 2007;50:653–65.
66. Bhatia N, Bhagat H, Sen I. Cricoid pressure: where do we stand? J Anaesthesiol Clin Pharmacol. 2014;30:3–6.
67. Ralph SJ, Wareham CA. Rupture of the oesophagus during cricoid pressure. Anaesthesia. 1991;46:40–1.
68. Heath KJ, Palmer M, Fletcher SJ. Fracture of the cricoid cartilage after Sellick's manoeuvre. Br J Anaesth. 1996;76:877–8.
69. Mechlin MW, Hurford WE. Emergency tracheal intubation: techniques and outcomes. Respir Care. 2014;59:881–92.
70. Boylan JF, Kavanagh BP. Emergency airway management: competence versus expertise? Anesthesiology. 2008;109:945–7.
71. Kovacs G, Law JA, Ross J, Tallon J, MacQuarrie K, Petrie D, Campbell S, Soder C. Acute airway management in the emergency department by non-anesthesiologists. Can J Anaesth. 2004;51:174–80.
72. Walls RM, Brown CA, Bair AE, Pallin DJ, NEAR II Investigators. Emergency airway management: a multi-center report of 8937 emergency department intubations. J Emerg Med. 2011;41:347–54.
73. Hutchison I, Lawlor M, Skinner D. ABC of major trauma. Major maxillofacial injuries. BMJ. 1990;301:595–9.
74. Hall CE, Shutt LE. Nasotracheal intubation for head and neck surgery. Anesthesia. 2003;58:249–56.
75. Muzzi DA, Losasso TJ, Cucchiara RF. Complication from a nasopharyngeal airway in a patient with a basilar skull fracture. Anesthesiology. 1991;74:366–8.
76. Barak M, Bahouth H, Leiser Y, Abu El-Naaj I. Airway management of the patient with maxillofacial trauma: review of the literature and suggested clinical approach. Biomed Res Int. 2015;2015:724032.
77. Talving P, DuBose J, Inaba K, Demetriades D. Conversion of emergent cricothyrotomy to tracheotomy in trauma patients. Arch Surg. 2010;145:87–91.
78. Vashishta A, Sharma S, Chugh A, Jain D, Gupta N, Bihani U. Submental intubation: a useful adjunct in panfacial trauma. Natl J Maxillofac Surg. 2010;1:74–7.
79. Schütz P, Hamed HH. Submental intubation versus tracheostomy in maxillofacial trauma patients. J Oral Maxillofac Surg. 2008;66:1404–9.
80. Eisemann B, Eisemann M, Rizvi M, Urata MM, Lypka MA. Defining the role for submental intubation. J Clin Anesth. 2014;26:238–42.
81. de Toledo GL, Bueno SC, Mesquita RA, Amaral MB. Complications from submental endotracheal intubation: a prospective study and literature review. Dent Traumatol. 2013;29:197–202.

82. Mittal G, Mittal RK, Katyal S, Uppal S, Mittal V. Airway management in maxillofacial trauma: do we really need tracheostomy/submental intubation. J Clin Diagn Res. 2014;8:77–9.
83. Cavallone LF, Vannucci A. Extubation of the difficult airway and extubation failure. Anesth Analg. 2013;116:368–83.
84. Popat M, Mitchell V, Dravid R, Patel A, Swampillai C, Higgs A. Difficult Airway Society Extubation Guidelines Group. Difficult Airway Society Guidelines for the management of tracheal extubation. Anaesthesia. 2012;67:318–40.
85. Peterson GN, Domino B, Caplan RA, Posner KL, Lee LA, Cheney FW. Management of the difficult airway: a closed claims analysis. Anesthesiology. 2005;103:33–9.
86. Jahromi HE, Gholami M, Rezaei F. A randomized double-blinded placebo controlled study of four interventions for the prevention of postoperative nausea and vomiting in maxillofacial trauma surgery. J Craniofac Surg. 2013;24:e623–7.

Emergency Resuscitation Procedures in Major Trauma: Operative Techniques

11

Paolo Aseni, Sharon Henry, and Thomas Scalea

Key Points

- The primary care of injured patients is performed emergently by a variety of healthcare practitioners such as emergency physicians, surgeons, and anesthesiologists.
- Complications of emergency surgical procedures are common and can be the source of considerable morbidity and mortality rate although can be minimized if meticulous techniques are adopted.
- Orotracheal intubation is the standard method of airway control following injury; however surgical airway control (cricothyroidotomy and percutaneous tracheostomy) can be required in 1–2% of patients.
- Pleural decompression is a common procedure following major injury and can be a lifesaving procedure; although it is relatively simple, complications can occur if attention to detail is not used.
- Pericardial window and transdiaphragmatic pericardial window at the time of laparotomy are diagnostic and potential temporarily therapeutic procedures in patients who may have hemopericardium.
- A median sternotomy is the ideal incision to access the heart and the anterior mediastinal great vessels.
- The most rapid method of accessing the chest is via an anterolateral left thoracotomy: this incision can be performed rapidly and is versatile, as it can be brought across the sternum into a clamshell thoracotomy.
- Obtaining hemostasis in patients who are bleeding in the pelvis following major pelvic fractures can be challenging: pelvic packing can be lifesaving.
- Aortic occlusion can be achieved with REBOA which can provide temporary control of hemorrhage almost anywhere in the body.

P. Aseni (✉)
Dipartimento di Emergenza Urgenza ASST Grande Ospedale Metropolitano Niguarda, Milan, Italy

S. Henry · T. Scalea
R Adams Cowley Shock Trauma Center, University of Maryland School of Medicine,
Baltimore, MD, USA

P. Aseni et al. (eds.), *Operative Techniques and Recent Advances in Acute Care and Emergency Surgery*,
https://doi.org/10.1007/978-3-319-95114-0_11

11.1 Introduction

The care of injured patients often requires invasive procedures. Depending on the circumstance, these may be performed by emergency physicians, surgeons, or a variety of other healthcare practitioners. They vary from simple to very complicated. Regardless of the level of complexity, they must often be performed emergently. Complications are relatively common and can be the source of considerable morbidity and even mortality. This can be minimized if they are done with meticulous technique. This chapter will describe the common procedures done during the resuscitation of a badly injured patient. We will strive to provide a practical approach to those who deal with injured patients in the hope that this will aid those practitioners and ultimately the patients [1–3].

11.2 Surgical Airway Control

11.2.1 Orotracheal Intubation

Orotracheal intubation is the standard method of airway control following injury. However, 1–2% of hospital intubations fail. Failure is less common as advanced airway techniques such as video laryngoscopy and use of rapid sequence intubation have become more common. Regardless, in a small number of cases, a surgical airway is required. Attention must be paid to cervical spine immobilization in patients with blunt trauma [4, 5].

11.2.2 Cricothyroidotomy

The airway is usually accessed via the cricothyroid membrane. This structure is closest to the skin, making it attractive for emergency airway access. While surgical cricothyroidotomy is most often performed as emergency surgical airway, needle cricothyroidotomy is also an option. However, in children, the cricoid ring is the narrowest part of the airway, and airway stenosis can follow surgical airway at that location. Thus, in children, cricothyroidotomy should be avoided.

11.2.2.1 Needle Cricothyroidotomy

Technique: Quickly prep the skin, if time allows. Stabilize the thyroid cartilage with the non-dominant hand. Locate the cricothyroid membrane, and insert a 12- or 14-gauge cannula through the skin and membrane at an angle of about 45° directing the needle caudad (Fig. 11.1). Aspirating while advancing the cannula confirms entering the airway. Advance the cannula an additional 5 mm and slide the catheter over the needle into the trachea. Attach the catheter to a ventilation device, if possible to a high-pressure jet ventilator, and begin oxygenation

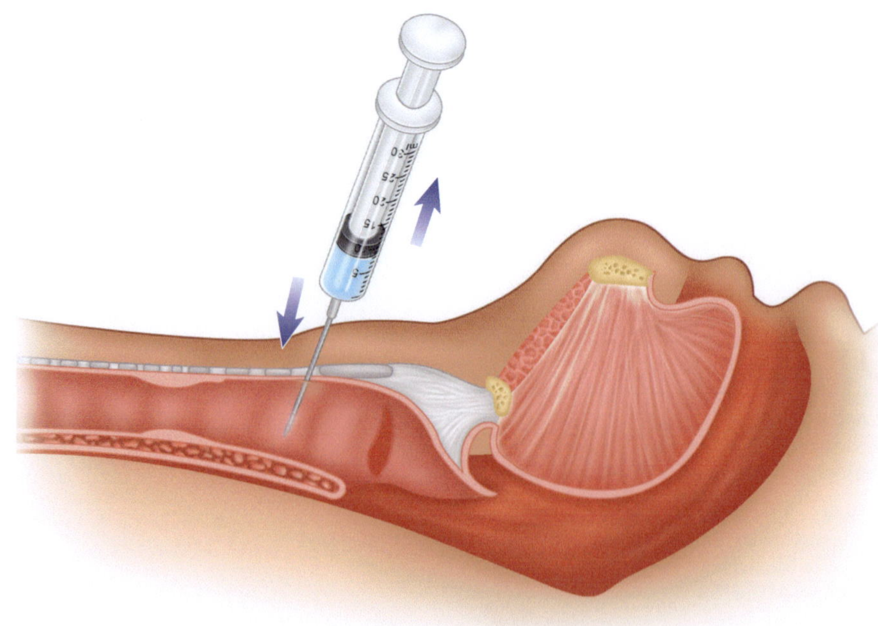

Fig. 11.1 Needle cricothyroidotomy. Position of the adult patient by hyperextending the neck unless c-spine concerns mandate neutral positioning. Insert the catheter/needle into the cricothyroid space at an angle of about 45° directing the needle caudad. Maintain suction with the syringe until air freely flows into the syringe or until bubbles are noted

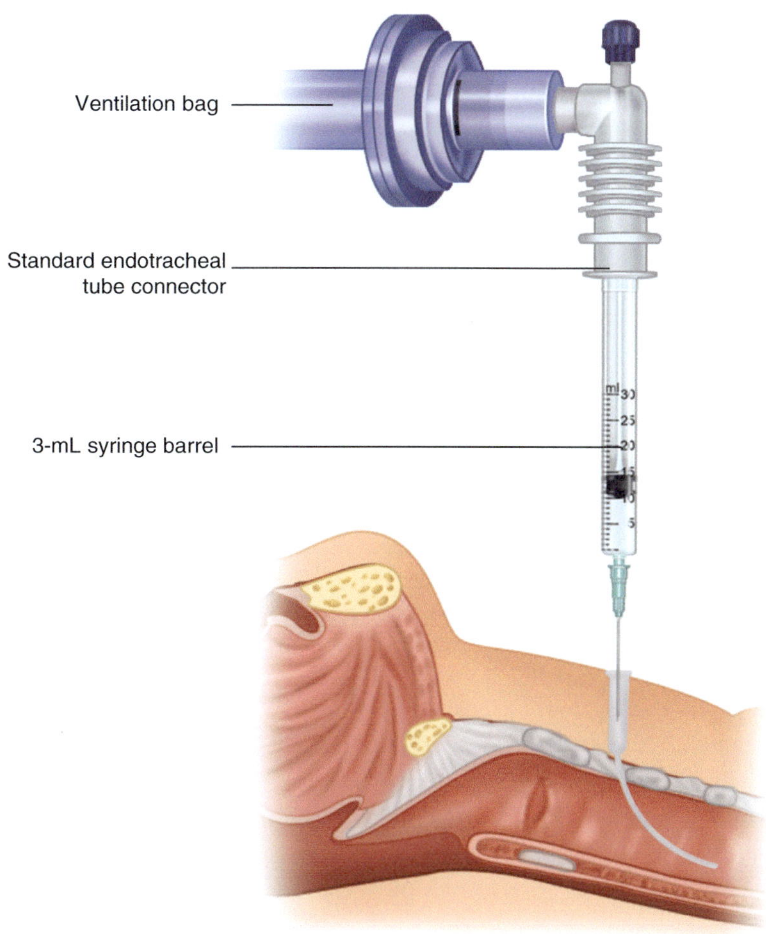

Fig. 11.2 Needle cricothyroidotomy. Attach a mechanism (**a**) to the small cannula and provide high flow oxygen through the cannula and begin oxygenation. Due to the small caliber of the catheter, a ventilation by a pressurized stream of oxygen or jet ventilation is required

(Fig. 11.2). Hold the catheter firmly in place at all times to reduce the chance of kinking or dislodgment. Complications are catheter kinking, obstruction of the cannula, poor efficacy of ventilation [6], malpositioning, and subcutaneous emphysema. In needle cricothyroidotomy, ventilation by a pressurized stream of oxygen is required. Because the catheter has a small diameter, it is less effective in providing adequate ventilation and should be used only as a temporizing measure before surgical cricothyroidotomy or tracheostomy.

11.2.2.2 Surgical Cricothyroidotomy

This technique is preferred in adults and children over the age of 12 years when the surgical airway is needed. The larger size of the tube makes it vastly preferable to needle cricothyroidotomy. While this is a relatively simple procedure, complications can be common. If complications occur, they can be devastating. Because of the potential complications of cricothyroidotomy, such as subglottic stenosis, a cricothyroidotomy should be converted to a tracheostomy if airway access is needed for more than 48–72 h.

Technique: The skin is prepped if time allows. The cricothyroid membrane is identified between the thyroid cartilage and cricoid cartilage. If the patient is awake and if time allows, infiltrating the skin with lidocaine with epinephrine can be helpful. The larynx is stabilized with the non-dominant hand, and a vertical incision is made (Fig. 11.3). The incision can be lengthened later if exposure is difficult. The subcutaneous tissue is incised sharply. Clamps can be placed onto the subcutaneous tissue, and the clamps elevated toward the ceiling. This both promotes hemostasis and allows the clamps to be used as retractors to bring the cricothyroid membrane more fully into view. The membrane is incised horizontally. The opening can be dilated using the handle of the scalpel, a small clamp, or even the operator's little finger. The use of a tracheal spreader should be avoided, as vigorous spreading can cause damage to the cricoid membrane or laryngeal contents. A tracheostomy tube or small endotracheal tube (ETT n.6) is inserted into the airway (Fig. 11.4). Endotracheal tubes are advantageous as it allows the operator to set the angle of the tube where the angle is set on all

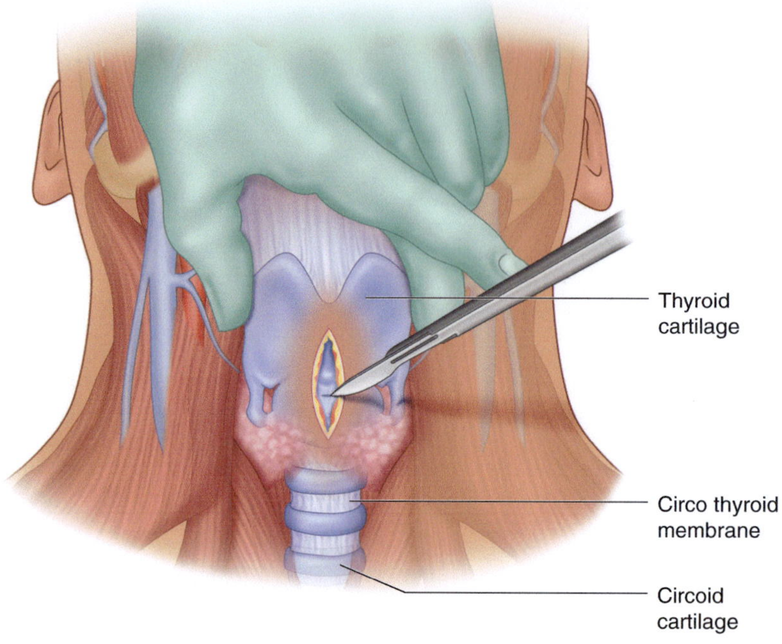

Fig. 11.3 Surgical cricothyroidotomy. The larynx is stabilized with the non-dominant hand, and a vertical incision is made

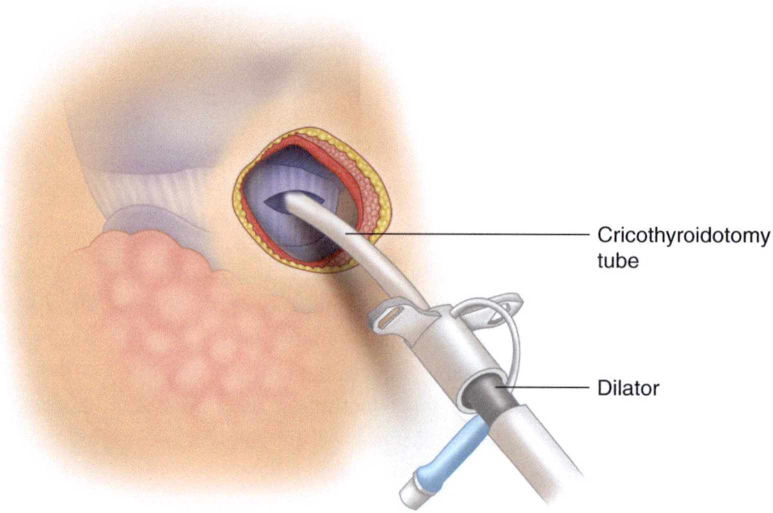

Fig. 11.4 Surgical cricothyroidotomy: the membrane is incised horizontally and a small endotracheal tube is inserted into the airway

commercially available tracheostomy tubes. A stylet can be helpful to place the endotracheal tube. Regardless of the tube used, it should be inserted only enough to be sure the cuff has been placed into the airway. Confirm placement with a CO_2 detector and begin ventilating. Complications occur in 15–20% of patients and include injury to the thyroid or cricoid cartilage, aspiration, retrograde intubation of the airway, main stem intubation, posterior airway perforation, bleeding in the airway or subcutaneous tissue, or inadvertent placement of the tube outside of the airway [7].

11.2.3 Percutaneous Tracheostomy

While formal tracheostomy is generally reserved for more permanent airway control (Fig. 11.5), in some cases, emergency tracheostomy makes sense. While this technique has been shown to be efficacious, it should only be attempted in an emergency by skilled and well-trained surgeons. In some patients, cricothyroidotomy is contraindicated. In those cases, emergency tracheostomy can be lifesaving. Several options exist for emergency

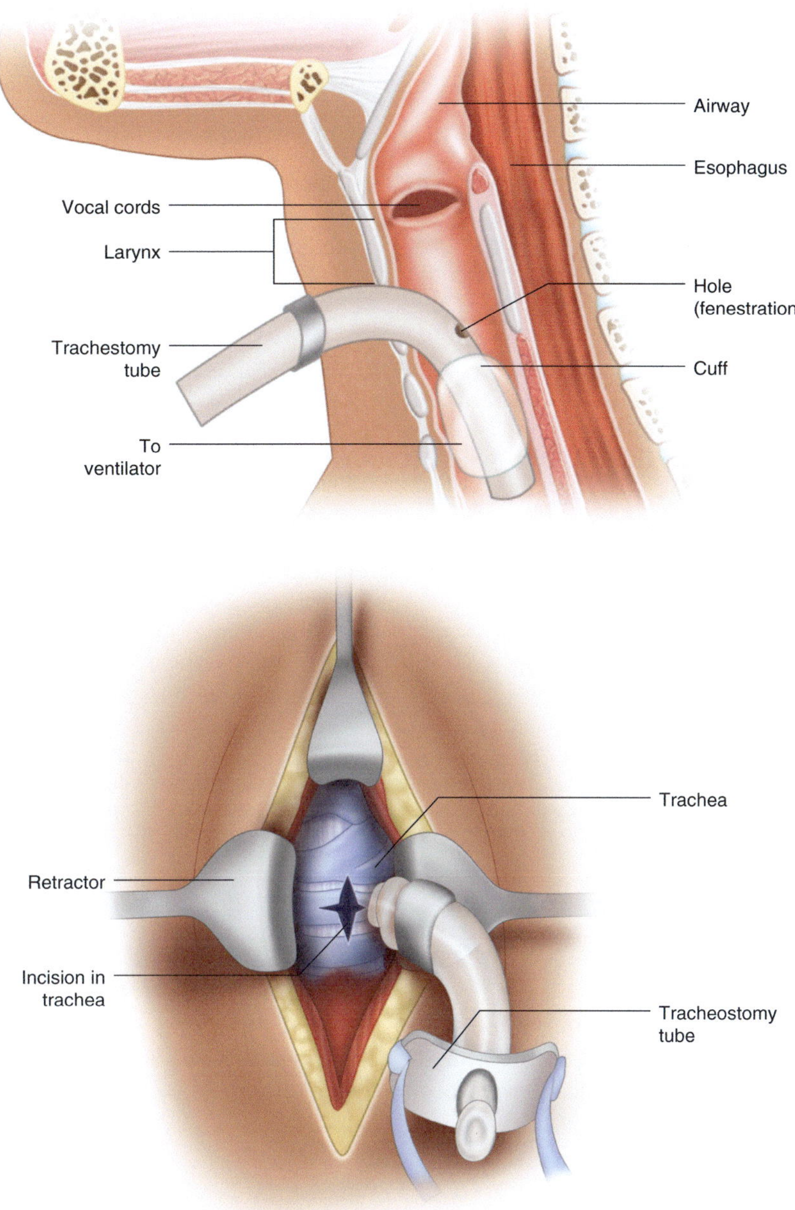

Fig. 11.5 Open tracheostomy

percutaneous tracheostomy, the Ciaglia and Griggs methods [8].

Technique: All techniques are based on the use of a needle guidewire to gain airway access. However, each method requires unique equipment and follows a different intraoperative procedural sequence (Fig. 11.6). Regardless of the particular method selected, several principles are always used. The skin is infiltrated with local anesthetic with epinephrine and prepped, if possible. A vertical or horizontal incision is made, and the subcutaneous tissues divided down to the pretracheal fascia. The trachea is entered below the second ring, stabilizing the trachea. The tracheal opening is dilated, using commercial dilators if the surgeon prefers the tracheostomy tube can be inserted over a guide wire or simply directly through the tracheal opening. The tracheostomy tube is secured and the patient ventilated. Complications are virtually the same as with cricothyroidotomy [9, 10].

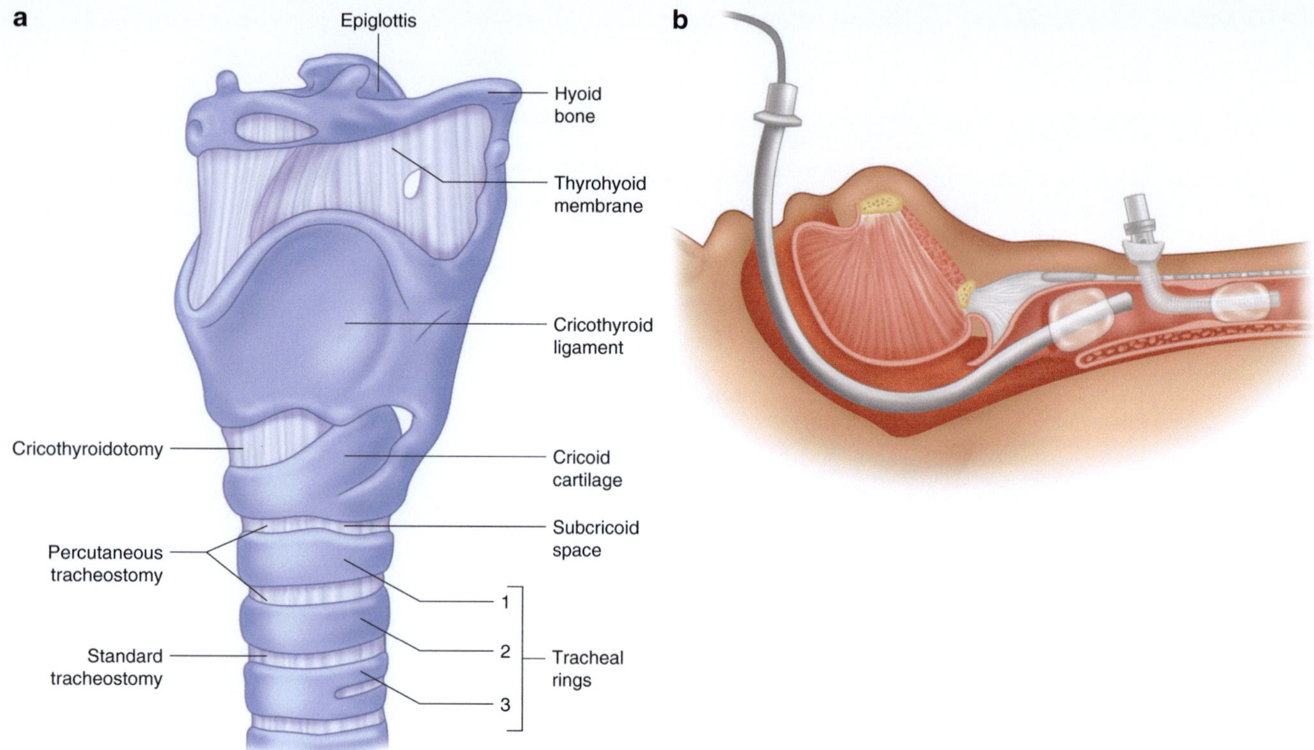

Fig. 11.6 Percutaneous tracheostomy. (**a**) Anatomy of the larynx and trachea. (**b**) Percutaneous tracheostomy techniques are based on the use of a needle guidewire to gain airway access. However, each method requires unique equipment and follows a different intraoperative procedural sequence

11.3 Pleural Decompression

Pleural decompression is a common procedure following major injury and can be lifesaving [11]. Although it is relatively simple, complications can occur if attention to detail is not used.

11.3.1 Needle Decompression

Needle decompression of tension pneumothorax is the common procedure in the prehospital phase of care. However, needle decompression can also be used in the emergency department, particularly if no one is immediately available to place a chest tube. It is important to gauge the thickness of the chest wall before attempting needle decompression. Unfortunately, many of the attempts at needle decompression in the field fail because the needle never actually enters the chest cavity.

Technique: Two sites can be used for needle decompression. The second intercostal space in the midclavicular line and the fifth intercostal space in the midaxillary line are both acceptable (Fig. 11.7). The skin is infiltrated with local anesthetic. A 14- or 16-gauge needle attached to a 10 mL syringe is generally used. The operator should hit the rib with the needle and then climb over the top of the rib aspirating. It is necessary to access the pleural cavity at the top of the costal margin to avoid damage to the intercostal vessels. Once air is aspirated, the needle can be advanced a few millimeters further to be sure that the plural cavity is decompressed. In the case of a tension pneumothorax, entering the pleural cavity should produce a rush of air.

Complications include bleeding, creating a pneumothorax, or failure because the chest cavity is not entered. Iatrogenic injury to major blood vessels, the heart, and the pulmonary vasculature has been reported. If the cause of hemodynamic compromise is a hemothorax, not a pneumothorax, needle decompression will do little to help.

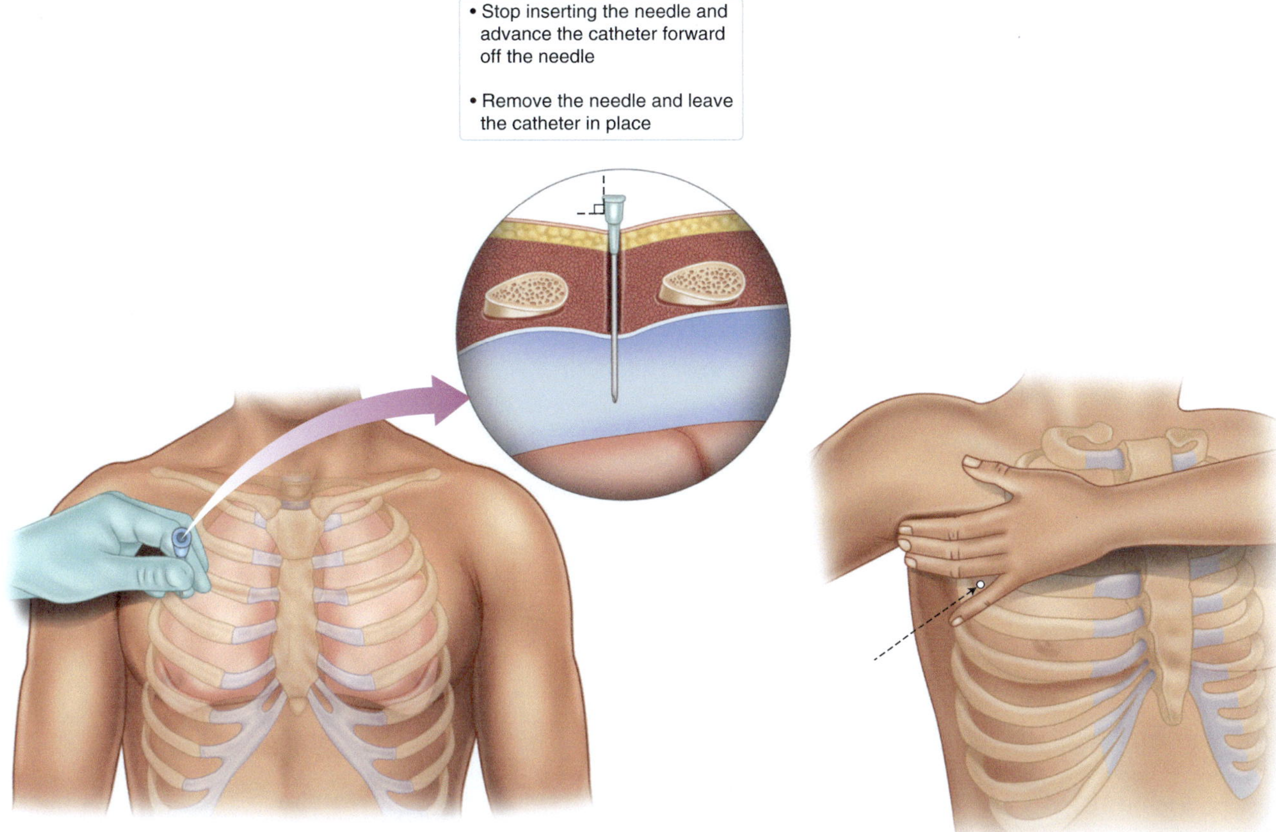

Fig. 11.7 Needle decompression for tension pneumothorax: the second intercostal space in the midclavicular line and the fifth intercostal space in the midaxillary line are both acceptable

11.3.2 Tube Thoracostomy

Placement of a chest tube is one of the most common lifesaving procedures performed in patients after injury [12]. While this is a relatively simple procedure, it is, in fact, a surgical procedure that requires expertise. Unfortunately, since it is thought to be simple, it is often performed by a relatively junior member of the trauma team. If a junior surgeon or emergency physician is to perform this procedure, careful supervision is mandatory to be sure the procedure is carried out effectively and with as little pain to the patient as possible.

Tube thoracostomy can be performed in several locations. While textbooks often recommend the fifth or sixth intercostal space in the midaxillary line, it is entirely reasonable to pick the thinnest portion of the chest wall with a lateral approach. International guidelines suggest the insertion for the chest drain in the fifth intercostal space or above, around the midaxillary line. A triangle of safety with its apex in the axilla has been described: (1) the anterior boarder of the latissimus dorsi, (2) lateral boarder of the pectoralis major, and (3) imaginary horizontal line from the nipple (Fig. 11.8).

There is often discussion about the appropriate size of tube that should be used. Many favor larger tubes if there is a hemothorax and smaller tubes or even a pigtail catheter for pure pneumothoraces. In fact, there is no data that supports larger tubes to drain hemothoraces. Free blood will likely come out via any sized tube inserted. If the hemothorax has clotted, it will not be able to be evacuated, regardless of the size of the tube.

Technique: The patient is positioned with the ipsilateral arm raised above the head, if at all possible. The area is widely prepped and draped unless the procedure is being performed to treat an immediately life-threatening condition. The skin is infiltrated with local anesthetic with epinephrine. A field block infiltrating a circle several inches in diameter provides the best pain relief. A skin incision is made parallel to the rib where the tube is to be inserted. The subcutaneous tissue can be bluntly dissected down to the rib. Additional local anesthetic

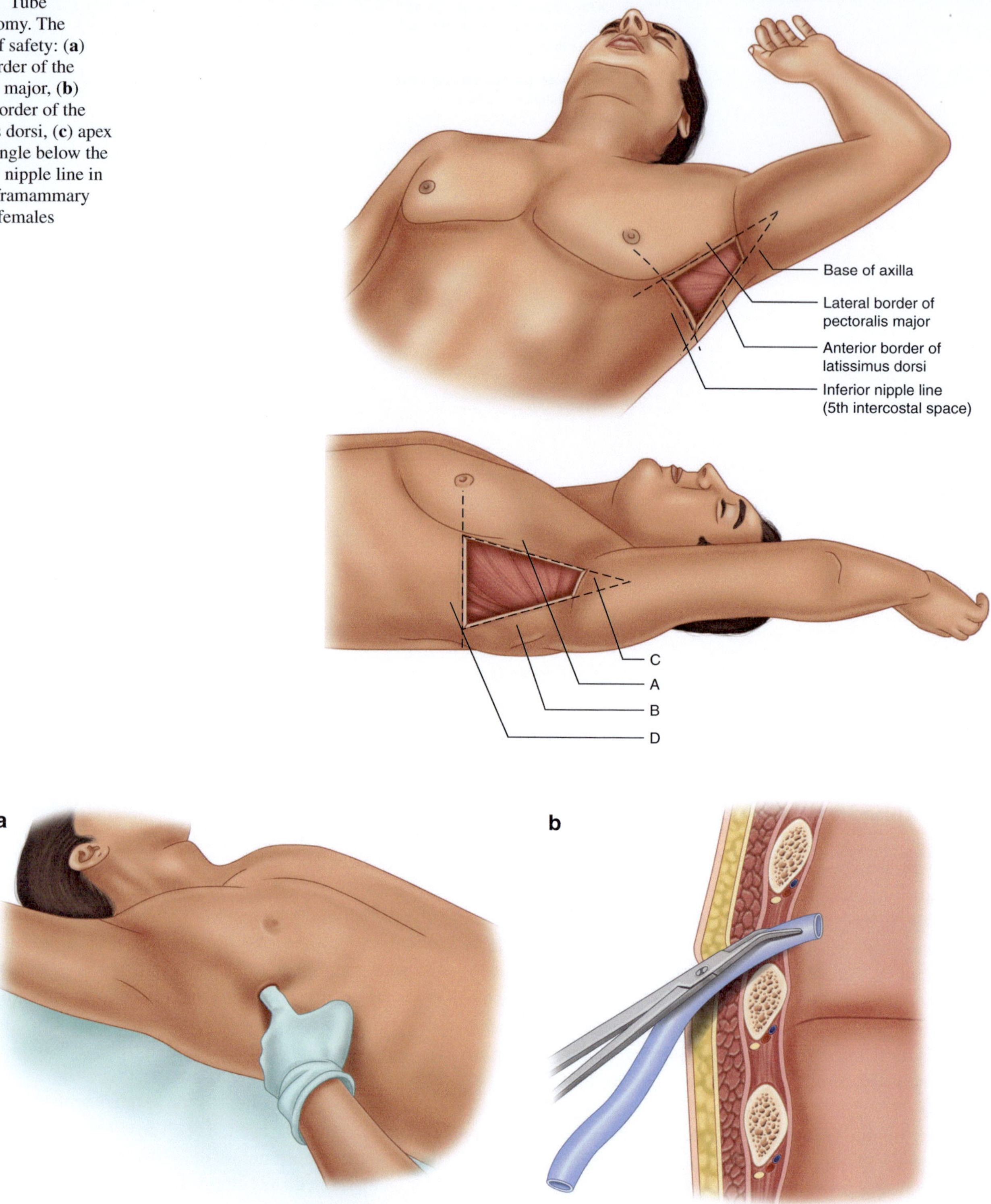

Fig. 11.8 Tube thoracostomy. The triangle of safety: (**a**) lateral border of the pectoralis major, (**b**) anterior border of the latissimus dorsi, (**c**) apex of the triangle below the axilla, (**d**) nipple line in males, inframammary crease in females

Fig. 11.9 Chest tube thoracostomy. (**a**) A finger is then inserted into the chest to be sure the chest has been entered and to evaluate for adhesions between the lung and the chest wall. (**b**) A clamp can be used to gently introduce the tube into the chest cavity

can be used to infiltrate the periosteum of the rib and the pleura. A clamp then can be used to dissect the tissue of the upper border of the rib and enter the pleura. Air or blood usually is expelled upon entering the pleural cavity.

The clamp should be used to dilate the opening in the pleura. A finger is then inserted into the chest to be sure the chest has been entered and to evaluate for adhesions between the lung and the chest wall (Fig. 11.9). The chest tube should be measured to estimate the length of the tube that needs to be inserted. The tube should be directed posteriorly and superiorly. A clamp can be used to gently introduce the tube into the chest cavity. A clamp should also be placed on the distal tube. The chest tube is inserted to a chest drainage system and the distal clamp removed. The tube is secured to the skin with a heavy nonabsorbable suture. A dry dressing is applied and a chest X-ray obtained to evaluate adequacy of tube placement.

Complications include iatrogenic injury to the intercostal vessels; poor positioning, including positioning the tube in the fissure of the lung or outside of the chest cavity, and an injury to underlying viscera, particularly the lung. Continued high output of blood or a large air leak should alert the surgeon that thoracotomy may be necessary.

11.4 Pericardial Window

Creating a pericardial window is a diagnostic and potential temporarily therapeutic procedure in patients who may have hemopericardium. Several options exist to perform this procedure. If it is carried out in conjunction with exploratory laparotomy, a transdiaphragmatic window can be performed. If done as a solo diagnostic procedure, it is usually done via a subxiphoid approach [13, 14].

A pericardial window involves excision of a portion of the pericardium, allowing any blood and/or fluid to drain from the pericardial space. As the pericardium is inelastic, only a small amount of blood or fluid is necessary to produce tamponade, if it accumulates quickly. Diagnostic pericardial window takes some time. Therefore, it is only appropriate in patients who are hemodynamically stable. Those in extremis with suspected pericardial tamponade are best served with alternative procedures such as emergency left thoracotomy or sternotomy.

11.4.1 Transdiaphragmatic Pericardial Window

Pericardial window can be performed at the time of laparotomy. As the surgeon is already in the abdomen, the additional time it takes to perform this procedure is quite short. This can be especially useful in a patient with penetrating thoracoabdominal injury near the mediastinum, particularly in patients who have multiple trajectories, making identification of missile tracts difficult.

Technique: The left lobe of the liver should be mobilized by incising the left triangular ligament and retracted. The pericardium can be located by identifying the cardiac pulsation through the diaphragm. The diaphragm should then be divided using the cautery as close to the midline as possible. The pericardium can be identified by its pearl gray color. The pericardium is then grasped with several fine clamps and a small hole made in it. We like to make the pericardiotomy large enough to see the heart beating. It is possible to inadvertently open the pleura instead of the pericardium. Seeing a beating heart documents the pericardium has, in fact, been opened. If there is blood in the pericardium, most surgeons then proceed with sternotomy. If it is negative, a single Vicryl suture can be used to close the pericardium and diaphragm in a single layer.

Complications include iatrogenic injury to the heart, pericardial infection, and injury to the left lobe of the liver.

11.4.2 Subxiphoid Pericardial Window

When a patient may have transpericardial injury and does not require either thoracotomy or laparotomy, a subxiphoid pericardial window can diagnose cardiac injury. This should only be done in patients who are stable. As even stable patients with hemopericardium can decompensate quickly after induction of anesthesia, it is often wise to prep and drape the patient before they are anesthetized. That way, if they develop hypotension, the window can be aborted, and the surgeon proceeds directly to sternotomy.

Technique: A midline incision is made over the lower xiphoid process and onto the midline of the abdominal wall. The subcutaneous tissue and fascia are divided. We find it helpful to dissect the xiphoid process out and amputate it, usually using a pair of bone shears or a rib cutter. The space above the fascia and behind the sternum can then be dissected. It is imperative that hemostasis be meticulous. Opening the pericardium in a bloody field

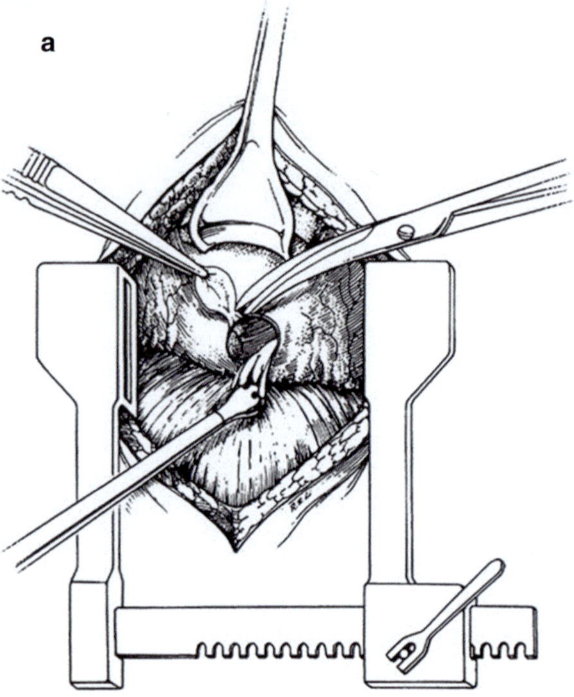

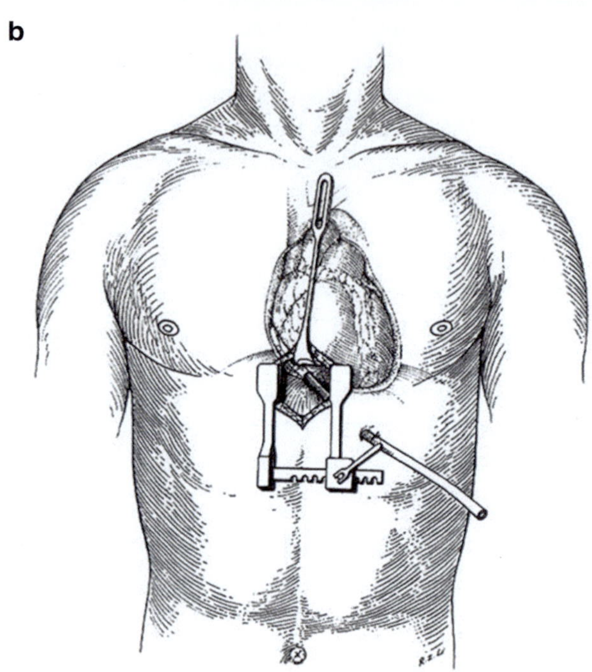

Fig. 11.10 Subxiphoid pericardial window: (**a**) With the transdiaphragmatic approach, the pericardium is grasped with two clamps and a hole cut in it. (**b**) A drain can be left in place(Reproduced with permission from Elesevier in: Moores DW et al. Subxiphoid pericardial drainage for pericardial tamponade. J Thorac Cardiovas Surg:109:546-51, 1995)

risks confusing clear pericardial fluid for a hemopericardium. The pericardium can be identified by its characteristic color. As with the transdiaphragmatic approach, the pericardium is grasped with two fine clamps and a hole cut in it (Fig. 11.10). The beating heart should be visualized. The surgeon then either proceeds with sternotomy or can close the pericardium with a Vicryl suture, depending on the findings.

Complications are similar to a transdiaphragmatic window. Sternal osteomyelitis can occur with deep wound infections.

11.5 Accessing the Mediastinum

The mediastinum occupies the space between the two hemithoraces. The heart and great vessels occupy the anterior mediastinum, and the aorta, trachea, and esophagus are located in the posterior mediastinum. Different incisions are used to access each structure. Additionally, different incision may be used to access different parts of the same structure. For instance, the upper cervical trachea may be accessed through a mini-sternotomy, while the more distal trachea is approached through a posterolateral thoracotomy.

11.5.1 Median Sternotomy

A median sternotomy is the ideal incision to access the heart and the anterior mediastinal great vessels [15]. It can be accomplished quickly, though it requires equipment that is not always readily assessable in every operating room. It is simple and should be in the armamentarium of every surgeon caring for injured patients. A sternotomy can be used for emergency mediastinal exploration, even in patients who are hypotensive. It can also be extended into the neck or along the clavicle to increase exposure.

Technique: A midline incision is made from the suprasternal notch down to the xiphoid process. This is extended down through the subcutaneous tissue on to the sternum. The interclavicular ligament located at the suprasternal notch is divided (Fig. 11.11). This gives the surgeon access to the superior mediastinum. We favor bluntly dissecting

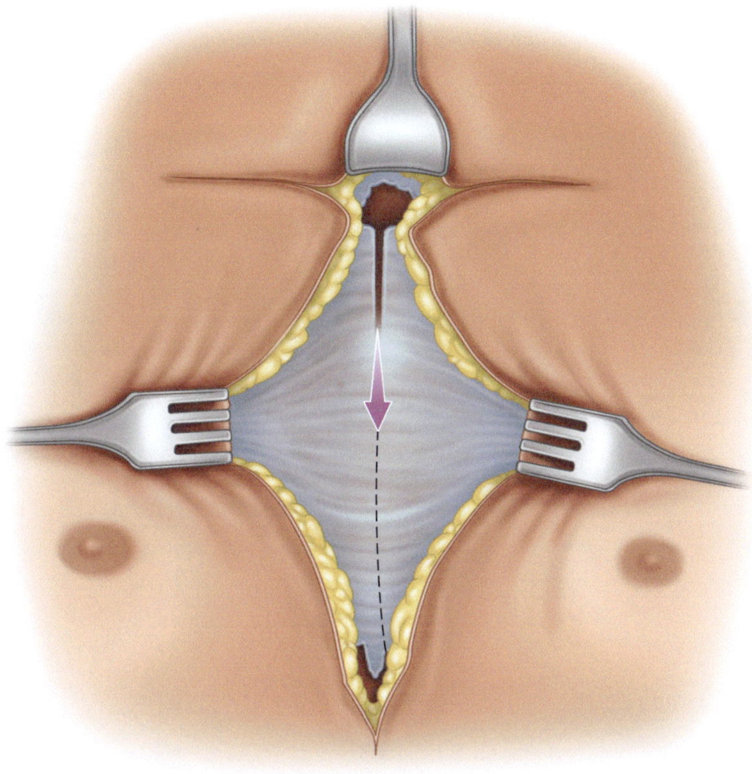

Fig. 11.11 Median sternotomy. A midline incision is made from the suprasternal notch down to the xiphoid process. This is extended down through the subcutaneous tissue on to the sternum. The interclavicular ligament located at the suprasternal notch is divided

the mediastinal tissues off the superior sternum. The same maneuver can be performed at the level of the xiphoid, making sternal division as safe as possible. It is important to dissect the suprasternal notch free of surrounding attachments. This allows the surgeon to insert a finger behind the manubrium and clear the areolar attachments. This maneuver is important to sweep the left brachiocephalic vein and the pleura free from the back of the manubrium. Once the back of the manubrium has been cleared, the midline should be identified and scored with the cautery. The sternum may then be divided from top to bottom or from bottom to top, depending on personal preferences of the surgeon. A standard pneumatic or electrical powered saw is generally used. The lungs should be deflated during the sternotomy to avoid entering the pleural cavity. It is essential to divide the sternum in the midline. Dividing the manubrium can occasionally be difficult; in such case, the Lebsche knife can be useful.

Once the sternum is divided, a sternal retractor should be placed (Fig. 11.12). A rapid exploration should help to find the source of hemorrhage and/or areas of major injury. The pericardium is then divided in the midline. The pericardial edges can be retracted off the midline by placing some pericardial "tack-up" stitches, securing them to the sternal retractor. Using gentle manipulation, all surfaces of the heart can be examined. The anterior mediastinal structures can be identified starting with the aortic arch. The left brachiocephalic vein is the structure encountered first. Injury of the left brachiocephalic vein is the major risk to the division of the upper sternum, and care should be taken to avoid damage to it, though it can be ligated and divided without consequence.

A sternotomy can be extended into the neck using a standard sternocleidomastoid incision. This gives access to the takeoff of the carotid arteries. It can also be extended along the clavicle to give better access to the subclavian arteries, particularly on the right side (Fig. 11.13). A median sternotomy combined with unilateral left or right anterior thoracotomy, which is called hemiclamshell incision, can allow a better surgical control of the anterior mediastinum as well as of right or left hemithorax (Fig. 11.14). Finally, a mini-sternotomy can be performed

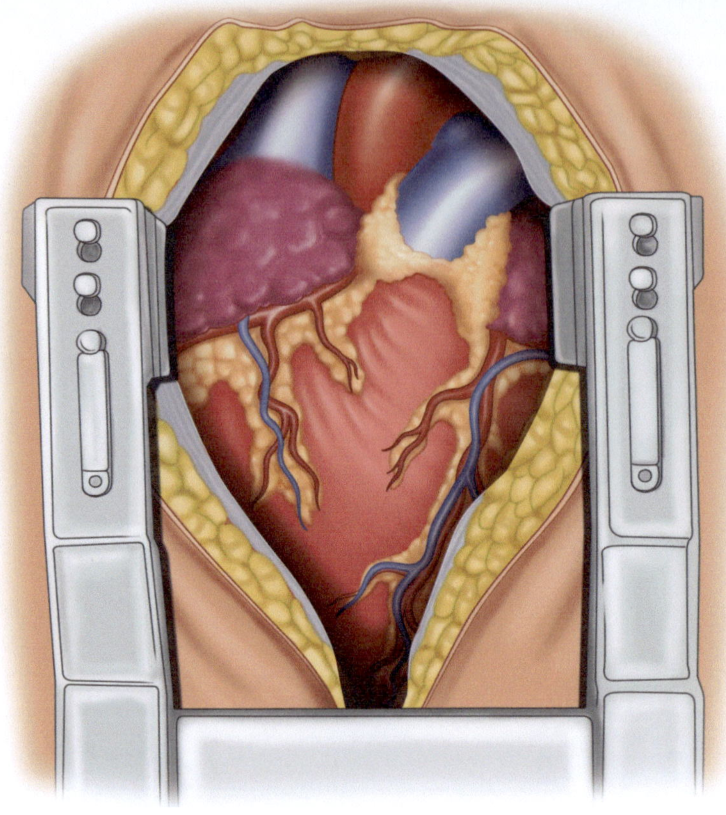

Fig. 11.12 Once the sternum is divided, a Finocchietto sternal retractor should be placed

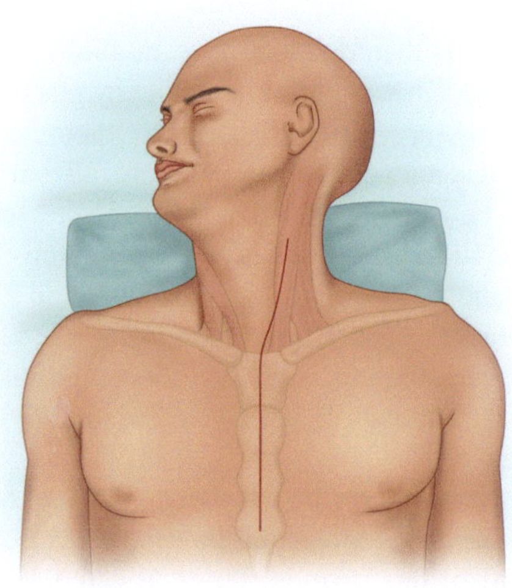

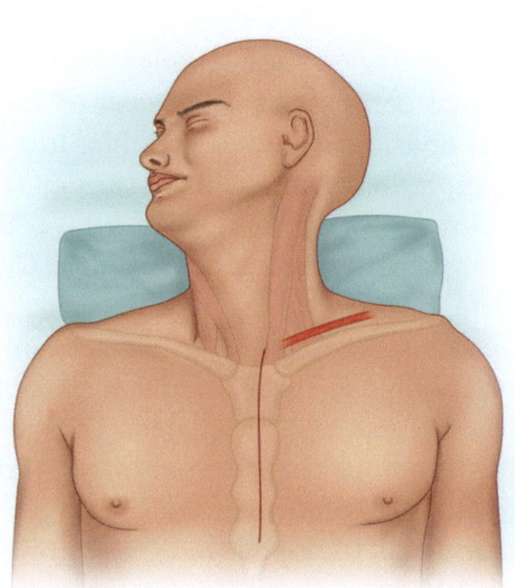

Fig. 11.13 A sternotomy can be extended into the neck using a standard sternocleidomastoid incision. This gives access to the takeoff of the carotid arteries. It can also be extended along the right or left clavicle to give better access to the subclavian arteries

if the surgeon only requires access to the upper mediastinal structures. The upper sternum is divided down through the manubrium. A pediatric Finochietto retractor can be placed to separate the sternal edges. This gives great access to the innominate artery and can be combined with a periclavicular incision on the right to access the proximal right subclavian artery.

11.6 Accessing the Chest

11.6.1 Posterolateral Thoracotomy

A posterolateral thoracotomy (Fig. 11.15) is the ideal incision to explore and repair injuries in the posterior mediastinum. It requires placing the patient in a full lateral position. This inci-

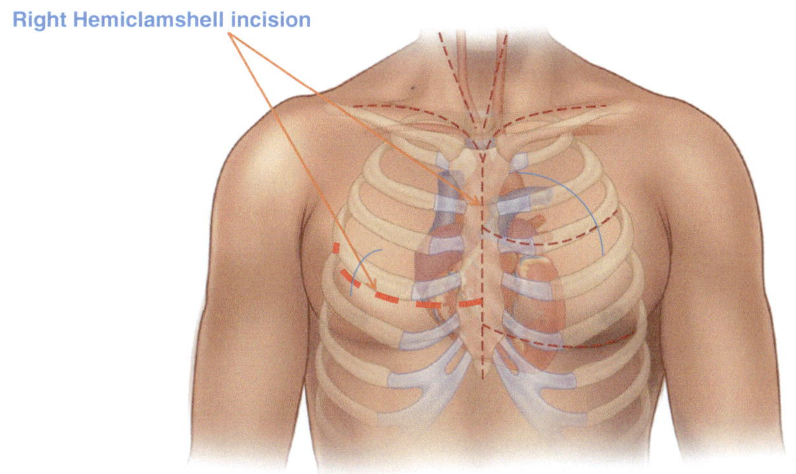

Fig. 11.14 A median sternotomy can be not only extended into the neck using a standard sternocleidomastoid incision but can also be combined with unilateral left or right anterior thoracotomy, which is called hemiclamshell incision; hemiclamshell incision can allow a better surgical control of the anterior mediastinum as well as of the right or left hemithorax

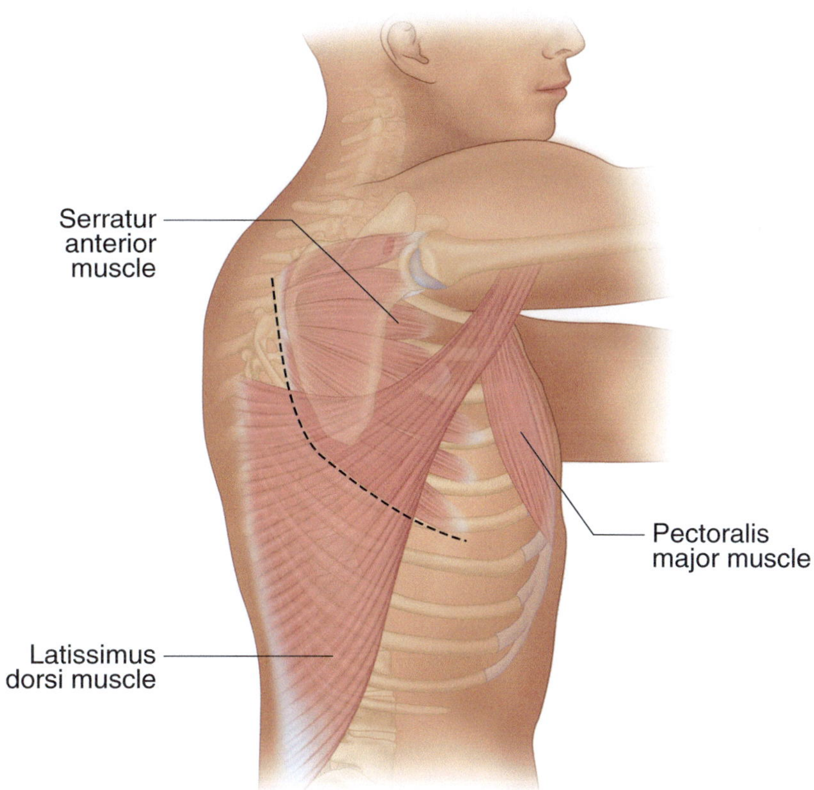

Fig. 11.15 Posterolateral thoracotomy is the ideal incision to explore and repair injuries in the posterior mediastinum. It requires placing the patient in a full lateral position

sion is not particularly versatile as it cannot be extended to explore other areas of the chest and/or abdomen. As such, it is useful only in stable patients who have injuries in the posterior mediastinum already diagnosed. The level of thoracotomy will be determined by the injury [15–17]. For instance, the typical blunt aortic injury is approached via a fifth or sixth interspace left thoracotomy. An injury to the trachea, it is approached via the right side, often in the fourth interspace.

Technique: A double lumen endotracheal tube is preferable in such patients. This allows the lung to be deflated, which improves exposure of the hemithorax once the chest is entered. The patient is then positioned in the full lateral position. The skin, subcutaneous tissue, and muscles are serially divided. The surgeon dissects down on to the chest wall and mobilizes the scapula. That allows the surgeon to count the ribs and enter the chest in the appropriate interspace. The lung is mobilized by dividing the inferior pulmonary ligament. On the right side, the azygous vein can be doubly ligated and divided to allow exposure. With the lung deflated, and the chest fully opened, the surgeon should be able to identify virtually any injury within the chest. The pleura may need to be divided in order to fully explore structures like the trachea, esophagus, and aorta.

11.6.2 Left Anterolateral Thoracotomy and Bilateral Anterior Thoracotomies (Clamshell Incision)

The most rapid method of accessing the chest is via an anterolateral left thoracotomy (Fig. 11.16).

This incision can be performed rapidly and is versatile, as it can be brought across the sternum into a clamshell thoracotomy. The surgeon can repair virtually any injury via the clamshell incision. The versatility and rapidity make anterolateral thoracotomy the ideal incision for chest exploration in a hemodynamically unstable patient.

Emergency department thoracotomy (EDT) is often performed for patients who present with cardiac arrest and/or those in extremis following penetrating chest trauma [18, 19]. In such patients, EDT offers the only option to save a life. Because of the nature of the patients, survival rates after EDT are relatively low. There has been much debate in the literature as to the appropriate setting for EDT. In general, the mechanism and location of the injury, combined with presence or absence of vital signs and signs of life, dictate whether EDT is appropriate. Some groups have published guidelines for EDT which are summarized in Table 11.1.

Technique: In general, the patient is placed supine. In the operating room, placing several folded sheets underneath the shoulder and back elevates the lateral thorax and can be helpful. The left arm can be raised above the head if desired. Airway control should be obtained simultaneously with the thoracotomy when EDT is being performed.

A curvilinear incision is made over the fifth rib beginning at the left margin of sternum and extending up into the posterior axillary line. In a female, the breast should be retracted, and the incision should follow the left inframammary crease. In a male, the incision is placed just inferior to the left nipple. The incision should be brought down through the subcutaneous tissue and muscles onto the chest wall. The interspace that is going to be used to enter the chest should then be selected, and the chest cavity entered over the superior portion of the rib to avoid injury to the intercostal vessels. A Finochietto retractor is generally used to spread the ribs. The retractor should be placed with the handle downward to permit extension of the incision as needed. The lung is then mobilized by incising the inferior pulmonary ligament.

Injuries to the lung and/or intercostal vessels can often be repaired via an anterolateral thoracotomy. However, injuries to the heart or complex injuries to the mediastinal vasculature

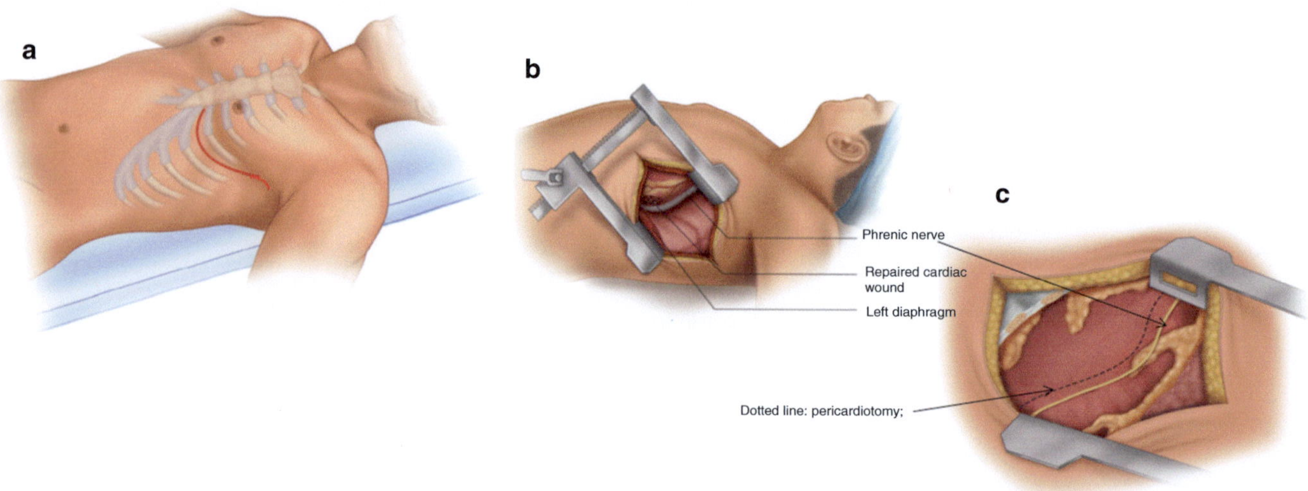

Fig. 11.16 Emergency department thoracotomy. (**a**) A curvilinear incision is made over the fifth rib beginning at the left border of the sternum and extending up into the posterior axillary line. (**b**) The phrenic nerve is visible along the lateral aspect of the pericardium. (**c**) Pericardiotomy is performed in the midline to avoid damage to the left phrenic nerve

Table 11.1 Indications for EDT are reported differently: widely or less accepted, questionable or uncertain indications

Indications for EDT
– Widely accepted: penetrating thoracic injury with the following conditions:
• Previously witnessed cardiac activity (prehospital or in-hospital)
• Unresponsive hypotension (systolic blood pressure [SBP] <70 mmHg) despite vigorous resuscitation
– Less accepted: blunt thoracic injury with the following conditions:
• Previously witnessed cardiac activity (prehospital or in-hospital)
• Rapid exsanguination from the chest tube (>1500 mL immediately returned)
• Unresponsive hypotension (SBP <70 mmHg) despite vigorous resuscitation
– American College of Surgeons Committee on trauma indications for EDT
• Precordial wound in a patient with prehospital cardiac arrest
• Trauma patient with cardiac arrest after arrival to ED
• Profound hypotension (<70 mmHg) in a patient with a truncal wound who is either unconscious or an operating room is unavailable
– *Questionable or uncertain indications*
• Penetrating nonthoracic injury (e.g., abdominal, peripheral) with traumatic arrest with previously witnessed cardiac activity (prehospital or in-hospital)
• Blunt thoracic injuries with traumatic arrest with previously witnessed cardiac activity

require additional exposure. In those cases, extending the thoracotomy across the sternum into a clamshell incision is wise. The clamshell incision is shaped like a curved "W" and is typically performed in the anatomic skin/rib groove below the breasts (Fig. 11.17). The incision is then brought across the sternum into the contralateral hemithorax. The sternum is divided with a Lebsche knife or Gigli saw. It is important to remember to ligate the internal mammary vessels. In patients in profound shock or those with cardiac arrest, these vessels will not be bleeding at the time of clamshell thoracotomy. However, as the patient is resuscitated, the internal mammary arteries will bleed impressively. A second rib spreader can be placed to aid in the exposure of both chest cavities.

When necessary, pericardiotomy can be performed. Ideally, this is performed in the midline, and the pericardium widely opened. This avoids damage to the phrenic nerves which are located literally on each side of the pericardium. The aorta can be cross-clamped, if desired. It can be difficult to distinguish the flaccid aorta from the esophagus. Placing a nasogastric tube can be helpful. The mediastinal pleura must be widely divided in order to isolate the aorta. It is necessary to truly isolate the descening thoracic aorta, usually on the operator's finger in order to reliably cross-clamp the vessel. Blindly inserting the clamp almost never is successful. The aorta is bluntly dissected anteriorly. The descending thoracic aorta can then be bluntly mobilized off the prevertebral fascia. With the aortic circumference completely mobilized, the cross-clamp can be easily placed.

For patients who have sustained a cardiac arrest, open CPR is necessary. In general, the pericardium is widely opened and the heart is delivered out of the pericardium. A hinged maneuver (clapping motion of the hands) is generally used (Fig. 11.18).

The surgeon provides internal cardiac massage using the palm of their hands, with one hand being placed posterior and the other anterior to the heart. The motion should force blood out of the heart, into the pulmonary vessels and the aorta. Using the palms minimizes the risk of iatrogenic injury to the heart [20].

Major hemorrhage from the pulmonary hilum requires immediate control. There are several maneuvers which can be helpful. The simplest is finger control. If that is successful, the patient should be immediately taken to the operating room for more formal exploration. Twisting the lung on the hilar vessels will occlude both the pulmonary artery and pulmonary vein. This requires mobilization of the inferior pulmonary ligament to be successful. While this can be effective, maintaining the lung twisted can be difficult, and this limits visualization when trying to identify the area of hemorrhage. Finally, simply placing a soft, non-crushing vascular clamp across the hilum can be effective. One must take care to not damage the bronchus during this maneuver. Regardless of the method selected, occluding the pulmonary vessels produces a marked increase in pulmonary vascular resistance. This is not tolerated well in patients who are badly hypotensive and is often followed by cardiac arrest.

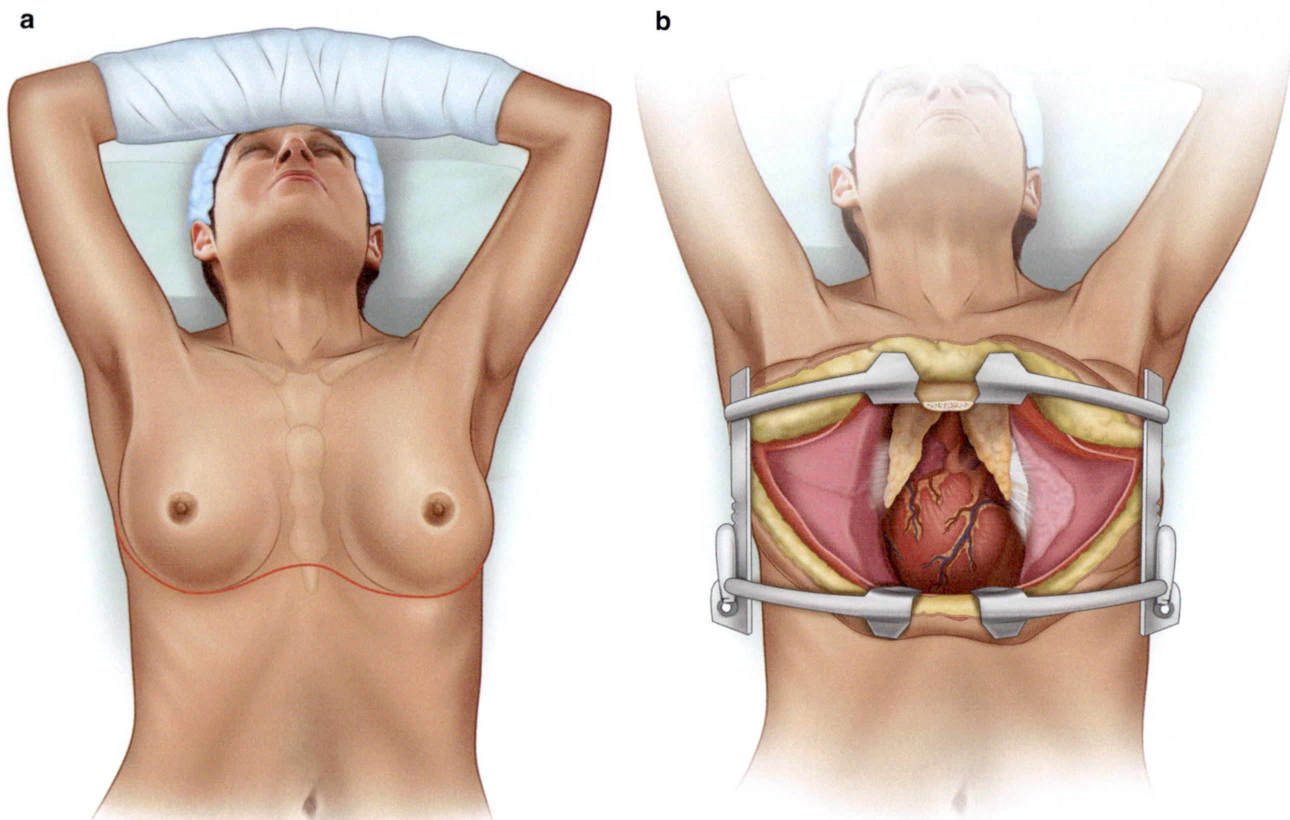

Fig. 11.17 Bilateral anterior thoracotomies or clamshell incision: (**a**) this is shaped like a curved "W" and is typically performed in the anatomic skin/rib groove below the breasts; it offers a wide exposure of anterior mediastinum and the chest (**b**)

11.7 Pelvic Packing

Obtaining hemostasis in patients who are bleeding in the pelvis following major pelvic fractures can be challenging. Direct operative exploration via a laparotomy is almost always doomed to failure. Much of the bleeding may be coming from venous sources. In addition, arterial injuries are often located deep in the pelvis and are not accessible via direct exploration. Angiographic embolization is an extremely attractive method for obtaining pelvic hemostasis. This allows the angiographer to precisely identify the site of hemorrhage and arrest hemorrhage, using a variety of hemostatic materials. However, some patients don't have the ability to tolerate the amount of time it takes to mobilize the embolization team. In those patients, pelvic packing can be lifesaving [21].

As most patients with major pelvic fracture hemorrhage have suffered open book fractures, pelvic packing should be combined with some maneuver that closes down the pelvic volume. Examples include tying a bed sheet around the patient, use of commercially available pelvic binders, and/or placement of a pelvic external fixator. These compressive devices are often placed in the emergency department. If the patient does not respond, pelvic packing is often the next step utilized.

Technique: In the operating room, the abdomen and perineum are prepped and draped. The pelvis can be packed via a midline incision or via a Pfannenstiel incision. Regardless of the incision used, it is important to not enter the peritoneal cavity. The intact peritoneum is very helpful to use to obtain pressure to tamponade pelvic hemorrhage. The rectus muscles can be divided in the midline (Fig. 11.19). Alternatively, they can be divided transversely to give access to the pelvic cavity. In those cases, however, incisional hernia is relatively common.

Whichever compressive device has been used, it may need to be adjusted in order to get access to the pelvis for

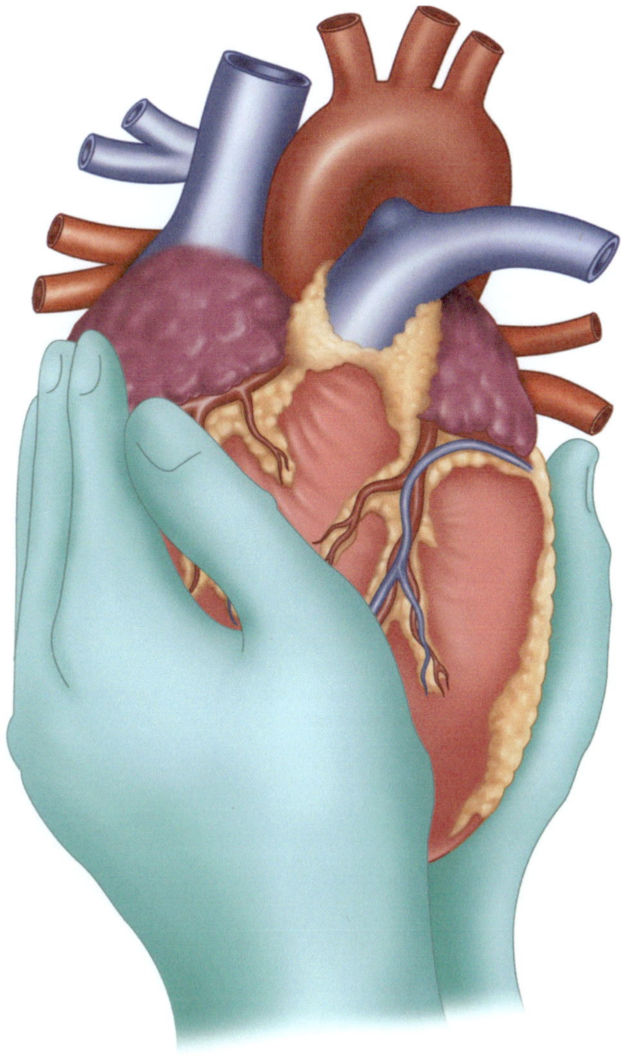

Fig. 11.18 Bimanual internal cardiac massage during cardiac arrest: a hinged clapping motion of the hands to compress the hearth from the apex toward the aortic root. Fingertip pressure should be avoided

packing. Placing a second bed sheet or binder lower on the upper thighs allows reduction of the trochanters, which should keep the pelvis reduced. If an external fixator has been placed, the anterior bars can be rotated to give access to the lower abdominal wall. The devices can be replaced, as needed once pelvic packing has been accomplished.

Once the pelvis is entered, the hematoma should be evacuated as completely as possible. Retractors should be placed and the pelvis explored. Occasionally, the surgeon encounters bleeding vessels, which can be suture ligated. They can do a great deal to stop pelvic hemorrhage. If none are seen, the pelvis should then be packed. Various methods exist. Some groups advocate placing three rolled-up laparotomy pads on either side of the pelvis (Fig. 11.20). While this is often sufficient, in patients with large public space hemorrhage, three lap pads may not suffice. Our preference is to use whatever number of lap pads that is necessary to achieve tight pelvic packing. This may take six or eight. Packing with hemostatic material is also an alternative. Use of commercially available hemostatic gauze may be preferable.

Once pelvic hemostasis is obtained, the pelvis can be closed. Some close the fascia over the packing to add additional tamponade effect. Closing the skin over the packing should achieve similar results. Finally, placing a temporary vacuum dressing over the pelvic packing allows the ICU team to monitor any additional bleeding in the pelvis.

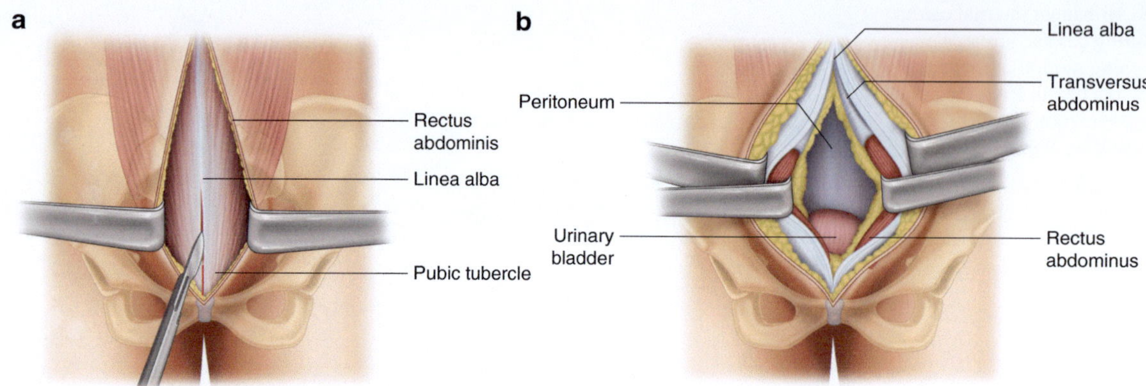

Fig. 11.19 Extraperitoneal packing: (**a**) the rectus muscles are divided in the midline; (**b**) both bellies of the rectus abdominis muscle are gently retracted laterally

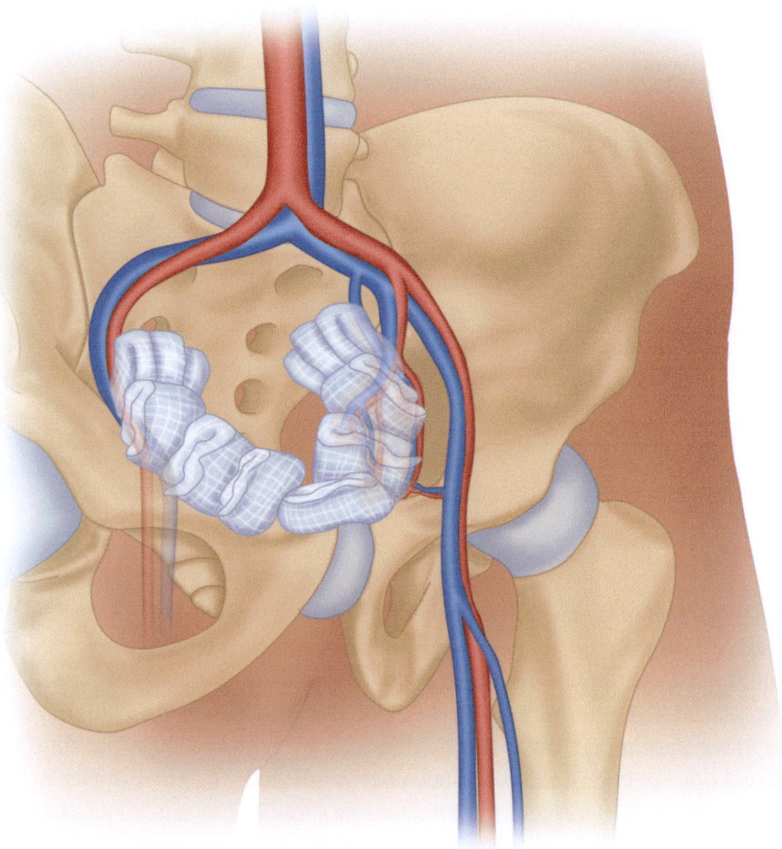

Fig. 11.20 Extraperitoneal pelvic packing: the retroperitoneal space is filled with three rolled-up laparotomy pads on either side of the pelvis to create a good pressure on both sides of the retroperitoneal region

11.8 Resuscitative Balloon Occlusion of the Aorta (REBOA)

REBOA was first described in 1954 by Dr. Carl Hughes who used it on three patients in the Korean War. The technology was so crude that the technique never became popular [22]. However, more recently, the technology has become increasingly sophisticated so that this has become clinical reality. The technique was first popularized for use in vascular surgery patients but is now commonly used in trauma patients in several major institutions in the United States.

Aortic occlusion provides temporary control of hemorrhage almost anywhere in the body. Traditionally, this was done using an open technique, either via left thoracotomy or laparotomy. REBOA is a minimally invasive technique where a transfemoral balloon catheter is inserted and threaded proximally in the aorta (Fig. 11.21). The balloon can then be inflated successfully, occluding the aorta. This is most commonly used to temporize intraabdominal hemorrhage or pelvic fracture bleeding. Several algorithms have been developed describing various zones for REBOA use (Fig. 11.22). Many questions still exist, such as how long the balloon can be left inflated, whether that is different in the various zones, and, ultimately, whether use of this technique actually saves lives. Much more work will be necessary before these answers are definitively known.

Technique: Patients in whom use of the REBOA may be useful should be identified as early as possible. We prefer to use the right femoral artery for REBOA insertion, if at all possible. Thus, insertion of a percutaneous right femoral arterial line early is ideal in patients who may benefit from deploying the REBOA.

If an arterial line has been placed, this can be exchanged in order to place the REBOA. If not, the femoral artery must be cannulated. If the femoral pulses are palpable, a percutaneous technique can be used. Ultrasound guidance can be very helpful. However, in approximately 50% of cases, the artery cannot be accessed percutaneously and a cutdown is necessary. It is imperative to place the REBOA into the common femoral arteries. Placement into the superficial femoral artery risks iatrogenic injury that requires repair and/or revascularization.

The original REBOA catheter was placed via a 12 French introducer. An Amplatz wire is fed into a standard arterial catheter, regardless of how the catheter was placed. The catheter is removed and the 12 French introducer placed. The introducer only needs to be placed in far enough to allow placement of the REBOA, usually into the common iliac artery. The Amplatz guide wire is left in place. A decision is made as to which zone in which the REBOA balloon will be inflated and the balloon and catheter inserted over the guide wire to the appropriate length. The balloon is then inflated. Radiographic confirmation is ideal and may be obtained via ultrasound or a plain X-ray. X-ray confirmation is especially easy if the balloon has been inflated with contrast material. The size of the introducer requires open exploration and repair of the femoral artery when the introducer is removed.

More recently, a smaller catheter has become commercially available. The ER REBOA (Prytime) is a smaller catheter placed via a 7 French introducer system. The introducer system is placed; no guide wire is required. The catheter can then be placed via the smaller introducer and the balloon inflated. When the balloon is deflated, the catheter can be removed. The smaller size of the introducer system does not require open repair. Holding pressure for 10–15 min is usually sufficient to obtain hemostasis.

Complications include insertion site vascular injury, compartment syndrome, and all of the effects of aortic occlusion, particularly if the balloon is inflated for a prolonged period of time. As this is a new technique, the exact incidence of complications is not yet known.

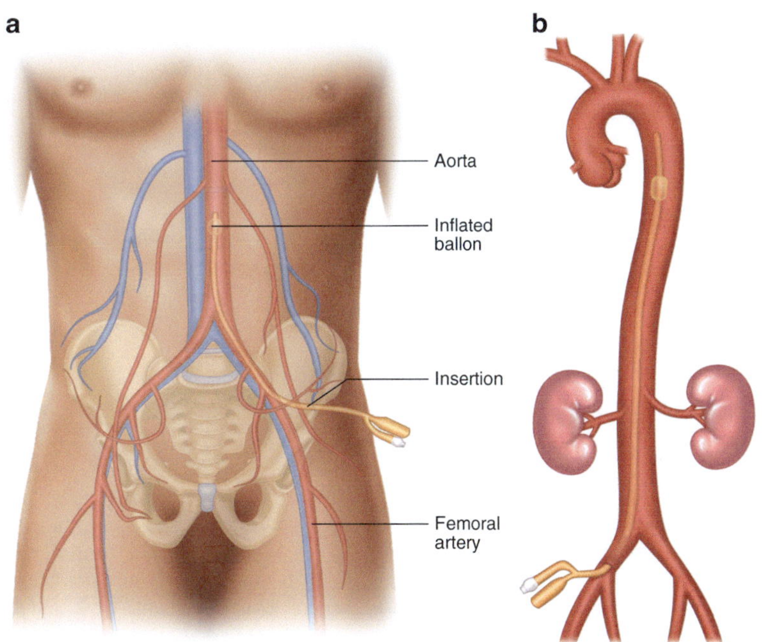

Fig. 11.21 REBOA (resuscitative endovascular balloon occlusion of the aorta). This technique involves rapidly placing a flexible catheter into the femoral artery, maneuvering it into the aorta and inflating the balloon at its tip. The balloon inflated in the abdominal aorta (**a**) and in the thoracic aorta (**b**)

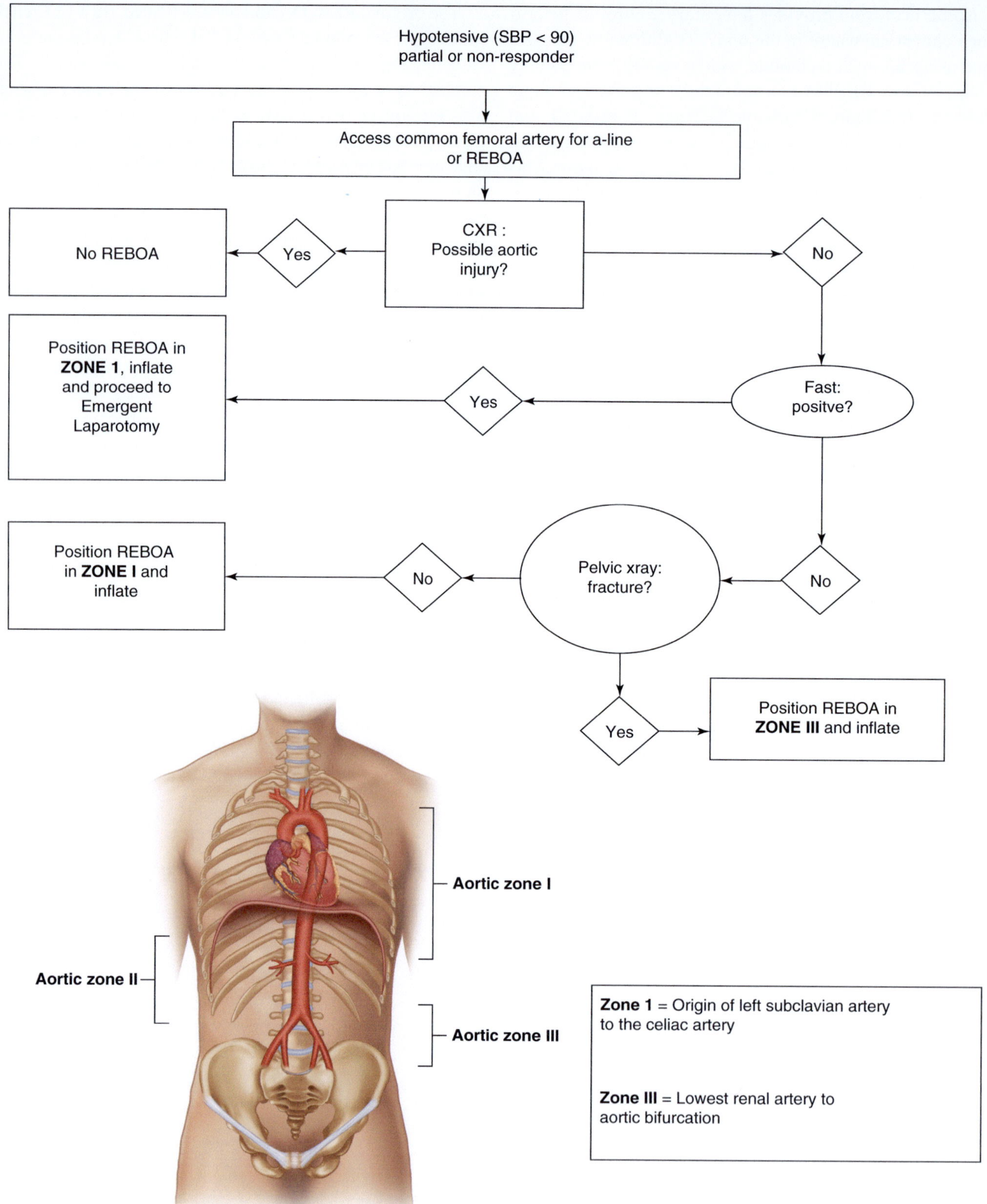

Fig. 11.22 Aortic zones in relation to REBOA: Zone I: extends from the origin of the left subclavian artery to the celiac artery and is a potential zone of occlusion. In this case, a larger diameter balloon and a longer sheath will be advanced into the thoracic aorta. Zone II: extends from the celiac artery to the lowest renal artery and is a no-occlusion zone. Zone III: exists from the lowest renal artery to the aortic bifurcation where REBOA may provide particular utility for instances of pelvic and junctional femoral (contralateral) hemorrhage

References

1. American College of Surgeons Committee. Advanced trauma life support instructor manual. 6th ed. Chicago: American College of Surgeons; 1997.
2. Scalea TM, editor. The shock trauma manual of operative techniques. New York: Springer; 2015. https://doi.org/10.1007/978-1-4939-2371-7_19.
3. Fingerhut A, Leppäniemi A, Coimbra R, Peitzman AB, Scalea TM, Voigli EJ, editors. Emergency surgery course (ESC®) manual. New York: Springer; 2016.
4. Li J, Murphy-Lavoie H, Bugas C, Martinez J, Preston C. Complications of emergency intubation with and without paralysis. Am J Emerg Med. 1999;17:141–3.
5. Jain U, McCunn M, Smith CE, Pittet JF. Management of the traumatized airway. Anesthesiology. 2016;124:199–206.
6. Scrase I, Woollard M. Needle vs surgical cricothyroidotomy: a short cut to effective ventilation. Anaesthesia. 2006;61:962–74.
7. Hsiao J, Pacheco-Fowler V. Videos in clinical medicine. Cricothyroidotomy. N Engl J Med. 2008;358(22):e25.
8. Park H, Kent J, Joshi M, Zhu S, Bochicchio GV, Henry S, Scalea T. Percutaneous versus open tracheostomy: comparison of procedures and surgical site infections. Surg Infect. 2013;14:21–3.
9. Freeman BD, Morris PE. Tracheostomy practice in adults with acute respiratory failure. Crit Care Med. 2012;40:2890–6.
10. Cools-Lartigue J, Aboalsaud A, Gill H, Ferri L. Evolution of percutaneous dilatational tracheostomy—a review of current techniques and their pitfalls. World J Surg. 2013;37:1633–46.
11. Fitzgerald M, Mackenzie CF, Marasco S, Hoyle R, Kossmann T. Pleural decompression and drainage during trauma reception and resuscitation. Injury. 2008;39:9–20.
12. Meredith JW, Hoth JJ. Thoracic trauma: when and how to intervene. Surg Clin North Am. 2007;87(1):95–118. vii.
13. Stranch EW, Zarzaur BL, Savage SA. Thinking outside the box: re-evaluating the approach to penetrating cardiac injuries. Eur J Trauma Emerg Surg. 2016. [Epub ahead of print].
14. Mayer HJ. Transdiaphragmatic pericardial window: a new approach. J Cardiovasc Surg. 1993;34(2):173–5.
15. Marshall M. Thoracic incisions. In: Kaiser LR, Kron IL, Spray TL, editors. Mastery of cardiothoracic surgery. 2nd ed. Philadelphia, PA: Lippincott Williams & Wilkins; 2006. p. 28–33.
16. O'Connor JV, DuBose JJ, Scalea TM. Damage-control thoracic surgery: management and outcomes. J Trauma Acute Care Surg. 2014;77(5):660–5.
17. Onat S, Ulku R, Avci A, Ates G, Ozcelik C. Urgent thoracotomy for penetrating chest trauma: analysis of 158 patients of a single center. Injury. 2011;42:900–4.
18. Seamon MJ, Haut ER, et al. Emergency department thoracotomy. J Trauma. 2015;79:159–73.
19. Simms ER, Flaris AN, Franchino X, Thomas MS, Caillot J-L, Voiglio EJ. Bilateral anterior thoracotomy (clamshell incision) is the ideal emergency thoracotomy incision: an anatomic study. World J Surg. 2013;37:1277–85.
20. Hunt PA, Greaves I, Owens WA. Emergency thoracotomy in thoracic trauma-a review. Injury. 2006;37:1–19. Epub 2005 Apr 20.
21. Filiberto DM, Fox AD. Preperitoneal pelvic packing: technique and outcomes. Int J Surg. 2016;33(Pt B):222–4.
22. Qasim Z, Brenner M, Menaker J, Scalea T. Resuscitative endovascular balloon occlusion of the aorta. Resuscitation. 2015;96:275–9.

Modern Management of Maxillofacial Injuries

12

Gabriele Canzi, Davide Sozzi, and Alberto Bozzetti

Key Points

- Bleeding after facial trauma is often self-limiting and life-threatening only in 1.4–11% of all severe facial injuries. Its prompt identification and timely management play a major role in ensuring safe access to airways and in avoiding increased blood loss with hemodynamic worsening.
- Trauma surgeons should become increasingly confident with local hemostatic measures, which are fast effective in facial bleeding control and hemodynamic stabilization, delaying definitive treatments according to the damage control strategies.
- Each patient requiring total body or brain CT, with concomitant external evidence of facial involvement, must be studied with thin-slice CT scan and additional tridimensional reconstruction, especially in middle third, orbital, cranial base, or panfacial involvement.
- In modern trauma centers, diagnostic arteriography and superselective embolization (by coaxial microcatheter) is the gold standard definitive treatment of facial hemorrhages which are refractory to local measures.
- When ABC priorities are dealt with, visual-threatening conditions have to be detected early and promptly managed. They occur in 0.56–6% of facial fractures and orbital compartment syndrome is the most common one. Anterior orbitotomy by lateral canthotomy and inferior cantholysis is an easier, faster, and more effective decompressive treatment.

G. Canzi (✉)
Maxillofacial Departmental Structure, the Emergency Department, ASST Grande Ospedale Metropolitano Niguarda, Milan, Italy
e-mail: gabriele.canzi@ospedaleniguarda.it

D. Sozzi
ASST Monza San Gerardo Hospital, and the Department of Medicine and Surgery, School of Medicine, University of Milano-Bicocca, Milan, Italy
e-mail: davide.sozzi@unimib.it

A. Bozzetti
Maxillofacial Departmental Structure, the Emergency Department, ASST Grande Ospedale Metropolitano Niguarda, Milan, Italy

ASST Monza San Gerardo Hospital, and the Department of Medicine and Surgery, School of Medicine, University of Milano-Bicocca, Milan, Italy
e-mail: alberto.bozzetti@unimib.it

P. Aseni et al. (eds.), *Operative Techniques and Recent Advances in Acute Care and Emergency Surgery*,
https://doi.org/10.1007/978-3-319-95114-0_12

12.1 Introduction

The importance of maxillofacial involvement in early management of trauma emergencies, following ATLS principles, lies in the matter that this life-threatening area is close to airways and the brain.

Moderate bleeding caused by facial trauma is frequent, but it is rarely one of the main causes of hemodynamic instability.

In addition, facial injuries are characteristically exposed for loss of specific sensory function, as in the case of visual involvement. This is another kind of emergency, as do as limb-threatening injuries, that must be promptly recognized and managed.

Other functional and morphological traumatic alterations, extremely relevant in facial trauma, are rarely a real priority.

Strict modern legislation regarding protection devices reduced overall incidence of facial injuries in road traffic accidents [1]; on the other hand, complex lesions increased because of a relatively greater number of high energy dynamics. However, most facial fractures occur in daily activities, followed by sports injuries and assaults. Self-inflicted lesions still remain less frequent but potentially devastating.

In 2016, according to the Niguarda Trauma Center Register in Milan, maxillofacial involvement concerns up to 25% of major trauma patients admitted to ER.

This demands an increased familiarity of trauma surgeons with identification and management of maxillofacial emergencies, among patients with multi-districtual and concomitant traumatic injuries.

12.2 Airways and Breathing

AB management (previously discussed in Chap. 10) can become exceedingly complex in facial trauma, because of bilateral and displaced mandibular fractures with glossoptosis, backward maxillary fractures with palatopharyngeal obstruction, oral swelling and hematomas, foreign bodies, missing teeth and dental prosthesis, and pharyngeal bleeding [2, 3].

Alcohol, drugs, and concomitant brain injury can cause nausea and vomiting and reduce protective reflexes. Laryngotracheal injury can further complicate definitive airways (orotracheal and nasotracheal intubation, surgical airway) which must be chosen in patients with facial bleeding to suggest aspiration over supraglottic devices.

In complex cranio-maxillofacial trauma, cervical spine fractures should always be considered unless it is proven otherwise. Their incidence ranges from 1 to 10% of all facial trauma [4]. Every attempt to protect airways needs to take this into account and must be performed with in-line stabilization; either can be hampered by hard cervical collar maintenance.

12.3 Circulation

12.3.1 Clinical Assessment

Bleeding after facial trauma is often self-limiting, particularly in patients with hypotension caused by concomitant hemorrhages from other sources. Thus, real life-threatening hemorrhages from facial fractures are very infrequent (from 1.4 to 11% of severe facial trauma) [5, 6].

Although a facial injury is the most noticeable, it rarely is an effective lifesaving priority [7].

Prompt identification and fast management of craniofacial bleeding play a primary role in ensuring safe access to airways and in avoiding increased blood loss, in the presence of other significant body lesions, with hemodynamic worsening.

However, its improvement, as well as fast local hemostasis, should never interfere with the team comprehensive acute care work-up, in patients with concomitant and multiple trauma injuries.

In any case, major trauma must be considered an evolving problem, and patients, after stabilization, have to be periodically reassessed to confirm treatment effectiveness, i.e., after normal hemodynamic parameters have been recovered.

Clinical evaluation starts by assessing specific evaluation about hemorrhagic risk, based on trauma dynamic analysis and then injury presumption, as well as the pharmacological and pathological anamnesis highlighting conditions which may lead to persistent bleeding.

12.3.2 Diagnosis

Assessment in emergency room during primary survey is mainly clinically oriented to identify bleeding coming from soft tissues deep wounds, anterior epistaxis, and oral hemorrhages.

The supine position can mask posterior bleeding from oral or anterior nasal laceration, accumulated in the pharyngeal space. They have to be discovered through inspection and continuous suction of the pharynx, at the same time as the oral cavity evaluation to exclude possible displaced jaw fractures or mucosal lacerations.

Relatively conscious patients can blow blood stagnant in the pharynx, especially in moderate bleeding which can remain misdiagnosed for a long time with the late onset of vomiting and further risk for airways and "unclear" cervical lesions.

During the secondary survey, traditional radiology is obviously not indicated in complex facial fractures. Each patient who requires total body or brain CT, with concomitant external evidence of facial involvement, must be studied with thin-slice CT scan with additional tridimensional reconstruction. This is diagnostic gold standard especially in patients with middle third, orbital, cranial base, or panfacial involvement. Contrast medium is unnecessary and no other additional information is given. Logically only stable or stabilized patients must be subject to CT.

12.3.3 Operative Management

12.3.3.1 Local Measures

Generally, local hemostatic measures are fast-acting in bleeding control and hemodynamic stabilization and allow diagnostic prosecution and patient transfer toward the IC unit, delaying definitive treatments according to damage control strategies.

Bleeding from deep, soft tissue wounds can be rapidly controlled by direct compression or by clamping any visible major vessel laceration. Wide and deep scalp flaps can be managed with compressive dressing or with handheld packing, 1-2/0 poly-filament stitches, or with temporary positioning of a Backhaus towel clamp.

In obvious middle third involvement with epistaxis, we recommend immediate anterior nasal packing with hemostatic self-expanding lubricated tampons (Merocel®, Rapid Rhino®) (Fig. 12.1a).

In this way, we can anticipate direct hemostasis of anterior nasal lacerations of the Kiesselbach plexus, which are the most frequent causes of epistaxis (Fig. 12.1b).

During pharyngeal inspection, we can so appreciate the end of bleeding from posterior choanae or, alternatively, discriminate necessity of conversion into anterior-posterior nasal packing. That is rarely indicated in case of blood origin from posterior nasal space or cranial base fractures, accumulated in sphenoidal sinuses.

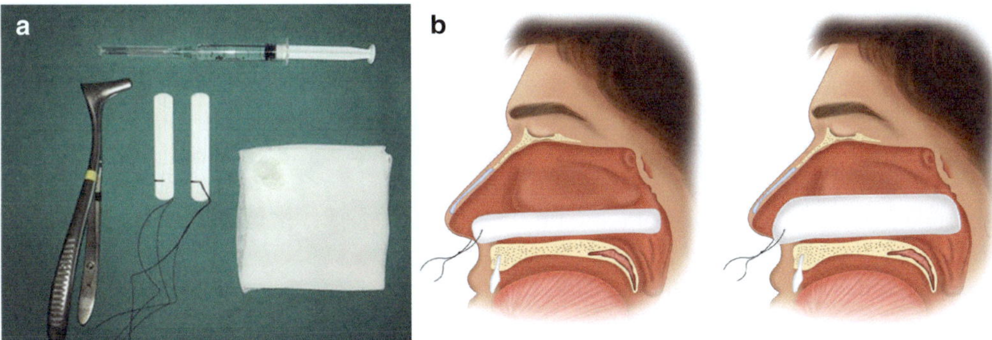

Fig. 12.1 (**a**) Devices needed to perform anterior nasal packing: nasal speculum and hemostatic nasal tampons. (**b**) Anatomic positioning of self-expanding nasal tampons in anterior nasal packing; note the anterior security ligature

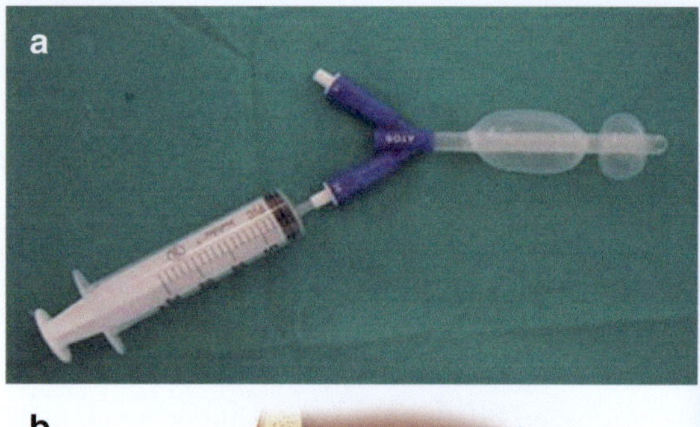

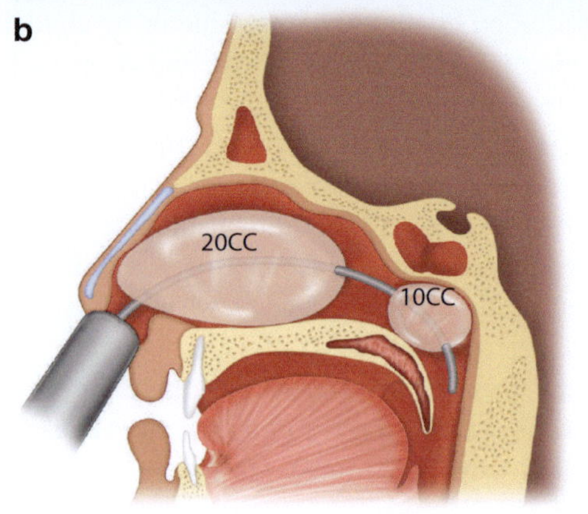

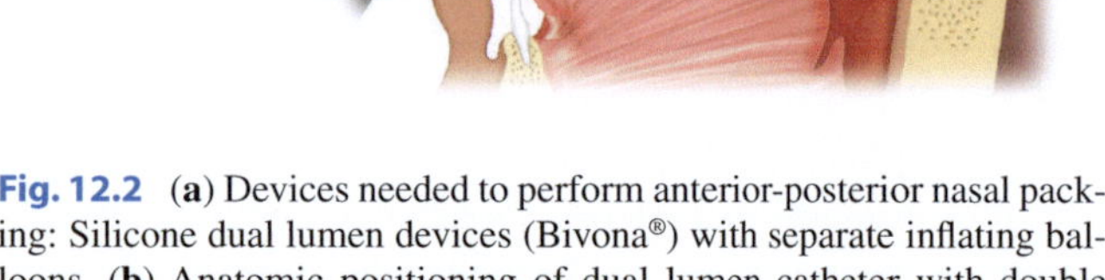

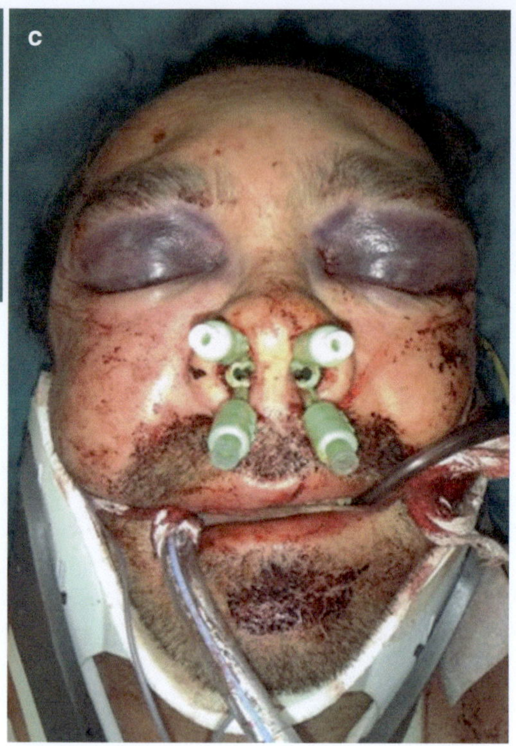

Fig. 12.2 (**a**) Devices needed to perform anterior-posterior nasal packing: Silicone dual lumen devices (Bivona®) with separate inflating balloons. (**b**) Anatomic positioning of dual lumen catheter with double balloons; note the posterior balloon positioned beyond the posterior choana. (**c**) Clinical example of bilateral anterior-posterior nasal packing with this kind of device

In case of profuse rhino-oropharyngeal bleeding, if anterior-posterior nasal packing is immediately necessary, we suggest the use of modern silicone dual lumen devices (Bivona®), which can variably inflate (with air or physiological solution) separate balloons for the anterior and posterior nasal spaces (Fig. 12.2a).

Their positioning is fast, easy, and effective, with few reports in literature about its accidental intracranial ectopic placement, in patients with concomitant skull base injuries [8].

This enhances prudential attitude and formal contraindication in those patients with this kind of lesions that, however, more than any others, could benefit from these devices to save time toward definitive control of bleeding.

In our experience correct device positioning, if necessary to control copious bleeding, is a safety maneuver also in patients with cranial base fractures.

First clinicians have to adequately consider direction of nasal floor in supine patients, possibly with displaced upper jaw fractures. Safe position of silicone double-balloon catheter needs to slide onto this anatomic guide. When the posterior wall of pharynx is reached with the tip of the device, the posterior balloon (smaller in volume) is inflated first and progressively, keeping on hand the device and feeling a downward traction back to the choana (Fig. 12.2b).

If this helpful feeling is not clearly perceived, the device must be removed and positioning starts over. In difficult cases, an upper oropharyngeal tight packing with gauzes could temporarily replace posterior nasal packing.

After that, a gentle pulling of the silicone catheter allows one to anchor the choana and could help for forward reduction of backward dislocated LeFort maxillary fractures.

Concomitant upper jaw reduction is recommended with anterior balloon inflation that otherwise could worsen bone disimpaction and bleeding [6].

Finally, the anterior balloon (bigger in volume) is inflated until a patient-specific volume, needed to fulfill anterior nasal cavity until bleeding stops.

In the majority of cases, this procedure is performed bilaterally, and only after complete stabilization of vital

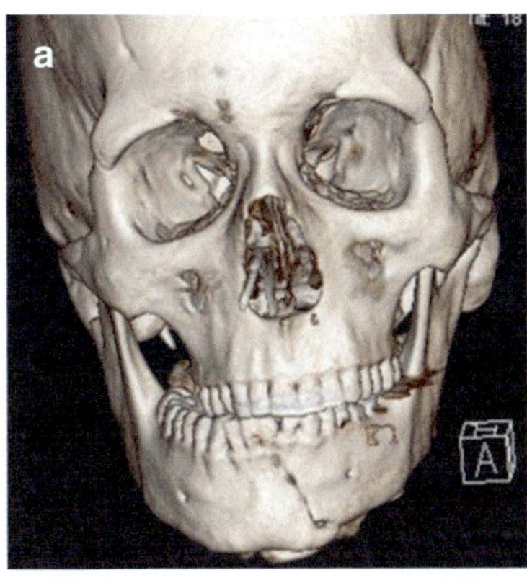

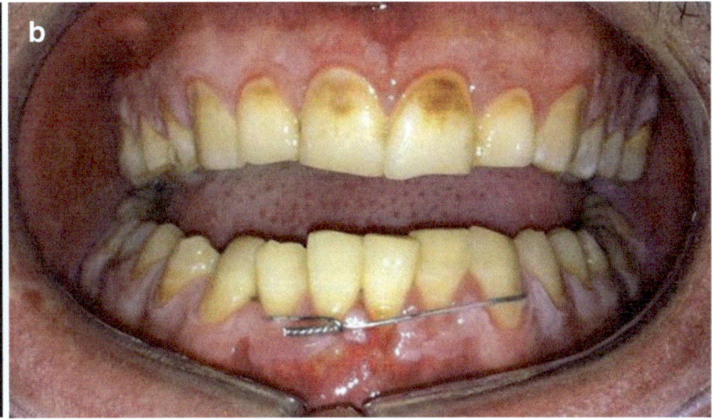

Fig. 12.3 (**a**) Unstable fracture of mandibular symphysis. (**b**) Temporary stabilization with iron interdental ligature, after manual reduction. Three teeth on the right and two teeth on the left of the fracture site were utilized

parameters and thin-slice CT scan analysis can one of the two be progressively removed (Fig. 12.2c).

If silicone devices with double balloons are unavailable, posterior nasal packing could be similarly made using a silicone urinary Foley catheter. Then traditional anterior nasal packing with tampons is completed.

After temporary control of external and pharyngeal bleeding, proceed with oral cavity inspection with adequate field illumination, rigid tongue depressors, and large caliber—high flow rigid aspirators.

Mobile dental prosthesis must be removed, and empty dental alveolus checked, suggesting that teeth are avulsed and have to be located and removed with forceps to avoid pharyngeal dislocations.

Systematic oral cavity evaluation starts with upper and lower vestibular fornix inspection, moving to gingival mucosa, cheeks, and palate. After comes meticulous and bilateral inspection of the floor of the mouth, base of the tongue, and mobile tongue.

Not only do mucosal lacerations have to be checked, which are potential expressions of corresponding bone fractures, but so do oral floor of mouth hematomas since active bleeding could push back the tongue base causing impending airway obstruction.

All wounds beneath the submucosal plane have to be treated with temporary hemostatic suture with 3-4/0 catgut suture.

Plane reconstruction of muscle involvement or full thickness wounds could be delayed until stable vital parameters are guaranteed, complying with ATLS priorities in a time-saving manner.

Oral cavity inspection also allows identifying any bony exposure, corresponding to displaced fractures of the mandible or alveolar processes of upper and lower jaws. Bone margins can bleed with inadequate response to local manual compression, although they are rarely the main cause of real hemorrhages.

In these cases, definitive hemostasis is achieved with fracture reduction and temporary stabilization.

Fractures of tooth-bearing lower jaw segments could be stabilized with steel interdental ligatures, placed between mesial and distal teeth across the fracture site. Steel ligatures positioning between teeth just corresponding to the fracture is unadvisable because the ligatures often lose stability with an increased risk of avulsion and bleeding relapse.

At least the second ones on both fracture side are generally chosen. Steel wire is first passed between the teeth in a vestibular-to-lingual way and then in the opposite way, lingual-to-vestibular, on the other side. This creates a loop that embraces the internal surface of selected teeth, and it is secured by twisting the wire forceps in outer position, holding together two bone fragments (Fig. 12.3a, b).

This temporary stabilization also reduces pain and could help to protect airways, by keeping forward reduced bilateral mandibular fractures.

If there are no concomitant upper jaw fractures, this maneuver is performed, after gross manual reduction of bone fragments, keeping the patient in his individual occlusion (maximal intercuspidation between upper and lower dental arches). It allows further reduction with bone margin compression and hemostatic optimization.

In partially edentulous patients or multiple traumatic teeth avulsion, stabilization can be achieved with dental arch bars positioning that involves at least three elements for each side.

Upper alveolar fractures with bleeding from margins are managed similarly with manual reduction and temporary steel ligature.

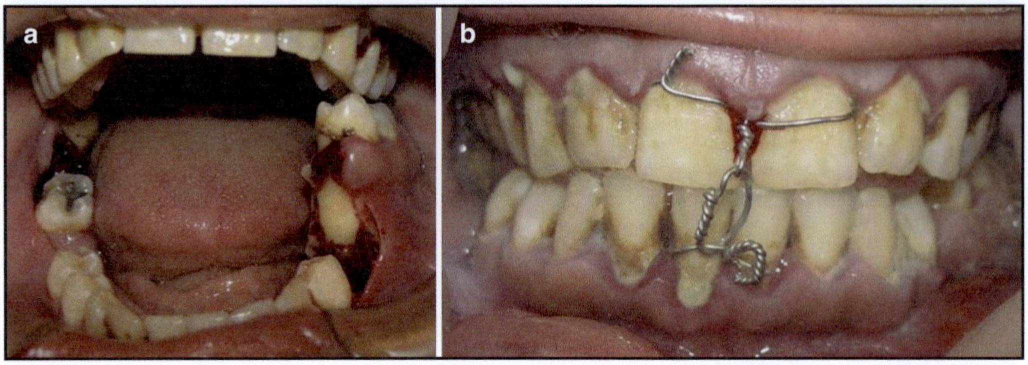

Fig. 12.4 (a) Bilaterally displaced fractures of the posterior mandibular body, with exposition, mucosal laceration, and bleeding. (b) Faster stabilization with intermaxillary fixation, performed by matching single median upper and lower interdental ligatures; oral cavity and orotracheal accesses are now avoided

Bleeding originating from mandibular angle fractures or LeFort fractures of the upper jaw needs reduction and stabilization with intermaxillary fixation (IMF) with arch bars or interdental ligatures (Fig. 12.4a, b).

IMF positioning obviously interferes with oral cavity inspection and access to airways. Thus, its use is recommended only in patients with definitive airways (nasotracheal or surgical, orotracheal if tube can be placed in retromolar or edentulous sites).

In patients with bleeding from displaced midfacial fractures and no definitive airways, a mouth prop can help to maintain reduction.

In the emergency room, the need for fracture stabilization with a time-consuming procedure (i.e., plate and screws positioning or external fixation) is extremely rare.

At this stage, oronasal bleeding must be controlled, and acute care surgeon can go back to soft tissue laceration, previously temporarily treated with packing or compressive dressing.

Major vessel damages must be clipped or ligated if not already done; each wound could be managed with diathermy or faster full thickness (including the aponeurosis layer in scalp lacerations) running suture, and each definitive treatment must be ideally delayed.

All tasks (identification of bleeding points, hemostasis, and efficacy observation) should be performed in a few minutes, as should further "C"-control of hemorrhages, without any delays for the workflow of the team.

At this time no specific diagnostic imaging is needed, and every maneuver is based on clinical evidence.

12.3.3.2 Definitive Control of Bleeding

These local hemostatic measures are adequate to manage facial bleeding in most trauma patients [9]. The rule is: "When hypovolemic shock is present, facial injuries are unlikely to be the sole cause" [10, 11].

However, massive facial hemorrhage has been reported to occur in up to 10% complex facial injuries [5, 6, 12, 13] and can cause itself hypovolemic shock in only 1.4% of these cases [9, 14], but the calculated mortality rate is 20.21% of these cases [9].

It is in major midface and panfacial injuries that blood loss can quickly become significant and refractory to local measures [15]; these account for 2–4% of all facial bleeding that arise from the maxillary artery or its branches, ethmoidal artery, ophthalmic artery, or Vidian branch of internal carotid artery [4] or rarely from skull base fractures with direct internal carotid artery involvement [16, 17].

Literature has identified anterior-posterior nasal packing as the initial management; it controls bleeding in 29% of patients and reduces it in another 44% of patients [10, 15, 18].

This would allow obtaining hemodynamic response to volemic resuscitation, necessary to go on with diagnostic tools or toward the definitive treatment of bleeding.

Historically the life-threatening facial bleeding which was refractory to local measures was managed with external carotid artery ligation [19], but internal and external carotid arteries are associated with extensive collateral circulation and bilateral communication, leading to faster relapse of bleeding [13].

Point of artery ligation is critical and by ligating the external carotid artery at its origin is ineffective in controlling hemorrhage, due to its extensive collateral circulation [9].

Thus, the artery ligation must be done bilaterally [20] or just corresponding to the bleeding point, in order to reduce relapses from collateral recruitment [16, 21].

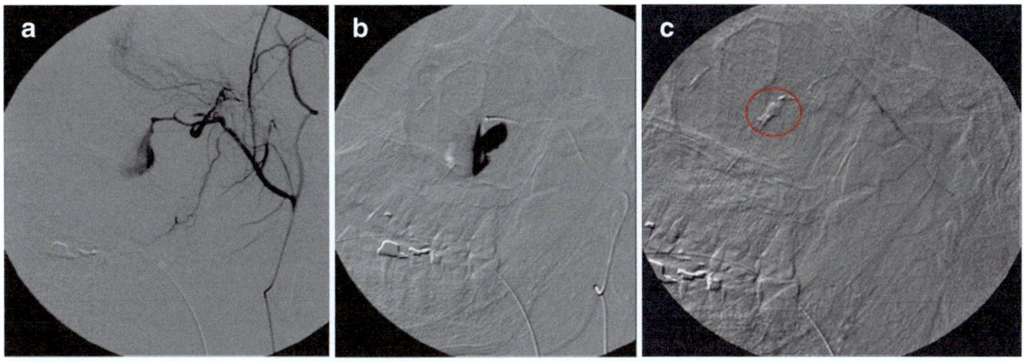

Fig. 12.5 (**a**) Right internal maxillary artery selective arteriography in complex middle third facial fracture with epistaxis refractory to local measures. Note extravasation of contrast medium into right maxillary sinus, coming from small ramification of internal maxillary artery. (**b**) 2F coaxial microcatheter reaching exactly the bleeding point. (**c**) Cyanoacrylate-Lipiodol deposit after bilateral arteriographic control to exclude any remaining bleeding

Sakamoto et al. found that catheter balloon tamponades and external carotid ligation cannot respond in over 72% to massive epistaxis [22].

In 70% of cases of traumatic intractable epistaxis, the internal maxillary artery, or one of its branches, is injured [9, 23]. That's why transantral ligation of the internal maxillary artery was described [24, 25].

Nevertheless, the anatomy complexity of the bony midface can make direct ligation of the bleeding point virtually impossible, especially in patients with torrential bleeding, nasal tamponade, and unclear neck involvement [13, 26].

For the same reasons angio-CT has no role in diagnostic work-up of facial hemorrhages which are refractory to local measures; peripheric small caliber ramification of facial vessels and bone comminution in naso-sinusal complex fractures make contrast blush unidentifiable. Thus, angio-CT remains time-consuming and it is usually skipped, proceeding with the angiographic suite. Also, preliminary and comprehensive evaluation of supra-aortic vessel anatomy could be better studied by arteriography.

A diagnostic arteriography and superselective embolization, aided by a coaxial microcatheter, has definitively replaced external carotid artery ligation in modern trauma centers, where this approach is available [4, 9, 13, 18, 27–30] (Fig. 12.5).

Transarterial embolization of internal maxillary artery for intractable epistaxis was first reported by Sokoloff et al. in 1974 [31]; since then many reports have suggested a success rate between 70 and 100%. The resolution of bleeding was often immediate and stable [5, 9–11, 13, 18, 22–24, 27, 32, 33].

The advantages are a less invasive procedure, faster control of bleeding even from multiple and surgically inaccessible points, more distal (ideally exactly at bleeding point) and definitive treatment, and repeatability.

Another advantage described was the feasibility in local anesthesia, useful in hemodynamically unstable patients; but we know that 93% of this kind of facially injured patients will require definitive airways [9].

In patients who are hypersensitive to iodine and in case of ethmoidal arteries embolization, this treatment is not always feasible.

When used early, endovascular embolization is associated with high survival rates and low incidence of complications [18, 32].

Complications include fever, pain, trismus, cerebrovascular accidents, blindness, facial nerve palsy, seizures, soft tissue swelling, or necrosis. The overall complication rate is around 3–27% but most complications were minor and transient [33].

The femoral artery is cannulated with a 5F diagnostic catheter equipped with a coaxial microcatheter for superselective embolization; materials generally used for hemostasis are cyanoacrylate 1:3 with Lipiodol glue and PVA particles (150–200 or 250–300 μm) or a platinum micro-coil. The former is preferred in patients with direct identification of the bleeding point; the latter are the choices in on-field hemostasis when an angiography cannot identify a specific vascular lesion.

A formal preoperative bilateral internal-external diagnostic carotid arteriography is advisable; a post-procedure CT scan is recommended.

12.3.3.3 End-Point-Guided Resuscitation

Also in maxillofacial trauma management, damage control surgery is part of a strategy in which permissive resuscitation

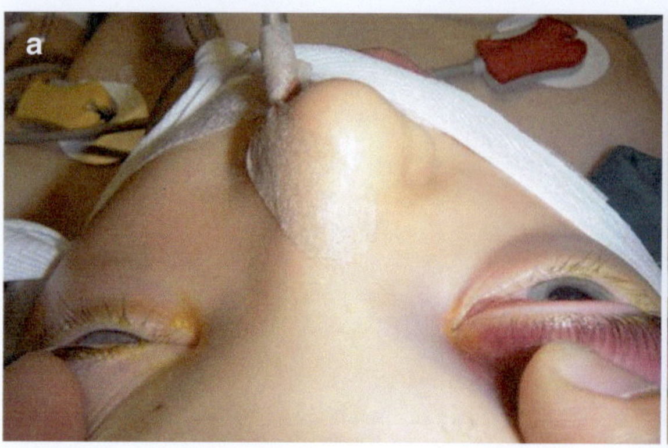
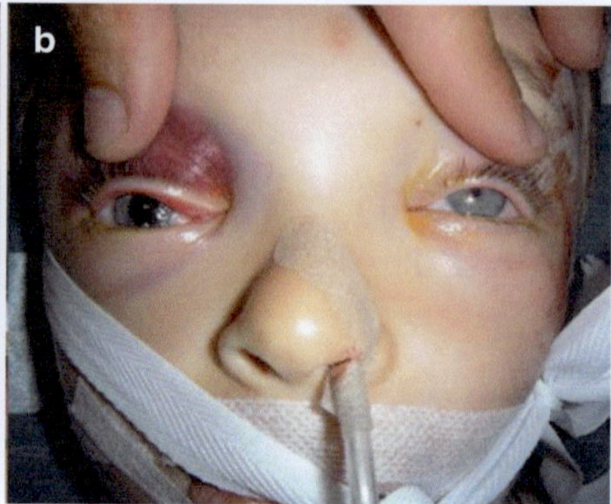

Fig. 12.6 (**a**) Right eye post-traumatic tense proptosis in an unconscious-intubated patient, due to right orbital compartment syndrome (upper retrobulbar hematoma). (**b**) Right eye caudal dystopia and a reagent right mydriasis in the same patient, confirming clinical suspicion of orbital compartment syndrome

with targeted hypotension, early recognition of coagulopathy, and thromboelastography-guided point of care are equally necessary.

As in bleeding from extra-facial sites, the ideal systolic target is permissive value of 80 mmHg; bleeding may recommence as the blood pressure improves during resuscitation.

But every facial trauma suggests a cranial trauma until this is excluded. For this reason, general safety 100 mmHg value is preferred.

12.4 Eyes and Visual-Threatening Injuries

12.4.1 Clinical Assessment

When ABC priorities have been dealt with, other treatments for facial injuries might be delayed for at least 24 h, but visual-threatening conditions have to be rapidly detected and promptly managed [34]. This kind of approach can be resumed in the "ABCDEyes" work-up [35], performed toward the end of the primary survey.

Visual-threatening injuries are reported to occur in between 0.56 and 6% of facial fractures. Middle and upper thirds injuries are obviously those of interest [35].

In addition to direct eyeball injuries and loss of globe protection from adnexal wound laceration (see Chap. 13), the main causes of loss of vision are orbital compartment syndrome and traumatic optic neuropathy [36, 37].

Orbital contents are enclosed by a continuous cone-shaped fascial envelope (Tenon's capsule) which reaches the eyelids and their bony insertions anteriorly [38].

The orbit anatomy creates a "closed room" with four bony walls and a fifth, soft but strong, anterior wall made of a fibrocartilaginous (septo-tarsal) structure, fixed by firm medial and lateral canthal ligaments. This anterior semiflexible wall resembles the orbit to other body sites prone to compartment syndrome [35, 38].

Another orbital anatomic peculiarity is the absence of lymphatic vessels; only inferior and superior ophthalmic veins can drain fluid form the orbit.

Physiological intraorbital pressure is about 3–6 mmHg; orbital perfusion pressure (to the retina and optic nerve) is the result of a difference between mean arterial pressure and this interstitial pressure value [39].

12.4.2 Diagnosis

Any causes of increased orbital contents volume (blood, swelling, emphysema, brain herniation) or blow-in bony fracture can raise intraorbital pressure until it reaches critical points, thus causing hypoperfusion or ischemia [40]. With similarities to traumatic brain injuries, mean arterial pressure critical reduction (hypovolemic shock, surgery, vasodilatation, or acute "pump" failure) can exasperate this equilibrium [35, 39].

If left untreated, damage becomes irreversible in 60–120 min [35, 41–43]. For this reason, early recognition and rapid management of orbital compartment syndrome is mandatory, although this must not interfere with any ongoing investigation and resuscitation.

Clinical signs are the best indicators of the onset of orbital compartment syndrome: progressive decrease of visual acuity with an enlarged blind spot on the visual field, red color

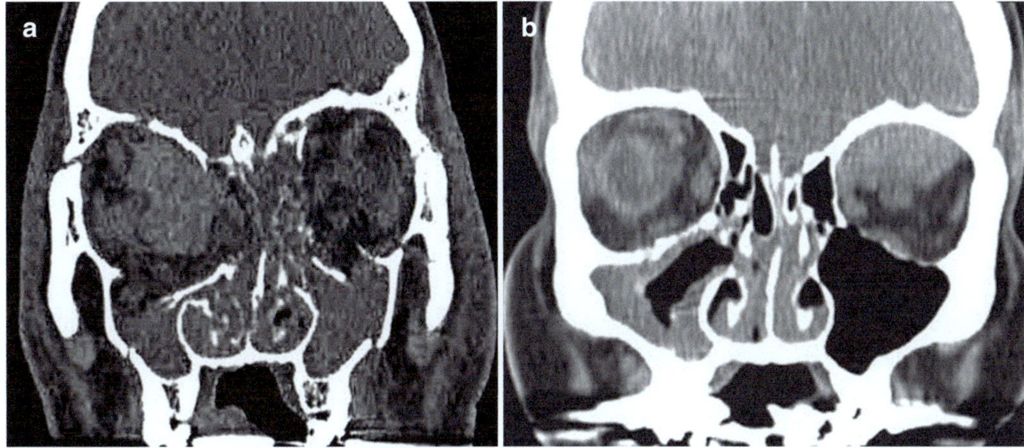

Fig. 12.7 (**a**) CT example of right superomedial intra-extraconal retrobulbar hematoma, coming from ciliary and ethmoidal arteries together. (**b**) CT demonstration of left upper extraconal retrobulbar hematomas, corresponding to linear fracture of left orbital roof

desaturation, tense proptosis resistant to manual retropulsion, relative afferent pupillary defect (RAPD) or Marcus Gunn pupil, orbital pain, ophthalmoplegia, conjunctival hemorrhages, and fundus oculi alterations are the most important of them [35, 40, 42, 44].

The crucial question to keep in mind is "Can the patient see?"

Any other signs could be trimmed down if no deterioration in visual acuity is shown after repeated evaluation.

Most of the patients have an altered consciousness, so proptosis, RAPD (Fig. 12.6a, b), and fundus alterations are the only clinical finding which can determine whether patients possibly need urgent treatment [35].

Proptosis has been reported to occur in up to 3% of blunt head injuries [45]. Acute traumatic proptosis may arise from blow-in fractures, retrobulbar hematoma, massive emphysema, and generalized retrobulbar swelling (accentuated in prolonged prone position or massive fluid resuscitation) [46].

In most cases proptosis is mild, and no active intervention is urgently required, other than regular reassessment [35] until its maximum expression (generally about 36 h after injury) [39, 42].

Warning is given in the presence of a "hard-stone" protruding eyeball which is resistant to reduction at gentle palpation (to avoid any uveal tissue prolapse from possible globe lacerations) compared with a non-injured site.

Emphysema is rarely the sole cause of compartment syndrome; in its presence, retinal ischemia occurs if intraorbital pressure values exceed a mean arterial pressure of 60–70 mmHg [46].

Retrobulbar hemorrhage, occurring in 0.3–1% of patients with orbitozygomatic fractures [36, 47], and generalized retrobulbar swelling are the most common causes of proptosis [39, 42]. Blow-in fractures can precipitate reducing orbital room volume.

Retrobulbar hemorrhages can be intra- or extraconal; the former are worse in prognosis because they originate from central retinal and ciliary arteries [35, 39] (Fig. 12.7ba9); their overall incidence of blindness is as high as 48% [47]. Extraconal ones derive from bony fractures, infra- or supraorbital artery damage, or muscle lacerations and are the main targets of surgical drainage (Fig. 12.7b).

As previously described the diagnosis of retrobulbar hematoma is primarily clinic, and in unconsciousness patients the presence of RAPD is one of the most sensitive indicators of aggressive urgent management needs [35, 42, 48].

Pupillary light reaction is a component of "D-disabilities" neurologic examination; it can be misinterpreted in the presence of direct injury of the globe (and ciliary muscle), alcohol, drugs, opiates, and paralyzing agents [12, 35].

Anisocoria is not a consequence of damage to the anterior visual pathway; even after unilateral cutting of the optic nerve, pupils remain symmetrical.

A reliable test for a primary diagnosis of optic nerve damage is the swinging flashlight test [49]: Just a "sluggish" response, although subjective, is accurate indicator of visual impairment [35].

In other words, only a brisk reaction to direct and consensual light stimuli in a round, concentric pupil can be a reliable way to exclude the necessity of emergency intervention [35].

Particular care is required in elderly patients, in which mild dilated and fixed pupil in a red-eye can be justified by an underling acute-angle glaucoma that can be worsened by drugs [35, 42].

A formal ophthalmologic evaluation is indicated in every patient with middle-upper third facial trauma; emergent examination is formally necessary only in patients with visual-threatening suspicion. It's imperative therefore to exclude sclero-conjunctival laceration, corneal wound, vitreous hemorrhages, retinal detachment, acute-angle glaucoma presence, lens dislocation, and hyphema before performing emergency surgical decompression.

Fundus evaluation is not just required to detect optic atrophy, which can be seen 4–17 days after injury, but also to check retinal vascularization (i.e., hemorrhages or venous congestion) [42].

Before starting surgical treatment, the real cause of proptosis should be ideally defined with CT. Any patient requiring a brain CT, who has suspected periorbital or ocular injuries, should undergo imaging of orbits at the same time [35].

Only a CT scan can identify the real etiology of orbital compartment syndrome.

Retrobulbar hematomas need to be evacuated with specific site incision [35, 38]; orbital compartment syndrome caused by swelling, diffuse bleeding into retrobulbar fat, or emphysema can be managed with a time-saving damage control anterior orbitotomy.

In case of blood collection, a CT also allows surgeons to choose the best (direct) access to drain it [39, 42]; generally, lateral (upper or lower lid) accesses are considered safer, and a precise preoperative imaging-guided strategy is important to avoid roaming in traumatized orbital anatomy.

In patients who are unstable or unresponsive to resuscitation, in whom the CT is skipped, and the patients sent to the operating room, lateral canthotomy with inferior cantholysis is the choice to save time also in case of an endoorbital hematoma. Definitive evacuation may be postponed to after a subsequent diagnostic phase [36, 42].

Clinical suspicion is particularly difficult in unconscious patients, in whom visual acuity deterioration cannot be proved. In hemodynamically stable patients, tonometry with portable devices, B-scan sonography [50], and flash-evoked visual potentials [42, 49, 51] are more useful than funduscopy, because the onset of anatomic alterations of the papilla needs time (7–14 days).

Tonometry, measured with portable device, is widely indicated in literature [35, 44, 47]. Normal intraocular pressure (IOP) is 10–20 mmHg and may give some indications of intraorbital (retrobulbar) pressure, though it doesn't precisely reflect its measure [44, 47, 52].

Comparative measurements on both sides are indicated [39].

In a proptosed eye, an IOP of around 40 mmHg or more indicates critical ischemia and the need for emergent treatment [42, 44, 53].

Flash visual evoked potentials have been reliable in checking the integrity of the visual pathway even in unconscious patients; unfortunately, the equipment is cumbersome for an emergency room [35, 50, 54].

They are useful also in traumatic optic neuropathy (TON), which can occur in 0.5–2% of head injuries, 2.5% of midface fractures, and 10% of major craniofacial injuries [36, 37, 55].

TON must be suspected after trauma with visual loss and RAPD without direct globe involvement [37].

Most commonly the optic nerve is damaged posterior to the entry point of central retinal vessels, presenting a normal optic disk appearance. If damaged anterior to this point, the disk conversely will appear swollen with retinal hemorrhages [56].

TON can be direct or indirect, by the transmission of forces from a distant site; also it can be primary (with immediate sharing of retinal ganglion cell axons) or secondary (due to swelling of the nerve within inflexible orbital apex).

12.4.3 Operative Management

There are few emergency sight-saving procedures: anterior orbitotomy by lateral canthotomy and inferior cantholysis, protection of the globe following loss of eyelid integrity, irrigation if chemical injury is suspected, orbital apex decompression (via intracranial approach or by endoscopy), and hematoma evacuation [35].

Anterior orbitotomy by lateral canthotomy and inferior cantholysis (defined as surgical disinsertion of inferior crus of lateral canthal tendon) is the gold standard decompressive treatment to obtain a significative intraorbital pressure reduction [35, 36, 38, 39, 42, 43, 53]. Unfortunately this effect is transient in setting of continuous bleeding [52, 57].

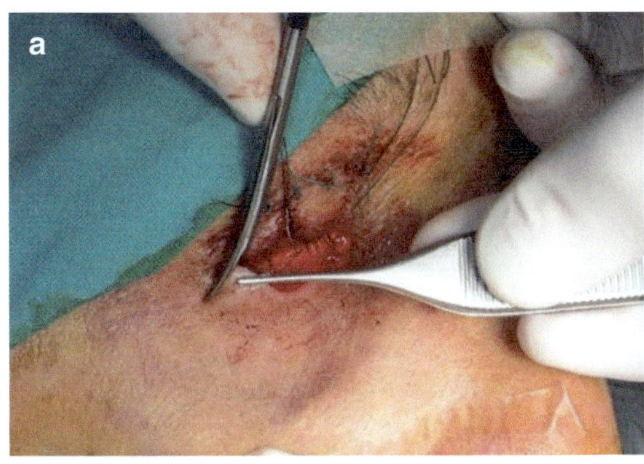

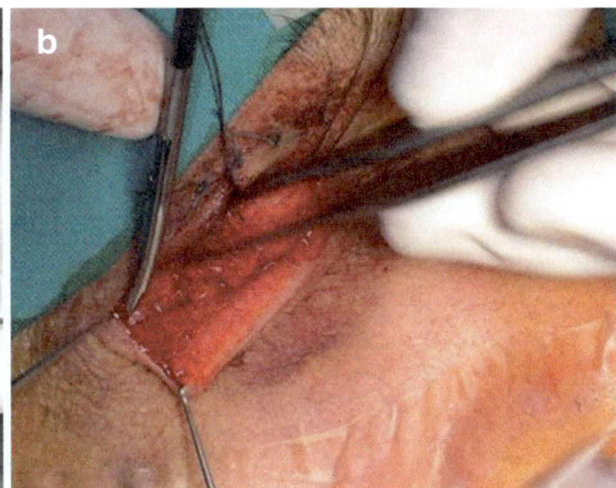

Fig. 12.8 (**a**) Right anterior orbitotomy by lateral canthotomy performed with a single, full thickness, 7 mm cut of the lower lid, leaving about 1 mm of the inferior crus inserted laterally. (**b**) Eversion of the loosened right lower lid facilitates septal plane dissection and its longitudinal incision (septolysis). Note also orbital fat herniation, meaning effective in intraorbital pressure release

Original technique can be done in the ER, with local anesthesia, and is carried out first by placing an artery clip at the lateral canthus, between the upper and lower lids, crushing the tissue beneath. Lateral canthal tendon incision is made horizontally at this level with iris scissors, with a length of 5–8 mm; the inferior lateral crus of lateral canthal tendon is then completely disinserted, resulting in a totally mobile lower lid. The lateral canthal incision can be sutured later or commonly left to granulate [38, 53].

Some authors suggest additional septolysis in a suborbicularis muscle plane, to improve intraorbital pressure reduction up to 70% of the initial value, superior cantholysis, or endoscopic medial/inferior bony walls decompression (further 17% reduction in intraocular pressure from peak level) [44, 58, 59].

Our modified technique consists in a single, full thickness, 5–8 mm cut of the lower lid (skin, muscle, septo-tarsal and conjunctival plane) placed as laterally as needed to leave about 1 mm of the inferior crus inserted. Eversion of the loosened lower lid facilitates septal plane dissection and its longitudinal incision (septolysis). Landmark 5/0 nylon stitches are placed on the "gray line", both medially and laterally to the incision, to facilitate postponed canthal repositioning and suture that always must be performed for better aesthetic results (Fig. 12.8).

To evacuate a superior-superolateral hematoma, generally a superior lid skin incision (in correspondence with the lateral third of orbito-palpebral sulcus, where levator palpebrae aponeurosis is not represented) and a supraorbicularis dissection straight to orbital margin is the safe way; bony margin is less than 15 mm from the skin incision, and here we can enter the orbital space to reach the blood collection (Fig. 12.9). A capillary drain can be placed for some days, skin secured with a single stitch, and the skin wound is sutured with 5-6/0 single nylon stitches or running suture.

Some authors suggest a lateral eyebrow incision, effective for lateral fluid collection but less ergonomic to reach orbital roof [60].

In the case of an inferior-inferolateral hematoma, a traditional subciliary approach is used; proptosis generally hind transconjunctival approach if no lateral canthotomy is prepared.

Hayter and Sugar in 1991 proposed a useful orbital post-surgical observation chart in which pain, acuity, proptosis, direct light reflex, and pupil size are carried out at 15-min intervals for the first 2 h, then at 30-min intervals for the next 4 h, and then hourly until further notice [61].

12.4.4 Nonoperative Management

In orbital compartment syndrome, additional medical treatment with acetazolamide 500 mg, either intravenous or intramuscular, and rapid infusion of 20% mannitol or corticosteroids should not delay surgery, and postoperative therapy is not indicated especially in patients with concomitant severe head trauma [43].

In traumatic optic neuropathy, primary injury is unavoidable, whereas minimizing secondary injuries is the rationale for every treatment. Despite this, no statistically significant benefit was demonstrated over conservative management, with either corticosteroid or surgical (intracranial or endoscopic) optic canal decompression [37, 62–65].

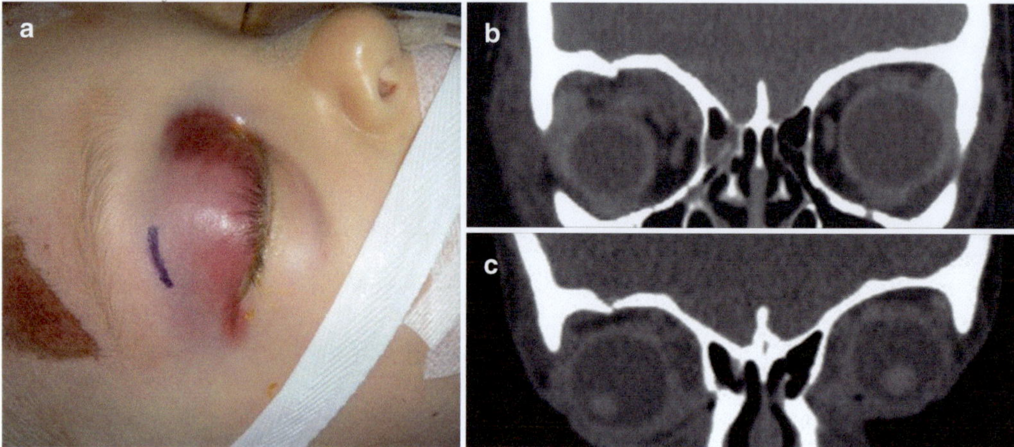

Fig. 12.9 (**a**) Lateral right upper lid 10 mm skin incision, to evacuate a retrobulbar hematoma coming from orbital roof fracture. Swelling can make it difficult to position the incision properly, just corresponding to orbito-palpebral sulcus; a contralateral one could be used as reference for normal distance to palpebral margin. (**b**) Preoperative CT location of retrobulbar hematoma, needed to choose the best ("straight to") access. (**c**) Postoperative CT control of complete surgical evacuation

TON has a high spontaneous visual recovery rate up to 40–60% when managed conservatively; patients with direct optic nerve injury and no light perception at presentation have a poorer prognosis [37, 55].

Furthermore 40–70% of patients with traumatic optic neuropathy have loss of consciousness associated [37, 62], and CRASH trial revealed an increased risk of death in head trauma patients treated with steroids [37, 63, 66]; thus they remain unadvisable.

12.4.5 Special Part: Orbital Trapdoor-Type Fractures in Children

The last traumatic orbital urgency that must be discussed is wall fractures with entrapment of orbital contents. It's called a trapdoor-type fracture and generally involves the orbital floor.

This type of fracture is frequent in children because of their bone elasticity.

The direct transmission of forces from bone rims ("buckling theory") or the eyeball, via intraorbital soft tissues ("hydraulic theory"), can cause green-stick thinner orbital wall fracture that can allow orbital soft tissue herniation. Subsequent spontaneous elastic bone repositioning, pivoting around a bony hinge, entraps them and causes restricted eye movement with diplopia, pain during limited up-gaze, minimal conjunctival response ("white-eyed blowout" fractures, Fig. 12.10a), and sympathetic reflex activation.

The oculo-cardiac (Aschner-Dagnini) reflex is an infrequently observed subtype of trigemino-vagal reflex, and its clinical characteristics can include headache, gastric hypermobility with vomiting, apnea, bradycardia until asystole (1:3500), and arterial hypotension [67].

In unconscious patients clinical findings may be reduced to a restricted duction and traction test; it consists in a forced upward and downward eye movement, tested with forceps pinching rectus muscles insertion.

The relative paucity of clinical signs may delay diagnosis and compromise the result.

CT findings are equally poor and consist of a linear orbital floor fracture, without bone displacement, and a minimal amount of soft tissue lying below, outside the orbit, downward into the maxillary sinus ("teardrop sign") with a double-density sign representing a rim of hemorrhagic mucosa surrounding entrapped periorbital fat (Fig. 12.10b).

Definitive treatment is a specialized skill, but early recognition and timely resolution are strongly associated with significantly better outcomes [68].

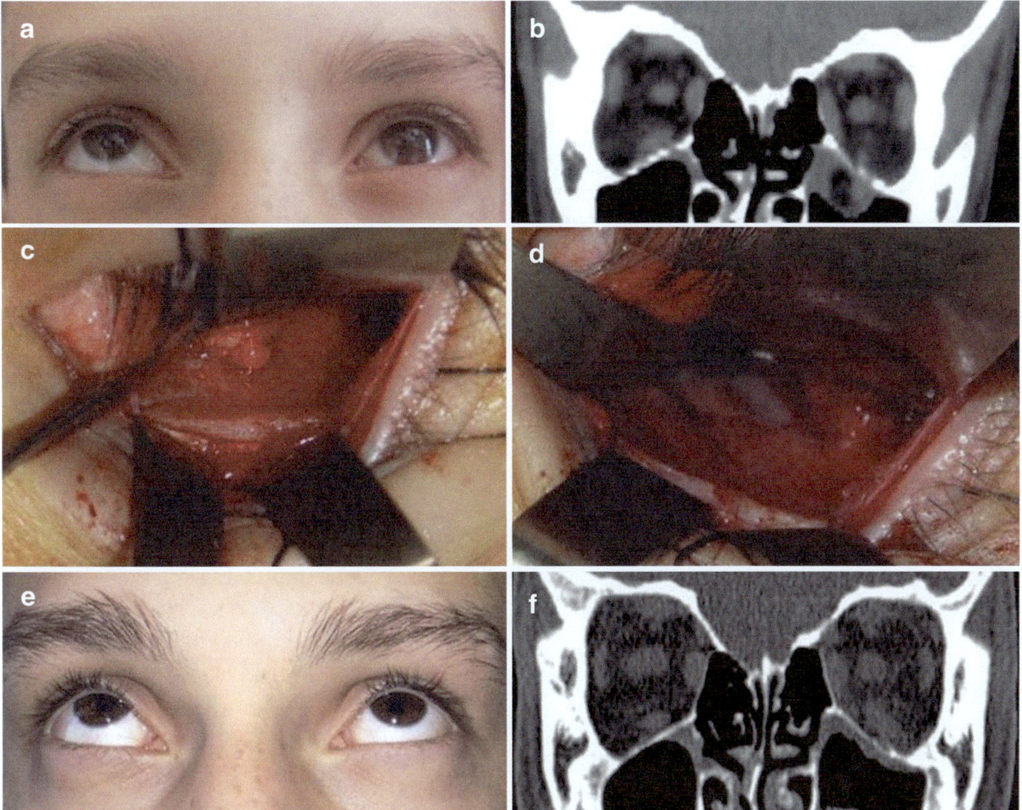

Fig. 12.10 (**a**) Left "white-eyed" trapdoor-type fracture of orbital floor, in 7-year-old boy with restricted eye movement, diplopia, pain during limited up-gaze, and minimal conjunctival response. (**b**) Preoperative CT showing "teardrop" with "double-density" sign. (**c**) Intraoperative picture in transconjunctival access and left orbital floor exploration; note herniation and entrapment of orbital content within the fracture. (**d**) Intraoperative picture of the same procedure, after reduction of end orbital tissue herniation; careful bone fragment repositioning avoids necessity of any further reconstruction, with a prefect continuity of orbital floor anatomy. (**e**) Postsurgical clinical resolution of any ocular movement restriction. (**f**) Postoperative CT control confirming proper reduction of soft tissue herniation and straight continuity of the left orbital floor reduced

In case of doubt and stable/conscious patients, orthoptic evaluation with Hess-Lancaster test could give adjunctive information.

The resolution of an oculo-cardiac reflex could be a life-saving emergency; however urgent muscular freeing avoids tissue ischemia and fibrosis causing irreversible scarring with persistent diplopia.

Surgery is done under general anesthesia, usually with lower lid transconjunctival-preseptal approach to inferior orbital rim and orbital floor. Subperiosteal dissection allows soft tissue reduction, after gentle bone fragment mobilization. In pediatric patients, careful bone repositioning, generally, makes any further reconstruction unnecessary (Fig. 12.10c, d, f).

Conjunctival incision is generally closed with single or running sutures with 7/0 resorbable poly-filament suture. An intraoperative postreduction forced duction test must show a release of any ocular movement restriction.

Clinical signs generally have an immediate resolution (Fig. 12.10e), and the patient could be followed with the previously described Hayter and Sugar orbital postsurgical observation chart [61].

Case Scenario

A 21-year-old male who fell from about 15 m. Paramedics found him conscious, with profuse epistaxis and oral bleeding, evident traumatic facial involvement, and abdominal pain.

Hemodynamically stable, in less than 15 min, he was admitted to trauma center ER, and airways were immediately secured with the orotracheal tube. E-FAST and thorax and pelvic X-rays showed free fluid collected in the abdomen, complex pelvic "open-book" fracture, and right pneumothorax with mild mediastinum shift. Hemodynamics worsened, so a pelvic binder was positioned and transfusion protocol contemporary was started.

1. What's the priority?
   A. To control orofacial bleeding
   B. Get CT scan of the face because of possible eyes involvement with threatening visual lesions
   C. Thorax drainage and simultaneous anterior nasal packing positioning
   D. Remove pelvic binder and perform extraperitoneal abdominal packing

Hemodynamic stability was gained and patient could be transferred to CT to get total body triphasic examination.

2. What to do about facial imaging?
   A. Facial examination must be postponed because of relative stability of hemodynamic. Only the brain, thorax, and abdomen are priorities in emergency setting.
   B. Facial fractures could be studied with traditional X-rays, during pelvic and thoracic evaluation at primary survey.
   C. Brain TC 5 mm slices allow to properly evaluate facial fracture at the same time.
   D. Thin-slice (1 mm or less) facial CT scan is the gold standard in middle third/orbital/complex facial fractures; its acquisition never significantly increases diagnostic time.

CT showed bilateral lung contusion, hepatic laceration, left kidney artery dissection, active arterial blushing from left gluteal artery, a complex pelvic fracture, and the presence of subdiaphragmatic free air. Contemporary facial CT demonstrated multifragmentary comminuted fracture of the middle third (with bilateral maxillary sinus involvement and maxillary intrusion) and mandibular symphyseal fracture.

Oropharyngeal inspection revealed a mild but persistent posterior epistaxis, despite bilateral anterior nasal packing.

3. How to get better local hemostatic control?
   A. Increasing the volume of bilateral anterior nasal packing
   B. With diathermocoagulation of nasal mucosa with nasal speculum and suction
   C. Performing anterior-posterior nasal packing with silicone dual lumen devices with separate inflating balloons
   D. Removing anterior nasal packing and performing oropharyngeal packing with gauzes

Patient then went to OR to perform damage control laparotomy, angiography, and embolization of left gluteal artery and pelvic anterior external fixation.

4. What else about facial fractures?
   A. Bleeding from jaw fractures into oral cavity may be treated conservatively with nonoperative management, until definitive surgery, because this is rarely a cause of hemodynamic instability.
   B. Facial fractures need to be treated immediately because they are exposed and bleeding.
   C. Facial damage control (manual reduction and temporary stabilization with iron wiring of bone fractures and suture of intra-extraoral wounds) must be done quickly and simultaneously to other maneuvers.
   D. Facial damage control always must follow neurosurgical and thoracoabdominal emergency surgery.

Patient was therefore transferred to IC unit; at 16 h from admission, his systolic blood pressure raised up to normal level and moderate but persistent rhinopharyngeal bleeding starts over.

5. What's definitive control of facial bleeding?
   A. Bilateral surgical ligation of external carotid arteries to prevent collateral circulation and bleeding relapse
   B. Diagnostic angiography and superselective embolization with coaxial microcatheter
   C. Angio-CT scan demonstration of maxillary artery involvement and its transantral endoscopic ligation
   D. To reduce systolic pressure resuscitation target (permissive resuscitation) to allow spontaneous hemostasis

Please see Chap. 58 for the correct answer.

References

1. Boffano P, Roccia F, Zavattero E, Dediol E, Uglešić V, Kovačič Ž, Vesnaver A, Konstantinović VS, Petrović M, Stephens J, Kanzaria A, Bhatti N, Holmes S, Pechalova PF, Bakardjiev AG, Malanchuk VA, Kopchak AV, Galteland P, Mjøen E, Skjelbred P, Koudougou C, Mouallem G, Corre P, Løes S, Lekven N, Laverick S, Gordon P, Tamme T, Akermann S, Karagozoglu KH, Kommers SC, Forouzanfar T. European Maxillofacial Trauma (EURMAT) project: a multicentre and prospective study. J Craniomaxillofac Surg. 2015;43:62–70.
2. Hutchinson I, Lawlor M, Skinner D. ABC of major trauma. Major maxillofacial injuries. Br Med J. 1990;301:595–9.
3. Perry M, Morris C. Advanced trauma life support (ATLS) and facial trauma: can one size fit all? Part 2: ATLS, maxillofacial injuries and airway management dilemmas. Int J Oral Maxillofac Surg. 2008;37:309–20.
4. Jose A, Nagori SA, Agarwal B, Bhutia O, Roychoudhury A. Management of maxillofacial trauma in emergency: an update of challenges and controversies. J Emerg Trauma Shock. 2016;9:73–80.
5. Ardekian L, Samet N, Shoshani Y, Taicher S. Life-threatening bleeding following maxillofacial trauma. J Craniomaxillofac Surg. 1993;21:336–8.
6. Perry M, O'Hare J, Porter G. Advanced Trauma Life Support (ATLS) and facial trauma: can one size fit all? Part 3: hypovolaemia and facial injuries in the multiply injured patient. Int J Oral Maxillofac Surg. 2008;37:405–14.
7. Ceallaigh PO, Ekanaykaee K, Beirne CJ, Patton DW. Diagnosis and management of common maxillofacial injuries in the emergency department. Part 1: advanced trauma life support. Emerg Med J. 2006;23:796–7.
8. Veeravagu A, Joseph R, Jiang B, Lober RM, Ludwig C, Torres R, Singh H. Traumatic epistaxis: skull base defects, intracranial complications and neurosurgical considerations. Int J Surg Case Rep. 2013;4:656–61.
9. Khanna S, Dagum AB. A critical review of the literature and an evidence-based approach for life-threatening hemorrhage in maxillofacial surgery. Ann Plast Surg. 2012;69:474–8.
10. Bynoe RP, Kerwin AJ, Parker HH 3rd, Nottingham JM, Bell RM, Yost MJ, Close TC, Hudson ER, Sheridan DJ, Wade MD. Maxillofacial injuries and life-threatening hemorrhage: treatment with transcatheter arterial embolization. J Trauma. 2003;55:74–9.
11. Tung TC, Tseng WS, Chen CT, Lai JP, Chen YR. Acute life-threatening injuries in facial fracture patients: a review of 1,025 patients. J Trauma. 2000;49:420–4.
12. Perry M, Dancey A, Mireskandari K, Oakley P, Davies S, Cameron M. Emergency care in facial trauma—a maxillofacial and ophthalmic perspective. Injury. 2005;36:875–96.
13. Ho K, Hutter JJ, Eskridge J, Khan U, Boorer CJ, Hopper RA, Deva AK. The management of life-threatening haemorrhage following blunt facial trauma. J Plast Reconstr Aesthet Surg. 2006;59:1257–62.
14. Gwyn PP, Carraway JH, Horton CE, Adamson JE, Mladick RA. Facial fractures—associated injuries and complications. Plast Reconstr Surg. 1971;47:225–30.
15. Shimoyama T, Kaneko T, Horie N. Initial management of massive oral bleeding after midfacial fracture. J Trauma. 2003;54:332–6; discussion 336.
16. Singam P, Thanabalan J, Mohammed Z. Superselective embolisation for control of intractable epistaxis from maxillary artery injury. Biomed Imaging Interv J. 2011;7:1–3.
17. Al-Jehani HM, Alwadaani HA, Almolani FM. Traumatic intracranial internal carotid artery pseudoaneurysm presenting as epistaxis treated by endovascular coiling. Neurosciences (Riyadh). 2016;21:60–3.
18. Cogbill TH, Cothren CC, Ahearn MK, Cullinane DC, Kaups KL, Scalea TM, Maggio L, Brasel KJ, Harrison PB, Patel NY, Moore EE, Jurkovich GJ, Ross SE. Management of maxillofacial injuries with severe oronasal hemorrhage: a multicenter perspective. J Trauma. 2008;65:994–9.
19. Waldron J, Stafford N. Ligation of the external carotid artery for severe epistaxis. J Otolaryngol. 1992;21:249–51.

20. Zachariades N, Rallis G, Papademetriou G, Papakosta V, Spanomichos G, Souelem M. Embolization for the treatment of pseudoaneurysm and transection of facial vessels. Oral Surg Oral Med Oral Pathol Oral Radiol Endod. 2001;92:491–4.
21. Lynham AJ, Hirst JP, Cosson JA, Chapman PJ, McEniery P. Emergency department management of maxillofacial trauma. Emerg Med Australas. 2004;16:7–12.
22. Sakamoto T, Yagi K, Hiraide A, Takasu A, Kinoshita Y, Iwai A, Yoshioka T, Sugimoto T. Transcatheter embolization in the treatment of massive bleeding due to maxillofacial injury. J Trauma. 1988;28(6):840–3.
23. Gamanagatti S, Prasad TV, Kumar A, Singhal M, Sagar S. Angioembolisation in maxillofacial trauma: an initial experience in a tertiary care center. J Maxillofac Oral Surg. 2016;15:59–66.
24. Buchanan RT, Holtmann B. Severe epistaxis in facial fractures. Plast Reconstr Surg. 1983;71:768–71.
25. Rockey JG, Anand R. A critical audit of the surgical management of intractable epistaxis using sphenopalatine artery ligation/diathermy. Rhinology. 2002;40:147–9.
26. Srinivasan V, Sherman IW, O'Sullivan G. Surgical management of intractable epistaxis: audit of results. J Laryngol Otol. 2000;114:697–700.
27. Baqain ZH, Thakkar C, Kalavrezos N. Superselective embolization for control of facial haemorrhage. Injury. 2004;35:435–8.
28. Goddard JC, Reiter ER. Inpatient management of epistaxis: outcomes and cost. Otolaryngol Head Neck Surg. 2005;132: 707–12.
29. Zhang C, Xie X, You C, Mao B, Wang C, He M, Sun H. Endovascular treatment of traumatic pseudoaneurysm presenting as intractable epistaxis. Korean J Radiol. 2010;11:603–11.
30. Radvany MG, Gailloud P. Endovascular management of neurovascular arterial injuries in the face and neck. Semin Intervent Radiol. 2010;27:44–54.
31. Sokoloff J, Wickbom I, McDonald D, Brahme F, Goergen TC, Goldberger LE. Therapeutic percutaneous embolization in intractable epistaxis. Radiology. 1974;111:285–7.
32. Liao CC, Hsu YP, Chen CT, Tseng YY. Transarterial embolization for intractable oronasal hemorrhage associated with craniofacial trauma: evaluation of prognostic factors. J Trauma. 2007;63:827–30.
33. Scaramuzzi N, Walsh RM, Brennan P, Walsh M. Treatment of intractable epistaxis using arterial embolization. Clin Otolaryngol Allied Sci. 2001;26:307–9.
34. Perry M. Advanced Trauma Life Support (ATLS) and facial trauma: can one size fit all? Part 1: dilemmas in the management of the multiply injured patient with coexisting facial injuries. Int J Oral Maxillofac Surg. 2008;37:209–14.
35. Perry M, Moutray T. Advanced Trauma Life Support (ATLS) and facial trauma: can one size fit all? Part 4: 'can the patient see?' Timely diagnosis, dilemmas and pitfalls in the multiply injured, poorly responsive/unresponsive patient. Int J Oral Maxillofac Surg. 2008;37:505–14.
36. McClenaghan FC, Ezra DG, Holmes SB. Mechanisms and management of vision loss following orbital and facial trauma. Curr Opin Ophthalmol. 2011;22:426–31.
37. Steinsapir KD, Goldberg RA. Traumatic optic neuropathy: an evolving understanding. Am J Ophthalmol. 2011;151:928–33.
38. Winterton JV, Patel K, Mizen KD. Review of management options for a retrobulbar hemorrhage. J Oral Maxillofac Surg. 2007;65:296–9.
39. Allen M, Perry M, Burns F. When is a retrobulbar haemorrhage not a retrobulbar haemorrhage? Int J Oral Maxillofac Surg. 2010;39:1045–9.
40. Popat H, Doyle PT, Davies SJ. Blindness following retrobulbar haemorrhage—it can be prevented. Br J Oral Maxillofac Surg. 2007;45:163–4.
41. Hislop WS, Dutton GN, Douglas PS. Treatment of retrobulbar haemorrhage in accident and emergency departments. Br J Oral Maxillofac Surg. 1996;34:289–92.
42. Perry M. Acute proptosis in trauma: retrobulbar hemorrhage or orbital compartment syndrome—does it really matter? J Oral Maxillofac Surg. 2008;66(9):1913–20.
43. Soare S, Foletti JM, Gallucci A, Collet C, Guyot L, Chossegros C. Update on orbital decompression as emergency treatment of traumatic blindness. J Craniomaxillofac Surg. 2015;43: 1000–3.
44. Mohammadi F, Rashan A, Psaltis A, Janisewicz A, Li P, El-Sawy T, Nayak JV. Intraocular pressure changes in emergent surgical decompression of orbital compartment syndrome. JAMA Otolaryngol Head Neck Surg. 2015;141:562–5.
45. Kulkarni AR, Aggarwal SP, Kulkarni RR, Deshpande MD, Walimbe PB, Labhsetwar AS. Ocular manifestations of head injury: a clinical study. Eye (Lond). 2005;19:1257–63.
46. Linberg JV. Orbital compartment syndromes following trauma. Adv Ophthalmic Plast Reconstr Surg. 1987;6:51–62.
47. Fattahi T, Brewer K, Retana A, Ogledzki M. Incidence of retrobulbar hemorrhage in the emergency department. J Oral Maxillofac Surg. 2014;72:2500–2.
48. Chen YA, Singhal D, Chen YR, Chen CT. Management of acute traumatic retrobulbar haematomas: a 10-year retrospective review. J Plast Reconstr Aesthet Surg. 2012;65:1325–30.
49. Schumann P, Kokemüller H, Tavassol F, Lindhorst D, Lemound J, Essig H, Rücker M, Gellrich NC. Optic nerve monitoring. Craniomaxillofac Trauma Reconstr. 2013;6:75–86.
50. Kniess CK, Fong TC, Reilly AJ, Laoteppitaks C. Early detection of traumatic retrobulbar hemorrhage using bedside ocular ultrasound. J Emerg Med. 2015;49:58–60.
51. Cornelius CP, Altenmüller E, Ehrenfeld M. The use of flash visual evoked potentials in the early diagnosis of suspected optic nerve lesions due to craniofacial trauma. J Craniomaxillofac Surg. 1996;24:1–11.
52. Zoumalan CI, Bullock JD, Warwar RE, McCulley TJ. Evaluation of intraocular and orbital pressure in the management of orbital hemorrhage: an experimental model. Arch Ophthalmol. 2008;126:1257–60.
53. Goodall KL, Brahma A, Bates A, Leatherbarrow B. Lateral canthotomy and inferior cantholysis: an effective method of urgent orbital decompression for sight threatening acute retrobulbar haemorrhage. Injury. 1999;30:485–90.
54. Ikejiri M, Adachi-Usami E, Mizota A, Tsuyama Y, Miyauchi O, Suehiro S. Pattern visual evoked potentials in traumatic optic neuropathy. Ophthalmologica. 2002;216:415–9.
55. Steinsapir KD, Goldberg RA. Traumatic optic neuropathy: a critical update. Comp Ophtalmol Update. 2005;6:11–21.
56. Warner N, Eggenberger E. Traumatic optic neuropathy: a review of the current literature. Curr Opin Ophthalmol. 2010;21:459–62.
57. Sun MT, Chan WO, Selva D. Traumatic orbital compartment syndrome: importance of the lateral canthomy and cantholysis. Emerg Med Australas. 2014;26:274–8.
58. Oester AE Jr, Fowler BT, Fleming JC. Inferior orbital septum release compared with lateral canthotomy and cantholysis in the management of orbital compartment syndrome. Ophthal Plast Reconstr Surg. 2012;28:40–3.
59. Haubner F, Jägle H, Nunes DP, Schleder S, Cvetkova N, Kühnel T, Gassner HG. Orbital compartment: effects of emergent canthotomy and cantholysis. Eur Arch Otorhinolaryngol. 2015;272: 479–83.
60. Ghufoor K, Sandhu G, Sutcliffe J. Delayed onset of retrobulbar haemorrhage following severe head injury: a case report and review. Injury. 1998;29:139–41.
61. Hayter JP, Sugar AW. An orbital observation chart. Br J Oral Maxillofac Surg. 1991;29:77–9.

62. Steinsapir KD. Treatment of traumatic optic neuropathy with high-dose corticosteroid. J Neuroophthalmol. 2006;26:65–7.
63. Yu-Wai-Man P, Griffiths PG. Steroids for traumatic optic neuropathy.Cochrane Database Syst Rev. 2011;(19):CD006032. https://doi.org/10.1002/14651858.CD006032.pub3.
64. Levin LA, Beck RW, Joseph MP, Seiff S, Kraker R. The treatment of traumatic optic neuropathy: the International Optic Nerve Trauma Study. Ophthalmology. 1999;106:1268–77.
65. Lee V, Ford RL, Xing W, Bunce C, Foot B. Surveillance of traumatic optic neuropathy in the UK. Eye (Lond). 2010;24:240–50.
66. Edwards P, Arango M, Balica L, Cottingham R, El-Sayed H, Farrell B, Fernandes J, Gogichaisvili T, Golden N, Hartzenberg B, Husain M, Ulloa MI, Jerbi Z, Khamis H, Komolafe E, Laloë V, Lomas G, Ludwig S, Mazairac G, Muñoz Sanchéz Mde L, Nasi L, Olldashi F, Plunkett P, Roberts I, Sandercock P, Shakur H, Soler C, Stocker R, Svoboda P, Trenkler S, Venkataramana NK, Wasserberg J, Yates D, Yutthakasemsunt S, CRASH trial collaborators. Final results of MRC CRASH, a randomised placebo-controlled trial of intravenous corticosteroid in adults with head injury-outcomes at 6 months. Lancet. 2005;365:1957–9.
67. Sires BS, Stanley RB Jr, Levine LM. Oculocardiac reflex caused by orbital floor trapdoor fracture: an indication for urgent repair. Arch Ophthalmol. 1998;116:955–6.
68. Gerbino G, Roccia F, Bianchi FA, Zavattero E. Surgical management of orbital trapdoor fracture in a pediatric population. J Oral Maxillofac Surg. 2010;68:1310–6.

Modern Management of Ophthalmic Injuries

13

Paolo Arpa, Marco Azzolini, and Luca Biraghi

Key Points

- *The use of a standardized terminology can avoid ambiguity in the management of traumatized eyes.*
- *The OTS (ocular trauma score) has a predictive accuracy of approximately 80%, which means that it will be accurate 4 out of 5 times.*
- Intraocular tissue prolapse should be suspected in all open globe injuries. The wound may remain hidden!
- *The* primary goal is to achieve a watertight globe and to maintain structural integrity of the anterior segment and/or of the eyeball.
- *Ophthalmic imaging is mandatory when an IOFB is suspected.*
- *In most cases the condition of the retina determines the outcome of an injury.*
- Primary lens removal should be considered at all times because vitreoretinal complications are expected in 50% of eyes with lens trauma and the retinal visualization is mandatory after a severe trauma.

13.1 Introduction

Ocular trauma is a leading cause of monocular visual loss and often affects young individuals, especially the pediatric groups. Great advances have been attained on the management of ocular injuries under the guidelines of the retrospective reviews; of great importance seems to make a consensus on the terminology classification, evaluation, and surgery.

P. Arpa (✉) · M. Azzolini · L. Biraghi
U.O. Oculistica, Ospedale San Gerardo, ASST Monza, Monza, Italy
e-mail: marcoazzolini@libero.it

13.2 Terminology and Classification of Ocular Trauma

Mechanical trauma can cause extensive damage to the orbit, eyeballs, adnexa, and optic nerve, other than the eyeball. It is essential for the ophthalmologists and non-ophthalmologists to use a standardized classification system of terminology and assessment.

13.2.1 Birmingham Eye Trauma Terminology (BETT) [1, 2]

BETT is currently applied by most of worldwide ophthalmic organizations. Figure 13.1: the key point of this system is to make distinct definitions referring to the globe, instead of the specific tissue, for tissue stands for the location. However, often there are more complicated injuries: for instance, a patient fall on a sharp object may suffer a laceration, which is a common type of penetrating injury, with a concomitant rupture (i.e., loss of eye tissue) with varying degrees of contusion to the retina. In such example, ocular rupture, as the most serious injury type, is the most appropriate description.

The anatomic region involved in the injury, for example, lacerated or ruptured, provides additional information that is important for injury prognosis.

- Zone 1 injury involves the cornea and limbus.
- Zone 2 injury refers to a rupture or laceration located in the anterior 5 mm of the sclera that doesn't extend into the retina.
- Zone 3 injury describes a full-thickness sclera laceration or rupture found more posterior than 5 mm from the limbus.

P. Aseni et al. (eds.), *Operative Techniques and Recent Advances in Acute Care and Emergency Surgery*,
https://doi.org/10.1007/978-3-319-95114-0_13

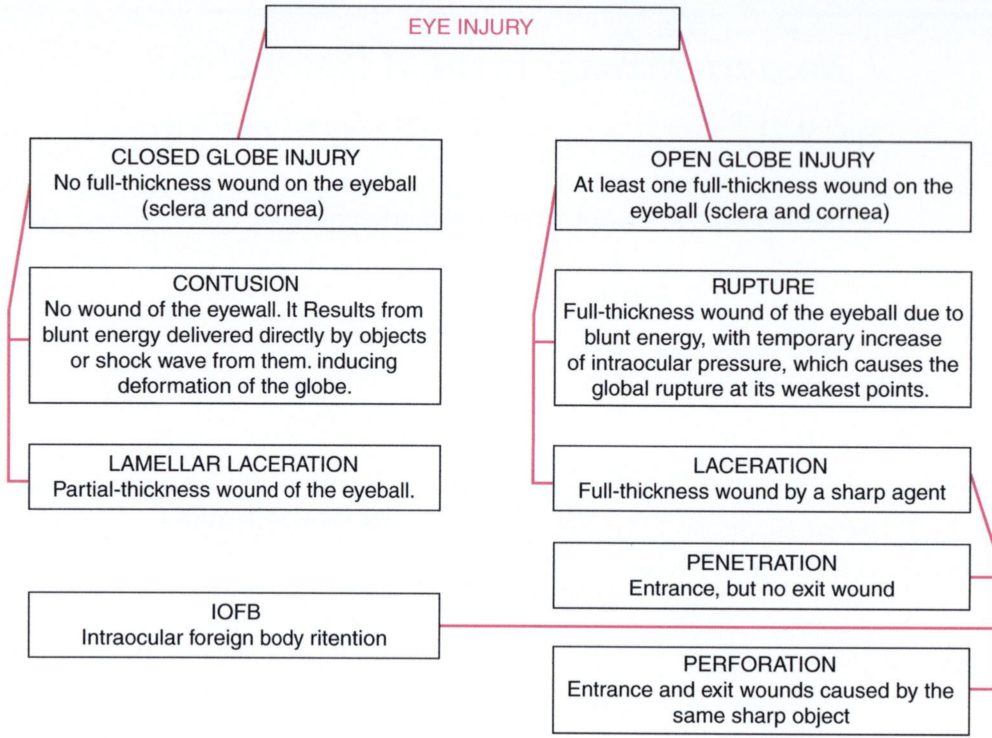

Fig. 13.1 Classification of eye injuries in BETT with terms and definitions. Modified from Kuhn [2]

Table 13.1 Computational method for deriving the OTS score

Initial visual factor	Raw points
Initial raw score (based on initial visual acuity)	NPL = 60
	PL or HM = 70
	1/200–19/200 = 80
	20/200–20/50 = 90
	20/40 = 100
Globe rupture	−23
Endophthalmitis	−17
Perforating injury	−14
Retinal detachment	−11
Relative afferent pupillary defect (RAPD)	−10
Raw score sum = sum of raw points	

NPL nil perception of light, *PL* perception of light, *HM* hand movements

Table 13.2 Estimated probability of follow-up visual acuity category at 6 months

Raw score sum	OTS score	NPL (%)	PL/ HM (%)	1/200–19/200 (%)	20/200–20/50 (%)	≥20/40 (%)
0–44	1	73	17	7	2	1
45–65	2	28	26	18	13	15
66–80	3	2	11	15	28	44
81–91	4	1	2	2	21	74
92–100	5	0	1	2	5	92

NPL nil perception of light, *PL* perception of light, *HM* hand movements

13.2.2 Ocular Trauma Score (OTS) [3, 4]

In cases of serious eye trauma, it is invaluable for both patient and ophthalmologist to obtain, as early as possible, reliable information regarding the expected outcome of the injury. The Ocular Trauma Classification Group analyzed more than 100 variables for over 2500 eye injuries recorded in the United States and Hungarian Eye Injury Registries in order to identify the best predictors of outcome at 6 months after injury. From this, they developed the ocular trauma score (OTS), which is used to predict the visual outcome of patients after open globe ocular trauma. Tables 13.1 and 13.2: OTS range from 1 (most severe injury and worst prognosis at 6-month follow-up) to 5 (least severe injury and least poor prognosis at 6 months). Each score is associated with a range of predicted post-injury visual acuities.

13.3 Epidemiology of Ocular Trauma

Basing on selected data reported in the last 20 years on the United States Eye Injury Registry (USEIR), which collected over than 18,000 cases requiring hospitalization, the eye traumas are the first cause of monocular blindness (40%) in the Western countries and the second reason for enucleation of the eyeball. Over two million eye injuries are estimated to occur in the USA each year. The incidence is about 400/100,000, with a male-female ratio of 5:5, with special preference for young people; the closed globe injury occurrences are fourfold higher than open globe ones.

The first reason for eye trauma is work accident, accounting for 25% of cases (although decreasing due to the introduction of accident prevention regulations), followed by violence, sports, and domestic accidents. Recent epidemiological data confirm the home has now surpassed the workplace as the most common site for serious ocular injury.

13.4 General Considerations

Each case of serious ocular trauma requires a thorough history taking and careful clinical examination that is crucial in the proper assessment and management. Ocular trauma may be isolated or occur in the context of polytrauma. Systemic evaluation of the patient with attention to vital signs, mental status, and serious or life-threatening non-ocular trauma is indispensable before proceeding with ocular evaluation. This triaging process will direct the decision whether the patient should be evaluated in a general trauma center or in a specialized eye emergency room.

An accurate history taking of the injury must be collected: the mechanism of injury and circumstances of the incident as reported by the patient should be reported. Blunt trauma usually results in different pathophysiologic processes compared with trauma by sharp objects, and the differentiation can guide clinical examination and management. For instance, blunt trauma may result in an occult open globe injury (ruptured globe) where the wound site may be hidden by bleeding underneath an intact bulbar conjunctiva or is situated posterior to the insertion of the extraocular muscles (EOMs); on the contrary, the laceration site is usually more visible on slit lamp examination when ocular trauma is inflicted by a sharp object.

The mechanism of injury may also a presence of a foreign body be suspected. Furthermore, the physical setting of trauma may influence the prognosis and final visual outcome, since open globe injuries in a rural setting have a much higher rate of intraocular infection and endophthalmitis [5]. Determining the exact time of injury and the time span between trauma and presentation is also imperative in planning the intervention, particularly in open globe injuries, since a more conservative approach may be employed in certain cases (such as small self-sealing corneal wounds) in which the eye has been quiescently stable for a relatively long period. Moreover, complications such as angle recession glaucoma can often develop years following ocular contusion [6].

A prompt clinical and functional evaluation, including visual acuity testing, fundus examination (and/or B-scan echography if the dioptric means are opaque), and diagnostic imaging, must be performed.

Upon initial presentation, placement of a protective eye shield and avoidance of eye patching are strongly recommended when open globe injury is suspected. Visual acuity of both eyes should be assessed. Inspection of the external appearance of the face and periocular tissues may help to determine the extent of the injury. For example, gross enophthalmos and periorbital ecchymosis may be the manifestations of an orbital wall fracture, and lacerations involving the eyelid margin are often associated with corneoscleral lacerations and open globe injuries.

Gross inspection may also reveal the presence of a visible foreign body on the ocular surface, prolapse of uveal tissue and/or other intraocular contents, or pupillary deformity. These observations often suggest, or confirm, the presence of an open globe injury. The presence of large periorbital ecchymosis or eyelid edema may preclude adequate ocular examination, and obtaining imaging studies directly in cases in which open globe injuries cannot be ruled out is safer than exerting undue pressure on the globe to open the eyelids.

13.5 Anterior Segment Trauma

Mechanical ocular trauma involving the anterior segment may result in damage to the conjunctiva, cornea, limbus, anterior chamber angle, iris, lens, and ciliary body. The mechanism of trauma (closed or open, blunt, penetrating, or perforating), force and extent of trauma, and whether a foreign body is involved determine the consequences of the trauma. The treatment modalities employed and the final visual outcome are also dependent upon these trauma variables.

13.6 Cornea

13.6.1 Mechanical Trauma

The cornea is involved in >50% of all serious mechanical ocular trauma, and 52% of corneal injuries involve full-thickness lacerations. Partial-thickness wound is treated only with medications, while full-thickness corneal lacerations are considered a surgical emergency due to the risk of endophthalmitis, the frequent presence of intraocular tissue prolapse, and the possible concomitance of scleral wounds.

Small self-sealing wounds may be treated with topical antibiotics alone, whereas slightly larger wounds may be treated with bandage contact lenses. Corneal gluing can successfully close mild corneal wounds without uveal prolapse. Fibrin glue or isobutyl cyanoacrylate, often applied under a contact lens, may be used to close partial-thickness corneal lacerations and corneal penetrations <2 mm. In case of large epithelial defects, amniotic membrane may be used: it provides mechanical protection, helps with reepithelialization, and helps to stop inflammation. The membrane can be sutured upon small penetrating wounds and covered with a contact lens. Also, this technique is applicable to cases of simple corneal penetrations. Larger wounds or loss of corneal tissue requires surgical management.

Single-point sutures with nylon 10/0 and curved needle are the traditional way to repair corneal lacerations (often it is also necessary to remove or reposition displaced internal ocular tissues). The wound must be closed with anterior and posterior edges apposed, without rendering overrides or underrides between the edges of the wound. Near full-thickness interrupted suture bites are ideal for wound closure: in the pupillary field, sutures should be shorter and widely spaced, while in the periphery longer and tighter sutures may be placed, to preserve centrally the natural curvature of the cornea and to reduce iatrogenic astigmatism; corneal sutures should reach 90–95% of the stromal thickness, almost 1.5–2 mm in length and of equal depth on each side; irregular sutures create internal wound gape, whereas sutures of unequal length and depth on each side of the wound result in wound override (Fig. 13.2).

For a wound that is less stable, a viscoelastic or air bubble may be injected into the anterior chamber preferably through a separate limbal paracentesis incision. For corneoscleral lacerations, the first suture steps should start at the limbus, the corneal, and scleral proceeding from there.

In case of wounds with loss of corneal tissue, lamellar or penetrating corneal transplantation has been described to not only reform globe integrity and decrease risk of infection but also achieve clear visual axis [7–17].

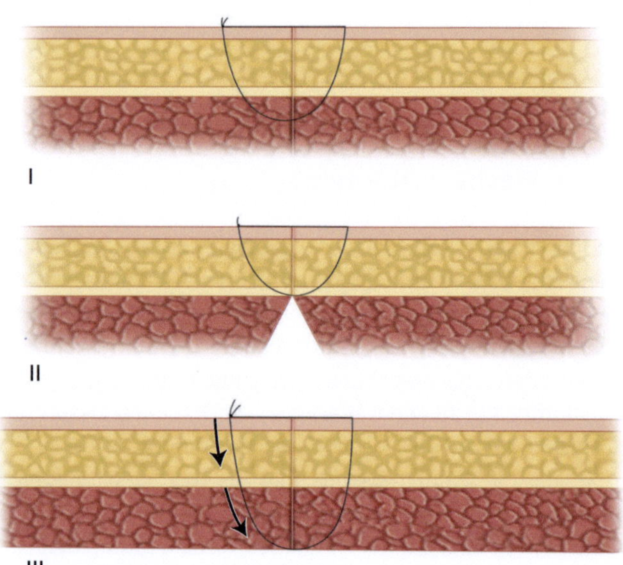

Fig. 13.2 (I) Deep suture placement equidistant from the wound margins gives excellent wound approximation. (II) Shallow sutures create internal wound gape. (III) Full-thickness sutures may create a conduit for microbial invasion

13.6.2 Chemical Trauma

The cornea is the typical main site of chemical eye injuries that may lead to blindness if not properly treated. Alkaline agents (i.e., ammonia, lye, magnesium hydroxide) penetrate ocular tissues rapidly and continue to do so, causing severe damage; acids (i.e., sulfuric, sulfurous, hydrofluoric, acetic) cause proteins to coagulate on corneal epithelium and stroma and precipitate out quickly, which limits ocular penetration. Both alkalines and acids cause ocular surface epithelial cells to die upon contact; penetration of alkalines and acids into corneal stroma result in keratocyte death and loss of corneal clarity. Time of penetration into the anterior chamber varies (immediate for ammonia); it can result in secondary glaucoma, cataract, hypotony, and phthisis bulbi.

The management includes prompt and copious irrigation, to minimize duration of contact between chemical and the eye in order to protect limbal stem cells: irrigate for 15–30 min; evert upper lid; irrigate fornices. Check pH after irrigation; continue until pH 7.0. Then debride necrotic corneal and conjunctival epithelium, and administer topical and oral antibiotic therapy. The second level treatment may include limbal cell transplantation, amniotic membrane implant, and penetrating keratoplasty [18–20].

13.7 Iris

Iris involvement is frequent in mechanical ocular trauma, both closed and open injuries. Closed globe injuries may produce mydriasis due to iris sphincter rupture, while open globe injuries (whether due to severe blunt or penetrating/perforating trauma) may cause iris laceration; iris prolapse through corneal, limbal, scleral, or corneoscleral wounds; traumatic aniridia; and iridodialysis.

13.7.1 Traumatic Mydriasis

Often asymptomatic, so treatment is not mandatory in the absence of visually disturbing or cosmetic problems. In mild cases, miotic agents and/or cosmetic contact lenses usually fix the problem. Otherwise, surgical correction of traumatic mydriasis is considered.

First, a radial cut of the iris, from the periphery to the pupillary margin at the point of sphincter rupture, is made with iris scissor; then, bring the two ends of the pupillary border apposed with a permanent 10–0 polypropylene suture (Figs. 13.3 and 13.4). The procedure is repeated distally

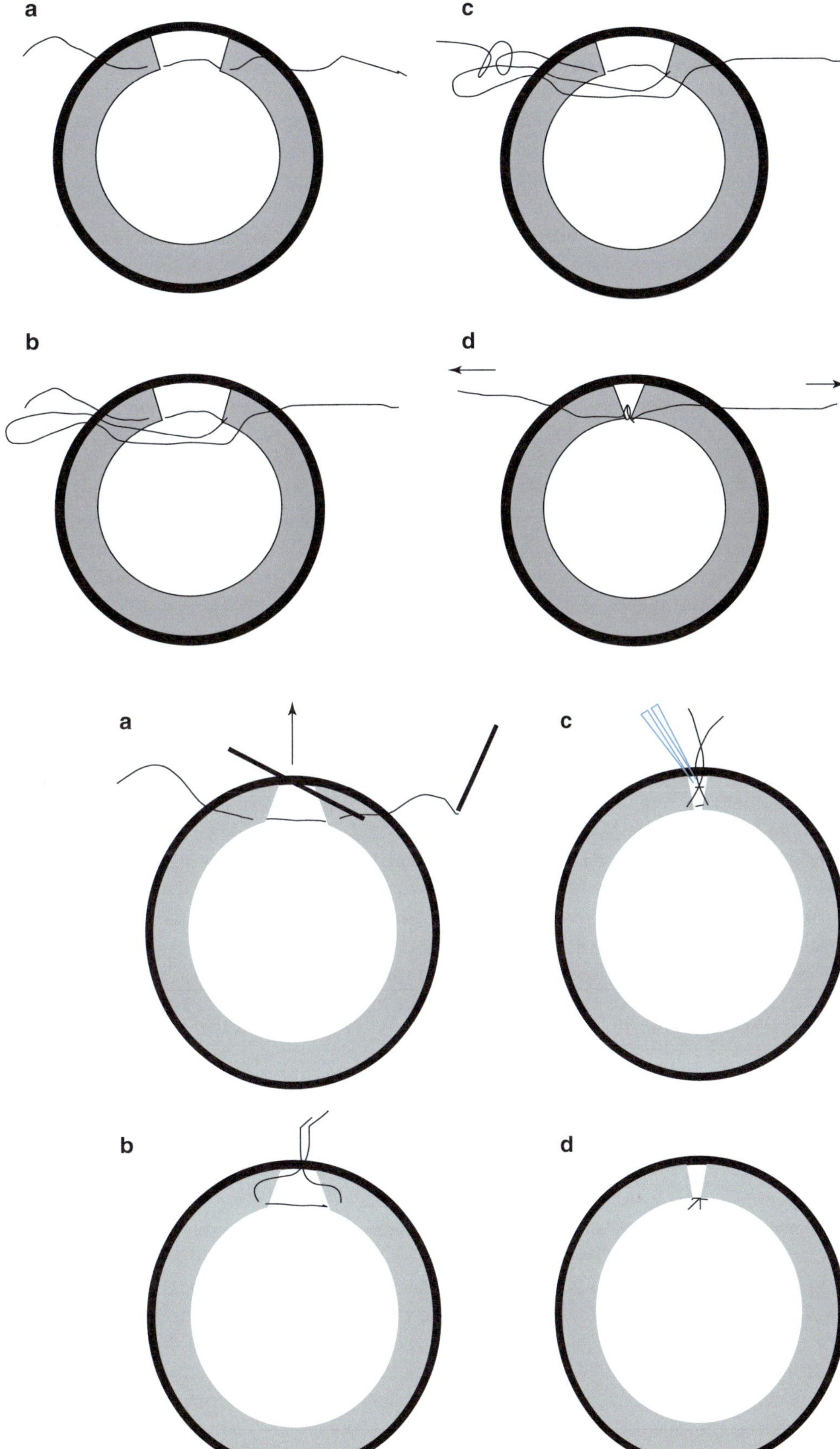

Fig. 13.3 Siepser slipknot technique. (**a**) Two opposing side ports are made, and a 10-0 suture is passed from the first paracentesis, through the two edges of the iris laceration and from the second side port incision. (**b**) The needle is cut and a large loop of suture is pulled out of the entry side port incision with a hook. (**c**) A double-throw slipknot is made by tying the loop around the free suture end. (**d**) The knot is slid into the anterior chamber by pulling the two suture ends firmly. The process is repeated to form a square knot. The suture ends are trimmed using intraocular scissors

Fig. 13.4 McCannel iris suture technique. (**a**) Creation of two opposing side ports, passage of a single-armed 10-0 suture through the two edges of the iris, and cutting off needle. (**b**) Exteriorization of the two suture ends through a third paracentesis. (**c**) Suture ends tied extraocularly and cut. (**d**) Sutured iris ends reposited intraocularly along the length of the radial iris cut. The same technique can be applied to iris lacerations [21–24].

13.7.2 Iris Prolapse

Iris prolapse occurs secondary to an open globe injury, through corneal, limbal, or scleral lacerations.

It is fundamental an early management of iris prolapse, as a delayed management may induce iridocorneal adhesions with ischemia and necrosis of the iris tissue, endophthalmitis, surface epithelialization and epithelial downgrowth, and secondary glaucoma.

Topical and systemic antibiotics should be considered on presentation; intracameral antibiotics may be used to minimize the risk of endophthalmitis.

The extent and the site of the prolapse, together with anterior chamber depth, and accessibility of the prolapsed iris tissue, determine the best surgical technique. For peripheral prolapses with the anterior chamber relatively formed, the management forecasts intracameral administration of miotic agents (e.g., acetylcholine) through a side port incision with gentle stroking of the prolapsed iris tissue back into the eye. When iris is prolapsed through a central corneal wound, intracameral injection of mydriatic agents (e.g., epinephrine) may help. When pupil changes alone fail, intracameral injection of viscoelastic agents through a paracentesis incision, to mechanically dislodge and reposit the prolapsed iris tissue, with a spatula, can be attempted. Care should be exercised to not exert undue force on the iris root which can result in iatrogenic iridodialysis.

When iris prolapse lasts for more than 48 h, it should be examined to detect signs of necrosis or epithelialization. Any unviable iris tissue should be excised without pulling excessively on viable iris. The native wound is then treated to restore globe integrity.

13.7.3 Iridodialysis

Iridodialysis represents detachment of the iris root from its ciliary insertion. Iridodialysis can result from blunt or penetrating ocular trauma, or it may be iatrogenic during intraocular surgery. Small iridodialyses or those adequately covered by the upper eyelid are usually asymptomatic. Symptoms of larger iridodialyses include monocular diplopia and glare. When small, iridodialysis can be managed with frequent instillation of mydriatic eye drops (e.g., atropine) and/or dark sunglasses to reduce light-induced miosis. These measures may result in spontaneous reattachment. Several surgical techniques have been described to correct large iridodialyses. Any vitreous strands prolapsing through the iridodialysis defect should be cut prior to suture placement. The most widely used techniques use the McCannel technique [25].

13.8 Lens

Mechanical ocular trauma can damage the crystalline lens by inducing loss of transparency (cataract), loss of position (subluxation, dislocation, or extrusion), or both.

The treatment of traumatic cataract or lens dislocation, like that of all other forms of crystalline lens pathology, is surgical. Extraction of age-related cataract is relatively simple and carries a great success rate; surgical treatment of traumatic cataract can be more technically challenging, and outcomes are generally less favorable; this is mainly due to reduced visibility due to coexisting ocular media lesions; loss of anterior chamber volume and uveal prolapse; difficult capsulorhexis for traumatic capsular injury; loss of contrast due to vitreous hemorrhage, loose zonular support, and poor view; zonular and/or capsular damage with vitreous prolapse; and loss of nuclear masses in the vitreous chamber.

Preoperative evaluation of traumatic cataract is therefore important in order to determine globe integrity status (a corneal, limbal, or scleral laceration must be addressed before management of the traumatic cataract), visual significance of cataract, intraocular pressure, anterior and posterior chamber status (volume, blood, lens material, etc.) or vitreous prolapse, lens integrity (anterior or posterior capsular lesions secondary to penetrating trauma) and position (dislocation in anterior or vitreous chamber, subluxation with zonular looseness), retina status (B-scan echography if fundus is not visible), and presence of intraocular foreign bodies.

13.8.1 Timing of Surgery

Primary cataract surgery to address traumatic cataract, at the same time of wound repair, has many advantages over secondary surgery:

- Faster visual rehabilitation
- Earlier elimination of lens-induced inflammation, particularly when the anterior lens capsule has been breached
- Avoidance or definitive treatment of lens-induced intraocular pressure (IOP) elevation including phacomorphic, phacoanaphylactic, lens particle, or lens subluxation/dislocation-associated (e.g., pupillary block) glaucomas
- Allowing prompt examination of the posterior segment
- Elimination of undue vitreous traction on the retina when vitreous prolapse or traction is present that may lead to a retinal detachment

Surgery may be deferred if the cataract is presumed to be visually insignificant, particularly in the absence of coexisting ocular injuries requiring surgery, or when particular surgical needs are present.

13.8.2 Type of Surgical Technique

Primary closure of globe lacerations, when present, is the first step in the management of traumatic cataract, since a formed globe is necessary for safe cataract removal. It is better to perform cataract surgery via a separate corneal incision than the existing traumatic corneal wound. Ophthalmic viscoelastic devices (OVDs) or an anterior chamber maintainer should be employed to keep the globe formed at all times. The anterior chamber should be washed from hyphema and any floating lens particles; limbal vitrectomy should also be performed when vitreous strands are visible anteriorly. The pupil should be dilated using iris retractors or pupil-dilating rings if the pupil is tight.

Important factors to consider when determining the method of cataract removal are amount of zonular support, posterior capsule integrity, and visibility of the lens. In cases in which zonular support is thought to be sufficient, cataract should be removed through an anterior (limbal) approach. Capsulorhexis can be challenging in the traumatic cataract: exert minimal pressure on the lens using a pair of capsulorhexis forceps or a cystotome needle in order to avoid further weakening of the zonules. The capsulorhexis should start away from the presumed area of zonular weakness. Partial capsulorhexis may be done, followed by insertion of capsule retractors to support the area of zonular loss.

Capsular tension rings or ring segments can be used. It is possible to use capsular microscissors (which insert through a paracentesis) if the anterior capsule is torn to achieve a continuous, curvilinear capsulorhexis.

Phacoemulsification (with low vacuum and aspiration settings to avoid anterior chamber fluctuation and prevent further zonular damage) is the preferred technique when the posterior capsule is intact and adequate zonular support is present.

The surgeon needs to be ready to switch to vitrectomy if vitreous prolapse is detected. In the presence of vitreous prolapse or a large tear in the posterior capsule, pars plana lensectomy/vitrectomy is the procedure of choice. The pars plana approach, while requires special expertise and equipment, is preferred to corneal or limbal approaches when vitrectomy is planned.

In young children, performing primary posterior capsulotomy and anterior vitrectomy is indicated due to the high rate of posterior capsule opacification. Anterior and posterior lens capsules are very elastic in young children, and standard continuous curvilinear capsulorhexis (CCC) is technically challenging.

13.8.3 Intraocular Lens (IOL) Implantation

Preservation of anterior and/or posterior capsular support is an important aim of surgery. However, achieving adequate capsular support is not always simple, especially when the degree of zonular loss is significant or when pars plana lensectomy/vitrectomy is employed. When enough anterior and posterior capsular support is present, it is best to perform in-the-bag implantation. Three-piece foldable IOLs provide more tensile strength. Moreover, the optic of a three-piece lens can be captured in the bag with placement of the haptics in the sulcus to provide additional tensile support. Sulcus implantation of a three-piece foldable IOL is indicated when the capsular support available is not enough to permit in-the-bag implantation.

If no enough capsular support permissive of IOL implantation in the bag or in sulcus or when such positioning may result in a significant IOL tilt with or without the use of capsular tension rings, the use of an angle-supported anterior chamber IOL, sulcus-sutured posterior chamber IOL, or iris-fixated IOL is indicated. A peripheral iridectomy using the vitrectomy system is recommended to prevent pupillary block glaucoma. This is achieved by introducing the vitrector into the anterior chamber at the 12 or 9 o'clock position with the port facing down, cutting rate initially set to zero, and an aspiration pressure of 300 mmHg.

In cases of traumatic coexisting aniridia, a black diaphragm tinted IOL may be implanted. Sutureless sulcus fixation of IOLs can be achieved with the utility of scleral flaps, limbus parallel tunnels, or both.

Intraocular lens (IOL) power calculation poses a challenge in cases of traumatic cataract, since biometry may be difficult. However, biometry from the contralateral eye may be used in such cases.

Timing of IOL implantation in traumatic cataract has been a controversial issue. Several studies demonstrated favorable results of primary IOL implantation. However, complications such as uveitis, synechiae, pupillary capture, retinal detachment, and other posterior segment complications have been described. Moreover, IOL implantation is sometimes deferred in pediatric patients due to sizing and refractive factors, although it may guard against the development of amblyopia, especially in children in whom contact lens wear is not suitable. In general, primary IOL implantation is better avoided in the following conditions: children younger than 1 year of age, highly myopic patients, large corneal lacerations in which a corneal transplant might be planned, high risk of endophthalmitis, aniridia, and retinal detachment with high likelihood of proliferative vitreoretinopathy [26–39].

13.9 Posterior Segment

Ocular trauma involving the posterior segment may damage the retina, choroid, optic nerve, and vitreous leading to permanent visual loss.

According to the United States Eye Injury Registry, the rate of vitreoretinal involvement among all injuries is 44%.

Among all retinal injuries, the most important complications of severe ocular traumas are:

- Hemorrhage: 35%
- Macular hole: 0.07%
- Commotio retinae: 9%
- Retinal detachment: 26%

Traumatic optic neuropathy is another common consequence of blunt trauma, occurring in about 5% of head trauma.

There is no specific treatment for traumatic optic neuropathy.

Vitreoretinal surgery is required most of the times in the management of posterior segment trauma because of visibility issues, to remove media opacities (hemorrhages), to reestablish ocular integrity, to treat retinal detachment, and to prevent complications and scar formation (PVR).

Post-traumatic proliferative vitreoretinopathy (PVR) prevents success in many cases of rhegmatogenous retinal detachment and especially in open globe injuries with secondary retinal detachment. The timing of PVR occurrence depends on the type of injury, presenting early in perforating injuries followed by ruptures and IOFB. It is reported to occur in up to 40% of eyes after serious trauma.

An open globe should be closed as soon as possible, possibly within hours.

If there's no intraocular foreign body or infection, the surgeon can delay the secondary intervention to 1 week later, because this period of time allows for natural hemostasis, improves corneal edema, and induces posterior vitreous separation and liquefaction of any hemorrhage, while still in time to prevent post-traumatic proliferative vitreoretinopathy (PVR).

The techniques for treating PVR and retinal detachment are the same as for treatment of rhegmatogenous retinal detachment (scleral buckle or vitrectomy, even with mini-invasive technique 23-25-27 gauge).

For eyes with serious posterior segment trauma, silicone oil is the preferred tamponade.

Endolaser cerclage is highly recommended in eyes undergoing vitrectomy for trauma, because it creates a new ora serrata [40, 41].

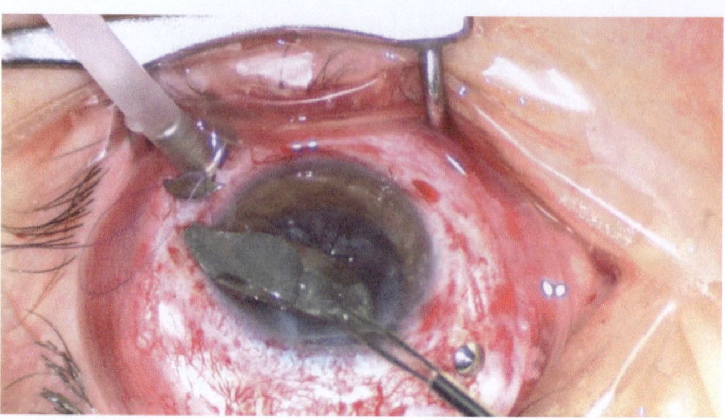

Fig. 13.5 Metallic intraocular foreign body (drill bit) just removed from the posterior segment of the eye with vitreoretinal forceps after vitrectomy and lens removal

13.10 Intraocular Foreign Bodies (IOFB)

An IOFB is an ophthalmic emergency because it causes mechanical damage but also brings pathogenic microorganisms into the eyes, leading to endophthalmitis, which seriously could compromise final visual acuity (Fig. 13.5).

These reasons make IOFBs one of the leading causes of monocular blindness, accounting for about 6% of the ocular trauma commonly seen in young adult males.

IOFB can be classified into metallic foreign bodies (active metals like iron, copper, etc. and inert metals) and nonmetallic foreign bodies (glasses, stones, wood).

Metallic foreign bodies, especially active metals, may make severe damage to the eyes within a short time due to its toxicity (siderosis or chalcosis).

Wooden foreign bodies and vegetable matter have a great chance of causing endophthalmitis.

The longer foreign bodies stay in the eyes, the greater damage they make.

X-ray examination is a traditional diagnostic method for IOFBs and is easy to have one.

Foreign bodies with high density, such as metals, stones, and glasses, can be clearly depicted by X-ray.

Computed tomography (CT), with its high resolution, is considered to be the gold standard for the diagnosis of IOFBs especially for diagnosing small metallic foreign bodies and nonmetallic ones, even though it is not always easy to access.

MRI is contraindicated in the suspicion of metallic IOFB.

The purpose of emergency surgery is to close the wound of the eye, reconstruct the anterior chamber, recover, and maintain the intraocular pressure, and in case of IOFBs, they should be removed as early as possible.

Vitrectomy allows removal of vitreous opacities, repairs tissue damages, and provides microbiologic specimens when endophthalmitis is suspected.

According to recent studies, 58% IOFB are located in the posterior segment, 13–24% in anterior segment, 7–10% in lens, 25–48% in vitreous, 16–44% in retina, 52% in both retina and choroid, and 0–15% subretinally [42–51].

13.11 Endophthalmitis

The incidence of endophthalmitis after open globe injury is 5–14%.

Traumatic endophthalmitis constitutes approximately 10–30% of all infectious endophthalmitis cases. It is more common in males (85%).

Risk factors for the development of traumatic endophthalmitis are:

- 24 h of delay in primary wound closure
- Presence of an IOFB
- Rural setting
- Rupture of the lens capsule

The relatively poor visual prognosis of traumatic endophthalmitis is due to the higher frequency of organisms that are more virulent than those in postoperative cases, the associated trauma, and the frequent delay in diagnosis and in the initiation of treatment due to masquerading signs that usually accompany the trauma.

The microbiology of traumatic endophthalmitis is significantly different from that in other categories.

Infections with more than one organism are common (15–48%).

Gram-positive bacteria such as *Streptococcus* and *Staphylococcus* species account for 75% of isolates in both the adult and pediatric age groups. There is a high incidence of *Bacillus* species (20%) and then Gram-negative bacteria (10%) and fungi (8.3%) [52–54].

Systemic antibiotics, although not confirmed in a randomized prospective study, may reduce the incidence of endophthalmitis in eyes with open globe injury.

13.11.1 Treatment Options

Topical	Vancomycin 50 mg/mL every hour
	Ceftazidime 50 mg/mL every hour
	Gentamicin/tobramycin 14 mg/mL
	Cefazolin 50 mg/mL
	Ciprofloxacin 0.3% every hour
	Moxifloxacin 0.5% every hour
	Gatifloxacin 0.3% every hour
Subconjunctival	Vancomycin 25 mg
	Ceftazidime 100 mg
	Dexamethasone 12 mg
Oral	Ciprofloxacin 750 mg twice daily
	Levofloxacin 500 mg once daily
	Moxifloxacin 400 mg once daily
	Voriconazole 6 mg/kg/day
	Fluconazole 400–1600 mg/day
Intravenous	Vancomycin 1 g every 12 h
	Ceftazidime 1 g every 8 h
	Amikacin 200–400 μg/mL
	Amphotericin B 0.6–1 mg/kg/day
	Voriconazole 6 mg/kg/day
	Fluconazole 400–1600 mg/day
Intravitreal	Vancomycin 1 mg/0.1 mL
	Ceftazidime 2.25 mg/0.1 mL
	Amikacin 0.4 mg/0.1 mL
	Piperacillin/tazobactam 250 μg/0.1 mL
	Amphotericin B 5 μg/0.1 mL
	Voriconazole 0.05–0.1 mg/0.1 mL
	Dexamethasone 0.4 mg/0.1 mL
Intraocular infusion	Vancomycin 0.2 mg/mL
	Ceftazidime 0.45 mg/mL
	Amikacin 0.08 mg/mL
	Gentamicin/tobramycin 0.08 mg/mL
	Amphotericin B 0.02 mg/mL

The ideal antibiotic regimen remains controversial.

Systemic antibiotics used simultaneously with topical antibiotics are considered standard of care by the ocular traumatologists. Our preference is intravenous ceftazidime which provides good Gram-negative coverage and has a good safety profile and good intravitreal penetration or oral ciprofloxacin for its good intravitreal penetration. In addition to systemic antibiotics, subconjunctival and topical antibiotics with a cycloplegic agent are used widely. *Antifungal prophylaxis* for open globe repairs is generally not recommended in the absence of clinical and microbiologic evidence for fungal infection [55–62].

The treatment of traumatic endophthalmitis remains early vitrectomy: in our hospital we use silicone oil at the completion of vitrectomy, reducing the postoperative complications without causing recurrence of the infection or concentrating the infecting organisms in the proximity of the inferior retina or the macular region. The eyes are irrigated with a solution containing antibiotics during vitrectomy (vancomycin hydrochloride diluted in the irrigating bottle), but we do not leave antibiotics in the vitreous once the silicone oil has been implanted.

Steroid therapy is controversial. There is no consensus on the use of steroids in post-traumatic endophthalmitis. Treatment of the infection with antibiotics, especially in Gram-negative organisms, leads to the release of endotoxins which can exacerbate the ocular damage. Corticosteroids may be beneficial to control inflammation and infection-related tissue injuries [63].

13.12 Severe Traumatic Eyes with No Light Perception

When a severe trauma, in particular an open globe one, results in the loss of light perception, it is well established that the treatment gives a poor outcome (Fig. 13.6).

In the ocular trauma score (OTS), 74% of patients with no light perception after open globe injury were irreversible. Painful bulbar phthisis and sympathetic ophthalmia in the other eye may also arise.

Most ophthalmologists agree that the primary management of traumatic eye with open globe and blindness should be to repair rather than enucleation or evisceration. The reasons are as follows: the assessment of blindness is a subjective measure and may be affected by psychological status; loss of light perception may be caused by severe optic media opacity, optic nerve injury by optic canal fracture, massive chorioretinal or suprachoroidal hemorrhage, ophthalmic artery occlusion, or central retinal artery occlusion; severe vitreous hemorrhage can block the light. The loss of light perception after open globe injury may be transient. Salehi-Had reported that in 88 cases with open globe injury and the presenting vision was NLP, 23 (26.1%) spontaneously recover to at least light perception after primary repair.

For the prevention of sympathetic ophthalmia, enucleation is traditionally recommended, within 2 weeks from the trauma. Actually, its incidence is very low, and most patients can still retain good vision with proper treatment, corticosteroid, and immunomodulators.

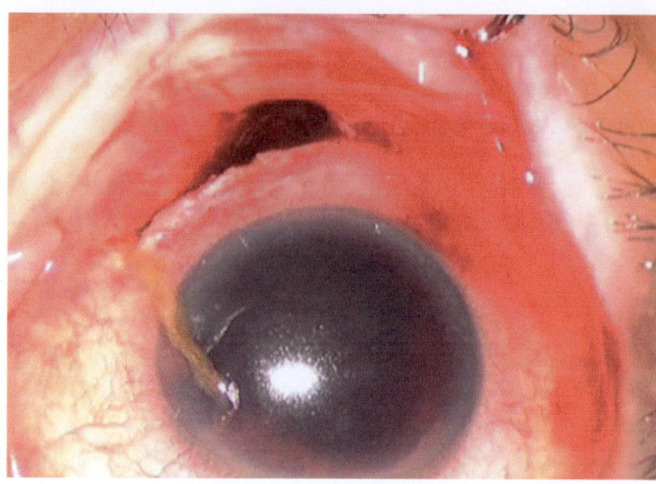

Fig. 13.6 Open globe injury with zone 2 rupture of the eyeball and prolapse of internal tissue of the eye

The surgical technique of severely traumatized eyes may be challenging, long, and complex, with anterior and posterior segment techniques combined (i.e., penetrating keratoplasty, cataract extraction, and vitrectomy with retinal reattachment); however, 23–88.9% of patients regained light perception after vitreoretinal surgery, and up to 33.4% of the patients could gain vision equal or better than 1/10 Snellen visual acuity [4, 64–72].

Case Scenario

A 36-year-old male presented with right eye pain immediately after pounding a metal object, having felt a strike in the orbital region. The vision was normal but a "red line" compared in the upper temporal conjunctiva.

At presentation, the anterior segment was normal with only a subconjunctival hemorrhage, no apparent conjunctival lesions, and negative fluorescein exploration; visual acuity was 20/20. The lens was clear. The ophthalmologist observed the fundus under pupil dilation, revealing the presence of a metallic foreign body lying on the retinal plan, with no other traumatic pathologies. B-scan echography was performed, confirming the presence of the intraocular foreign body.

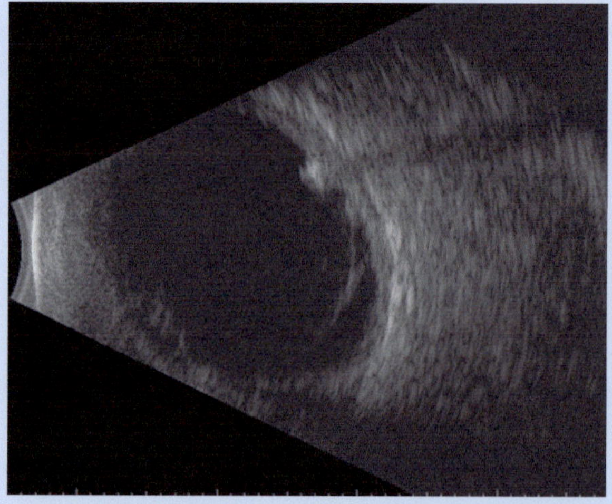

Antibiotic coverage was prescribed, and an emergency surgical exploration was performed. Limbal conjunctival peritomy was performed, revealing a self-sealing scleral full-thickness radial wound, 1 mm long, 2 mm posterior to the limbus. Safety scleral polypropylene suture was applied, and conjunctiva repositioned with fibrin glue.

The patient was strictly observed to detect signs of infection, and 24 h after the first one, 23-gauge vitreoretinal surgery was performed to remove the foreign body (the 10-o'clock sclerotomy needed to be enlarged with removal of the trocar to allow for the foreign body to be extracted by magnetic vitreous forceps). No retinopexy or internal tamponade was necessary, and in the postoperative follow-up, no cataract or ocular infection developed, and vision was restored to 20/20.

Questions

1. Would orbital imaging have been useful in this case?
   A. No
   B. Yes, but no MR if metallic foreign bodies were suspected
   C. Yes, both MR and CT
2. Which are the specific complications of metallic intraocular foreign bodies?
   A. No specific complications
   B. Metallosis, due to toxicity of the IOFB, arousing in a few days
   C. Metallosis, arousing after at least 2 weeks

Please see Chap. 58 for the correct answer.

References

1. Kuhn F, Morris R, Witherspoon CD, Heimann K, Jeffers JB, Treister G. A standardized classifi cation of ocular trauma. Ophthalmology. 1996;103(2):240–3.
2. Kuhn F. Ocular traumatology. Berlin Heidelberg: Springer; 2008.
3. Bullock JD, Warwar RE. A system for classifying mechanical injuries of the eye (globe). Am J Ophthalmol. 1998;125(4):565–6.
4. Kuhn F, Maisiak R, Mann L, Mester V, Morris R, Witherspoon CD. The ocular trauma score (OTS). Ophthalmol Clin N Am. 2002;15(2):163–5.
5. Boldt HC, Pulido JS, Blodi CF, et al. Rural endophthalmitis. Ophthalmology. 1989;96(12):1722–6.
6. Bai HQ, Yao L, Wang DB, et al. Causes and treatments of traumatic secondary glaucoma. Eur J Ophthalmol. 2009;19(2):201–6.
7. Hamill MB. Corneal and scleral trauma. Ophthalmol Clin N Am. 2002;15:185–94.
8. Liu ML, Chang YS, Tseng SH, et al. Major pediatric ocular trauma in Taiwan. J Pediatr Ophthalmol Strabismus. 2010;47:88–95.
9. Kiire C, Srinivasan S, Stoddart MG. A novel use of fibrin glue in the treatment of a partial thickness corneal laceration. Br J Ophthalmol. 2010;94:810–1.
10. Alio JL, Rodriguez AE, Martinez LM. Bovine pericardium membrane (Tutopatch) combined with solid platelet-rich plasma for the management of perforated corneal ulcers. Cornea. 2013;32:619–24.
11. Said DG, Nubile M, Alomar T, et al. Histologic features of transplanted amniotic membrane: implications for corneal wound healing. Ophthalmology. 2009;116:1287–95.
12. Chan E, Shah AN, O'Brart DP. "Swiss roll" amniotic membrane technique for the management of corneal perforations. Cornea. 2011;30:838–41.
13. Rowsey JJ, Hays JC. Refractive reconstruction for acute eye injuries. Ophthalmic Surg. 1984;15:569–74.
14. Hussin HM, Biswas S, Majid M, et al. A novel technique to treat traumatic corneal perforation in a case of presumed brittle cornea syndrome. Br J Ophthalmol. 2007;91:399.
15. Bhatt PR, Lim LT, Ramaesh K. Therapeutic deep lamellar keratoplasty for corneal perforations. Eye (Lond). 2007;21:1168–73.
16. Jang JH, Chang SD. Tectonic deep anterior lamellar keratoplasty in impending corneal perforation using cryopreserved cornea. Korean J Ophthalmol. 2011;25:132–5.
17. Savino G, Colucci D, Giannico MI, et al. Amniotic membrane transplantation associated with a corneal patch in a paediatric corneal perforation. Acta Ophthalmol. 2010;88:e15–6.
18. Dua HS, King AJ, Joseph A. A new classification of ocular surface burns. Br J Ophthalmol. 2001;85:1379–83.
19. Davis AR, Ali QK, Aclimandos WA, Hunter PA. Topical steroid use in the treatment of ocular alkali burns. Br J Ophthalmol. 1997;81:732–4. [PMCID: PMC1722301] [PubMed: 9422923].
20. Sing P, Tyagi M, Kumar Y. Ocular chemical injuries and their management. Oman J Ophthalmol. 2013;6(2):83–6.
21. Siepser SB. The closed chamber slipping suture technique for iris repair. Ann Ophthalmol. 1994;26(3):71–2.
22. Barlow A, Weiner HL. Traumatic iridodialysis; its surgical correction. Arch Ophthalmol. 1945;34:292–4.
23. McCannel MA. A retrievable suture idea for anterior uveal problems. Ophthalmic Surg. 1976;7(2):98–103.
24. Wachler BB, Krueger RR. Double-armed McCannell suture for repair of traumatic iridodialysis. Am J Ophthalmol. 1996;122(1):109–10.
25. Romem M, Singer L. Traumatic aniridia. Br J Ophthalmol. 1973;57(8):613–4.
26. Mester V, Kuhn F. Lens. In: Kuhn F, Pieramici D, editors. Ocular trauma principles and practice. New York: Thieme New York; 2002.
27. McElvanney AM, Talbot EM. Posterior chamber lens implantation combined with pars plana vitrectomy. J Cataract Refract Surg. 1997;23(1):106–10.
28. Chang DF. Single versus three piece acrylic IOLs. Br J Ophthalmol. 2004;88(6):727–8.
29. Rubsamen PE, Irvin WD, McCuen BW 2nd, et al. Primary intraocular lens implantation in the setting of penetrating ocular trauma. Ophthalmology. 1995;102(1):101–7.
30. Holt DG, Young J, Stagg B, Ambati BK. Anterior chamber intraocular lens, sutured posterior chamber intraocular lens, or glued intraocular lens: where do we stand? Curr Opin Ophthalmol. 2012;23(1):62–7.
31. Li J, Yuan G, Ying L, et al. Modified implantation of black diaphragm intraocular lens in traumatic aniridia. J Cataract Refract Surg. 2013;39(6):822–5.
32. Guell JL, Verdaguer P, Elies D, et al. Secondary irisclaw anterior chamber lens implantation in patients with aphakia without capsular support. Br J Ophthalmol. 2014;98(5):658–63.

33. Teng H, Zhang H, Tian F, et al. Artisan iris claw intraocular lens implantation for the correction of aphakia after pars plana vitrectomy. Zhonghua Yan Ke Za Zhi. 2014;50(2):89–94.
34. Por YM, Lavin MJ. Techniques of intraocular lens suspension in the absence of capsular/zonular support. Surv Ophthalmol. 2005;50(5):429–62.
35. Bowman RJ, Yorston D, Wood M, et al. Primary intraocular lens implantation for penetrating lens trauma in Africa. Ophthalmology. 1998;105(9):1770–4.
36. Pavlovic S. Primary intraocular lens implantation during pars plana vitrectomy and intraretinal foreign body removal. Retina. 1999;19(5):430–6.
37. Eckstein M, Vijayalakshmi P, Killedar M, et al. Use of intraocular lenses in children with traumatic cataract in south India. Br J Ophthalmol. 1998;82(8):911–5.
38. Malukiewicz-Wisniewska G, Kaluzny J, Lesiewska-Junk H, Eliks I. Intraocular lens implantation in children and youth. J Pediatr Ophthalmol Strabismus. 1999;36(3):129–33.
39. Nihalani BR, VanderVeen DK. Technological advances in pediatric cataract surgery. Semin Ophthalmol. 2010;25(5–6):271.
40. Cardillo JA, Stout JT, LaBree L, Azen SP, Omphroy L, Cui JZ, Kimura H, Hinton DR, Ryan SJ. Post-traumatic proliferative vitreoretinopathy. The epidemiologic profile, onset, risk factors, and visual outcome. Ophthalmology. 1997;104:1166–73.
41. May DR, Kuhn FP, Morris RE, et al. The epidemiology of serious eye injuries from the United States Eye Injury Registry. Graefes Arch Clin Exp Ophthalmol. 2000;238:153–7.
42. Adesanya OO, Dawkins DM. Intraorbital wooden foreign body (IOFB): mimicking air on CT. Emerg Radiol. 2007;14:45–9.
43. Rubinstein A, Riddell CE, Kafi l-Hussain N, et al. Self-inserted intraorbital foreign bodies. Ophthal Plast Reconstr Surg. 2005;21:156–7.
44. Pinto A, Brunese L, Daniele S, et al. Role of computed tomography in the assessment of intraorbital foreign bodies. Semin Ultrasound CT MR. 2012;33:392–5.
45. Parke DW 3rd, Pathengay A, Flynn HW, et al. Risk factors for endophthalmitis and retinal detachment with retained intraocular foreign bodies. J Ophthalmol. 2012;2012:758526.
46. Affeldt JC, Flynn HW, Forster RK, et al. Microbial endophthalmitis resulting from ocular trauma. Ophthalmology. 1987;94:407–13.
47. Ahmed Y, Schimel AM, Pathengay A, et al. Endophthalmitis following open-globe injuries. Eye. 2012;26:212–7.
48. Parke DW 3rd, Flynn HW Jr, Fisher YL. Management of intraocular foreign bodies: a clinical flight plan. Can J Ophthalmol. 2013;48:8–12.
49. Yeh S, Colyer MH, Weichel ED. Current trends in the management of intraocular foreign bodies. Curr Opin Ophthalmol. 2008;19:225–33.
50. Singh R, Bhalekar S, Dogra MR, Gupta A. 23-gauge vitrectomy with intraocular foreign body removal via the limbus: an alternative approach for select cases. Indian J Ophthalmol. 2014;62:707–10.
51. Huang Z, Chen L, Zeng Y, Lin C. Clinical features of perforating eye injuries complicated with intraocular foreign bodies located at the posterior global wall. Eye Sci. 2013;28:180–4.
52. Reynolds DS, Flynn HW Jr. Endophthalmitis after penetrating ocular trauma. Curr Opin Ophthalmol. 1997;8:32–8.
53. Brinton GS, Topping TM, Hyndiuk RA, Aaberg TM, Reeser FH, Abrams GW. Traumatic endophthalmitis. Arch Ophthalmol. 1984;102:547–50.
54. Affeldt JC, Flynn HW Jr, Forest RK, Mandelbaum S, Clarckson JG, Jarras GD. Microbial endophthalmitis resulting from ocular trauma. Ophthalmology. 1987;94:404–13.
55. Irvine D, Flynn HW Jr, Miller D, Pflugfelder S. Endophthalmitis caused by gram-negative organisms. Arch Ophthalmol. 1992;110:1450–4.
56. Donahue SP, Kowalski RP, Eller AW, DeVaro JM, Jewart BH. Empiric treatment of endophthalmitis; are aminoglycosides necessary? Arch Ophthalmol. 1994;112:45–7.
57. Campochiaro PA, Green WR. Toxicity of intravitreal ceftazidime in primate retina. Arch Ophthalmol. 1992;110:1625–9.
58. Aguilar HE, Meredith TA, Shaarawy A, Kincaid M, Dick J. Vitreous cavity penetration of ceftazidime after intravenous administration. Retina. 1995;15:154–9.
59. Walstad RA, Bilka S, Thurmann-Neilsen E, Halvorsen TB. The penetration of ceftazidime into the inflamed rabbit eye. Scand J Infect Dis. 1987;19:131–5.
60. Karen G, Ahalel A, Bartov E, et al. The intravitreal penetration of orally administered Ciprofloxacin in humans. Invest Ophthalmol Vis Sci. 1991;32:2388–92.
61. Rubenstein E, Goldfarb J, Keren G, Blumenthal M, Triester G. The penetration of gentamicin into the vitreous humor. Invest Ophthalmol Vis Sci. 1983;24:637–9.
62. El-massry A, Meredith TA, Aguilar HE, et al. Aminoglycoside levels in the rabbit vitreal cavity after intravenous administration. Am J Ophthalmol. 1996;122:684–9.
63. Schulman JA, Peyman GA. Intravitreal corticosteroids as an adjunct in the treatment of bacterial and fungal endophthalmitis. A review. Retina. 1992;12:336–40.
64. Agrawal R, et al. Controversies in ocular trauma classification and management: review. Int Ophthalmol. 2013;33(4):435–45.
65. Morris R, Kuhn F, Witherspoon CD. Management of the opaque media eye with no light perception. In: Alfaro III DV, Liggett PE, editors. Vitreoretinal surgery of the injured eye. Philadelphia: Lippincott Raven; 1999. p. 113–24.
66. Abrams GW, Knighton RW. Falsely extinguished bright-flash electroretinogram. Its association with dense vitreous hemorrhage. Arch Ophthalmol. 1982;100(9):1427–9.
67. Salehi-Had H, et al. Visual outcomes of vitreoretinal surgery in eyes with severe open-globe injury presenting with no-light-perception vision. Graefes Arch Clin Exp Ophthalmol. 2009;247(4):477–83.
68. Chan CK, Chhablani J, Freeman WR. Prognostic indicators for no light perception after open-globe injury: eye injury vitrectomy study. Am J Ophthalmol. 2012;153(4):777, author reply 778.
69. Chu DS, Foster CS. Sympathetic ophthalmia. Int Ophthalmol Clin. 2002;42(3):179–85.
70. Albert DM, Diaz-Rohena R. A historical review of sympathetic ophthalmia and its epidemiology. Surv Ophthalmol. 1989;34(1):1–14.
71. Galor A, et al. Sympathetic ophthalmia: incidence of ocular complications and vision loss in the sympathizing eye. Am J Ophthalmol. 2009;148(5):704–10.e2.
72. Heidari E, Taheri N. Surgical treatment of severely traumatized eyes with no light perception. Retina. 2010;30(2):294–9.

Advances in Traumatic Brain Injury Care: A Problem-Solving Approach for a Heterogeneous Syndrome

14

Arturo Chieregato

Key Points

- The day of the injury is probably more important than the subsequent phase because delays and secondary damage must be prevented as far as possible.
- Concepts concerning the care of intracranial pressure can be translated in the emergency phase if intracranial hypertension is suspected.
- In a well-established inclusive trauma system, moderate TBI patients without evolving lesions not always need to be centralized.
- Arterial pressure management should be titrated to the patient's age and extracranial lesions.
- The indications to intracranial pressure monitoring should be personalized on the basis of the heterogeneity of TBI.
- Today in high-income countries, new TBI patients are more frequently elderly.
- Aged patients suffer more frequently focal lesions but benefit from less elevated intracranial pressure. They need good general medical care more than specialized therapies.
- Therapies for refractory intracranial hypertension, before to be applied, must take account of the extent of diffuse axonal injury and focal lesions which could damage brain connectivity.
- Last-tier therapies should be considered in the light of the patient's best interest, expected disability/quality of life, estimated life expectancy, and social sustainability.

A. Chieregato (✉)
Neurorianimazione, ASST Grande Ospedale Metropolitano Niguarda, Milan, Italy
e-mail: arturo.chieregato@ospedaleniguarda.it

14.1 Extra-Hospital Care: Patients with Pupils Dilated and Unreactive to Light

Patients in coma and with pupil abnormalities (dilated and unreactive to light) usually present with a low Glasgow coma scale (GCS) score. While in some cases dilated pupils may be due to direct contusion of the eye (more frequently the injury is monolateral, and the pupil is unreactive to light) or to sympathetic activation (in such case the pupils are bilaterally dilated and reactive), in most of these patients, the dilated unreactive pupil is a sign of transtentorial herniation (TTH) (i.e., an enlarging supratentorial mass or diffuse swelling that displaces the brain downward through the tentorial notch, compromising the midbrain and also the brainstem lower levels). Transtentorial herniation, if left untreated, is associated with brain death; in fact TTH is due to high levels of intracranial pressure (which per se is a cause of global brain ischemia). Furthermore, TTH, for regional effects, causes the compression of the perforators of the midbrain, so leading to intra-axial ischemia. Even the large cerebral conduct arteries (mainly posterior cerebral artery) can be distorted consequently leading to territorial infarct. Although potentially catastrophic, brain herniation is a dynamic process that can be at least temporarily, and sometime definitively, reversed. After intubation, sedation, and ventilation, we can expect the pupils to constrict and become reactive again in some patients. Occult hypercarbia can be solved, or pupil dilatation due to it can be reversed by opioid treatment. However, if at least one pupil remains dilated, unreactive, and insensitive to sedation, with normal ventilation, immediate action to lower suspected intracranial hypertension should be considered [1]. The simplest approach is hyperventilation—raising the rate of mechanical ventilation and, if necessary, even the tidal volume. However, one must always bear in mind that in patients with hemorrhagic shock, ventilation and hyperventilation can induce or worsen hypotension. An alternative, together with or after hyperventilation, is to inject hypertonic saline

P. Aseni et al. (eds.), *Operative Techniques and Recent Advances in Acute Care and Emergency Surgery*,
https://doi.org/10.1007/978-3-319-95114-0_14

(especially in hypotensive patients) or high-dose mannitol (doses >1 g/kg) in a very short time (5 min) [2]. Early follow-up suggests that all these therapies are potentially useful mostly in patients with a mass lesion, to gain time before surgery. The importance of the negative outcome associated with tentorial herniation probably justifies these aggressive therapies, although intracranial hypertension can only be suspected in this phase, but not measured. The severity of the picture and the devastating consequences of brain herniation suggest aggressive management even at the cost of some potential collateral effect.

14.2 Extra-Hospital Care: Intubation

Several studies have failed to show any benefit of extra-hospital intubation. The operator's skill is probably important, just as much as the time needed to get the patient to the trauma center (TC). However, when trials were standardized for severity or randomized, the most severe patients seemed to benefit from extra-hospital intubation done by specialized teams. To improve the efficacy of intubation, it has been suggested to use anesthetic drugs to minimize hypotension (e.g., ketamine, midazolam, and fentanyl). Finally, after having applied at least 5 cm H_2O PEEP, any induced hypotension can be minimized, aiming for normocapnia.

14.3 Extra-Hospital Care: Agitation

Agitation may be the only symptom of TBI when a frontal contusion is developing. This is one of the lessons learned from following patients in the early few hours. The natural history of agitation in some cases reflects also the decline of consciousness in response to the increase in intracranial pressure (ICP) associated with the evolution of intraparenchymal focal lesions. Since neurological monitoring is essential, sedatives like benzodiazepine or propofol are not recommended in these patients subtype because they preclude a neurological evaluation. The drugs of choice are antipsychotics.

14.4 Extra-Hospital Care: Centralization of Patients

Trauma systems differ appreciably between countries. Most regional trauma systems in the United States are based on the "exclusive" design (the trauma center, encouraging direct admission, excludes the other hospital in the same territory). However, this precludes the participation of non-TC acute care facilities in the treatment of less severe trauma patients, so the expertise in these centers can fall below critical levels. By contrast, in Europe, which is more urbanized and has a higher density of hospitals, an "inclusive" model is more frequently adopted, encompassing non-TC hospitals caring chiefly for less severe trauma (level II TC—spokes) [3, 4]. In this system, level I TCs (hubs) play a key role in the trauma system organization. They directly admit the most severe patients and secondarily receive those who were too severe at first admission to a level II TC or who deteriorate after admission to a level II center. The inclusive system is challenging for extra-hospital care because the decision on where to transport the patient has to be taken in the field. Factors like evidence of high-velocity impact, abnormalities in Glasgow coma scale (GCS) score not due to hypotension or hypoxia, external lesion to the scalp with abnormal GCS, multiple injuries (e.g., fractures of the arms and legs or of the spinal column) with external bleeding, or pediatric age suggest direct centralization to the nearest level I TC. At night, and in countries where one cannot always count on helicopter support, a valid option is to transfer the patient to the nearest level II TC able and equipped to stop bleeding. Similarly, patients with isolated alteration of GCS suggesting mild or moderate TBI could be initially admitted to a level II TC spoke (without neurosurgery facilities) where a first computed tomography (CT) can be done and submitted by telemedicine to the hub hospital.

14.5 Secondary Referral to a Trauma Center

Independently from protocols, missing evaluations, or practical reasons (such as poor access), some patients with more complex injuries are frequently admitted from the field to level II TCs without neurosurgery facilities. Examples are polytrauma patients with potentially evolving associated lesions both in the brain as well as outside the brain (e.g., a small temporal extradural hematoma and bleeding from kidney injury). In other cases, patients with an initial GCS suggesting moderate TBI, a first CT scan in the level II TC hospital showing focal lesions (intraparenchymal) or traumatic subarachnoid hemorrhage (e.g., scissural) may suggest the risk of a dangerous progression [5, 6]. Such lesions can evolve in the hemorrhagic core within 48 h, and the surrounding edema can expand in the next few days [7]. Frequently in elderly patients, these findings are associated with medications increasing the risk of progression (e.g., antiplatelet drugs). Depending on the local resources and policy, it may be preferable to centralize these all these subtypes patients. The flexible resources of the level I TC, however, need to be titrated even to a certain rate of over-centralization.

14.6 Management of Moderate TBI in Non-neurosurgical Hospitals

Over-centralization is a form of over-treatment and can reduce the efficiency of the TC for patients who really need acute trauma care. Furthermore, in some patients, for whom the benefit of centralization is questionable, there is also the risk of iatrogenic interventions due to overdiagnosis/overtreatment, which is naturally more probable in the hub center. There is evidence that well-cared-for patients with moderate TBI, mostly elderly, can be followed up remotely by the neurosurgeon and managed in a regular medical ward in a level I TC without neurosurgery facilities, improving the efficiency of the trauma system without affecting the care of the individual patient [8].

14.7 Transport of Patients Secondarily Referred to a Trauma Center

Transport from a peripheral hospital to a TC is still a problem. Medical teams engaged in the interhospital transport are rarely dedicated and involved in continuous quality improvement. Patients centralized who show neurological worsening and/or are scheduled for emergency surgery and/or with CT findings suggestive of intracranial hypertension should probably be intubated, sedated, and ventilated to reduce the progression toward severe intracranial hypertension as well as to reduce the risk of hypoventilation and inhalation. Ambulance or helicopter should be equipped with ECG and an automatic ventilator, syringe pumps, ETCO2, and SpO2 recording equipment.

Continuous infusion of a short-lasting sedative (midazolam, propofol) and opioids (remifentanil, fentanyl) is suggested, while boluses are discouraged because they can induce hypotension and an unstable levels of sedation depth. Initial care and transport of severe patients in whom intracranial hypertension is suspected should not be influenced by the fear of impeding neurological examination, and deep anesthesia should be induced. Delays in intubation or fighting the ventilator or spontaneous breathing after intubation must not be tolerated just to permit neurological evaluation [9]. It is the job of the level I TC to start a neurological examination as soon as possible once mass lesions have been removed and bleeding, hypoxia or hypothermia, and other problem situations have been stabilized.

Even in industrialized countries, health system resources are limited, so hospital networks are one of the possible ways to ensure highly specialized care [10]. To allow that, well-established networks probably will need specialized teams dedicated to inter-hospital transfer to reduce delays and secondary damage potentially associated with transport.

14.8 Admission to the Trauma Center: The Multiple-Injured Patient with Bleeding

The management of patients with combined TBI and bleeding remains difficult. Today a compromise is permissible to achieve acceptable cerebral perfusion without excessively increasing extra-cerebral bleeding. Many experts suggest RBC and fresh frozen plasma support until bleeding is stopped. Otherwise, the restoration of arterial pressure is postponed until the bleeding has been stopped. In the TBI patient, the systolic arterial pressure target should anyway be between 90 and 110 mmHg. The suggested upper levels however may well not be appropriate for an elderly patient, expecially in those who suffer of chronic arterial hypertension.

14.9 Admission to the Trauma Center: Patients Using Anticoagulants or Antiplatelets

Patients using oral coagulants are at high risk of CT evolution and of a worse outcome. For vitamin K antagonist-associated TBI, 3- or 4-factor prothrombin complex concentrates (PCCs) rather than fresh frozen plasma are recommended for patients with INR >1.4. More difficult is the management of new oral anticoagulants, and clinicians are encouraged to keep up to date on this fast-moving field. In patients with novel oral anticoagulant-associated trauma who present within 2 h of ingestion, activated charcoal is recommended. Idarucizumab, a humanized monoclonal antibody fragment against dabigatran (direct thrombin inhibitor), is approved for emergency situations. Administer activated PCC (50 U/kg) or 4-factor PCC (50 U/kg) to TBI patients taking direct thrombin inhibitors if idarucizumab is not available or if the hemorrhage is associated with a direct thrombin inhibitor other than dabigatran. For patients using factor Xa inhibitor, 4-factor PCC or aPCC is preferred over recombinant FVIIa because of the lower risk of adverse thrombotic events.

In patients using antiplatelet drugs, platelet transfusion should not be considered for those who will not need surgery. For TBI patients with aspirin or ADP inhibitor who will require a neurosurgical procedure platelet function testing is recommended before platelet transfusion, and in patients with normal function, no transfusion is needed. If platelet function testing is not readily available, empiric platelet transfusion may be a reasonable decision.

A single dose of desmopressin (DDAVP) (0.4 mcg/kg IV) in TBI patients with hemorrhagic lesions associated with aspirin/COX-1 inhibitors or ADP receptor inhibitors is suggested by experts, though not yet well supported by evidence.

14.10 Admission to the Trauma Center: Neurological Examination of the Multiple-Injured Patient

As already stated above, intubation, deep sedation, analgesia, and muscle paralysis are still suggested during the transport of patients with multiple injuries from the field to the TC and also during the first hours when a CT scan and primary stabilization are done. Except for patients with impending brain herniation and those already directed toward the operating room for emergency craniotomy for mass evacuation, in all other cases, a neurological examination is always advisable [11–13]. The post-stabilization GCS remains useful for prognosis and serves as the initial reference basis for evaluation of the patient and for planning prolonged intubation and whether or not to monitor ICP. Furthermore, some patients arriving intubated and ventilated or with impaired consciousness due to hypoxia and hypotension can have their severity overestimated if a clinical neurological examination is not done. Young patients with diffuse injury may be overestimated as having brain swelling, from only looking at the CT scan, and in these cases, neurological evaluation could be useful to reduce the risk of over-treatment [14]. Similarly, in patients with isolated extradural hematoma (EDH) or subdural hematoma (SDH), the neurological findings, evaluated post their surgical removal, could well be better than expected or better than what can be seen before surgery.

To avoid pain, shivering, and fighting with the ventilator, a baseline infusion of opioids is recommended to facilitate neurological evaluation. Patients with focal injuries (mainly frontal, bifrontal), elderly, or drug-/alcohol-addicted can be frequently agitated, and combative consequently antipsychotic drugs are useful to permit a more reliable neurological evaluation especially once hypnotics are discontinued.

14.11 Admission to the Trauma Center: The Multiple-Injured Patient with Simultaneous Cerebral and Extracerebral Emergencies

Patients with manageable concomitant life-threatening cerebral lesions for whom surgery is indicated (e.g., EDH or SDH) and active bleeding (spleen, liver, pelvis, vascular injury) are not frequent (in our own experience less than 5%). In such cases, however, only prompt diagnosis and intervention can avoid death and minimize secondary cerebral damage. Other factors that can play a critical role are the logistic facilities of the emergency department to reduce the patient's transport and the availability of two surgical teams to operate simultaneously or in a closely coordinated manner on the head and on the source of bleeding. A portable CT scanner, and intrasurgical echography to follow the progression of the mass during craniotomy, can be helpful in conditions when stopping bleeding is priority.

14.12 Primary External Decompression

Primary external decompression is recommended for patients who are expected to achieve a favorable outcome. It is mandatory when brain bulging impedes closure of the dura. However, in cases without this obstacle, it is probably preferable to close the vault with the bone. Then, if there is refractory intracranial hypertension in the next few days, the bone flap can be definitively removed. In fact, external decompression may per se be a source of complications, delaying recovery, and anyway it is always an extra cost for the healthcare system or for the patient [15].

14.13 Indications to Measure Intracranial Pressure

Intracranial pressure (ICP) monitoring is indicated in patients in whom high ICP (HICP) is expected, when this can be considered potentially harmful and when ICP treatments are likely to improve the outcome [16, 17]. However, in some of the most severe patients, even if HICP is expected, monitoring may not be useful either because the treatment is not efficient or because further causes of brain damage (damage in connectivity) preclude an acceptable recovery. For example, patients with GCS 3 with bilateral unreactive pupils and diffuse brain swelling or a not-evacuated mass lesion will probably have HICP, but ICP-guided management is not going to help much.

In patients with diffuse injury without swelling and intraparenchymal lesion and high motor GCS ratings, ICP monitoring can probably be omitted. However, if ICP is measured, the risk of over-treatment due to monitoring-guided therapy must be considered and avoided. In contrast, patients with lesions not immediately evacuated and potentially evolving are, independently from the GCS rating, of potential interest for ICP monitoring. In patients who underwent immediate craniotomy and primary decompression, ICP should be measured because occult HICP can be underestimated and external herniation could damage the brain at the border of the decompression.

14.14 Which Method Is Best for Measuring Intracranial Pressure?

Today the first choice for ICP monitoring is an electronic parenchymal device. Intraventricular drainage can be considered as part of a second level in a staircase ICP protocol if cerebrospinal fluid drainage is likely to lower ICP. However, external ventricular drainage is not without risk for focal hemorrhages during insertion and, more importantly, for ventriculitis.

14.15 The Management of High Intracranial Pressure

There is evidence that in the first few weeks post-injury, mortality is associated with and probably frequently related to intracranial hypertension. However, it is not clear whether there is a relationship between high, sublethal ICP and unfavorable outcomes. ICU care is directed toward minimizing HICP and reducing extracranial complications associated with coma. In the past few years, some RCT [18] and observational studies [19–21] have suggested that strict control of ICP using a personalized protocol seems to give a patient outcome similar to protocols not including ICP measurement. One possible explanation could be that complications due to therapies for intracranial hypertension overwhelmed the potential benefit from ICP control.

There is a general agreement about the staircase approach. As described by Stocchetti (2014) [22, 23], "The level of therapy in patients with raised intracranial pressure is increased step by step, with more aggressive interventions when there is no response. The sequence of interventions may vary among different institutions; every intervention is associated with adverse effects." According to this strategy, the first one uses the therapies with the lowest potential complications, and only once ICP has become refractory to the first-line therapies is it recommended to use hypothermia, barbiturates, and secondary decompression. Before starting a treatment or raising the level of treatment, the physician and team should establish the cause of the ICP elevation—is it reversible, is it really dangerous, and what are the costs of potential side effects of further therapies? ICP fluctuations are normal in TBI patients like in healthy subjects, and compulsive treatment of "abnormal" high ICP is discouraged. For example, "hyperemia waves" [24] have to be partly accepted or treated gently. Conversely, plateau waves [24], which are usually due to exhausted brain compliance, can acutely kill the patient, causing immediate brain herniation. As previously stated, in elderly people brain compliance is higher, and probably the causes of HICP are less likely to induce harmful levels of ICP [25].

14.16 Thresholds for Managing High Intracranial Pressure

Probably the ICP threshold of 20 mmHg is too low, except for patients with temporal lobe hematoma or diencephalic lesions. Today there is an increasing propensity to raise the threshold for treatment (e.g., 25 mmHg) and to tolerate longer-lasting ICP elevation or fluctuation before further raising the therapeutic levels.

14.17 Medical Management

One of the cornerstones in medical management is avoiding oversedation. Once ICP is stable, we recommend reducing or stopping sedation, and titrate it again. Early enteral feeding is now the established best way to support nutrition. Early passive mobilization is also one of the milestones for preventing pulmonary complications. For infections, some centers prefer immediate short-term antibiotic prophylaxis against early pneumonia due to common sensitive pathogens, while other centers opt for a wait-and-see strategy [15] combined with procalcitonin determination. Though there is considerable variability among centers, there is a tendency toward early tracheostomy as it can reduce the length of stay and the severity of pneumonia. Once aggressive therapies like hypothermia and barbiturates are employed, early tracheostomy can probably help reduce the associated medical complications.

Fever is a frequent problem in ICU care and is a cause of HICP. In the last decade, we have observed the spread of low-dose diclofenac infusion, which has the advantage of the low cumulative doses (reducing renal and gastric complications) and the weak impact on arterial pressure, thanks to the continuous infusion [26].

Glycemic control has now resettled at a higher level (150–200 g/L) than before. Tight control can put the patient at risk of disastrous episodes of hypoglycemia. Furthermore, there is evidence of an obstacle to glucose diffusion from the capillaries to the cells in penumbra areas (e.g., ischemic tissue potentially destined for infarction but not yet irreversibly injured) [27]. This could make the neurons more sensitive to lower-to-normal glucose levels, affecting their viability.

14.18 Not Only ICP but CPP Too

Besides ICP, cerebral perfusion pressure (CPP) is another target for management. The main factor is deciding on the "naturally" appropriate CPP. Here one has to consider aging and the severity of previous arterial hypertension. Young patients have physiologically low pressure, so their CPP end point could be accepted as 40–60 mmHg, depending on their age; 60–70 mmHg should be right for a normal adult, and above 70 but below 90 mmHg for older or hypertensive patients. A bedside check of the ICP/CPP relationship can help detect passive/active patterns to estimate cerebral autoregulation and brain compliance. Patients with pericontusional areas could be at a higher risk of regional cerebral blood flow dropping because of the deranged microcirculation, and in such cases, CPP should be more tightly controlled [28].

14.19 Indications for Secondary Decompression

Indications for secondary decompression are still under investigation [29, 30]. As just a very rudimental approach, for patients in whom intracranial hypertension is associated with diffuse multiple lesions [31, 32] or who have lesions in areas more involved in the brain connectivity [33], it is probably opportune to recall that decompression saves lives but increases the risk of vegetative state or lower severe disability. Conversely, in patients in whom a focal lesion, and its associated edema, is the main cause of refractory HICP, secondary decompression should be indicated because a disability due to a focal deficit could leave a more acceptable outcome [34].

14.20 Indications for MRI at the Beginning of the Acute Phase

In patients in whom CT scans show diffuse brain injury, an MRI is recommended during the acute phase. For these subtype of patients, besides the neurological examination, MRI can be helpful for planning early management (sedation schedule or long recovery, waiting for extubation or early tracheostomy, giving family more information). MRI may be useful even for patients in whom there is the suspicion of lesion(s) due to severe and diffuse axonal injury potentially affecting connectivity. In fact in such patients, therapies for refractory HICP could potentially warrant survival but not an acceptable quality of life.

14.21 Indications for MRI at the End of the Acute Phase

In most patients, an MRI at the end of the acute phase will also be useful to predict defects in neurological function and help plan the most appropriate rehabilitation. The mapping of the location and extent of focal lesions (T2 flair) could help the prediction of motor impairment or language deficits. The discrimination of the type of edema surrounding the intraparenchymal lesions by means of diffusion MRI could help to detect vasogenic edema, which could be potentially reversible. This latter knowledge could help to reduce the risk of self-fulfilling negative prophecy concerning patient disability. Conversely, diffusion tensor imaging (DTI) could help to predict, in the next few months after trauma, the extent of any eventual damage of connectivity and therefore to plan a cognitive, in addition to a motor one, rehabilitation plan.

Finally, there is growing evidence which suggests that even patients with mild TBI can be affected by diffuse axonal injuries. This perspective is not infrequently perceived enough due to the frequently elevated high GCS and the initial negative CT scan. With the aim to miminize any underestimation, young patients, usually victims of high-speed road traffic accidents, admitted to the ICUs more for the burden of the extracranial lesions, could be considered for MRI even if CT scan was negative. The MRI should be otherwise highly suggested if the CT was positive for thin traumatic subdural hemorrhage or for gliding contusions. The MRI in such patients could be relevant for their future life. Infact, while in next months after injury, most of them are usually concentrated on further surgical procedure (e.g., orthopedic, maxilla-facial, plastic) and on motor rehabilitation, the under-recognition of subtle damage of brain connectivity can lead to frustrating, even because not expected and explained, handicaps once they return to their normal activity.

14.22 Elderly Patients

Aging is one of the most firmly established, important factors affecting late outcome in TBI patients [25, 35–37]. Elderly patients have a higher frequency of acute SDH subdural hematoma and intraparenchymal lesions, but those who survive the first few days are at less risk of intracranial hypertension, due to their better cranial compliance. The care of these patients can be surgical but even conservative if the lesions do not exert a mass effect. Therefore, the medical care of systemic complications becomes very closely related to the outcome. While death in the ICU is no more frequent than among young people, in the few months after discharge, mortality among elderly patients is high. Nevertheless, aged patients who survive with disabilities (e.g., limited function of arms or legs, speech or language difficulties, loss of thinking ability) may find their quality of life acceptable on account of their different outlook on life, and anyway the expected life span is intrinsically lower. Social and family support is extremely important to foster recovery, and all this information should be recorded in the acute phase to help in the search for the best individual patient plan.

14.23 Young Patients with Severe Brain Damage

In general, young patients are likely to enjoy a definitely better outcome than elderly ones. That encourages clinicians to apply aggressive therapies to control HICP though in fact this is the main cause of death in the ICU. However, frequently HICP is associated with multiple brain lesions, intra-axial brainstem lesions, thalamic lesions, or lesions of the corpus callosum [31, 32] suggesting diffuse axonal injury, which can heavily damage connectivity [33]. This often precludes an acceptable patient outcome. The message is that while doctors can manage even extremely high ICP, this cannot ensure any improvement of structural damage governing connectivity. Thus from a more personal patient-neighbors-social-oriented point of view, the care of young patients with extreme lesions can lead to unacceptable long-lasting disability or a persistent vegetative state.

14.24 After the Acute Phase, One or Two ICUs, One or Two Hospitals, Rehabilitation Outside Acute Hospitals?

Ideally, continuity of care should be ensured in the hospital where the initial acute care was given. Therefore, immediately after discharge from the ICU, patients can be managed in a lower-intensity ward present in the same hospital, and physiotherapy should be rapidly shifted from passive to active. Finally, the physiatrist and cognitive psychologist must be informed of the patient's history, brain damage, and potential for recovery and plan the most cost-effective care individually for each patient as early as possible. However, especially in a hospital that is part of a clinical network, the level I TC can be primarily dedicated to acute care, while the other hospitals can be involved in the long-term care, nearer to patients and the family home. In such cases, it is important for the family's perception, and probably also for the patient's continuity of care, that the ICU and in general these other hospital(s), selected to accept the patients for the transition, should be involved not only in the process of top-down patient allocation but also in a well-established and regularly updated clinical network [10, 38].

14.25 Follow-Up

Every TC should be organized for outpatient follow-up [39]. This organizational model can not only serve for benchmarking across other centers or over the years in the same center but can also boost knowledge of the relationships between anatomo-clinical findings in the acute phase (e.g., GCS, pupils, CT scan, evoked potentials, etc.) and improve prognostic ability. Follow-up means one can observe the consequence of trauma on patients and their families, in terms of quality of life, social integration, and economic consequences. It can also provide useful information for understanding how psychological aspects like post-traumatic stress disorder and resilience develop and evolve. Finally, specific syndromes associated with initial findings and managements can be followed up, for example, post-traumatic hydrocephalus, sunken skin flap syndrome [40], craniocerebral liquoral fistulae, and post-traumatic epilepsy. ICU procedures too can be monitored: the persistence or not of a tracheotomy and its follow-up after removal of the cannula. Features associated with systemic involvement, incidence of multiresistant bacteria, bronchiectasis, corneal lesions, skin ulcers, acquired muscle weakness, CRIMYNE (CRitical Illness MYopathy and NEuropathy) [17], weight loss, hypothalamic insufficiency, acquired arterial hypertension, and acquired chronic renal failure can all be useful sources of feedback for future patients.

Last but not least, the 6–12-month ambulatory clinics, done by the same team involved in the acute phase, could disclose patients who have not been scheduled for an appropriate rehabilitation program. In such cases, the ambulatory visit by the acute hospital could help to recover a new more appropriate rehabilitation process. Finally, follow-up ambulatory clinics are useful to reinforce the confidence and the self-appreciation of physicians, nurses, and all carers involved in the acute phase.

Case Scenario

A 50-year-old female bicycler was admitted to a level II trauma center in a hospital without neurosurgery facilities after an accident with a car. The accident occurred in the daytime. In the field, the GCS was 10 but subsequently improved to 14. At the hospital, a small left temporo-polar extradural hematoma (EDH) was found. A body CT scan showed the left kidney was fractured, with a retroperitoneal hematoma and signs of active bleeding. Systolic arterial pressure was 130 mmHg, and hemoglobin 11.1 g/dL.

The level I TC hub was contacted, and the patient was centralized sedated, intubated and ventilated, and carried by helicopter (overall duration of the trip, 30 min). At the level I TC the brain CT scan was repeated and indicated enlargement of the EDH. Hemoglobin at arrival was 9.7 g/dL and systolic arterial pressure stable. Echography showed the kidney hematoma was enlarged too. The patient underwent combined surgery with two surgical teams, one on the kidney (nephrectomy) and one for the brain (EDH evacuation).

On day 4 post-injury, the patient was transferred to a regular ward, with no appreciable neurological deficits.

1. Was it appropriate to admit the patient to the level II trauma center?

A. No, because initial GCS was 10 (correct)
B. Yes
C. No, because it was a high energy impact
D. No, because initial GCS was low and the energy impact was high

Only the team who managed the patient in the field really know her full picture and trauma scenario, but it seems evident that direct centralization to a level I TC was justified.

2. The level II trauma center had the surgical resources to operate the kidney. Do you believe the transfer was appropriate with active bleeding?

A. Yes, because two lesions were in potential evolution (correct).
B. No, because to deal with the bleeding should be more important for survival.
C. Angiography preferred before transfer.
D. Both brain and kidney evolution could be followed in the level II trauma center.

The patient was considered hemodynamically stable, so considering the potential progression of the EDH which could be not be cared for at the level II TC, and the short transfer time, it was preferable to centralize the patient.

3. Was the combined surgical intervention mandatory?

A. Yes, because the EDH was rapidly evolving (correct).
B. No, the hemodynamics were stable, so nephrectomy could be deferred.
C. The nephrectomy should be done first.
D. There is too little information to answer this question.

An expanding mass in the temporal fossa risks inducing sudden tentorial herniation. The rate of progression of the EDH was appreciable, and the patient was not properly evaluable (intubated and ventilated).

Please see Chap. 58 for the correct answer.

References

1. Stocchetti N, Maas AI, Chieregato A, van der Plas AA. Hyperventilation in head injury: a review. Chest. 2005;127(5):1812–27. Review. PubMed PMID: 15888864.
2. Chieregato A, Venditto A, Russo E, Martino C, Bini G. Aggressive medical management of acute traumatic subdural hematomas before emergency craniotomy in patients presenting with bilateral unreactive pupils. A cohort study. Acta Neurochir (Wien). 2017; https://doi.org/10.1007/s00701-017-3190-4. PubMed PMID: 28435989.
3. Chiara O, Cimbanassi S. Organized trauma care: does volume matter and do trauma centers save lives? Curr Opin Crit Care. 2003;9(6):510–4. Review. PubMed PMID: 14639071.
4. Chieregato A, Volpi A, Gordini G, Ventura C, Barozzi M, Caspani MLR, Fabbri A, Ferrari AM, Ferri E, Giugni A, Marino M, Martino C, Pizzamiglio M, Ravaldini M, Russo E, Trabucco L, Trombetti S, De Palma R. How health service delivery guides the allocation of major trauma patients in the intensive care units of the inclusive (hub and spoke) trauma system of the Emilia Romagna Region (Italy). A cross-sectional study. BMJ Open. 2017;7(9):e016415. https://doi.org/10.1136/bmjopen-2017-016415. PubMed PMID: 28965094; PubMed Central PMCID: PMC5640142.
5. Chieregato A, Fainardi E, Morselli-Labate AM, Antonelli V, Compagnone C, Targa L, Kraus J, Servadei F. Factors associated with neurological outcome and lesion progression in traumatic subarachnoid hemorrhage patients. Neurosurgery. 2005;56(4):671–80; discussion 671–80. PubMed PMID: 15792505.
6. Fainardi E, Chieregato A, Antonelli V, Fagioli L, Servadei F. Time course of CT evolution in traumatic subarachnoid haemorrhage: a study of 141 patients. Acta Neurochir (Wien). 2004;146(3):257–63; discussion 263. PubMed PMID: 15015048.
7. Servadei F, Murray GD, Penny K, Teasdale GM, Dearden M, Iannotti F, Lapierre F, Maas AJ, Karimi A, Ohman J, Persson L, Stocchetti N, Trojanowski T, Unterberg A. The value of the "worst" computed tomographic scan in clinical studies of moderate and severe head injury. European Brain Injury Consortium. Neurosurgery. 2000;46(1):70–5; discussion 75–7. PubMed PMID: 10626937.
8. Fabbri A, Servadei F, Marchesini G, Stein SC, Vandelli A. Observational approach to subjects with mild-to-moderate head injury and initial non-neurosurgical lesions. J Neurol Neurosurg Psychiatry. 2008;79(10):1180–5. PubMed PMID: 18356255.
9. Chieregato A, Martino C, Pransani V, Nori G, Russo E, Noto A, Simini B. Classification of a traumatic brain injury: the Glasgow Coma scale is not enough. Acta Anaesthesiol Scand. 2010;54(6):696–702. https://doi.org/10.1111/j.1399-6576.2010.02234.x. PubMed PMID: 20397980.
10. Suntharalingam G, Handy J, Walsh A. Regionalisation of critical care: can we sustain an intensive care unit in every hospital? Anaesthesia. 2014;69(10):1069–73. https://doi.org/10.1111/anae.12810. Erratum in: Anaesthesia. 2014;69(11):1298. PubMed PMID: 25204233.
11. Sharshar T, Citerio G, Andrews PJ, Chieregato A, Latronico N, Menon DK, Puybasset L, Sandroni C, Stevens RD. Neurological examination of critically ill patients: a pragmatic approach. Report of an ESICM expert panel. Intensive Care Med. 2014;40(4):484–95. https://doi.org/10.1007/s00134-014-3214-y. PubMed PMID: 24522878.
12. Menon DK, Schwab K, Wright DW, Maas AI. Demographics and Clinical Assessment Working Group of the International and Interagency Initiative toward Common Data Elements for Research on Traumatic Brain Injury and Psychological Health. Position statement: definition of traumatic brain injury. Arch Phys Med Rehabil. 2010;91(11):1637–40. https://doi.org/10.1016/j.apmr.2010.05.017. Review. PubMed PMID: 21044706.
13. Saatman KE, Duhaime AC, Bullock R, Maas AI, Valadka A, Manley GT, Team WS, Members AP. Classification of traumatic brain injury for targeted therapies. J Neurotrauma. 2008;25(7):719–38. PubMed PMID: 18627252; PubMed Central PMCID: PMC2721779.
14. Stocchetti N, Pagan F, Calappi E, Canavesi K, Beretta L, Citerio G, Cormio M, Colombo A. Inaccurate early assessment of neurological severity in head injury. J Neurotrauma. 2004;21(9):1131–40. PubMed PMID: 15453984.
15. Chieregato A, Malacarne P, Cocciolo F, Ravaldini M, Russo E, Viaggi B, Giardino M, Rossi C, Simini B, Bertolini G. Aggressive versus conservative antibiotic use to prevent and treat ventilator-associated pneumonia in patients with severe traumatic brain injury: comparison of two case series. Minerva Anesthesiol. 2017;83(6):553–62. https://doi.org/10.23736/S0375-9393.17.11068-0. PubMed PMID: 28275224.
16. Stocchetti N, Picetti E, Berardino M, Buki A, Chesnut RM, Fountas KN, Horn P, Hutchinson PJ, Iaccarino C, Kolias AG, Koskinen LO, Latronico N, Maas AI, Payen JF, Rosenthal G, Sahuquillo J, Signoretti S, Soustiel JF, Servadei F. Clinical applications of

intracranial pressure monitoring in traumatic brain injury: report of the Milan consensus conference. Acta Neurochir (Wien). 2014;156(8):1615–22. https://doi.org/10.1007/s00701-014-2127-4. PubMed PMID: 24849391.

17. Latronico N, Bolton CF. Critical illness polyneuropathy and myopathy: a major cause of muscle weakness and paralysis. Lancet Neurol. 2011;10(10):931–41. https://doi.org/10.1016/S1474-4422(11)70178-8. Review. PubMed PMID: 21939902.
18. Chesnut RM, Temkin N, Carney N, Dikmen S, Rondina C, Videtta W, Petroni G, Lujan S, Pridgeon J, Barber J, Machamer J, Chaddock K, Celix JM, Cherner M, Hendrix T. A trial of intracranial-pressure monitoring in traumatic brain injury. N Engl J Med. 2012;367(26):2471–81. https://doi.org/10.1056/NEJMoa1207363. PubMed PMID: 23234472; PubMed Central PMCID: PMC3565432.
19. Cremer OL, van Dijk GW, van Wensen E, Brekelmans GJ, Moons KG, Leenen LP, Kalkman CJ. Effect of intracranial pressure monitoring and targeted intensive care on functional outcome after severe head injury. Crit Care Med. 2005;33(10):2207–13. PubMed PMID: 16215372.
20. Maas AI, Schouten JW, Stocchetti N, Bullock R, Ghajar J. Questioning the value of intracranial pressure (ICP) monitoring in patients with brain injuries. J Trauma. 2008;65(4):966–7. PubMed PMID: 18849824.
21. Shafi S, Diaz-Arrastia R, Madden C, Gentilello L. Intracranial pressure monitoring in brain-injured patients is associated with worsening of survival. J Trauma. 2008;64(2):335–40. https://doi.org/10.1097/TA.0b013e31815dd017. PubMed PMID 18301195.
22. Stocchetti N, Maas AI. Traumatic intracranial hypertension. N Engl J Med. 2014;370(22):2121–30. https://doi.org/10.1056/NEJMra1208708. Review. PubMed PMID: 24869722.
23. Stocchetti N, Zanaboni C, Colombo A, Citerio G, Beretta L, Ghisoni L, Zanier ER, Canavesi K. Refractory intracranial hypertension and "second-tier" therapies in traumatic brain injury. Intensive Care Med. 2008;34(3):461–7. PubMed PMID: 18066523.
24. Czosnyka M, Smielewski P, Piechnik S, Schmidt EA, Al-Rawi PG, Kirkpatrick PJ, Pickard JD. Hemodynamic characterization of intracranial pressure plateau waves in head-injury patients. J Neurosurg. 1999;91(1):11–9. PubMed PMID: 10389874.
25. Stocchetti N, Paternò R, Citerio G, Beretta L, Colombo A. Traumatic brain injury in an aging population. J Neurotrauma. 2012;29(6):1119–25. https://doi.org/10.1089/neu.2011.1995. PubMed PMID: 22220762.
26. Cormio M, Citerio G. Continuous low dose diclofenac sodium infusion to control fever in neurosurgical critical care. Neurocrit Care. 2007;6(2):82–9. PubMed PMID: 17522789.
27. Magnoni S, Tedesco C, Carbonara M, Pluderi M, Colombo A, Stocchetti N. Relationship between systemic glucose and cerebral glucose is preserved in patients with severe traumatic brain injury, but glucose delivery to the brain may become limited when oxidative metabolism is impaired: implications for glycemic control. Crit Care Med. 2012;40(6):1785–91. https://doi.org/10.1097/CCM.0b013e318246bd45.
28. Nordström CH, Reinstrup P, Xu W, Gärdenfors A, Ungerstedt U. Assessment of the lower limit for cerebral perfusion pressure in severe head injuries by bedside monitoring of regional energy metabolism. Anesthesiology. 2003;98(4):809–14. PubMed PMID: 12657839.
29. Cooper DJ, Rosenfeld JV, Murray L, Arabi YM, Davies AR, D'Urso P, Kossmann T, Ponsford J, Seppelt I, Reilly P, Wolfe R, DECRA Trial Investigators; Australian and New Zealand Intensive Care Society Clinical Trials Group. Decompressive craniectomy in diffuse traumatic brain injury. N Engl J Med. 2011;364(16):1493–502. PubMed PMID: 21434843.
30. Hutchinson PJ, Kolias AG, Timofeev IS, Corteen EA, Czosnyka M, Timothy J, Anderson I, Bulters DO, Belli A, Eynon CA, Wadley J, Mendelow AD, Mitchell PM, Wilson MH, Critchley G, Sahuquillo J, Unterberg A, Servadei F, Teasdale GM, Pickard JD, Menon DK, Murray GD, Kirkpatrick PJ, Collaborators RESCUET. Trial of decompressive craniectomy for traumatic intracranial hypertension. N Engl J Med. 2016;375(12):1119–30. https://doi.org/10.1056/NEJMoa1605215. PubMed PMID:27602507.
31. Adams JH, Jennett B, McLellan DR, Murray LS, Graham DI. The neuropathology of the vegetative state after head injury. J Clin Pathol. 1999;52(11):804–6. PubMed PMID: 10690167; PubMed Central PMCID: PMC501589.
32. Graham DI, Maxwell WL, Adams JH, Jennett B. Novel aspects of the neuropathology of the vegetative state after blunt head injury. Prog Brain Res. 2005;150:445–55. PubMed PMID: 16186041.
33. Sharp DJ, Scott G, Leech R. Network dysfunction after traumatic brain injury. Nat Rev Neurol. 2014;10(3):156–66. https://doi.org/10.1038/nrneurol.2014.15. Review. PubMed PMID: 24514870.
34. Geurts M, Macleod MR, van Thiel GJ, van Gijn J, Kappelle LJ, van der Worp HB. End-of-life decisions in patients with severe acute brain injury. Lancet Neurol. 2014;13(5):515–24. https://doi.org/10.1016/S1474-4422(14)70030-4. Review. PubMed PMID: 24675048.
35. Hukkelhoven CW, Steyerberg EW, Rampen AJ, Farace E, Habbema JD, Marshall LF, Murray GD, Maas AI. Patient age and outcome following severe traumatic brain injury: an analysis of 5600 patients. J Neurosurg. 2003;99(4):666–73. Review. PubMed PMID: 14567601.
36. Stocchetti N, Carbonara M, Citerio G, Ercole A, Skrifvars MB, Smielewski P, Zoerle T, Menon DK. Severe traumatic brain injury: targeted management in the intensive care unit. Lancet Neurol. 2017;16(6):452–64. https://doi.org/10.1016/S1474-4422(17)30118-7. Review. PubMed PMID: 28504109.
37. Maas AI, Stocchetti N, Bullock R. Moderate and severe traumatic brain injury in adults. Lancet Neurol. 2008;7(8):728–41. Review. PubMed PMID: 18635021.
38. Chieregato A, Paci G, Portolani L, Ravaldini M, Fabbri C, Martino C, Russo E, Simini B. Satisfaction of patients' next of kin in a 'Hub & Spoke' ICU network. Anaesthesia. 2014;69(10):1117–26. https://doi.org/10.1111/anae.12806. PubMed PMID: 25204238.
39. Stocchetti N, Zanier ER. Chronic impact of traumatic brain injury on outcome and quality of life: a narrative review. Crit Care. 2016;20(1):148. https://doi.org/10.1186/s13054-016-1318-1. Review. PubMed PMID: 27323708; PubMed Central PMCID: PMC4915181.
40. Chieregato A. The syndrome of the sunken skin flap: a neglected potentially reversible phenomenon affecting recovery after decompressive craniotomy. Intensive Care Med. 2006;32(10):1668–9. PubMed PMID: 16917776.

Emergent Management of Neck Trauma

15

Benjamin D. Nicholson, Ron Medzon, and Niels K. Rathlev

Key Points

- Vertebral artery injuries are commonly associated with cervical spine fractures. Have a low threshold to do vascular studies in patients with c-spine fractures.
- CT angiography is the study of choice to rule out vascular traumatic injury.
- CT is the study of choice to rule out c-spine fractures. Plain films are not sensitive enough.
- CTA is a sensitive test for disruption of the airway in penetrating trauma. A negative test with high clinical suspicion requires bronchoscopy.
- CT is sensitive for penetrating esophageal injuries. A negative test with high clinical suspicion requires a gastrografin swallow study and/or esophagoscopy.
- CTA is the diagnostic test of choice in the stable penetrating neck-injured patient. Zone 2 injuries no longer require immediate surgical exploration.
- The cervical collar may be removed to manage trauma to the neck in gunshot wounds to the neck without neurological signs. Follow-up c-spine CT is recommended, as stable c-spine fractures may be present.
- Strangulation can cause tracheal and vascular injuries even without a fall. Keep a low threshold for CTA in these cases.

15.1 Introduction

Members of the trauma team must be prepared to recognize and evaluate traumatic injuries to the neck during the initial evaluation of a trauma patient and intervene to decisively manage these potentially life-threatening injuries. Often, the approach begins with consideration of the mechanism involved in the traumatic event, and injuries associated with the mechanism are anticipated. The same approach will be followed in this chapter, and each injury mechanism section will then consider injuries grouped by the three main components of the neck: aerodigestive, vascular, and spinal. Airway injuries require a high index of suspicion and prompt management in all trauma patients. However, the anatomic distortions that accompany severe neck trauma require providers to proceed in an organized and stepwise process potentially through the entire range of airway adjuncts to ensure the ultimate goal of oxygenation and ventilation. Esophageal injuries are not easily evaluated during the initial trauma survey but must be identified early, as delays beyond 24 h are associated with significant increase in mortality [1]. Arterial and venous injuries have both immediate and long-term associated morbidity and mortality and may require advanced imaging to evaluate, prognose, and plan interventions. Active hemorrhage from the neck must be managed in the initial trauma resuscitation as patients are bridged to definitive surgical or interventional radiology approaches to achieving hemostasis. High spinal cord injuries remain devastating

B. D. Nicholson
Department of Emergency Medicine, Boston University School of Medicine—Boston Medical Center, Boston, MA, USA
e-mail: Benjamin.nicholson@bmc.org

R. Medzon (✉)
Department of Emergency Medicine, Solomont Center for Clinical Simulation and Nursing Education, Boston University School of Medicine—Boston Medical Center, Boston, MA, USA
e-mail: ron.medzon@bmc.org

N. K. Rathlev
Department of Emergency Medicine, University of Massachusetts Medical School-Baystate and Baystate Health, Worcester, MA, USA
e-mail: Niels.Rathlev@baystatehealth.org

P. Aseni et al. (eds.), *Operative Techniques and Recent Advances in Acute Care and Emergency Surgery*,
https://doi.org/10.1007/978-3-319-95114-0_15

injuries. Patients with an unstable cervical spine must be identified and efforts undertaken to prevent additional spinal cord injury.

15.2 Blunt Injuries

15.2.1 Blunt Aerodigestive Injuries

15.2.1.1 Epidemiology

Blunt aerodigestive trauma remains rare. A large review of 11,663 blunt trauma patients only identified 40 (0.34%) cases of laryngotracheal trauma and 9 (0.08%) cases of esophageal injury [2]. Other large reviews have found incidences closer to 1% [3]. As a result, providers must remain vigilant as many injuries present subtly without evidence of overt injury.

Motor vehicle collisions are thought to be one of the more common blunt mechanisms of aerodigestive injury. Padded dash syndrome has previously been described prior to the widespread use of seatbelts [4]. In these cases, unrestrained patients involved in a collision would continue forward with their neck hyperextended, striking it on the steering wheel or dashboard. This results in fracture of tracheal rings. The esophagus may also be injured as the hyperextended neck stretches the esophagus and upon collision compresses it between the cervical vertebrae and the trachea, resulting in tears in the muscular wall. Blunt chest trauma in a patient who fully inhales prior to the traumatic event may significantly raise his or her intrathoracic pressure and when this force is transmitted to a closed glottis, resulting in trachea rupture. Other common mechanisms include direct blows during athletic events such as hockey pucks or balls propelled at high velocities. Assaults with fists, feet, or objects may also focus kinetic energy on the trachea.

Clothesline injuries are a unique group of injuries that often have devastating consequences. Force is applied as a partially circumferential band that may crush the trachea and cause fractures of the tracheal rings. As the patient continues moving through the wire, often while riding a motorized vehicle, the wire will be dragged up the neck and over the head. This may result in distraction injury particularly when it reaches the mandible and hyperextends the neck [5].

15.2.1.2 Clinical Presentation

Establishing the mechanism of injury through a thorough history, either from the patient or emergency medical services providers, is paramount to the initial evaluation of a patient with neck trauma. Blunt traumatic injuries to the aerodigestive tract range from benign injuries requiring brief observation to significant distortion of the trachea with airway compromise. Esophageal injuries often present subtly and may be easily missed. Delay in recognition of these injuries results significantly in increased mortality [1].

Prompt evaluation of the airway following blunt neck trauma is paramount. Signs and symptoms vary greatly and relate to the degree of injury and the location. Partial transection of the trachea creates a one-way valve during spontaneous respirations and allows air to exit through the defect into the surrounding subcutaneous tissue. If the defect is small enough or the surrounding tissue adherent, there may be limited difficulty for the patient to spontaneously breathe. Patients who have been intubated in the prehospital environment prior to imaging must be met with particular caution as case reports have identified endotracheal tubes in the mediastinum, soft tissue of the neck, and the esophagus. Post-intubation, providers may miss injuries because the endotracheal tube has crossed the defect, and the patient ventilates easily without significant leak. Greene and Stark evaluated cervical tracheal injuries and identified a relationship between the injury being above or below the glottis and the associated signs of injury. Those injured above the glottis had changes in voice, difficulty swallowing, subcutaneous air, and progressive obstruction of the airway. In contrast, injuries below the glottis had signs of more lower airway injury including persistent air leak from chest tubes or endotracheal tubes and hemoptysis [6]. The increasing use of anticoagulants in the outpatient setting has led to rare cases of delayed airway compromise due to expanding neck hematomas after minor neck injury [7].

Esophageal injuries are easily missed as the focus is on the airway during the initial evaluation. Gastric tubes are often blindly placed in the emergency department prior to imaging, and later finding the tube outside of the gastrointestinal tract may be the first evidence of an injury. Therefore, a high index of suspicion based on the mechanism and associated injuries including complete transection of the trachea or posterior wall disruption of the trachea should raise suspicion for an esophageal injury. Blood return from the gastric tube is neither sensitive nor specific but should raise concern in the right clinical context. Pain with swallowing and chest pain are also early symptoms. The eponym Hamman's sign refers to the auscultation of crepitus or a popping sound that changes throughout the cardiac cycle classically as a result of mediastinal emphysema [8].

15.2.1.3 Diagnostic Evaluation

High-resolution computed tomography (CT) imaging has radically changed the approach to the evaluation of blunt neck trauma and is now the standard in the initial evaluation of blunt neck trauma. Figure 15.1 outlines the diagnostic pathway for these patients. CT imaging has largely supplanted the use of plain films, though significant aerodigestive injuries can be diagnosed with lateral soft tissue neck X-rays [9]. Chest X-ray during the initial trauma room evaluation may raise suspicion for an aerodigestive injury when there is evidence of pneumomediastinum or pneumothorax

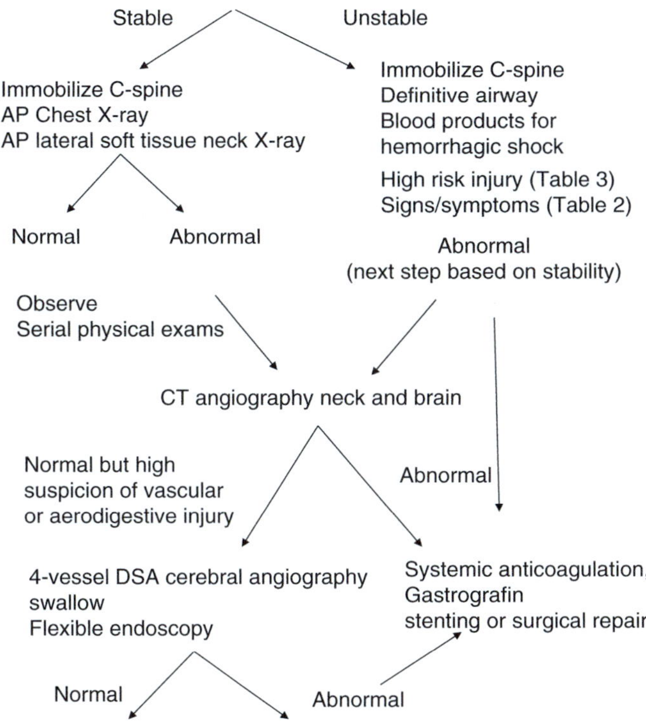

Fig. 15.1 Diagnostic evaluation of blunt neck trauma

without overlying chest injury. However, for hemodynamically stable patients, CT imaging remains paramount and guides decisions about operative repair.

Chen and colleagues investigated the accuracy of CT in the evaluation of tracheal rupture utilizing a cadaver model and trauma room patient controls. With a sensitivity of 85% for the detection of tracheal injury, including directly visualizing the tracheal injury in 71% of cases, the authors concluded that CT was a useful modality for screening trauma patients with pneumomediastinum and selecting those patients who should undergo early bronchoscopy [10]. Moriwaki et al. found that adding three-dimensional reconstruction to the CT evaluation of tracheal injuries was useful and accurately identified the location of injuries seen on bronchoscopy [11]. Airway patency and the need for emergent intubation often dictate the ability to adequately perform direct evaluation of the upper airway. In patients who do not require urgent intubation, fiber-optic nasopharyngoscopy remains useful for evaluating vocal cord function and the extent of injury to the upper airway. In conjunction with the upper airway evaluation, bronchoscopy should be considered to evaluate the subglottic larynx. Table 15.1 reviews a proposed management strategy system for laryngeal injuries which Schaefer and Brown developed based on CT imaging and endoscopy [12].

Imaging modalities to evaluate the esophagus include direct visualization with esophagoscopy and indirect methods that utilize an ionizing imaging study with a contrast agent, generally gastrografin. Computed tomography remains a valuable tool in the initial evaluation of these patients and aids in the detection of associated injuries including disruption of the posterior trachea. Such injuries should significantly raise the concern for esophageal injury and additional studies should be performed even when screening studies are negative.

15.2.2 Blunt Vascular Injuries

15.2.2.1 Epidemiology

Blunt vascular injuries (BVI) of the neck are identified in 0.24–1% of all major blunt trauma patients [13–17]. Motor vehicle collisions and motorcycle crashes are noted to be particularly common mechanisms of injury for BVI. Falls, pedestrians struck by a vehicle, and assaults are also commonly identified mechanisms [17–19]. These injuries remain devastating with a reported 28–40% mortality in some studies and 80% morbidity in those patients identified after neurologic symptoms develop [20, 21].

Blunt vascular injuries result from stretching of the vessel and disruption of the vessel wall. These tears are thought to occur after the vessel is stretched beyond its elastic capacity, through either a hyperflexion, hyperextension, or rotational force. Direct blows may result in vessel disruption, but the mechanism is again likely related to local stretching of the vessel beyond its capacity to deform. Partial tears of the intima expose the thrombogenic subendothelium and promote the formation of a thrombus [22]. Complete disruption of the vessel is possible and, in the case of carotid artery injury, rapidly fatal. In less severe injuries, thrombus formation that completely occludes a vessel is often not clinically evident due to collateral flow; however, partial thrombus that embolizes will produce a diffuse ischemic stroke. BVI may also lead to pseudoaneurysms, arteriovenous fistula formation, and dissections. Identifying these injuries early remains paramount to reducing morbidity and mortality [21].

15.2.2.2 Clinical Presentation

Trauma team members must identify significant vascular injury early in a patient's hospitalization to avoid serious adverse events. While some patients may present with frank uncontrollable hemorrhage and hemodynamic instability, often there are only subtle clues on the history and physical exam to alert providers to impending instability. So-called hard (Table 15.2) and soft (Table 15.3) signs have been described to both raise clinical suspicion for injury and aid in the decision to take a patient immediately to the operating room. Hard signs describe physical exam findings that indicate a high likelihood of the need for early surgical intervention. Providers should examine a patient for evidence of severe hemorrhage such as pulsatile bleeding or an expanding

Table 15.1 Classification system for laryngeal injuries based on a combination of CT scanning and endoscopy [62]

Group	Symptoms	Signs	Management
1.	Minor airway symptoms	Minor laryngeal hematoma or laceration	Steroids, antibiotics, voice rest, humidification, anti-reflux meds, observation
2.	Compromised airway	Worse edema, hematoma mucosal disruption, non-displaced fractures	Intubation/tracheotomy steroids, antibiotics, pan endoscopy
3.	Compromised airway	Massive edema, large mucosal lacerations	Panendoscopy, open repair with stenting, ±tracheotomy
4.	Compromised airway	More severe than group 3 disruption anterior larynx unstable fracture, 2 or more fracture lines, severe mucosal injury	Panendoscopy, open repair with stenting, tracheotomy
5.	Compromised airway	Complete laryngotracheal separation	Intubation/tracheotomy, pan endoscopy, reconstruction, restoration, or resection with end-to-end anastomosis ±stenting

Shaeffer's approach to management of laryngeal trauma

Table 15.2 Hard signs

Hard signs
Expanding hematoma
Active uncontrollable hemorrhage
Pulsatile hematoma
Airway compromise
Hemorrhagic shock
Neurologic deficit
Massive subcutaneous air

Table 15.3 Soft signs

Soft signs
Hemoptysis
Dyspnea
Voice change
Non-expanding hematoma

hematoma. Pulse deficit, while not sensitive, should be noted if present. Injuries that create flaps of the intimal layer, dissections, or pseudoaneurysms are nonocclusive, and a pulse deficit will not be present. A bruit or thrill raises the concern that a traumatic arteriovenous fistula has developed.

Soft signs are not as predictive of vascular injury as these signs, such as hypotension, shock, non-pulsatile hematoma, are present in many patients without significant vascular injury. Neurologic deficit is also considered a soft sign, and traumatic brain injury must be distinguished from neurologic insult as a result of decreased flow or thromboembolic event due to a vascular injury. When considering neurologic deficits, providers should consider the time course. In the case of thromboembolic events, patients may have no symptoms until minutes to hours after the event and then develop stroke-like symptoms such as aphasia or loss of motor function. Similar delays occur when there is a non-functioning circle of Willis, and a vascular insult results in a low-flow state to a portion of the brain. If this occurs after frank vessel transection, these symptoms will occur early post-injury; however, if it results from expanding thrombus formation, a longer delay to symptom onset can be expected.

History and physical exam alone, prior to the onset of neurologic deficits, are insufficient to definitively rule out blunt cerebrovascular injury [23]. McKevitt et al. found that only 40% of blunt vascular neck injuries were suspected during the initial evaluation [21]. Unfortunately, patients are typically diagnosed with a vascular injury after the onset of neurologic deficits or a stroke [13]. Part of this challenge comes from these patients often not having isolated neck trauma. These concurrent injuries draw the traumatologist's attention away from the neck, and providers attribute the patient's hemodynamic and neurologic state to an injury outside the neck. Further clouding the evaluation, head and major thoracic injuries, both common entities in blunt trauma patients, are associated with a significantly increased risk of blunt cerebrovascular injury [21]. Both the Eastern and Western Trauma Associations of the United States endorse definitive diagnostic testing, even in asymptomatic patients, with any of the high-risk characteristics listed in Table 15.4 [24–27]. With this aggressive approach, Miller and colleagues diagnosed 79% of carotid artery and all vertebral artery injuries prior to the onset of ischemic neurologic deficits [17].

The vast majority of patients with blunt vertebral artery injury have concurrent cervical spine injury. Associated carotid injuries are also common [19]. Miller et al. found that 33% of patients with cervical spine fracture screened for vascular injury had a vertebral artery injury [17]. Transverse foramen fractures may have up to an 88% rate of vertebral artery injury [28]. Unfortunately, many of these studies have slim enrollment due to the overall uncommon nature of these injuries. As a result, rates of injury may be misleading, but overall trends likely hold.

15.2.2.3 Diagnostic Evaluation

The gold standard remains four-vessel biplanar cerebral angiography (FVCA) [20]. It allows providers to detect dissection and pseudoaneurysm formation. Occlusive thrombus and transection are also clearly demonstrated. Prior evaluations of FVCA have found that injuries missed on angiography do not generally require repair, and mortality is exceedingly low in this population [29, 30]. Unfortunately,

Table 15.4 High-risk criteria for blunt cerebrovascular injury (endorsed by both the Eastern and Western Trauma Associations of the United States)

Symptomatic patients
Arterial hemorrhage from the neck, mouth, nose, or ear
Cervical hematoma
Cervical bruit <50 years of age
Focal or lateralizing neurologic deficit (e.g., hemiparesis, transient ischemic attack, Horner's syndrome, vertebrobasilar insufficiency)
Major thoracic trauma
Asymptomatic patients
Severe cervical hyperextension/rotation or hyperflexion
Severe facial trauma including bilateral facial, complex midface LeFort and subcondylar fractures
Basilar skull fracture involving the carotid canal
Blunt head injury with diffuse axonal injury and Glasgow Coma Score <6
Cervical vertebral body or transverse foramen fracture, any fracture at C1–C3 level, subluxation, or ligamentous injury
Near-hanging with cerebral anoxia
Clothesline-type injury or seat belt abrasion with significant cervical pain, swelling, or altered mental status

Table 15.5 Classification system for blunt carotid artery injuries based on the angiographic findings [22]

Injury grade	Findings on imaging
1	Dissection or luminal irregularity with <25% narrowing of lumen
2	Raised intimal flap, intraluminal thrombus, dissection, or intraluminal hematoma with ≥25% narrowing of lumen
3	Pseudoaneurysm
4	Occlusion
5	Transection with active extravasation

Developed by and Biffl and colleagues 1999
Biffl WL, Moore EE, Offner PJ, Brega KE, Franciose RJ, Burch JM. Blunt carotid arterial injuries: implications of a new grading scale. J Trauma. 1999;47(5):845–53

FVCA is not rapidly available, requires special resources and providers, and has associated complications. Table 15.5 outlines a system Biffl and colleagues developed to classify angiographic findings in blunt carotid artery injury [22]. The broad categories remain useful in both predicting outcome and guiding therapy.

Multi-detector CT angiography (CTA) has gained widespread availability and likely performs comparably with FVCA. Eight or greater multi-slice (multi-detector) CTA should be considered the minimum for acceptable images. CTA with four or fewer slice capabilities lacks the required sensitivity and specificity for providers to make sound decisions of its results [20]. Direct comparison of newer CT scanners supports this recommendation with reported sensitivity of 97.7% and specificity of 100% [31]. Other studies have not found such impressive results, but the missed injuries were patients in the low-risk Biffl classification grade 1 [32]. Patients stable enough to undergo initial imaging should have a CTA performed if risk factors and clinical suspicion raise the concern for vascular injury. This approach decreases the time to diagnosis and the rate of stroke compared to the historic approach of screening with FVCA [33]. Limitations with CTA remain and, in some cases, make the images suboptimal or unusable. As expected, this impacts the sensitivity of this screening modality [34]. The limitations of metal fragment artifact are less common than in patients with ballistic injuries, and despite its limitations, this technology remains appealing for the blunt trauma population.

Magnetic resonance angiography (MRA) lacks appreciable added benefit to the screening of blunt neck trauma. Prior studies have found that it lacks sufficient sensitivity and specificity [35]. Given the ever-improving image quality and availability of CTA, the added cost, time, and limited availability of MRA make it a poor study for the evaluation of blunt vascular injuries. Duplex ultrasound is also a poor study for screening and is not recommended [20]. It is limited to evaluating the common and external carotid arteries only. It is highly operator dependent, and injuries with uninterrupted flow (dissection, pseudoaneurysm formation) may be missed. In the era of ever-improving CTA, FVCA, MRA, and duplex ultrasound should be considered secondary modalities.

15.2.3 Blunt Cervical Spine Injuries

The possibility of cervical spine injury must be considered in any multiple trauma patient. Hyperflexion/extension and rotation of the cervical spine precipitate many cord injuries by creating unstable bony and ligamentous injuries. This occurs when the head moves rapidly in a particular direction causing extra stress on the spine. Cervical spine injury should be considered in any blunt injury mechanism, particularly those with concurrent head injuries. Hanging and strangulation will be considered in a separate section.

Plain radiographs lack the sensitivity and specificity necessary to confidently diagnose injuries to the cervical spine. Two primary decision rules, National Emergency X-Radiography Utilization Study (NEXUS) criteria for cervical spine imaging and the Canadian C-Spine Rule, were created to determine which patients are sufficiently low risk for injury that they can be safely evaluated without cervical spine imaging. NEXUS criteria require providers to answer negatively to five questions, listed in Table 15.6 [36]. The Canadian C-Spine Rule was derived as a series of three questions, outlined in Table 15.7 [37]. Both rules have high sensitivities at the expense of limited specificity. Unlike NEXUS, the Canadian C-Spine Rule includes an age cutoff of 65, above which it is not validated. More recent evidence has

Table 15.6 NEXUS criteria [36]

NEXUS (National Emergency X-ray Utilization Study) criteria for clearing the cervical spine without imaging. If none of the findings below are present, a patient may be safely evaluated without cervical spine imaging
1. Midline spinal tenderness
2. Focal neurological deficit
3. Intoxication
4. Distracting injury
5. Focal neurological deficit

Table 15.7 Canadian C-Spine Rule [37]

Exclusion criteria:
1. Age 65 years or older
2. Paresthesias
3. Dangerous mechanism (fall from greater than 3 ft (1 m)/5 stairs, axial load, high-speed motor vehicle collision/rollover/ejection, bicycle collision, motorized recreational vehicle)
Low-risk criteria:
1. Sitting position in the ED
2. Ambulatory at any time
3. Delayed (not immediate onset) neck pain
4. No midline tenderness
5. Simple rear-end motor vehicle collision (MVC), not simple if pushed into traffic, hit by bus/large truck, rollover, hit by high-speed vehicle
At least one low-risk criteria present:
1. Patient is able to rotate head 45° to the left and right
Patients do not require c-spine imaging if they fulfill any one of the low-risk criteria and are able to perform head rotation of 45° to the left and right

questioned the validity of NEXUS application to those over 65 years of age as well, and NEXUS may lack the sensitivity to safely exclude these patients [38]. A more prudent approach given the decreased risk of radiation exposure and resulting malignancy with age is a more liberal approach to imaging in those patients over the age of 65.

In those who fail the decision rule or have concerning high-risk features, the initial imaging modality of choice is CT scan. Unfortunately, concern remains that CT may not effectively rule out patients, and those with persistent pain on palpation or range of motion of the neck must have an MRI to evaluate for ligamentous injury and a potentially unstable cervical spine. Inaba et al. recently challenged this belief with an assessment of patients who failed the NEXUS decision rule and underwent CT scanning. The three patients with clinically important c-spine injuries who were missed on CT scan all had a focal neurologic deficit and may be sensitive enough to rule out injury without the need for further imaging [39]. The Eastern Association for the Surgery of Trauma (EAST) has also recently released a conditional recommendation for the removal of cervical collars after a negative high-quality CT scan in obtunded patients [40]. The data pool for the meta-analysis was low, yet there are no documented negative outcomes in any obtunded trauma patients whose collars were removed after a normal CT. While it may be premature for institutions to change their imaging policy, it would appear that CT of the cervical spine may ultimately be sufficient to clear both trauma patients with persistent pain and no neurological symptoms, as well as obtunded patients with normal scans.

15.3 Penetrating Injuries

15.3.1 Penetrating Aerodigestive Injuries

15.3.1.1 Epidemiology

Penetrating aerodigestive injuries are most commonly the result of gunshot or stab wounds, likely due to gunshot and stab wounds being the most common forms of penetrating trauma. Overall, these wounds remain extremely rare with one large center identifying only 10 cases out of 12,789 consecutive blunt and penetrating trauma patients presenting over 8 years. Most of these patients required emergent operative management [41].

15.3.1.2 Clinical Presentation

Presenting symptoms vary depending on the structures damaged. In patients with disruption of the trachea, change in voice, dyspnea, and progressive deterioration of the airway may occur. Penetrating wounds also result in injury to surrounding vascular structures, and patients with known vascular injury must be carefully observed for expanding hematomas that may progress to airway obstruction. Concurrent vascular and airway injuries may allow communication between the two structures, and patients who survive to the emergency department will have significant hemorrhage into the trachea that is difficult to control prior to the operating room, and these are often nonsurvivable injuries. Hemoptysis was seen rarely in a large review, but its presence in isolated neck injury should raise serious concerns [42].

It is anatomically challenging for patients to have an isolated penetrating injury to the esophagus; however, given its relatively central location, it must be considered in any patient in whom the likely trajectory of the penetrating object crosses the central plane. As with blunt trauma, these injuries must be detected early as delays result in mediastinal infections and significant mortality [43]. Patients going directly to the operating room for exploration may have less morbidity compared with those who undergo exhaustive preoperative evaluation [44]. Greene et al. found odynophagia, severe chest pain, hematemesis, and dysphagia to be sensitive for esophageal injury [6]. The neck should be palpated for crepitance, and plain X-rays of the chest that include the neck should be reviewed for subcutaneous emphysema or evidence of mediastinal free air.

15.3.1.3 Diagnostic Evaluation

Figure 15.2 outlines a diagnostic approach to penetrating neck injuries. Initial evaluation should include a chest X-ray as part of routine imaging during the initial evaluation and resuscitation of a trauma patient. Evidence of subcutaneous free air should alert providers to an aerodigestive injury. While trajectories of penetrating objects are difficult to predict, any patient with an isolated neck injury who is found to have a pneumothorax on screening X-ray should raise significant concern for an aerodigestive injury. Stable patients should undergo further imaging to define injuries and plan operative management. Unstable patients should have their airway secured and aerodigestive injuries evaluated further in the operating room.

The ever-improving image quality and accessibility of CTA make this the preferred initial imaging study. CTA accurately evaluates for disruption of the tracheal wall and allows for surgical planning [10]. The addition of three-dimensional reconstructions further improves visualization of complex injuries. Despite the advancements in CT, bronchoscopy remains the gold standard, and institutional policies should be followed regarding the decision to routinely screen with bronchoscopy. If suspicion remains high after a negative CT, bronchoscopy should be pursued.

Extrapulmonary air is easily identified on CT and is useful in raising suspicion for an esophageal injury, especially when it is found within the mediastinum (Fig. 15.3). Weigelt et al. evaluated the utility of barium swallow and endoscopy in a series of stable patients with penetrating neck trauma and found all cases of esophageal injury were identified when a combination of both modalities was employed [45]. Recently, CT esophagography has emerged as a sensitive and specific screening test that will likely replace barium swallow studies and may significantly reduce the need for flexible or rigid endoscopy. Conradie and Gebremariam reported 95% sensitivity and 85.4 and 91.5% specificity for two independent and blinded radiologists reviewing the studies. False positives were noted when the study was performed concurrently with CTA [46]. While this imaging modality is exciting, enough literature evaluating its sensitivity and specificity is lacking; therefore, providers should obtain a combination of gastrografin swallow and endoscopy if suspicion remains high for esophageal injury despite a negative CT [47].

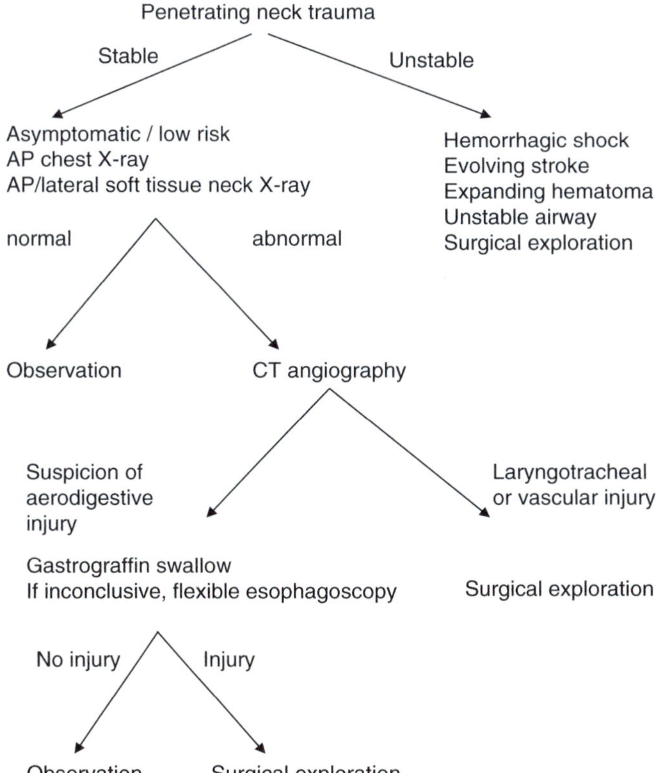

Fig. 15.2 Diagnostic evaluation for penetrating neck trauma

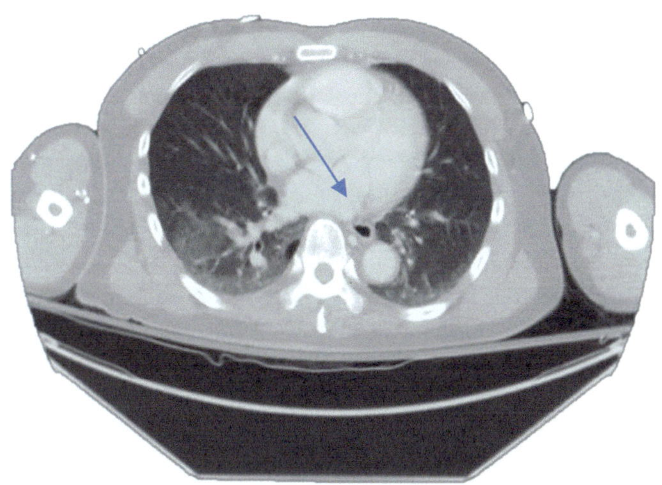

Fig. 15.3 CT image with free air. CT thorax reveals free air in the mediastinum (arrow). Also noted are pulmonary contusions bilaterally posteriorly

15.3.2 Penetrating Vascular Injuries

15.3.2.1 Epidemiology

As with other types of penetrating neck trauma, penetrating vascular injuries are most commonly the result of gunshot and stab wounds. In the civilian environment, these are commonly the result of interpersonal violence and involve handguns in comparison with the military experience involving higher-energy rifles. Mortality has been estimated at 3–6% [48].

15.3.2.2 Clinical Presentation

Vascular injuries resulting from penetrating trauma may be rapidly fatal and must be identified early in a patient's hospital course. The "hard" and "soft" signs discussed in the blunt vascular injury section should be reviewed in all cases of penetrating neck trauma and may assist the clinician in identifying those patients who should undergo additional investigation for a vascular injury (see Tables 15.2 and 15.3). Penetrating injuries vary greatly and may range from injury to the adventitia alone to frank transection with exsanguination. Given the tight confines of the neck, vascular injuries may result in expanding hematomas with compression effects on surrounding structures producing respiratory symptoms (change in voice, tracheal deviation) or neurologic symptoms (cervical plexopathy). Isolated injuries to the neck that produce hemodynamic instability without neurologic symptoms (indicating a high spinal cord injury) should initially be assumed to result from significant injury to the vascular bed. Of special note, isolated jugular injuries often tamponade prior to intervention, and these injuries may not be recognized on initial exam [49].

15.3.2.3 Diagnostic Evaluation

The principles reviewed above in the blunt vascular section generally apply to the approach for the diagnostic evaluation of penetrating injuries. Hemodynamically unstable patients should be taken urgently to the operating theater for neck exploration. Historically, surgical exploration was conducted for all penetrating wounds that violated the platysma in zone 2. As a result of improved imaging modalities and additional techniques for more conservative management of vascular neck injuries, this dogmatic approach is no longer practiced when a selective approach is feasible. While unstable patients still require operative evaluation for a vascular injury, stable patients should first undergo imaging to identify injuries that are amenable to both surgical and nonsurgical techniques.

The widespread availability of CT has allowed clinicians to rapidly image patients. In series of penetrating neck injuries, the sensitivity of CT angiography is 90–100% compared with conventional angiography and surgical exploration [50, 51]. Others have observed that multi-slice helical computed tomography angiography (MCTA) may provide 100% sensitivity for the detection of all vascular and aerodigestive injuries making this an excellent screening test [52]. CT angiography (CTA) evaluates the vessels and provides information about the wound trajectory; the study may raise suspicion for vascular injury when ballistic fragments or the trajectory are within 5 mm of a major vessel [53]. CTA may show frank extravasation of contrast material, pseudoaneurysm formation with evidence of an irregular vessel wall, or occlusion with a lack of contrast visualized distal to the injury.

15.3.3 Penetrating Cervical Spine Injuries

Cervical injuries as a result of penetrating trauma with a normal neurologic exam are unlikely to be unstable. Published reports of patients with an unstable cervical spine due to stab wounds have not been identified, and it remains unlikely that an attacker would have the physical strength necessary to fracture the cervical spine in such a way as to create an unstable injury. Gunshot wounds that create an unstable cervical spine require disruption of the column in two places and must traverse or injure the spinal cord. Medzon and colleagues reviewed 14 years of patient records and found no gunshot wounds to the face or neck that created an unstable cervical spine without neurologic signs on presentation. There were three neurologically intact patients identified who did have stable cervical spine fractures after gunshot wounds to the face [54]. Additionally, a large review of gunshot wounds to the head found no cases of cervical spine injury [55]. Despite these findings, CT scan of the neck remains important during the evaluation of the traumatically injured patient. However, it appears that cervical injuries are rare, and any injury without neurologic deficit is likely stable. Therefore, providers should treat the patient's airway compromise or vascular injury as needed and remove the cervical collar if necessary. Once stabilized or access is no longer needed, the collar should be replaced until CT evaluation of the spine is obtained to ensure no occult fractures exist.

15.4 Strangulation

Strangulation represents a broad range of mechanisms that ultimately result in the application of force around the neck. The injuries that result from strangulation are related to the manner in which the force is applied and the rate of application, the duration of application, and the vector of the force. Commonly encountered strangulation categories include hangings, strangulation with a ligature device, manual choking with hands, and excessive manipulation of the neck as may occur during chiropractor manipulation. Four primary mechanisms of death have been described: carotid body compression with resulting dysrhythmia; obstruction of blood flow into the brain through carotid artery compression; obstruction of blood flow out of the brain resulting in cerebral congestion, loss of consciousness, and either increased pressure against the ligature device obstructing respirations and resulting in asphyxia or prolonged cerebral congestion from continued vascular outflow obstruction and decreased ability to allow blood into the brain resulting in a fatal prolonged fall in the cerebral perfusion pressure; and asphyxiation due to tracheal compression. Jugular venous obstruction takes the least amount of force and is likely the most common. Asphyxiation through tracheal compression requires sufficient force to fracture the trachea. Carotid compression takes more force than jugular compression and is difficult to produce without associated jugular obstruction. Carotid body reflex stimulation rates are difficult to determine [56].

Hangings in which a person falls from a significant distance may cause cervical fractures with spinal cord injuries resulting in apnea, but these are less frequently encountered.

15.4.1 Aerodigestive Injuries

15.4.1.1 Special Considerations in Strangulation

Suspension hangings without an associated fall may result in injury to the pharynx with fractures of the thyroid cartilage being most frequently observed. This risk may increase as the patient ages, likely related to ossification of the thyroid cartilage [57]. A large series failed to find any injury to the cricoid cartilage, and again the injuries were isolated to the thyroid cartilage and hyoid bone [58]. Unlike clothesline injuries that may cause a shearing injury to the trachea, suspension strangulation appears to apply forceful pressure that fractures higher airway structures. This has important clinical implications for those patients who require a surgical airway approach as it makes these patients more amenable to a cricothyroidotomy compared with clothesline injuries in which transection and distraction may result in a complete separation of the upper pharynx from the lower trachea [5].

15.4.2 Vascular Injuries

15.4.2.1 Special Considerations in Strangulation

Patients who present after a suspension hanging may sustain vascular injuries. One series of 175 patients noted 32 (18.3%) with a vascular injury. Injuries were more common on the ipsilateral side of the ligature knot, and the proposed mechanism of injury is traction on the vessel resulting in intimal tears or perivascular hematomas and not a result of direct pressure on the vessel [57]. An additional large review of suspension hangings found tearing of the carotid adventitia in 21.7% of cases, and providers must remain vigilant for these injuries. This review found a low incidence of jugular injuries (2.2%), and it has been hypothesized that this is due to the venous vascular bed having more elastic fibers that allow for greater traction without injury [58].

15.4.3 Cervical Spine Injuries

15.4.3.1 Special Considerations in Strangulation

Cervical spine injuries in strangulation depend greatly on the associated fall. For those patients strangulated without a fall, either in a choke hold or hanged in a standing or seated position, there is decreased risk of cervical spine injury. However, one review of hangings did find three patients with anterior subluxation of C6–C7, but all were over the age of 60, and all had the ligature knot under the mandible in an anterior position, indicating a hyperextension stretching mechanism [57]. Others have noted a low incidence of C2 fractures [58]. Regardless of the cervical level involved, these injuries are relatively infrequent in suspension hangings. In contrast, patients who have fallen from any distance into the ligature may sustain significant spinal injuries.

15.5 Management

15.5.1 Aerodigestive Injuries

Airway injuries necessitate early definitive control of the injured airway with endotracheal intubation being the preferred method. Isolated airway injuries that have been secured can then be taken to the operating room for planned repair. If a cervical collar is in place, particularly in blunt trauma, a second provider should perform in-line cervical stabilization to minimize movement of the cervical spine during laryngoscopy. However, the decision to intubate remains one of clinical judgment. Clear indications include severely altered mental status, inability to protect the upper airway, or expectation that the clinical course likely involves deterioration with failure of the patient's ability to control his or her airway. Patients with severe vascular injury and expanding or large hematoma should raise concern for eventual airway impingement and be managed definitively during the initial resuscitation.

Rapid sequence intubation (RSI) with the use of a sedative and paralytic remains the standard approach. Succinylcholine was studied in patients with a penetrating neck injury and found to be safe and allow a high degree of success. Of the 39 patients who underwent RSI, clinicians had a 100% success rate. Three out of 12 had failure of fiberoptic intubation by otolaryngology but were successfully intubated with RSI [59]. Other paralytic agents including rocuronium and vecuronium are safe and effective agents with the caveat of prolonged duration of action. Sedatives should be selected and dosage given to maintain hemodynamic stability. Etomidate provides rapid onset of sedation and minimal hemodynamic impact.

In patients with significant facial trauma, heavy bleeding into the oropharynx, or distortion of the upper airway anatomy, clinicians should anticipate a difficult airway. It is paramount that clinicians understand and practice alternative methods for securing the airway. In the case of heavy bleeding, the use of constant suction throughout laryngoscopy may improve the view. The head of the bed should remain elevated and not flat as blood will rapidly fill the airway, obscure the view, and fill the lower airway. Clinicians should consider sedative only intubation to allow patients to maintain some protection of their airway. Ketamine provides a dissociative state in which patients continue to breath and is an excellent choice. Fiber-optic intubation and video laryngoscopy are appealing modalities, but blood often obscures the lens and makes visualization impossible. A gum-elastic bougie provides tactile information as it is inserted and should be considered in all patients with airway injury. As it is inserted, it is possible to feel the tracheal rings. When inserted deeply, it will stop at the carina and confirm being in the airway. If it is inadvertently placed in the esophagus, it will continue without interruption, and the tracheal rings will not be felt. The bougie may even allow providers to perform blind intubation through a wound tract when other methods have failed [60].

Tracheal transection presents unique challenges as the endotracheal tube may exist through the defect and enter the surrounding tissue, mediastinum, or in the case of combined tracheal and esophageal injury, it may enter the esophagus distally. These patients are some of the most challenging airway cases, and it is important to emphasize that the goal of airway management during initial resuscitation is to provide oxygenation and ventilation. In cases of failed intubation, the use of supraglottic devices should be considered. While these devices do not provide a secure airway, they may be used to bridge to definitive therapy and provide oxygenation and ventilation as a surgical approach is undertaken.

Ultimately a stepwise approach is necessary, and providers should begin managing each airway with a systematic thoughtful assessment of what backup maneuvers will be utilized if intubation fails. Such a stepwise approach was described in the case of complete tracheal transection and partial esophageal injury that ultimately allowed a child to have an endotracheal tube blindly pass through the proximal esophagus, exit the esophageal defect, and enter the trachea distally through the transection [5]. A surgical airway, either cricothyroidotomy or tracheostomy, is the final approach to airway management. However, in the event of tracheal injury, these techniques may be challenging, and early consultation with otolaryngology should be considered. Concurrent use of methods to maintain oxygenation and ventilation during the surgical procedure will support the best possible neurologic outcome.

15.5.2 Vascular Injuries

Vascular injuries should be managed with the initial goal of achieving hemostasis in any unstable patient. Venous bleeding including the jugular veins may often be managed with ligation. However, if the patient is stable and time allows, primary surgical repair is preferred over graft placement or ligation. Carotid artery injuries should be repaired if possible. In patients with a non-functioning circle of Willis, carotid ligation may result in decreased cerebral blood flow and infarction.

In stable patients who undergo imaging, the degree of injury dictates the approach. Biffl and colleagues described the grading system in Table 15.5 based on angiography findings and proposed treatment strategies [22]. Much of the therapy depends on selective surgical intervention and early anticoagulation. Surgical options include resection, thrombectomy, and vessel ligation. Anticoagulation has reduced both the morbidity and mortality of these injuries [19]. Early detection and anticoagulation of vertebral artery injuries have demonstrated significant improvement in the rate of strokes with Miller et al. finding a 0% incidence of stroke when this approach was taken compared to historic rates of 14% [17]. Endovascular techniques are rapidly advancing and may replace open repair. Continued research and technique mastery are required.

15.5.3 Cervical Spine Injuries

The management of cervical spine injuries depends on prompt recognition and early cervical motion limitation with a rigid cervical collar. While these collars do not prevent movement of the cervical spine, they should be utilized to provide cervical support pending formal surgical means of cervical motion restriction, including placement of a halo vest.

Intubation, both in the emergency department and perioperatively, may require the removal of the cervical collar, but providers should remain vigilant to minimize any extension of the cervical spine and provide in-line traction. Evidence suggests that without manual stabilization, direct laryngoscopy produces 10–11° of head extension during intubation [61]. Patients should be logrolled with a provider manually stabilizing the cervical spine whenever the patient is moved. Alert patients should be engaged throughout their hospitalization as active participants in their care and reminded to limit any movement of their neck.

Case Scenario

A 57-year-old male construction worker falls two floors into the basement of a house onto a concrete surface. It is unclear if he has had loss of consciousness, but on arrival emergency services find him alert and oriented, with an occipital hematoma and stable vital signs. On arrival to the emergency department, he has a cervical collar in place. Vitals are 137/74, heart rate 95, and oxygen saturation of 97% on room air. He is complaining of difficulty breathing. On exam the hematoma is noted as well as a laceration to his chin; breath sounds are symmetric. He has two large-bore IVs placed. Anteroposterior chest X-ray reveals a widened mediastinum. FAST exam is negative.

1. What is the most appropriate next step in the management of this patient?
   A. Intubate prior to further studies to protect his airway.
   B. Cervical spine X-ray in the trauma bay.
   C. CT brain, CT cervical spine, and CT thorax, abdomen, and pelvis.
   D. CT brain, CT cervical spine, CTA neck and thorax, and CT abdomen and pelvis.
2. CT scan reveals free air in the mediastinum. Further evaluation should include:
   A. Esophagoscopy
   B. Bronchoscopy
   C. Immediate intubation
   D. A and B
3. His CT of the cervical spine reveals no fracture of the cervical spine.
   A. If pain persists in the midline, he requires an MRI of the c-spine.
   B. His collar may be removed even if he has midline pain and tenderness.
   C. His collar must remain in place according to EAST guidelines.
   D. Regardless of midline pain, the collar should remain in place and MRI performed.
4. Which of the following physical exam findings, if present, would be considered hard findings concerning for vascular injury?
   A. Hypotension
   B. Pulsatile mass in the neck
   C. Right-sided weakness in the arm and leg
   D. Obvious large hematoma in the anterior neck

Please see Chap. 58 for the correct answer.

References

1. Kaman L, Iqbal J, Kundil B, Kochhar R. Management of esophageal perforation in adults. Gastroenterol Res. 2010;3(6):235–44.
2. Demetriades D, Velmahos GG, Asensio JA. Cervical pharyngoesophageal and laryngotracheal injuries. World J Surg. 2001;25(8):1044–8.
3. Vassiliu P, Baker J, Henderson S, Alo K, Velmahos G, Demetriades D. Aerodigestive injuries of the neck. Am Surg. 2001;67(1):75–9.
4. Butler RM, Moser FH. The padded dash syndrome: blunt trauma to the larynx and trachea. Laryngoscope. 1968;78(7):1172–82.
5. Nicholson B, Dhindsa H, Seay L. Pediatric blunt neck trauma causing esophageal and complete tracheal transection. Prehosp Emerg Care. 2017;21(2):257–62.
6. Greene R, Stark P. Trauma of the larynx and trachea. Radiol Clin North Am. 1978;16(2):309–20.
7. Keogh IJ. Critical airway compromise caused by neck hematoma. Clin Otolaryngol. 2002;27:244–5.
8. Enguidanos L, Pfleiderer A, Smith W, Ramkumar S. Pneumomediastinum secondary to an apparently trivial stab wound to the neck: the value of the Hamman's sign and thorough radiological investigation. Emerg Med J. 2005;22(3):230–1.
9. Spencer JA, Rogers CE, Westaby S. Clinico-radiological correlates in rupture of the major airways. Clin Radiol. 1991;43(6):371–6.
10. Chen JD, Shanmuganathan K, Mirvis SE, et al. Using CT to diagnose tracheal rupture. AJR Am J Roentgenol. 2001;176(5):1273–80.
11. Moriwaki Y, Sugiyama M, Matsuda G, et al. Usefulness of the 3-dimensionally reconstructed computed tomography imaging for diagnosis of the site of tracheal injury (3D-tracheography). World J Surg. 2005;29(1):102–5.
12. Schaefer SD, Brown OE. Selective application of CT in the management of laryngeal trauma. Laryngoscope. 1983;93:1473–5.
13. Fabian TC, Patton JH Jr, Croce MA, et al. Blunt carotid injury: importance of early diagnosis and anticoagulant, vol. 223; 1996. p. 513–25.
14. WL B, Moore EE, Ryu RK, et al. The unrecognized epidemic of blunt carotid arterial injuries: early diagnosis improves neurologic outcome. Ann Surg. 1998;228:462–70.
15. Kerwin AJ, Bynoe RP, Murray J, et al. Screening for blunt carotid and vertebral artery injuries is justified. J Trauma Inj Infect Crit Care. 2001;51:308–14.
16. Rozycki GS, Tremblay L, Feliciano DV, et al. A prospective study for the detection of vascular injury in adult and pediatric patients with cervicothoracic seat belt signs. J Trauma Inj Infect Crit Care. 2002;52:618–24.
17. Miller PR, Fabian TC, Croce MA, et al. Screening for blunt cerebrovascular injuries: analysis of diagnostic modalities and outcomes. Ann Surg. 2002;236:386–95.
18. Biffl WL, Moore EE, Offner PJ, et al. Optimizing screening for blunt cerebrovascular injuries. Am J Surg. 1999;178:517–22.
19. Biffl WL, Moore EE, Elliott JP, et al. The devastating potential of blunt vertebral artery injuries. Ann Surg. 2000;231:672–81.
20. Bromberg WJ, Collier BC, Diebel LN, et al. Blunt cerebrovascular injury practice management guidelines: the Eastern Association for the Surgery of Trauma. J Trauma. 2010;68(2):471–7.
21. McKevitt EC, Kirkpatrick AW, Vertesi L, et al. Blunt vascular neck injuries: diagnosis and outcomes of extracranial vessel injury. J Trauma. 2002;53:472–6.
22. Biffl WL, Moore EE, Offner PJ, et al. Blunt carotid arterial injuries: implications of a new grading scale. J Trauma. 1999;47:845–53.
23. Carrillo EH, Osborne DL, Spain DA, et al. Blunt carotid artery injuries: difficulties with the diagnosis prior to neurologic event. J Trauma Inj Infect Crit Care. 1999;46:1120–5.
24. Franz RW, Willette PA, Wood MJ, et al. A systematic review and meta-analysis of diagnostic screening criteria for blunt cerebrovascular injuries. J Am Coll Surg. 2012;214:313.
25. Burlew CC, Biffl WL, Moore EE, Barnett CC, Johnson JL, Bensard DD. J Trauma Acute Care Surg. 2012;72(2):330–5; discussion 336–7, quiz 539.
26. Biffl WL, Cothren CC, Moore EE, et al. Western Trauma Association critical decisions in trauma: screening for and treatment of blunt cerebrovascular injuries. J Trauma. 2009;67:1150.
27. Mundinger GS, Dorafshar AH, Gilson MM, et al. Blunt-mechanism facial fracture patterns associated with internal carotid artery injuries: recommendations for additional screening criteria based on analysis of 4,398 patients. J Oral Maxillofac Surg. 2013;71:2092.

28. Woodring JH, Lee C, Duncan V. Transverse process fractures of the cervical vertebrae: are they insignificant? J Trauma. 1993;34(6):797–802.
29. Snyder WH, Thal ER, Bridges RA, et al. The validity of normal arteriograms in penetrating trauma. Arch Surg. 1978;113:424.
30. Rathlev NK. Penetrating neck trauma: mandatory versus selective exploration. J Emerg Med. 1990;8:75–8.
31. Eastman AL, Chason DP, Perez CL, Mcanulty AL, Minei JP. Computed tomographic angiography for the diagnosis of blunt cervical vascular injury: is it ready for primetime? J Trauma. 2006;60(5):925–9.
32. Paulus EM, Fabian TC, Savage SA, et al. Blunt cerebrovascular injury screening with 64-channel multidetector computed tomography: more slices finally cut it. J Trauma Acute Care Surg. 2014;76(2):279–83.
33. Eastman AL, Muraliraj V, Sperry JL, Minei JP. CTA-based screening reduces time to diagnosis and stroke rate in blunt cervical vascular injury. J Trauma. 2009;67(3):551–6.
34. Malhotra AK, Camacho M, Ivatury RR, et al. Computed tomographic angiography for the diagnosis of blunt carotid/vertebral artery injury: a note of caution. Ann Surg. 2007;246(4):632–42.
35. Biffl WL, Ray CE Jr, Moore EE, et al. Noninvasive diagnosis of blunt cerebrovascular injuries: a preliminary report. J Trauma. 2002;53:850–6.
36. Hoffman JR, Mower WR, Wolfson AB, Todd KH, Zucker MI. Validity of a set of clinical criteria to rule out injury to the cervical spine in patients with blunt trauma. National Emergency X-Radiography Utilization Study Group. N Engl J Med. 2000;343(2):94–9.
37. Stiell IG, Wells GA, Vandemheen KL, et al. The Canadian C-spine rule for radiography in alert and stable trauma patients. JAMA. 2001;286(15):1841–8.
38. Paykin G, O'Reilly G, Ackland HM, Mitra B. The NEXUS criteria are insufficient to exclude cervical spine fractures in older blunt trauma patients. Injury. 2017;48(5):1020–4.
39. Inaba K, Byerly S, Bush LD, et al. Cervical spinal clearance: a prospective Western Trauma Association Multi-institutional Trial. J Trauma Acute Care Surg. 2016;81(6):1122–30.
40. Patel MB, Humble SS, Cullinane DC, et al. Cervical spine collar clearance in the obtunded adult blunt trauma patient: a systematic review and practice management guideline from the Eastern Association for the Surgery of Trauma. J Trauma Acute Care Surg. 2015;78(2):430–41.
41. Huh J, Milliken JC, Chen JC. Management of tracheobronchial injuries following blunt and penetrating trauma. Am Surg. 1997;63(10):896–9.
42. Kelly JP, Webb WR, Moulder PV, Everson C, Burch BH, Lindsey ES. Management of airway trauma. I: Tracheobronchial injuries. Ann Thorac Surg. 1985;40(6):551–5.
43. Asensio JA, Berne J, Demetriades D, et al. Penetrating esophageal injuries: time interval of safety for preoperative evaluation—how long is safe? J Trauma. 1997;43(2):319–24.
44. Asensio JA, Chahwan S, Forno W, et al. Penetrating esophageal injuries: multicenter study of the American Association for the Surgery of Trauma. J Trauma. 2001;50(2):289–96.
45. Weigelt JA, Thal ER, Snyder WH 3rd. Diagnosis of penetrating cervical esophageal injuries. Am J Surg. 1987;154(6):619–22.
46. Conradie WJ, Gebremariam FA. Can computed tomography esophagography reliably diagnose traumatic penetrating upper digestive tract injuries? Clin Imaging. 2015;39(6):1039–45.
47. Feliciano DV. Penetrating cervical trauma. "Current concepts in penetrating trauma", IATSIC Symposium, International Surgical Society, Helsinki, Finland, August 25-29, 2013. World J Surg. 2015;39(6):1363–72.
48. Burgess CA, Dale OT, Almeyda R, Corbridge RJ. An evidence based review of the assessment and management of penetrating neck trauma. Clin Otolaryngol. 2012;37(1):44–52.
49. Kumar SR, Weaver FA, Yellin AE. Cervical vascular injuries: carotid and jugular venous injuries. Surg Clin North Am. 2001;81(6):1331–44, xii–xiii.
50. LeBlang SD, Nunez DB, Rivas LA, et al. Helical computed tomographic angiography in penetrating neck trauma. Emerg Radiol. 1997;4:200–6.
51. Munera F, Soto JA, Palacio D, et al. Diagnosis of arterial injuries caused by penetrating trauma to the neck: comparison of helical CT angiography and conventional angiography. Radiology. 2000;216:356–62.
52. Inaba K, Munera F, Mckenney M, et al. Prospective evaluation of screening multislice helical computed tomographic angiography in the initial evaluation of penetrating neck injuries. J Trauma. 2006;61(1):144–9.
53. Saito N, Hito R, Burke PA, Sakai O. Imaging of penetrating injuries of the head and neck: current practice at a level I trauma center in the United States. Keio J Med. 2014;63(2):23–33.
54. Medzon R, Rothenhaus T, Bono CM, et al. Stability of the cervical spine after gunshot wounds to the head and neck. Spine. 2005;30(20):2274–9.
55. Lanoix R, Gupta R, Leak L, Pierre J. C-spine injury associated with gunshot wounds to the head: retrospective study and literature review. J Trauma. 2000;49(5):860–3.
56. Hawley DA, Mcclane GE, Strack GB. A review of 300 attempted strangulation cases part III: injuries in fatal cases. J Emerg Med. 2001;21(3):317–22.
57. Nikolic S, Micic J, Atanasijevic T, Djokic V, Djonic D. Analysis of neck injuries in hanging. Am J Forensic Med Pathol. 2003;24(2):179–82.
58. Suárez-Peñaranda JM, Alvarez T, Miguéns X, et al. Characterization of lesions in hanging deaths. J Forensic Sci. 2008;53(3):720–3.
59. Mandavia DP, Qualls S, Rokos I. Emergency airway management in penetrating neck injury. Ann Emerg Med. 2000;35(3):221–5.
60. Steinfeldt J, Bey TA, Rich JM. Use of a gum elastic bougie (GEB) in a zone II penetrating neck trauma: a case report. J Emerg Med. 2003;24(3):267–70.
61. Hastings RH, Vigil AC, Hanna R, Yang BY, Sartoris DJ. Cervical spine movement during laryngoscopy with the Bullard, Macintosh, and Miller laryngoscopes. Anesthesiology. 1995;82(4):859–69.
62. Omakobia E, Micallef A. Approach to the patient with external laryngeal trauma: the Schaefer Classification. Otolaryngol (Sunnyvale). 2016;6:230. https://doi.org/10.4172/2161-119X.1000230.

Vascular Injuries of the Neck

16

Stefano Pirrelli, Pietro Quaretti, Lorenzo Moramarco, Vittorio Arici, Antonio Bozzani, and Riccardo Corti

Key Points

- If direct pressure is unable to minimize significant active bleeding, focused attempts with balloon catheter tamponade may be of benefit.
- Hope for the best, but prepare for the worst: plan for the unexpected, such as the need for emergent, proximal, or distal exposure by including the chest and jaw in the surgical field.
- Obtain a preoperative chest X-ray to evaluate for mediastinal widening, suggesting proximal vascular injury as these may change operative planning in an unstable patient.
- Avoid pressure dressings as a means of temporary vascular control. Temporary vascular control is better achieved with direct digital pressure.
- Jaw dislocation, clavicular head resection, and surgical access to the distal segments of the vertebral arteries are time-consuming and require significant expertise and are unlikely to benefit an unstable, actively bleeding patient. Consider then first catheter-based techniques or balloon tamponade for Zone III lesions.
- Similarly, Zone I lesions can be effectively managed endovascularly.
- A hybrid approach may be the best solution for vascular injury in difficult-to-expose areas and may combine operative or balloon tamponade followed with catheter therapy.

16.1 Background

Vascular injuries of the neck have been historically studied in times of war. The earliest recording of a repair of a vascular trauma was in 1552 when Ambroise Paré ligated both common carotid artery and jugular vein of a soldier causing aphasia and hemiparesis. Later in 1803 John Gibson Fleming successfully ligated the common carotid artery with no negative sequelae.

The neck is a complex anatomical region because in a small space, there are numerous critical aerodigestive, neurological, and vascular structures. Blunt and penetrating trauma to the neck can result in life-threatening injuries that demand immediate attention and intervention. The management of neck trauma requires the expertise of many different specialties including emergency medicine, trauma surgery, interventional radiology, ear, nose, and throat, thoracic, and vascular surgery. A quick diagnosis and prompt treatment are mandatory to reduce mortality and morbidity of these

S. Pirrelli (✉)
Chief Unit of Vascular Surgery, Cardiothoracovascular Department, Asst Mantova, Ospedale Carlo Poma, Mantova, Italy
e-mail: stefano.pirrelli@asst-mantova.it

P. Quaretti · L. Moramarco · R. Corti
Interventional Radiology Unit, Foundation IRCCS Policlinico San Matteo, Pavia, Italy
e-mail: p.quaretti@smatteo.pv.it; l.moramarco@smatteo.pv.it; riccardo.corti01@universitadipavia.it

V. Arici · A. Bozzani
Vascular Surgery Unit, Foundation IRCCS Policlinico San Matteo, Pavia, Italy
e-mail: a.bozzani@smatteo.pv.it

P. Aseni et al. (eds.), *Operative Techniques and Recent Advances in Acute Care and Emergency Surgery*,
https://doi.org/10.1007/978-3-319-95114-0_16

complex injuries. The management of neck injuries has changed dramatically over the last 30 years with modern imaging techniques, from a mandatory exploration of all wounds that penetrated the platysma to an increasingly selective approach. Technological advances in interventional radiology and endovascular procedures allow identification and management of potentially life-threatening injuries while saving many patients from surgery.

16.2 Epidemiology

The frequency, the pathogenic mechanisms, and the severity of vascular trauma of the neck are different in civil or military data. The military database reports that carotid artery injuries represent approximately 5% of all arterial lesions, and the vast majority of these injuries are penetrating, though gunshot wounds were found to be much less common because military weaponry tends to be of high velocity and more likely to be fatal.

The overall incidence of civilian vascular injury from trauma is 1.6% for adults and 0.6% for pediatric patients, which is significantly lower than the 6–12% incidence of combat casualties [1–3]. The civilian traumatic injuries of the neck vessels are relatively uncommon, accounting for 5–10% of all vascular injuries, and are caused mainly by penetrating mechanisms, although the blunt trauma is probably underestimated because related symptoms are often vague and not recognized. The prevalence of vascular injury in the neck is 20% with penetrating trauma and approximately 1% in blunt trauma. The incidence of arterial injury in patients with penetrating neck wounds is 12–13%, while that of venous injury is 18–19% [4–6]. According to the 2009 National Trauma Databank, penetrating neck trauma represented only 1.04% of all injuries reported that year [7]. McConnell and Trunkey combined data from 16 papers from 1963 through 1990 to estimate the frequencies of various kinds of injuries in a total of 2495 patients. According to their findings, aerodigestive tract as a group were the most frequently injured organs, with 10% of the study group having injuries in the larynx or trachea. 9.6% of patients had pharyngeal or esophageal injuries. 9.0% of patients had internal jugular vein injuries. The carotid artery was the most commonly injured artery, with the injury occurring in 6.7% of patients. Interestingly, the spinal cord was injured in only 3.0% of patients in this study. Other less common areas of injury included the subclavian artery (2.2%), vertebral artery (1.3%), brachial plexus (1.9%), cranial nerves 9 and 10 (9%), and the thoracic duct (<0.1%) [8].

Typically, patients with penetrating injuries to the neck vessels are young. Although these lesions are rare, unfortunately, they are characterized by high mortality and morbidity. Mortality is, in most series, between 5 and 40% and is not only caused by massive bleeding but also secondary damage to the aerodigestive tract (e.g., airway compression from a large expanding hematoma). The main cause of morbidity is represented by persistent neurological consequences that are reported in up to 80% of patients. Currently, spinal cord injuries and thrombosis of the common and internal carotid arteries account for 50% of all deaths attributable to blunt and penetrating neck trauma [9]. Decreased transport times and improved prehospital care are resulting in more severely injured patients with significant vascular injury reaching a hospital alive, and the ratio of prehospital to in-hospital deaths has decreased from 1.5 to less than 0.5.

Venous injuries to the internal jugular vein occur in 20% of penetrating neck trauma, and subclavian vein injuries occur in 50% of penetrating subclavian injuries [10, 11].

The cervical vessels are involved in about 25% of patients with blunt head and neck trauma. However, blunt cervical vascular injuries (extracranial carotid and vertebral arteries) have been considered rare with a reported incidence of 0.33–0.45% among patients admitted to trauma centers that aggressively screen for these injuries. The internal carotid artery is involved in more than 90% of the injuries, most commonly its distal parts. The injuries of the vertebral artery are less common (incidence of less than 1%) because they are well protected by osseous structures. Bilateral injuries occur in approximately 15% of all patients [4]. Their incidence is difficult to quantify because many remain asymptomatic, or symptoms may be attributed to the associated injury. They are to be suspected in the case of several cervical hyperextension/rotation or hyperflexion, or near hanging resulting in cerebral anoxia, or the presence of seatbelt abrasion or other soft tissue injury of the anterior neck, or basilar skull fracture, or cervical vertebral body fracture or distraction injury.

Although these injuries are rare, the morbidity and mortality rates are significantly higher than penetrating trauma (20–30%). Besides, 37–58% of patients develop permanent neurologic deficits attributable to central nervous system ischemia.

Blunt venous injuries are extremely rare and should be considered with sternal and clavicle fractures.

16.3 Causes and Mechanisms

In evaluating the injuries of the neck, the mechanism of the trauma must also be carefully considered: blunt versus penetrating, knife versus gunshot wound, and small-caliber gunshot versus high-power gunshot wound.

16.3.1 Penetrating Trauma

The most common mechanism for cervical vascular injuries is penetrating trauma, and the degree of tissue damage is highly dependent on the mechanism and energy of the injury. Thus high-velocity injuries result in greater damage because of the exponentially larger amounts of energy being transmitted to the tissue (velocity is squared). The type of penetrating trauma is most often stab wounds by knives, but other mechanisms are high- or low-velocity projectile and gunshot wounds and bone fragments from fractures. The wounding power of a gun is proportional to the caliber (diameter) of the weapon's muzzle. Firearms are classified by their caliber and muzzle velocity. High-velocity wounds to the head and neck produced by rifles or close-range gunshot blasts produce severe and often fatal damage. A combination of bullet's velocity, as well as the kinetic energy transferred to structures upon entry, causes a devastating shock-wave effect to the surrounding tissues, creating a zone of injury up to 30 times the size of the missile. Low-velocity weapons are responsible for most civilian injuries and include various handguns or pistols. Low-velocity missiles, produced by handguns, long-range birdshots, or buckshots cause limited damage along the projectile path. Brennan et al. reported that significant injury occurred in fewer than 50% of low-energy wounds. The common carotid artery is the most frequently injured major artery (Table 16.1).

The vessel lesion secondary to penetrating trauma is most frequently a laceration, a perforation, or a contusion. The complete transection is less frequent and almost always fatal, except in cases of retraction and thrombosis of the arterial stump, thus alleviating the hemorrhage. A secondary phenomenon to the arterial trauma of the neck is represented by vasospasm that occurs immediately after the injury and may cause a cerebral hypoperfusion. Less frequently penetrating neck trauma can cause arteriovenous fistula or a pseudoaneurysm.

16.3.2 Blunt Trauma

Blunt trauma to the cervical vessels is thought to be less than 0.5% of all blunt traumas of the body, but recent reports indicate that many blunt vascular injuries go undetected.

Common mechanisms of injury associated with blunt trauma include motor vehicle crash (41–70%), direct cervical blow (10–20%), automobile versus pedestrian (12–18%), falls from height (5–15%), and hanging events (5%). Most common associated injuries at the time of diagnosis include closed-head injuries (50–65%), facial fractures (60%), cervical spine fractures (50%), and thoracic injuries (40–51%) [4, 12, 13]. Furthermore, other causes of neck vascular blunt trauma are any athletic endeavor, chiropractic manipulation, visiting the hairdresser, and rapid head turning.

Table 16.1 Site of injury

Major vessels		
Arteries (10–15%)	Common carotid artery	73%
	Internal carotid artery	22%
	External carotid artery	5%
Veins (15–25%)	External jugular	50%
	Internal jugular	50%
Other organs	Digestive tract	5–15%
	Airway	4–12%
	Major nerves	3–8%

Vascular structures are stretched over the cervical spine, and shearing forces create intimal tears in the vessel wall and can cause embolism or dissection and thrombotic occlusion [14]. Other possible consequences are false aneurysm development, complete disruption of the internal carotid at the base of the skull, and the carotid dissection.

Other mechanisms associated with vertebral artery injuries are intraoral trauma, dislocated fractures, and cervical spine trauma. Some 33% of cervical spine fractures are associated with a vertebral artery injury after excluding simple spinous process fractures. Fractures involving the transverse foramen are present in 78% of these patients, whereas subluxation is associated with most of the remaining injuries. At least one of these bony injuries is present in 92% of patients who have vertebral artery injury [15]. Summarily, there are distinguishable three pathogenic mechanisms underlying these vascular lesions:

- Extreme hyperextension and rotation (Fig. 16.1).
- A direct blow to the vessel.
- Vessel trauma by adjacent bone fractures.

16.3.3 Iatrogenic Trauma

Several series have identified major increases in iatrogenic trauma from percutaneous endovascular or endoscopic procedures, accounting for up to half of all vessel injuries in some centers. Iatrogenic arterial injuries are increasingly common and are seen in the context of attempts for central venous access and surgery. Despite training and experience, the installation of such catheters is not risk-free. Inadvertent arterial puncture with a small needle is usually benign and occurs in 5% of cases (0–11%). Much more morbid complications from arterial misplacement of large-caliber cannula have an incidence of 0.1–0.8%. The incidence of arterial puncture is higher with attempted internal jugular versus subclavian access (3% vs. 0.5%) [16]. These complications include hematoma, which can potentially expand and obstruct the airway, hemothorax, pseudoaneurysm, arteriovenous fistula, and stroke [17, 18].

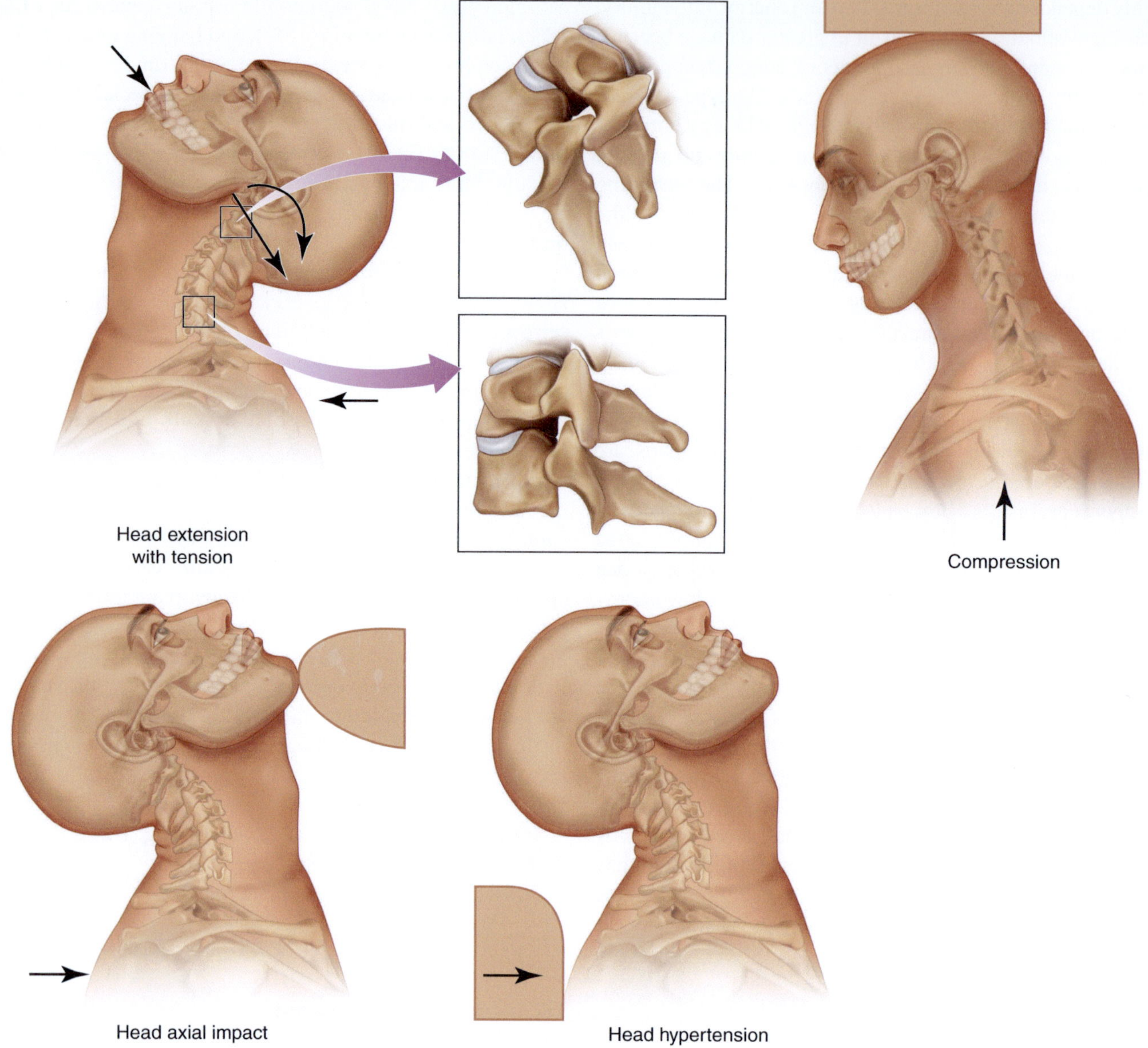

Fig. 16.1 Pathogenic mechanisms of blunt vascular trauma of the neck

16.4 Classification

Monson and colleagues described the most widely accepted anatomic classification of penetrating neck injuries by dividing the neck into three anatomic zones anterior to the sternocleidomastoid muscle [19]:

- Zone I is the area from the cricoid cartilage to the clavicles. It contains the inferior trachea and esophagus and the vessels of the root of the neck: the brachiocephalic trunk, the subclavian arteries, the common carotid arteries, the thyrocervical trunk, and the corresponding veins, as well as the thoracic duct, thyroid gland, and spinal cord.
- Zone II is the area from the cricoid cartilage to the angle of the mandible. It contains the common carotid arteries; the internal and external carotid arteries; the internal jugular veins; the larynx; the hypopharynx; the cranial nerves 10, 11, and 12; and the spinal cord.
- Zone III is the area from the angle of the mandible to the base of the skull. It contains the carotid arteries, the vertebral arteries, the internal jugular veins, the pharynx, multiple cranial nerves, and the spinal cord (Fig. 16.2).

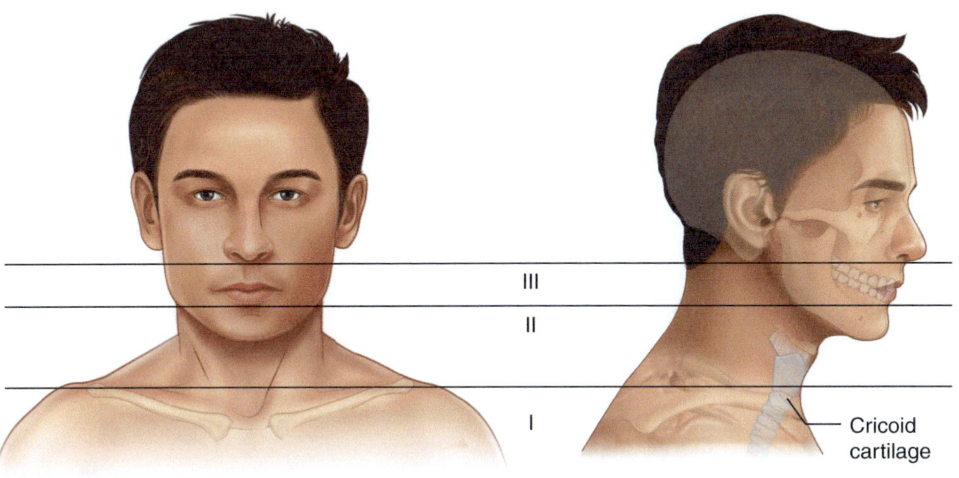

Fig. 16.2 Classical anatomic classification into three zones described by Monson et al. [19]

Table 16.2 Denver grading scale for blunt carotid artery injury

Grade	Angiographic findings	Prognosis	Treatment
I	Vessel wall irregularity or dissection with <25% of luminal diameter	Good, 7% progress	Systemic anticoagulation controversial
II	Raised intimal flap, thrombus, dissection, or hematoma >25% of luminal diameter	Fair with treatment, 70% progress	Systemic anticoagulation
III	Pseudoaneurysm	Requires intervention	Surgery or stenting
IV	Total vessel occlusion	Outcome assured at the time of diagnosis	Systemic anticoagulation
V	Transection	Very poor, high mortality	Surgery

Bell et al. found in a review of their hospital's experience that of injuries penetrating the platysma, 64% were Zone II injuries, whereas 16% and 20% were in zones I and III, respectively [20].

Classically, Zone II injuries that penetrate deep to the platysma have been managed with immediate operative exploration. In contrast, Zone I and III injuries, as a result of their anatomic inaccessibility, have traditionally been evacuated more selectively.

Biffl and colleagues developed a classification system for blunt carotid artery injuries based on the angiographic findings (Table 16.2). The system is successfully used to guide further management [14].

16.5 Diagnosis

The clinical picture is variable, and its expression clearly affects the diagnosis and the latency time for a treatment. In emergency and in subacute phase neurological pictures range from asymptomatic to symptomatic with focal or global signs, coma, or shock states, which impair a neurological evaluation. In cases of external hemorrhage and/or airway compression, the picture is clearly of extreme urgency due to hemodynamic instability and/or acute respiratory failure; the possibility of complementary investigations is nothing as the immediate goal is hemostasis, which can be carried out by compression and therefore, in an emergency, surgically. In such cases the conduct rests solely on timing and decisiveness; the analysis of the topography of the entry orifice (and possibly output), of the anamnestic survey on the dynamics of the event and the nature, and of the trajectory of the injurious agent is fundamental. The clinical presentation can have a broad spectrum of symptoms in correlation with both the intensity of the trauma and the presence of concomitant cranial lesions and the specific pattern of the lesion varying from lesion of one layer (dissection with intramural hematoma), two layers (pseudoaneurysm), to all layers (rupture). Sometimes the signs are more discrete, thus forming a subacute picture with hemodynamic stability. Pathognomonic signs are a pulsating or slow-release hematoma, a bruit, and a central variable neurological deficit (transient or permanent). Even a nearby organ injury is highly evocative. However, even in the absence of such signs, a vascular lesion diagnosis should be made if the reconstruction of the injured agent's path, its nature, and the traumatic event dynamics let him suppose. Such attitudes, for some overemphasis, rest on the rationality that in the case of negative exploration, morbidity is similar to that of patients under observation.

Various typologies of lesions can be detected in vascular neck injuries in correlation with the trauma mechanism: blunt or penetrating. CT, MR, and conventional angiography findings share some common signs such as progressive vessel tapering, occlusion, or the presence of a thrombus or intimal flap. Multiplanar reconstructions and MIPs from CT or MR data sets are mandatory to assess the extent of the lesion better. Arteriovenous fistulas can be seen with either blunt or penetrating trauma and are the result of the dissection or laceration of an artery located near a venous structure [21]. The CT scan gives the possibility to have a four-vessel evaluation in a lesser time. Ultrasound examination also is attractive for the lower invasivity is not used for medicolegal aspects depending on the need to document the lesions with a non-operator dependency and the difficulties in evaluating the vertebral and intracranial vessels. MRI has limited use in trauma patients due to the incompatibility with monitoring equipment, the duration of the exam, and difficult accessibility to the patient. Although digital subtraction angiography (DSA) historically was the preferred method for evaluating patients with possible vascular injuries, it has been largely replaced by CTA due to its speed, noninvasive nature, accuracy, and widespread availability [23]. When compared outright with conventional angiography, CTA was found to have a sensitivity of 90%, a specificity of 100%, and a negative-predictive value of 98% in penetrating trauma. When patients are followed for clinically significant CAI in penetrating trauma, CTA has a sensitivity of 100% [22]. DSA is however preferred in cases in which the hemodynamic instability of the patient requires fast treatment, and the mechanism of trauma suggests a lesion prone to endovascular diagnosis and treatment. In those cases, the angiographic aspects can appear as a progressive narrowing (Case 2 Fi a) or a complete occlusion [24]. Early venous filling and enlargement of draining veins are both worrisome for arteriovenous fistula. The importance of identifying these injuries lies in their prognostic value for the development of cerebrovascular accident (CVA) [25]. Venous injuries are more commonly clinically silent when compared with arterial injuries, and injuries of peripheral branches of the cervical veins are often treated conservatively. Therefore imaging should be focused on the identification of more clinically significant injuries [26].

16.6 Treatment

16.6.1 Historical Perspective

The first case of treatment of a cervical vascular injury is attributed to Ambroise Paré (1510–1590), who ligated the carotid artery and jugular vein of a stabbed French soldier [27]. Since then, ligation remained the unique treatment of open carotid trauma for centuries, and until the WW2, penetrating wounds to the neck were managed conservatively unless in the presence of active life-threatening hemorrhage. In these cases, neck arteries were ligated, with a resulting stroke rate around 30%. Surgical [28, 29] repair was first attempted and shown to be feasible during the Korean conflict: over 11 cases of carotid injuries, 4 were repaired directly or by vein interposition [30]. In 1956 Fogelman et al. reported the first civilian series of 100 cases, which showed the benefit of direct arterial repair in comparison with ligation and the direct relationship to the time between injury and repair [31]. The first attempts to introduce endovascular techniques in vascular trauma of the neck were proposed in the late 1980s [32], and endovascular repair represents up to date the treatment of choice for proximal (Zone I) and distal (Zone III) lesions.

16.6.2 Patient Assessment

The first evaluation should consider the Advanced Trauma Life Support (ATLS) guidelines for the management of penetrating neck injuries. These guidelines establish priorities in diagnostics and treatment of life-threatening injuries [33]. Control of hemorrhage is the major topic after airway management. In several cases, external bleeding can easily be controlled by direct pressure. However, in certain anatomical locations as the base of the skull and behind the clavicle, direct pressure is difficult to achieve. In this situation, the use of a finger or a balloon catheter may be helpful. Blind clamping should be avoided for the potential damage to other structures and because it is rarely effective. Consider that up to 10% of penetrating neck injuries involve the airway: this compromise may be due to direct trauma and large hematoma compressing the airway or airway edema. A pathognomonic sign of airway injury is air bubbling through a neck injury. Precisely, systemic status of the patients (hemodynamic stability) is crucial to decide for immediate treatment or imaging assessment. Initial evaluation must focus on the presence of *hard signs* that are mostly related to vessel injuries and demand immediate intervention: expanding and/or pulsatile hematoma, brisk bleeding, bruit, or thrill. The hard signs are usually associated with pulse deficit and cerebral ischemia with neurological signs or symptoms [34]. Other findings in the absence of "hard signs" can be included among the *soft signs*: hemoptysis/hematemesis, oropharyngeal blood, nonexpanding hematoma, dysphonia/dysphagia, subcutaneous or mediastinal emphysema, and focal neurologic deficits. A more selective approach is mandatory for these patients that can undergo imaging assessment. The Western Trauma Association (WTA) algorithm (Fig. 16.3) for penetrating trauma (2013) recommends a selective approach: patients with hard signs should undergo airway stabilization and tamponade and proceed to operative exploration, and likewise, patients who are symptomatic with Zone II injuries should undergo early operative exploration. In the absence of hard signs or major injury, all Zone I and III

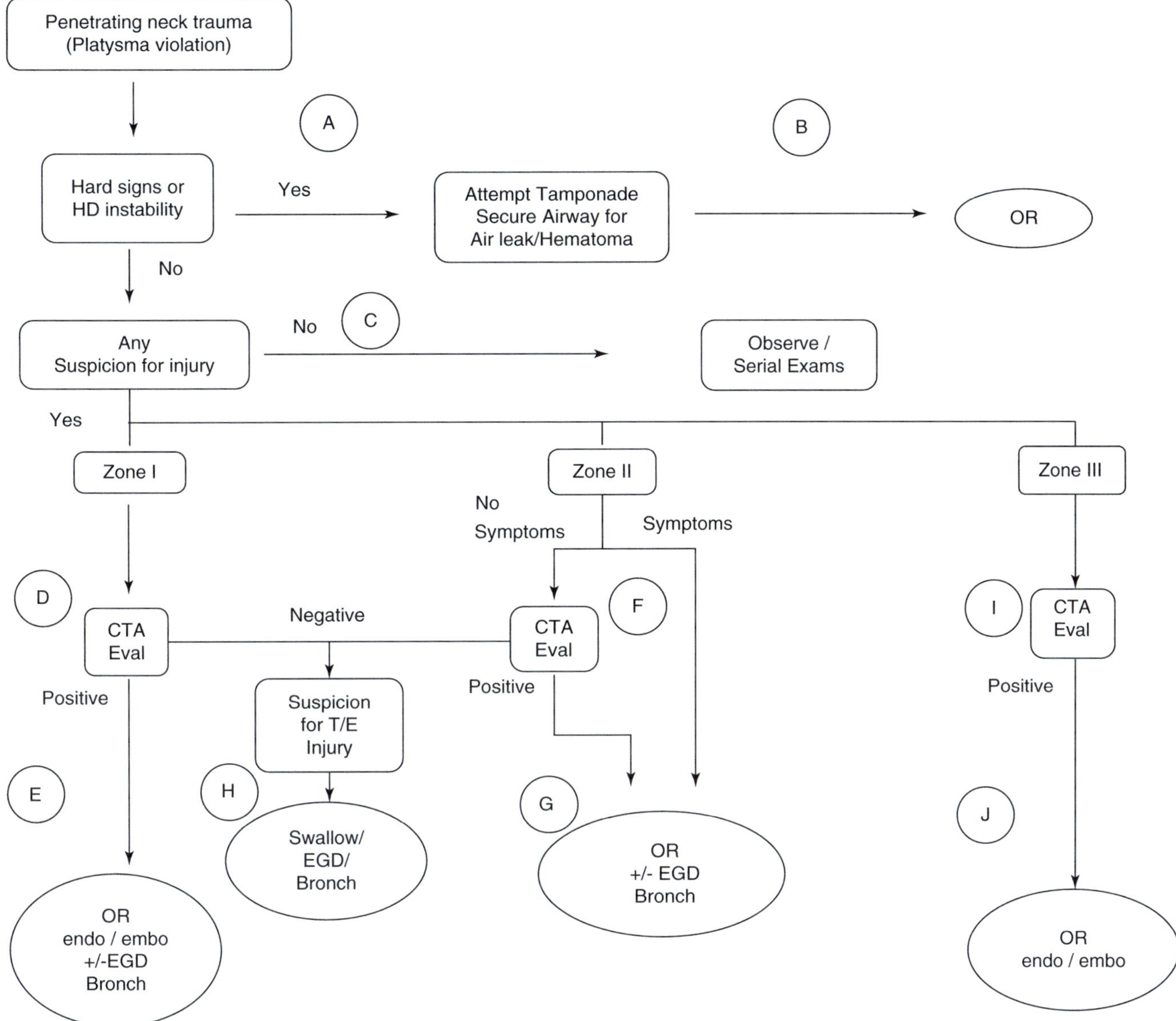

Fig. 16.3 The Western Trauma Association management algorithm for penetrating neck trauma (Sperry et al. [35])

injuries and asymptomatic Zone II injuries should undergo diagnostic imaging [35]. It is important to consider that patients with negative imaging but positive physical examination still need surgical exploration (Table 16.3).

The classical topographic division of the neck is widely accepted for the first assessment of the injury. The neck is divided into three zones: *Zone I* extends from the sternal notch to the cricoid cartilage and includes the thoracic outlet vasculature, proximal carotids and vertebral arteries, the trachea, esophagus, spinal cord, thoracic duct, and cervical nerve trunks. *Zone II* is the largest and therefore the most affected one; it is more accessible and easier to evaluate, thus suitable for simple and fast surgical exposure. It extends from the cricoid cartilage to the angle of the mandible and includes the carotid bifurcation, internal jugular vein, vagus nerve, upper trachea, and the larynx. Eventually, *Zone III* is superior to the angle of the mandible [36].

16.6.3 Surgical Techniques

Emergent surgical exploration is mandatory in the presence of hard clinical signs. While surgical approach in Zone II is relatively easy, Zone III requires mandibular dislocation (with nasal intubation) and possible mastoid fracture, which are time-consuming procedures; in the same way Zone I approach considers clavicular fracture or dislocation and/or sternotomy, equally morbid and time-consuming. In the latter cases, an endovascular approach should be preferable.

Table 16.3 Indications for immediate exploration (hard signs)

Shock	*Systemic*
Unstable vital signs	
Large amount of blood loss	*Hemorrhagic/vascular*
Continued bleeding	
Pulsatile bleed	
Expanding hematoma	
Hemoptysis or hematemesis (severe)	
Bruit	
Absent or diminished pulse	
Hemothorax	
Airway obstruction	*Respiratory*
Air blowing from wound	

16.6.3.1 Preparation

The patient should be placed in a prone position with both arms tucked in if possible. The operative field should include the lower jaw, all the anterior and lateral surfaces of the neck, the supraclavicular fossa, and the entire anterior chest. When cervical spine is cleared preoperatively, a shoulder roll will improve neck extension. The head should be slightly turned to the contralateral side for the standard anterior sternocleidomastoid incision or maintained straight midline if a collar incision is required. The groin and both thighs are prepared and draped for possible saphenous vein harvest. Type of incision is determined by the location of suspected injuries. High Zone III injuries resulting in distal carotid artery lesion can be very problematic in exposure and control: anterior subluxation of the mandible allows to gain only 2 cm.

16.6.3.2 Approach

In Fig. 16.4 the typical incisions are depicted. Neck exploration is typically done through an incision on the anterior border of the sternocleidomastoid. This incision allows rapid exposure and control of the vasculature and can be extended into a sternotomy or laterally on the superior edge of the clavicula if necessary.

A supraclavicular incision may be indicated for exposure of Zone I and can be combined with resection of the head of the clavicle or a trap-door sternotomy to extend exposure toward the mediastinum. If extension is needed proximally, the incision should curve posteriorly toward the mastoid process to avoid damage to the mandibular branch of the facial nerve. The platysma is divided along the same plane as the skin incision exposing the sternocleidomastoid muscle. The vascular sheath underlies the medial border of the sternocleidomastoid. The muscle is retracted laterally exposing the vascular sheath. The omohyoid muscle and facial vein cross the carotid. Dividing them will allow the exposure of the common carotid and its bifurcation. The internal jugular vein, vagus nerve, and carotid artery are all exposed with the same technique. The hypoglossal nerve runs perpendicular to the carotid near the level of the bifurcation and must be preserved to avoid deviation of the tongue toward the ipsilateral side. Unilateral hypoglossal nerve injury may be asymptomatic but can result in difficulty with mastication, speech, and swallowing. Visualization of vascular structures may be difficult in cases of ongoing hemorrhage, and proximal control may require access in the chest. For distal and proximal lesions, placement of Fogarty balloon to provide blood loss control can be lifesaving during surgical isolation maneuvers.

16.6.3.3 Carotid Artery Injury (CAI)

Asensio has reported an incidence of 11–13% CAI for all penetrating neck injuries [37]. According to the literature, the carotid artery segment that is most frequently involved is the common carotid (73%), followed by the internal carotid (22%), and finally the external carotid (5%) [38]. When a common or internal carotid arterial injury is identified by neck exploration, current consensus agrees that primary repair of the artery is preferred to ligation, irrespective of any abnormality in focal preoperative neurologic examination findings [35]. Once proximal and distal control is secured, a Fogarty balloon catheter is carefully passed to remove any thrombus, and both proximal and distal ends are flushed with heparinized saline. The use of 5000 units of heparin systematically is recommended in this type of injuries. A monofilament polypropylene suture 5 or 6–0 size is used with appropriate vascular technique. When possible, primary repair is the best choice, and direct arteriorrhaphy should be attempted. However, in injuries with extensive destruction of the carotid artery, resection of the involved segment should be done followed by reconstruction of the artery. Except for tangential CAI, transected ends of the artery retract, making the repair difficult. For small CAI, interrupted suture is usually possible. Larger laceration requires running suture. Care must be taken to inspect for and repair any intimal flap at this time: this can often be done by incorporating the intimal defect into the suture. Also, care must be taken not to narrow the vessel lumen with the suture; if needed be, vein patch angioplasty is recommended. End-to-end direct anastomosis can be done if there is no sign of tension [39]. Otherwise, the interposition of a saphenous vein graft should be performed. When the saphenous vein is not available, a PTFE graft can be used in order to restore blood flow. Regardless of the size, lesions of the external carotid artery need to be treated once diagnosis is made, as they can rapidly expand and cause stroke, nerve impingement, pain, and cosmetic disfigurement. Surgical exploration with ligation is considered the definitive treatment because hemostasis can be effectively achieved, and the mass effect is promptly resolved by evacuating the hematoma.

16.6.3.4 Vertebral Artery Injury (VAI)

VAIs are uncommon (about from 1 to 7.4%), and usually they are not life-threatening, but associated vascular injuries

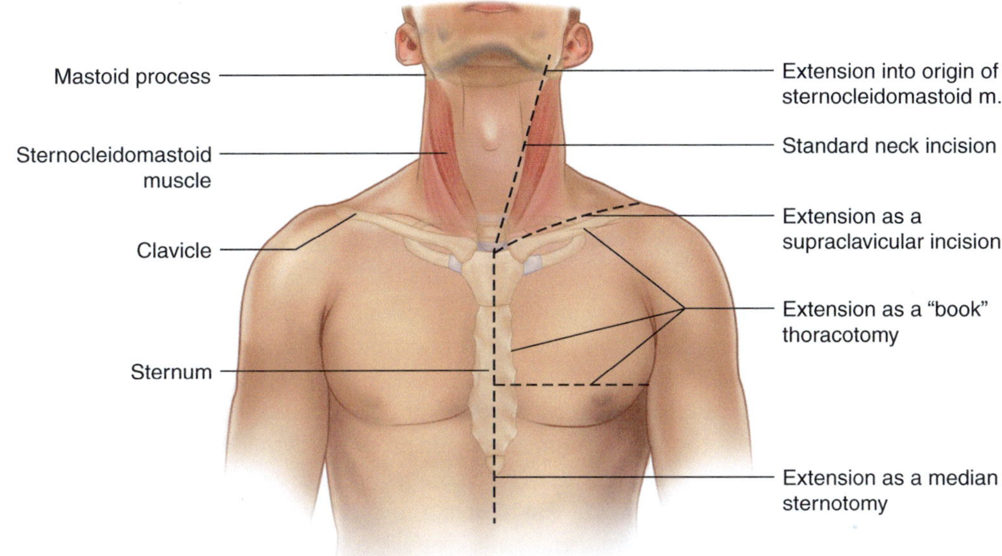

Fig. 16.4 Typical incisions are depicted. Neck exploration is typically done through an incision on the anterior border of the sternocleidomastoid. This incision allows rapid exposure and control of the vasculature and can be extended into a sternotomy or laterally on the superior edge of the clavicula if necessary

occur in a range from 13 to 19% [40]. The management of traumatic VAIs is controversial since no Level I and limited Level II evidence exists to guide treatment. Observation, antithrombotic therapy, endovascular management, and rarely surgery are the treatment options available for these injuries. The most controversial issue of management is the treatment of the asymptomatic casualty with a VAI. Many surgeons believe that these casualties should be treated with aggressive anticoagulation, but no consensus has been reached on the ideal type of therapy (anticoagulation vs. antiplatelet), and recent evidence suggests equivalent effects. The vast majority of VAIs does not require any treatment or are treated with angiography [41]. The surgical management of these injuries is reserved for patients with active bleeding or when endovascular treatment had failed. Proximal vascular control of the vertebral artery can be achieved at the base of the neck where it origins from the subclavian artery through a supraclavicular incision followed by transection of the clavicular attachment of the sternocleidomastoid muscle. By retracting the subclavian vein caudally and the anterior scalene muscle laterally, the vertebral artery can be found in the superior/posterior wall of the ascending subclavian artery. The intertransversarial portion of the vertebral artery is achieved by a standard pre-sternocleidomastoid incision. The *longus colli* muscle is found deep in the neck and should be removed from the bony structures. The anterior arm of one or more vertebral transverse process must be resected to expose the vertebral artery. Vertebral artery injuries can be challenging, and for these difficult-to-access injuries, external bone wax compression can provide temporary control of bleeding, potentially allowing time for definitive surgical control of bleeding or allowing time for endovascular techniques to obtain definitive control of bleeding, if required. Alternatively, proximal ligation at the vessel's origin or insertion of a Fogarty catheter into the proximal vertebral artery for occlusive control may be performed. Exposure of the distal vertebral artery requires subspecialty expertise. The vertebral artery can be safely ligated without major complications. Special care must be taken in order to avoid injury to the nerves. It is important to remark that the preferred approach of these injuries is endovascular for the intricacy of the surgical approach.

16.6.3.5 Vein Injury

Most jugular venous injuries are unrecognized without exploration due to the low-pressure venous system. The majority of jugular venous injuries can be safely managed conservatively. In those with significant hemorrhage or that are found at exploration, ligation can be performed with low risk.

16.6.4 Endovascular Techniques

Endovascular management has become the standard approach for Zones I and III, especially for lesions resulting from blunt trauma. In 1999 Biffl et al. proposed an angiographic classification of carotid and vertebral artery traumatic lesion to guide treatment strategy useful both for blunt and open or iatrogenic trauma (Table 16.4). Grade II and III lesions are best treated endovascularly. Grade IV lesions, in which the vessel is completely occluded, are more challenging for endovascular techniques, because crossing the lesion may be highly time-consuming or impossible. Grade V lesions (transection with extravasation) are rarely treated by the endovascular approach, as those patients are addressed to immediate surgical exploration. Possible techniques are balloon occlusion, embolization, stenting, stent-assisted coil

Table 16.4 Angiographic grading system to stratify lesions and guide treatment strategy [14]

Vascular injury grading system	
Grade I	Intimal irregularity with <25% narrowing
Grade II	Dissection/intramural hematoma with >25% narrowing
Grade III	Pseudoaneurysm
Grade IV	Occlusion
Grade V	Transection with extravasation

embolization, stent grafting, and thrombin injection. Treatment strategy varies with the type of lesion (dissection vs. pseudoaneurysm) and location [42].

Flow-limiting dissection requires invasive treatment due to risk of stroke. The aim is to close the intimal tear and press the flap to the wall, in order to increase true lumen diameter and allow adequate brain perfusion. This can be achieved by placing a stent across the lesion: bare-metal self-expandable stents are the preferred option to treat dissections [43].

Due to its pathophysiology, stent grafting is now the preferred option for the treatment of pseudoaneurysm, because the vessel wall defect can be effectively sealed by the endoprostheses, resulting in complete exclusion and thrombosis of the pseudoaneurysm. Balloon-expandable stents are not suited for the common and extracranial internal carotid arteries because they are subjected to increased external compression, which can lead to strut damage and stent occlusion. The preference is to use covered self-expandable stents, which are more flexible and less likely to be damaged by external compression. The Viabahn™ stent (W. L. Gore and Associates), which is a PTFE-covered nitinol self-expandable stent, shows best results because it is nonporous and avoids type IV endoleak. When treating lesions involving the carotid bifurcation, there is potential risk of pseudoaneurysm refueling through the external carotid artery: coil embolization is advisable to avoid type II endoleak [44]. Postprocedural dual antiplatelet therapy with clopidogrel and close follow-up is recommended to reduce the risk of acute occlusion.

Endovascular management has reached an important role in external carotid artery injury for lesions that are not easily surgically accessible and for cosmetic reasons. Embolization is performed in most of the lesions, utilizing different embolic agents. Coils are the most common agents followed by cyanoacrylate. Other agents are foam, microparticles, thrombin, and polyvinyl alcohol. Given the rich collateral circulation of the external carotid artery territory and small size of its branches, embolization is a safe and effective way to treat these pseudoaneurysms. Coil embolization is associated with the lowest complication rate among the embolic agents, while cyanoacrylate had the highest. Most complications come from the innumerous anastomoses between the external and internal carotid arteries that can lead to nontarget embolization of intracranial branches, resulting in stroke or blindness. Therefore, 0.018-in. detachable coils delivered through a micro-catheter represent an appropriate choice for this task [45].

Because of its theoretical risk of future rupture or distal embolism, vertebral artery pseudoaneurysms are usually treated aggressively regardless of the presence of symptoms with coil embolization or with covered stents. Lower-profile stenting devices and improved endovascular techniques have been demonstrated to be effective in the management of VAIs specifically in the areas of the vertebral artery where they are difficult to access [41].

16.7 Complications

Complications after treatment can relate to hematoma, pneumothorax resulting from violation of airways or the apical lung, infection, and iatrogenic injury to the cranial nerves in the neck. Operative drains should remain in place until output decreases. Series evaluating a mandatory exploration strategy result in 50–68% negative exploration, suggesting avoidable perioperative morbidity [46].

Clinical Images and Case Scenarios

Clinical images: Case 1.

See Figs. 16.5, 16.6, 16.7, 16.8, 16.9, 16.10 and 16.11.

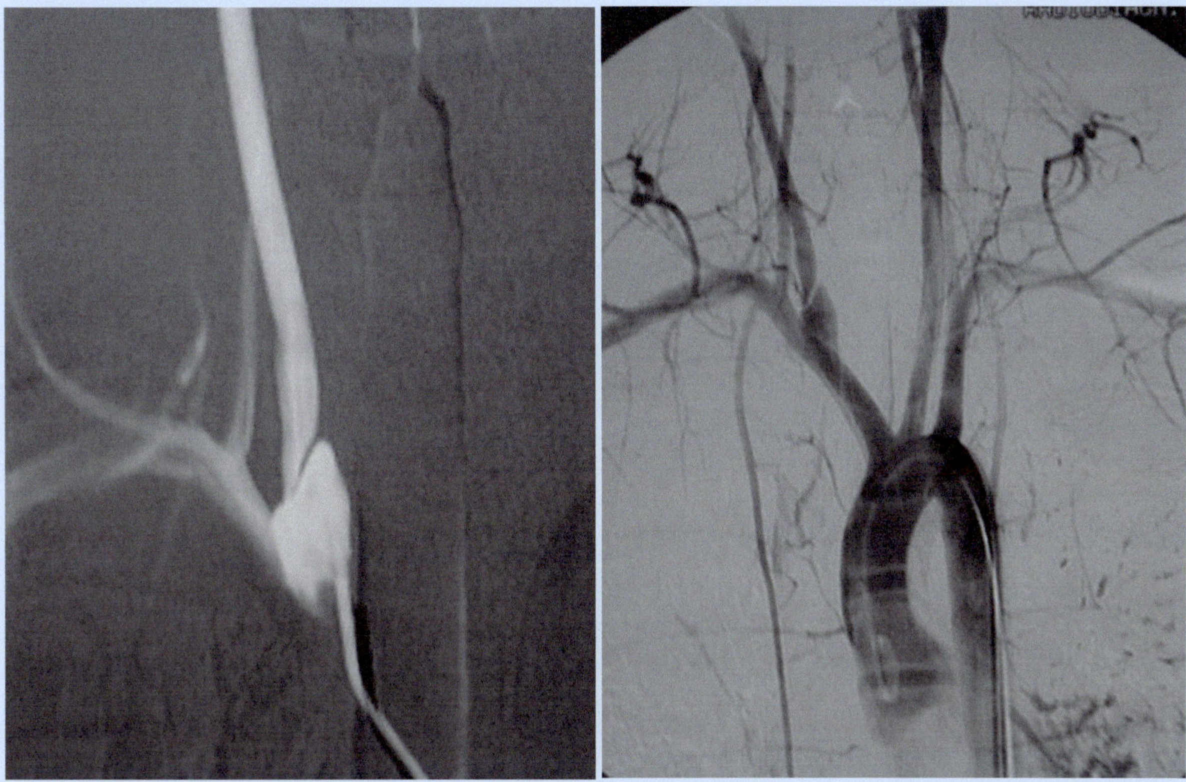

Figs. 16.5 and 16.6 Preoperative digital subtraction angiography (DSA) of posttraumatic dissection and subsequent aneurysm of the origin of the right common carotid artery

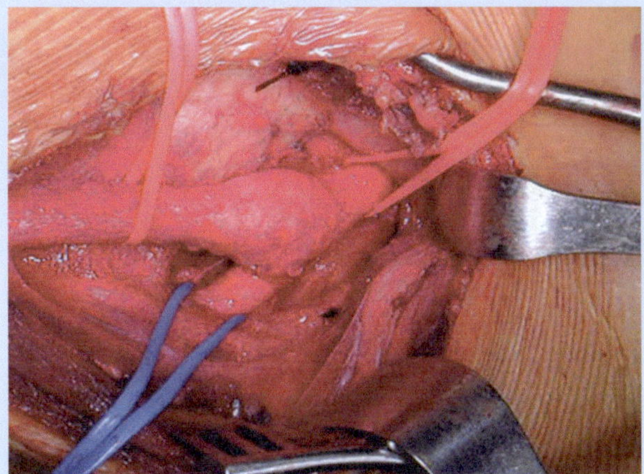

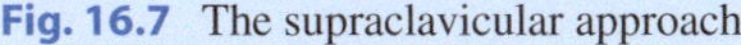

Fig. 16.7 The supraclavicular approach

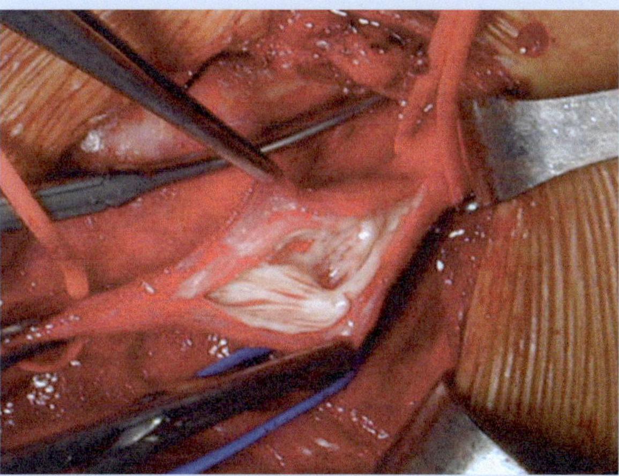

Fig. 16.8 Aneurysm opening with dissection exposure

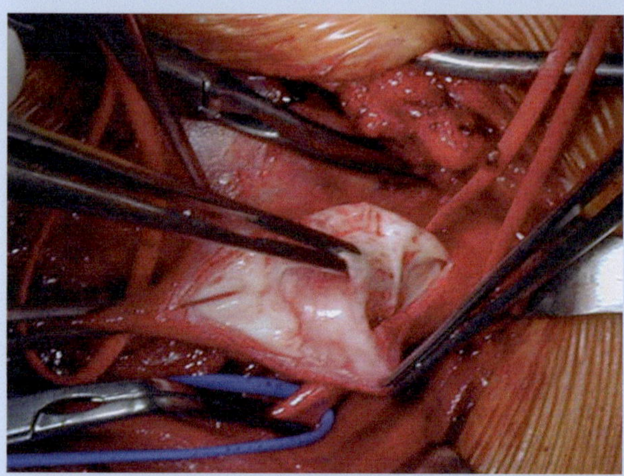

Fig. 16.9 Dissection flap removal and fixation

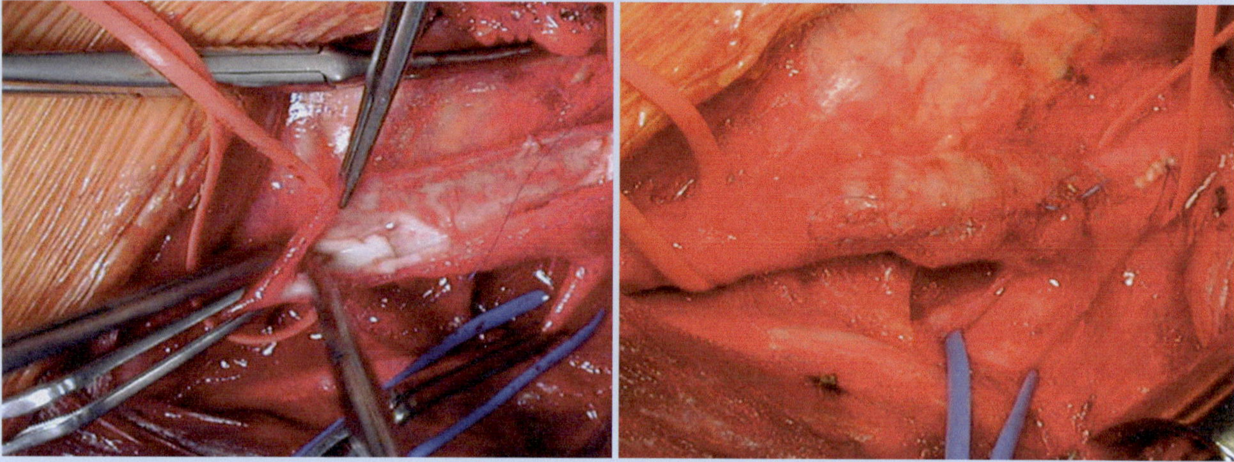

Figs. 16.10 and 16.11 Tailoring with direct running suture

Auto-evaluation test:

1. Trauma to a vessel bifurcation is better treated by:
   A. Surgical approach.
   B. Endo approach.
   C. Both.
2. Surgical treatment can include:
   A. Direct repair.
   B. Graft interposition.
   C. Vein interposition.
   D. All the above answers are correct.

Clinical images: Case 2.

See Figs. 16.12, 16.13 and 16.14.

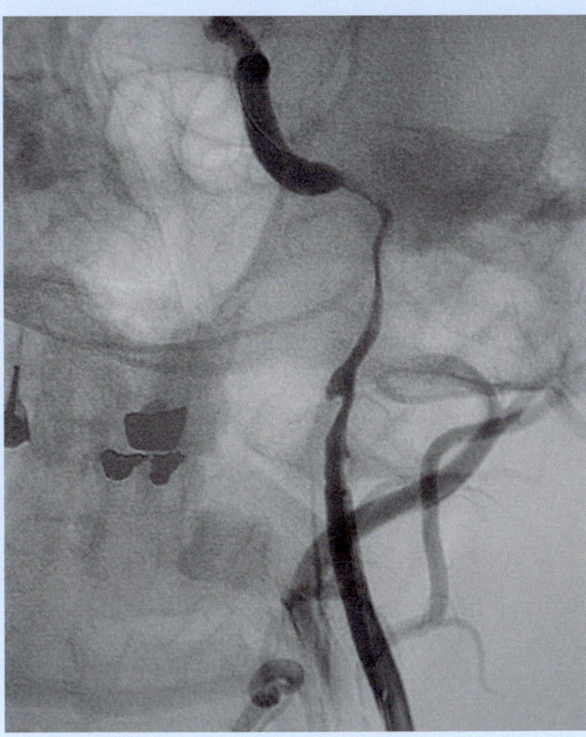

Fig. 16.12 Blunt neck trauma with internal carotid artery symptomatic dissection. Pre-procedural DSA angiogram showing dramatic narrowing of internal carotid lumen

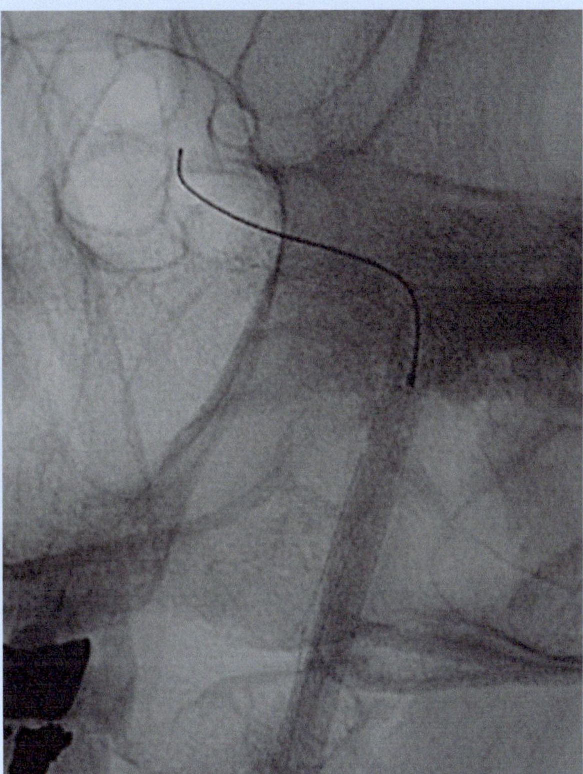

Fig. 16.13 Stenting with dissection sealing

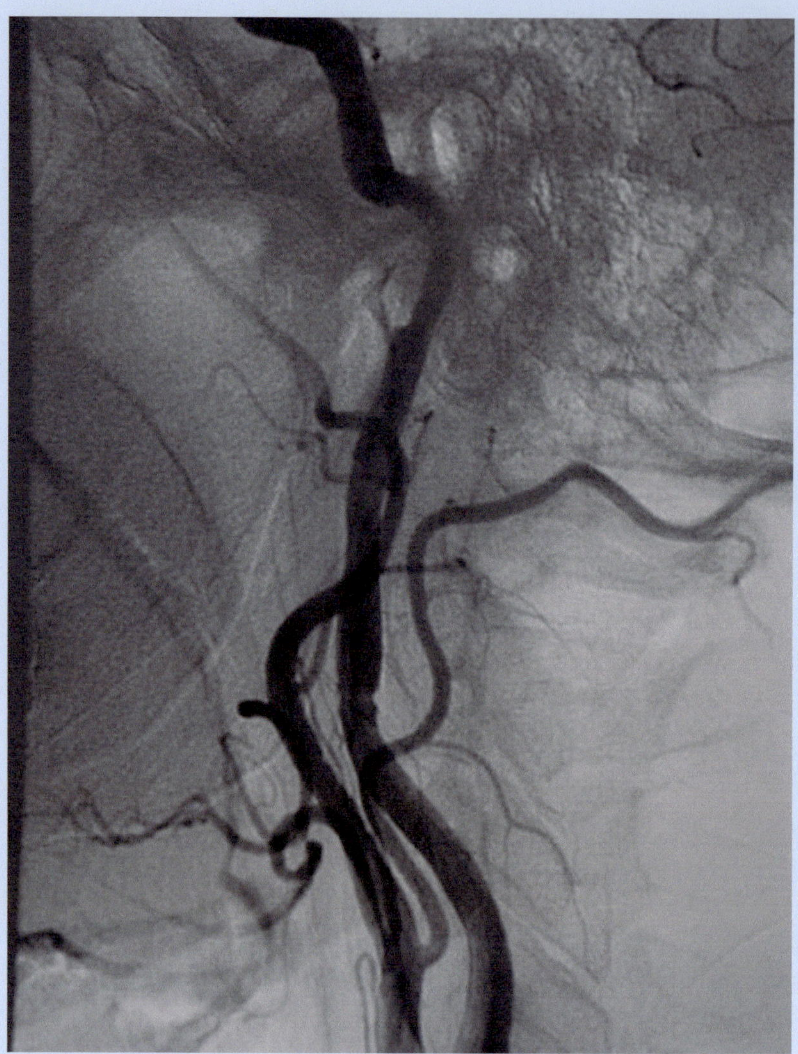

Fig. 16.14 Completion angiography showing lumen patency complete restoration

Auto-evaluation test:

1. DSA's most common aspect of dissection is:
   A. Narrowing of the vessel.
   B. Extravasation.
   C. Venous rapid filling.

Clinical images: Case 3.

See Figs. 16.15, 16.16, 16.17 and 16.18.

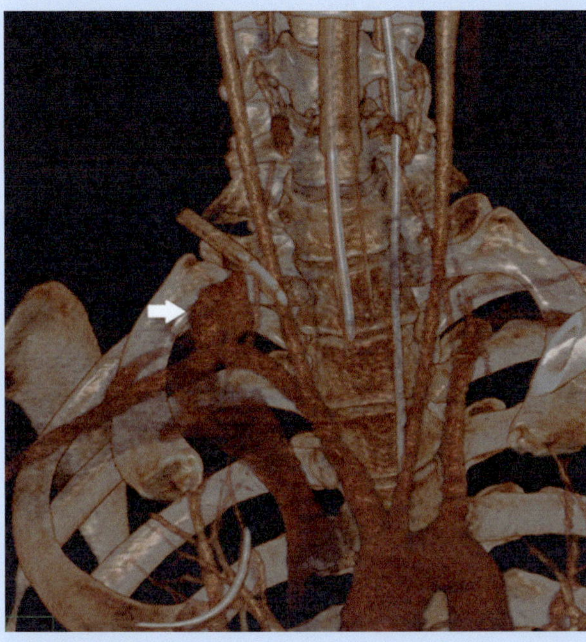

Fig. 16.15 A subclavian pseudoaneurysm (arrow) showed at volume rendering CTA subsequent to car accident in a 45-year-old male

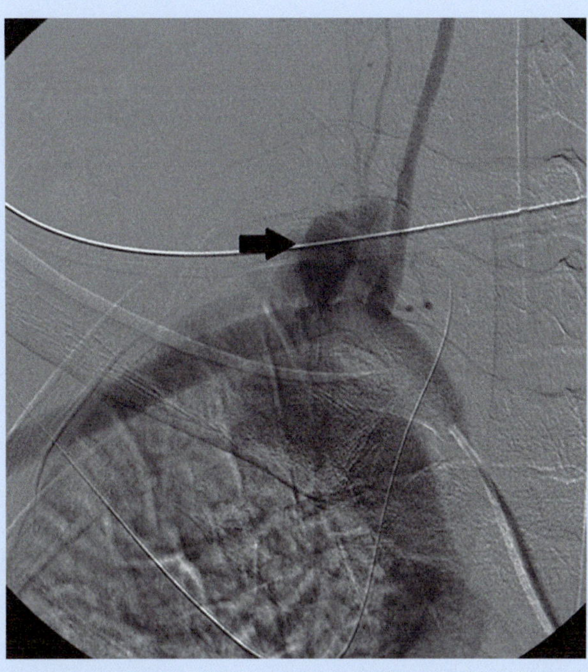

Fig. 16.16 Preliminary angiography pointed out the pseudoaneurysm of the right subclavian artery (arrow) proximal to the vertebral artery ostium. The early evidence of the right subclavian vein was due to a posttraumatic arteriovenous fistula

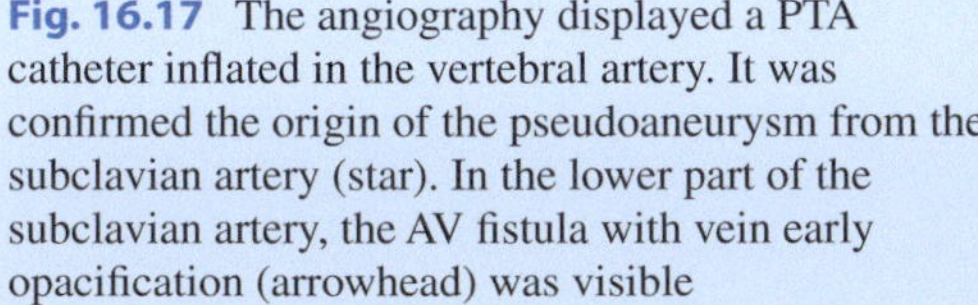

Fig. 16.17 The angiography displayed a PTA catheter inflated in the vertebral artery. It was confirmed the origin of the pseudoaneurysm from the subclavian artery (star). In the lower part of the subclavian artery, the AV fistula with vein early opacification (arrowhead) was visible

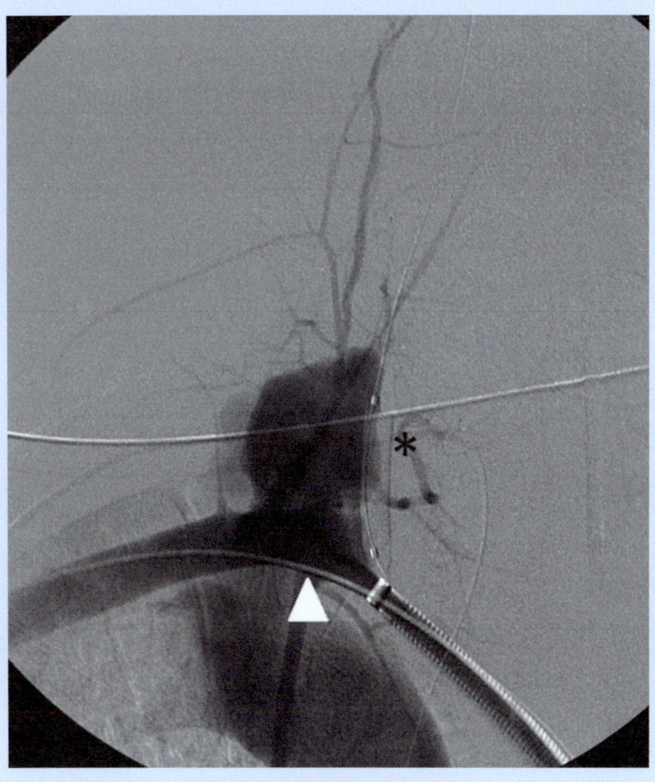

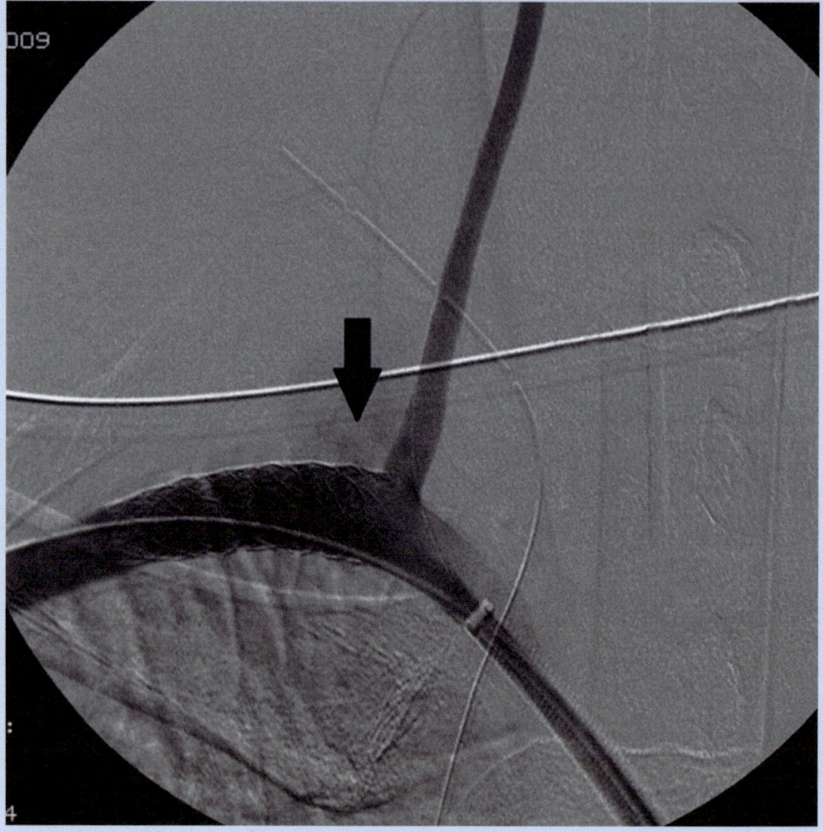

Fig. 16.18 Completion angiography demonstrated balloon-expandable ePTFE stent graft placement (arrow) in the subclavian artery with maintained patency of the subclavian and vertebral arteries with contrast media stagnation in the pseudoaneurysm sac and arteriovenous fistula exclusion without early venous opacification

Auto-evaluation test for Case 3:

1. Endovascular treatment of a pseudoaneurysm must be done with:
   A. Brachial approach.
   B. Femoral approach.
   C. Venous and arterial approach.

Case Scenario No. 1.

A 65-year-old male underwent planned central venous catheter (CVC) placement in the right jugular vein. After the US-guided placement, the patient presented neurological symptoms, and a CT was performed (Fig. 16.19).

A large-diameter central venous catheter was inserted into the right vertebral artery (arrow) with the distal end into the aortic arch. 3D volume rendering posterior and anterior views confirmed the entry point of the central venous catheter arrow and the tip in the aortic arch (Figs. 16.20 and 16.21, arrow).

A preliminary angiography through a right femoral artery approach confirmed the CVC insertion at the proximal tract of the right vertebral artery (Fig. 16.22, arrow) and the patency of the right carotid and vertebral arteries.

The decision taken was to implant a self-expandable ePTFE stent graft (5x25mm) placement (arrowhead) in the vertebral artery (Fig. 16.23).

In the final angiogram (Fig. 16.24), it is possible to appreciate the CVC removal and the absence of contrast media extravasation and the patency of the vertebral artery.

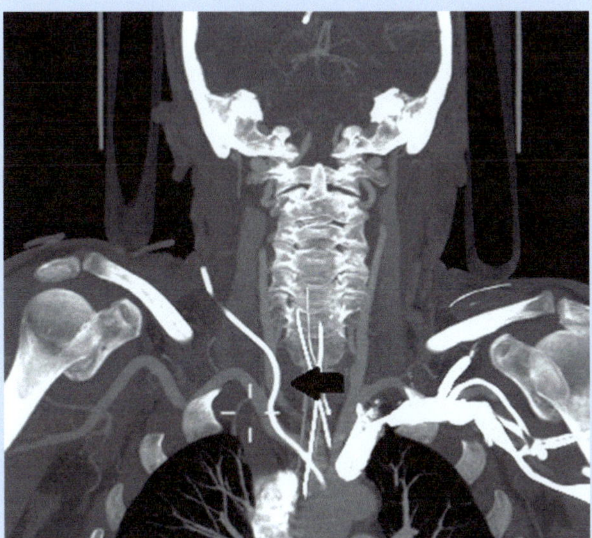

Fig. 16.19

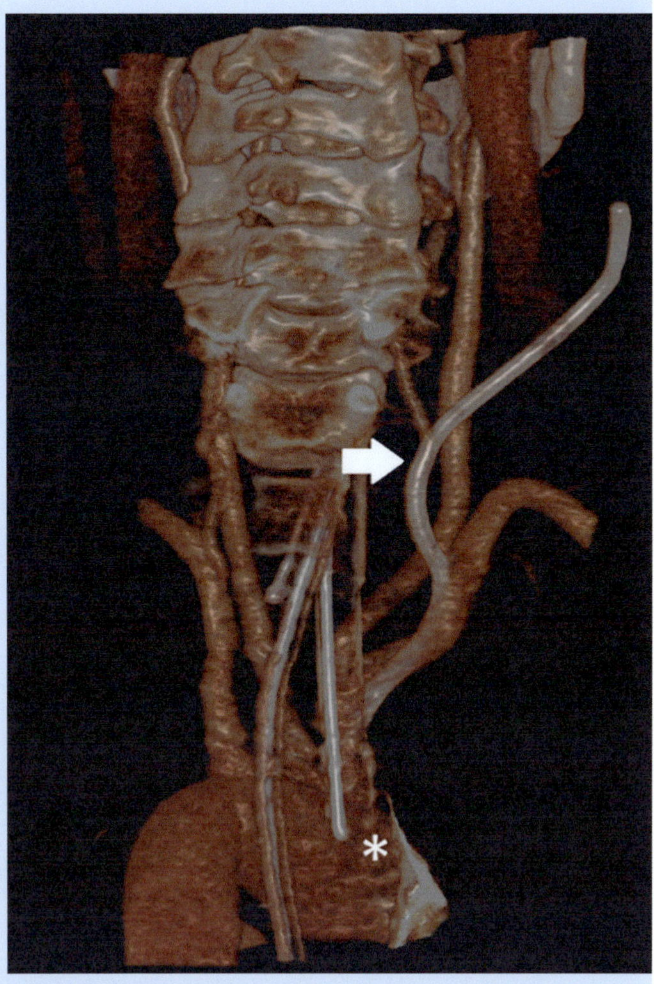

Fig. 16.20

Case Scenario No. 2.

A 49-year-old male underwent ECMO placement for acute respiratory failure. US-guided cannulation of the right jugular vein was performed to ECMO catheter insertion. Immediate hemodynamic instability occurred due to massive hemothorax.

Preliminary venography showed the laceration of the right internal jugular vein (IJV) (arrow) at the catheter ECMO entry site in the right jugular vein (Fig. 16.25, arrowhead).

A self-expandable ePTFE stent graft was placed in the IJV and released (Fig. 16.26).

Completion venography confirmed vein reconstruction (Fig. 16.27, star) without contrast media extravasation and recovery of hemodynamic stability.

CT follow-up at 1 week (Fig. 16.28) showed stent graft in the jugular vein.

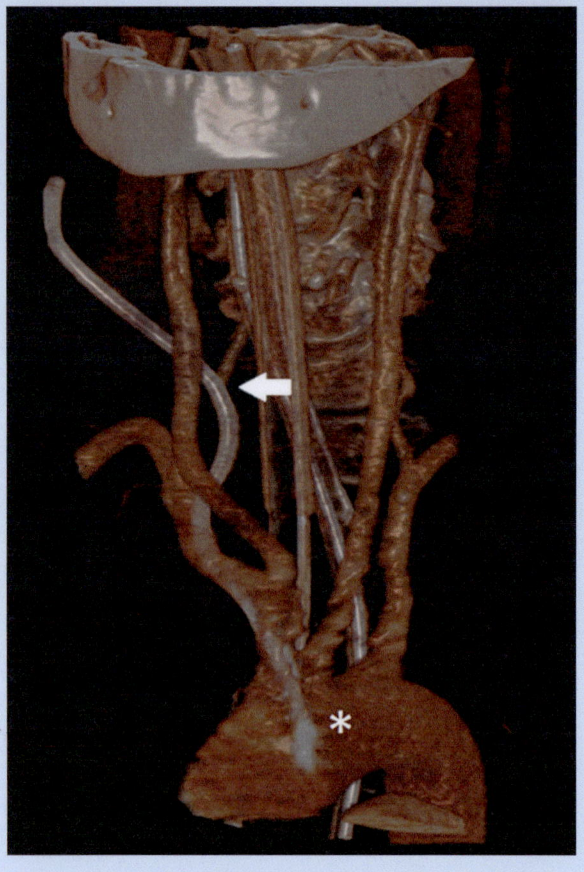

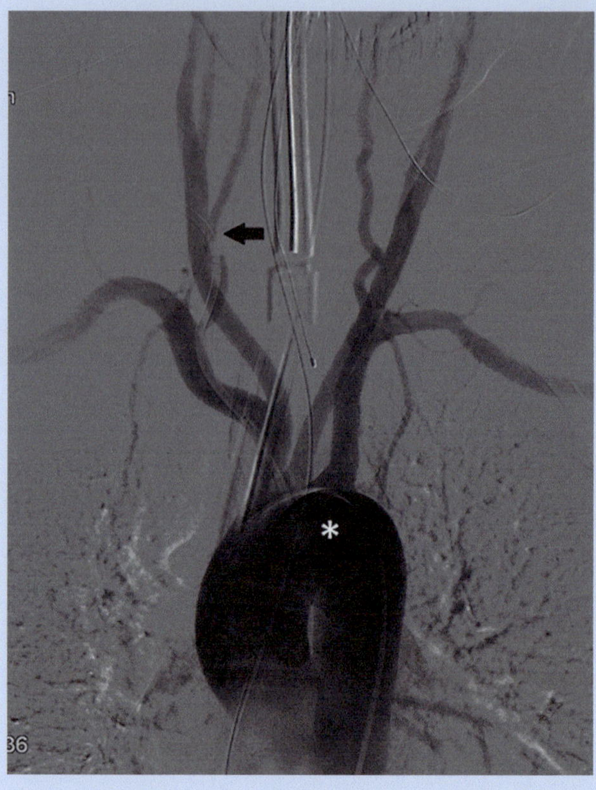

Fig. 16.22

Fig. 16.21

Case Scenario No. 3.

A 32-year-old stable female was admitted to the emergency ward after a firearm trauma of the neck.

Preliminary angiography in different projections. Multiple foreign bodies were evident (Fig. 16.29).

It showed multiple pseudoaneurysms of the right common carotid artery (Fig. 16.30, star) and a giant pseudoaneurysm of the right external carotid artery (Fig. 16.31, arrow).

The arteriography of the vertebral artery demonstrated the presence of an arteriovenous fistula with connection between the vertebral artery and vertebral vein (Fig. 16.32, arrowhead).

Embolization of the external carotid artery giant pseudoaneurysm with detachable coils (Fig. 16.33, arrow).

Postembolization angiography showed pseudoaneurysm exclusion (arrow). Presence of multiple pseudoaneurysm of the CCA (Fig. 16.34, star).

Self-expandable stent placed in the right CCA to reduce pseudoaneurysm direct blood flow (Fig. 16.35, star).

Self-expandable ePTFE stent graft (5 × 25 mm) placed in the vertebral artery in the 6 months follow-up angiography showed complete exclusion of the arteriovenous fistula and the patency of the vertebral artery (Fig. 16.36, arrowhead). Exclusion of both external carotid artery and CCA multiple pseudoaneurysms was confirmed (Fig. 16.37, star).

Please see Chap. 58 for the correct answer.

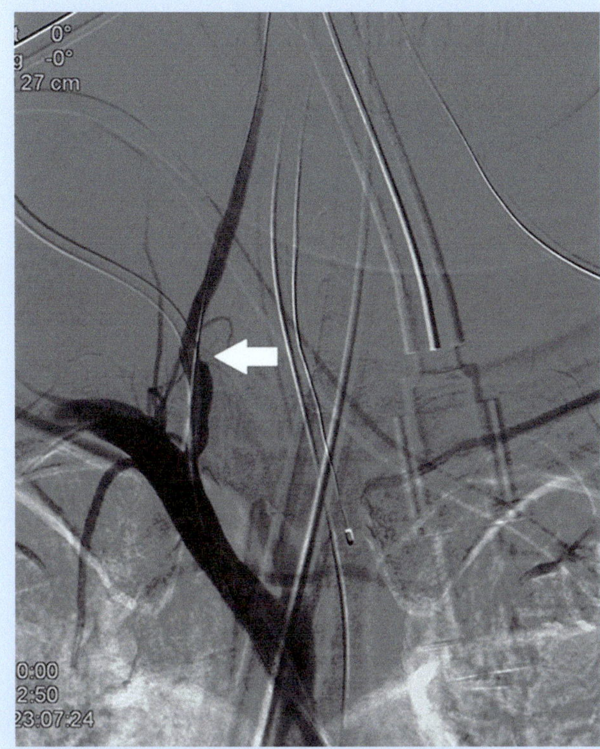

Fig. 16.23

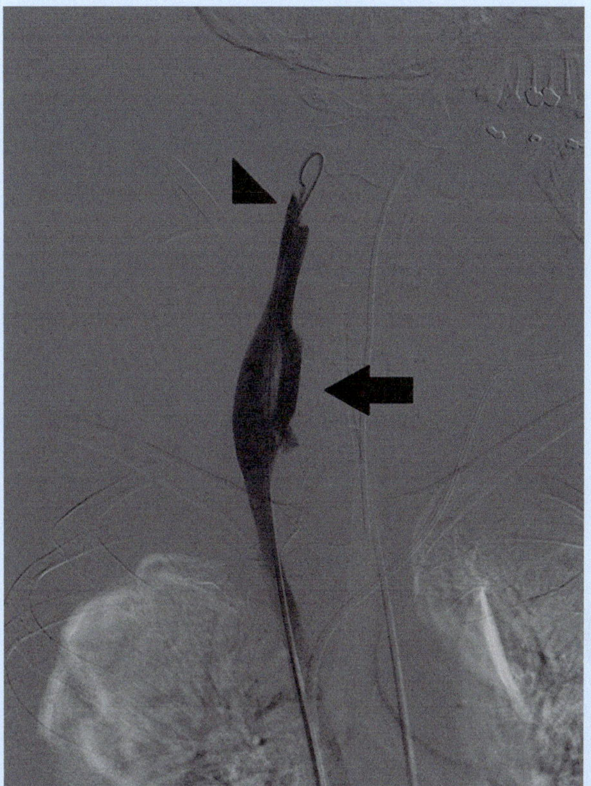
Fig. 16.25

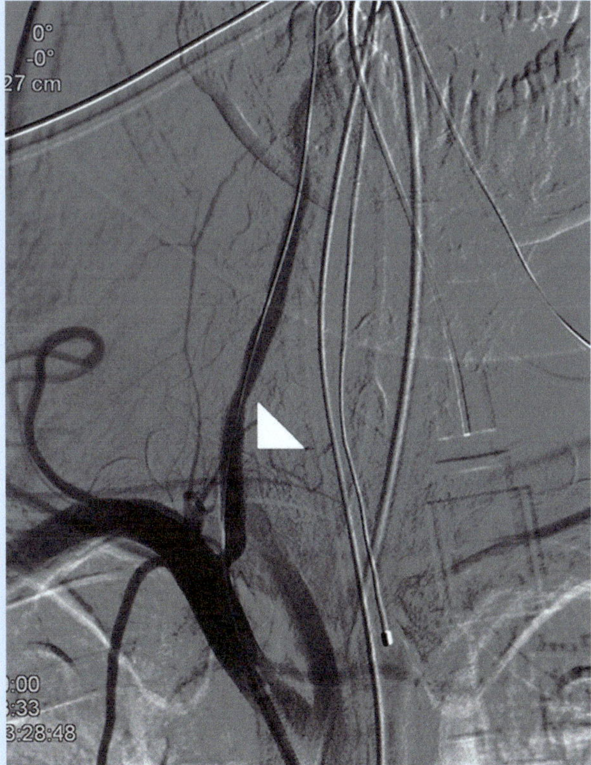

Fig. 16.24

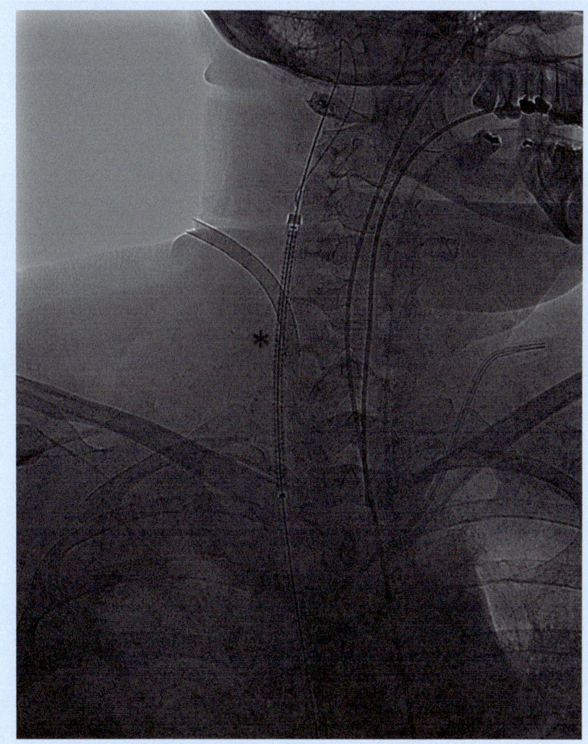
Fig. 16.26

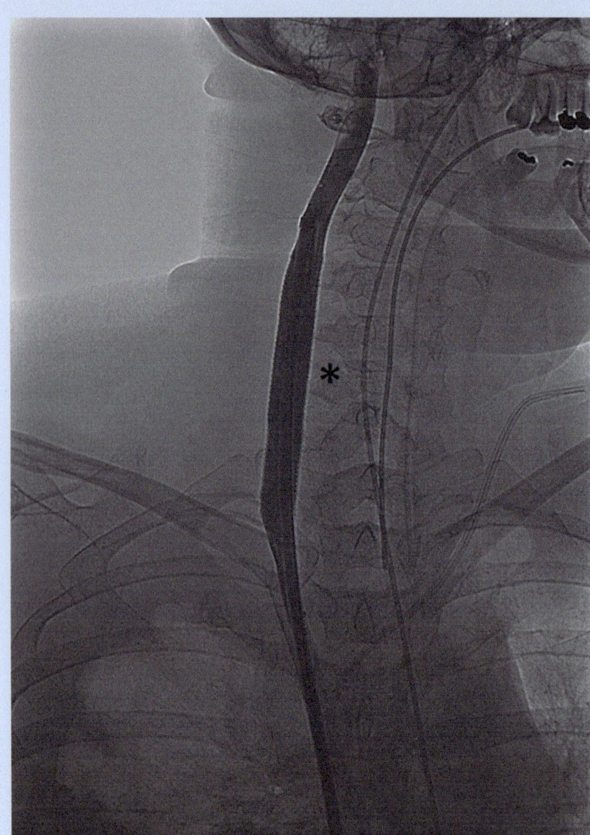

Fig. 16.27

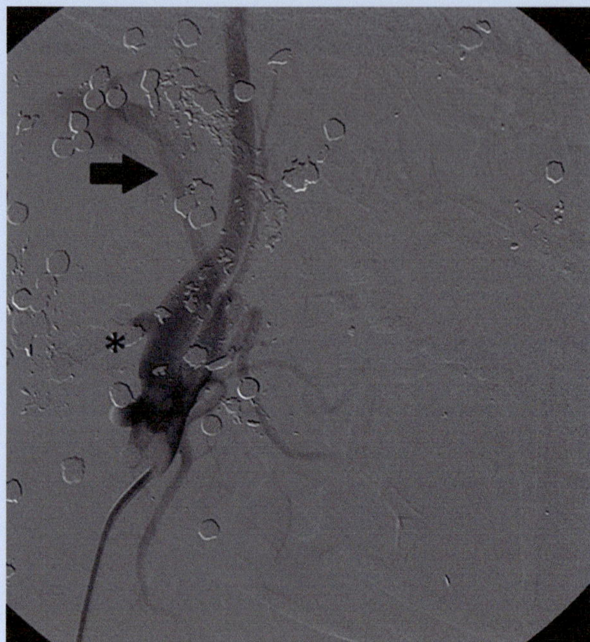

Fig. 16.29

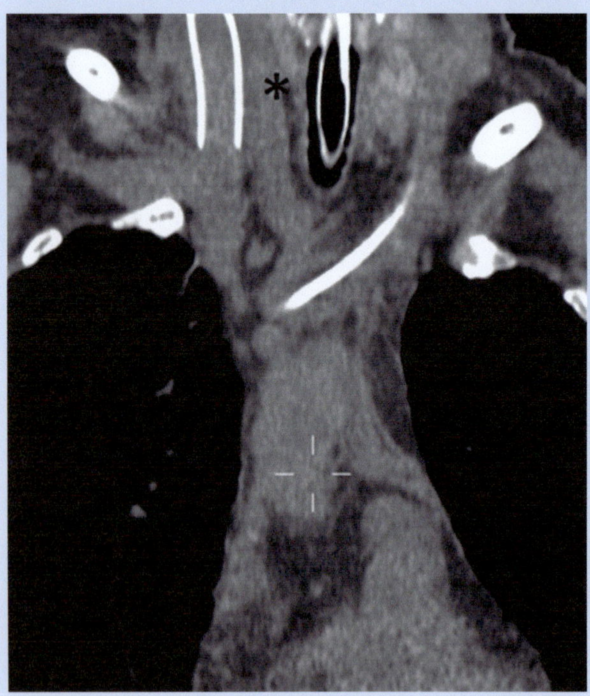

Fig. 16.28

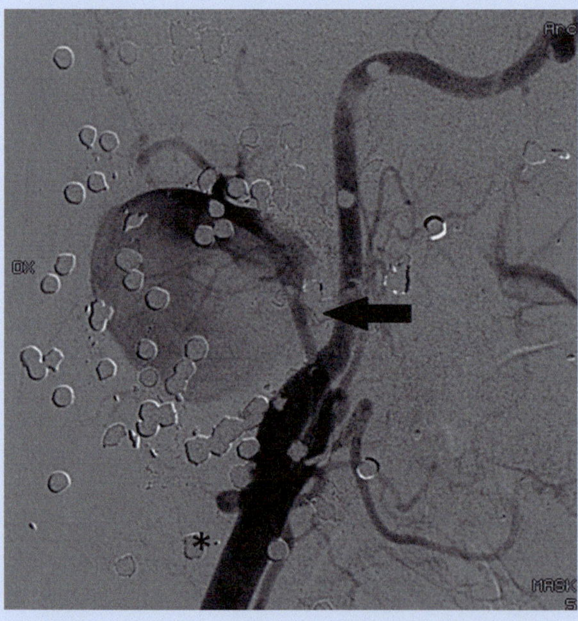

Fig. 16.30

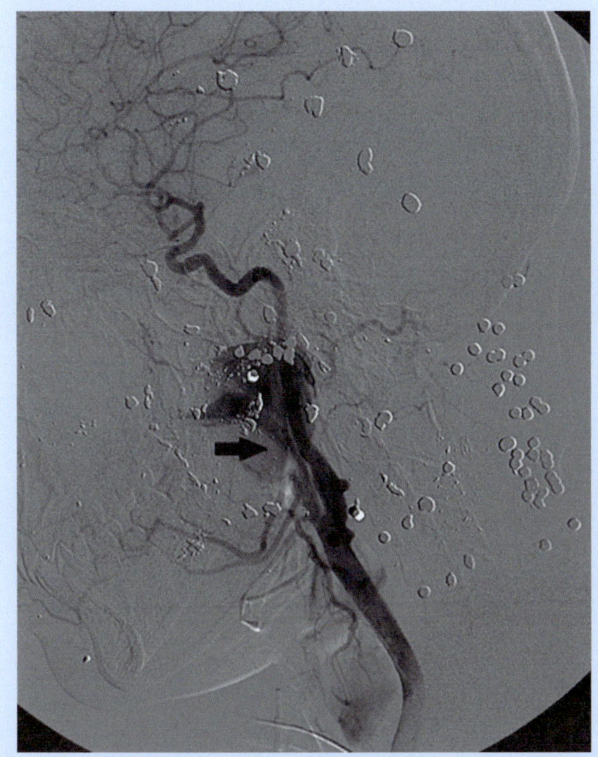

Fig. 16.31

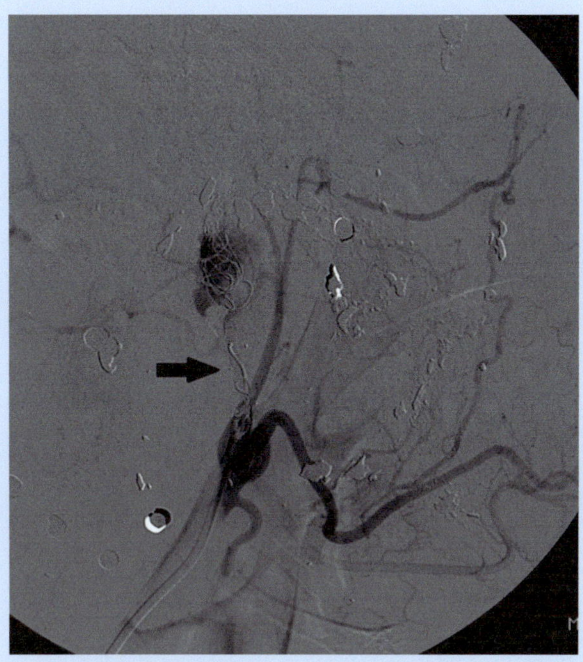

Fig. 16.33

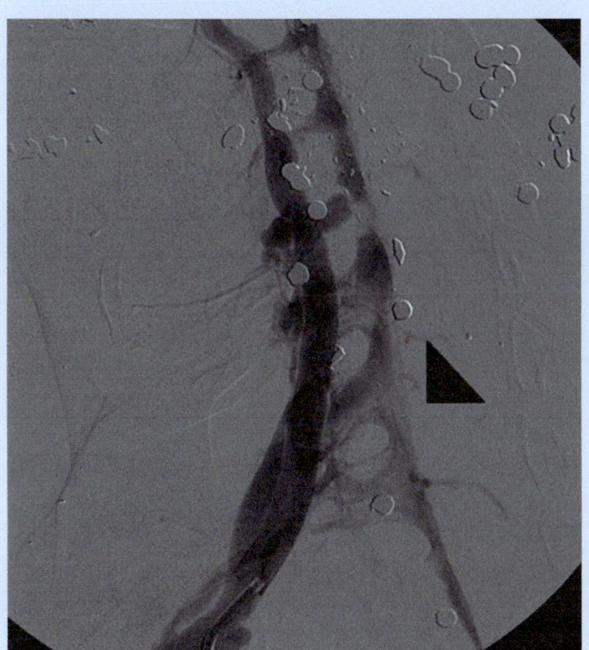

Fig. 16.32

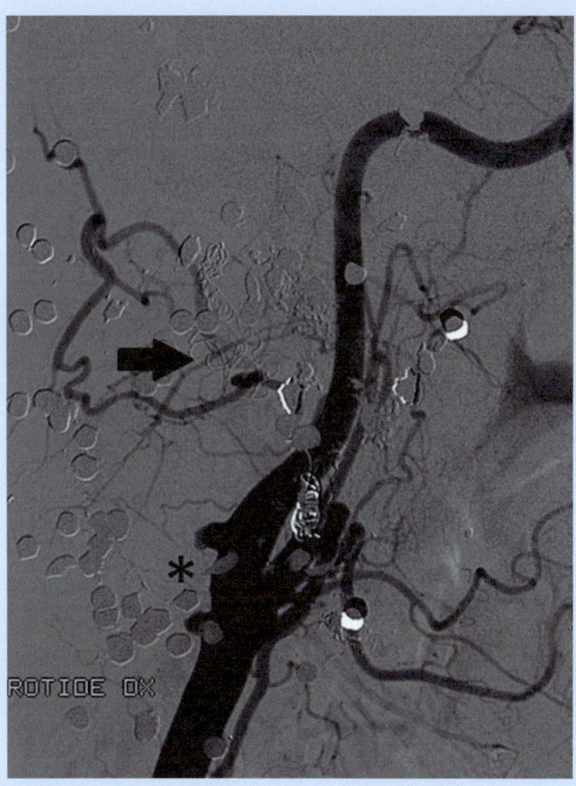

Fig. 16.34

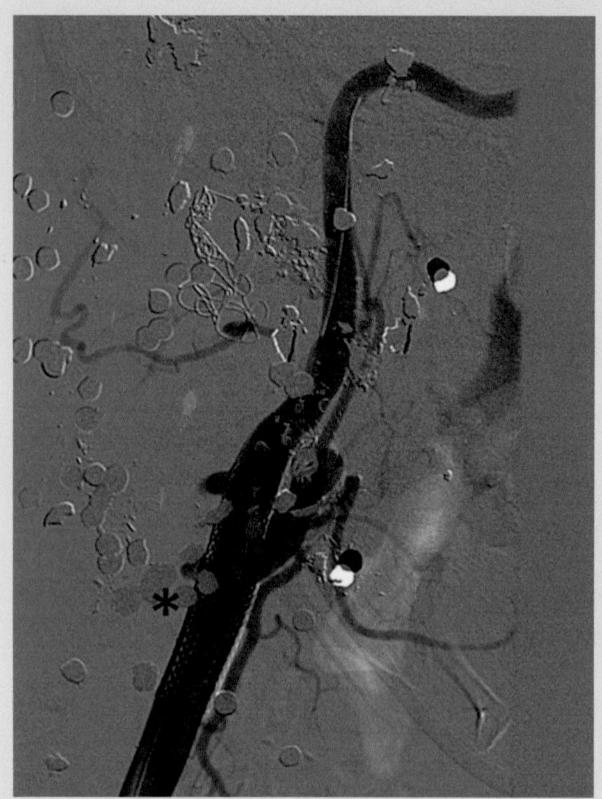

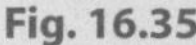

Fig. 16.35

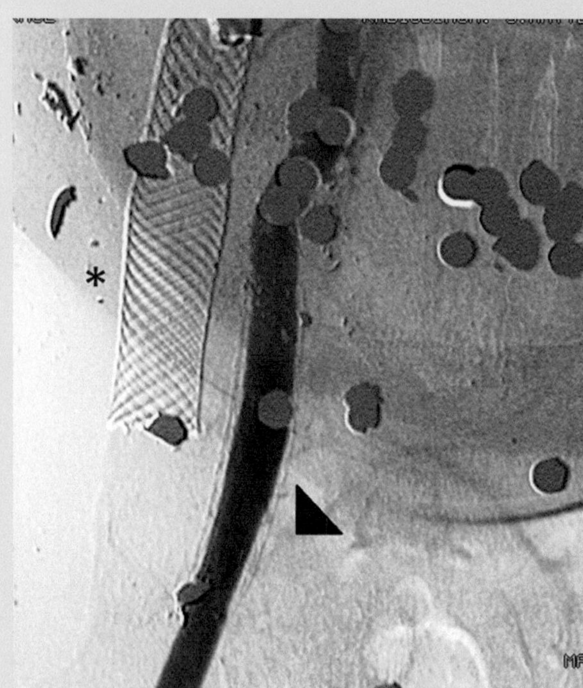

Fig. 16.36

Fig. 16.37

References

1. White JM, Stannard A, Burkhardt GE, Eastridge BJ, Blackbourne LH, Rasmussen TE. The epidemiology of vascular injury in the wars in Iraq and Afghanistan. Ann Surg. 2011;253:1184–9.
2. MacLeod JB1, Cohn SM, Johnson EW, McKenney MG. Trauma deaths in the first hour: are they all unsalvageable injuries? Am J Surg. 2007;193:195–9.
3. Rasmussen TE, Clouse WD, Jenkins DH, Peck MA, Eliason JL, Smith DL. The use of temporary vascular shunts as a damage control adjunct in the management of wartime vascular injury. J Trauma. 2006;61:8–12.
4. Fabian TC, Patton JH Jr, Croce MA, Minard G, Kudsk KA, Pritchard FE. Blunt carotid injury: importance of early diagnosis and anticoagulant therapy. Ann Surg. 1996;223:513–22.
5. Duke BJ, Ryu RK, Coldwell DM, Brega KE. Treatment of blunt injury to the carotid artery by using endovascular stents: an early experience. J Neurosurg. 1997;87:825–9.
6. Punjabi AP, Plaisier BR, Haug RH, Malangoni MA. Diagnosis and management of blunt carotid artery injury in oral and maxillofacial surgery. J Oral Maxillofac Surg. 1997;55:1388–95.
7. National Trauma DataBank. American College of Surgeons—Committee on Trauma, Chicago, IL, 2009.
8. McConnell DB, Trunkey DD. Management of penetrating trauma to the neck. Adv Surg. 1994;27:97–123.
9. Carducci B, Lowe RA, Dalsey W. Penetrating neck trauma: consensus and controversies. Ann Emerg Med. 1986;15:208–15.
10. Davis JW, Holbrook TL, Hoyt DB, Mackersie RC, Field TO Jr, Shackford SR. Blunt carotid artery dissection: incidence, associated injuries, screening, and treatment. J Trauma. 1990;30:1514–7.
11. Biffl WL, Ray CE Jr, Moore EE, Franciose RJ, Aly S, Heyrosa MG, Johnson JL, Burch JM. Treatment-related outcomes from blunt cerebrovascular injuries: importance of routine follow-up arteriography. Ann Surg. 2002;235:699–706.
12. Biffl WL, Moore EE, Ryu RK, Offner PJ, Novak Z, Coldwell DM, Franciose RJ, Burch JM. The unrecognized epidemic of blunt carotid arterial injuries: early diagnosis improves neurologic outcome. Ann Surg. 1998;228:462–70.
13. Berne JD, Norwood SH, McAuley CE, Vallina VL, Creath RG, McLarty J. The high morbidity of blunt cerebrovascular injury in an unscreened population: more evidence of the need for mandatory screening protocols. J Am Coll Surg. 2001;192:314–21.
14. Biffl WL, Moore EE, Offner PJ, Brega KE, Franciose RJ, Burch JM. Blunt carotid arterial injuries: implications of a new grading scale. J Trauma. 1999;47:845–53.
15. Miller PR, Fabian TC, Croce MA, Cagiannos C, Williams JS, Vang M, Qaisi WG, Felker RE, Timmons SD. Prospective screening for blunt cerebrovascular injuries: analysis of diagnostic modalities and outcomes. Ann Surg. 2002;236:386–95.
16. Ruesch S, Walder B, Tramer MR. Complications of central venous catheters: internal jugular versus subclavian access a systematic review. Crit Care Med. 2002;30:454e60.
17. Golden LR. Incidence and management of large-bore introducer sheath puncture of the carotid artery. J Cardiothorac Vasc Anesth. 1995;9:425–8.
18. Reuber M, Dunkley LA, Turton EP, Bell MD, Bamford JM. Stroke after internal jugular venous cannulation. Acta Neurol Scand. 2002;105:235–9.
19. Monson DO, Saletta JD, Freeark RJ. Carotid vertebral trauma. J Trauma. 1969;9:987–99.
20. Bell RB, Osborn T, Dierks EJ, Potter BE, Long WB. Management of penetrating neck injuries: a new paradigm for civilian trauma. J Oral Maxillofac Surg. 2007;65:691–705.
21. Kohler R, Vargas MI, Masterson K, Lovblad KO, Pereira VM, Becker M. CT and MR angiography features of traumatic vascular injuries of the neck. Am J Roentgenol. 2011;196:W800–9.
22. Bleazard S, Riccelli L. Imaging of traumatic vascular injuries in the neck. Semin Roentgenol. 2006;41:237–9.
23. Uyeda JW, Anderson SW, Sakai O, Soto JA. CT angiography in trauma. Radiol Clin N Am. 2010;48:423–38.
24. Chokshi FH, Munera F, Rivas LA, Henry RP, Quencer RM. 64-MDCT angiography of blunt vascular injuries of the neck. AJR. 2011;196:W309–15.
25. Biffl WL, Moore EE, Offner PJ, Burch JM. Blunt carotid and vertebral arterial injuries. World J Surg. 2001;25:1036–43.
26. Saito N, Hito R, Burke PA, Sakai O. Imaging of penetrating injuries of the head and neck: current practice at a level 1 trauma center in the US. Keio J Med. 2014;63(2):23–33.
27. Key G, editor. The Apologie and treatise of Ambroise Paré containing the voyages made into divers places with many writings upon surgery. London: Falcon Education Books; 1957.
28. Makin GH. Injuries to the blood vessels. In: Official history of the great war medical services: surgery of the war, vol. 2. London: His Majesty's Stationery Office; 1922. p. 170e296.
29. Lawrence KB, Shefts LM, McDaniel JR. Wounds of the common carotid arteries: report of seventeen cases from World War II. Am J Surg. 1948;76:29e37.
30. Hughes CW. Arterial repair during the Korean war. Ann Surg. 1958;147:555e61.
31. Fogelman MJ, Stewart RD. Penetrating wounds of the neck. Am J Surg. 1956;91:581e96.
32. Higashida RT, Halbach VV, Tsai FY, Norman D, Pribram HF, Mehringer CM, Hieshima GB. Interventional neurovascular treatment of traumatic carotid and vertebral artery lesions: results in 234 cases. Am J Roentgenol. 1989;153(3):577–82.
33. ATLS Subcommittee; American College of Surgeons' Committee on Trauma; International ATLS Working Group. Advanced trauma life support (ATLS®): the ninth edition. J Trauma Acute Care Surg. 2013;74(5):1363–6.
34. Demetriades D, Theodorou D, Cornwell E, Beme TV, Asensio JA, Belzberg H, Velmahos G, Weaver F, Yellin A. Evaluation of penetrating injuries of the neck: prospective study of 223 patients. World J Surg. 1997;21(1):41–8.
35. Sperry JL, Moore EE, Coimbra R, Croce M, Davis JW, Karmy-Jones R, McIntyre RC Jr, Moore FA, Malhotra A, Shatz DV, Biffl WL. Western Trauma Association critical decisions in trauma: penetrating neck trauma. J Trauma Acute Care Surg. 2013;75(6): 936–40.
36. Demetriades D, Asensio JA, Velmahos G, Thal E. Complex penetrating neck injuries. In: Asensio JA, Demetriades D, Berne TV (eds). W.B. Saunders Co., Philadelphia. Surg Clin North Am. 1996;76(4): 685–724.
37. Asensio JA, Valenziano CP, Falcone RE, Grosh JD. Management of penetrating neck injuries. Surg Clin North Am. 1991;71(2): 267–96.
38. Asensio JA, Vu T, Mazzini F, Herrerias F, Pust GD, Sciarretta J, Chandler J, Verde JM, Menendez P, Sanchez JM, Petrone P, Marini C. Penetrating carotid artery: uncommon complex and lethal injuries. Eur J Trauma Emerg Surg. 2011;37(5):429–37.
39. Ivatury RR, Stoner MC. Penetrating cervical vascular injury. In: Rich NM, Mattox KL, Hirshberg A, editors. Vascular trauma. 2nd ed. Philadelphia: Elsevier Saunders; 2004. p. 223–40.
40. Rowe V, Petrone P, García-Nuñez LM, Asensio JA. Carotid, vertebral artery, and jugular venous injuries. In: Asensio JA, Trunkey D, editors. Current therapy of trauma and surgical critical care. 5th ed. Philadelphia: Mosby/Elsevier; 2008. p. 203–6.
41. Greer LT, Kuehn RB, Gillespie DL, White PW, Bell RS, Armonda RA, Fox CJ. Contemporary management of combat-related vertebral artery injuries. J Trauma Acute Care Surg. 2013;74(3):818–24.
42. Lee TS, Ducic Y, Gordin E, Stroman D. Management of carotid artery trauma. Craniomaxillofac Trauma Reconstr. 2014;7:175–89.

43. Pham MH, Rahme RJ, Arnaout O, et al. Endovascular stenting of extracranial carotid and vertebral artery dissections: a systematic review of the literature. Neurosurgery. 2011;68:856–66.
44. Yamada R, Miller C, Guimaraes M, Schnōltz C. Overview of endovascular management of traumatic carotid lesions. Determining appropriate intervention based on lesion severity and patient characteristics. Endov Today. 2016;15(1):79–82.
45. Dolati P, Eichberg D, Thomas A, Ogilvy C. Aneurysms of the external carotid artery and its branch vessels: a case report, pooled data analysis, and current treatment strategies. J Neurosurg Sci. 2015. [published online ahead of print September 25, 2015].
46. Buchanan LS. Neck. In: The shock trauma manual of operative techniques. New York: Springer; 2015. p. 3–12.

Update on Traumatic Spinal Cord Injury

17

Carolina Rouanet and Gisele Sampaio Silva

Key Points

- Traumatic spinal cord injury (TSCI) is a devastating disease, with great morbidity and high costs.
- TSCI is insufficiently reported worldwide with a global prevalence ranging between 236 and 1009 per million.
- Goals in the management of SCI patients include reducing primary neurological damage and preventing secondary damage.
- In patients with injuries above the sixth thoracic vertebra (Th6), there will be not only sensory and motor disturbances but also cardiovascular, thermoregulatory, urinary, gastrointestinal, sexual, and respiratory/ bronchopulmonary disturbances due to the interruption of the descending sympathetic pathways.
- Patients with lesions below Th6 will have preserved sympathetic/parasympathetic responses.
- Respiratory complications are the main cause of morbidity and mortality in the acute phase of SCI, with atelectasis, pneumonia, and respiratory failure being the most common.
- The lack of diaphragm function, previous cardiopulmonary disease, tachypnea at admission, advanced age, copious sputum, pneumonia, and major lobe collapse are predictive for the need of mechanical ventilation.
- Neurogenic shock with profound hypotension and bradycardia due to interruption of sympathetic tone and an unopposed intact vagal tone is a major acute complication after SCI.
- Patients with high cervical and complete lesions are at more risk for cardiovascular instability and more frequently need vasopressor support.
- Early surgical decompression may lead to better outcomes than late decompression, with the neuroprotective effect thus varying with time elapsed since the trauma.
- All recent studies fail to demonstrate a real benefit of the IV methylprednisolone use as part of treatment for acute SCI.
- Cell-based therapies are promising modalities of neuroregenerative treatments.

17.1 Epidemiology

Traumatic spinal cord injury (TSCI) is insufficiently reported worldwide, with its prevalence probably being underestimated. The range of global prevalence is between 236 and 1009 per million. Most of the data come from North America, Western Europe, and Australia. Regarding its incidence, in North America, it is estimated to be 39 per million, in Canada 15 per million, and Australia 16 per million. In these regions, road traffic car accidents are the major cause of TSCI. In Western Europe, the falls predominate, probably due to the older-aged population. Another important etiology in North America and South America is violence/self-harm (especially firearm-related injuries). In Brazil, rates of SCI resulting from gunshots were as high as 37% [1].

Direct lifetime costs can be as high as \$1.1–\$4.6 million per patient in North America, with devastating consequences for patients and their families [2].

Regarding mortality, also little is known. Ten-year mortality following TSCI in the USA seems to be 16,2%, in Canada 10,7%, and Australia 14,3%. Developed countries have significantly better survival rates than undeveloped countries [1].

C. Rouanet (✉) · G. S. Silva
Neurology and Neurosurgery Department, Federal University of São Paulo, São Paulo, Brazil

P. Aseni et al. (eds.), *Operative Techniques and Recent Advances in Acute Care and Emergency Surgery*, https://doi.org/10.1007/978-3-319-95114-0_17

17.2 Pathophysiology

The primary initial injury starts with an abrupt trauma to the spine that leads to fractures and/or dislocation of the vertebra. The displaced bone fragments, disc material, and tension forces lead to mechanical injury to the spinal cord as a consequence of compression, laceration, distraction, and shearing. Seconds after the primary lesion, a sequence of pathological events that will last up to several weeks start, which is called the secondary injury. The initial damage to the microvasculature results in progressive edema, ischemia and the beginning of a pro-apoptotic signaling. With the disruption of the blood-spinal barrier, there is an influx of inflammatory cells, cytokines, and vasoactive peptides and release of coagulation factors. There is thrombosis, spasm of the microvessels, worsening of the ischemia, generation of oxygen free radical, and excess of glutamate release, and then a serious energetic crisis is installed and self-perpetuated. Cytotoxic edema occurs.

The regeneration is impaired by physical barriers with the loss of parenchymal volume and the formation of cystic cavities, and also by the deposition of fibroblasts that promote a distortion of the structural framework. Also, the family of inhibitory proteins that bind to the Nogo receptor found on regenerating axons lead to activation of the Rho pathway, which inhibits neurite outgrowth. Together, all those mechanisms contribute to the impaired spinal cord regeneration [2–4] (see Fig. 17.1).

Goals in the management of SCI patients include reducing primary neurological damage and preventing secondary damage. The aim of neuroprotective therapies is to limit the extent of the acute neural injury, while the goal of neuroregenerative therapies is to facilitate neuronal outgrowth.

17.3 Clinical/Neurological Presentation

Clinical presentation will depend on the extent, level, and type of the lesion. Injuries above the sixth thoracic vertebra (Th6) will interrupt or disturb the descending sympathetic pathways from the sympathetic trunk, which travel from the first thoracic vertebra (Th1) until the second lumbar vertebra (L2). As consequences, there will be lack of inhibition of parasympathetic pathways, resulting in stimulation of vagus nerve and increased parasympathetic tone below the injury level. There will be not only sensory and motor disturbances but also cardiovascular (mainly hypotension with profound bradycardia and atrioventricular nodal block), thermoregulatory, urinary, gastrointestinal, sexual, and respiratory/bronchopulmonary disturbances. Lesions below Th6 will have preserved sympathetic/parasympathetic responses [5, 6].

Regarding motor and sensorial presentation, the most common injury is central cord syndrome. It is typically due to a hyperextension injury that causes a buckling of the ligamentum flavum and a cord contusion. There is a loss of cervical motor function with sparing of lower limb strength (somatotopic organization, with the upper extremity motor fibers being the most medial).

Brown-Sequard syndrome (hemiplegia with ipsilateral loss of light touch and proprioception and contralateral loss of pain and temperature) is typically due to traumatic hemisection of the spinal cord and is more common with penetrating injuries.

Anterior cord syndrome is rare after trauma but can occur when axial compression and burst fractures cause retropulsion of vertebral body and bone fragments dislodge into the

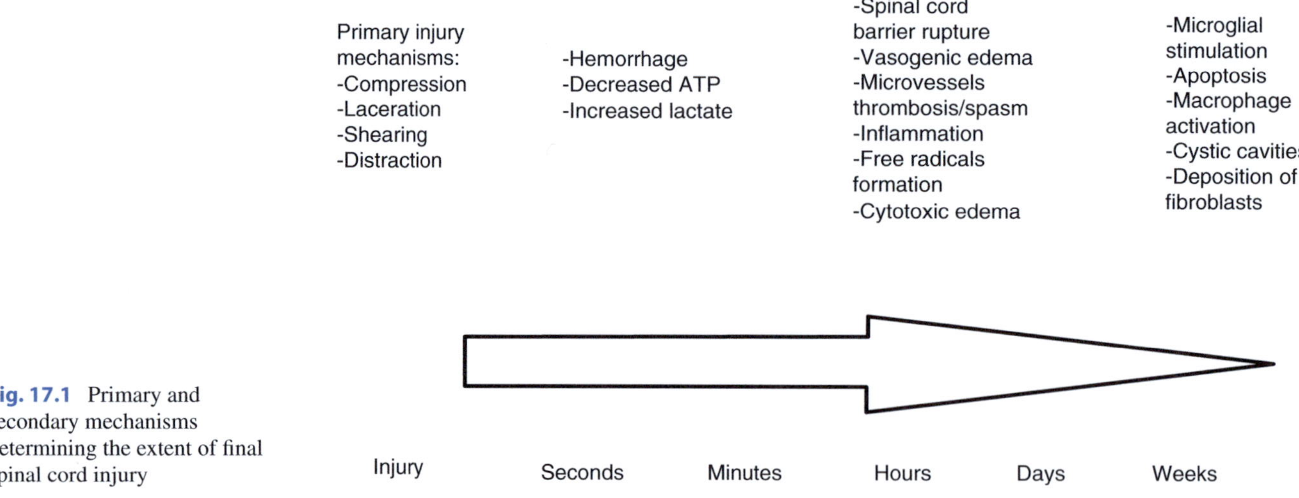

Fig. 17.1 Primary and secondary mechanisms determining the extent of final spinal cord injury

Central cord syndrome

Descending Tracts (Motor)
Ascending Tracts (Sensory)
Lateral Corticospinal Tract (Motor)
Doral Columns (Deep touch, Propioception, Vibration)
Lateral Spinothalamic Tract (Pain, Temperature)
Ventral Corticospinal Tract (Motor)
Ventral Spinothalamic Tract (Light touch)

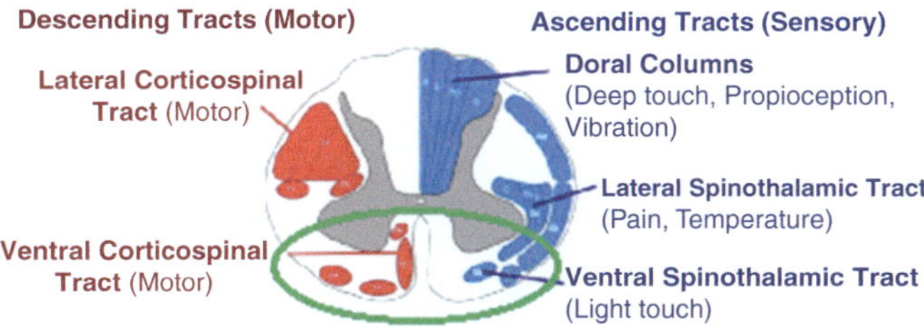

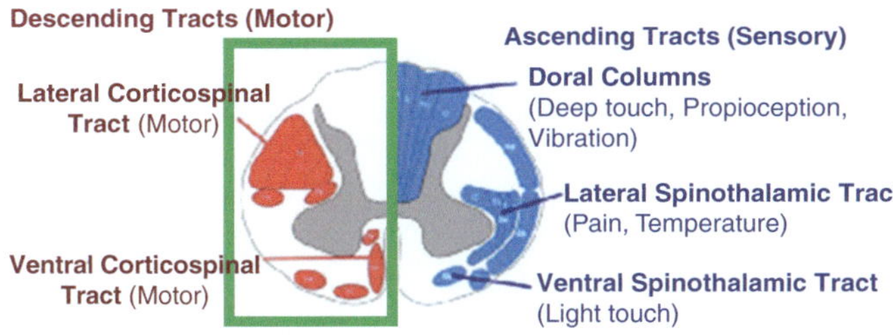

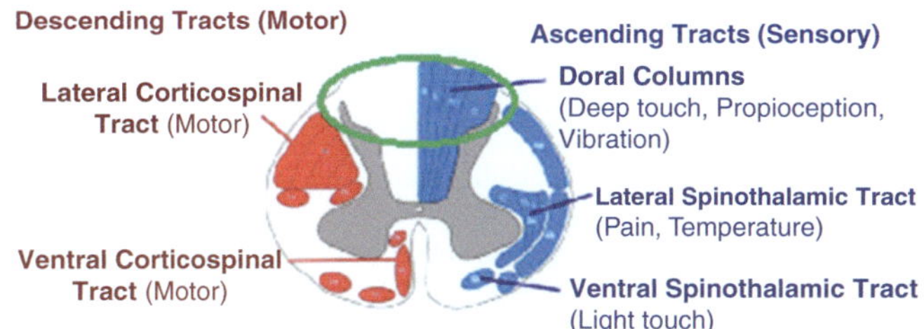

Fig. 17.2 Schematic depiction of major cord syndromes

anterior portion of the cord. There is disruption of corticospinal and spinothalamic tracts, with sparing of dorsal columns.

Posterior cord syndrome is also rare following trauma and results in the loss of proprioception with preservation of motor function and pain, temperature, and light touch functions (see Fig. 17.2).

Cauda equina syndrome is usually caused by the retropulsion of bone fragments in the lumbosacral region, with lower spinal nerve root compression. There are lower back and limb pain, bowel and bladder dysfunction, saddle anesthesia, decreased rectal tone and contraction, absent or decreased "anal wink," or bulbocavernosus reflex [6].

The complete neurological exam is always of major importance, but in the context of TSCI, the recommended preferred tool for neurological and functional classification is the American Spinal Injury Association (ASIA). It is important as a way to standardize the evaluation and the follow-up, as well as it has a role in predicting the patient's prognosis.

It consists of the motor and sensitive components.

The sensitive exam comprises testing each of the 28 dermatomes (from C2 to S4–5) on the right and left sides. Light touch and pinprick sensation are also tested. Each modality scores from 0 to 2 on a three-point scale, with 0 being absent and 2 normal/intact.

The motor exam comprises testing of muscle functions corresponding to ten paired myotomes (C5–T1 and L2–S1). Voluntary external anal sphincter must also be tested. The strength is graded from 0 to 5, according to the Medical Research Council (MRC) grading system.

The most caudal segment with antigravity muscle function strength and intact sensation corresponds to the injury level (see Fig. 17.3).

After this evaluation, the ASIA Impairment Scale should be determined, which is as follows:

- Complete. The absence of sensory or motor functions in sacral segments S4–S5.

  Poor prognosis: 85% will not regain function, and only 3% of those who improve have a useful function.
- Sensory incomplete. Sensory function preserved below the injury level, including S4–S5. No motor is preserved more than three levels below the motor level on each side of the body.

  54% patients regain function.
- Motor complete. Motor function preserved below the neurological level, with more than half of the muscles below the level of injury with grade <3.

  86% of patients regain function.
- Motor incomplete. Motor function preserved below the neurological level, with at least half of the muscles below the level of injury with grade >3.
- Normal. Sensorial and motor functions are normal in all segments tested [3, 7, 8].

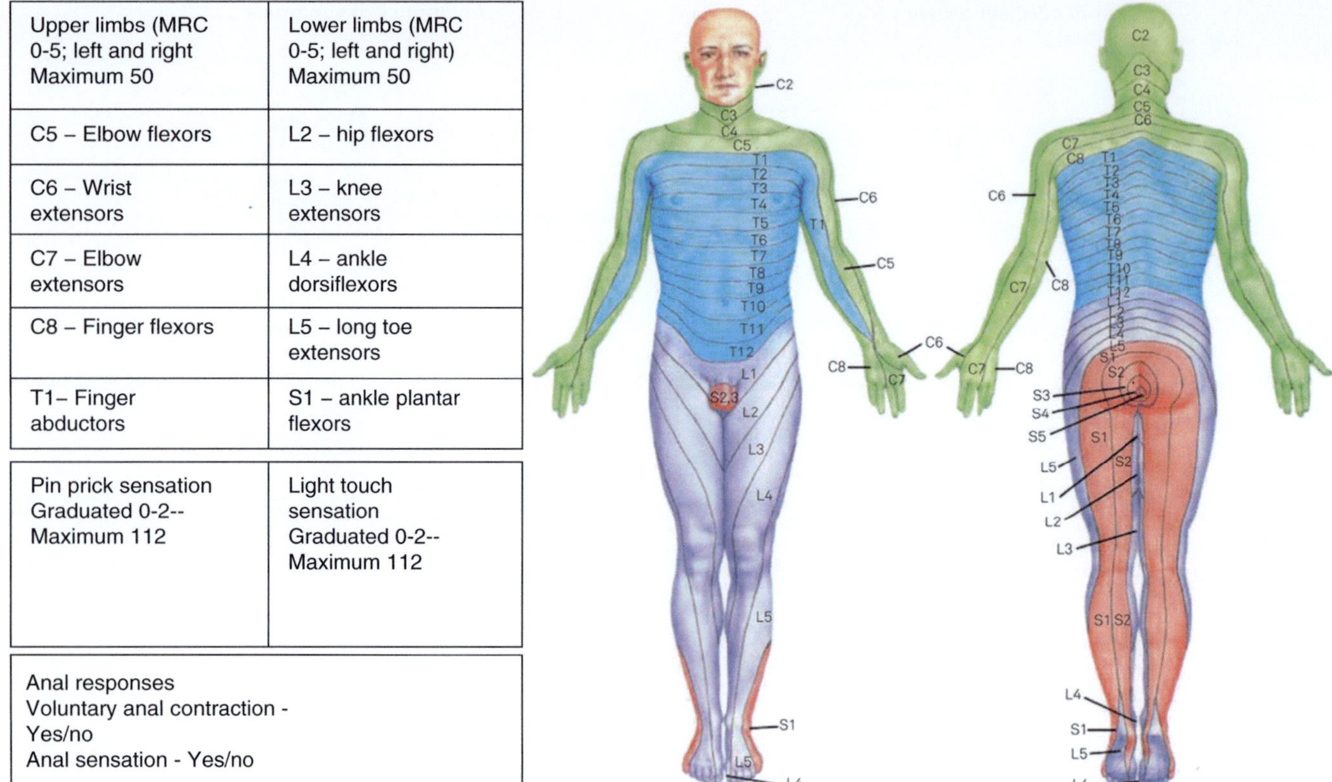

Upper limbs (MRC 0-5; left and right Maximum 50	Lower limbs (MRC 0-5; left and right) Maximum 50
C5 – Elbow flexors	L2 – hip flexors
C6 – Wrist extensors	L3 – knee extensors
C7 – Elbow extensors	L4 – ankle dorsiflexors
C8 – Finger flexors	L5 – long toe extensors
T1– Finger abductors	S1 – ankle plantar flexors

Pin prick sensation Graduated 0-2-- Maximum 112	Light touch sensation Graduated 0-2-- Maximum 112

Anal responses
Voluntary anal contraction - Yes/no
Anal sensation - Yes/no

Fig. 17.3 Steps required for the motor (left) and sensory (right) examination for American Spinal Injury Association (ASIA) neurological classification of spinal cord injury

17.4 Acute Complications

Neurogenic shock is a major acute complication after SCI. It consists of profound hypotension and bradycardia due to the interruption of sympathetic tone and an unopposed intact vagal tone, as previously mentioned. It is estimated to occur in 19,3% of cervical, 7% in thoracic, and 3% in lumbar injuries. Blood loss due to polytrauma may contribute to the shock. Some studies report that 16% of patients with neurogenic shock will develop cardiac arrest.

Other cardiovascular complications may occur as a consequence of the disturbed autonomic nervous system. Irregularities of cardiac rhythm such as bradyarrhythmias, supraventricular ectopic beats, and ventricular ectopic beats may occur. Orthostatic hypotension happens in up to 74% of the patients. There is an association with heart disease (OR 2,72) and stroke (OR 3,72)

Respiratory complications are the main cause of morbidity and mortality in the acute phase of SCI, with atelectasis (36,4%), pneumonia (31,4%), and respiratory failure (22,6%) being the most common. Regarding the level of the injury, 84% of patients with injuries above C4 and 60% of those with injuries from C5 to C8 will experience airway issues. In those with injuries from Th1 to Th12, 65% may have severe respiratory complications as well. A reduced vital capacity, retention of secretions, and autonomic dysfunction all play a role. See "Airway Management" for further discussion and explanation.

Abnormal temperature regulation is another well-described phenomenon after SCI, especially in cervical and high thoracic injuries. Poikilothermia, fluctuating temperature, hypothermia, and hyperthermia may happen.

Bladder and bowel issues frequently also occur. In the acute phase, they are frequently hypotonic [5].

17.5 Imaging

According to the last SCI guideline, a radiographic study of the spinal cord is mandatory to those who complain of neck pain and spinal tenderness, who have neurological focal deficits related to the spine, and who cannot be properly evaluated (the ones who are unconscious, not cooperative, or intoxicated) [9].

There are two protocols available that estimate the risk of a patient having a cervical fracture/subluxation/dislocation, in order to identify those who don't need a spinal imaging. The first is the National Emergency X-Radiography Utilization Study (NEXUS). It consists of five criteria: no posterior midline cervical tenderness, no intoxication, normal mental status, no other painful injuries, and no neurological deficits. Patients that meet all these criteria have a low risk of cervical injury, and imaging can be waived, with a sensitivity of 99% and a negative predictive value of 99.9% [10]. The second protocol is the Canadian C-Spine Rule, which consists of three questions: the presence of a high risk factor that mandates radiography (age >65 years, dangerous trauma mechanism, paresthesia in extremities), the presence of low risk factors allowing safe assessment of the range of motion, and the ability of performing neck rotation 45° to the left and right. It has a sensitivity of 100% and a specificity of 42,5% [11].

A three-view spinal X-ray (anteroposterior, odontoid, and lateral views) or, whenever possible, a computed tomography (CT) should be ordered (the CT is superior to the X-ray) [9].

A magnetic resonance imaging (MRI) should be obtained, when feasible, in the first 48 h after the trauma. It allows a good visualization of spinal cord edema, blood products, ongoing compression, ligamentous and disc injury, and displacement of the vertebral column. It helps to predict the outcome and classify the injury severity. Intraspinal hemorrhage longer than 1 cm is associated with poor recovery, as well as 3 cm or more of longitudinal T2 signal change (related to diffuse edema). A normal initial MRI is a marker of good prognosis.

However, we still face limitations concerning prognostication. New emerging MRI techniques may improve this issue. A technique called diffusion tensor imaging (DTI) reflects axonal integrity, magnetization transfer (MT) and myelin water fraction (MWF) correlate with myelin quantity, and magnetic resonance spectroscopy (MRS) measures the concentration of molecules that reflect cell loss. Those are investigational but promising techniques for the future [12].

17.6 Cardiovascular Management

As previously mentioned, hypotension is common after TSCI. Its consequences have not been studied in a controlled prospective way, although, there is convincing evidence that it worsens secondary injury by reducing spinal cord flow and perfusion. The current recommendation is to strictly avoid hypotension and to maintain mean arterial pressure (MAP) at 85–90 mmHg for 7 days after injury (level III evidence). Volemia should be kept normal or slightly elevated by the use of fluids and vasopressors. The patients should be monitored in an intensive care unit (ICU), and an arterial line should be placed. Those with high cervical and complete lesions are at more risk for cardiovascular instability and more frequently need vasopressor support [9, 13].

The most used drugs in this context are norepinephrine, phenylephrine, dopamine, dobutamine, and vasopressin. Norepinephrine acts through alpha and beta receptors and leads to both increased cardiac contractility and peripheral vasoconstriction. Phenylephrine acts just through alpha receptors and has just arterial vasoconstriction effect. Dopamine answer depends on the dosage used: in low dosage, it has just beta-receptor effect, leading to inotropic and chronotropic answers, and in high dosages, it also has strong alpha-receptor effect with peripheral vasoconstriction. Dobutamine has an inotropic effect (and has to be used with caution as it can cause mild vasodilation) and vasopressin and just vasoconstriction effect. There is no clear superiority in one vasopressor over the others. The choice should be made according to the clinical context, and the decision should be individually tailored.

Sometimes the injury level can help in guiding the decision. In cervical and high thoracic lesions that present with both bradycardia and hypotension, dopamine or norepinephrine may be good options. In low thoracic lesions, where the hypotension is just the result of peripheral vasodilation, phenylephrine is a reasonable choice.

It is important to notice that there is an elevated rate of side effects with the use of vasopressors, with some series describing up to 70%. The most common side effects are tachycardia, bradycardia, new-onset atrial fibrillation, changes of ST in the electrocardiogram, and elevated troponin. In older-aged patients, norepinephrine and phenylephrine seem safer than dopamine [14–16].

All these findings have led to a non-inferiority trial that is currently recruiting patients, the "Mean Arterial Blood Pressure for Treatment for Acute Spinal Cord Injury." It is comparing the avoidance of hypotension (MAP ≥ 65 mmHg) versus the induction of hypertension (MAP ≥ 85 mmHg) [17].

17.7 Airway Management

Respiratory complications are really prevalent in patients with TSCI.

The respiratory muscles comprise the diaphragm, the intercostal and accessory muscles, and the muscles of the abdomen. The degree of failure usually worsens as the injury is more rostral and complete. There are reduced lung volumes and flow rates. Complete lesions above the third cervical level (C3) lead to paralysis of diaphragmatic (innervation from C3 to C5), intercostal, and abdominal muscles and are virtually incompatible with life in the absence of mechanical ventilatory support. In patients with high cervical but incomplete lesions or cervical lesions bellow C5, neural control of diaphragm is preserved, and spontaneous ventilation can be possible. Paradoxical breathing can happen—the abdominal wall retracts during inspiration and protrudes during expiration [18].

The lack of diaphragm function, previous cardiopulmonary disease, tachypnea at admission, advanced age, copious sputum, pneumonia, and major lobe collapse are predictive for the need of mechanical ventilation [12].

The two most important predictive markers for the need of intubation are the level of the injury and the ASIA classification. Intubation should be done in an elective way, since urgent intubation when there is respiratory distress increases the risk of neurological damage. Neck hyperextension should be avoided, as well as rotation or other movements of the neck. When possible, awake, fiber-optic intubation should be preferred. When fiber-optic laryngoscope or bronchoscope is unavailable, in-line stabilization without traction is an alternative.

In those patients that can be managed conservatively, lung function should be strictly monitored. A reduction in current volume to less than 15 mL/kg, a maximum inspiratory pressure below −20 cmH_2O or/and, an increase in pCO_2 are indicative of the need for intubation.

It is important to keep in mind some particularities of the TSCI patients, which do not apply to other patients from general ICUs, or even from neuro-ICU—in high-level injuries—ventilation will depend almost exclusively on the diaphragm (responsible for 90% of the tidal volume); coughing is impaired so there is accumulation of secretions; also there is increased production of secretions secondary to autonomic dysfunction, which facilitates the onset of atelectasis. In up to 60% of patients, there is also associated lung trauma [18].

Regarding ventilator weaning, success rates are low, with only 40% of those with lesions above C4 being extubated. Predictors of the need for tracheostomy are ASIA A lesions, the extent of the lesion smoking, and previous lung disease. The literature suggests that early tracheostomy (within 7–10 days) may facilitate pulmonary management, with shorter duration of mechanical ventilation, decreased laryngotracheal complications, and faster ICU discharge [19].

17.8 Decompressive Surgery

The aim of surgical decompression is to relieve the pressure caused by the progressive edema and hemorrhage that develops after the initial trauma, worsening secondary damage and spinal ischemia. Rational existed to believe that early decompression would lead to better outcomes than late decompression, with the neuroprotective effect thus varying with time elapsed since the trauma.

The STASCIS trial ("The Surgical Timing in Acute Spinal Cord Injury"), published in 2012, evaluated this issue, and, in a prospective, observational way concluded that surgery performed before 24 h was safe, did not lead to major complication rates, and was associated with better neurological outcomes than late surgery (>24 h) [20]. After that, other studies were published with similar results, even after adjustment to preoperative neurological status and neurological level [21].

With that, the concept of "time is spine" has emerged, and nowadays recommendation is that decompressive surgery should be performed in the first 24 h after trauma. We still do not know, however, which patients will benefit the most from the early intervention strategy. Probably, a more individual approach will be necessary for the future.

The SCI-POEM is an ongoing observational and prospective trial, still recruiting participants, that aims to compare an ultra-early approach (surgery within the first 12 h) versus from 12 h until 14 days. The primary outcome is the change in ASIA lower extremity motor score [22].

17.9 Intravenous Methylprednisolone

Methylprednisolone (MP), a synthetic corticosteroid with minimal mineralocorticoid activity, has anti-inflammatory effects by upregulating anti-inflammatory factors, suppressing migration of polymorphonuclear cells and fibroblasts, reducing capillary permeability, stabilizing lysosomes at a cellular level, decreasing oxidative stress, and enhancing cell survival. Animal studies have reported improvement in functional outcome after steroid treatment. With this rationale, since the 1980s trials have been conducted trying to demonstrate in vivo benefits of methylprednisolone in TSCI [23].

The first trial conducted, the NASCIS I ("National Acute Spinal Cord Injury Study I"), examined the efficacy of high-dose methylprednisolone (1000 mg bolus and daily thereafter for 10 days) compared with a standard dose (100 mg bolus and daily thereafter for 10 days). It is important to notice that both groups received corticosteroids. The neurological outcome was measured by motor function, response to pinprick, and light touch. At 6 weeks and 6 months, recovery rates were almost identical in both groups, but wound infection rate was significantly higher in the high-dose group. The case fatality rate did not reach statistically significant difference, even though fatality was three times higher in the 1000 mg group [24].

The second trial was the NASCIS II that evaluated efficacy and safety of MP 30 mg/kg bolus followed by 5.4 mg/kg/h infusion per 23 h versus naloxone 5.4 mg/kg bolus, followed by 4 mg/kg infusion per 23 h versus placebo. Motor and sensory outcomes were evaluated in 6 weeks and 6 months. The group treated with corticosteroids until 8 h of the trauma had significant improvement in motor, pinprick sensation, and touch. Those treated with naloxone or MP after 8 h did not have any benefit. There were more wound infections and gastrointestinal bleeding, but they did not reach statistical significance [25].

The third trial was the NASCIS III, compared MP for 24 h, MP for 48 h or tirilazad mesylate for 48 h, all in patients until 8 h from trauma. All patients received initially a 30 mg/kg bolus of MP, followed by an infusion of 5.4 mg/kg for 24 or 48 h, depending on the group. Those in the tirilazad group received 2.5 mg/kg bolus infusion or doses every 6 h for 48 h. Main outcome measures were motor recovery and chance in functionality. There were better outcomes for those who received MP for 48 h and started the drug between 3 and 8 h after injury. However, sepsis and pneumonia rates were also elevated [26].

With those studies, despite the results were not robust at all and despite the lack of evidence, MP was used in large scale for many years. Until 2002 guideline, MP for 24 or 48 h was considered a therapeutic option with the knowledge that harmful side effects can occur, and with the caveat that there was insufficient evidence on the subject.

All the studies that came after fail to demonstrate real benefits of the MP use. The last consensus does not recommend it as part of treatment for acute SCI [9].

A recently published meta-analysis and systematic review reinforce this recommendation since pooled evidence from multiple randomized controlled trials and observational studies did not demonstrate significant long-term benefits and demonstrated increased rates of gastrointestinal bleeding. Strong recommendations, however, are not warranted since confidence in the effect estimated is limited [27].

17.10 Neuroprotective Therapies

Several drugs have been evaluated as potential candidates for neuroprotection in TSCI. The aim of neuroprotection is to preserve injured tissue and reduce secondary insult, by targeting components of the pathophysiologic cascade [2–4].

Herein we will review the drugs evaluated in clinical trials and those which are underway at the moment (see Table 17.1).

Table 17.1 Drugs evaluated as potential candidates for neuroprotection in TSCI

Drug	Purposed mechanism	Evidence for use
Naloxone [25]	Blockage of neurotoxic effect of endogenous opioid dynorphin A	No evidence of improvement (NASCIS II)
Nimodipine [28]	Calcium channel blocker, prevents activation of apoptotic enzymes and blocks release of glutamate	No evidence of improvement
Tirilazad mesylate [26]	Attenuates peroxidation of neuronal membrane	No evidence of improvement (NASCIS III)
GM1 ganglioside [29]	Enhance axonal regeneration, prevention of apoptosis, anti-excitotoxic activity	No longer recommended (it was until 2002 guideline)—no evidence of improvement
Riluzole [30]	Sodium channel blocker, decreases glutamate release and enhances uptake	"Riluzole in Spinal Cord Injury Study" (RISCIS)—currently recruiting patients (phase II/III trial)
Minocycline [31]	Anti-inflammatory properties—inhibition of TNF alpha, IL-1beta, COX-2, NOS, and microglial activation; decreases lesion size and neuron loss	"Minocycline in Acute Spinal Cord Injury" (MASC)—currently recruiting patients (phase III)
Fibroblast growth factor (FGF) [32]	Reduces excitotoxic activity, cell death, and oxygen free radical production	Results pending from a phase I/II study
Cytokine granulocyte colony-stimulating factor (G-CSF) [33, 34]	Inhibits TNF-alpha and IL-1beta, promotes cell survival	Benefits shown in two nonrandomized studies
Magnesium [35]	Decreases neurotoxicity and inflammation	Phase I trial did not show benefits

TNF-alpha tumor necrosis factor alpha, *COX-2* cyclooxygenase-2, *NOS* nitric oxide synthase

17.11 Neuroregenerative Therapies

Neuroregenerative strategies are being the subject of numerous studies worldwide. They use endogenous and exogenous repair mechanisms that aim to surpass barriers to recovery, such as the loss of architectural framework, cystic cavitations, astroglial scarring, and inhibitory molecular signaling.

The Rho-ROCK pathway is associated with inhibition of neurite outgrowth. It is activated by chondroitin sulfate proteoglycans (CSGPs), myelin-associated glycoproteins (MAGs), oligodendrocyte-myelin glycoprotein (OMgp), and neurite outgrowth inhibitor-A (NOGO-A). There are multiple attempts in developing drugs to interrupt this signaling cascade (anti-Nogo-A antibody, epidural paste with direct Rho inhibition properties). Chondroitinase ABC is also under evaluation as an attempt to degrade the CSGPs in the glial scar, therefore avoiding the abovementioned inhibitory cascade to start.

Cell-based therapies are promising modalities of neuroregenerative treatments. Embryonic stem cells and induced pluripotent stem cells are theoretically capable of regenerating lost neural circuits, remyelinating axons, modulating the inflammatory response, and modifying the microenvironment. Schwan cells are also capable of remyelinating central and peripheral nervous system axons and seem to reduce cystic cavitation. Olfactory ensheathing cells are potent phagocytes and have shown to enhance axonal regeneration and remyelination. Finally, mesenchymal stem cells and multipotent stromal cells have the capacity of differentiating into connective tissue lineages and can modulate local inflammatory response. There are several ongoing trials and studies trying to establish benefits with those cell therapies [2, 4].

Until now, however, it should be noticed that the neuroregenerative therapies remain experimental, and not yet formally recommended.

17.12 Final Remarks

TSCI is a devastating disease, with great morbidity and high costs. There is still a lot to be done, but advances that can impact on long-term prognosis have occurred in the last years. Neuroprotective and neuroregenerative strategies seem to be the future of care for those patients and probably work better when done together. Pending trial results are eagerly awaited.

References

1. Cripps RA, Lee BB, Wing P, et al. A global map for traumatic spinal cord injury epidemiology: towards a living data repository for injury prevention. Spinal Cord. 2011;49:493–501.
2. Ahuja CS, Martin AR, Fehlings MG. Recent advances in managing spinal cord injury secondary to trauma. F1000 Res. 2016;5(F1000 Faculty Rev):1017.
3. Rouanet C, Reges D, Rocha R, et al. Traumatic spinal cord injury: current concepts and treatment update. Arq Neuropsiquiatr. 2017;75(6):387–93.
4. Wilson JR, Forgione N, Fehlings MG. Emerging therapies for acute traumatic spinal cord injury. CMAJ. 2013;185(6):485–92.
5. Hagen EM. Acute complications of spinal cord injuries. World J Orthop. 2015;6(1):17–23.
6. Stein DM, Sheth KN. Management of acute spinal cord injury. Continuum (Minneap Minn). 2015;21(1):159–87.
7. Kirshblum SC, Burns SP, Biering-Sorensen F, Donovan W, Graves DE, Jha A, et al. International standards for neurological classification of spinal cord injury (revised 2011). J Spinal Cord Med. 2011;34(6):535–46.
8. Le CT, Price M. Survival from spinal cord injury. J Chronic Dis. 1982;35(6):487–92.
9. Hadley MN, Walters BC, Aarabi B, Dhall SS, Gelb DE, Harrigan MR, et al. Update guidelines for the management of acute cervical spine and spinal cord injury. Neurosurgery. 2013;72(Suppl 3):1.
10. Hoffman JR, Mower WR, Wolfson AB, Todd KH, Zucker MI. Validity of a set of clinical criteria to rule out injury to the cervical spine in patients with blunt trauma. N Engl J Med. 2000;343(2):94–9.
11. Stiell IG, Wells GA, Vandemheen KL, Clement CM, Lesiuk H, De Maio VJ, et al. The Canadian C-spine rule for radiography in alert and stable trauma patients. JAMA. 2001;286(15):1841–8.
12. Krishna V, Andrews H, Varma A, Mintzer J, Kindy MS, et al. Spinal cord injury: how can we improve its classification and quantification of its severity and prognosis? J Neurotrauma. 2014;31:215–27.
13. Casha S, Christie S. A systematic review of intensive cardiopulmonary management after spinal cord injury. J Neurotrauma. 2011;28(8):1479–95.
14. Ploumis A, Yadlapalli N, Fehlings MG, Kwon BK, Vaccaro AR. A systematic review of the evidence supporting a role for vasopressor in acute SCI. Spinal Cord. 2010;48:356–62.
15. Inoue T, Manley GT, Patel N, Whetstone WD. Medical and surgical management after spinal cord injury: vasopressor usage, early surgeries, and complications. J Neurotrama. 2014;31:284–91.
16. Readdy WJ, Dhall SS. Vasopressor administration in spinal cord injury: should me apply a universal standard to all injury patterns? Neural Regen Res. 2016;11(3):420–1.
17. Jacobs WB. Mean arterial blood pressure treatment for acute spinal cord injury (MAPS). Clinical Trialsgov. NCT 02232165.
18. Vazquez RG, Sedes PR, Farina MM, Marques AM, Velasco EF. Respiratory management in the patient with spinal cord injury. Biomed Res Int. 2013;2013:168757.
19. Choi HJ, Paeng SH, Kim ST, Lee KS, Kim MS, Jung YT. The effectiveness of early tracheostomy in cervical spinal cord injury patients. J Korean Neurosurg Soc. 2013;54:220–4.
20. Fehlings MG, Vaccaro A, Wilson JR, Singh A, Cadotte D W, Harrop JS, et al. Early versus delayed decompression for traumatic cervical spinal cord injury: results of the Surgical Timing in Acute Spinal Cord Injury Study (STASCIS). PLoS One. 2012;7(1):e32037.
21. Wilson JR, Singh A, Craven C, Verrier MC, Drew B, Ahn H, et al. Early versus late surgery for traumatic spinal cord injury: the results of a prospective Canadian cohort study. Spinal Cord. 2012;50(11):840–3.
22. AOSpine Europe. Surgical treatment for spinal cord injury(SCI-POEM). Clinical Trials.gov. NCT 01674764; 2012.
23. Anwar MA, Shehabi TSA, Eid AH. Inflammogenesis of secondary spinal cord injury. Front Cell Neurosci. 2016;10(98):1–24.
24. Bracken MB, Collins WF, Freeman DF, Shepard MJ, Wagner FW, Silten RM, et al. Efficacy of methylprednisolone in acute spinal cord injury. JAMA. 1984;251(1):45–52.
25. Bracken MB, Shepard MJ, Collins WF, Holford TR, Young W, Baskin DS, et al. A randomized, controlled trial of methylprednisolone or naloxone in the treatment of acute spinal cord injury: results of the Second National Acute Spinal Cord Injury Study. N Engl J Med. 1990;322(20):1405–11.
26. Bracken MB, Shepard MJ, Holford TR, Leo-Summers L, Aldrich EF, Fazl M, et al. Administration of methylprednisolone for 24 or 48hours or tirilazad mesylate for 48 hours in the treatment of acute spinal cord injury: results of the Third National Acute Spinal Cord Injury Randomized Controlled Trial. JAMA. 1997;277(20):1597–604.
27. Evaniew N, Belley-Côté EP, Fallah N, Noonan VK, Rivers CS, Dvorak MF. Methylprednisolone for the treatment of patients with acute spinal cord injuries: a systematic review and meta-analysis. J Neurotrauma. 2016;33(5):468–81.
28. Petitjean ME, Pointillart V, Dixmerias F, Wiart L, Sztark F, Lassié P, et al. [Medical treatment of spinal cord injury in the acute stage]. Ann Fr Anesth Reanim. 1998;17(2):115–22.
29. Geisler FH, Coleman WP, Grieco G, Poonian D. The Sygen multicenter acute spinal cord injury study. Spine. 2001;26(24 Suppl):87–98.
30. AOSpine North America Research Network. Riluzole in spinal cord injury study (RISCIS). Clinical Trials.gov. NCT 01597518.
31. Rick Hansen Institute. Minocycline in acute spinal cord injury(MASC). Clinical Trials.gov. NCT 01828203.
32. Daiichi Sankyo Inc. Study to evaluate the efficacy, safety, and pharmacokinetics of SUN13837 injection in adult subjects with Acute Spinal Cord Injury (ASCI). Clinical Trials.gov. NCT01502631.
33. Kamiya K, Koda M, Furuya T, Kato K, Takahashi H, Sakuma T, et al. Neuroprotective therapy with granulocyte colony-stimulating factor in acute spinal cord injury: a comparison with high-dose with methylprednisolone as a historical control. Eur Spine J. 2015;24(5):963–7.
34. Takahashi H, Yamazaki M, Okawa A, Sakuma T, Kato K, Hashimoto M, et al. Neuroprotective therapy using granulocyte colony-stimulating factor for acute spinal cord injury: a phase I/IIa clinical trial. Eur Spine J. 2012;21(12):2580–7.
35. Streijger F, Lee JH, Monouchehri N, Okon EB, Tigchelaar S, et al. The evaluation of magnesium chloride within a polyethylene glycol formulation in a porcine model of acute spinal cord injury. J Neurotrauma. 2016;33(24):2202–16.

18 Modern Strategies for the Management of High-Energy Pelvic Fractures in the Twenty-First Century

Philip F. Stahel and Ernest E. Moore

Key Points

- High-energy pelvic ring disruptions continue to represent a global cause of preventable post-injury mortality from exsanguinating retroperitoneal hemorrhage.
- The application of pelvic binders is recommended as an early measure to stabilize the pelvic ring and decrease the amount of pelvic hemorrhage in the prehospital setting.
- Serum lactate and base deficit are sensitive tests for early recognition of the extent of traumatic hemorrhage and "hidden shock" in patients with pelvic ring disruptions.
- Injury mechanism-based classification systems of pelvic fractures are essential for understanding the severity of injury and to provide a guide for therapeutic decision-making.
- Resuscitative endovascular balloon occlusion of the aorta (REBOA) represents an effective and rapid bedside procedure for temporary bleeding control in hypotensive patients with hemodynamically unstable pelvic fractures.
- A protocolized approach of early external fixation with direct preperitoneal pelvic packing and delayed angioembolization in case of ongoing hemodynamic instability has been shown to significantly reduce post-injury mortality from acute exsanguinating hemorrhage.
- Recently published international expert consensus guidelines provide standardized algorithms for multidisciplinary care and classification-based decision-making toward improving outcomes of patients with severe pelvic ring disruptions.
- Resuscitated trauma patients are managed by delayed definitive reconstruction of the pelvic ring with conversion from external to internal fixation during a physiological "time window of opportunity."
- Definitive pelvic ring fixation is performed subsequent to successful resuscitation using standardized anterior and posterior surgical approaches.

18.1 History of Pelvic Fracture Management

The modern history of pelvic fracture management begins with the seminal work of Joseph-François Malgaigne (1806–1865), a French surgeon and world-renowned medical historian who published multiple influential textbooks on the management strategies of fractures and joint dislocations [1]. The eponym *Malgaigne's fracture* relates to the first historic description of a "vertical shear" pelvic ring injury with bilateral sacroiliac joint dislocations and associated anterior fractures of the pubic rami [2]. Malgaigne described the injury as a "double fracture" of the anterior and posterior pelvic ring, with displacement of the hemipelvis and shortening of the affected extremity. Malgaigne documented that vertically displaced pelvic fractures were often accompanied by impairment or complete loss of lower extremity function, and he advocated for a closed reduction maneuver, aided by vaginal and/or rectal palpation, followed by traction in a pelvic sling for a minimum of 45–50 days. Malgaigne also noted that many patients would not survive this severe injury and understood that there was a significant association between this fracture pattern, bleeding, and visceral injuries. The more fortunate patients who survived the initial injury remained at signifi-

P. F. Stahel (✉)
Rocky Vista University, College of Osteopathic Medicine, Parker, CO, USA

E. E. Moore
Department of Surgery, University of Colorado, School of Medicine, Denver Health Medical Center, Denver, CO, USA
e-mail: Ernest.Moore@dhha.org

P. Aseni et al. (eds.), *Operative Techniques and Recent Advances in Acute Care and Emergency Surgery*,
https://doi.org/10.1007/978-3-319-95114-0_18

cant risk of delayed suppuration and sepsis, which was likely the result of contaminated open fracture wounds and associated visceral injuries [2].

In parallel to Malgaigne's seminal work in France, a British surgeon named Charles Hewitt Moore (1821–1870) conducted similar research on pelvic ring disruptions in England [3]. In one of his case reports published in 1851, Dr. Moore described the deforming forces of a severe pelvic ring injury associated with a femoral head protrusion through an acetabular fracture, and he described the pelvic fracture pattern in excruciating scientific detail by emphasizing the nature of the underlying vectors related to the impacting and deforming forces (Fig. 18.1).

In 1895, the introduction of X-ray technology by Wilhelm Conrad Röntgen (1845–1923) dramatically improved the diagnostic accuracy and classification of pelvic ring injuries and allowed to monitor the healing process. The classic non-operative measures of pelvic ring injury management by application of skeletal traction (Fig. 18.2) were further refined by Sir Frank Wild Holdsworth (1904–1969) in England [4]. In a landmark article from 1948, Dr. Holdsworth reported a 10-year experience on 50 patients with traumatic pelvic ring disruptions in which he provided a first report on the modern equivalents of the "open-book" pattern, the "crescent" lateral compression pattern, and the "vertical shear" injury type [2]. Based on the surrogate marker for functional recovery related to the patients' ability of returning to previous employment, Holdsworth noted that pure sacroiliac joint dislocations had a poor prognosis, as fewer than half of these patients returned to their previous work. In contrast, nearly all of the patients with injuries involving a fracture of the ilium or sacrum returned to heavy labor. Thus, Holdsworth's landmark article provided a first "crude" classification of pelvic ring injuries, predictive of post-injury outcomes [2].

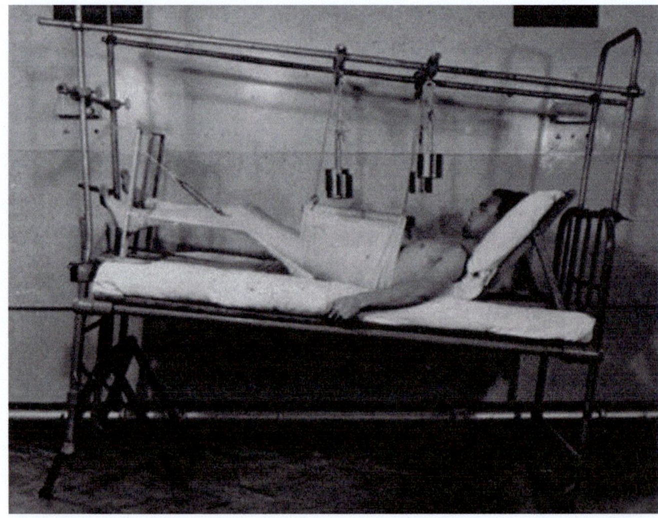

Fig. 18.2 Original photograph depicting the concept of skeletal traction for treatment of a pelvic ring injury in Sir Frank Wild Holdsworth's original publication (1948)

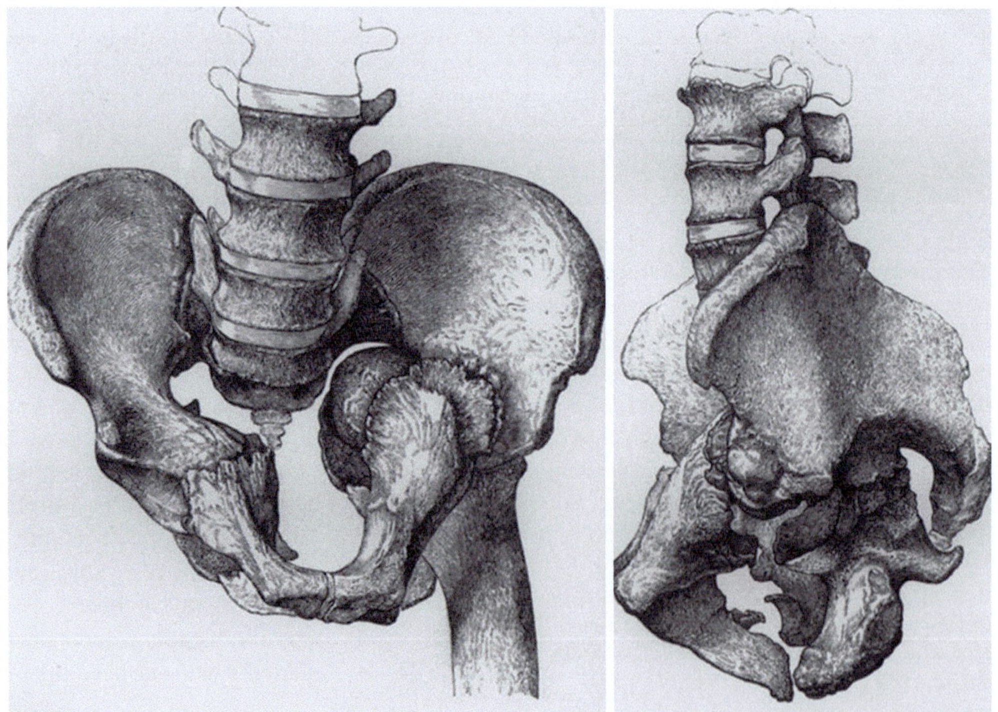

Fig. 18.1 Original graphic artwork from Charles Hewitt Moore's historic article "An account of a case of fracture and distortion of the pelvis, combined with an unusual form of dislocation of the femur" (1851)

18.2 The Evolution of Pelvic Fracture Classification

The first clinically relevant systematic classification of pelvic fractures, based on the mechanism of injury, was described in 1961 by Pennal and Sutherland [5, 6]. This system defines three distinct categories of pelvic ring injuries, (1) avulsion fractures, (2) "stable" fractures, and (3) "unstable" fractures, and attempts to correlate injury severity with outcomes. In 1980, Pennal and Tile introduced the aspect of fracture stability to the original Pennal/Sutherland classification and incorporated mechanisms and vectors of injury [6]. The Pennal/Tile classification furthermore served as a basis for therapeutic decision-making and management protocols of pelvic ring injuries. Currently used classification systems are largely based on the seminal publications by Tile, Pennal, and Sutherland [7]. In essence, the AO/OTA classification for pelvic ring injuries is based on Marvin Tile's original classification system [8]. Similarly, the classification by Young and Burgess is reflective of the original Pennal/Sutherland description [9]. Both the Tile and Young and Burgess classification systems are still widely used in the twenty-first century for decision-making and guidance of therapeutic protocols in the acute management of patients with pelvic ring disruptions. A comparison of the three most widely used classification systems for pelvic ring injuries is shown in Fig. 18.3.

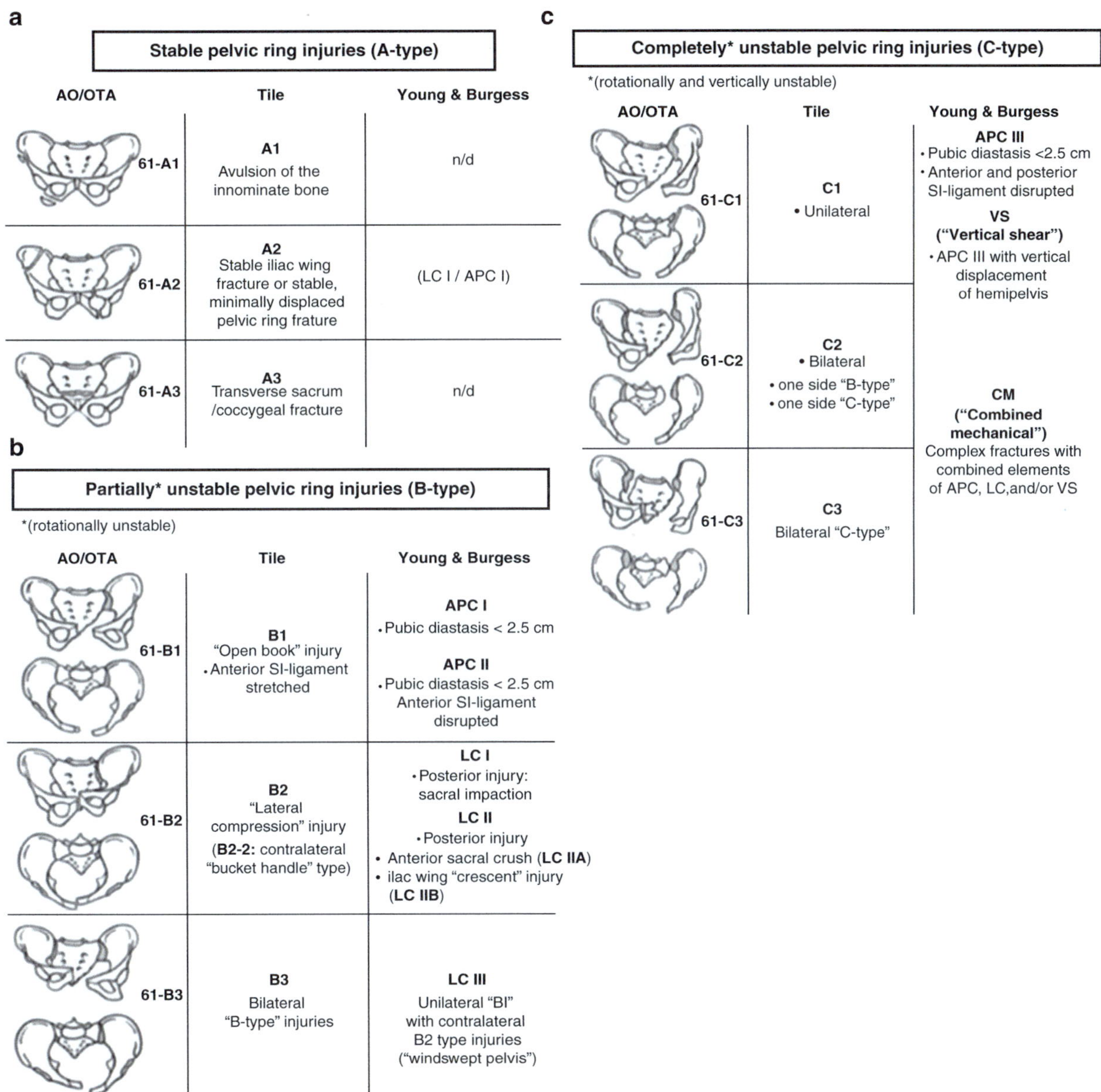

Fig. 18.3 Comparison of the prevalent classification systems for pelvic ring injuries, based on injury mechanism and pelvic ring stability. (Marsh JL, *et al.* Fracture and dislocation classification compendium - 2007: Orthopaedic Trauma Association classification, database and outcomes committee. *J Orthop Trauma* 2007, 21:S1–133). The drawings of the pelvic images were kindly provided by Ms. Marianne Peters, Berlin, Germany. The use of the AO/OTA classification is reprinted with permission

18.3 Mechanism-Based Classification Systems

The biomechanical stability of the pelvic ring relies on the integrity of the pubic symphysis and the posterior ligamentous complex. High-energy translational, rotational, and vertical shearing forces are required to disrupt the integrity and stability of the pelvic ring, leading to potentially exsanguinating retroperitoneal hemorrhage from venous presacral and paravesical plexus and cancellous bone from associated sacral fractures [10]. The vector of the impacting force has been shown to drive specific patterns of pelvic ring disruptions and determine their underlying extent of biomechanical instability and risk of associated bleeding [11]. In the twenty-first century, the most widely used classification systems that serve as a basis for therapeutic decision-making include (1) the alpha-numeric AO/OTA classification, (2) the historic classification by Marvin Tile, and (3) the mechanistic classification by Young and Burgess (Fig. 18.3).

The mechanistic classification system by Young and Burgess appears to represent the most clinically relevant system in the acute trauma setting by reflecting injury severity and taking into account the three main vectors of impacting forces, as well as any combination of multiple injury vectors [6, 12]. In brief, *anteroposterior compression (APC)* mechanisms induce a gradual disruption of the pubic symphysis with an external rotation deformity of the injured hemipelvis ("open book"), leading to hinging forces on the sacroiliac (SI) joints and consecutive disruption of the anterior and posterior SI ligaments. In contrast, *lateral compression (LC)* injuries lead to an internal rotation deformity of the injured hemipelvis and to gradual disruption of the SI ligament complex by compressing forces, as opposed to the tensile forces resulting from APC injuries. While most high-energy pelvic ring injuries are based on predicted APC- and LC-type mechanisms, a rare yet more lethal entity is represented by *vertical shear (VS)* injuries due to massive axial loading forces, including high-speed acceleration/deceleration collisions and falls from significant heights. Vertical shear injuries are characterized by a complete unilateral disruption of the anterior and posterior pelvic ring, leading to external rotation and vertical translation of the injured hemipelvis. Any injury mechanism with multiple vectors which do not follow the standard mechanisms of APC, LC, or VS forces can be classified as a *combined mechanism (CM)* injury which is typically highly unstable and associated with major retroperitoneal hemorrhage [13, 14].

A shortcoming of the conventional classification systems discussed above is related to the lack of a predictive correlation between the purely anatomic and mechanistic criteria with the physiologic and hemodynamic response in patients with pelvic ring disruptions. To overcome this limitation, the *World Society of Emergency Surgery* (WSES) recently published a new classification [15] which is based on a combination of the anatomic/mechanistic classification by Young and Burgess in conjunction with hemodynamic stability based on ATLS® guidelines. Based on these combined criteria, the new WSES classification stratifies pelvic ring injuries into three grades of severity:

1. *Minor* pelvic ring injuries (*WSES grade 1*): Mechanically (APC-1, LC-1) and hemodynamically stable injury patterns.
2. *Moderate* pelvic ring injuries: Mechanically unstable (*WSES grade 2*, LC-2, LC-3, APC-2, APC-3; *WSES grade 3*, VS or CM) with hemodynamic stability and/or adequate response to resuscitation ("responders").
3. *Severe* pelvic ring injuries (*WSES grade 4*): Any hemodynamically unstable injury pattern with patients at risk for acute exsanguinating hemorrhage, independent of the mechanistic fracture classification ("non-responders").

Based on this new anatomic/physiologic classification, the WSES recently published international expert consensus guidelines [15] to provide a classification-based decision-making algorithm for the management of patients with bleeding pelvic fractures (Fig. 18.4).

18.4 The Role of Pelvic Binders in the Prehospital Setting

The application of pelvic binders is a life-saving measure for acute bleeding control in patients with unstable pelvic ring disruptions [15]. Systematic reviews have demonstrated the effectiveness of pelvic binders in the temporary restoration of adequate blood pressure in hemodynamically unstable pelvic ring disruptions [16]. In a large database analysis of the German Pelvic Trauma Registry, the application of pelvic binders has been associated with a lower incidence of exsanguinating pelvic hemorrhage compared to the use of sheets. Placement of the pelvic binder at the level of the greater trochanter was shown to improve pelvic ring stability in human cadaveric studies. As the long-term ramifications of pelvic binders remain unclear at present, including the potential risk of soft-tissue complications from prolonged compression, the general recommendation is to remove pelvic binders as soon as physiologically justifiable and to consider replacing binders by early external pelvic fixation [15].

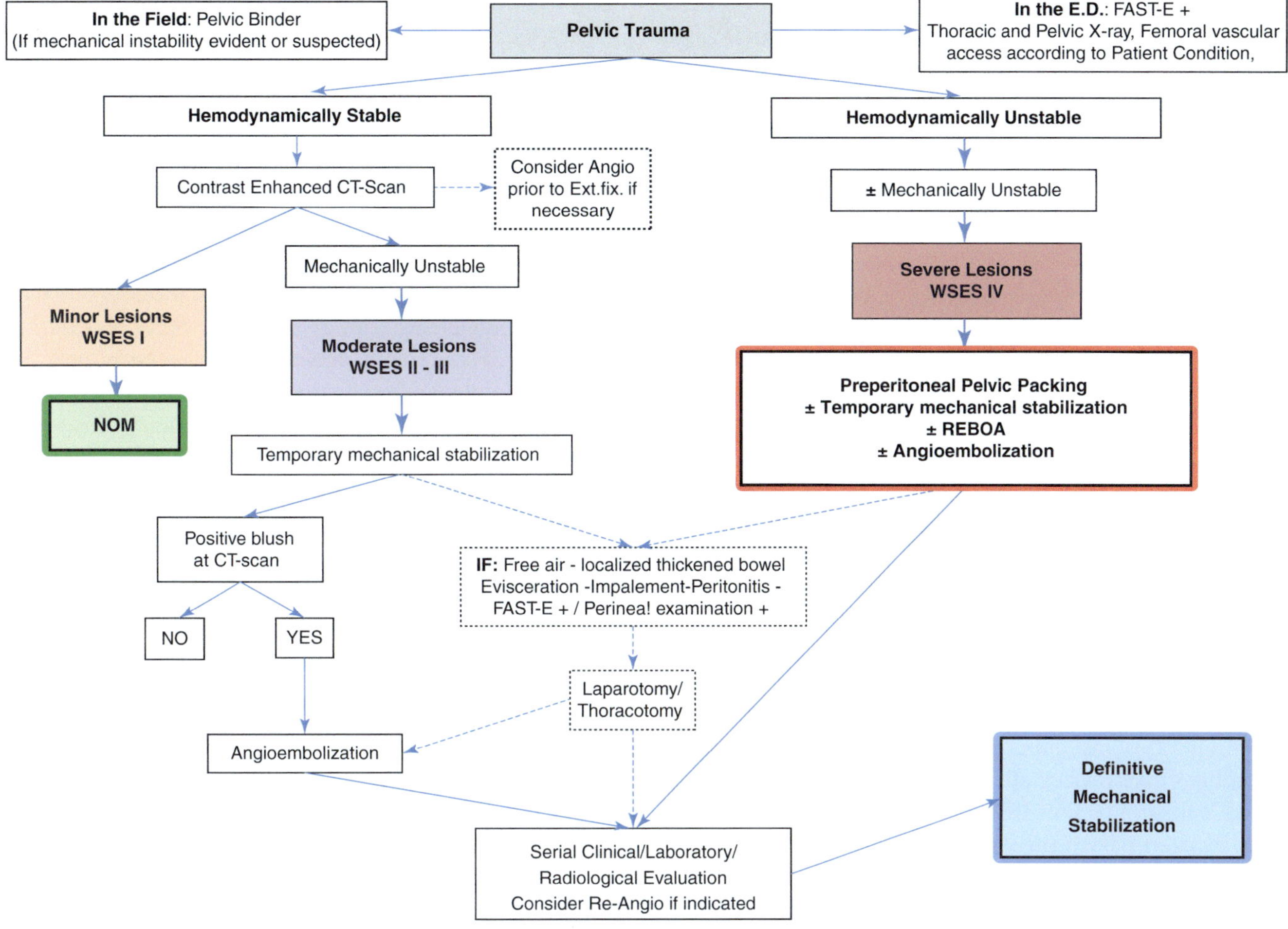

Fig. 18.4 International consensus algorithm for the management of acute pelvic ring injuries by the World Society for Emergency Surgery (WSES). Adapted with permission from Coccolini F. et al., *World J. Emerg. Surg.* 2017, 12:5

18.5 Acute Resuscitation Strategies for Bleeding Pelvic Fractures

High-energy pelvic ring disruptions represent a major source of life-threatening hemorrhage and potentially preventable post-injury mortality [14]. For patients with hemodynamically unstable pelvic ring injuries, survival depends on the early recognition and control of the associated retroperitoneal hemorrhage. The initial diagnostic workup in the emergency department (ED) is guided by standardized guidelines, including the "Advanced Trauma Life Support" (ATLS®) protocol [17]. About one third of all patients with complex pelvic ring disruptions are coagulopathic on admission, which is associated with significantly increased post-injury mortality [10]. The early presence of post-injury coagulopathy is best determined with bedside "point-of-care" testing by thrombelastography (TEG) or rotational thromboelastometry (ROTEM) [18]. These real-time diagnostic methods allow for a targeted resuscitation from traumatic-hemorrhagic shock and coagulopathy with blood products and improved post-injury survival rates [19]. In this regard, a recent randomized prospective trial revealed that the use of goal-directed, TEG-guided resuscitation strategies resulted in improved post-injury survival rates compared to standard mass transfusion protocols guided by conventional laboratory testing [20].

Serum lactate and base deficit represent sensitive markers for early recognition of occult hemorrhage and "hidden shock" [21]. The amount of lactate produced by anaerobic glycolysis is an indirect marker of oxygen debt, tissue hypoperfusion, and the severity of hemorrhagic shock, and base deficit values derived from arterial blood gas analysis provide an indirect estimation of global tissue acidosis from impaired tissue perfusion [21]. A landmark study from the 1990s on multiply injured patients correlated lactate clearance with survival [22]. The study results demonstrated a 100% survival rate in patients whose lactate levels returned to the normal range (≤2 mmol/L) within 24 h, whereas survival decreased to just above 10% in those patients with elevated lactate levels above 2 mmol/L for more than 48 h post-injury [22]. Similar to the predictive value of lactate levels, the initial base deficit has been established as a potent independent predictor of mortality in patients with traumatic-hemorrhagic shock [23]. The extent of base deficit has been stratified into three categories of severity (mild, −3 to −5 mEq/L; moderate, −6 to −9 mEq/L; severe, <−10 mEq/L), and a significant correlation has been demonstrated between the admission base deficit and transfusion requirements within the first 24 h and the risk of posttraumatic organ failure and post-injury death [23].

In patients with exsanguinating hemorrhage in extremis, a resuscitative "ED thoracotomy" (EDT) with cross-clamping of the aorta has been proven effective for bridging the time to the operating room until definitive surgical bleeding control [24]. More recently, bedside endovascular techniques in the ED have provided an alternative to aortic cross-clamping, e.g., with the resurgence of a resuscitative endovascular balloon occlusion of the aorta (REBOA) procedure for temporary hemorrhage control in hypotensive patients with a systolic blood pressure <80 mmHg on presentation [25]. The intuitive advantages of endovascular techniques over resuscitative thoracotomies have to be balanced against a technical learning curve for REBOA with an associated risk of severe iatrogenic complications [26]. Radiologic imaging is used to confirm proper catheter placement in aortic zone III (Fig. 18.5). Patients are then immediately taken to the operating room for surgical bleeding control, including external fixation and pelvic packing, if indicated [14, 15].

18.6 External Fixation of the Pelvic Ring

As part of acute "damage control" resuscitation strategies, any unstable pelvic ring injury with associated disruption of posterior element instability (WSES grades 2 and 3), particularly in conjunction with hemodynamic instability (WSES grade 4), should be considered for temporary external pelvic fixation [15]. In essence, pelvic external fixation represents a crucial resuscitative tool for acute hemorrhage control, as retroperitoneal bleeding is decreased after closure and reduction of the pelvic ring with adjunctive stability by external fixation [11]. Furthermore, pelvic packing has been shown to be effective only in conjunction with external fixation, in order to provide a counterpressure from the pelvic ring to the applied lap sponges in the retroperitoneal space [27–29]. From a technical decision-making perspective, most APC- or LC-equivalent injury patterns are preferably stabilized by anterior external fixation, either through the iliac crest route or through a fluoroscopy-guided supraacetabular route [11]. Either technique has distinct advantages and limitations, as previously described [11]. Anterior pelvic external fixation allows for a closed reduction of the externally malrotated hemipelvis in APC-2 and APC-3 injuries ("close the book"), and for a provisional reduction and retention of the internally malrotated hemipelvis in LC-2 and LC-3 injury patterns. In contrast to the fast application of a "damage control" iliac crest frame, the supraacetabular route for external fixation allows for improved stability of the external fixator frame, however, at the price of requiring strict fluoroscopy-guided pin placement with dedicated views of the supraacetabular corridor. In contrast to APC- and LC-injury patterns, vertical shear (VS) injuries inadequately stabilized by anterior exter-

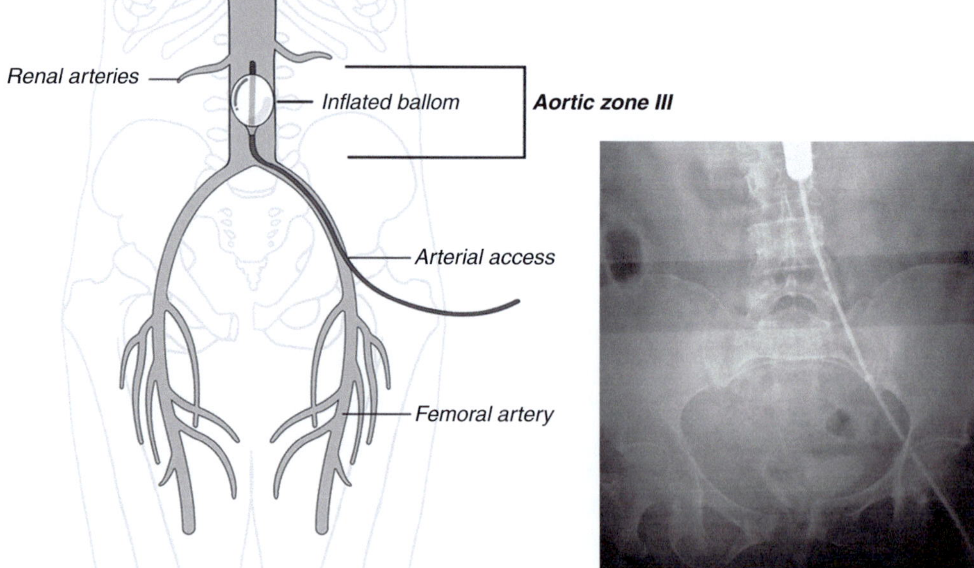

Fig. 18.5 Technique of REBOA placement in aortic zone III for temporary bleeding control in hemodynamically unstable pelvic ring disruptions. The graph and the pelvic radiograph depict a scenario of an unstable anteroposterior compression pelvic ring disruption in a hypotensive patient with retroperitoneal hemorrhage. © Phil Stahel & Ernest E. Moore, 2017

nal fixation frames, due to the complete instability of the posterior elements through the iliosacral joint. For these rare injury patterns, the pelvic "C-clamp" has been shown to provide temporary stabilization of the posterior pelvic elements and to effectively control associated retroperitoneal hemorrhage [30–32]. However, the use of a C-clamp should be restricted to selected indications (VS injuries with exsanguinating hemorrhage) and to adequately trained orthopedic trauma surgeons in order to mitigate the risk of serious intraoperative complications associated with inconsiderate C-clamp application [33].

18.7 Direct Preperitoneal Pelvic Packing

Traumatic hemorrhage from pelvic ring disruptions originates in large part from venous bleeding sources, and less than 10% of all cases are due to arterial bleeding amenable to early angioembolization [34]. As a matter of fact, recent studies have shown that the traditional ATLS-guided management of hemodynamically unstable pelvic ring injuries with angioembolization as the primary means of acute hemorrhage control results in poor patient outcomes and is associated with mortality rates over 40% in patients with hemodynamically unstable pelvic ring injuries [35]. These insights provide a strong rationale for pelvic packing as a first-line approach for early bleeding control in the retroperitoneal space [36]. The concept of pelvic packing was initially described in the 1980s and 1990s in Hannover, Germany, and Zurich, Switzerland, as a technique of transabdominal open pelvic packing through a "damage control" explorative laparotomy [30, 37]. These early studies demonstrated that severely injured patients with associated pelvic ring injuries have improved outcomes by early surgical "damage control" intervention, including temporary external fixation of unstable pelvic fractures, transabdominal pelvic packing, and surgical bleeding control [31]. The pelvic packing technique was later modified in Denver, Colorado, to a concept of "direct" preperitoneal pelvic packing (PPP) by applying a distinct surgical technique through a suprapubic midline incision that allows packing directly into the space of Retzius, without the necessity of opening the retroperitoneal compartment through a laparotomy [38]. When using the new PPP technique, a midline laparotomy can still be performed through a separate proximal midline incision, if a laparotomy is indicated simultaneously for the management of associated intraabdominal bleeding sources [28]. Importantly, the technique of using two separate midline incisions for pelvic packing and explorative laparotomy appears to be safe with regard to the potential risk of postoperative infections subsequent to pelvic de-packing and delayed definitive orthopedic fracture fixation [39]. Recent studies demonstrated that the pelvic packing protocol incorporated as part of a standardized institutional guidelines led to a significant decrease in blood product utilization and to improved patient outcomes [27, 29, 36]. Indeed, the current literature supports the notion that pelvic packing represents an effective technique for acute hemorrhage control that is associated with a significantly reduced mortality compared to conventional measures without pelvic packing [14, 15]. In addition, we have recently demonstrated that the PPP technique can be performed effectively and fast, within less than 10 min "skin-to-skin" [40]. In patients with ongoing hemorrhage and blood product transfusion requirements subsequent to pelvic packing, delayed angioembolization has been recommended as an adjunct to pelvic packing, which appears indicated in the small selected cohort of patients with ongoing hemorrhage from arterial sources [14]. Very recent data from our own 11-year institutional experience with protocolized pelvic packing on a cohort of 138 consecutive patients revealed that the post-injury mortality from acute exsanguinating pelvic hemorrhage was reduced to 2% after resuscitative measures that include PPP and external pelvic fixation [36].

18.8 Surgical Approaches for Pelvic Fracture Fixation

Standard surgical approaches for pelvic fracture fixation are described in meticulous technical detail in a variety of dedicated textbooks in the field, and this chapter will only provide a brief overview on the most frequent surgical approaches for the sake of comprehensiveness [41]. The use of a radiolucent operating table is generally recommended for procedures in supine position, to allow unrestricted visualization with intraoperative fluoroscopy, including inlet/outlet views of the pelvic ring, dedicated obturator and iliac oblique views, and a combination of those images. In prone position, a Jackson spine table offers excellent access to the posterior pelvic ring. All patients should have an indwelling urinary catheter placed preoperatively to decompress and protect the bladder throughout the surgical procedure.

The *Pfannenstiel approach* is one of the most widely used approaches to the anterior pelvic ring and is ideal for visualization of the pubic symphysis for the management of "open-book" anterior pelvic ring disruptions and unstable lateral compression-type injuries. A horizontal (straight or slightly curved) incision of 10–15 cm length is made two fingers proximal to the pubic symphysis and centered on the midline which is marked proximally to the umbilicus for orientation (Fig. 18.6). Retroperitoneal packing for acute hemorrhage control may also be performed through this approach which is, however, preferably performed as a vertical incision in the acute setting of "damage control" management of unstable pelvic ring injuries. The linea alba is identified and opened

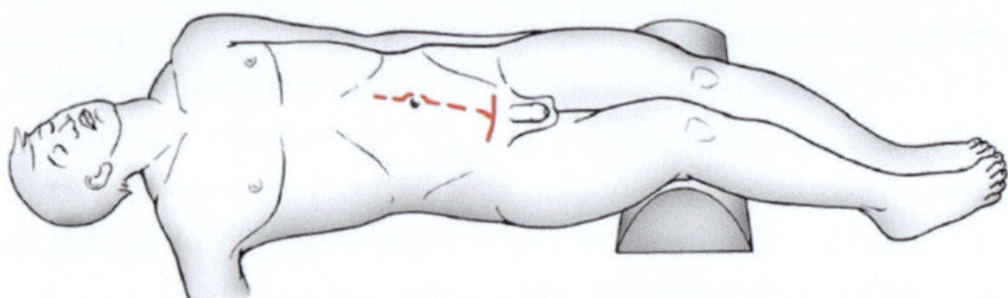

Fig. 18.6 Anterior "Pfannenstiel" approach for anterior pelvic ring fixation. An inferior median laparotomy can be chosen alternatively in cases with concomitant intra-abdominal injuries and/or in case of a preceding incision for preperitoneal pelvic packing (dashed line). The drawing was kindly provided by Ms. Marianne Peters (Berlin, Germany)

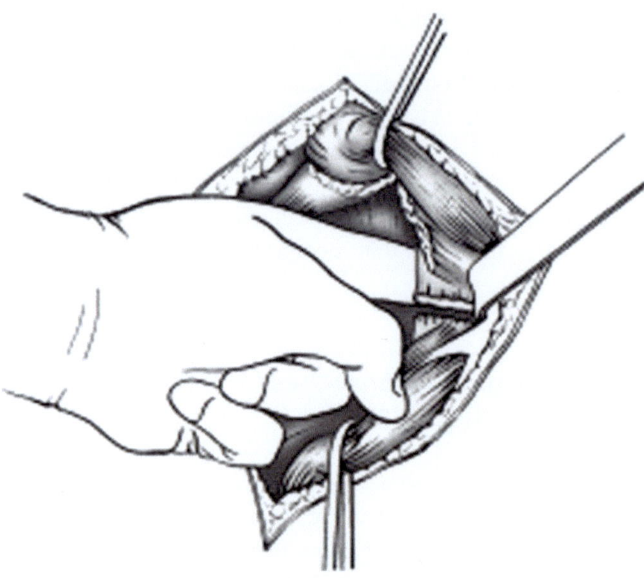

Fig. 18.7 Anterior "Pfannenstiel" approach for anterior pelvic ring fixation. Digital palpation of the space of Retzius allows for intraoperative control of fracture reduction. The drawing was kindly provided by Ms. Marianne Peters (Berlin, Germany)

longitudinally and extended distally all the way to the pubic symphysis. The retroperitoneal space of Retzius is opened in a careful blunt dissection technique through the rectus sheath, with careful digital mobilization of the bladder to avoid an iatrogenic bladder injury (Fig. 18.7). One or two lap sponges are placed behind a wide malleable retractor for protection of the bladder throughout the case. Exposure of the pubic tubercles is performed bilaterally by subperiosteal dissection. The tubercles are used as landmarks for pubic symphysis plate application and for the intraoperative use of pointed reduction clamps. The reduction clamps can also be placed on the medial side of the obturator foramen for closure of pubic symphysis disruptions. Two Hohmann retractors are placed bilaterally in a subperiosteal fashion under the superior pubic rami bilaterally to retract the rectus muscles for improved visualization. Care is taken to avoid detaching the rectus insertion by using a strict subperiosteal dissection technique, and repair of the rectus muscles and insertion in case of identified traumatic rectus tears. Anterior pelvic ring fixation is typically performed using 3.5 mm reconstruction plates. Once adequate fracture reduction and fixation is ascertained with dedicated fluoroscopy views and direct inspection and palpation of the anterior pelvic ring, lap sponges are removed and counted prior to wound closure. Integrity of the bladder and adequate hemostasis are ascertained prior to wound closure which occurs by secure repair of the rectus muscles, followed by fascial closure of the midline, subcutaneous closure, and stapling of the skin. Surgical drains are typically not needed in the authors' experience.

A *modified Stoppa approach* is sometimes preferred over the standard Pfannenstiel approach whenever a more lateral dissection is needed for anterior pelvic ring fixation. This represents an extension of the Pfannenstiel approach that allows for lateral visualization of the pubic rami, pelvic brim, and quadrilateral plate in case of acetabular fracture fixation. The incision for the modified Stoppa approach is similar to the Pfannenstiel approach. A visualization and ligation of the "corona mortis" is performed to avoid intraoperative bleeding from an accidental intraoperative vascular injury. The obturator vessels and nerve are visualized and protected throughout the case. This approach can be combined with an anterior approach to the iliosacral joint if an open reduction and anterior plate fixation is indicated.

The anterolateral *Olerud approach* or first window of the ilioinguinal *Letournel approach* allows for exposure of the iliac wing and anterior iliosacral joint. This approach can be used in conjunction with a modified Stoppa approach for reduction and fixation of iliac wing fractures, transiliosacral "crescent" fractures, and SI joint injuries. A curved skin incision is made parallel to the iliac crest, beginning approximately 5 cm dorsal to the anterior superior iliac spine (ASIS) and continuing for an additional 5 cm ventromedially along the line of the inguinal ligament (Fig. 18.8). After deepening the skin incision through the subcutaneous fat, the aponeurosis of the oblique external abdominal muscle is exposed and detached from the iliac crest in a subperiosteal fashion. The lateral cutaneous femoral nerve runs ventrally to the anterior superior iliac crest and should be spared throughout the case. The abdominal muscles are released with a Cobb elevator

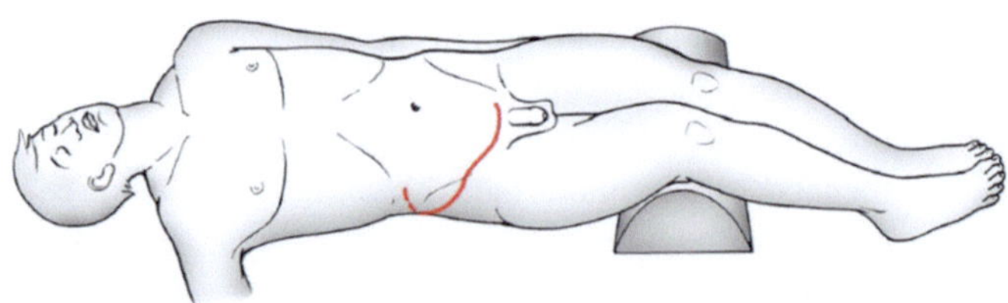

Fig. 18.8 Anterolateral approach to the iliac wing and anterior SI joint. The Olerud approach corresponds to the first window of the ilioinguinal Letournel approach, which can be expanded accordingly. The drawing was kindly provided by Ms. Marianne Peters (Berlin, Germany)

Fig. 18.9 Intraoperative structures of the anterolateral approach: (*1*) Arcus iliopectineus, (*2*) Lateral cutaneous femoral nerve, (*3*) Femoral nerve (on the psoas muscle), (*4*) External iliac artery (red) and vein, (*5*) Spermatic cord. The drawings were kindly provided by Ms. Marianne Peters (Berlin, Germany)

from the brim of the iliac wing to expose the inner table of the pelvis. The origin of the sartorius and rectus femoris is preserved throughout the case. Bleeding from nutrient vessels from the ilium is controlled by topical application of bone wax. The iliosacral joint is exposed by retracting the iliacus and psoas muscles medially. Care has to be taken not to induce an indirect shearing injury to the lumbosacral plexus by inconsiderate placement of retractors. After fracture reduction and fixation, typically using 3.5 mm lag screws and reconstruction plates, the wound is closed by repair of the gluteal muscles and tensor fascia lata to the iliac wing and abdominal fascia. The subcutaneous tissue is closed in layers and the skin is closed with staples. Surgical drains are typically not needed in the authors' experience. The anterolateral Olerud approach can be extended anteriorly and medially through the "classical" three windows of the ilioinguinal Letournel approach (Fig. 18.9) which is mainly indicated for fixation of acetabular fractures and rarely used in the management of acute pelvic ring disruptions.

Posterior approaches are typically indicated for fixation of lateral sacral fractures and iliosacral injuries (Fig. 18.10). The posterior approach is at increased risk for significant soft tissue injuries with a risk for wound breakdown and surgical site infections due to the thin posterior soft tissue envelope and frequent presence of associated degloving injuries (e.g., Morel-Lavallée lesion).

Patients are placed prone on a well-padded Jackson spine table. A longitudinal skin incision is performed medial to the posterior superior iliac spine. After subcutaneous dissection, the lumbosacral fascia is exposed and incised. The gluteus maximus is then carefully detached from the iliac crest.

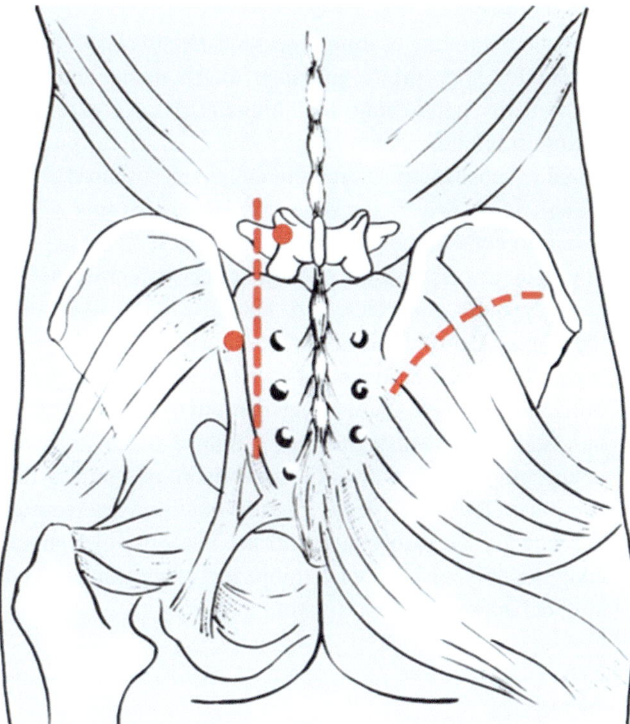

Fig. 18.10 Posterior approaches to the sacrum and SI joint. The red dots mark the starting points for pedicle screws in the case of posterior lumbopelvic fixation (L5 pedicle and PSIS). The drawing was kindly provided by Ms. Marianne Peters (Berlin, Germany)

Reflecting the muscle laterally and distally, the gluteus medius und piriformis muscles are exposed. The gluteus medius muscle is incised and elevated carefully from the outer wall of the ilium. Posteriorly and inferiorly, the mobilization of the gluteus maximus muscle is limited by the inferior gluteal neurovascular structures penetrating this muscle through the deep surface after surrounding the piriformis muscle inferiorly. Digital control of the anterior sacroiliac joint might be necessary by palpation through the greater sciatic notch to ascertain adequate intraoperative reduction. Posterior tension band plating is typically performed by the use of 4.5 mm reconstruction plates. Wound closure occurs in layers of the lumbosacral fascia and subcutaneous tissue, with a preferred use of sutures instead of staples for skin closure, to decrease the risk of skin irritation and wound breakdown. Surgical drains are typically not needed in the authors' experience.

A widely used alternative to open posterior approaches is represented by closed reduction and *percutaneous transiliosacral screw fixation*. This technique can be performed either in prone or supine position on a radiolucent table. A perfect surgical "corridor" has to be ascertained under fluoroscopic guidance with dedicated inlet and outlet views, as widely described in the pertinent literature in the field.

Conclusion

The understanding of injury mechanism and classification allows for appropriate guidance in the management of high-energy pelvic ring disruptions at risk for exsanguinating traumatic hemorrhagic shock. Current international consensus guidelines are based on classification-driven decision-making algorithms which take into consideration the anatomic/mechanistic aspects of pelvic ring disruptions in conjunction with physiologic/hemodynamic variables and response to resuscitative measures. A protocolized approach of early pelvic packing and external fixation, followed by delayed angioembolization in case of ongoing hemodynamic instability, has been shown to significantly reduce the historically unacceptably high mortality from severe pelvic ring disruptions. Definitive pelvic fracture fixation is performed subsequent to resuscitation from hemorrhagic shock, coagulopathy, and associated injuries, using standardized surgical approaches and fixation techniques.

References

1. Peltier LF. Joseph Francois Malgaigne and Malgaigne's fracture. Surgery. 1958;44(4):777–84.
2. Stahel PF, Hammerberg EM. History of pelvic fracture management: a review. World J Emerg Surg. 2016;11:18.
3. Brand RA. Biographical sketch: Charles Hewitt Moore, FRCS (1821-1870). Clin Orthop Relat Res. 2012;470(8):2075–6.
4. Brand RA. Biographical sketch: Frank Wild Holdsworth, FRCS (1904-1969). Clin Orthop Relat Res. 2012;470(8):2083–4.
5. Young JW, Resnik CS. Fracture of the pelvis: current concepts of classification. AJR Am J Roentgenol. 1990;155(6):1169–75.
6. Fakler JKM, Stahel PF, Lundy DW. Classification of pelvic ring injuries. In: Smith WR, Ziran BH, Morgan SJ, editors. Fractures of the pelvis and acetabulum. New York: Informa Healthcare; 2007. p. 11–25.
7. Tile M. Acute pelvic fractures: I. Causation and classification. J Am Acad Orthop Surg. 1996;4(3):143–51.
8. Marsh JL, Slongo TF, Agel J, et al. Fracture and dislocation classification compendium—2007: Orthopaedic Trauma Association classification, database and outcomes committee. J Orthop Trauma. 2007;21(10 Suppl):S1–133.
9. Osterhoff G, Scheyerer MJ, Fritz Y, Bouaicha S, Wanner GA, Simmen HP, Werner CM. Comparing the predictive value of the pelvic ring injury classification systems by Tile and by Young and Burgess. Injury. 2014;45(4):742–7.
10. Mauffrey C, Cuellar DO 3rd, Pieracci F, Hak DJ, Hammerberg EM, Stahel PF, Burlew CC, Moore EE. Strategies for the management of haemorrhage following pelvic fractures and associated trauma-induced coagulopathy. Bone Joint J. 2014;96-B(9):1143–54.
11. Stahel PF, Mauffrey C, Smith WR, McKean J, Hao J, Burlew CC, Moore EE. External fixation for acute pelvic ring injuries: decision making and technical options. J Trauma Acute Care Surg. 2013;75(5):882–7.
12. Alton TB, Gee AO. Classifications in brief: Young and Burgess classification of pelvic ring injuries. Clin Orthop Relat Res. 2014;472(8):2338–42.
13. Halawi MJ. Pelvic ring injuries: Emergency assessment and management. J Clin Orthop Trauma. 2015;6(4):252–8.
14. Stahel PF, Burlew CC, Moore EE. Current trends in the management of hemodynamically unstable pelvic ring injuries. Curr Opin Crit Care. 2017;23(6):511–9.
15. Coccolini F, Stahel PF, Montori G, et al. Pelvic trauma: WSES classification and guidelines. World J Emerg Surg. 2017;12:5.
16. Bakhshayesh P, Boutefnouchet T, Totterman A. Effectiveness of non invasive external pelvic compression: a systematic review of the literature. Scand J Trauma Resusc Emerg Med. 2016;24:73.
17. Stahel PF, Heyde CE, Wyrwich W, Ertel W. Current concepts of polytrauma management: from ATLS to "damage control". Orthopade. 2005;34(9):823–36.
18. Kashuk JL, Moore EE, Sawyer M, et al. Postinjury coagulopathy management: goal directed resuscitation via POC thrombelastography. Ann Surg. 2010;251(4):604–14.
19. Stahel PF, Moore EE, Schreier SL, Flierl MA, Kashuk JL. Transfusion strategies in postinjury coagulopathy. Curr Opin Anaesthesiol. 2009;22(2):289–98.
20. Gonzalez E, Moore EE, Moore HB, et al. Goal-directed hemostatic resuscitation of trauma-induced coagulopathy: a pragmatic randomized clinical trial comparing a viscoelastic assay to conventional coagulation assays. Ann Surg. 2016;263(6):1051–9.
21. Rossaint R, Bouillon B, Cerny V, et al. Management of bleeding following major trauma: an updated European guideline. Crit Care. 2010;14(2):R52.
22. Abramson D, Scalea TM, Hitchcock R, Trooskin SZ, Henry SM, Greenspan J. Lactate clearance and survival following injury. J Trauma. 1993;35(4):584–8; discussion 588–589.
23. Davis JW, Parks SN, Kaups KL, Gladen HE, O'Donnell-Nicol S. Admission base deficit predicts transfusion requirements and risk of complications. J Trauma. 1996;41(5):769–74.
24. Burlew CC, Moore EE, Moore FA, Coimbra R, McIntyre RC Jr, Davis JW, Sperry J, Biffl WL. Western Trauma Association critical decisions in trauma: resuscitative thoracotomy. J Trauma Acute Care Surg. 2012;73(6):1359–63.
25. Manzano Nunez R, Naranjo MP, Foianini E, Ferrada P, Rincon E, Garcia-Perdomo HA, Burbano P, Herrera JP, Garcia AF, Ordonez CA. A meta-analysis of resuscitative endovascular balloon occlusion of the aorta (REBOA) or open aortic cross-clamping by

resuscitative thoracotomy in non-compressible torso hemorrhage patients. World J Emerg Surg. 2017;12:30.
26. Davidson AJ, Russo RM, Reva VA, et al. The pitfalls of REBOA: risk factors and mitigation strategies. J Trauma Acute Care Surg. 2018;84(1):192–202.
27. Osborn PM, Smith WR, Moore EE, Cothren CC, Morgan SJ, Williams AE, Stahel PF. Direct retroperitoneal pelvic packing versus pelvic angiography: a comparison of two management protocols for haemodynamically unstable pelvic fractures. Injury. 2009;40(1):54–60.
28. Burlew CC, Moore EE, Smith WR, Johnson JL, Biffl WL, Barnett CC, Stahel PF. Preperitoneal pelvic packing/external fixation with secondary angioembolization: optimal care for life-threatening hemorrhage from unstable pelvic fractures. J Am Coll Surg. 2011;212(4):628–35; discussion 627–635
29. Chiara O, di Fratta E, Mariani A, Michaela B, Prestini L, Sammartano F, Cimbanassi S. Efficacy of extra-peritoneal pelvic packing in hemodynamically unstable pelvic fractures, a Propensity Score Analysis. World J Emerg Surg. 2016;11:22.
30. Pohlemann T, Culemann U, Gansslen A, Tscherne H. Severe pelvic injury with pelvic mass hemorrhage: determining severity of hemorrhage and clinical experience with emergency stabilization. Unfallchirurg. 1996;99(10):734–43.
31. Ertel W, Keel M, Eid K, Platz A, Trentz O. Control of severe hemorrhage using C-clamp and pelvic packing in multiply injured patients with pelvic ring disruption. J Orthop Trauma. 2001;15(7):468–74.
32. Lustenberger T, Meier C, Benninger E, Lenzlinger PM, Keel MJ. C-clamp and pelvic packing for control of hemorrhage in patients with pelvic ring disruption. J Emerg Trauma Shock. 2011;4(4):477–82.
33. Koller H, Balogh ZJ. Single training session for first time pelvic C-clamp users: correct pin placement and frame assembly. Injury. 2012;43(4):436–9.
34. Suzuki T, Smith WR, Moore EE. Pelvic packing or angiography: competitive or complementary? Injury. 2009;40(4):343–53.
35. Hou Z, Smith WR, Strohecker KA, Bowen TR, Irgit K, Baro SM, Morgan SJ. Hemodynamically unstable pelvic fracture management by advanced trauma life support guidelines results in high mortality. Orthopedics. 2012;35(3):e319–24.
36. Burlew CC, Moore EE, Stahel PF, Geddes AE, Wagenaar AE, Pieracci FM, Fox CJ, Campion EM, Johnson JL, Mauffrey C. Preperitoneal pelvic packing reduces mortality in patients with life-threatening hemorrhage due to unstable pelvic fractures. J Trauma Acute Care Surg. 2017;82(2):233–42.
37. Platz A, Friedl HP, Kohler A, Trentz O. Surgical management of severe pelvic crush injuries. Helv Chir Acta. 1992;58(6):925–9.
38. Smith WR, Moore EE, Osborn P, Agudelo JF, Morgan SJ, Parekh AA, Cothren C. Retroperitoneal packing as a resuscitation technique for hemodynamically unstable patients with pelvic fractures: report of two representative cases and a description of technique. J Trauma. 2005;59(6):1510–4.
39. Glass NE, Burlew CC, Hahnhaussen J, Weckbach S, Pieracci FM, Moore EE, Stahel PF. Early definitive fracture fixation is safely performed in the presence of an open abdomen in multiply injured patients. J Orthop Trauma. 2017;31(12):624–30.
40. Moore EE, Burlew CC, Pieracci F, Stahel PF. Preperitoneal pelvic packing for acute hemorrhage control. https://www.vumedi.com/video/pelvic-packing-surgery-live-real-time-instructional-video/. Accessed 15 Dec 2017.
41. Fakler JKM, Pallister I, Stahel PF. Surgical approaches for pelvic ring injuries. In: Smith WR, Ziran BH, Morgan SJ, editors. Fractures of the pelvis and acetabulum. New York: Informa Healthcare; 2007. p. 87–98.

Chest Wall and Diaphragmatic Injuries

19

Filippo Antonacci, Stephane Renaud, Alessandra Mazzucco, Giulio Orlandoni, and Nicola Santelmo

Key Points

- Multidisciplinary management of thoracic trauma improves outcome.
- Main indications for osteosynthesis: flail chest, chest wall instability and paradoxical respiration, chest wall deformity, difficult weaning from mechanical ventilation.
- 3D chest CT to localize fracture and plan adequate incision.
- Always rule out a diaphragmatic injury in penetrating thoracoabdominal trauma.
- Abdominal approach for acute diaphragmatic injuries; thoracic or abdominal approach for chronic lesions, but when adhesions in the upper chest are expected, thoracotomy is preferable.

19.1 Chest Wall Injuries

19.1.1 Brief Introduction

Thoracic trauma is the second leading cause of death in case of trauma, after head trauma. Rib fractures are one of the most common injuries affecting trauma patients, occurring in approximately 10% of all cases [1], and they are associated with a mortality of 3–13% [2]. Frequent complications of this condition are pneumonia, prolonged ventilator time, prolonged hospitalization, and chronic debilitating pain [2, 3]. It has been shown that a greater number of rib fractures are associated with an increased risk of complications, particularly in older patients [4].

Optimal treatment of rib fractures has not been established; in particular, the role of surgery is a matter of debate.

19.1.2 Brief Initial Clinical Assessment

Rib fractures are the most common injuries associated with blunt thoracic trauma, and the most common mechanisms of injury are related to direct impact causing fractures in the interested area [5]. The majority of these injuries are a consequence of motor vehicle accidents or falls.

The ribs from the fourth to the tenth are most commonly fractured, and ribs 1–3 are associated with nerve or vascular injury, while lower ribs (10th to 12th) are often associated with abdominal injuries [3, 6].

Flail chest is a condition in which three or more consecutive ribs are fractured in two sites, causing paradoxical respiration. It is now understood that respiratory failure, associated with this condition, is caused by underlying pulmonary contusion [7].

It has been described that more than four rib fractures have a mortality of 10%, while if more than eight ribs are fractured, mortality increases to 34%. In patients older than 65 years old who die following thoracic trauma, rib fractures are the cause of death in 56% of the cases [4].

Lung parenchymal lesions and pleural and vascular injuries are frequently seen in association with rib fractures and are described in another chapter of this textbook.

Sternal fractures are observed mainly following motor vehicle accidents and are a marker of major trauma. An ECG together with serum troponin level should be evaluated to rule out a cardiac injury. Cardiac ultrasound should be performed when increased troponin or ECG alterations are evident [6].

F. Antonacci (✉) · A. Mazzucco · G. Orlandoni
Department of Thoracic Surgery, Fondazione IRCCS Policlinico San Matteo, Pavia, Italy
e-mail: G.Orlandoni@smatteo.pv.it

S. Renaud
Department of Thoracic Surgery, Institut Lorrain Du Coeur Et Des Vaisseaux Louis Mathieu, Nancy University Hospital, Nancy, France

N. Santelmo
Department of Thoracic Surgery, Strasbourg University Hospital, Strasbourg, France
e-mail: Nicola.SANTELMO@chru-strasbourg.fr

P. Aseni et al. (eds.), *Operative Techniques and Recent Advances in Acute Care and Emergency Surgery*,
https://doi.org/10.1007/978-3-319-95114-0_19

The scapula requires considerable force to fracture; consequently, it is a marker of severe chest trauma, and associated injuries are present in 80–98% of cases. Management in most of the cases is conservative [5].

Clavicle fractures often present isolated to other chest wall fractures; management is conservative in the majority of cases [5].

On clinical examination, pain is the most common symptom; it can be associated with ecchymosis, subcutaneous emphysema, and deformity of the chest wall [3, 6, 8]. Pain can be severe, limiting a patient's cough, causing sputum retention and eventually pneumonia.

Chest X-ray shows the presence of fractures, with a sensitivity of 50% [9], but CT is more sensitive and is able to quantify and localize the lesions exactly. Moreover, since rib fractures are associated with other important injuries in 50% of the cases, CT may reveal other major lesions [10]. When surgical stabilization is indicated, three-dimensional CT reconstruction may help to choose the best approach.

Ultrasound is an essential tool in case of hemodynamically unstable patients to diagnose pneumothorax or hemothorax, but in case of stable patients, chest X-ray and CT are the gold standards to evaluate the presence and the extent of injuries [11].

19.1.3 Non-operative Management

It has been shown that patients affected by rib fractures who were followed by a multidisciplinary team including pain service, respiratory team, and physiotherapist had an improved outcome consisting of decreased ICU and hospital length of stay, pneumonia, and mortality.

Aggressive pulmonary toilet, positive airway pressure system, incentive spirometry, and coughing to encourage volume expansion are essential adjuncts in the treatment of these patients [2].

Pain control is one of the mainstays of non-operative treatment to optimize chest wall mechanics. This can be achieved with i.v. analgesics, but it has been shown that regional anesthesia is much more effective. Optimization of the analgesia in thoracic trauma is an essential component of the therapy, because it reduces the risk of morbidity, like atelectasis, pneumonia, respiratory failure, and mortality [2].

Regional anesthesia can be delivered in different ways:

- Epidural analgesia consists of injecting opioid and/or local anesthetic agents into the epidural space at the thoracic level.
- Thoracic paravertebral blockade produces unilateral segmental somatic and sympathetic nerve blockade because the local anesthetics are injected into the paravertebral space, which contains spinal nerves and preganglionic sympathetic nerves. The local anesthetics can be injected as a single-shot procedure or with placement of a catheter for a continuous block.
- Intercostal nerve block is a single or continuous injection of local anesthetics into the intercostal space, where the intercostal nerve is located.
- Intrapleural analgesia involves placement of local anesthetic agents into the pleural space, which blocks multiple unilateral dermatomes.

It has been shown that epidural catheters are the preferred technique with optimal pain relief but at the same time can be technically difficult to place, are contraindicated in patients with coagulopathy or spinal injury, may induce hypotension, and may have major complications (hematoma and abscess of the epidural space) [12].

Thoracic paravertebral blockade is technically easier compared to epidural and with the widespread use of ultrasound may become the ideal technique [13].

Intercostal nerve blocks can give good results in terms of pain control but have a short effect (6/8 h) and need to be repeated several times [2].

The disadvantages of intrapleural analgesia are the loss of anesthetic through the chest tubes, impaired absorption in the presence of hemothorax, and higher risk of local anesthetic systemic toxicity [14].

The effects of the techniques mentioned above, excluding epidural analgesia, have not been rigorously investigated in patients affected by chest wall fractures.

A multimodal analgesic strategy, which incorporates different regional techniques and systemic analgesics, may improve management of pain related to blunt thoracic trauma [2].

Ventilation is another important treatment modality for rib fracture management. According to EAST (Eastern Association for the Surgery of Trauma) practice management guidelines, mechanical ventilation, in the absence of respiratory failure, solely to treat chest wall instability should be avoided. Patients should be separated from the ventilator as soon as possible, and noninvasive ventilation should be included in the ventilator management [15].

Patients treated with continuous positive airway pressure (CPAP) compared to intubated patients have a shorter ICU and hospital stay and a lower risk of developing complications, in particular, pneumonia [2].

19.1.4 Operative Management

Management of rib fractures traditionally consisted in intubation and positive pressure ventilation. Surgical fixation has regained interest in the last few years following a few studies showing an improved outcome in operated patients compared to those conservatively managed and the development of new materials to fix the fractures.

Surgical treatment aims to improve the respiratory mechanics, reduce pain, and prevent pulmonary restriction that can be associated with chest wall deformity.

Three randomized controlled studies, comparing operative versus conservative treatment of flail chest, were published.

Tanaka and colleagues [16] published a series of 37 patients, 18 of which were surgically treated with Judet struts. They showed shorter time of mechanical ventilation (10.8 vs. 18.3 days), lower incidence of pulmonary complications (24% vs. 77%), and a shorter ICU stay (16.5 vs. 26.8 days) for the patients submitted to surgery compared to those conservatively managed.

Even Granetzny et al. [17] demonstrated that surgical fixation of a flail segment is of great value for this post-traumatic pathology. Analyzing 40 patients, equally divided between surgical and conservative approach, they concluded that operative internal fixation achieves stability of the thoracic cage without deformity of the chest wall (5% vs. 45%), lower pulmonary morbidity (5% vs. 50%) and mortality rate (10% vs. 15%), and minor restrictive impairment.

More recently Marasco et al. [18], in a series of 46 patients, showed that the 23 patients who underwent operative repair of flail chest had a reduced duration of ICU stay (324 h vs. 448 h) and a lower requirement for mechanical ventilation, if the duration of the latter was analyzed from the time of operation. Moreover, the patients in the surgical group demonstrated a cost saving for the hospital of $14.443 per patient.

To summarize, the advantage of surgery compared to conservative treatment resides in the reduction of mechanical ventilation, ICU and overall hospital stay, pneumonia risk, and chronic pain and improved long-term respiratory function.

According to recent literature, even if not universally accepted, indications for surgery are flail chest, chest wall instability and paradoxical respiration, chest wall deformity, difficult weaning from mechanical ventilation, uncontrolled pain, thoracotomy done for other reasons, pseudoarthrosis with chronic non-union, and pain [4].

Regarding the timing of surgery, it has been proposed that patients should be operated within 72 h of injury. Once inflammation and callus formation have initiated, it can be difficult to repair the fractures. In the medium term, surgery can be performed when it is evident that the patient cannot be weaned from the ventilator. In the long term, surgical fixation is performed in case of chronic non-union [1, 4].

Lung contusions associated with rib fractures or flail chest are conditions in which surgical fixation is debated.

A study described the effect of surgical repair of rib fractures in the presence and absence of lung contusion. It was noted that patients with contusions did not benefit from surgical repair compared to those without contusions. It was shown that surgery may have a role in case of flail chest without lung contusion or when progressive collapse of the thorax is evident during weaning from the respirator after resolution of contusions. Worse outcomes in patients operated with associated pulmonary contusions are explained by the fact that surgery may improve chest wall mechanics, but it does not resolve the underlying pulmonary condition [19].

To resume, selected patients with respiratory failure related to rib fractures, likely those with underlying preserved parenchyma, may benefit from intervention.

When surgery is indicated, chest CT with 3D reconstruction may be helpful to exactly localize the fractures and plan the incision [3] (Figs. 19.1 and 19.2).

Surgical approach depends on the localization of injuries and has to provide adequate exposure, with respect to muscle fibers, optimizes cosmesis, and is tailored according to the site of fracture.

Anterior fractures may be exposed with the patient supine, performing an oblique incision along the mammary fold and raising the pectoral muscle. This will give access to the anterior aspect of the fourth to sixth ribs. In case of anterior flail chest, a bilateral anterior thoracotomy allows access to both sides of the sternum [1].

Lateral fractures can be dealt with a thoracotomy along the anterior border of the latissimus dorsi muscle which is raised, and fibers of the serratus anterior are split, thus exposing the ribs. This approach allows targeted incisions in cor-

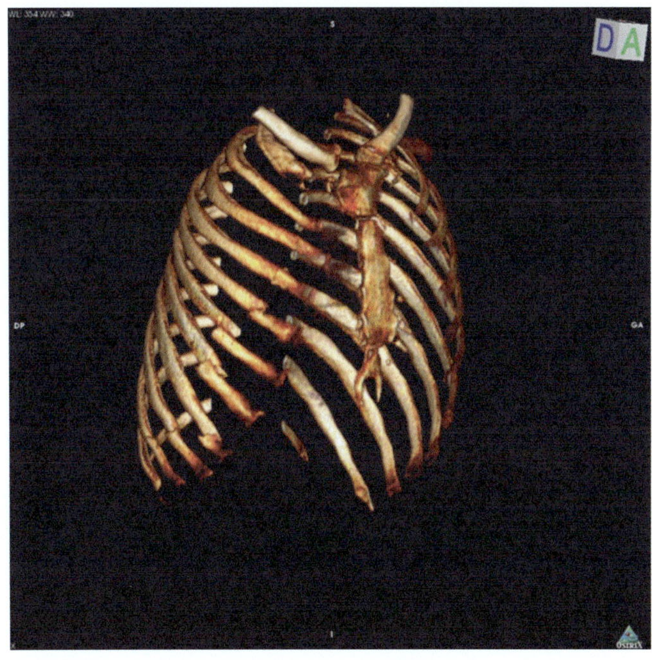

Fig. 19.1 Preoperative 3D CT reconstruction following blunt thoracic trauma showing exact localization of rib fractures

respondence to the different fractures reducing invasiveness to a minimum [1].

Posterior fractures are the most difficult to treat due to proximity to the transverse process. A Paulson incision can be performed to raise a latissimus dorsi flap and adequately expose the posterior aspect of the chest wall; alternatively, a classical posterolateral thoracotomy may be utilized [1] (Fig. 19.3).

If no evident pleuroparenchymal lesions are evidenced by preoperative investigations, the pleural cavity may be preserved from surgical access, or a VATS can be performed to adequately explore and drain the pleura.

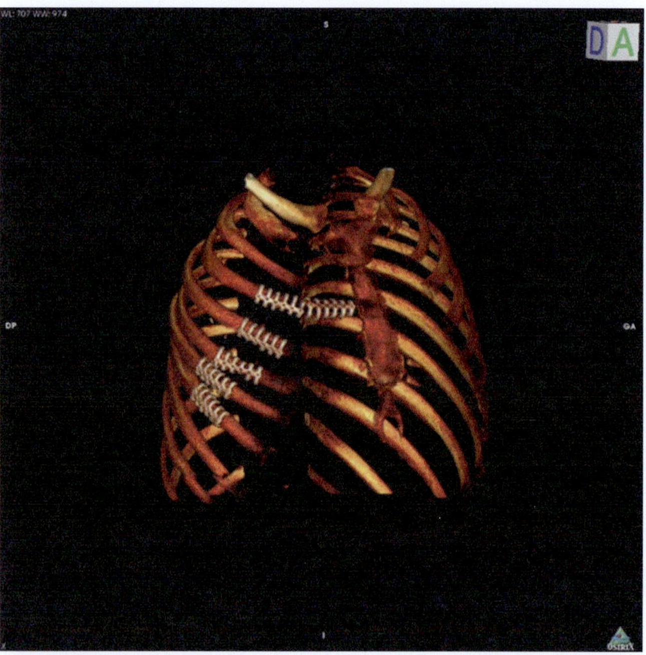

Fig. 19.2 Postoperative 3D CT reconstruction showing fixation of fractured ribs

Concerning the selection of ribs for repair, upper and lower ribs (1, 2, 11, and 12) can be left as their repair does not confer any benefit to ventilation, except in case of marked displacement, vascular involvement, or intractable pain. Posterior fractures (>2.5 cm) from transverse process should not be repaired [1]. Finally, all fractures, within the exposure of the surgical field, should be repaired.

Regarding the material used to repair ribs, there is no consensus and a variety of hardware exists. The choice of the equipment for osteosynthesis depends on the surgeon's preference.

Most current evidence shows the use of outer cortical plate with bicortical screws or malleable claw attachments (clips). The first allows stabilization without nerve impingement by fixing the plate on the anterior face of the ribs with bicortical screws. Clips provide greater stabilization by grabbing the ribs above and below while spanning the fracture without screws [3] (Figs. 19.4, 19.5, and 19.6).

Another device consists in U-plate which grasps the ribs on the superior surface and spans the fracture; screws secure the plate anteriorly and posteriorly sparing the intercostal nerve.

Intramedullary splints have a risk of migration and do not assure rotational stability [3].

Metallic wires offer a valid alternative when appropriate material is not available for rib fixation.

When loss of substance or comminuted fractures are present, and a suitable site to lock the plate is not found, a system with clips fixed at the two ends of the ribs attached to a bar has been developed allowing a bridging of the defect and stabilization [4] (Fig. 19.7).

Fig. 19.3 Posterolateral thoracotomy, latissimus dorsi muscle has been raised and longitudinally incised for fixation of multiple rib fractures with clips

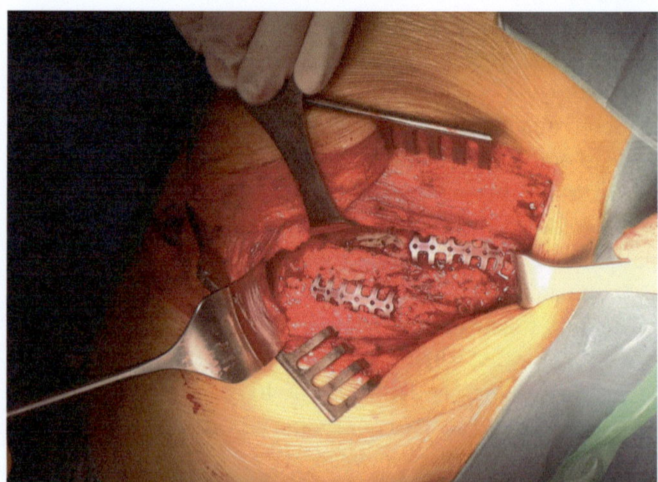

Fig. 19.4 Posterolateral thoracotomy, latissimus dorsi muscle has been anteriorly displaced for fixation of rib fractures with clips

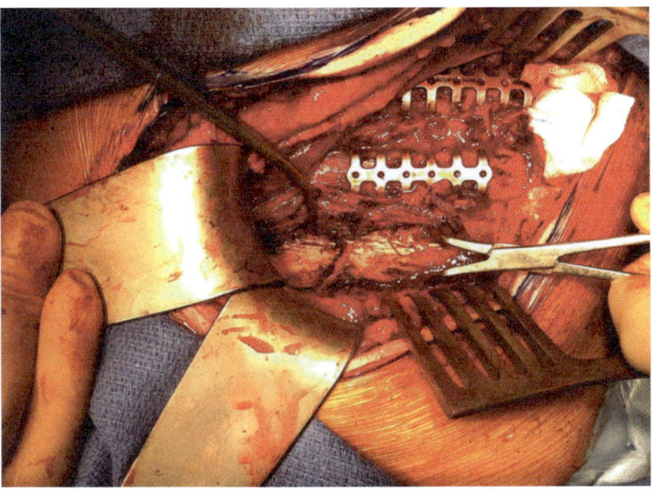

Fig. 19.5 Two clips have already been secured; a rib is cleaned of muscular tissue and fracture is exposed, ready to be fixed

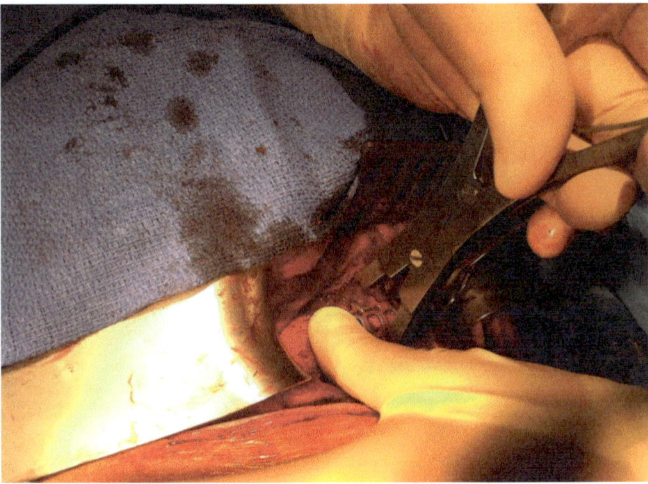

Fig. 19.6 Clip is secured and rib fracture fixed

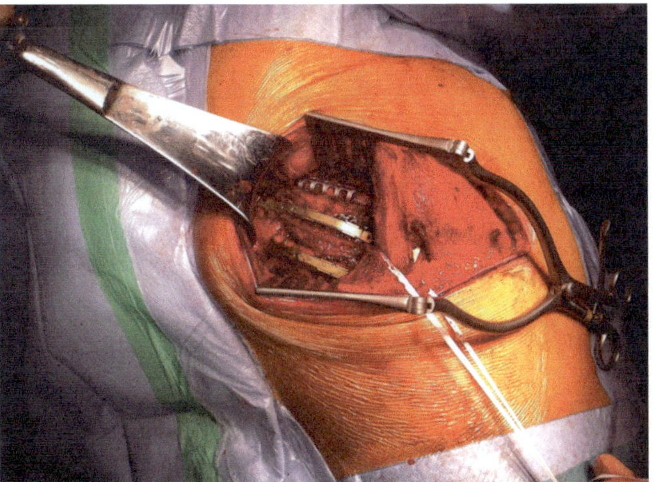

Fig. 19.7 Bars positioned for rib fractures with loss of substance

At last, even resorbable material is available, but permanent plates offer superior strength and reliability [1].

Authors' preference goes to clips in case of simple fractures and bars when loss of substance is present; nevertheless, there is still insufficient evidence to support a fixation system over the others; further studies are necessary in order to define the optimal tool.

19.2 Diaphragmatic Injuries

19.2.1 Brief Introduction

Diaphragmatic injuries have been reported in 0.8–20% of patients hospitalized for blunt trauma and in 3.4–47% [20] of patients sustaining a penetrating thoracoabdominal trauma [21]. Mechanism of injury may be a dissipation of energy from the abdominopelvic cavity to the chest in case of blunt trauma or penetrating thoracoabdominal trauma. These result in a laceration of the diaphragm, causing a hernia, that can be diagnosed in the acute setting or remain silent for months or years.

19.2.2 Brief Clinical Assessment

Traumatic diaphragmatic hernia consists of intraperitoneal structures in the chest after a traumatic event. Regarding blunt trauma, two-thirds of diaphragmatic injuries develop on the left side, probably due to the protective effect of the liver on the right side [20].

Traumatic diaphragmatic hernia, according to the time of clinical manifestation, is classified into three categories: acute, latent, and obstructive. The acute phase starts at the time of trauma and continues until the apparent recovery from the injuries incurred [22]. Afterward, the latent phase commences, and it may last for years with or without symptoms. In the obstructive phase, the herniated content develops ischemia, necrosis, or perforation [20].

Acutely, the stomach is more commonly found to migrate into the chest (48%), followed by the spleen (26%), small bowel, large bowel, and omentum (13%). Less frequently in case of a high-energy impact, a complete avulsion of the diaphragm with liver herniation can be observed [22].

Because of the significant force required to rupture the diaphragm, collateral injuries are frequently associated (lung, liver, spleen, stomach) with an overall mortality rate of 21% [23].

If a lesion is not diagnosed in the acute setting, a small diaphragmatic laceration may heal spontaneously; otherwise the hole may progressively enlarge, and intra-abdominal content migrates upward. This is explained by the negative pressure of the chest and the positive intra-abdominal pressure; moreover contraction of the diaphragm during respiration may distract tissue edges [22].

Acute traumatic diaphragmatic hernia is associated with symptoms like shoulder pain, epigastric pain, vomiting, or dyspnea. On clinical examination bowel sounds in the chest or absent breath sounds may be found [22].

Penetrating torso injuries, generally caused by gunshots or stabs, may potentially involve the diaphragm and adjacent structures in the chest or abdomen [21].

Regarding chronic traumatic diaphragmatic hernia, history of trauma is the key feature, and in the latent phase, the patient is asymptomatic, or symptoms may be vague and unspecific (nausea, vomiting, postprandial pain, intermittent obstructive symptoms, dyspnea). In the obstructive phase, signs of compromised viscera become evident with fever, tachycardia, increasing pain, and dehydration. This clinical picture may be a consequence of a volvulus, strangulation, or perforation [20].

Acutely, a chest X-ray may show a nasogastric tube on the left chest; supradiaphragmatic air-fluid levels identifying abdominal viscera in the chest are present in 25–49% of the cases. On the right side, a chest X-ray is less helpful since hollow viscera rarely migrate in the chest, and the contour of the liver mimics the diaphragmatic shadow [20].

CT has a reported sensitivity of 71–100% and a specificity of 75–100% in diagnosing a diaphragmatic laceration [20].

MRI is the best radiologic study to visualize the diaphragm, but its impracticality in the acute setting makes it a valuable tool mainly in the latent phase [20].

Laparoscopy or thoracoscopy has been proposed as a diagnostic tool in case of high suspicion of a diaphragmatic lesion, such as a left lower chest penetrating wound and no clinical or radiological signs of diaphragmatic laceration [20].

Another clinical entity that may be associated with trauma needs to be mentioned: diaphragmatic paralysis.

Diaphragmatic paralysis may be a consequence of penetrating injury with direct lesion of the phrenic nerve and cervical strain with traction injury to the phrenic nerve or following a blunt crush injury resulting in severe traction or stretching [24].

It clinically presents with gastrointestinal symptoms (nausea, vomiting, and pain secondary to gastric outlet obstruction in left-sided paralysis; gallbladder dysfunction in case of right-sided paralysis), respiratory symptoms (dyspnea, cough, poor exercise tolerance), and cardiac symptoms (palpitations, tachycardia, arrhythmias). On chest X-ray elevated hemidiaphragm is evident [24].

19.2.3 Management

Once a diagnosis of traumatic diaphragmatic hernia has been made, surgical repair of the defect is mandatory either in the acute or chronic setting.

In the acute setting, a laparotomic approach to repair the hernia is generally recommended considering the high probability of concurrent abdominal lesions [22] (Figs. 19.8 and 19.9).

If a thoracotomy is necessary to treat intrathoracic lesions such as a hemothorax or aerodigestive tract injury, the diaphragm can be repaired from the chest.

Chronic diaphragmatic hernia can be repaired either through a thoracotomy or a laparotomy [20].

Thoracotomy in the seventh or eighth intercostal space is generally performed. Perforation can be managed with this approach; to improve access to the abdominal cavity, it can be extended through the costal arch by adding a laparotomy (thoracoabdominal approach) or by incising the diaphragm

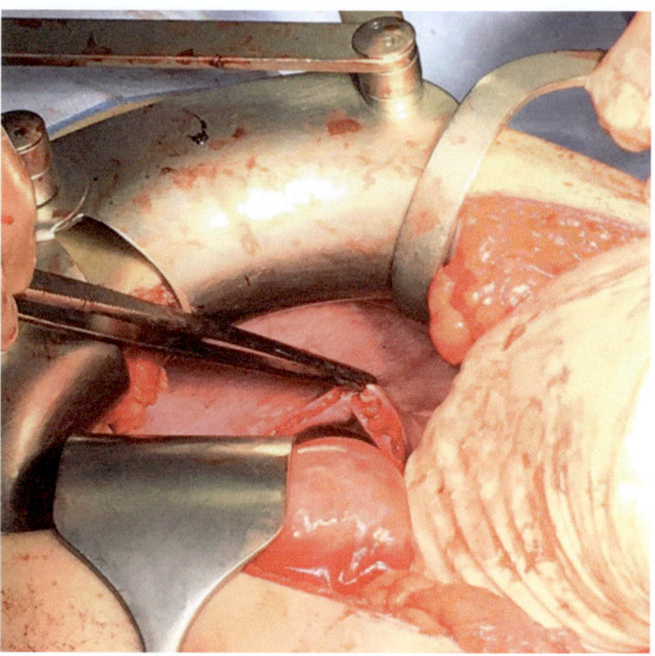

Fig. 19.8 Transabdominal approach for acute diaphragmatic hernia following blunt thoracoabdominal trauma. Viscera have been reduced in the abdomen, and diaphragmatic laceration is evidenced

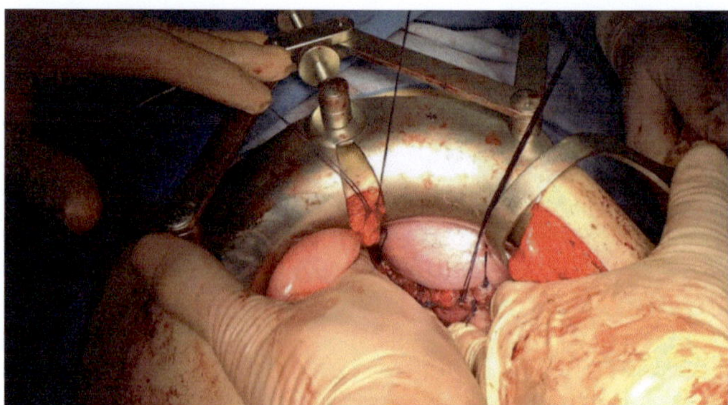

Fig. 19.9 Transabdominal approach for acute diaphragmatic hernia. Diaphragm is repaired with non-adsorbable interrupted sutures

circumferentially. Moreover a transthoracic approach allows a safer adhesiolysis of herniated tissue with the lung [20].

Even a thoracoscopic approach has been described, but the management of abdominal content may be demanding [20].

Transabdominal approach to repair diaphragmatic hernias has been widely used by several authors. Abdominal adhesions, resulting from the severe trauma that caused the diaphragmatic lesion, can be easily dealt with. In case of thoracic adhesions that can reach the upper portion of the chest, a second access may be necessary. An anterolateral thoracotomy, without changing the position of the patient, can be performed; nevertheless this incision allows a limited view of the posterior aspect of the chest; alternatively, a posterolateral thoracotomy can be done after having closed and turned the patient on the table [20].

Laparoscopic repair of a diaphragmatic hernia is also widely accepted with the limit that a defect larger than 10 cm or those extending through the esophageal hiatus may be better managed through a laparotomy [20].

Principles of operative technique, both in acute and chronic setting, consist in, after lysis of adhesions between abdominal viscera and thoracic structures, the reduction of herniated viscera. The diaphragmatic defect is exposed, and care is taken to avoid tension between the edges we intend to suture. Nonabsorbable interrupted sutures are used to close the defect. Following a running suture may be done on the top of the previous one to ensure the seal. The use of a prosthetic mesh to obtain a tension-free suture is accepted in case of long-standing noncomplicated diaphragmatic hernias [20].

In acute diaphragmatic hernias, the use of a mesh is not advised considering the risk of infection in case of concurrent visceral lesions. Moreover the edges are usually easily approached and prostheses are not necessary [22].

The outcome of patients with acute diaphragmatic injuries is related to associated lesions rather than the diaphragmatic injury itself. Reported mortality is between 18 and 40% depending on whether the mechanism of trauma is blunt or penetrating [22].

In chronic diaphragmatic hernia, patients operated in the latent phase have a mortality up to 10%, while in the obstructive phase, the reported morbidity is greater than 60% and mortality is 25–80% [20].

Surgical treatment of hemi-diaphragmatic paralysis is indicated in case of dyspnea or orthopnea and impairment of pulmonary function test [24]. In particular, the decrease of vital capacity is measured in the upright and supine positions [25].

The operation consists in the plication of the diaphragm to obtain a fixed, immobile structure improving the ability of accessory muscles to create a negative inspiratory pressure [25].

Surgery is performed through a posterolateral thoracotomy in the sixth, seventh, or eighth intercostal space, but even a thoracoscopic approach can be used [26]. Plication of the diaphragm consists in the placement of a series of nonadsorbable U-shaped sutures in the attenuated diaphragm. Redundant tissue can then be fixed to cover the previous suture. Obviously, care should be taken not to damage underlying abdominal viscera with the sutures [25].

References

1. Pieracci FM, Majercik S, Ali-Osman F, Ang D, Doben A, Edwards JG, French B, Gasparri M, Marasco S, Minshall C, Sarani B, Tisol W, VanBoerum DH, White TW. Consensus statement: surgical stabilization of rib fractures rib fracture colloquium clinical practice guidelines. Injury. 2017;48(2):307–21.
2. Galvagno SM Jr, Smith CE, Varon AJ, Hasenboehler EA, Sultan S, Shaefer G, To KB, Fox AD, Alley DE, Ditillo M, Joseph BA, Robinson BR, Haut ER. Pain management for blunt thoracic trauma: a joint practice management guideline from the Eastern Association for the Surgery of Trauma and Trauma Anesthesiology Society. J Trauma Acute Care Surg. 2016;81(5):936–51.
3. Senekjian L, Nirula R. Rib fracture fixation: indications and outcomes. Crit Care Clin. 2017;33(1):153–65.
4. Olland A, Renaud S, Reeb J, Guinard S, Jeitlinger J, Santelmo N, Falcoz PE, Massard G. Traitement chirurgical des traumatismes fermes du thorax et technique de l'osteosynthese costale. Encyclopedie Medico Chirurgicale, Techniques chirurgicales Thorax. 10.1016/S1241-8226(16)64626-1.
5. Kucharczuk JC, Cohen JE. Thoracic Trauma, Chapter 100. In Intensive Care Unit Manual, pp. 916–20.
6. Bailitz J, Hedayati T. Thoracic trauma. Emerg Med. 78:681–94.
7. Asensio JA, Trunkey DD. Thoracic injuries. In: Asensio JA, Trunkey DD, editors. Current therapy of trauma and surgical critical care. 2nd ed. New York: Elsevier; 2016. p. 205–28.
8. Bhavnagri SJ, Mohammed TL. When and how to image a suspected broken rib. Cleve Clin J Med. 2009;76(5):309–14.
9. Davis S, Affatato A. Blunt chest trauma: utility of radiological evaluation and effect on treatment patterns. Am J Emerg Med. 2006;24(4):482–6.
10. Peters S, Nicolas V, Heyer CM. Multidetector computed tomography-spectrum of blunt chest wall and lung injuries in polytraumatized patients. Clin Radiol. 2010;65(4):333–8. Epub 2010 Feb 12.
11. Griffith JF, Rainer TH, Ching AS, Law KL, Cocks RA, Metreweli C. Sonography compared with radiography in revealing acute rib fracture. Am J Roentgenol. 1999;173(6):1603–9.
12. Zaw AA, Murry J, Hoang D, Chen K, Louy C, Bloom MB, Melo N, Alban RF, Margulies DR, Ley EJ. Epidural analgesia after rib fractures. Am J Surg. 2015;81(10):950–4.
13. Mohta M, Verma P, Saxena AK, Sethi AK, Tyagi A, Girotra G. Prospective, randomized comparison of continuous thoracic epidural and thoracic paravertebral infusion in patients with unilateral multiple fractured ribs—a pilot study. J Trauma. 2009;66(4):1096–101.
14. Simon BJ, Cushman J, Barraco R, Lane V, Luchette FA, Miglietta M, Roccaforte DJ, Spector R. Pain management guidelines for blunt thoracic trauma; EAST Practice Management Guidelines Work Group. J Trauma. 2005;59(5):1256–67.
15. Kerwin AJ, Haut ER, Burns JB, Como JJ, Haider A, Stassen N, Dahm P, Eastern Association for the Surgery of Trauma Practice Management Guidelines Ad Hoc Committee. The Eastern Association of the Surgery of Trauma approach to practice management guideline development using Grading of Recommendations, Assessment, Development, and Evaluation (GRADE) methodology. J Trauma Acute Care Surg. 2012;73(5 Suppl 4):S283–7.

16. Tanaka H, Yukioka T, Yamaguti Y, Shimizu S, Goto H, Matsuda H, et al. Surgical stabilization of internal pneumatic stabilization? A prospective randomized study of management of severe flail chest patients. J Trauma. 2002;52:727–32; discussion 732.
17. Granetzny A, Abd El-Aal M, Emam E, Shalaby A, Boseila A. Surgical versus conservative treatment of flail chest. Evaluation of the pulmonary status. Interact Cardiovasc Thorac Surg. 2005;4:583–7.
18. Marasco SF, Davies AR, Cooper J, Varma D, Bennett V, Nevill R, et al. Prospective randomized controlled trial of operative rib fixation in traumatic flail chest. J Am Coll Surg. 2013;216: 924–32.
19. Voggenreiter G, Neudeck F, Aufmkolk M, Obertacke U, Schmit-Neuerburg KP. Operative chest wall stabilization in flail chest-outcomes of patients with or without pulmonary contusion. J Am Coll Surg. 1998;187:130–8.
20. Blitz M, Louie BE. Chronic traumatic diaphragmatic hernia. Thoracic Surg Clin. 2009;19(4):491–500.
21. Steyn E. Penetrating injuries to the diaphragm. In: Velmahos GC, Degiannis E, Doll D, editors. Penetrating trauma. Berlin: Springer; 2017.
22. Hanna WC, Ferri LE. Acute traumatic diaphragmatic injury. Thorac Surg Clin. 2009;19(4):485–9.
23. Dante Yeh D, Lee J. Trauma and blast injuries. In: Robert Mason V, Broaddus C, Martin T, et al., editors. Murray and Nadel's Textbook of respiratory medicine. 5th ed. Philadelphia: Saunders. p. 1354–66.
24. Dalshaug GB, Rothwell BC. Diaphragmatic paralysis following minor blunt trauma. J Trauma. 1999;47(2):413–5.
25. Ko MA, Darling GE. Acquired paralysis of the diaphragm. Thorac Surg Clin. 2009;19(4):501–10.
26. Groth AS, Andrade RS. Thoracic surgery clinics. Diaphragmatic Eventration. 2009;19(4):511–9.

Pleural, Lung and Tracheal Injuries

20

Francesco Guerrera, Filippo Antonacci, Stéphane Renaud, and Alberto Oliaro

Key Points

- Early diagnosis and immediate medical-surgical treatment are cornerstones of pleural, lung and airway injury management.
- Thoracentesis and chest tube placement are often enough on their own to save the lives of many thoracic trauma patients affected by pleural, lung or airway injuries.
- Correct localization of airway injuries allows choosing the best surgical approach.
- Tracheal injuries can be repaired with simple sutures in majority of cases.
- Extracorporeal life support is a valid tool in the treatment of airway injuries.

Table 20.1 Traumas and cause of death

Traumas	First cause of death (one to four decades of life)
Neoplasms	First cause of death (all decades)
Atherosclerosis	Second cause of death (all decades)
Traumas	Third cause of death (all decades)

Table 20.2 Decalogue

1. Assessment of injuries
2. Ensure airway patency and ventilation
3. Treatment of shock
4. Decompression of the pleural space
5. Pericardiocentesis
6. Identification of chest injuries on chest X-ray
7. Identification of abdominal injuries
8. Identification of intracranial injuries
9. Identification of spinal injuries
10. Identification of injuries to the musculoskeletal system

20.1 Introduction

Traumas are the leading cause of death in the first four decades of life.

Taking into account all age groups, only neoplasms and atherosclerotic disease surpass traumas as the prime cause of death (Table 20.1). Many patients die on arrival at the hospital, but many of them could be saved by early diagnosis and immediate medical-surgical treatment (Table 20.2).

Traumatic chest injuries may impair cardiorespiratory balance and breathing. Breathing brings atmospheric air into contact with the blood in order to facilitate the intake of oxygen and the transfer of carbon dioxide. Breathing involves three phases:

- Ventilation: mechanical phase whereby air is introduced into the alveoli.
- Diffusion: gases diffuse in both directions through the alveolar-capillary membrane.
- Perfusion: blood is conducted from the heart to the capillaries and vice versa.

A traumatic event may alter one or more breathing phases, determine a characteristic symptomatology and promote the possible onset of complications up to the point of acute respiratory failure.

We must not forget that following a chest trauma, a patient may report a rib fracture (primary lesion); as a complication, the rib fracture can determine a haemothorax (secondary

F. Guerrera · A. Oliaro
Department of Thoracic Surgery, Azienda Ospedaliera Universitaria Città della Salute e della Scienza di Torino, Torino, Italy
e-mail: alberto.oliaro@unito.it

F. Antonacci (✉)
Department of Thoracic Surgery, Fondazione IRCCS Policlinico San Matteo, Pavia, Italy

S. Renaud
Department of Thoracic Surgery, Institut Lorrain Du Coeur Et Des Vaisseaux Louis Mathieu, Nancy University Hospital, Nancy, France

P. Aseni et al. (eds.), *Operative Techniques and Recent Advances in Acute Care and Emergency Surgery*, https://doi.org/10.1007/978-3-319-95114-0_20

Table 20.3 Types of trauma injuries and immediate procedures

Immediately life-threatening injuries	Obstruction of airways Tension pneumothorax Open pneumothorax Rib flap Massive haemothorax Cardiac tamponade
Potentially lethal injuries	Pneumothorax Haemothorax Lung contusion Tracheobronchial rupture Closed cardiac trauma Traumatic aortic rupture Diaphragmatic rupture
Procedures	Thoracentesis Pericardiocentesis Positioning of pleural drain

lesion), and the haemothorax may evolve into pleural empyema (tertiary lesion). The importance of thoracentesis and pleural drainage: the physician must always have in mind this wise assertion regarding chest trauma patients: "Some chest trauma patients pass away without receiving first aid; others follow them without having received effective treatment; many can be healed by simple actions". The intention of this statement is to emphasize the concept that sometimes simple actions, such as thoracentesis or the placement of a pleural drain, are enough on their own to save the lives of many patients (Table 20.3).

20.2 Lung Injuries

20.2.1 Pulmonary Contusion

In the absence of lung parenchyma tearing, the most frequently observed occurrence is pulmonary contusion (PC) [1]. It may take place in 30–75% of patients affected by a major chest trauma [2]. PC is mostly observed in car accidents, due to the impact of the chest on the steering wheel, but it is commonly also seen in other blunt or penetrating trauma. An isolated PC is rarely observed and is commonly associated with other thoracic or extrathoracic lesions.

Following post-traumatic blood spillage and concomitant oedema, more or less extensive areas of alveolar consolidation are formed in the most peripheral areas of the lung parenchyma; a shunt occurs in these locations, as the lung is perfused but does not ventilate with consequent hypoxaemia (Fig. 20.1).

The standard chest radiography and computed tomography (CT) scans demonstrate isolated or multiple alveolar infiltrates, which could evolve in a consolidation of a lobe or of the entire lung [3, 4]. Associated symptoms are hypotension, tachypnoea, haemoptysis, dyspnoea and cyanosis.

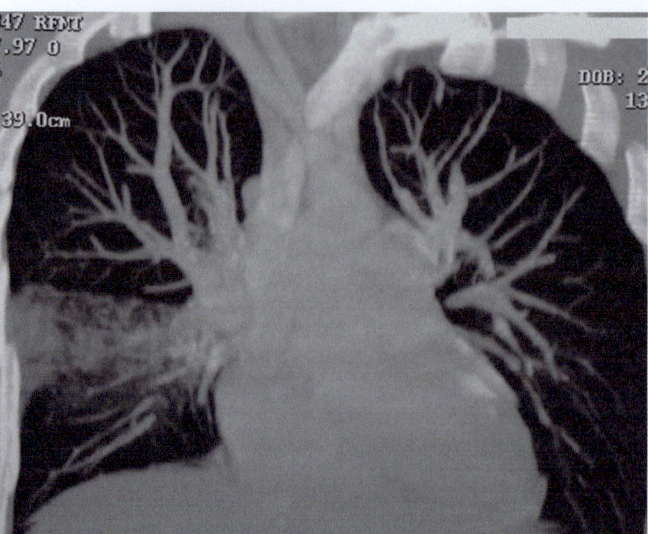

Fig. 20.1 Right lung contusion in closed chest trauma. Chest CT with front reconstruction highlights an area of right lung contusion in the presence of right rib fractures

20.2.1.1 Management

PC patient requires a careful monitoring because the evolution can be fast and life-threatening. Hypoxia, hyperventilation and resultant hypocapnia and respiratory alkalosis are commonly observed [5].

The treatment is medical and consists of chest physiotherapy, antibiotics and the use of anti-inflammatory drugs and membrane balance restorers (e.g. corticosteroids).

20.2.2 Pulmonary Laceration

Lung parenchymal lacerations are commonly observed after penetrating chest trauma, but they are also seen consequently to blunt trauma. In patients who have suffered cuts and puncture wounds, it is essential to observe the site of any chest wall (anterior, lateral, posterior) wound accurately and to understand the direction of the offending agent in order to consider the possibility of injuries to endo-thoracic and endo-abdominal organs. The execution of a chest and abdominal CT scan will highlight possible injuries related to the traumatic event.

In cuts and puncture wounds, in the right posterior chest wall, the most frequently observed injuries are due to sectioning of intercostal vessels and laceration of the lung parenchyma (Fig. 20.2). In case of cuts and puncture wounds located on the left posterior chest wall, in paravertebral location, a possible lesion of the thoracic aorta should always be considered (Fig. 20.3).

In view of the fact that the diaphragmatic dome may also be located at the level of the fifth intercostal space, in cuts and puncture wounds of the lateral chest wall, possible injury

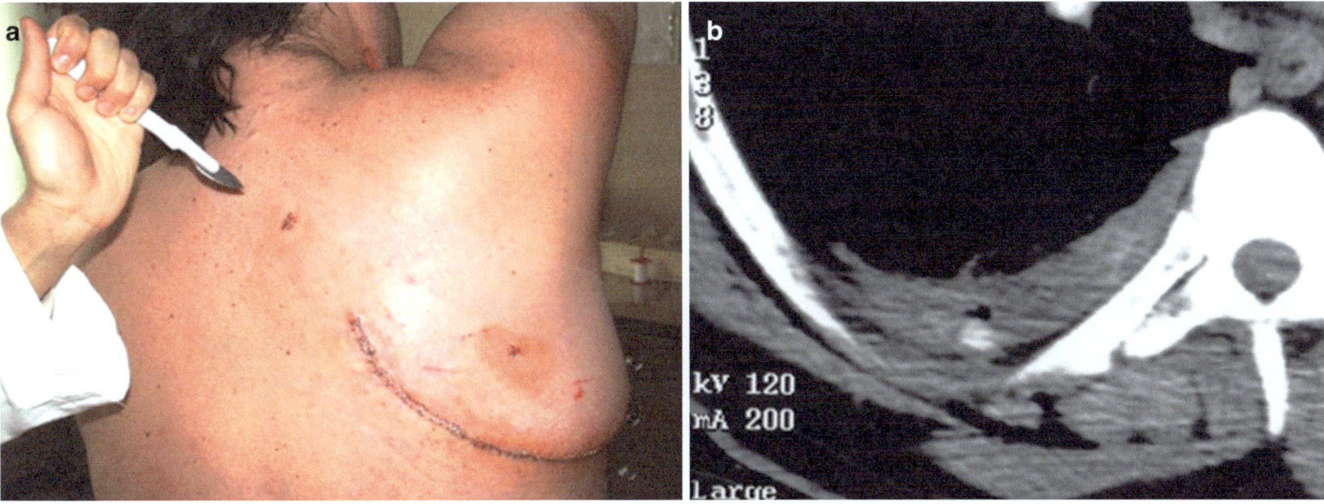

Fig. 20.2 (**a**) Cut and puncture wound right posterior chest wall: patient submitted to thoracotomy to control bleeding due to laceration of an intercostal artery. (**b**) Chest CT: presence of haemothorax caused by injured intercostal artery

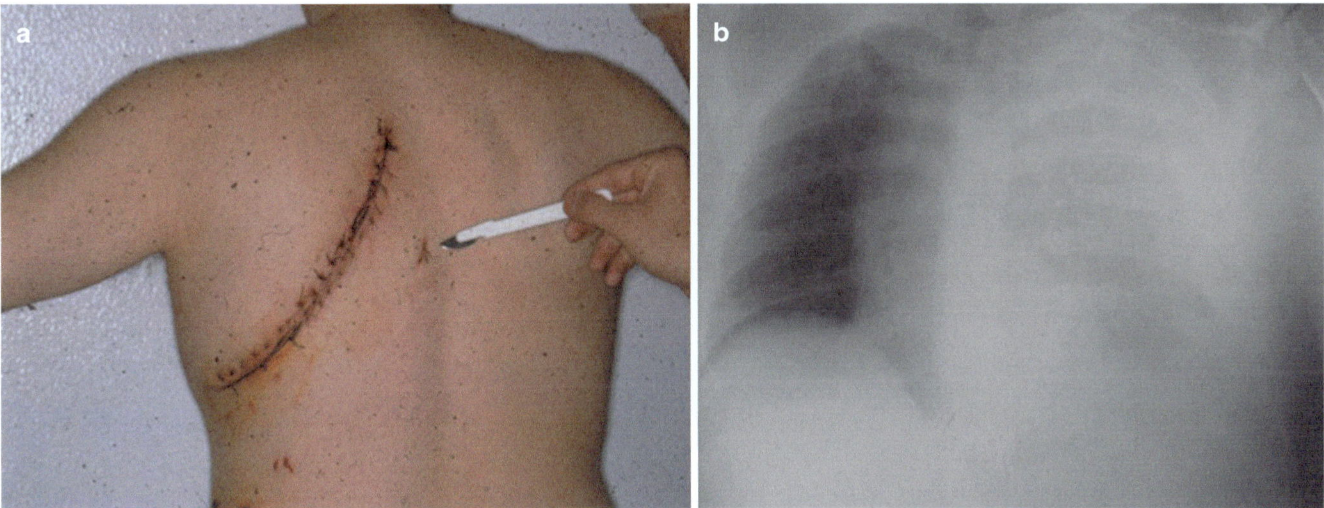

Fig. 20.3 (**a**) Cut and puncture wound to left posterior chest wall in the paravertebral site: patient submitted to thoracotomy to control bleeding due to laceration of two intercostal arteries close to where they emerge from the thoracic aorta and lacerations of the lung parenchyma. (**b**) Preoperative chest X-ray: massive opacification of the left hemithorax caused by massive haemothorax

to the diaphragmatic dome and to subdiaphragmatic organs should always be considered: the liver on the right, the stomach and spleen on the left must always be suspected, in addition to injuries to the pleural cavity. In fact, a wound involving the last intercostal spaces may determine a diaphragm injury in a percentage between 13 and 19% (Fig. 20.4).

In cuts and puncture wounds with retention of the offending object, generally a knife, it is essential not to remove the object before arriving at the ER as it might be of use in spontaneous haemostasis, and the physician, at admission to ER, can use the position of the foreign body to predict what injuries may be involved (chest wall, lung, diaphragm, pericardium, heart) (Figs. 20.5 and 20.6).

Lung parenchymal lacerations are commonly complicated by pneumothorax, haemothorax and pulmonary haematoma.

20.2.2.1 Management

Generally, complications of lung parenchymal lacerations require chest tube insertion. In cases of small pulmonary lacerations, it is usually the only treatment required.

Extensive lacerations or centrally located ones, involving wide blood effusions covering more or less extensive segments of lung parenchyma, should be sutured, stapled or wedged. Proceeding to a thoracotomy is usually required, but video-assisted thoracic surgery (VATS) has been suggested for initial management of pulmonary lacerations by some authors [6, 7].

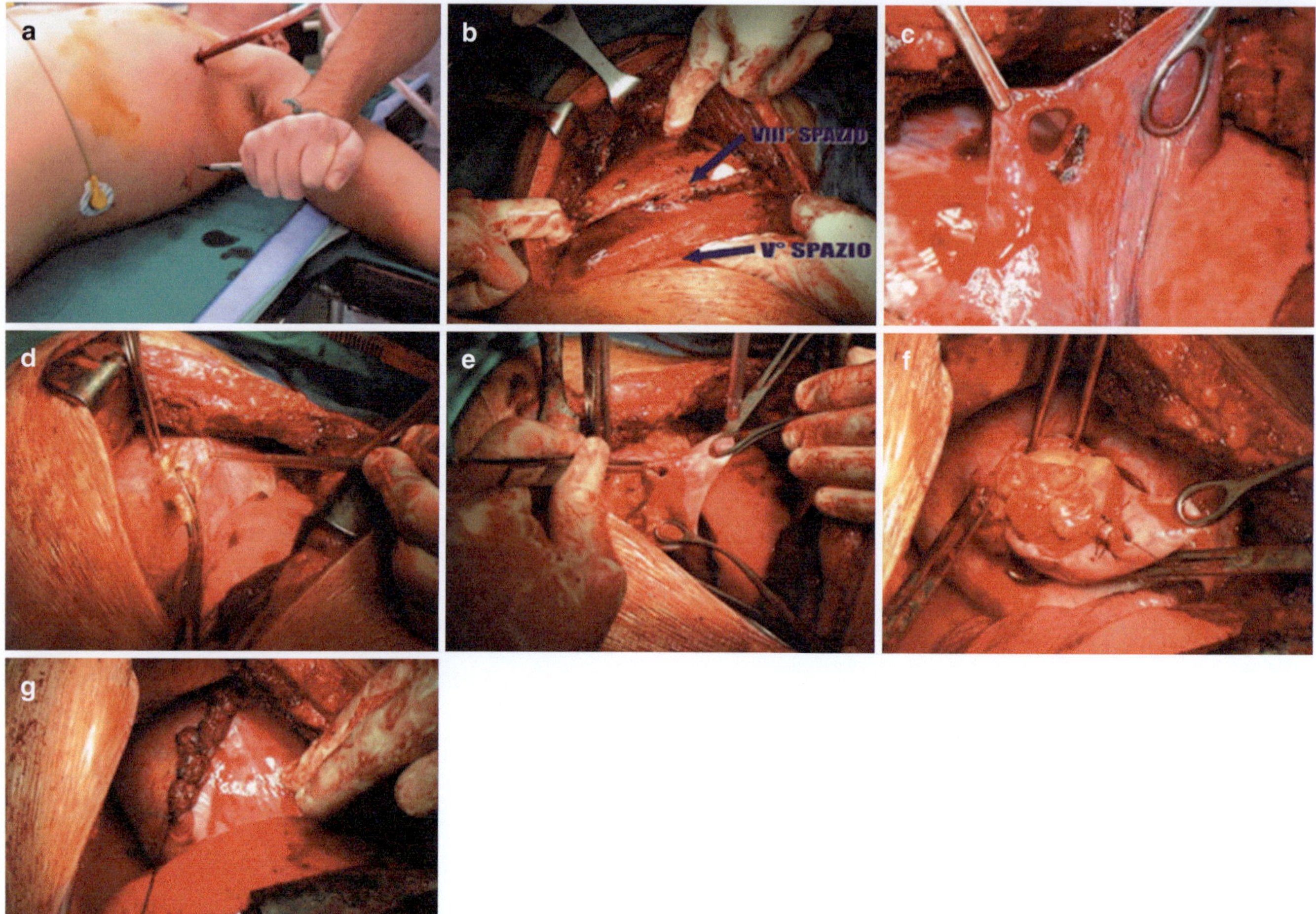

Fig. 20.4 (**a**) Cut and puncture wound (*arme blanche*) left lateral chest wall, at the level of the last intercostal spaces, in cranial-caudal direction. Presence of major haemothorax treated with a pleural drain. Suspecting a pleural cavity and diaphragm injury, the patient undergoes a left posterolateral thoracotomy. (**b**) Second access by pleurotomy at eighth intercostal space to examine any diaphragm lesions. (**c**) A lung injury is sutured. (**d**) Injury of the diaphragm. (**e**) The stomach presents a laceration due to a knife wound. (**f**) Stomach is sutured. (**g**) Diaphragm is sutured

If suturing of the lung parenchyma is not possible, anatomic lung resection (segmental resection, lobectomy) may be necessary.

20.2.2.2 Gunshot Wounds

In patients with gunshot wounds admitted to the emergency department, it is first necessary to determine how many bullet holes are involved, what direction the bullets came from and whether or not any are retained.

Precisely because of how it acts, a bullet can sometimes cause a lung injury that is then responsible for a haemopneumothorax that can be treated by inserting a pleural drain, if there is no massive loss of blood and air (Fig. 20.7), by suturing the parenchyma or by atypical resection during thoracotomy in the event of a substantial loss of blood and air (Fig. 20.8).

Multiple gunshot wounds with bullet retention require exploratory thoracotomy for the repair of injuries produced by the bullets and for the removal of the foreign bodies.

20.3 Pleural Injuries

Blunt trauma, cuts and puncture wounds, gunshot wounds, wounds from conventional and unconventional weapons and interruptions of continuity of the chest wall (traumatic thoracotomy) can lead to penetrating wounds through the chest wall associated with more or less serious injuries of the chest wall, lung and mediastinal organs.

Thus, in both open and closed chest trauma, the execution of chest CT scans could highlight possible pleural effusion or a pneumothorax related to the traumatic event.

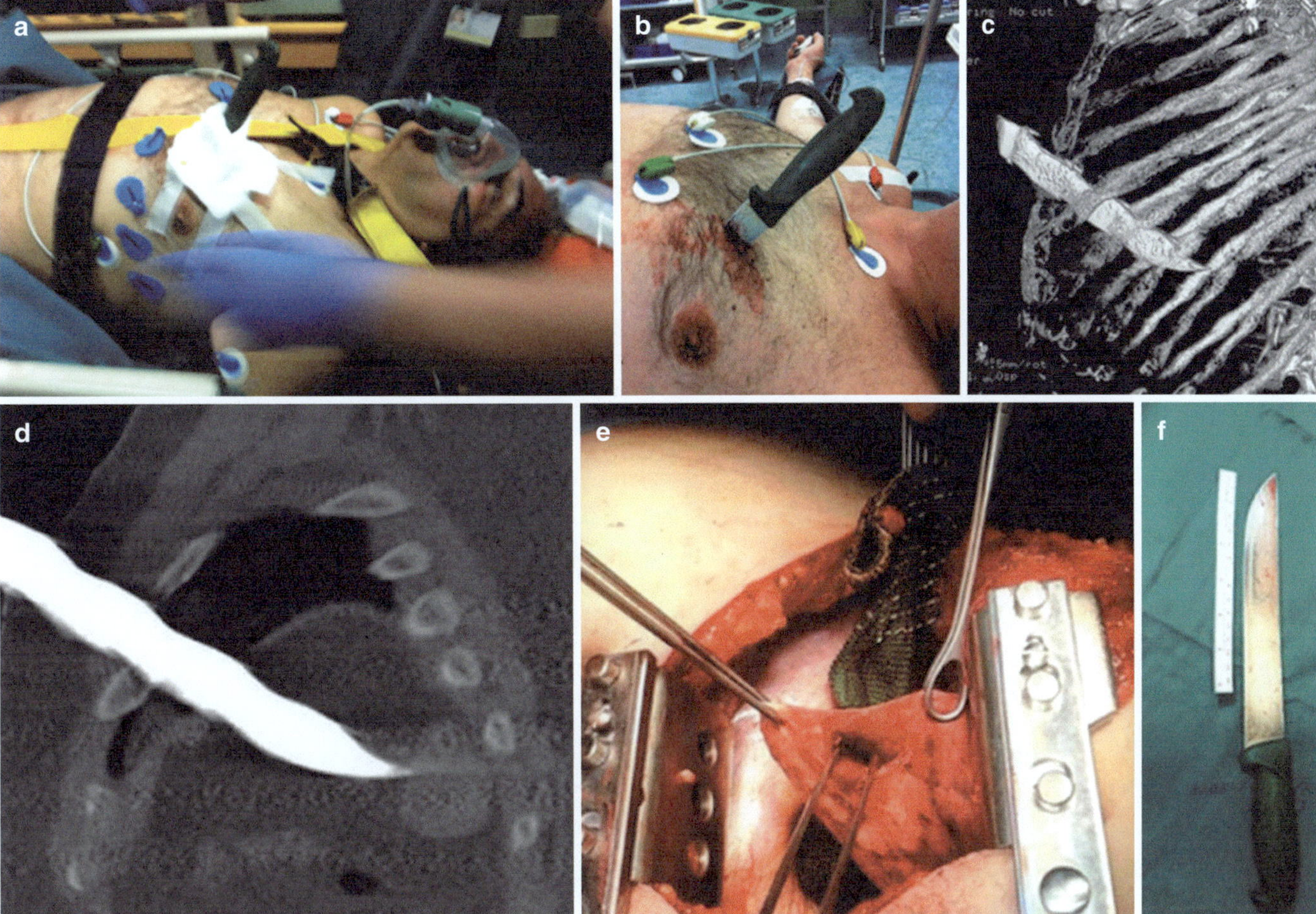

Fig. 20.5 (**a**) Knife wound with knife retained in the left pleural cavity. The patient in A&E presents a knife in the left pleural cavity. (**b**) After removal of the dressing applied urgently at the site of the traumatic event, the possible direction of the knife can be observed. (**c**) Chest CT highlights where the knife is located and a possible diaphragmatic injury. (**d**) CT reconstruction shows that the tip of the knife, after passing the left diaphragm, ends up below the diaphragm, in close proximity to the stomach and spleen. (**e**) Laparotomic access is used to explore the abdominal cavity where no stomach, spleen or colon injuries are observed. The left diaphragmatic dome and lung are sutured through a left posterolateral thoracotomy. (**f**) The removed knife

20.3.1 Haemothorax

Haemothorax is represented by the presence of blood in the pleural cavity.

Post-traumatic haemothorax in a closed chest trauma may be due to:

- Rib fractures
- Lung laceration
- Intercostal artery laceration
- Internal mammary artery laceration
- Azygos vein and superior vena cava laceration

As in the case of post-traumatic pneumothorax, haemothorax may occur hours after the traumatic event.

In diagnostic radiology, if the presence of a haemothorax is suspected from a standard chest X-ray, a chest CT with contrast medium must be performed. A haemothorax of modest entity (<500 mL) does not generally show up on a chest X-ray and can only be diagnosed by performing a chest CT.

20.3.1.1 Management

The haemothorax must be treated with a chest tube. Indeed, a stable haemothorax has a high risk to evolve into an empyema or a fibrothorax. In case of stable patients following the insertion of a chest tube for haemothorax, we propose the following algorithm (Fig. 20.9) [8]. If blood evacuated immediately after chest tube placement reaches an amount equal to or greater than 1500 mL, if blood loss of over

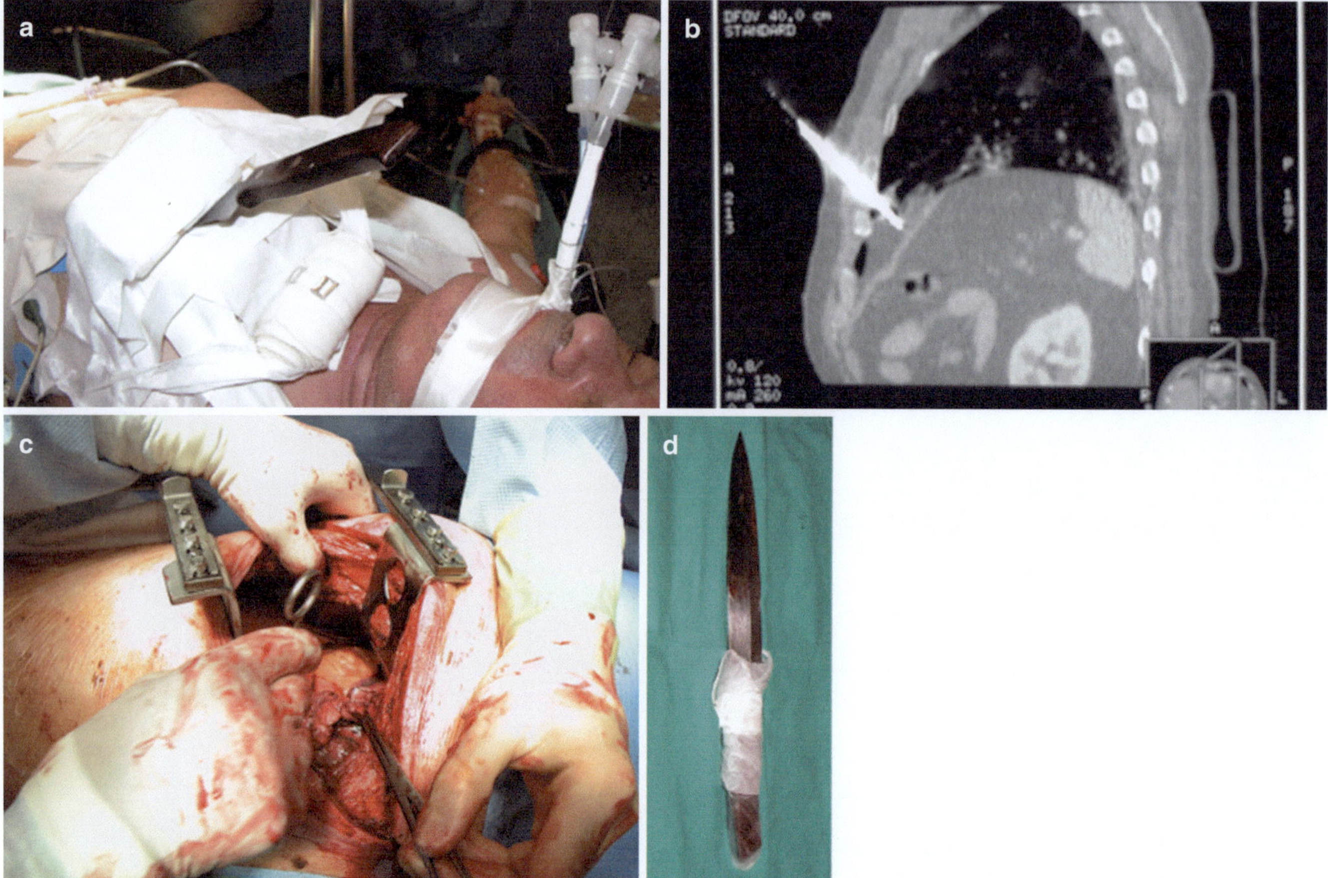

Fig. 20.6 Penetrating wound in the left pleural cavity with retained foreign body (knife) and injury to the diaphragm and lung. Upon arrival at the ER, after application of a compressive dressing by doctors from the call-out service, the patient presents a retained foreign body in the left pleural cavity. (**a**) Before removal of the knife, a chest CT is carried out. (**b**) Presence of foreign body in the pleural cavity with possible injury to the left hemidiaphragm. (**c**) After execution of left posterolateral thoracotomy, the knife is removed under visual control. It is possible to evaluate the injuries produced by the foreign body: in this case there was a laceration of the lung and diaphragm. (**d**) The removed knife

200 mL/h for 4 h, or in the case of haemodynamic instability, the execution of exploratory surgical procedures (by thoracotomy or thoracoscopy) or, eventually, a trans-catheter arterial embolization is indicated [9–11].

20.3.2 Pneumothorax

Pneumothorax is the presence of air in the pleural cavity.

Post-traumatic pneumothorax in closed chest trauma may be due to rib fracture, lung laceration, laceration or rupture of the tracheobronchial tree and laceration or rupture of the oesophagus. The air in the pleural cavity may result in a more or less complete collapse of the lung parenchyma with or without a shift of the mediastinum. A contralateral mediastinal shift is an indicator of tension pneumothorax: namely, air under pressure in the pleural cavity displaces the mediastinal structures contralaterally. The most serious consequence of this is the angle of the venae cavae, especially the inferior vena cava, with a reduction in systemic venous return and hypovolaemic shock. Tension pneumothorax is an emergency clinical situation which if not treated leads to the death of the patient within a few hours.

On the other hand, a penetrating chest wound causes a communication between the external environment and the pleural cavity. In the event of the passage remaining open, an open wound of this kind causes an open pneumothorax with air passing from the outside to the inside of the pleural space during each respiratory action (blowing wound). An open parietal breach, in fact, causes the so-called blowing wound from which air and blood bubbles exit from the pleural cavity at every respiratory action. To avoid this complication, it is always crucial to immediately transform every open chest trauma into a closed trauma at the site of the traumatic event using three-sided compression medication to avoid "mediastinal flutter" or the creation of a valve mechanism, the cause of "tension pneumothorax". Once the patient has been hospitalized, emergency surgery consisting of dressing the parietal

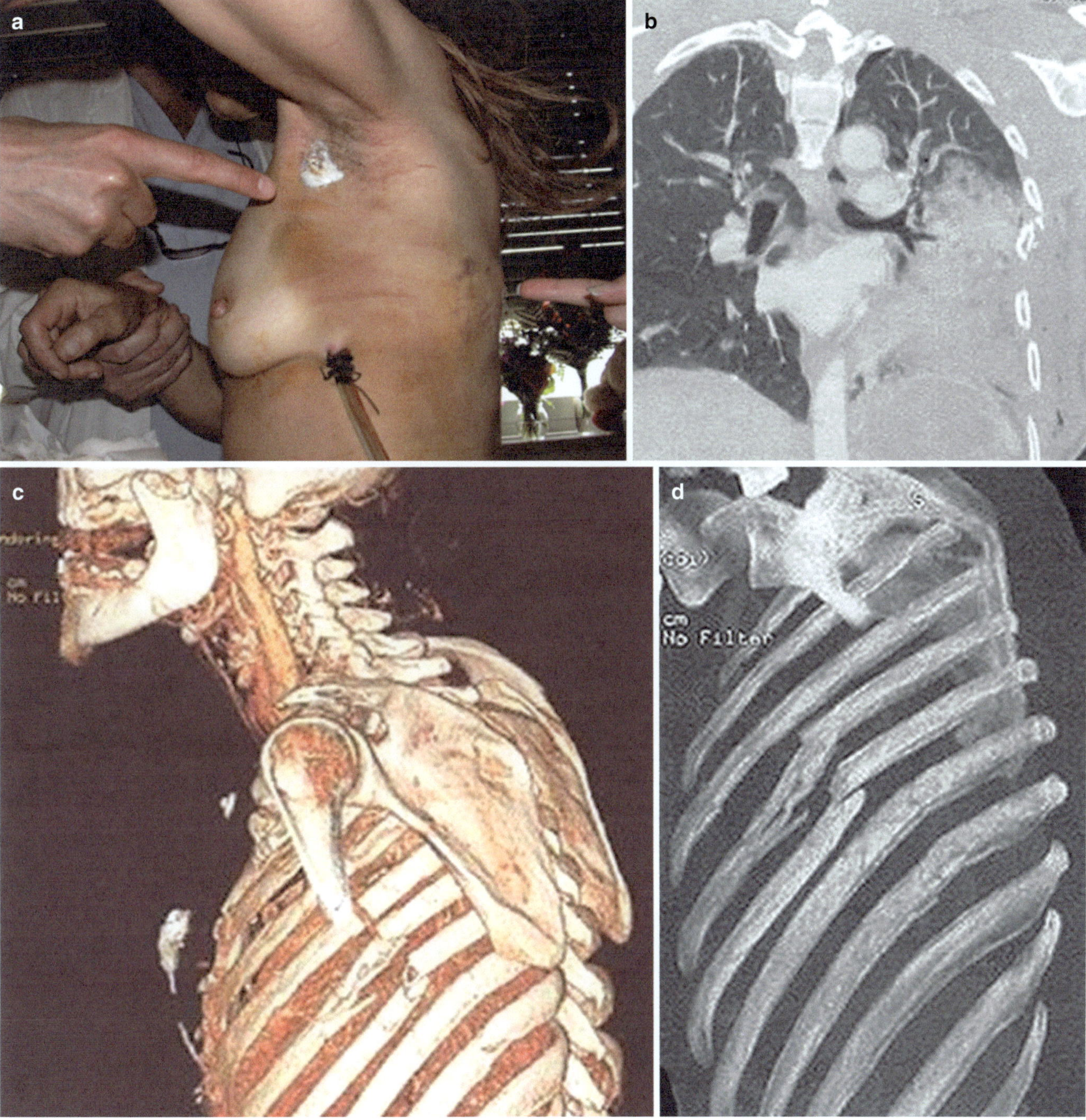

Fig. 20.7 Gunshot wound of the left hemithorax with fracture of two ribs and haemothorax of the left pleural cavity treated with a pleural drain. (**a**) The two fingers indicate the path of the bullet. (**b**) Chest CT: left pleural effusion. (**c**, **d**) Chest CT: the rib fractures determined by the force of the bullets are clear to see

solution of continuity and monitoring pulmonary and mediastinal intrapleural injuries will be indispensable in this pathology.

Post-traumatic pneumothorax can also occur several hours after the traumatic event: this eventuality should always be kept in mind when you observe a chest trauma with or without rib fractures. In fact, it should be remembered that pneumothorax could occur even in the absence of rib fractures.

20.3.2.1 Management

Post-traumatic pneumothorax therapy consists of the insertion of a chest tube into the pleural cavity and in the treatment of associated lesions or injuries.

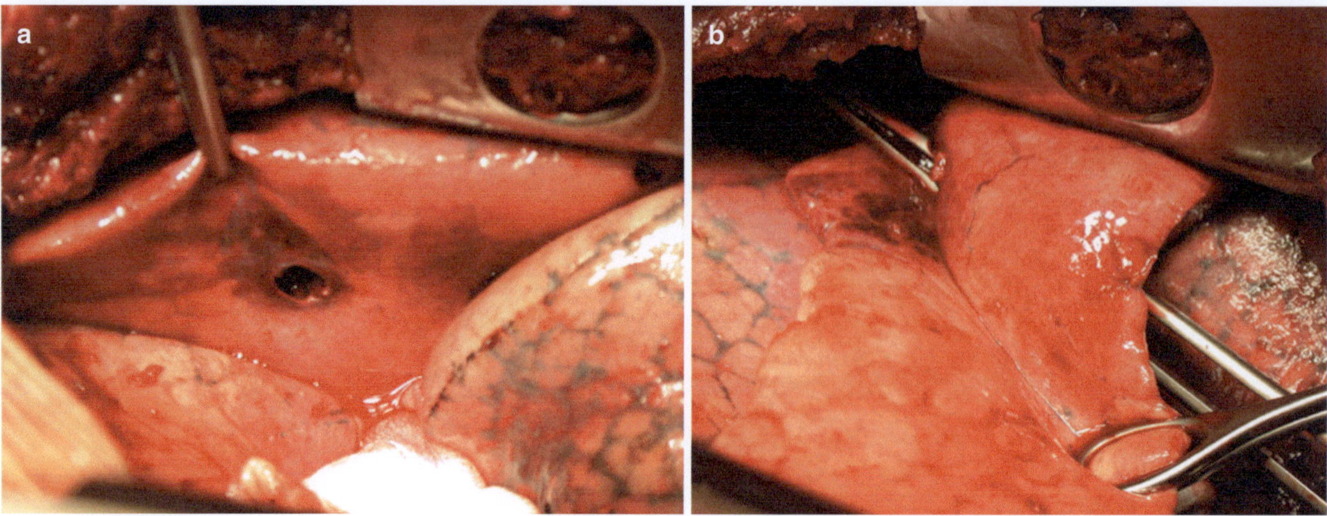

Fig. 20.8 (**a**) Gunshot wound piercing the lung parenchyma. (**b**) A forceps introduced in the path of the bullet highlights the wound passing through the lung parenchyma

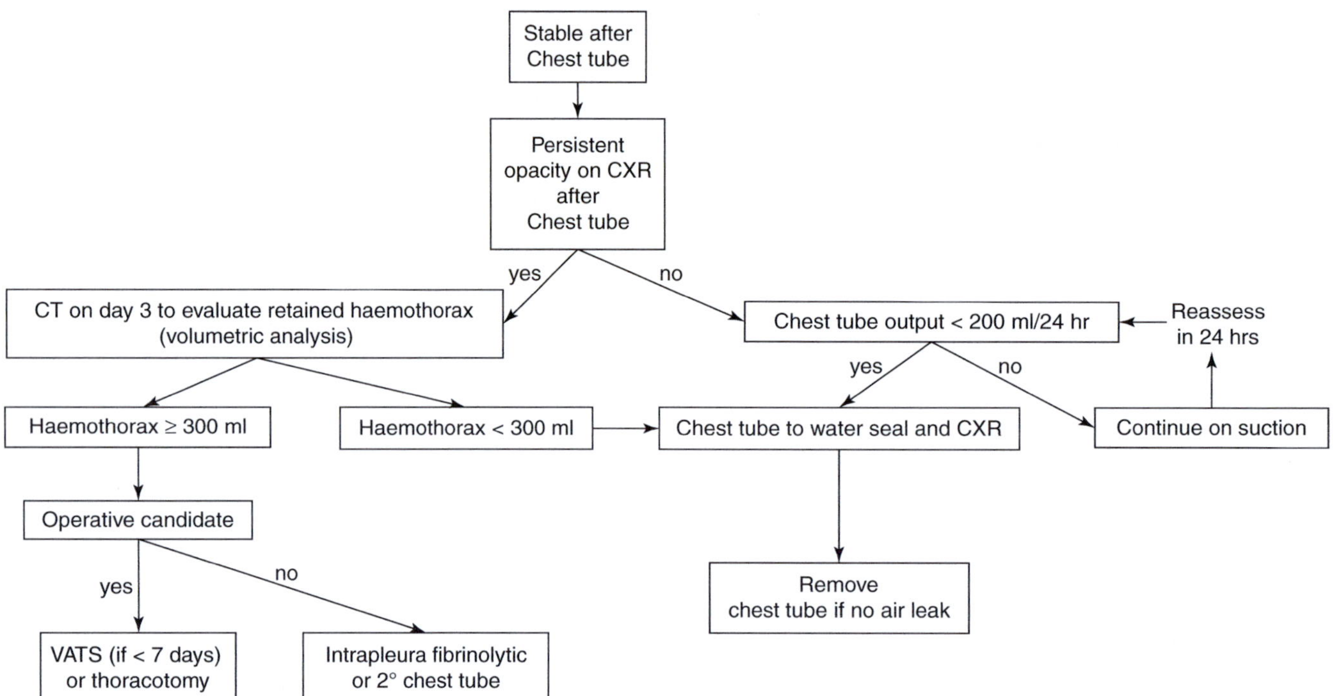

Fig. 20.9 Algorithm for patients with traumatic haemothorax [8] (from: Dennis BM et al. J Trauma Acute Care Surg 2017; 82: 728–732)

20.3.3 Chylothorax

Chylothorax is the presence of chyle in the pleural cavity. Chyle is defined as a "milky" effusion, containing chylomicrons and a high level of triglycerides (usually above 1.1 g/L) at the biochemical examination. Chylothorax should be differentiated from pseudo-chylothorax: both have a milky appearance, but the former present chylomicrons in pleural effusion and an increased level of triglyceride, while pseudo-chylothorax showed a high level of cholesterol, a low level of triglyceride and presence of cholesterol crystals in the absence of chylomicrons [12].

The side of post-traumatic chylothorax is correlated on the level of the injuries of thoracic duct: wound lower than T3–T4 generated a right chylothorax, while higher lesions generated a left pleural effusion [13].

Acute symptomatology of post-traumatic chylothorax is represented by dyspnoea, usually with rapid development.

20.3.3.1 Management

Traumatic injuries of the thoracic duct may resolve spontaneously. Nevertheless, the conservative management is complex and requires on one hand the maintenance of a correct nutritional status and on the other a reduction of lipid intake (usually by total parenteral nutrition) to reduce the chyle flow. Insertion of a chest tube into the pleural cavity is generally required in case of chylothorax of a vast entity. In the eventuality of a prolonged chyle leak without spontaneous resolution, surgical ligation of thoracic duct could be indicated. An alternative to thoracic duct ligation is chemical pleurodesis with talc.

20.4 Airway Injuries

Tracheobronchial rupture is a rare condition often not recognized at the time of trauma and, without early recognition and prompt intervention, frequently represents a life-threatening condition [14]. Airway patency may not be sufficient to breathe adequately and to allow a correct oxygenation. Moreover, intrathoracic tracheobronchial ruptures are commonly associated with other intra- or extrathoracic injuries: haemothorax, pneumothorax and diaphragm, oesophagus and great vessel, bone and facial and intraabdominal lesions [15–18]. Due to the concomitant severe injuries, the diagnosis of tracheobronchial rupture can be initially misled [19, 20]. Nevertheless, a traumatic tracheobronchial injury usually requires emergency surgery, and if misunderstood the pathology can lead to long-term cicatricial stenosis.

In the event of a pneumothorax, already treated with a pleural drain, with persistent lung collapse and with an air leak from the drain in the presence of subcutaneous (Fig. 20.10) and/or mediastinal emphysema, a tracheobronchial rupture must be suspected.

Subcutaneous emphysema is the presence of air in the loose tissue under the skin with detachment of anatomical layers. Normally there is no air in these locations, and when the air is found under the skin, it may have come from the lung, the pleural cavity, the tracheobronchial tree, the oesophagus or the external environment in the case of an open chest trauma. Mediastinal emphysema means the presence of air in the space between the two mediastinal pleurae (Fig. 20.11). Air is never present at this site, and when found it is due to the air coming from the lung, from the tracheobronchial tree or from the oesophagus. In chest X-ray, subcutaneous emphysema may sometimes conceal a possible pneumothorax because the presence of air under the skin determines a radiological image like a lung pattern (Fig. 20.12).

20.4.1 Management

The execution of a flexible fibre-optic bronchoscopy is fundamental for diagnosis to determine the extent of the injury (fissure, tear, rupture). Moreover, it can be used to assist intubation in critical patients [21, 22]. Rigid bronchoscopy is a well-established alternative procedure to assess the exact extension of tracheal or bronchial injuries and to clean the airways from secretions or blood [20]. In a critical patient, after initial invasive evaluation, definitive airway protection by oro-tracheal intubation, if possible performed guided by bronchoscopy, is fundamental [16, 20, 21]. Occasionally, like in case of massive trauma with alteration of laryngeal anatomy, tracheostomy represents the procedure of choice to protect the airway and subsequently perform the assessment of airway injuries [22–24].

Small tracheal or bronchial traumatic injuries (less than 2 cm) that do not necessitate positive ventilation resolve spontaneously [22, 25–27]. However, during conservative management a careful monitoring is mandatory for early detection of any clinical worsening to allow a prompt intervention [22].

In case of major traumatic tracheal injuries (larger than 2 cm), surgery is indicated with the aim to restore airway continuity [15, 21, 22]. The surgical techniques used to repair the airways are similar to those normally performed for resection and reconstruction of the trachea and bronchi in elective thoracic surgery [28]. Thus, expertise offered by thoracic surgery units represents the cornerstone of tracheobronchial injury management [20, 29].

Cervicotomy is the surgical approach of choice in case of cervical trachea injuries [20, 30]. Cervical trachea injuries following a tracheostomy can be repaired by enlarging the stoma on the anterior wall of the trachea and suturing the lesion from the inside of the lumen [31]. Manubriotomy can be performed to expose the middle third of the trachea as well as the innominate vein and artery [32]. In case of injuries to the distal third of the trachea, a right posterolateral thoracotomy is required; with this approach the right mainstem and proximal left mainstem bronchi are accessible [22, 28, 32]. If the injury involves the distal left mainstem bronchus, left posterolateral thoracotomy is indicated [32].

Finally, according to associated parenchymal, mediastinal and pleural injuries, median sternotomy and clamshell incision represent rational approaches [18].

Surgery consists of the debridement and primary repair with 3/0 or 4/0 interrupted sutures in case of simple lacerations. The suture may be covered with vital tissue: strap or sternocleidomastoid muscle in the cervical region, intercostal muscle, pericardial fat or pleural flap in the chest [32].

For mainstem bronchial disruption, repair should be attempted over pneumonectomy because of the high rate of mortality of the latter in the setting of trauma [32].

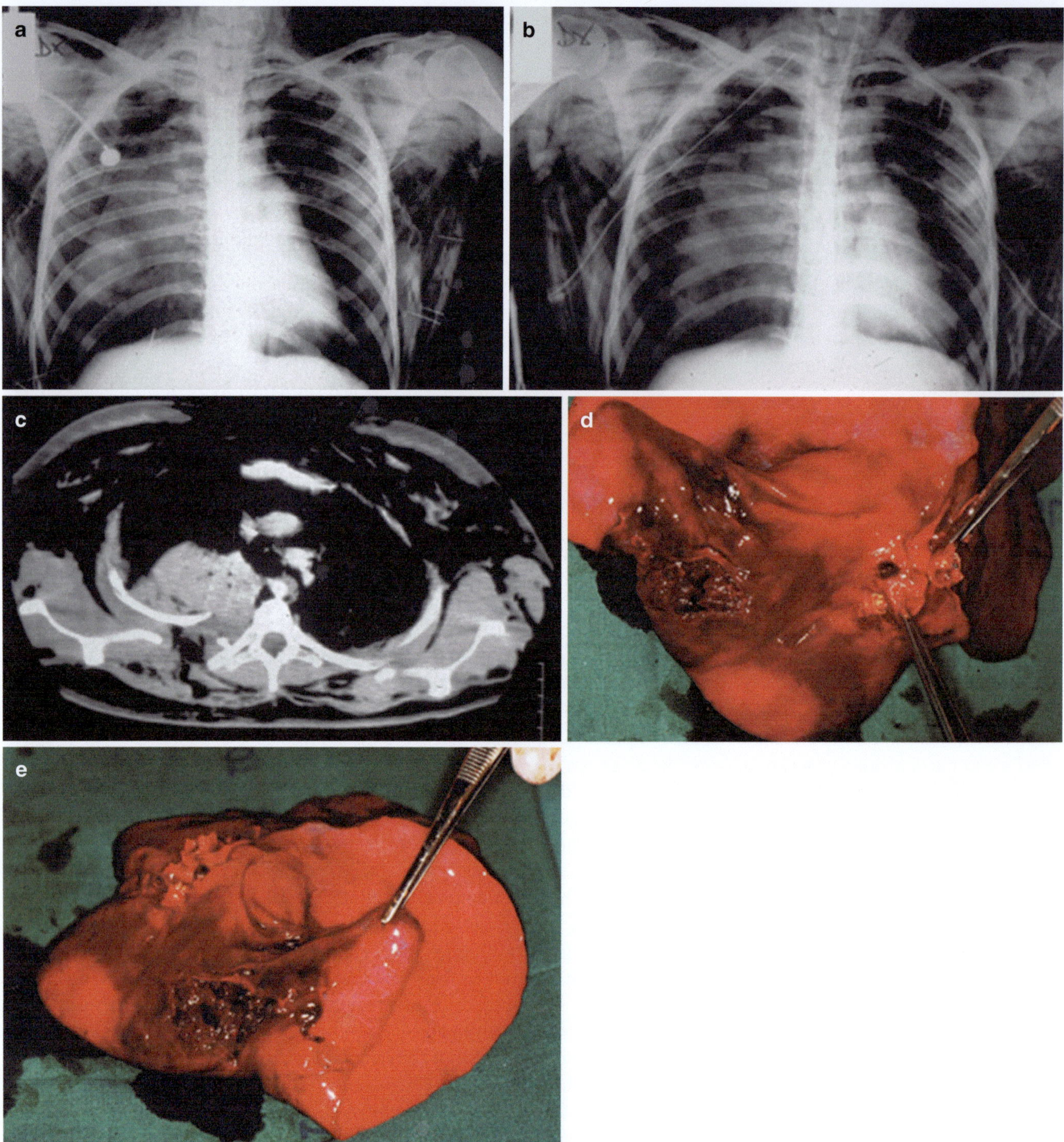

Fig. 20.10 Traumatic rupture of the intermediate bronchus in severe closed chest-abdominal trauma. (**a**) Chest X-ray at A&E: subcutaneous emphysema extending bilaterally to the chest wall, neck, face, multiple rib fractures on the right, bilateral pnx. (**b**) Chest X-ray at A&E after placement of left and right pleural drain: persisting right lung collapse with presence of major air loss from the right pleural drain. (**c**) Chest CT scan: presence of rib fragment in the parenchyma of the lower lobe of the right lung. (**d**) After emergency execution of right posterolateral thoracotomy, a disconnection of the middle lobar bronchus and the lower lobar bronchus from the intermediate bronchus is found. The operation ends with a right middle-lower bilobectomy. (**e**) The laceration of the lung parenchyma of the right lower lobe by a rib fragment is clearly evident

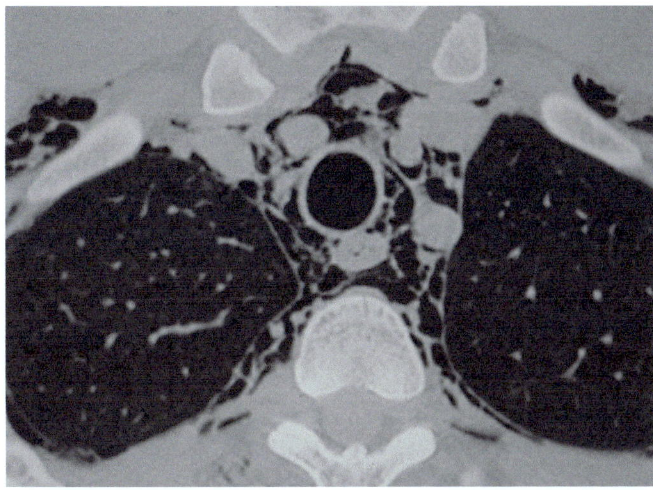

Fig. 20.11 Mediastinal emphysema. The chest CT highlights the presence of air in the loose mediastinal tissue. The trachea and oesophagus surrounded by air are clearly evident

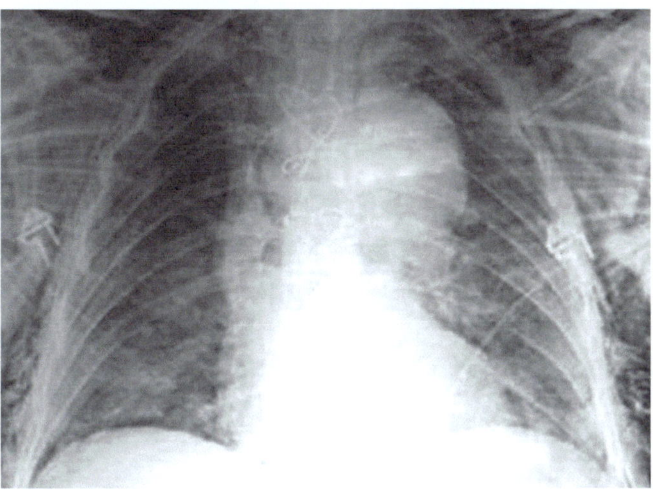

Fig. 20.12 Chest X-ray: presence of bilateral subcutaneous emphysema and mediastinal emphysema

Tracheal resection may be necessary in case of extensive damage not amenable of simple repair. This consists in a circumferential dissection only at the level of injured segment to maintain blood supply. Anastomosis is performed with adsorbable interrupted sutures. The oral endotracheal tube is retracted and the patient ventilated from the surgical field. Then the posterior wall is sutured. After completion of the posterior wall, ventilation is restored with the standard oral endotracheal tube, and the remaining sutures can be placed. Knots should be tied at the end and the suture may be protected with vital tissue [32].

If extensive resection of the trachea is required, release manoeuvers may be necessary to allow a tension-free suture [32].

20.4.2 New Trends in Recent Clinical Practice: ECMO in Trachea-Bronchial Rupture Management

Extracorporeal life support (ECLS) techniques are used to provide cardio- or respiratory support in cases of severe and refractory respiratory failure. Normally, they represent a "bridge" to transplantation or other treatment, but ECLS could also supply cardiorespiratory function until patient recovery. Extracorporeal membrane oxygenation (ECMO) is one of the most commonly used ECLS techniques in the thoracic domain. In particular, in thoracic surgery, ECMO is mainly used as a bridge to delayed surgical management or transplantation [33].

Nevertheless, complications due to haemorrhage on ECMO are commonly observed and can result in intracranial haemorrhage or cerebral infarction in traumatic patient [33–35].

As described above, traumatic tracheobronchial injuries may require an emergency surgical repair [15, 21, 22]. However, most of the patients present an unbalanced haemodynamic and respiratory function with a difficult management and, consequently, a high mortality rate [36, 37]. Similarly, patients with small airway injuries mendable by conservative management can present a critical clinical condition, and positive pressure ventilation should be avoided [22, 25–27].

Venovenous (VV) ECMO can supply extracorporeal respiratory support and could be applied to stabilize the patient, as a bridge to a delayed airway surgical repair [34, 35, 38]. In case a circulatory stabilization is required, arteriovenous (AV) ECMO should be preferred over VV-ECMO [33, 34].

Moreover, when a conservative management of a traumatic airway lesion is affordable, ECMO could be used to supply cardiorespiratory support and to reduce the use of positive pressure ventilation, to decrease complications of long-term ventilation and to allow patient self-respiration [39–41].

Finally, in recent years, the use of ECMO as intraoperative support for surgical repair of the tracheobronchial lesions has frequently been reported [38, 42–45]. Furthermore, ECMO represents an effective support in the postoperative period to avoid barotrauma after bronchial repair [38].

References

1. Wiot J. The radiographic manifestations of blunt chest trauma. JAMA. 1975;231:500–3.
2. Chopra P, Kroncke G, Berkoff H, et al. Pulmonary contusion: a problem in blunt chest trauma. Wis Med J. 1977;76:S1–3.
3. Wagner RB, Crawford WO Jr, Schimpf PP. Classification of parenchymal injuries of the lung. Radiology. 1998;167:77–82.
4. Stevens E, Templeton A. Traumatic nonpenetrating lung contusions. Radiology. 1965;85:247–52.
5. Erikson D, Shinozaki T, Beekman E, et al. Relationship of arterial blood gases and pulmonary radiographs to the degree of pulmonary contusion. J Trauma. 1971;11:689–94.
6. Abolhoda A, Livingston DH, Donahoo JS, et al. Diagnostic and therapeutic video assisted thoracic surgery (VATS) following chest trauma. Eur J Cardiothorac Surg. 1997;12:356–60.
7. Manlulu AV, Lee TW, Thung KH, et al. Current indications and results of VATS in the evaluation and management of hemodynamically stable thoracic injuries. Eur J Cardiothorac Surg. 2004;25:1048–53.
8. Dennis BM, Gondek SP, Guyer RA, et al. Use of an algorithm for patients with traumatic hemothorax reduces need for additional interventions. J Trauma Acute Care Surg. 2017;82(4):728–32.
9. Carrillo EH, Richardson JD. Thoracoscopy in the management of hemothorax and retained blood after trauma. Curr Opin Pulm Med. 1998;4:243–6.
10. Hagiwara A, Yanagawa Y, Kaneko N, et al. Indications for transcatheter arterial embolization in persistent hemothorax caused by blunt trauma. J Trauma. 2008;65:589–94.
11. Meyer DM, Jessen ME, Wait MA, et al. Early evacuation of traumatic retained hemothoraces using thoracoscopy: a prospective, randomized trial. Ann Thorac Surg. 1997;64(5):1396–400.
12. Staats BA, Ellefson RD, Budahn LL, et al. The lipoprotein profile of chylous and nonchylous pleural effusions. Mayo Clin Proc. 1980;55:700–4.
13. Hillerdal G. Effusions from lymphatic disruptions. In: Light RW, Lee YC, editors. Textbook of pleural diseases. London: Hodder Arnold; 2008. p. 393–4.
14. Kummer C, Netto FS, Rizoli S, et al. A review of traumatic airway injuries: potential implications for airway assessment and management. Injury. 2007;38:27–33.
15. Huh J, Milliken JC, Chen JC. Management of tracheobronchial injuries following blunt and penetrating trauma. Am Surg. 1997;63:896–9.
16. Lee RB. Traumatic injury of the cervico-thoracic trachea and major bronchi. Chest Surg Clin N Am. 1997;7:285–304.
17. Inci I, Ozçelik C, Taçyildiz I, et al. Penetrating chest injuries: unusually high incidence of high-velocity gunshot wounds in civilian practice. World J Surg. 1998;22:438–42.
18. Karmy-Jones R, Wood DE. Traumatic injury to the trachea and bronchus. Thorac Surg Clin. 2007;17:35–46.
19. Glazer ES, Meyerson SL. Delayed presentation and treatment of tracheobronchial injuries due to blunt trauma. J Surg Educ. 2008;65:302–8.
20. Farzanegan R, Alijanipour P, Akbarshahi H, et al. Major airways trauma, management and long term results. Ann Thorac Cardiovasc Surg. 2011;17:544–51.
21. Koletsis E, Prokakis C, Baltayiannis N, et al. Surgical decision making in tracheobronchial injuries on the basis of clinical evidences and the injury's anatomical setting: a retrospective analysis. Injury. 2012;43:1437–41.
22. Mussi A, Ambrogi MC, Ribechini A, et al. Acute major airway injuries: clinical features and management. Eur J Cardiothorac Surg. 2001;20:46–52.
23. Rossbach MM, Johnson SB, Gomez MA, et al. Management of major tracheobronchial injuries: a 28-year experience. Ann Thorac Surg. 1998;65:182–6.
24. Rathlev NK, Modzon R, Bracken ME. Evaluation and management of neck trauma. Emerg Med Clin North Am. 2007;25:679–94.
25. Gomez-Caro Andres A, Moradiellos Diez FJ, Ausin Herrero P, Kiaz-Hellin Gude V, Larru Cabrero E, de Miguel Porch E, et al. Successful conservative management in iatrogenic tracheobronchial injury. Ann Thorac Surg. 2005;79:1872–8.
26. Gomez-Caro A, Ausin P, Moradiellos FJ, et al. Role of conservative medical management of tracheobronchial injuries. J Trauma. 2006;61:1426–34.
27. Carretta A, Melloni G, Bandiera A, et al. Conservative and surgical treatment of acute posttraumatic tracheobronchial injuries. World J Surg. 2011;35:2568–74.
28. Bolukbas A, Schirren J. Parenchyma sparing bronchial sleeve resections in trauma, benign and malign diseases. Thorac Cardiovasc Surg. 2010;58:32–7.
29. Schneider T, Volz K, Dienemann H, et al. Incidence and treatment modalities of tracheobronchial injuries in Germany. Interact Cardiovasc Thorac Surg. 2009;8:571–6.
30. Angelillo-Mackinlay T. Transcervical repair of distal membranous tracheal laceration. Ann Thorac Surg. 1995;59:531–2.
31. Lee SK, Kim DH, Lee SK, et al. Does surgical repair still have a role for iatrogenic tracheobronchial rupture? Clinical analysis of a thoracic surgeon's opinion. Ann Thorac Cardiovasc Surg. 2016;22:348–53.
32. Majercik SD, Ng T, Adams CA, Cioffi WG. Tracheal injury and repair. In: Cioffi WG, Asensio JE, editors. Atlas of trauma/emergency surgical techniques (Chapter 8). New York: Elsevier. p. 82–92.
33. Reeb J, Olland A, Renaud S, et al. Vascular access for extracorporeal life support: tips and tricks. Thorac Dis. 2016;8(Suppl 4):S353–63.
34. Zhou R, Liu B, Al LK e. ECMO support for right main bronchial disruption in multiple trauma patient with brain injury—a case report and literature review. Perfusion. 2015;30(5):403–6.
35. Campione A, Agostini M, Portolan M, et al. Extracorporeal membrane oxygenation in respiratory failure for pulmonary contusion and bronchial disruption after trauma. J Thorac Cardiovasc Surg. 2007;133(6):1673–4.
36. Miñambres E, Burón J, Ballesteros MA, Llorca J, Muñoz P, González-Castro A. Tracheal rupture after endotracheal intubation: a literature systematic review. Eur J Cardiothorac Surg. 2009;35:1056–62.
37. Marty-Ané C-H, Picard E, Jonquet O, Mary H. Membranous tracheal rupture after endotracheal intubation. Ann Thorac Surg. 1995;60(5):1367–71.
38. Ballouhey Q, Fesseau R, Benouaich V, Léobon B. Benefits of extracorporeal membrane oxygenation for major blunt tracheobronchial trauma in the paediatric age group. Eur J Cardiothorac Surg. 2013;43(4):864–5.
39. Fuehner T, Kuehn C, Hadem J, Wiesner O, Gottlieb J, Tudorache I, et al. Extracorporeal membrane oxygenation in awake patients as bridge to lung transplantation. Am J Respir Crit Care Med. 2012;85:763–8.
40. Son BS, Cho WH, Kim CW. Conservative extracorporeal membrane oxygenation treatment in a tracheal injury: a case report. J Cardiothorac Surg. 2015;10:48.
41. Swol J, Fülling Y, Ull C, Bechtel M, Schildhauer TA. 48 h cessation of mechanical ventilation during venovenous extracorporeal membrane oxygenation in severe trauma: a case report. J Artif Organs. 2017;20(3):280–4. https://doi.org/10.1007/s10047-017-0949-6.

42. Nakagiri T, Inoue M, Nakagawa J, Okumura M. Blunt tracheal transection repair requiring open abdominal management. Ann Thorac Surg. 2011;92:2248–50.
43. Voelckel W, Wenzel V, Rieger M, Antretter H, Padosch S, Schobersberger W. Temporary extracorporeal membrane oxygenation in the treatment of acute traumatic lung injury. Can J Anaesth. 1998;45:1097–102.
44. Liu C, Lin Y, Du B, Liu L. Extracorporeal membrane oxygenation as a support for emergency bronchial reconstruction in a traumatic patient with severe hypoxaemia. Interact Cardiovasc Thorac Surg. 2014;19(4):699–701.
45. Korvenoja P, Pitkänen O, Berg E, Berg L. Veno-venous extracorporeal membrane oxygenation in surgery for bronchial repair. Ann Thorac Surg. 2008;86(4):1348–9.

Blunt Trauma to the Heart and Great Vessels

21

Antonino M. Grande and Paolo Aseni

Key Points

- Blunt cardiac injury comprehends a large spectrum of different injuries, including contusion, chamber rupture, and acute valvular disorders.
- Blunt cardiac injuries are not uncommon and often underdiagnosed and may cause significant morbidity and mortality; therefore, a high index of suspicion is fundamental for a prompt diagnosis.
- In all patients involved in a chest trauma, diagnostic workup must always include, after EKG and cardiac enzymes, echocardiography if specific disorders (i.e., tamponade or valvular disorders) are suspected.
- Observe patients with myocardial contusion for arrhythmias for 24–48 h.
- Surgical intervention must not be delayed once the diagnosis is suspected and the patient is hemodynamically unstable.

21.1 Blunt Cardiac Trauma

Patients with blunt cardiac injury (BCI) have a wide spectrum of clinical manifestation, ranging from clinically silent to life-threatening hemodynamic instability, depending mainly on the lesion site and severity, shifting from a mild contusion to deadly cardiac wall rupture. It is clear that prompt diagnosis is lifesaving, although it is often challenging. The heart is anatomically located within the thoracic cage that is formed by the sternum anteriorly, by the 12 pairs of ribs on either side, and by the vertebral column behind.

A BCI can occur during a deceleration trauma with a mechanism similar to thoracic rupture: the main strain is at the level of the aortic isthmus that is the least mobile portion of the thoracic aorta, "held down" by the ligamentum arteriosum. In the same manner, sudden high-velocity deceleration can determine a violent shift of the anterior portion of the heart producing different types of cardiac damages. Anyway, there are other causes of BCI: falls, accidental and criminal trauma, crush injuries, explosions, and unexpectedly several sports injuries that may occur with improper preparation or poor judgment. Therefore, different mechanisms may cause BCI: forceful blows to the chest (baseball, hockey puck, karate kicks) and a sudden compression between the sternum and the vertebral column which increases intraventricular volume and pressure (hydrostatic forces) [1].

Cardiac injuries. Following a blunt chest trauma, there is a wide range of possible cardiac injuries including cardiac contusion, cardiac concussion and dysrhythmic complications, wall rupture, pericardial involvement, valvular disruptions, and injury to the great vessels or the coronary arteries.

21.1.1 Cardiac Contusion

Cardiac contusion (CC) represents the most frequent injury to the heart after blunt chest trauma. CC is histologically characterized by myocardial hemorrhage, edema, and localized necrosis, and clinically there are wall motion alterations, loss of contractility, arrhythmias, and conduction abnormalities [2]. Any cardiac structure may be interested in various degrees of severity, alone or in combination depending on the type and violence of the trauma [1]. A prompt diagnosis is required in order to identify patients at elevated risk considering that in traumatic deaths cardiac injuries are often not diagnosed even in the presence of clinical

A. M. Grande (✉)
Department of Cardiac Surgery, IRCCS Fondazione Policlinico San Matteo, Pavia, Italy
e-mail: amgrande@libero.it

P. Aseni
Dipartimento di Emergenza Urgenza, ASST Grande Ospedale Metropolitano Niguarda, Milano, Italy

P. Aseni et al. (eds.), *Operative Techniques and Recent Advances in Acute Care and Emergency Surgery*,
https://doi.org/10.1007/978-3-319-95114-0_21

signs like hypotension, jugular vein distention, and hypoxia [3, 4] that can be easily masked in patients with multiple severe injuries. Myocardial necrosis is the most serious lesion, and it is determined by a direct cardiac trauma or by a coronary artery lesion causing an occlusion and myocardial damage. CC is the most diffuse injury after blunt trauma but its diagnosis, due to the variety of its subsequent myocardial infarction. The latter can also present an aneurismal evolution or pseudoaneurysm formation and rupture into the pericardial cavity determining cardiac tamponade and sudden death.

Diagnosis. While the more serious injuries are often very evident to the clinician on presentation, CC may be particularly difficult to diagnose, and appropriate management may be delayed. In Fig. 21.1 is represented an algorithm for diagnosis and management of patients with suspected BCI.

(a) History. Signs of cardiac heart failure or cardiogenic shock in the absence of cardiac disease suggest the presence of cardiac injury; therefore, in all polytrauma patients, getting accurate medical history is mandatory.
(b) Physical examination. Chest inspection is equally important for diagnosis: BCI should be highly suspected when chest wall bruising is present.
(c) Chest X-ray. Chest X-ray does not have specificity and sensitivity for CC diagnosis, but it is important to rule out fractured ribs and sternum and pleural effusion due to active bleeding. Anyway, an enlarged mediastinum may indicate a pericardial effusion. Therefore, an abnormal chest X-ray may raise suspicion for further investigation.
(d) ECG. ECG is more sensitive for lesions in the left ventricle than in the right; because the right ventricle is more frequently involved in blunt trauma (it is located anteriorly just behind the sternum), ECG as a diagnostic tool is controversial. Anyway, ST wave changes are the most frequent abnormalities and are related to concomitant hypoxia, hypovolemia, and electrolyte disturbances [5]; right bundle branch is the second most common abnormality. Dysrhythmias and ST elevation are more indicative of CC. ST segment elevations represent a real treatment challenge because they may be caused by either traumatic myocardial infarction (from coronary rupture, dissection, or thrombosis) or by myocardial contusion. In this clinical setting, it is useful to perform a coronary angiography. The most frequent dysrhythmia is sinus tachycardia, which is treated through volume resuscitation/transfusion and analgesia. Atrial fibrillation is the second most common dysrhythmia, which can be determined by alcohol or drug abuse, fluid shifts, electrolyte abnormalities, and/or catecholamine increase.

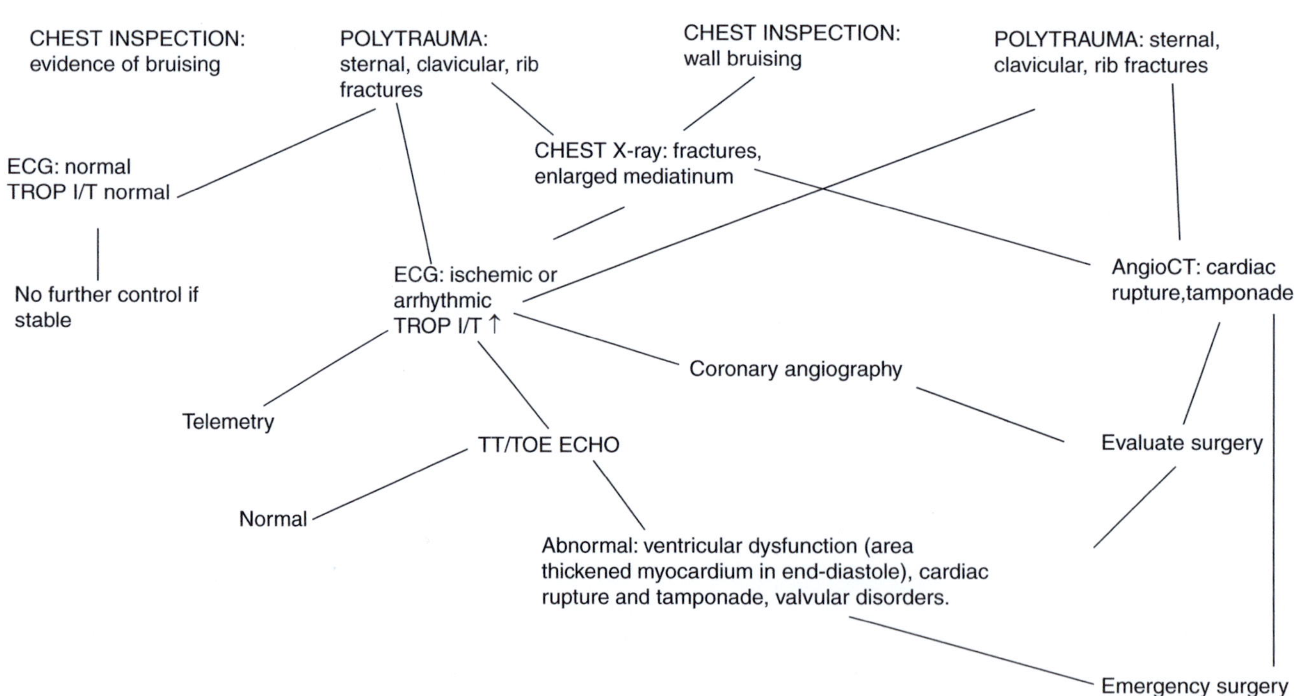

Fig. 21.1 Algorithm for diagnosis and management of patients with suspected blunt cardiac injury

(e) Cardiac markers. Creatine kinase-MB (CK-MB) is considered unreliable and non-specific especially in concomitant severe skeletal muscle, liver diaphragm, and intestinal lesions [6, 7]. Troponin T was found to be a very specific indicator (91%) for myocardial injury but with low sensitivity (31%) [8]. The sensitivity of troponin I varies from 23 to 100% [9, 10].
(f) Echocardiography. This is a noninvasive test fundamental for CC diagnosis. Transthoracic echocardiography (TTE) detects regional wall motion abnormalities, increased echo brightness, and increased end-diastolic wall thickness of the contused area [11, 12]. TTE can show pericardial effusion, cardiac tamponade, intracardiac shunts, and valvular function. Image acquisition in case of chest and lung lesions can be difficult; in these cases, transesophageal echocardiography (TOE) is superior to TTE for the diagnosis of CC [11, 13]. Ventricular thrombi are also associated with the regional wall motion abnormalities caused by myocardial contusion [14].
(g) Angio-computed tomography (angio-CT). Often the test is done in the emergency room in polytrauma patients, and it is possible to easily diagnose the most life-threatening cardiac injuries that necessitate immediate cardiac surgery.

Treatment. Life-threatening ventricular arrhythmias and cardiac failure in most cases occur within 24–48 h after blunt chest trauma. Therefore, hospitalization time for ECG monitoring can be short unless there are concomitant extracardiac injuries that would prolong hospital stay [15–18].

Hemodynamic unstable cases need immediate intensive care, inotropic support for pump failure, and fluid infusion for volume replacement. Emergency surgery is required in case of cardiac rupture, valvular lesions, and injuries to great vessels.

21.1.2 Cardiac Concussion or "Commotio Cordis"

Cardiac concussion is determined by a sudden, nonpenetrating, localized chest trauma that may result in almost simultaneous sudden death from a disruption to the conductive system. This setting is substantially different from CC as there is no evidence of morphologic lesion or preexisting cardiac disease [2]. Ventricular fibrillation and sudden death are triggered by a blunt trauma, often innocent and appearing unintentional blow to the chest without damage to the ribs, sternum, or heart [19]. Cardiac concussion represents the second cause of sudden death in young athletes [20]. The underlying pathophysiological mechanism is thought to be a high-velocity impact against the chest during ventricular repolarization determining an "R-on-T" phenomenon and ventricular fibrillation [21]. Immediate diagnosis and cardiopulmonary resuscitation may improve outcome.

21.1.3 Cardiac Wall Rupture and Pericardial Lacerations

Septal [22] and free wall ruptures are frequent: Right-sided chambers are more frequently involved though left-sided injuries, as well as multiple chamber ruptures, have been reported (Figs. 21.2 and 21.3). The main symptoms and signs in patients who had survived cardiac rupture are hypotension (100%); elevated central venous pressure (95%); tachycardia (89%); distended neck veins (80%); cyanosis of the head, neck, upper chest, and arms (76%); unresponsiveness (74%); distant heart sounds (61%); associated chest injuries (60%); and increased heart shadow on chest X-ray (59%) [23]. Anatomically, the venae cavae, the aorta, the pulmonary trunk, and the pulmonary arteries and veins firmly support the superior and posterior portion of the heart. During a deceleration trauma, the anterior portion of the heart is therefore shifted rapidly forward, and this movement may determine a laceration. That explains why cardiac lacerations are often recognized in the absence of sternal or costal fractures.

21.1.4 Case Scenario N. 1

We briefly report the case [24] of a right atrial rupture and concomitant pericardial tear in a 42-year-old man who was involved in an automobile accident and admitted to the emergency room in a conscious state, hemodynamically stable, tachypneic, and with severe epistaxis. Roentgenograms showed a nasal fracture, a fracture of the upper third of the sternum, two left rib fractures, and a widened mediastinum. Electrocardiography showed sinus tachycardia. Angio-CT showed anterior mediastinal hematoma and bleeding in the anterosuperior pericardial cavity (Fig. 21.4). Late sequential scans detected active bleeding in the anterosuperior pericardial portions that showed late contrast enhancement as do the great vessels (Fig. 21.5). This picture at first seemed to be consistent with an ascending aortic rupture. During angio-CT the patient suffered loss of consciousness. The patient was immediately intubated and transferred to the operating room for an emergency surgery. Extracorporeal circulation started using femoral vessel bypass; the sternum was then opened through a midline incision, and upon entering the pericardium, a 0.5-cm laceration of the right atrium was found (Fig. 21.6), which was sutured with polypropylene 4-0 sutures. The

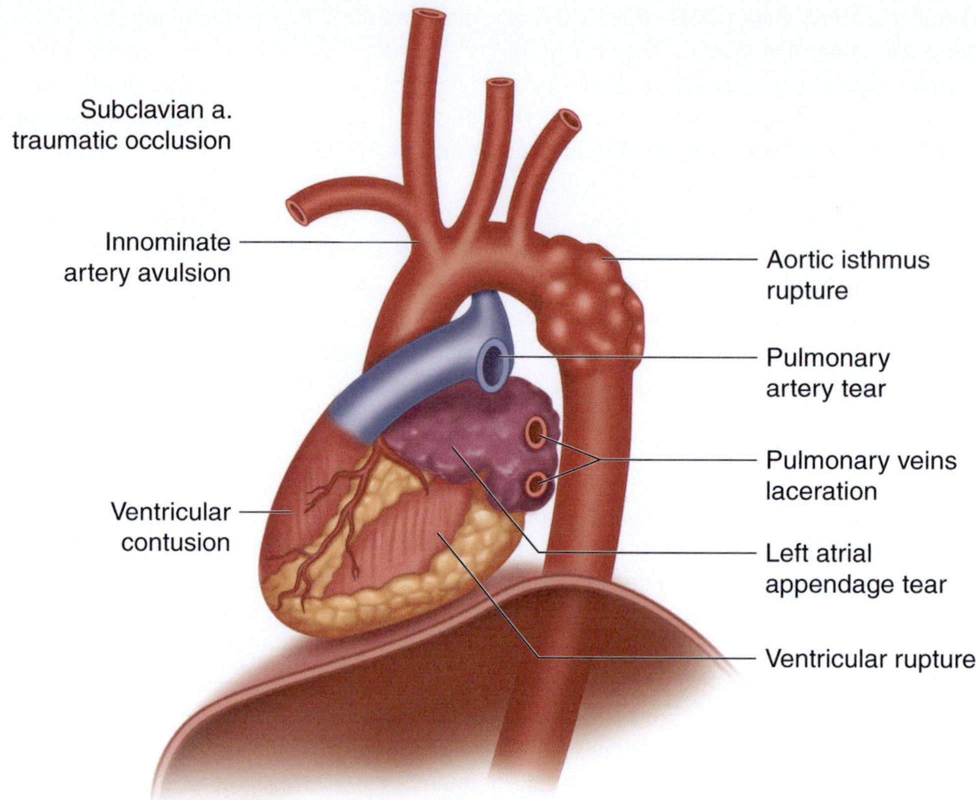

Fig. 21.2 Cardiovascular sites most commonly involved in blunt chest trauma

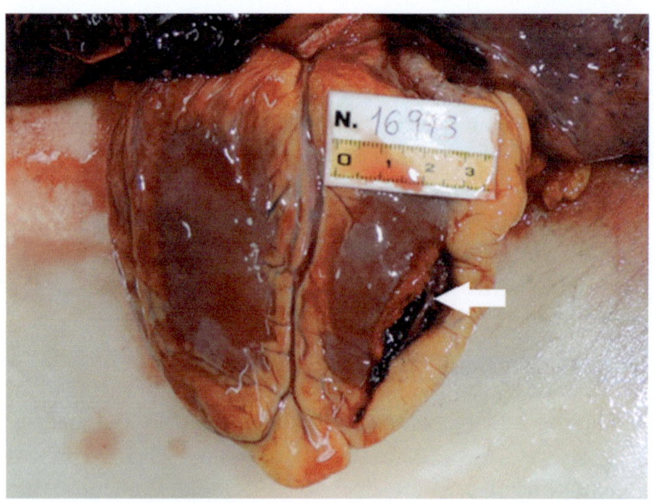

Fig. 21.3 Same case of Fig. 21.11 white arrow indicates a 3-cm wall rupture in the posterolateral surface of the right ventricle

pericardium also had wide lateral tear facing the superior and inferior venae cavae (Fig. 21.7). Both pulmonary hila showed congestion and hemorrhagic infiltration. The postoperative course was uneventful; the patient achieved complete functional recovery and 2 years later he is in the NYHA class I. The patient did not present cardiac tamponade because the pericardial tears determined hemothorax formation. It has been reported that 30% of cardiac ruptures are accompanied by pericardial lacerations which lead to hemothorax; on the remaining 70% of cases cardiac tamponade occurs [25]. It is fundamental to recognize concomitant pericardial effusion, even if those are small in amount, and hemothorax: We should suspect a cardiac rupture as the cause of hemothorax based on pericardial effusion. When hemothorax is present in patients with concomitant cardiac rupture and pericardial lacerations, the latter may prevent pericardial tamponade [26].

21.1.5 Cardiac Herniation

Cardiac herniation is a severe complication of pericardial rupture that may present a high mortality. The death is a direct consequence of torsion of inferior vena cava and great vessels that determine strangulation of the heart [27]. The pericardial rupture is in most cases longitudinal; left side tears are more frequent. In case of right herniation, if there is hemodynamic stability, in an attempt to restore the normal anatomic position, the patient is placed in left lateral decubitus [28]. Surgical intervention is usually performed through median sternotomy.

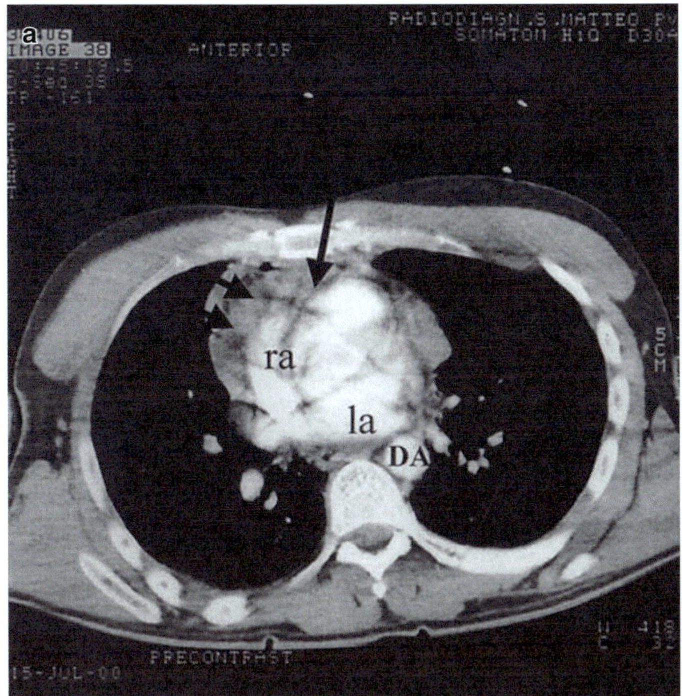

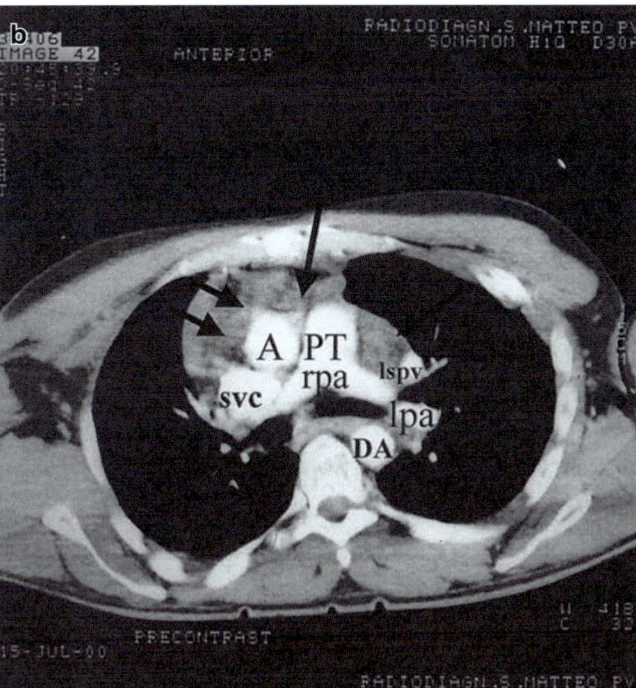

Fig. 21.4 Computed tomography angiogram. (**a**) The right atrium appears in apparent normal shape during first phases of contrast enhancement. An anterior mediastinal hematoma (arrows) is near the atrium, and a layer of fluid collection is in the right mediastinal pleura. (*DA* descending aorta, *la* left atrium, *ra* right atrium.) (**b**) Mediastinal hematoma (arrows) and anterosuperior portions of the pericardium with bleeding. The shape of the ascending aorta and the superior vena cava is normal. (*A* aorta, *lpa* left pulmonary artery, *lspv* left superior pulmonary vein, *PT* pulmonary trunk, *rpa* right pulmonary artery, *svc* superior vena cava). Reprinted from Grande AM, et al. Nonpetrating right atrial and pericardial trauma. Ann Thorac Surg 2003;76:923–6, permission from Elsevier [24]

21.1.6 Cardiac Valve Injury

Cardiac valve injury after blunt chest trauma is much less frequent than CC. Aortic valve injury is the most frequent followed by mitral and tricuspid valves. Rupture of cardiac valves after closed chest trauma may be determined by acute compression of the heart between the sternum and the vertebral column resulting in increased cardiac pressure [22]. Then, the heart, which is suspended in the mediastinum by the great vessels, can shift forward during a deceleration trauma, and the stress is localized, particularly at the atrial and valvular levels, causing lacerations of these structures. In addition, during deceleration, the blood inside the ventricles is violently moved against the valves that are closed at the moment of trauma, contributing to valvular damage. Atrioventricular valve apparatus lesions may occur in early systole during isovolumetric ventricular contraction when the deceleration forces can significantly increase intraventricular pressure: the result can be laceration of the chordae tendineae, papillary muscle rupture, and leaflet disruption [29]. Another mechanism of valvular injury, in most cases delayed, is a primitive papillary muscle contusion followed by necrosis and valve insufficiency [29].

A cardiac valve rupture should be suspected in patients who have experienced severe blunt trauma and then have developed congestive heart failure. The symptoms of valvular damage may appear immediately after the injury or after a relatively asymptomatic period of days or even years. In case of (a) history of trauma, (b) normal heart before trauma, and (c) sudden onset of valvular regurgitation, traumatic valvular injury should always be suspected in patients who present with heart murmurs after blunt chest trauma.

Aortic valve rupture. Aortic valvular injury usually presents with a sudden cardiovascular instability or cardiogenic shock. Acute mitral valve injury typically manifests itself as acute pulmonary edema and hypotension. These cases are handled by afterload reduction as a bridge to surgery.

21.1.7 Case Scenario N. 2

In Fig. 21.8 it is shown an aortic valve rupture after blunt trauma [30]: a 50-year-old man old man was admitted for severe aortic insufficiency 10 weeks after a motor vehicle accident where he sustained left scapular and humeral fractures. Shortly after the trauma, he started complaining

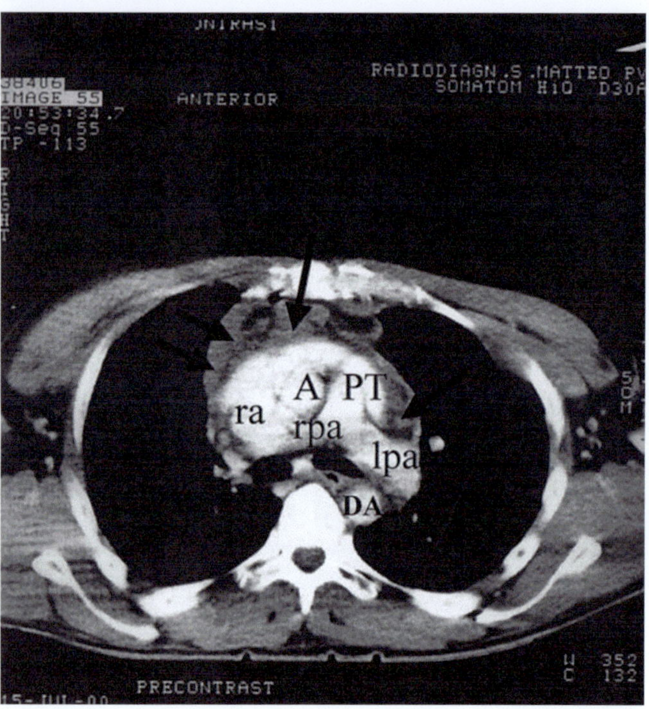

Fig. 21.5 Late scan demonstrates active bleeding in the anterosuperior pericardial portions, which show late contrast enhancement as great vessels. No active bleeding is in the mediastinal hematoma (arrows) and the right mediastinal pleural space. (*A* aorta, *DA* descending aorta, *lpa* left pulmonary artery, *PT* pulmonary trunk, *ra* right atrium, *rpa* right pulmonary artery). Reprinted from Grande AM, et al. Nonpetrating right atrial and pericardial trauma. Ann Thorac Surg 2003;76:923–6, permission from Elsevier [24]

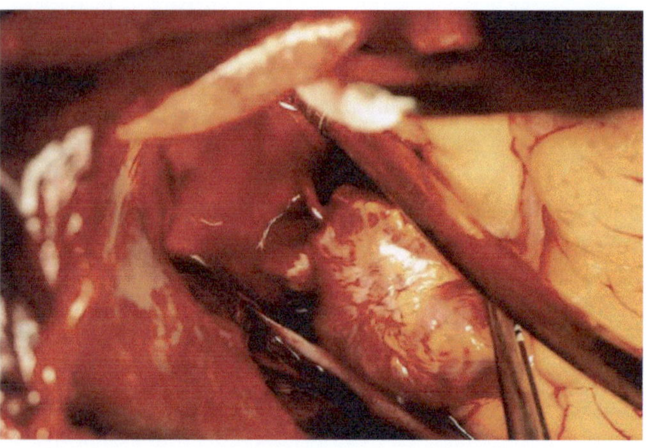

Fig. 21.6 Operative finding: right atrial laceration near the atriocaval junction. Reprinted from Grande AM, et al. Nonpetrating right atrial and pericardial trauma. Ann Thorac Surg 2003;76:923–6, permission from Elsevier [24]

precordial pain and shortness of breath. He had a Grade 4 diastolic murmur, heard along the left sternal border, and blood pressure was 130/50 mmHg; his chest X-ray showed left ventricular hypertrophy, and on ECG left ventricular hypertrophy and strain were present. TTE showed severe

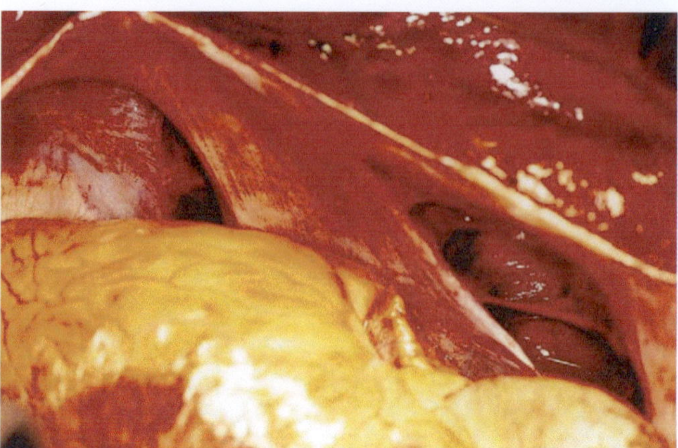

Fig. 21.7 Operative finding: wide pericardial lacerations of the pericardium on its lateral aspect facing the superior and inferior venae cavae. Reprinted from Grande AM, et al. Nonpetrating right atrial and pericardial trauma. Ann Thorac Surg 2003;76:923–6, permission from Elsevier [24]

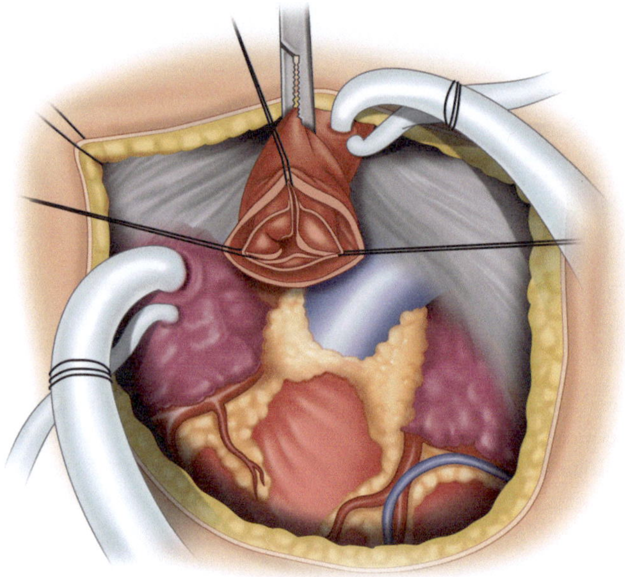

Fig. 21.8 Exposure of the aortic valve and tear in the non-coronary cusp after a motor vehicle accident sustained 10 weeks before

aortic regurgitation and prolapsed of non-coronary cusp into the left ventricle; left cardiac catheterization showed massive aortic insufficiency in diastole, left ventricular dilation, and diffuse hypokinesia.

The patient was immediately transferred to surgery. A median sternotomy was made, and after pericardial incision, the heart was exposed: the left ventricle appeared enlarged, and the ascending aorta was dilated. The patient was then connected to the extracorporeal circulation, the ascending aorta was clamped, and after the infusion of cardioplegic solution, the aortic valve was exposed through a transverse aortic incision. Cardioplegia was also infused into the coronary ostia. A laceration was found in the middle portion of the non-coronary cusp, extending from the edge to the aortic annulus (Fig. 21.8). Because of the absence of other lesions, a valvuloplasty was performed by suturing the defect with interrupted 6-0 polypropylene (Fig. 21.9). The patient's postoperative course was uneventful. After more than 6 years from the operation, he is doing well [31], and TTE has shown reduction of the left ventricular cavity (28 mm in systole and 47 mm in diastole) associated with an almost normal aortic valvular function; minimal aortic incompetence is demonstrated in Fig. 21.10.

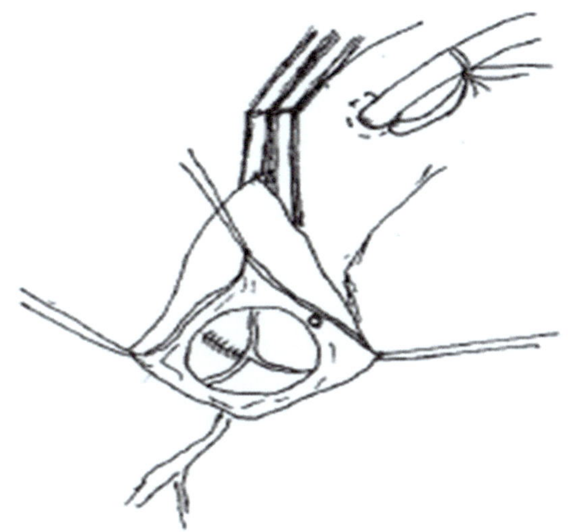

Fig. 21.9 Non-coronary cusp repair using interrupted 6-0 Polypropylene

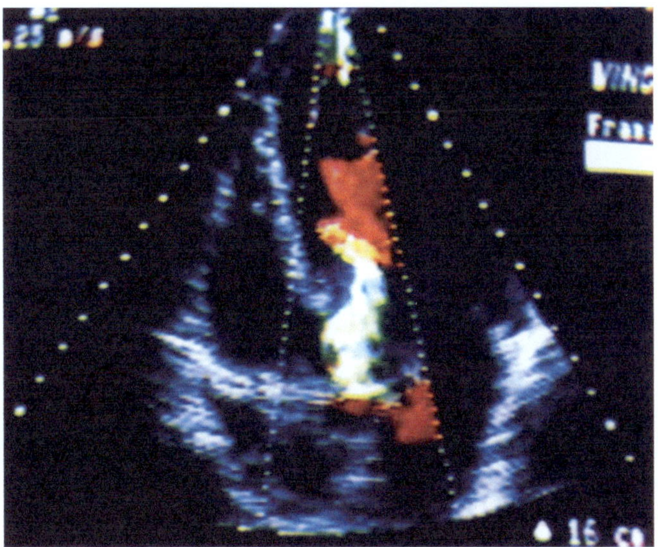

Fig. 21.10 The aortic valve shows minimal incompetence more than 6 years after repair procedure

21.1.8 Mitral Valve Rupture

Mitral valve injury after blunt chest trauma is rare, and in a literature review, since the earliest report in 1964, 82 cases were found [32].Traumatic mitral injury should always be supposed in the presence of acute heart failure in a patient with a history of blunt chest trauma. Patients present sudden pulmonary venous hypertension and frank pulmonary edema and acute respiratory distress syndrome. Often hypotension is erroneously attributed to hypovolemia secondary to other injuries. Anyway, the presence of new systolic murmur should be the clue to the diagnosis in a patient that had been in good health before the trauma. The most common mitral injuries are papillary muscle lesions, from contusion to rupture; the second cause of mitral injury is *chordae tendineae* rupture; the third cause is mitral valve leaflet injury [32]. In unstable patients and in case of refractory congestive heart failure, emergency surgery should be done. In stable patients and in case of important systemic injuries (especially pulmonary), surgery may be delayed until lesions have healed. Furthermore, extracorporeal circulation is necessary for valvular surgery, and the required anticoagulation may cause bleeding from other associated injuries.

21.1.9 Tricuspid Valve Rupture

The pathology is most of the times an anterior leaflet prolapse due to chordal or papillary muscle rupture with annular dilatation [33, 34]. However, the management ranges from medical therapy to surgical intervention in severe regurgitation; conservative surgery using reparative techniques can often successfully correct the defect and should always be attempted because repaired valves do not require anticoagulant therapy and present a lower risk of endocarditis and thromboembolism.

21.2 Thoracic Aorta and Arch Vessel Trauma

Blunt aortic rupture is addressed in Chap. 34 in "Acute Aortic Syndrome."

21.2.1 Traumatic Blunt Injuries of Great Vessels

In a healthy adult, who is between 70 and 80 kg, the estimated average blood volume is 4.7–5.0 L that is about equal to the amount of blood pumped from the heart each minute. Therefore, it is obvious that great vessel injuries (GVI) may

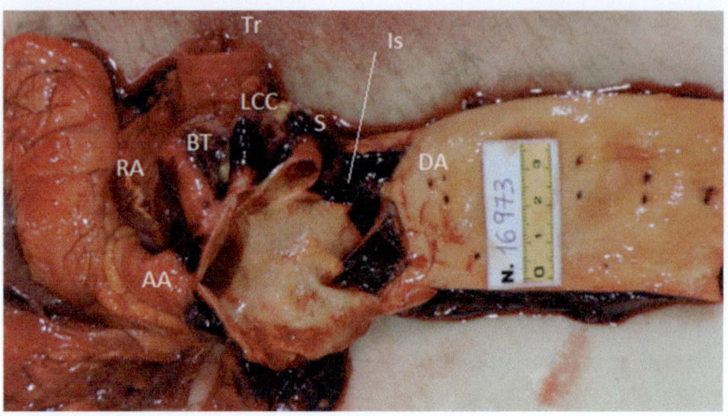

Fig. 21.11 Necropsy examination, aortic rupture in a 53-year-old man who was killed when the car he was driving ran into a stop sign and was struck by another vehicle: death was instantaneous and the man had a circumferential aortic isthmus and right ventricle ruptures. Note the hematoma; *RA* right atrium, *BT* brachiocephalic trunk, *LCC* left common carotid artery, *S* subclavian artery, *AA* ascending aorta, *DA* descending aorta, *Is* isthmus

be rapidly fatal. Blunt traumatic GVI chiefly occur in the aorta and is the second most common cause of trauma-related death in the USA after head injury [35] (Figs. 21.2 and 21.11). Except for traumatic aortic rupture, the incidence of GVI is lower.

The great vessels more frequently involved in blunt trauma are innominate artery and vein, subclavian artery and vein, left common carotid artery, pulmonary arteries and veins, azygous vein, and venae cavae. Innominate artery is the most frequently involved (in about 50% of cases), followed by subclavian and left common carotid arteries [36]. Injuries of the great venous structures and the pulmonary arteries are mainly due to penetrating trauma; anyway, blunt trauma lesions are uncommonly rare, because of their distensibility and low pressure.

21.2.1.1 Pathogenesis

Several theories try to explain GVI pathogenesis, but mainly deceleration and traction are involved. The aorta is held by the *ligamentum arteriosum*, the left main bronchus and the intercostal arteries; therefore, the most fragile aortic site is the isthmus, situated at the junction between the mobile aortic arch and the more fixed descending aorta: blunt aortic injury (BAI) in most cases occurs at the aortic isthmus, just distal to left subclavian artery. Horizontal deceleration determines shearing forces that in turn produce traction tears at isthmus level. Vertical deceleration shifts the heart inferiorly and into the left pleural cavity determining a sudden strain on the ascending aorta and/or the innominate artery [37]. Acute extension of the neck or traction on the shoulder can overstrain the arch arteries causing partial wall tears or complete rupture of the vessel that may produce vessel dissection, thrombosis, pseudoaneurysm, or copious blood loss [37].

Another mechanism of rupture may be a hydrostatic pressure increase inside the aorta due to a "water-hammer effect": after a rapid deceleration, the flow inside the aorta is suddenly stopped determining a high-pressure wave. The reflected wave produces a huge pressure increase that is greatest at the aortic arch [38], because of its curvature, and in the ascending aorta [39].

Furthermore, another modality of injury is the "osseous pinch" theory where the aorta is directly sheared between the bony structure of the anterior and posterior thoracic cage [40, 41].

21.2.1.2 Diagnosis

- Initial survey: Airway-breathing-circulation assessment (ABC) and concomitant treatment of life-threatening lesions. Check arterial saturation, and control external bleeding, expanding hematoma, presence of upper extremity pulse differential or arterial pulse absence, and differential upper extremities' blood pressure. Evidence of thrill or bruit may indicate vascular injury. Brachial plexus injury is often correlated with thoracic vessel lesions, especially the subclavian vein and artery [35].
- Second survey: Chest and pelvic X-ray and use of focused assessment with sonography for trauma (FAST). Evaluate clinical status and hemodynamic stability. Chest X-ray showing mediastinal enlargement strongly suggests an angio-CT. If possible, further imaging studies are requested; otherwise treatment is immediate surgery.
- Lactate and excess base deficit indicate shock and its intensity.

21.2.1.3 Treatment

While there is a continuous increase in the number of traumatic aortic ruptures treated by means of endovascular intervention, this approach is really limited in case of blunt injuries of the aortic arch vessels. With the exception of the subclavian artery, most of the lesions are proximal, where the arteries originate from the aortic arch [42, 43].

The choice of surgical incision must grant an adequate exposure, and in very unstable patients in most cases surgery is diagnostic and curative. There are mainly two surgical approaches to the chest: an anterolateral incision that can be extended through the midline (bilateral thoracotomy or "clamshell") and median sternotomy. Exposure is much better placing a bump under the patient's chest and extending the ipsilateral arm.

Median sternotomy, with clavicular or neck extension of the incision, is the most used approach for the majority of GVI (Fig. 21.12a). After sternotomy, the division of the left innominate vein will improve exposure. The innominate and left common carotid arteries are best approached via median sternotomy with a clavicular extension for handling sudden

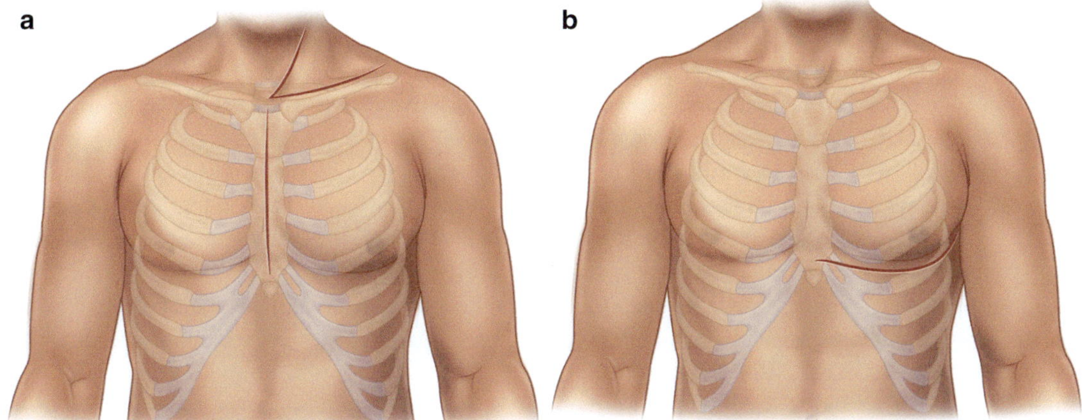

Fig. 21.12 Red lines indicate surgical incision for great vessel repair

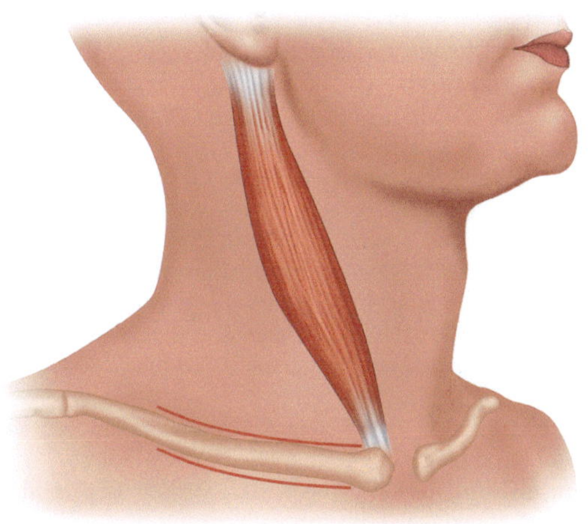

Fig. 21.13 Periclavicular incision: red lines show supra- and infraclavicular approaches

or unexpected situations. The left subclavian artery is approached through a median sternotomy with periclavicular extension of the incision. It is also described a periclavicular incision (Fig. 21.13), and a concomitant anterior thoracotomy in III or IV left intercostal space (Fig. 21.12b). Control of acute bleeding can be initially made using a side-biting vascular clamp until the vessel injured is dissected free.

(a) *Innominate artery.* Repairing innominate artery injuries, after debridement of contused or lacerated vessel, controlling proper orientation of vessels, the surgeon has several options:
   - At first, primary repair using sutures reinforced with pledgets.
   - Patch angioplasty.
   - Graft interposition: end-to-side anastomosis at the ascending aorta site and end-to-end in the distal innominate artery. At this point is possible the complete closure of the proximal portion of the innominate artery (Fig. 21.14). This procedure does not need cardiopulmonary bypass; for complex cases it is useful to monitor stump pressure to determine whether a shunt should be placed.

(b) *Left common carotid artery.* Primary repair is rare; in most cases vessel repair is performed using an interposition tube graft [44].

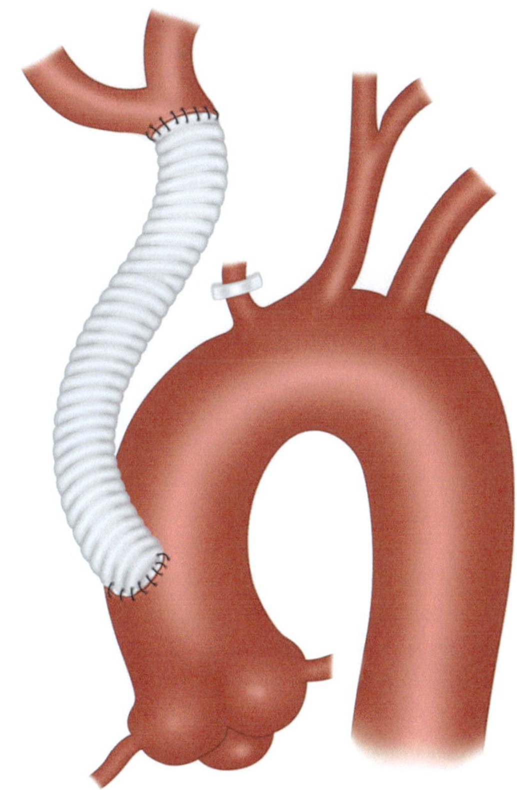

Fig. 21.14 Graft interposition: end-to-side anastomosis at the ascending aorta site and end-to-end in the distal innominate artery; complete closure of the proximal portion of the innominate artery

(c) *Subclavian artery.* Subclavian artery lesion is often associated with brachial plexus lesion and clavicular fracture. Repair is made through median sternotomy and often a periclavicular extension is necessary, supra- or infraclavicular (Fig. 21.13); subclavian artery blunt injuries are more distal and therefore are in most cases repaired by graft interposition. Arterial ligation is rarely necessary but can be lifesaving and the rich collateral flow reduces the risk of upper extremity [44].

At the end of the surgical repair, whichever technique was applied, patency should be confirmed by a palpable distal pulse and, for a better diagnosis, by intraoperative Doppler; the anastomosis should always be tension free.

(d) *Pulmonary artery and veins.* Pulmonary artery and vein lacerations (Fig. 21.2), also called deep pulmonary laceration (DPL), cause death very often before patient arrival in the emergency department [45]. Pulmonary artery injuries are very rare, the commonest site of non-penetrating injury is at the hilum level, and hemothorax is the main finding [46].

Pulmonary vein deceleration injury alone is rare and patients with this lesion can be falsely stable for a short period after trauma. The lesion causes severe bleeding in the pleural cavity from the pulmonary venous circulation at low pressure and impedance. Therefore, a pulmonary vein injury may bleed at a relatively slow rate, and the collapsed lung around the hilum with hemothorax may prevent immediate exsanguination, during chest drain clamping, allowing time for resuscitation, assessment, and surgery [47, 48]. Thoracotomy is the most often surgical approach, although median sternotomy may often offer a better exposure especially in massive bleeding [49]. As for exsanguinating abdominal injuries, the damage control technique can be the only possible approach to control massive bleeding from the pulmonary hilum, and stapled pneumonectomy can be done in a second stage when hemodynamic stability has been obtained. Damage control by packing the chest with laparotomy packs and closure of the chest seems much less effective than the abdominal packing. Quick vascular occlusion of the pulmonary hilum by Crawford or Satinsky clamps can be complex and ineffective due to the rigidity of the main bronchus. Pulmonary hilar twist of 180° can be easier and effective [50]. The twisted lung can be left in place similar to a retained clamp to maintain hemostasis, while the resuscitation maneuvers proceed. Once the lung has been twisted by 180°, the twisted position can be maintained by leaving the laparotomy packs at the apex, the base, and around the hilum.

The advantageous factors of low pulmonary vascular/atrial pressures and intrinsic lung clotting factors are neutralized by an immediate chest tube positioning, especially with suction applied. In case of hemothorax, chest drainage may determine massive exsanguination in a relatively stable patient. Delay in tube drainage for an hour or two while the patient is evaluated and an operating room made available is usually wiser [51]. When blood loss through the inserted chest tube is more than 500 mL in 30 min and >200 mL per hour, immediate surgery is mandatory [48]. Note that after thoracotomy the pulmonary vein lacerated should be straight away occluded in order to prevent air embolism [51].

References

1. RuDusky BM. Classification of myocardial contusion and blunt cardiac trauma. Angiology. 2007;58:610–3.
2. Marcolini EG, Keegan J. Blunt Cardiac Injury. Emerg Med Clin N Am. 2015;33:519–27.
3. Baum VC. The patient with cardiac trauma. J Cardiothorac Vasc Anesth. 2000;14:71–81.
4. Liedtke AJ, DeMuth WE Jr. Nonpenetrating cardiac injuries: a collective review. Am Heart J. 1973;86:687–97.
5. El-Chami MF, Nicholson W, Helmy T. Blunt cardiac trauma. J Emerg Med. 2008;35:127–33.
6. van Wijngaarden M, Karmy-Jones R, Talwar M, Simonetti V. Blunt cardiac injury: a 10 year institutional review. Injury. 1997;28:51–5.
7. Clancy K, Velopulos C, Bilaniuk JW, et al. Screening for blunt cardiac injury: an Eastern Association for the Surgery of trauma practice management guideline. J Trauma Acute Care Surg. 2012;73(5 Suppl 4):S301–6.
8. Ferjani M, Droc G, Dreux S, et al. Circulating cardiac troponin T in myocardial contusion. Chest. 1997;111:427–33.
9. Adams JE 3rd, Davila-Roman VG, Bessey PQ, et al. Improved detection of cardiac contusion with cardiac troponin I. Am Heart J. 1996;131(2):308–12.
10. Bertinchant JP, Polge A, Mohty D, et al. Evaluation of incidence, clinical significance, and prognostic value of circulating cardiac troponin I and T elevation in hemodynamically stable patients with suspected myocardial contusion after blunt chest trauma. J Trauma. 2000;48(5):924–31.
11. Garcia-Fernandez M, Lopez-Perez J, Perez-Castellano N, et al. Role of transesophageal echocardiography in the assessment of patients with blunt chest trauma: correlation of echocardiographic findings with the electrocardiogram and creatine kinase monoclonal antibody measurements. Am Heart J. 1998;135:476–81.
12. Skinner DL, Laing GL, Rodseth RN, Hardcastle TC, Muckart DJJ. Blunt cardiac injury in critically ill trauma patients: a single Centre experience. Injury. 2015;46:66–70.
13. Chirillo F, Totis O, Cavarzerani A, Bruni A, et al. Usefulness of transthoracic and transesophageal echocardiography in recognition and management of cardiovascular injuries after blunt chest trauma. Heart. 1996;75:301–6.
14. Dumesnil JG, Lentini S, Desanluier D. Vanishing posttraumatic left ventricular outflow tract thrombi. Ann Thorac Surg. 1994; 58:276.
15. Sybrandy KC, Cramer MJM, Burgersdijk C. Diagnosing cardiac contusion: old wisdom and new insights. Heart. 2003;89:485–9.
16. Salim A, Velmahos GC, Jindal A, Chan L, Vassiliu P, Belzberg H, et al. Clinically significant blunt cardiac trauma: role of serum troponin levels combined with electrocardiographic findings. J Trauma. 2001;50:237–43.

17. Karalis DG, Victor MF, Davis GA, McAllister MP, Covalesky VA, Ross JJ Jr, Foley RV, Kerstein MD, Chandrasekaran K. The role of echocardiography in blunt chest trauma: a transthoracic and transesophageal echocardiographic study. J Trauma. 1994;36:53–8.
18. Nagy KK, Krosner SM, Roberts RR, Joseph KT, Smith RF, Barrett J. Determining which patients require evaluation for blunt cardiac injury following blunt chest trauma. World J Surg. 2001;25: 108–11.
19. Maron BJ, Estes NA 3rd. Commotio cordis. N Engl J Med. 2010;362:917–27.
20. Maron BJ, Doerer JJ, Haas TS, Tiemey DM, Mueller FO. Sudden deaths in young competitive athletes: analysis of 1866 deaths in the United States, 1980-2006. Circulation. 2009;119:1085–92.
21. Link MS, Maron BJ, Wang PJ, VanderBrink BA, Zhu W, Estes NA 3rd. Upper and lower limits of vulnerability to sudden arrhythmic death with chest-wall impact (commotion cordis). Am J CollCardiol. 2003;41:99–104.
22. Aris A, Delgado LJ, Montiel J, Subirana MT. Multiple intracardiac lesions after blunt chest trauma. Ann Thorac Surg. 2000;70: 1692–4.
23. Leavitt BJ, Meyer JA, Morton JR, Clark DE, Herbert WE, Hiebert CA. Survival following nonpenetrating traumatic rupture of cardiac chambers. Ann Thorac Surg. 1987;44:532–5.
24. Grande AM, Rinaldi M, Pasquino S, Dore R, Viganò M. Nonpenetrating right atrial and pericardial trauma. Ann Thorac Surg. 2003;76:923–6.
25. Hamaji M, Kano S, Ishigami M, Mikuriya A, Kitano M, Matsuda M. Two cases of right atrial rupture due to blunt chest injury in teenaged drivers after motor vehicle accidents. Jpn J Cardiovasc Surg. 2006;35:295–8. https://doi.org/10.4326/jjcvs.35.144.
26. Oizumi H, Suzuki K, Hoshino H, Tatsumori T. A case report: hemothorax caused by rupture of the left atrial appendage. Surg Case Rep. 2016;2:142.
27. Restrepo CS, Gutierrez FR, Marmor-Vélez JA, Ocazionez D, Martinez-Jimenez S. Imaging patients with cardiac trauma. Radiographics. 2012;32:633–49.
28. Chughtai T, Chiavaras MM, Sharkey P, Shulman H, Miller HA. Pericardial rupture with cardiac herniation. Can J Surg. 2008;51:E1001–E102.
29. Grande AM, Rinaldi M, Alloni A, Viganò M. Traumatic tricuspid valve rupture treated by minimally invasive thoracotomy. Ital Heart J. 2003;4:888–90.
30. Grande AM, Vigna V, Bex JP. Valvular injuries resulting from blunt chest trauma. Tex Heart Inst J. 1985;12:261–4.
31. Bex JP, Grande A, Deveze JL. Traumatic aortic insufficiency. Ann Thorac Surg. 1991;51:694–5.
32. Pasquier M, Sierro C, Yersin B, Delay D, Carron P-N. Traumatic mitral valve injury after blunt chest trauma: a case report and review of the literature. J Trauma. 2010;68:243–6.
33. Maisano F, Lorusso R, Sandrelli L, Torracca L, Coletti G, La Canna G, Alfieri O. Valve repair for traumatic tricuspid regurgitation. Eur J Cardiothorac Surg. 1996;10:867–73.
34. Smith RS, Chang FC. Traumatic rupture of the aorta: still a lethal injury. Am J Surg. 1986;152:660–3.
35. Rosenberg JM, Bredenberg CE, Marvasti MA, Bucknam C, Conti C, Parker FB Jr. Blunt injuries to the aortic arch vessels. Ann Thorac Surg. 1989;48:508–13.
36. Pretre R, Chilcott M. Blunt trauma to the heart and great vessels. N Engl J Med. 1997;336:626–32.
37. Ray G, Liu YK, Davids N. Wall stress in curved aorta in blunt chest trauma. In: Proceedings of the 28th annual conference on engineering in medicine and biology. Alliance for Engineering in Medicine and Biology, Chevy Chase, MD; 1975.
38. Symbas P. Fundamentals of clinical cardiology: great vessel injury. Am Heart J. 1977;93:518–22.
39. Crass J, Cohen A, Motta A, Tomashefski JF, Wiesen EJ. A proposed new mechanism of traumatic aortic rupture: the osseous pinch. Radiology. 1990;176:645–9.
40. Richens D, Field M, Neale M, Oakley C. The mechanism of injury in blunt traumatic rupture of the aorta. Eur J Cardiothorac Surg. 2002;73:951–3.
41. Shaw AD, Milne AA, Christie J, Jenkins AM, Murie JA, Ruckley CV. Vascular trauma of the upper limb and associated nerve injuries. Injury. 1995;26:515–8.
42. Symbas JD, Halkos ME, Symbas PN. Rupture of the innominate artery from blunt trauma: current options for management. J Card Surg. 2005;20:455–9.
43. O'Connor JV, Byrne C, Scalea TM, Griffith BP, Neschis DG. Vascular injuries after blunt chest trauma: diagnosis and management. Scand J Trauma Resusc Emerg Med. 2009;17:42. https://doi.org/10.1186/1757-7241-17-42.
44. Nishiumi N, Maitani F, Tsurumi T, Kaga K, Iwasaki M, Inoue H. Blunt chest trauma with deep pulmonary laceration. Ann Thorac Surg. 2001;71:314–8.
45. Ambrose G, Barrett LO, Angus GLD, Absi T, Shaftan GW. Main pulmonary artery laceration after blunt trauma: accurate preoperative diagnosis. Ann Thorac Surg. 2000;70:955–7.
46. Varghese D, Patel H, Cameron EW, Robson M. Repair of pulmonary vein rupture after deceleration injury. Ann Thorac Surg. 2000;70:656–8.
47. Nwaejike N, Mosca R, Hooper TL, Soon SY. Surgical repair of pulmonary vein injury from blunt trauma. Ann R Coll Surg Engl. 2015;97(3):e34–6. https://doi.org/10.1308/003588414X14055925059714.
48. Ouda A, Kappert U, Ghazy T, Weise M, Ebner B, Tugtekin S-M, Matschke K. Isolated rupture of the right upper pulmonary vein: a blunt cardiac trauma case. Ann Thorac Surg. 2011;91:1267–9.
49. Pate JW. Invited commentary. Ann Thorac Surg. 2000;70:658.
50. Wilson A, Wall MJ Jr, Maxson R, Mattox K. The pulmonary hilum twist as a thoracic damage control procedure. Am J Surg. 2003;186:49–52.
51. Yee ES, Verrier ED, Thomas AN. Management of air embolism in blunt and penetrating lung trauma. J Thorac Cardiovasc Surg. 1983;85:661–8.

Penetrating Cardiac Injury

22

Antonino M. Grande and Alessandro Mazzola

Key Points

- Do not assume a straight line of missile's trajectory: surface injuries often do not correspond to missile trajectory.
- Do not assume "entry" vs. "exit" wounds.
- Do not rely on "probing" a wound missing the real trajectory and internal injuries.
- Do not rely on initial patient's hemodynamic stability.
- Consider that the diaphragm is a moving target and an injury that on first glance may look abdominal is actually thoracic.
- Think outside the "cardiac box."
- In case of impalement injuries, do not remove an impaled object from the wound but rather try to stabilize it.
- e-FAST should be done on all patient with suspected chest penetrating trauma: because bleeding is a dynamic status, e-FAST should be done every 15 min in the first hours until patient stabilization.
- In thoracic stab wound, if a cardiac injury is excluded, because the weapon can be aimed at any direction (Fig. 22.2), the knife wound may enter the diaphragm with the possibility of intraabdominal lesions.
- Protect always yourself and your staff against exposure to blood-borne pathogens during the emergency surgery.

A. M. Grande (✉)
Department of Cardiac Surgery, IRCCS Fondazione Policlinico San Matteo, Pavia, Italy
e-mail: amgrande@libero.it

A. Mazzola
Cardiac Surgery, IRCCS Multimedica Sesto S. Giovanni, Milano, Italy

22.1 Introduction

Penetrating cardiac injuries (PCIs) are exceedingly devastating lesions that represent a major surgical challenge because of a mortality rate ranging from 40 to 90% [1–11]. In PCI the right ventricle presents the injury site entry more often than the left ventricle because it is positioned anteriorly in the chest and makes up the largest part of the anterior surface [12].

Major and life-threatening chest injuries can be memorized as the "Deadly Dozen." The first six are lethal and require immediate evaluation and treatment during primary survey: airway obstruction, tension pneumothorax, cardiac tamponade, open pneumothorax, massive hemothorax, and flail chest. The second six are "hidden": thoracic aortic disruption, tracheobronchial disruption, myocardial contusion, traumatic diaphragmatic tear, esophageal disruption, and pulmonary contusion; the "hidden six" are potentially life-threatening injuries and should be diagnosed at a later survey [13, 14].

External wounds are necessarily examined and used as markers for internal injuries. The *cardiac box* is the area where all the penetrating trauma may determine an injury to the heart structures and the great vessels. The cardiac box is the area delimited superiorly by the sternal notch, laterally by the nipples, and inferiorly by the transpyloric line (a transverse line halfway between the xiphoid process and the umbilicus) (Fig. 22.1). Considering that the diaphragm is a moving target, an injury that on first glance may look abdominal is actually intrathoracic. In Table 22.1 the anatomical relationships with the "cardiac box" are shown.

Furthermore, thoracic injuries should be organized according to the site of the wounds or trajectory of the knife or missile [13]: (a) base of the neck into mediastinum or pleural cavity, (b) one pleural cavity into the mediastinum or spinal cord, (c) parasternal wound, and (d) two lateral chest wounds involving both pleural cavities and mediastinum (usually caused by gunshot wounds) (Fig. 22.2).

P. Aseni et al. (eds.), *Operative Techniques and Recent Advances in Acute Care and Emergency Surgery*,
https://doi.org/10.1007/978-3-319-95114-0_22

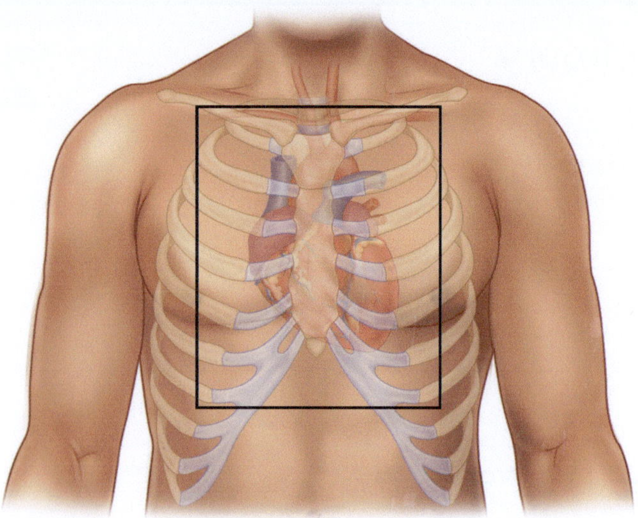

Fig. 22.1 The "cardiac box": the area is delimited superiorly by the sternal notch, laterally by the nipples, and inferiorly by a transverse line halfway between the xiphoid process and the umbilicus

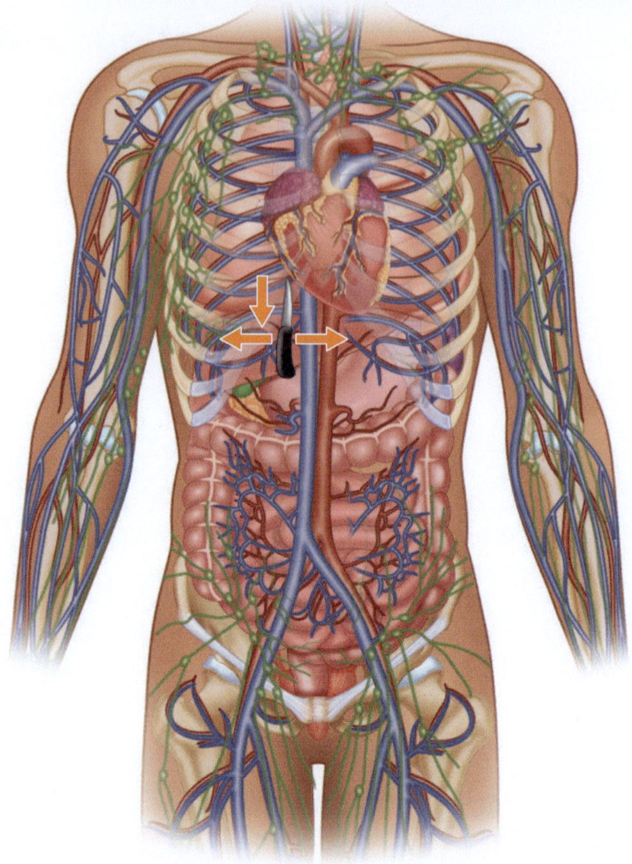

Fig. 22.2 Thoracic stab wound: in the picture the knife is headed superiorly but the blade can be aimed in any direction as shown by the arrows and an abdominal injury is possible

Table 22.1 Anatomical relationships with the "cardiac box"

Right hemithorax	*Left hemithorax*
Lung	Lung
Superior vena cava	Aorta
Azygos vein	Hemiazygos vein
Pulmonary arteries/veins	Pulmonary arteries/veins
Anterior mediastinum	*Posterior mediastinum*
Trachea	Aorta
Great vessels	Esophagus
Heart	Vertebral column
Anterior abdomen	*Back and flanks*
Stomach	Colon
Small bowel/transverse colon	Kidneys
Liver/porta hepatis	Ureters
Spleen	Pancreas
Mesentery	Aorta
Inferior vena cava	
Vertebral column	

22.2 Clinical Presentation

Penetrating cardiac wounds may show a large spectrum of signs and symptoms depending upon the severity of injuries and ranging from being asymptomatic to nonspecific mild or severe chest pain, shortness of breath, and cyanosis, hemoptysis, life-threatening arrhythmias, and hemodynamic instability secondary to cardiac tamponade and cardiac chambers' rupture [15]. One of the most recurrent signs in cardiac tamponade is jugular vein distension for increased venous pressure and the inability of the right ventricle to fill; anyway, cardiac tamponade may be misdiagnosed due to tachycardia, hypotension, and cold extremities for extreme vasoconstriction [15]. Furthermore, jugular distension may be absent for the deep hypotension rapid volume depletion for the copious hemorrhage. Other clinical signs of cardiac tamponade include: (a) *pulsus paradoxus*, a decrease ≥10 mmHg in systolic blood pressure during inspiration (due to a reduction in cardiac output for the increased negative intrathoracic pressure during inspiration), and (b) Kussmaul's sign, a rise in venous pressure during inspiration.

22.3 Diagnosis

In Fig. 22.3 it is shown an algorithm where *e-FAST* (extended focused assessment with sonography for trauma) is utilized for penetrating trauma to the torso when CT scan is not available or patient's conditions do not allow. FAST represents the preferred initial examination, because of its simplicity, rapidity, and accuracy: sensitivity of FAST for pericardial fluid finding is high with a reported sensitivity of 97–100% [16]. FAST is done at the scene of an accident and

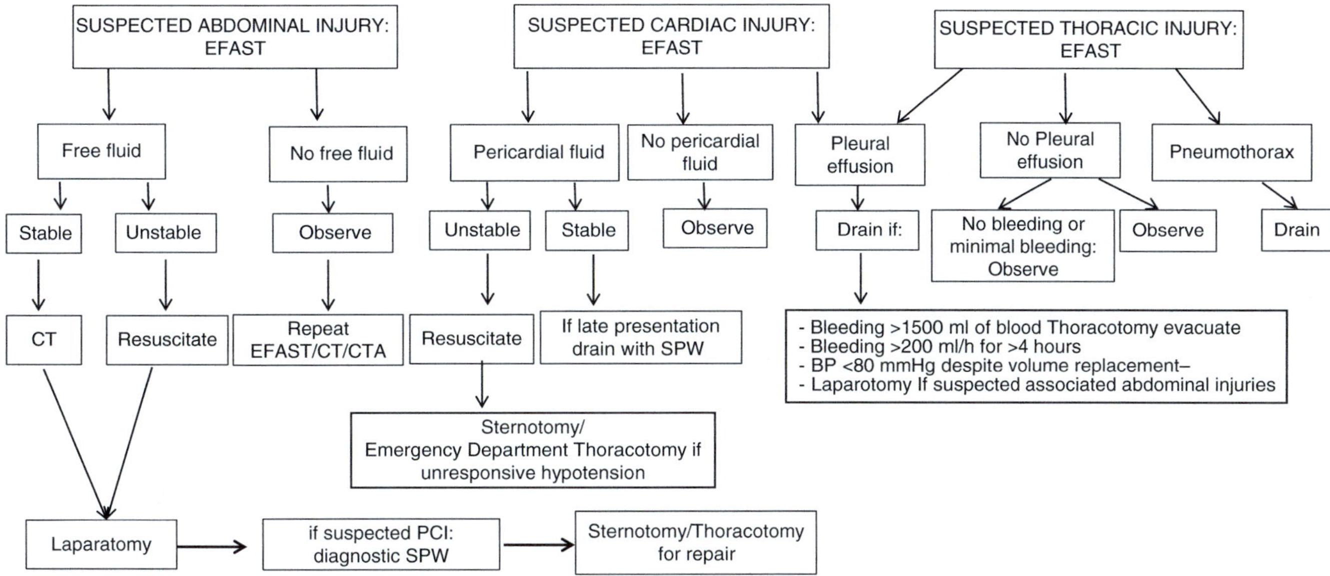

Fig. 22.3 Clinical-based e-FAST algorithm in penetrating trauma. SPW, Subxyphoid Pericardial Window; CT, Computed Tomography; CTA, Computed Tomography Angiography; PCI, Penetrating Cardiac Injury; E-FAST, Extended Focused Assessment with Sonography in Trauma. Reproduced from [20]

can be performed by both paramedics and physicians who were not familiar with the technique before attending a specific course. A negative exam does not exclude injuries, and the test should be repeated. Bowel gas may be a limitation, fluid in the bowel or stomach may be diagnosed for hemoperitoneum, and small amounts of fluid in pleural cavities may be missed (may be useful to take an upright scan). Since the intrathoracic and intra-abdominal bleeding is a dynamic status, FAST should be repeated every 15 min to monitor the patient, both before the patient's admittance and after in the emergency department (Fig. 22.4).

Chest X-ray it is important to check pneumothorax, hemothorax, cardiac enlargement, and bone fractures; furthermore, the exam can visualize bullets and ballistic fragments, providing information on their trajectories and organ involvement.

Computed tomography (CT) if available and/or hemodynamic conditions allow the exam, CT is the most important and useful diagnostic tool for studying patients with suspected cardiac and great vessel injuries.

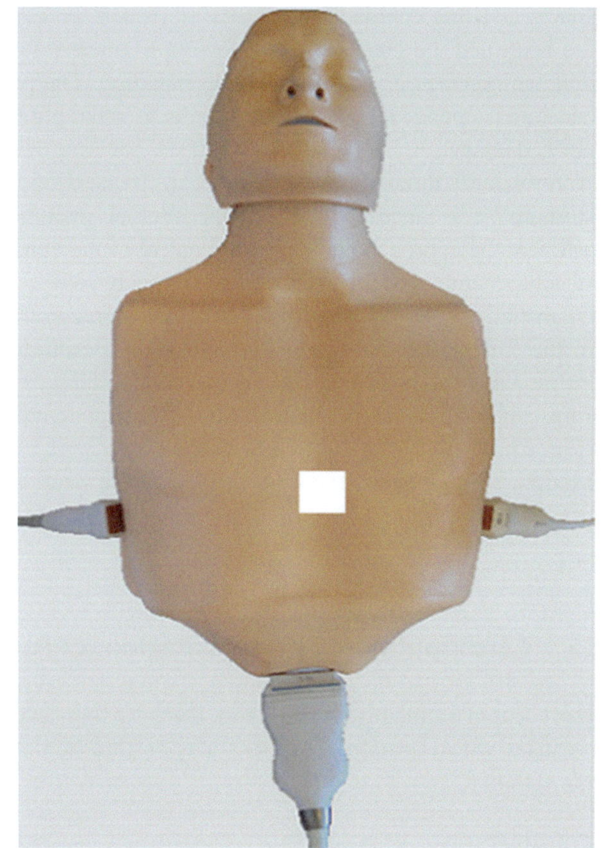

Fig. 22.4 e-FAST exam: Transducer positions for the abdominal and chest views; the white square represents the subxiphoid position of the transducer

22.4 Surgical Exposure

In the management of PCI, the first issue is the surgical approach choice.

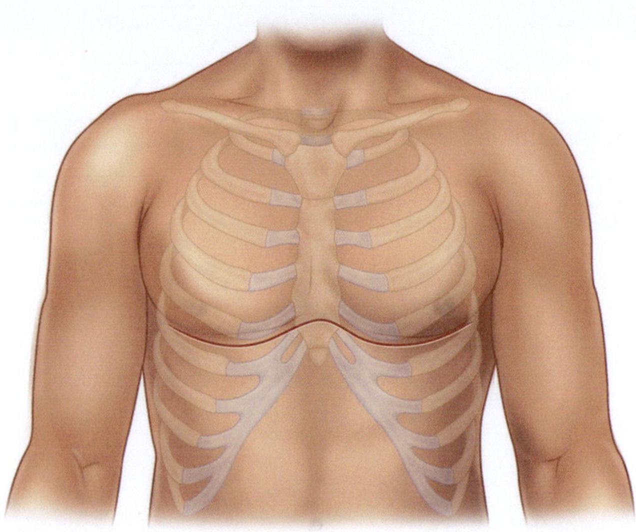

Fig. 22.5 Clamshell incision: bilateral thoracotomy and sternotomy in the fifth intercostal space; at sternotomy both internal thoracic arteries should be ligated

- Left anterolateral thoracotomy: it is the preferred incision in unstable patients and in case of cardiopulmonary arrest. The skin incision is performed in the fifth intercostal space, and this approach represents the fastest access to the heart and the great vessels, allowing to release a cardiac tamponade or to control copious bleeding. The pericardium is opened longitudinally in order to avoid phrenic nerve damage.
- Anterolateral thoracotomy extended by transecting the sternum: it is necessary to control internal mammary arteries; the approach allows better control of the cardiac structures and to establish cardiopulmonary bypass.
- Clamshell incision: bilateral anterolateral thoracotomies in the fifth intercostal space and transverse sternotomy. Pulmonary and hilar injuries are controlled. This exposure allows bleeding control in all chest cavities (Fig. 22.5).
- Median sternotomy is the best access for the heart and great vessels, particularly in stable patients.

22.5 Cardiopulmonary Resuscitation (CPR)

Observe that in traumatic cardiac arrest, there are four reversible causes whose prompt treatment may restore hemodynamic stability:

(a) Hypoxia.
(b) Hypovolemia.
(c) Cardiac tamponade.
(d) Tension pneumothorax.

- Left anterolateral thoracotomy in the fifth intercostal space. Open the pericardium longitudinally, avoid phrenic nerve damage, and start CPR using the two-handed technique that produces a better cardiac output and tissue perfusion. In case of uncontrollable hemorrhage, the cardiac chambers result empty and CPR ineffective. In this case, connect the patient to cardiopulmonary bypass (CPB).
- In case of marked hypotension and shock, the aorta is cross-clamped at the thoracic level: the rationale for clamping the aorta is to redistribute blood flow to the coronary vessels, lungs, and brain. Clamp time should ideally be 30 min or less. Cross-clamping is done ideally at the level of the diaphragm, to maximize spinal cord perfusion.
- Thoracotomy in uncontrollable abdominal bleeding: in case of massive hemorrhage in the lower torso, the descending thoracic aorta can be clamped by means of emergency thoracotomy.

22.6 Cardiac Repair

Damage control concept: permissive hypotension is now targeted, while aggressive resuscitation with high doses of inotropic drugs to restore normal blood pressure is ill-advised and is associated with increased bleeding and death. It is necessary to establish early empiric blood component therapy, caring for prevention and treatment of hypothermia and acidosis.

22.6.1 Silent Cardiac Wound

Keep in mind that any cardiac injury must be steadily studied and eventually surgically treated. This holds particularly true for patients that had a stab wound to the anterior chest, with initial little bleeding that later stops; these patients may show at arrival either normal physical exam or instrumental tests. Late cardiac tamponade for rebleeding and/or constrictive pericarditis has been described [17, 18]. Therefore, conservative management should be considered only after an adequate period of observation when all instrumental revaluations result negative. Utilize CPB in case of multi-chamber injuries in order to obtain a bloodless field and to facilitate repair. However, the heparin administered for extracorporeal circulation may be dangerous in these patients, and hemostasis time is consequently prolonged.

22.6.2 Atrial Injuries

In our experience, atrial bleeding can be controlled applying a Satinsky clamp and lesions repaired using 3.0 or 4.0 polypropylene monofilament suture in a running or interrupted fashion. When the atrial wall is thin, use 5.0 polypropylene, try to avoid positioning a clamp, and make a precise approximation of the wound edges, which helps minimize and redistribute tension across the wound preventing tears that may enlarge the original injury.

It is preferable to avoid the use of bioprosthetic material; if necessary employ patient's pericardial tissue.

22.6.3 Ventricular Injuries

Ventricular injuries can be controlled initially with direct finger pressure; the injuries can be repaired by digitally occluding the lesion while positioning either simple or horizontal mattress nonabsorbable sutures in polypropylene monofilament, 2.0–3.0 reinforced by Teflon strips [19] (Figs. 22.6 and 22.7). Apply the suture inserting the needle 3–4 mm from the wound edge; obtain an adequate tissue bite passing around the finger that is occluding the lesion. The needle should penetrate only through the myocardium avoiding the endocardium. Valvular and septal injuries are less often life-threatening, need CPB, and may be repaired in a second time after adequate patient's study.

In case of massive ventricular hemorrhage, a Foley catheter may be placed inside the injury trying to control bleeding (Fig. 22.8). Then, the lesion may be repaired applying stitches around the catheter. If profuse bleeding continues, repair must be accomplished establishing CPB, especially if there is no longer organized cardiac activity and internal cardiac massage is started.

22.6.3.1 Clinical Case N. 1

A 30-year-old man came to the emergency department with two gunshot wounds (GSW): one on the middle left finger and the other on the left nipple edge (N, left nipple). At arrival, he was hemodynamically stable and conscious, and heart and breath sounds were normal. The bullet hit initially the man's finger deflecting both the trajectory and the kinetic energy; then, the projectile penetrated in the heart directed from the apex to the posterior wall of the left ventricle (Figs. 22.6, 22.7, 22.9, 22.10, 22.11, 22.12, and 22.13). Postoperative period was uneventful and the patient was discharged a week later.

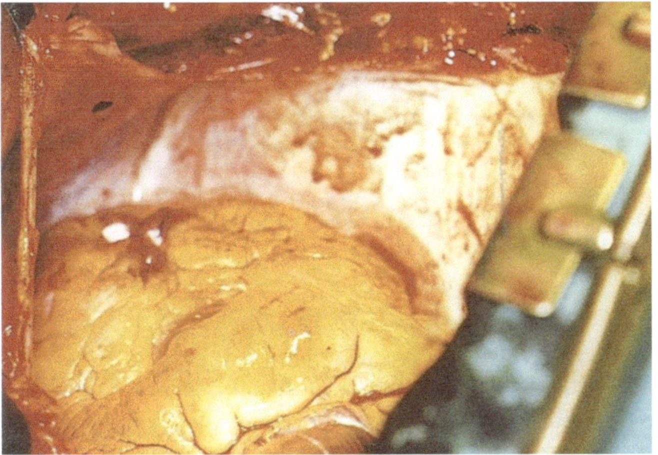

Fig. 22.6 Entrance GSW in the anterior surface of the right ventricle in a 54-year-old man; the GSW was repaired positioning simple stitches in monofilament 3.0 reinforced by Teflon strips

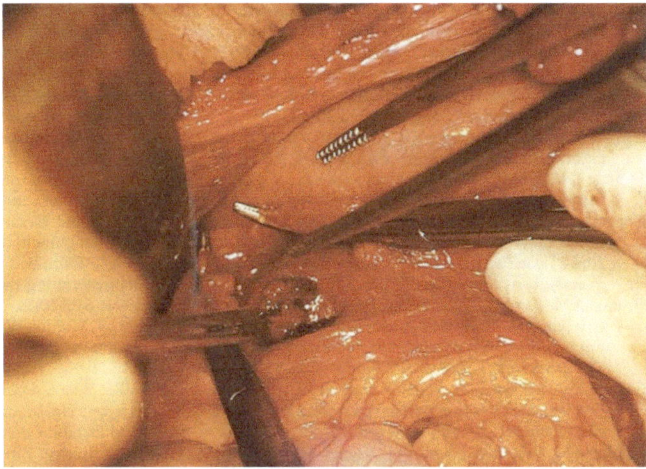

Fig. 22.7 Same patient Fig. 22.6. Exit GSW on the posterior wall of the right ventricle involving the posterior interventricular coronary artery. The patient was operated utilizing cardiopulmonary bypass and postoperative course was uneventful

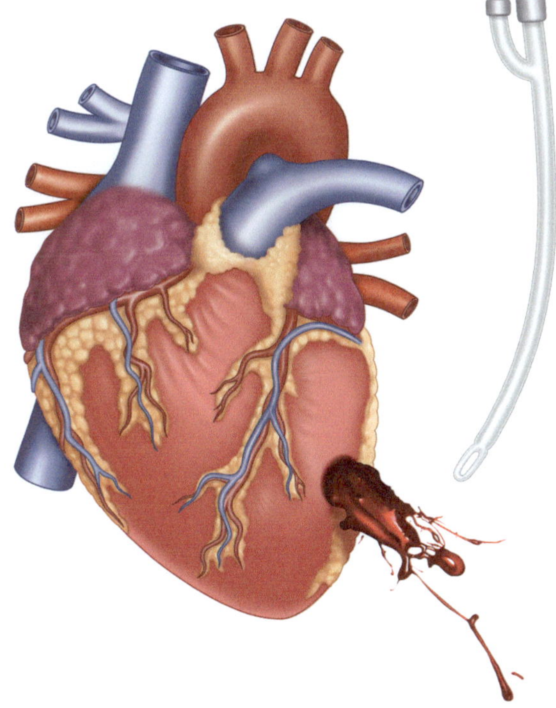

Fig. 22.8 A Foley catheter placed inside a ventricular injury to control bleeding. The lesion is repaired applying stitches around the catheter

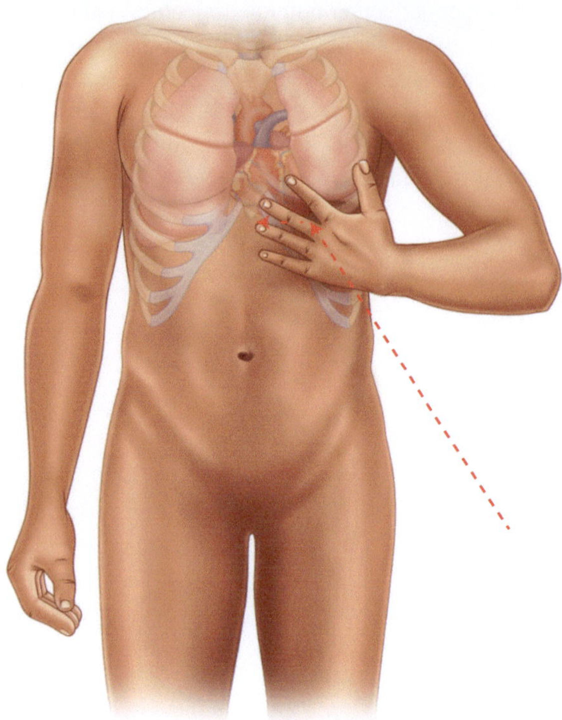

Fig. 22.9 Clinical case n.1 Bullet's trajectory: the left medium finger deflected the missile that, losing its kinetic energy, penetrated the left ventricle apex toward the posterior wall, within the thickness of the myocardium

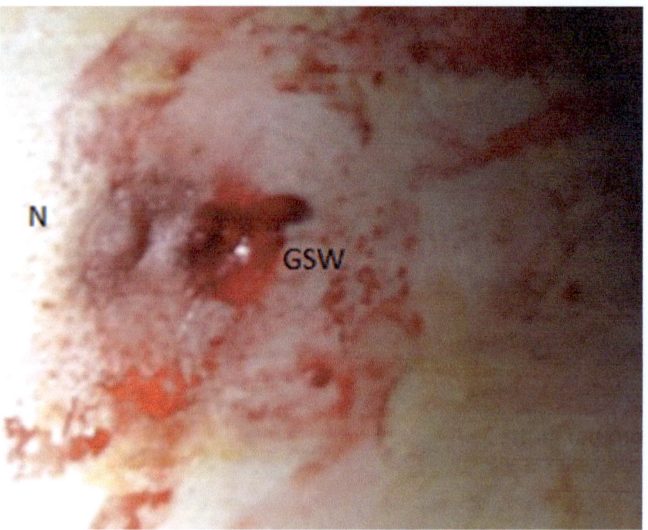

Fig. 22.10 Clinical case n.1. The bullet entry hole near the left nipple. Reproduced with permission from [19]

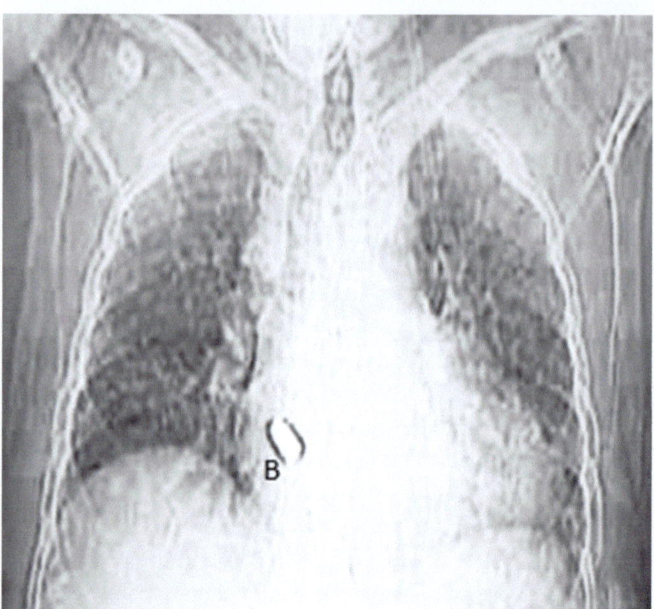

Fig. 22.11 Clinical case n.1. Same case of Fig. 22.9. Chest X-ray: B, bullet. Reproduced with permission from [19]

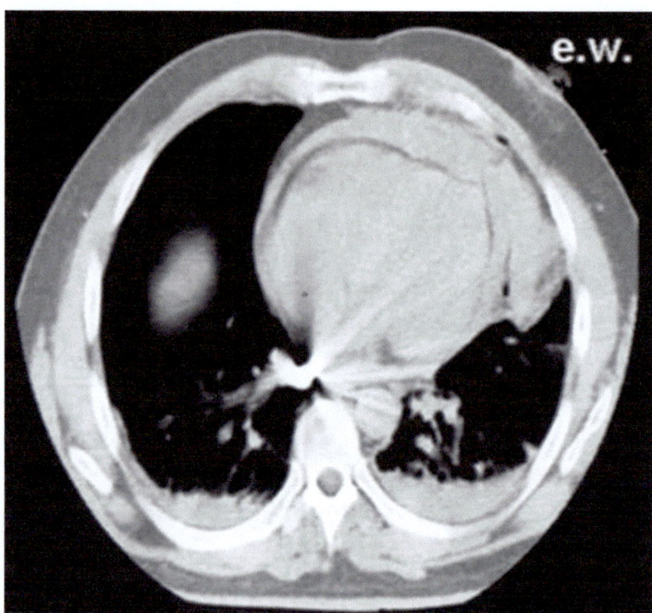

Fig. 22.12 Clinical case n. 1. Computed tomography of the chest visualizes bilateral hemothorax and a huge effusion inside the pericardium. Reproduced with permission from [19]

22.6.3.2 Clinical Case N. 2

A 57-year-old man who attempted suicide: three scissor stab wounds are visible medial to the left nipple. A left anterolateral thoracotomy was performed in the fourth intercostal space. Suture of one right ventricle lesion was obtained with polypropylene 4.0 reinforced by Teflon strip. Other cardiac wounds (CW) are observed on the anterior aspect of the right ventricle and near the course of the left anterior descending coronary artery. The patient recovered uneventfully, and on postoperative day 6, he was transferred to a psychiatric unit (Figs. 22.14, 22.15, and 22.16) [20].

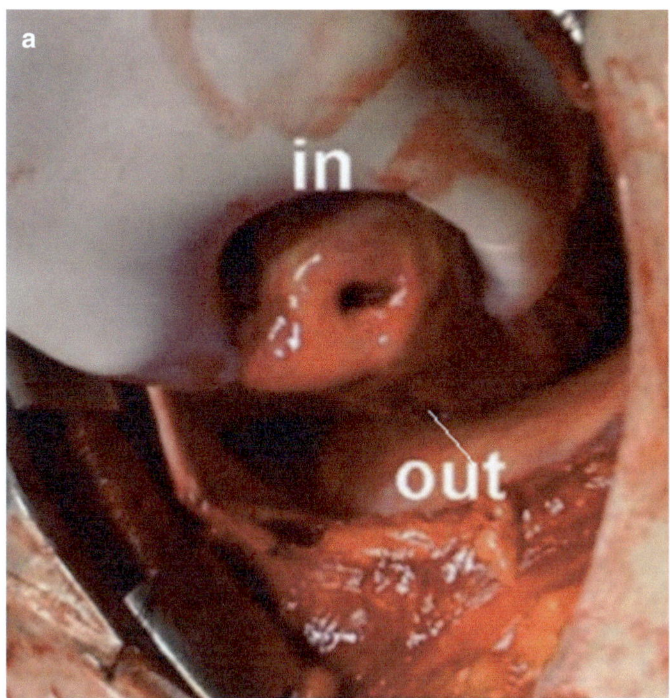

Fig. 22.13 Clinical case n. 1: Intraoperative images: (**a**) in the entry site wound in the left ventricular apex and the exit on the posterior surface, the lesion did not cause ventricular rupture; the bullet was found inside the pericardium; (**b**) the ventricular lesion was repaired with interrupted 3.0 monofilament stitches reinforced by Teflon strips. Reproduced with permission [19]

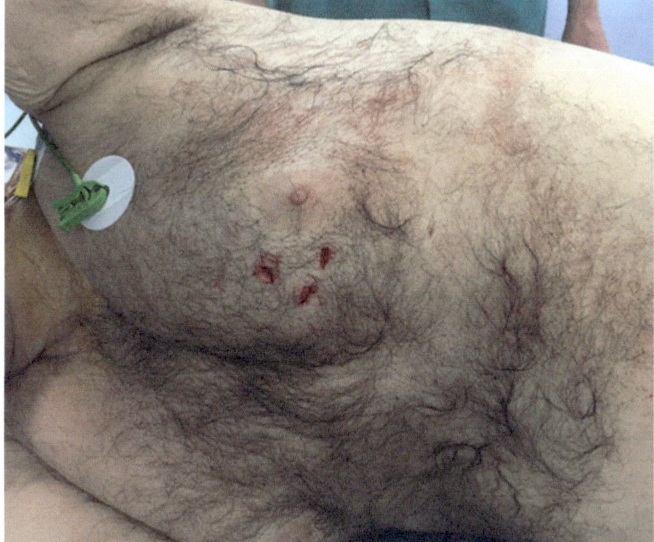

Fig. 22.14 Clinical case n.2. Self-inflicted scissor stab wounds. Reproduced from [20]

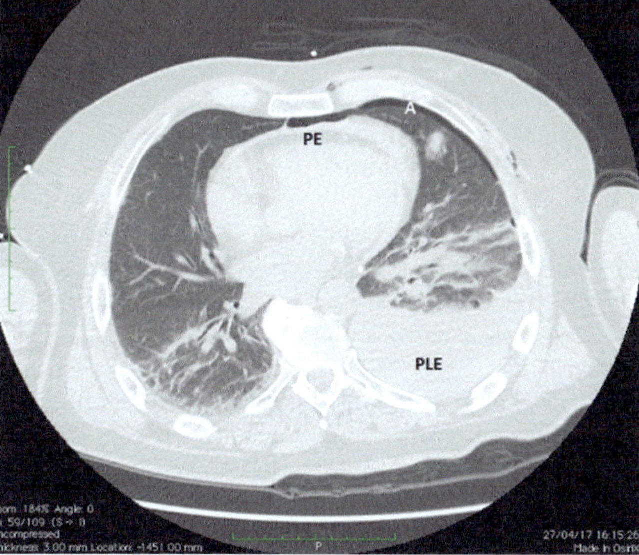

Fig. 22.15 Same case n. 2. Chest CT scan showing pericardial effusion (PE), a huge left pleural effusion (PLE), and air (A) in anterior mediastinum and anteriorly in the left pleural cavity. Reproduced from [20]

22.6.4 Coronary Arteries

Avoid main coronary arteries trying to apply the stitches laterally and deeply to the vessels. On the other hand, small and distal arteries can be ligated. At the end of the procedure, the pericardial cavity should be cleaned with warm saline solution and left open after placing mediastinal and thoracic drains.

22.6.5 Great Vessel Injuries

Injuries to the great vessels, either located in the chest or in the neck, in most cases require a median sternotomy in order to achieve an adequate hemostatic control of the proximal

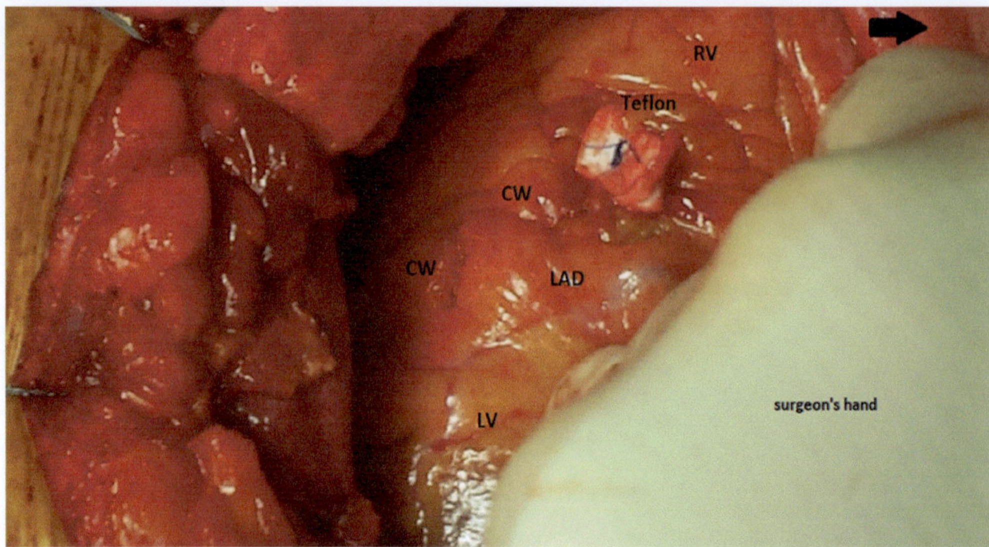

Fig. 22.16 Clinical case n. 2. Intraoperative picture; cardiac wounds (CW); right ventricle (RV); LAD, left anterior descending coronary artery; LV, left ventricle; the black arrow indicates patient's head

vessel involved. Stents and embolic coils are frequently utilized in these cases.

In case of cardiac death, when it is impossible to repair huge cardiac or great vessel injuries, it is important to consider venoarterial extracorporeal membrane oxygenation (ECMO) support for organ preservation; this system is employed to sustain organ perfusion, avoiding high-dose inotropic drugs and ischemic damage until organ retrieval for transplantation is accomplished [21].

22.6.6 Internal Mammary Injury Post-stab Wound

Clinical case n. 3. A 26-year-old man who was admitted in the emergency department after a stab wound, determined by a kitchen knife, in the second left intercostal space. At arrival he appeared eupneic (peripheral O2 saturation was 98%; arterial blood pressure was 120/80 mmHg), but he showed a progressive hemoglobin reduction (Hb 11 g/dL after 12 h); his chest X-ray showed a small pleural effusion in the left costophrenic angle. The patient was transferred to the pneumology department, and 2 days later his chest X-ray showed hemothorax with a Hb value dropped to 9.4 g/dL. A first attempt of thoracentesis resulted unsuccessful; he underwent chest angio-CT that showed massive hemothorax. A second thoracentesis was performed and 1 L of blood was drained. Four days later his chest X-ray was negative, and the patient was discharged and scheduled for a control a week later. Seven days later he complained of dyspnea and fever; his chest X-ray showed a recurrence of hemothorax. A new thoracentesis was performed and 1.2 L of hematic liquid was evacuated, but control X-ray showed the persistence of abundant hemothorax. The patient has undergone a new angio-CT that confirmed left hemothorax (Fig. 22.17) and showed, in second intercostal space, a left internal mammary artery pseudoaneurysm sac, 2 cm in diameter (Fig. 22.18). The pseudoaneurysm was removed through an anterior thoracotomy in the third intercostal space; postoperative course was uneventful, without recurrence. This case confirms that in patients receiving penetrating chest trauma with important hemothorax, surgical exploration is highly recommended [22].

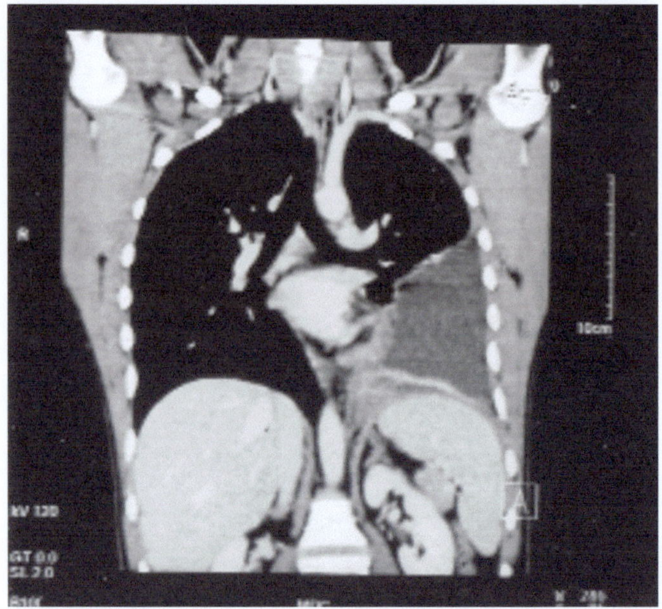

Fig. 22.17 Clinical case n. 3: Angio-CT scan showing important left hemothorax. Reproduced with permission from [22]

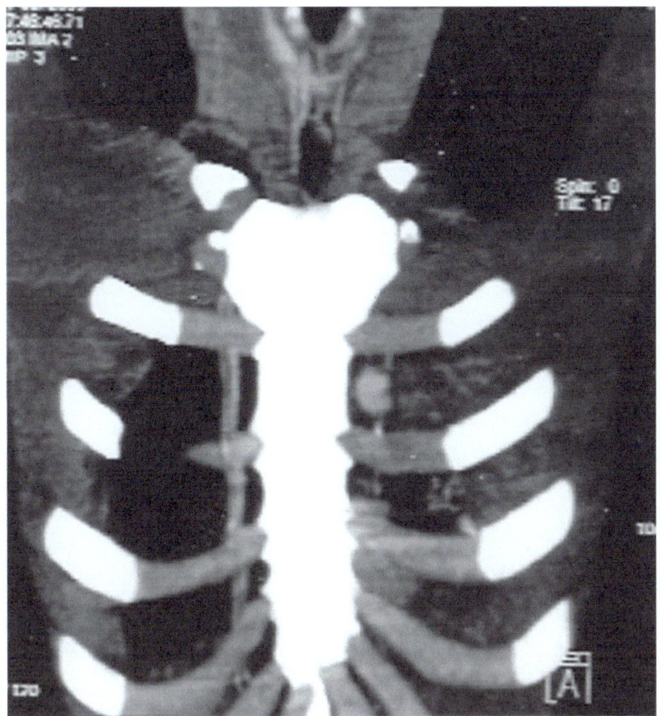

Fig. 22.18 Clinical case n. 3: Angio-CT scan showing a left internal mammary pseudoaneurysm in the second left intercostal space. Reproduced with permission from [22]

22.7 Iatrogenic Trauma to the Heart and Great Vessels

The rapid development and expansion of interventional cardiology have determined a contemporary rise in procedural complications that are frequently described. During diagnostic catheterization one of the most dreaded complications is an injury to a great vessel: carotid and brachiocephalic arteries and, in rare cases, the aortic arch. Endomyocardial biopsy may cause right ventricle perforation and tricuspid valve regurgitation. Pacemaker and defibrillator devices may cause cardiac chamber rupture.

Clinical case n. 4. A 45-year-old woman with dilated cardiomyopathy had an upgrade of a previously implanted pacemaker. A cardiac resynchronization therapy defibrillator (CRT-D) was implanted. Following procedure termination, the lady had a cardiac arrest and died despite resuscitation attempts. At autopsy about 180 cm^3 of blood and clots were found inside the pericardial cavity; ascending aorta showed a deep lesion, 2 mm in length, on the lateral aspect of the vessel, and about 3 cm above the valvular plane. Inspection of medial aspect of the right atrium showed the lead metal extremity implanted in the atrial wall, on average 2 mm thick [21] (Fig. 22.19). The pathogenetic mechanism determining the patient's death can be explained in this way: the active lead (Fig. 22.20), positioned in the medial aspect of the right atrium, perforated the thin atrial wall and damaged the lateral aspect of the aortic wall. The lead perforated the aortic wall, probably remaining inside the wall explaining why the device interrogation revealed normal function with lower pacing threshold (Fig. 22.21). The device was able to control the induced arrhythmias by means of DC shock. At this point, the active lead, positioned inside the aorta like a cork, slipped out causing cardiac tamponade and patient's death [23].

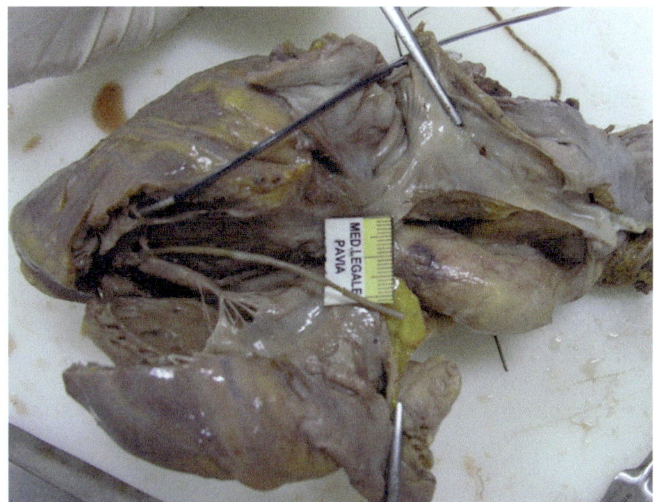

Fig. 22.19 Clinical case n. 4. At autopsy about 180 cm^3 of blood and clots were found inside the pericardial cavity; ascending aorta showed a deep lesion, 2 mm in length

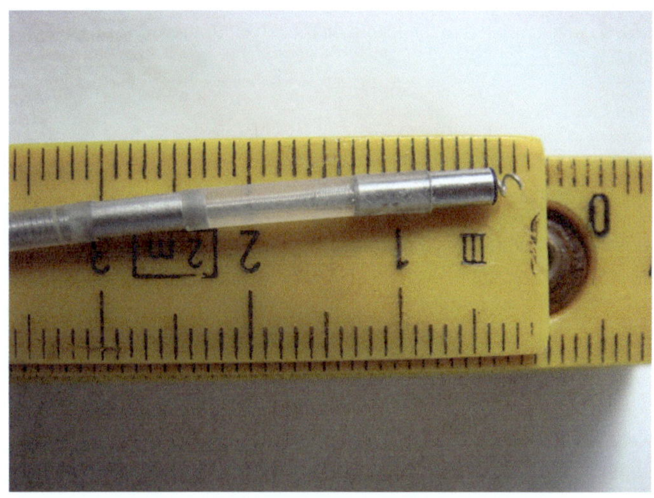

Fig. 22.20 Clinical case n. 4. Active electrode of the lead that pierced the right atrial appendage and determined aortic perforation

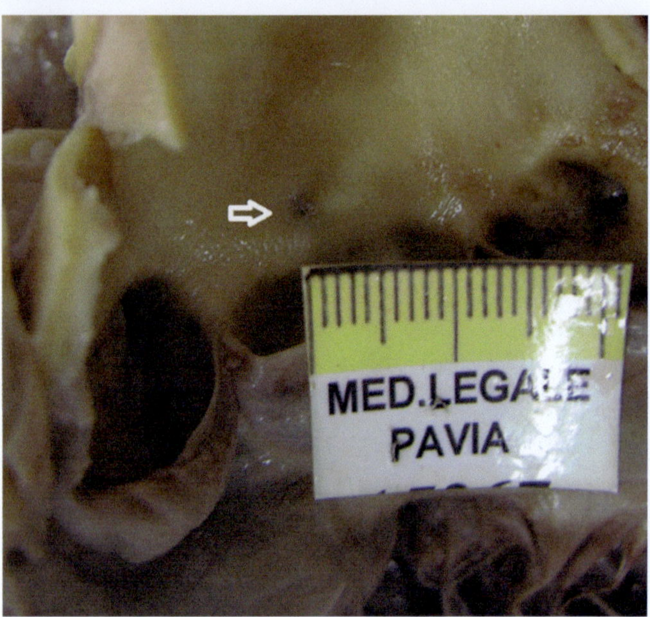

Fig. 22.21 Clinical case n. 4. Inside view of the ascending aorta: a pinpoint injury is noted 2 cm above the non-coronary cusp (white arrow) that is related to the lesion on the adventitial portion of the aorta shown in Fig. 22.19

Case Scenario

A 30-year-old man has been stabbed during a street brawl: he received a stab wound to the anterior chest. On his arrival in the emergency department, he is hemodynamically stable, heart sounds are normal, and breath sounds are equal bilaterally; vital signs are heart rate 120, arterial blood pressure 95/60 mmHg, respiratory rate 20, and oxygen saturation 95% on non-rebreather mask. He received 1 L of normal saline solution administered via an indwelling cannula inserted into a large vein in the antecubital fossa.

At inspection there is a 2 cm entrance wound just left of the midline of the chest in the lower sternal area. Chest X-ray did not show hemothorax or pneumothorax and the patient is conscious.

1. What are you going to do next?
   A. Order red blood cell transfusion.
   B. Perform transesophageal echocardiography.
   C. Require immediate surgery.
   D. Require FAST.

The patient is revaluated after 15 minutes; his arterial pressure is lower than 80 mmHg; he becomes diaphoretic, tachycardic, and tachypneic, showing a decreased level of consciousness; there is no time to perform a computed tomography angiography.

2. What are you going to do at this point?
   A. Require second FAST.
   B. Immediate surgery.
   C. Repeat chest X-ray.
   D. Intubate the patient.

The second FAST is positive showing a cardiac tamponade.

3. What would be the surgical approach?
   A. Pericardial window.
   B. Correct hypovolemia and hypoxia.
   C. Sternotomy.
   D. Left thoracotomy with or without transverse sternotomy (Emergency Department Thoracotomy).

Please see Chap. 58 for the correct answer.

References

1. Campbell NC, Thomson SR, Muckart DJ, Meumann CM, Van Middelkoop I, Botha JB. Review of 1198 cases of penetrating cardiac trauma. Br J Surg. 1997;84:1737–40.
2. Kish G, Kozloff L, Joseph WL, Adkins PC. Indications for early thoracotomy in the management of chest trauma. Ann Thorac Surg. 1976;22:23–8.
3. Demetriades D, van der Veen BW. Penetrating injuries of the heart: experience over two years in South Africa. J Trauma. 1983;23:1034–41.
4. Asensio JA, Soto SN, Forno W, Roldan G, Petrone P, Salim A, et al. Penetrating cardiac injuries: a complex challenge. Injury. 2001;32:533–43.
5. Asensio JA, Berne JD, Demetriades D, Chan L, Murray J, Falabella A, et al. One hundred five penetrating cardiac injuries: a 2-year prospective evaluation. J Trauma. 1998;44:1073–82.
6. Thourani VH, Feliciano DV, Cooper WA, Brady KM, Adams AB, Rozycki GS, et al. Penetrating cardiac trauma at an urban trauma center: a 22-year perspective. Am Surg. 1999;65:811–6.
7. Degiannis E, Loogna P, Doll D, Bonanno F, Bowley DM, Smith MD. Penetrating cardiac injuries: recent experience in South Africa. World J Surg. 2006;30:1258–64.
8. Gao JM, Gao YH, Wei GB, Liu GL, Tian XY, Hu P, et al. Penetrating cardiac wounds: principles for surgical management. World J Surg. 2004;28:1025–9.
9. Asensio JA, Stewart BM, Murray J, Fox AH, Falabella A, Gomez H, et al. Penetrating cardiac injuries. Surg Clin North Am. 1996;76:685–724.
10. Asensio JA, Murray J, Demetriades D, Berne J, Cornwell E, Velmahos G, et al. Penetrating cardiac injuries: a prospective study of variables predicting outcomes. J Am Coll Surg. 1998;186:24–34.
11. Demetriades D, Rabinowitz B, Markides N. Indications for thoracotomy in stab injuries of the chest: a prospective study of 543 patients. Br J Surg. 1986;73:888–90.
12. Restrepo CS, Gutierrez FR, Marmol-Velez JA, Ocazionez J, Martinez-Jimenez S. Imaging patients with cardiac trauma. Radiographics. 2012;32:633–49.
13. Burack JH, Kandil E, Sawas A, et al. Triage and outcome of patients with mediastinal penetrating trauma. Ann Thorac Surg. 2007;83:377–82.

14. Yamamoto L, Schroeder C, Morley D, Beliveau C. Thoracic trauma: the deadly dozen. Crit Care Nurs Q. 2005;28:22–40.
15. Agarwal D, Chandra S. Challenges in the diagnosis of blunt cardiac injuries. Indian J Surg. 2009;71:245–53.
16. Adams A, Fotiadis N, Chin JY, Sapsford W, Brohi K. A pictorial review of traumatic pericardial injuries. Insight Imaging. 2012;3:307–11.
17. Westphal LF, Lima LC, Jaber BA. Traumatic late cardiac tamponade: analysis of five cases. J Pneumol. 2000;26:241–4.
18. da Costa Medeiros BJ. Silent cardiac wound. J Cardiothorac Trauma. 2016;1:19–20.
19. Divisi D, Villani C, Di Tommaso S, Mazzola A. Fortunate finger deviation of a fatal heart bullet injury. Heart Views. 2010;11: 126–7.
20. Grande AM, Antonacci F, Aseni P. Penetrating cardiac wounds: A case report with management algorithm and review of the literature. Emerg Care J 2018; 14:14:63–7. https://doi.org/10.481/ecj.2018.7384.
21. Barrou B, Billault C, Nicolas-Robin. The use of extracorporeal membranous oxygenation in donors after cardiac death. Curr Opin Organ Transplant 2013;18:148–53.
22. Grande AM, Cattadori B, D'Armini AM, Viganò M. Post-traumatic pseudoaneurysm of internal mammary artery: a case report. G Chir 2006;27:377–9.
23. Grande AM, Fiore A. Merlano M, Buzzi F, Mazzola A. Aortic perforation due to cardiac resynchronization therapy defibrillator lead placement: Case report and medicolegal considerations. J Arrhythmia 2015;31:398–400.

Damage Control and Open Abdomen in Abdominal Injury

23

Antonio Tarasconi, Hariscine K. Abongwa, Gennaro Perrone, Giacomo Franzini, Arianna Birindelli, Edoardo Segalini, Federico Coccolini, Roberto Cirocchi, Alberto Casati, Gregorio Tugnoli, Fausto Catena, and Salomone Di Saverio

Key Points

- The term damage control describes a temporized surgical approach aimed to stop the lethal triad (hypothermia, coagulopathy, and acidosis) in patients with reduced physiological reserve.
- Acute care surgeons must be well aware of the pros and cons of OA and must use it wisely, not fearing to leave the abdomen open when is indicated and closing it as soon as possible.
- Physiology drives the strategy: if the patient has conserved physiological reserve, then a definitive treatment could be considered; on the contrary, if the physiological reserve is impaired, a temporized treatment is the best option.
- The role of the Temporary Abdominal Closure method (TAC) is critical, and some of the most dreadful OA complications could derive directly from an improper application of TAC methods.
- Open abdomen complications could be divided in medical and surgical and could be real surgical nightmares with mortality rates up to 40%. Prevention is the key.
- Every effort should be made to close the OA as soon as possible: it is demonstrated that after seven days of OA, the rate of complications increases and the rate of delayed primary fascial closure drops significantly.

23.1 Introduction

Even if it could seem a crazy behavior to someone, leaving the abdomen open after an emergent laparotomy could be beneficial for patient survival in some specific scenarios. The first attempts date back to the late nineteenth century, when Andrew J. McCosh described the use open abdomen (OA) for generalized peritonitis [1]. After that, Pringle described its application in trauma patients [2], and Ogilvie provided the first description of a temporary abdominal closure (TAC) system for OA management [3]. However, these pioneering applications of the OA led to tragic results, due to tremendous infective and hemorrhagic complications. The fathers of the modern OA are probably Stone [4] and Rotondo [5] who, in the last decades of the past century, rediscovered the use of abbreviated laparotomy and set the base for the development of the so-called damage control surgery (DCS). The huge advancements in acute care medicine and antibiotic therapy and the rising comprehension of the pathophysiology of trauma and abdominal compartment syndrome (ACS) made the open abdomen (OA) a cornerstone step of damage control surgery (DCS) [6].

Currently the advantages of OA and DCS in trauma patients are well known, but the exposure of the abdominal viscera to the outer environment brings with itself a great

A. Tarasconi · H. K. Abongwa · G. Perrone · G. Franzini (✉) · F. Catena
Emergency Surgery Department, Maggiore Hospital of Parma, University of Parma, Parma, Italy
e-mail: giacomo.franzini@studenti.unipr.it

A. Birindelli · E. Segalini · A. Casati · G. Tugnoli (✉)
Emergency Surgery and Trauma Surgery Unit, Maggiore Hospital Regional Emergency Surgery and Trauma Center—Bologna Local Health District AUSL Bologna, Bologna, Italy
e-mail: gregorio.tugnoli@ausl.bologna.it

F. Coccolini
Emergency and General Surgery Department, Papa Giovanni XXIII Hospital, Bergamo, Italy

R. Cirocchi
University of Perugia, Perugia, Italy

S. Di Saverio
Department of Surgery, Addenbrooke's Hospital, Cambridge University Hospitals NHS Foundation Trust, Cambridge, UK

P. Aseni et al. (eds.), *Operative Techniques and Recent Advances in Acute Care and Emergency Surgery*,
https://doi.org/10.1007/978-3-319-95114-0_23

burden of dreadful complications, the most feared and devastating being the arise of an enteroatmospheric fistula (EAF) whose mortality can still be as high as up to 40% [7, 8].

Presently accepted indications for OA [9–11] are the following: as part of DCS for trauma; for intra-abdominal hypertension or abdominal compartmental syndrome (ACS) not responsive to medical therapy; in case of acute mesenteric ischemia necessitating a surgical "second look" and when a safe primary abdominal closure results not possible, either because of massive visceral edema and retroperitoneal swelling or because of the loss of abdominal wall (traumatic or after necrotizing fasciitis). The use of AO in infected pancreatic necrosis and abdominal sepsis is still matter of debate, and comparative or randomized studies are lacking.

Acute care surgeons must be well aware of the pros and cons of OA and must use it wisely, not fearing to leave the abdomen open when is indicated and closing it as soon as possible.

23.2 Open Abdomen and Damage Control Surgery in Abdominal Trauma

The term damage control was borrowed from the US Army [12], to describe a temporized surgical approach aimed to stop the lethal triad (hypothermia, coagulopathy, and acidosis) in patients with reduced physiological reserve. In the last decades, the concept of damage control surgery (DCS) has changed the way abdominal injuries are treated, modifying the surgical approach from "early definitive treatment" to "bridge surgical therapy."

23.2.1 Definition and Rationale for Their Use

One of these "bridge surgeries" is the open abdomen (OA) in which the abdominal cavity is left open following an emergency laparotomy and, in order to maintain the abdominal domain and to prevent the exposure of viscera to the external environment, a temporary abdominal closure (TAC) system is set in place. The rationale of the use of OA in trauma patients is that it allows to rapidly terminate the surgical procedure and to promptly admit the patient to the ICU; furthermore, it expedites any further surgical re-exploration and prevents the onset of the abdominal compartment syndrome (ACS).

The DCS approach can thus be divided into four subsequent steps:

- DCS 0: is the immediate care of the traumatized patient, both on the field and later at the arrival to the ER. The ER triage is performed in the shock room and comprehends the usual ABCD assessment, blood tests, chest and pelvic x-rays, extended FAST, and a urine test whenever possible.
- DCS 1: takes place in the OR, and the aim of the surgeon must be the temporary control of life-threatening injuries (i.e., the control of hemorrhages and source of contamination). It ends with an OA after the placement of a TAC.
- DCS 2: at the end of the initial operation, the patient is then transferred to the ICU, and this phase is targeted for the restoration of patient's physiological reserve.
- DCS 3: is the definitive treatment of the injuries and should be performed once physiological restoration is complete; the end points of this phase are the definitive repair of the injuries and the definitive closure of the abdomen.

23.2.2 Physiology Drives the Strategy

Here comes the dilemma: should I temporize and leave the open abdomen or should I aim for a definitive surgery? To answer this question, multiple key points must be kept in mind. First of all, OA brings with itself a great burden of dreadful complications. Some indications of OA use in trauma patients are pretty straightforward and include the treatment of ACS, the need for a "second-look" operation (suspected bowel ischemia, vascular injuries treated with temporary measures such as temporary shunt, etc.), post-injury septic and grossly contaminated abdomen, and impossibility to close the abdomen because of partial or entire loss of the abdominal wall [11]. In every other case is the patient's physiology that drives the strategy: if the patient has conserved physiological reserve, then a definitive treatment could be considered; on the other hand, if the physiological reserve is impaired, a temporized treatment is the best option.

But which are the best indicators of reduced reserve? Recently, Mutschler et al. published the results of a study showing that base deficit (BD) and shock index (SI) could be used to predict the need for massive blood transfusion and poor outcome in trauma patients, thus becoming reliable indicators of the shock status of the patient [13, 14]. They divided the shock in four different categories (no shock, mild, moderate, and severe) on the base of BD and SI. According to their work, indicators of reduced physiological reserve could be considered a BD > 6.0 mmol/L or SI > 1.0 (moderate shock). Furthermore, a core temperature persistently <34 °C, an arterial pH < 7.2 and international normalized ratio or partial thromboplastin time lower than 50% of normal (indicators of coagulopathy), estimated blood loss greater than 4 L, transfusion requirement of more than 10 U of packed red blood cells, and lactate levels greater than 5 mmol/L are good indications for a temporized surgery [11, 15].

Additionally, OA could be beneficial for all those patients in which the onset of ACS is extremely likely. ACS is defined as sustained intra-abdominal pressure (IAP) >20 mmHg (with or without abdominal perfusion pressure < 60 mmHg) that is associated with a new organ dysfunction or failure [16], and an untreated post-injury ACS is an independent predictor of organ failure [17]. It easy to understand how any morbid situation that could lead to a volumetric increase of abdominal content or reduce the abdominal wall compliance is a predictor of ACS. Thus, risk factors for ACS in trauma patients are (1) increased intraluminal contents consequent to bowel posttraumatic dynamic ileus (pseudo-obstruction); (2) increased intra-retroperitoneal content, deriving from hemorrhage from organ or pelvic injury; (3) the presence of surgical packing or emergency surgery with packing procedures; (4) decreased abdominal wall compliance related to high body mass index or due to a third-degree burn of the abdominal wall; and (5) massive visceral swelling shadowing massive fluid/blood resuscitation [9]. IAP should ideally be measured at the end of the damage control operation and the abdomen should be left open if the IAP is greater than 12 mmHg [18]. Whenever one of these conditions is present, the application of OA could help prevent the onset of ACS and improve the final outcome. Furthermore, in case of increased IAP, all the medical procedures aimed to lower it should be applied: NG and rectal tube, negative fluid balance, sedation and neuromuscular blockade, prokinetics, supine position, etcetera. Once the patient is stabilized after DCS 1, other specialties should be on board for the patient management, especially the interventional radiologist that could perform angioembolization of further bleedings or percutaneous drainage of intra-abdominal fluid collections; both these procedures could help reducing the intra-abdominal content, thus lowering the IAP.

23.2.3 Temporary Abdominal Closure

The role of the TAC is critical, and some of the most dreadful OA complications could derive directly from an improper application of TAC methods. An extensive review of all the myriad of TAC described in literature goes beyond the intend of this chapter, but theoretically the ideal TAC should: (1) provide a barrier, protecting the abdominal viscera from outer environment; (2) be totally not traumatic on the abdominal viscera; (3) prevents the formation of adhesions between viscera and abdominal wall; (4) allow collection, quantification, and examination of abdominal fluids; (5) be quick and easy to apply; (6) allow easy access to the abdominal cavity for any further re-explorations; (7) ease nursing management; (8) prevent fascial retraction and be gentle with the fascia for the subsequent primary closure; (9) prevent the ACS; and (10) be cost-effective.

Surgical procedures and skills for OA management have progressed remarkably since the early attempts in the 1980s [19, 20], and currently the use of negative pressure wound therapy (NPWT) seems to be the best option [11, 21], especially in the setting of a septic abdomen, and could be associated with different kinds of fascial traction systems [22–24].

23.3 Open Abdomen Complications

Even if OA is proven to be beneficial in a selected cohort of patient, the exposure of abdominal content to the atmosphere is an unnatural condition that brings itself a great load of complications. OA complication could be synthetically divided in medical and surgical, where medical complications derive from the pathophysiology of a massive open abdominal wound and surgical complications are strictly related to the surgical maneuvers performed.

23.3.1 Medical Complications

Medical complications are (1) dehydration, electrolyte imbalance, and acid-base disturbances and (2) malnutrition and starvation.

23.3.1.1 Dehydration, Electrolyte Imbalance, and Acid-Base Disturbances

Massive fluid loss derives both from direct secretion and from augmented evaporation. At the beginning of the DCS era, the Bogotà bag (Fig. 23.1) and the skin-only closure were the most used TAC [25, 26]; these techniques do not allow the quantification of fluid losses and most of the time are not tight sealing. The application of NPWT is the best way to prevent this complication because it allows a correct quantification of fluid losses and completely isolates the open abdomen, reducing considerably the evaporation across the open wound [27]. This is even more important in the setting of ACS, where fluid overload must be avoided and fluid replacement should be meticulously balanced on the base of patient's fluid balance and an accurate volume status monitoring is mandatory.

23.3.1.2 Malnutrition and Starvation

Patients with OA are continuously in a hypercatabolic state related to the incessant activation of the systemic inflammatory response, promoted by the secretion of pro-inflammatory cytokines in the open abdominal wound. At the same time, the never-ending healing process consumes calories and proteins, and a high amount of nitrogen is lost from peritoneal fluid discharge. This combination explains the high risk of malnourishment and starvation typical of this population of patients. In this scenario, the appliance of a negative pressure TAC, which promotes the egress of peritoneal fluid with all the pro-inflammatory mediators, could help to reduce the

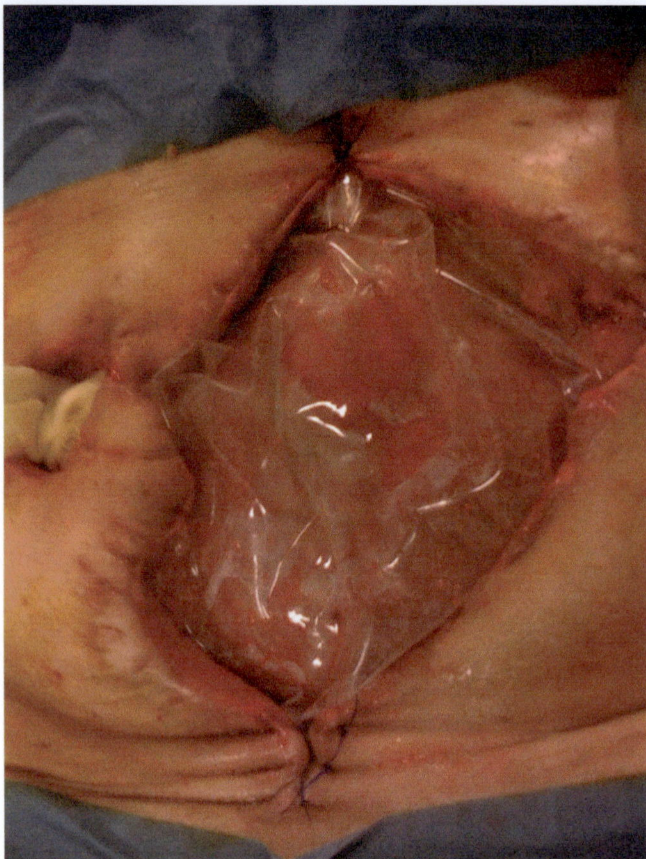

Fig. 23.1 The Bogotá bag is a sterile plastic bag used for closure of abdominal wounds. It is generally a sterilized, 3 L genitourinary irrigation bag that is sewn to the skin or fascia of the anterior abdominal wall. Its use was first described by Oswaldo Borraez while a resident in Bogotá, Colombia

systemic inflammatory response and slow the catabolic process [28]. Thus, the creation of a personalized nutritional plan and a correct initial nutritional assessment are of utmost importance. The establishment of a safe and effective feeding access is a critical step and could be either enteral or parenteral. An effective adequate total parenteral nutrition (TPN) usually necessitates of a central venous access, which could be easier to obtain compared to access for enteral nutrition (EN) that must be tailored to specific patient characteristics and to the presence of any EAF [29, 30]. Nevertheless, whenever feasible, enteral nutrition (EN) should be preferred for prolonged feeding, because its advantages in terms of reduced rate of infectious complications and preservation of the intestinal mucosal barrier are indisputable [27, 29, 31–39]. EN has the added aim of manipulating the stress response to injury and infection [40] and should be started as soon as possible to improve the patients outcome. Usually an addition of 2 g of nitrogen per liter of abdominal fluid lost is necessary to maintain a positive nitrogen balance [39], and supplementation of vitamins and trace elements is mandatory.

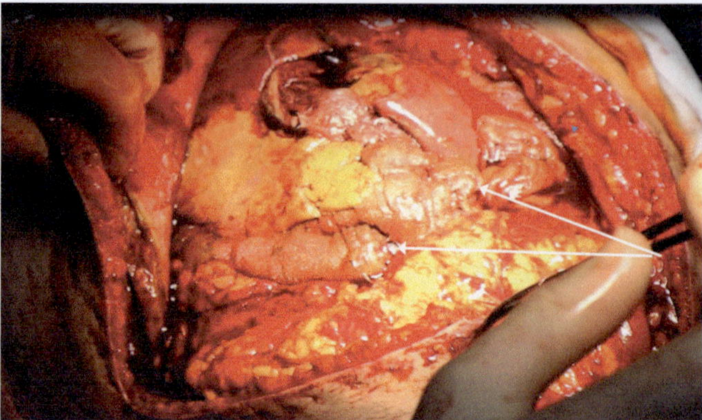

Fig. 23.2 "Enteroatmospheric" fistula represents the most feared complication in the open abdomen: two holes are evident in the mid-ileum without overlying soft tissue (arrows)

23.3.2 Surgical Complications

Surgical complications are (1) bleeding, (2) enteroatmospheric fistula (Fig. 23.2), (3) frozen abdomen (Fig. 23.3), and (4) planned ventral hernia.

23.3.2.1 Bleeding

Theoretically, the establishment of a negative pressure inside of the abdomen could increase the risk of hemorrhage. If active bleeding or coagulopathy are suspected, the optimal amount of negative pressure should be decreased to 75 mmHg or lower, for the first 48 h [11, 41].

23.3.2.2 Enteroatmospheric Fistula

The enteroatmospheric fistula (EAF) is a complication unique of the open abdomen and is an opening in the GI wall occurring in the setting of an open abdomen that creates a communication between the GI lumen and the external atmosphere. It has exclusive features that make its spontaneous closure extremely unlikely, as the absence of a fistula tract and the lack of well-vascularized surrounding tissue. Moreover, the presence of an EAF guarantees the presence of a continuous peritonitis, caused by the spillage of enteric content in the open peritoneal cavity.

It is recognized that a septic open abdomen is more fistula prone when compared to an OA for trauma [42–44]. Traumatic insults to the bowel are critical for the formation of EAF, as demonstrated by the evidence that the incidence of EAF increases with the increase in duration of OA [45] and shows a direct correlation with the number of surgical re-explorations [46–48]. In this scenario, adhesion of the bowel to the fascia may be a major cause of EAF: a proper placement of the TAC deep into the paracolic gutter could prevent these adhesions and subsequently reduce the risk of EAF. The best way to deal an EAF is still to prevent it. The acronym **FRIENDS (F** foreign body, **R** radiation, **I** infection

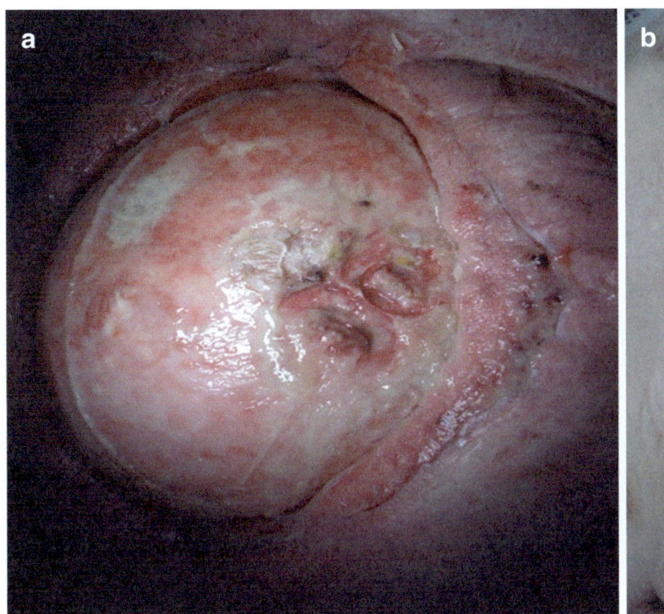

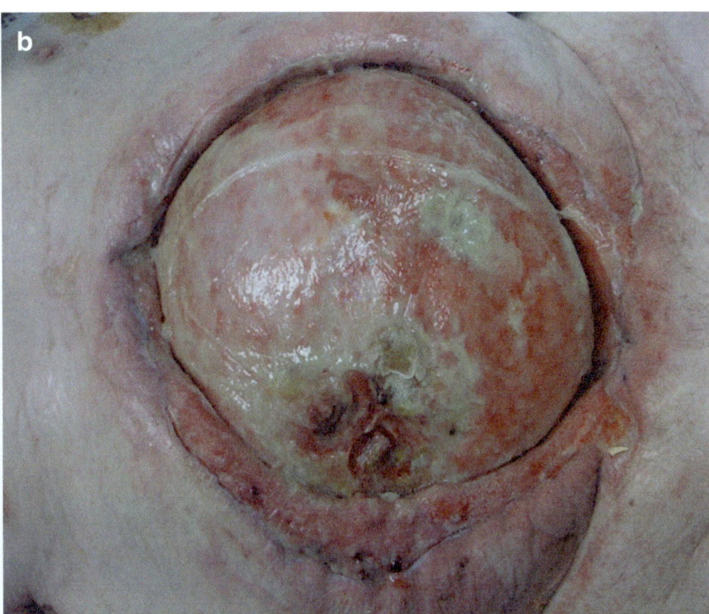

Fig. 23.3 The "frozen abdomen" (**a**) is a condition widely recognized after open abdomen where delayed wound closure appears as the only realistic alternative. Although early reconstruction is the target, a significant proportion of patients will develop adhesions between abdominal viscera and the anterolateral abdominal wall (**b**)

or inflammatory bowel disease, **E** epithelialization of fistula tract, **N** neoplasm, **D** distal obstruction, and **S** short tract <2 cm) summarizes the factors that are known to promote EAF development and maintenance; these conditions should be identified and addressed promptly. Another useful acronym is **SNAP** (**S** *sepsis and skin care*, **N** *nutrition*, **A** *anatomy*, and **P** *plan*) [49], which condense the key points of EAF management. Firstly, in the acute phase, **S**epsis control and **S**kin care (and wound care) are mandatory. **N**utritional support can be extremely challenging because EN can increase EAF output, and a reduction of fistula output could be tremendously helpful (consider the use of H_2 receptor antagonists, proton pump inhibitors [50], somatostatin and its analogs [34, 50–52]). The exact determination of **A**natomy of the EAF is mandatory for a proper management, because the exact determination of fistula location allows a correct quantification of fluid and electrolyte losses [37] and consent the determination of the total length of the remaining bowel available for absorption. For a proper EAF management, a well-conceived **P**lan, prepared by a multidisciplinary team, is of pivotal importance. In the best case scenario, the entire care of the patient until the resolution of the EAF should be in charge of the same team ("same team concept") [53].

The obvious best therapeutic option would be a proximal bowel diversion, but this option is almost invariably impossible. A throughout discussion of all the surgical techniques described so far in literature [54–81] goes far beyond the intent of this chapter. Recently Di Saverio et al., after performing an accurate literature review, created a clinical algorithm [82] and proposed a new classification of EAF [83], which could be extremely useful while dealing with EAF. Most of the management options are intended to be a bridge from the acute phase to a chronic phase, when patient has completely recovered and is fit for definitive fistula takedown and abdominal wall reconstruction. This condition usually requires at least 8–12 months.

23.3.2.3 Frozen Abdomen

The condition called frozen abdomen is the result of a prolonged OA and is characterized by the presence of dense adhesions that create a continuous layer of granulation tissue overlays the guts and fixing them into an inseparable single mass; every surgical maneuver is thus precluded and formation of EAF is relatively frequent in this situation. This scenario configures the grade 3 in Bjork's classification of OA revised by World Society of Abdominal Compartment Syndrome [84, 85]. The evolution of the OA with frozen abdomen is the formation of a huge ventral hernia.

Prevention is the key and is mainly based on TAC methods that contrast fascial retraction (i.e., NPWT with or without fascial traction systems); the use of instillation with NPWT seems to improve bowel loop moisture, reducing adhesions and increasing primary closure rates [11, 86]. The only option available for frozen abdomen management possibility is to promote the granulation of the exposed bowel. The effect of NPWT over a frozen abdomen can promote granulation over the viscera; the supposed association between negative pressure and EAF formation [87, 88] has been contradicted [21, 54, 89], but being gentle with the negative pressure is advisable [21]. Biological dressing and split-thickness skin graft [56–58] can speed up the epithelialization process and help to prevent traumatic damage to the exposed bowels.

23.3.2.4 Planned Ventral Hernia

At the beginning of the OA era, the usual management was to allow the open wound to granulate, creating a *planned ventral hernia*. However, this approach is associated with an increased risk of OA complications and also with an increased rate of hernia recurrence after surgical delayed fascial reconstruction compared to patients where primary fascial closure was achieved [90]. For this reason, the best treatment option nowadays is to close the abdomen as soon as possible. It is demonstrated that fascial retraction begins as early as day 3 [24], hence it is crucial to choose a TAC that could reduce fascial retraction from the very beginning of OA. NPWT has demonstrated a better tendency toward primary fascial closure when compared to other TAC methods, especially if associated with fascial traction systems [22, 23, 43]. The management of these huge planned ventral hernias is extremely challenging, and definitive surgical treatment should be performed only after the complete recovery of the patient (at least 6–12 months after initial surgery). Multiple approaches for definitive surgery have been described so far in literature [76, 91–95], and the definitive management of this condition brings with itself a great burden of morbidity and mortality that should not be ignored.

Conclusion

I thought it would be useful to discuss extensively the complications associated with OA, because some of them are extremely challenging to deal with and could greatly prolong the hospital stay; thus it is really important that a DCS strategy is applied only in those patients in whom the benefits certainly exceed its expected negative consequences.

Furthermore, the knowledge of the possible complications is crucial, because their prevention is still the best management option. Every effort should be made to close the OA as soon as possible, because it is demonstrated that after the first week of OA, the rate of complications increases dramatically [24, 45, 46, 96, 97] and the rate of delayed primary fascial closure drops significantly [47]. A recent meta-analysis demonstrated a mortality rate significantly lower in patients treated with NPWT versus patients without NPWT (28.5% versus 41.4%) [53]; this demonstrates again that the earlier the fascia is closed, the lower the complication rate became. Even if the choice of the right timing for abdominal closure is extremely hard and a safe primary closure could be prohibited in some cases, a primary fascial closure within the first week of OA is the best way to reduce the complication rate.

OA patients are extremely challenging and should be managed by multidisciplinary team formed by surgeons, anesthetists and ICU attendings, nutritionists, psychologists, and specialized nurses with specific expertise.

Case Scenario

A 54-year-old man is conducted to the emergency department after a motor vehicle crash (MVC). The hemodynamic appears unstable (BP 80/30, HR 125 bpm), E-FAST shows free abdominal fluid in all the windows explored and an arterial blood gas analysis demostrated altered parameters (pH 7.09, BE 16, Lac 6.9). The thoracic XR shows multiple rib fractures and parenchymal lung contusions on the right with no signs of pneumothorax; pelvic XR is negative.

1. What will you do?
   - A. Need for further information to obtain a correct diagnosis (perform thoraco-abdominal CT scan)
   - B. Immediate explorative laparotomy and perform damage control surgery
   - C. Proceed with DPL (diagnostic peritoneal lavage) to identify the characteristics of the free abdominal fluid
   - D. Close observation in ICU and abdominal CT scan 12 hours after the ER referral

2. You perform an immediate laparotomy without any further delay. Presence of gross hemoperitoneum (about 1500 ml) due to hepatic injury (S4–S5–S8, AIS AAST IV°). No evidence of further injuries to other abdominal organs.

   What is your next step?
   - A. Peri-hepatic packing and open abdomen treatment
   - B. Right hepatectomy extended to S4
   - C. Perform hemostasis at the site of hepatic bleeding with trans-parenchymal stitches and definitive closure of the abdomen
   - D. Accurate hemostasis and biliostasis of the hepatic injuries using argon beam cautery

3. You perform an immediate laparotomy without any further delay. Presence of gross fecal contamination due to a large blunt intestinal tear at rectosigmoid junction.

   What is your next step?
   - A. Sigmoidectomy with terminal colostomy (Hartmann's procedure) and primary abdominal closure
   - B. Primary suture of the sigmoid tear and built-up loop-ileostomy for protection of the intestinal repair

C. Resection of the intestinal tract involved in the injury (sigmoidectomy) without performing any anastomosis and open abdomen technique with planned second-look surgery within 48 h
D. Sigmoidectomy and immediate anastomosis by Knight-Griffen, with tubular drains in Douglas pouch

4. You perform an immediate laparotomy without any further delay and follow damage control surgery strategy leaving the abdomen open.

Which are the main risks related to this treatment?

A. Effective source control of the infection
B. Development of postoperative hernia defect
C. Enteroatmospheric fistula formation
D. B and C

Please see Chap. 58 for the correct answer.

References

1. Mccosh AJ. II. The treatment of general septic peritonitis. Ann Surg. 1897;25:687–97.
2. Pringle JH. V. Notes on the arrest of hepatic hemorrhage due to trauma. Ann Surg. 1908;48:541–9.
3. Ogilvie WH. The late complications of abdominal war-wounds. Lancet. 1940;2:253–6.
4. Stone HH, Strom PR, Mullins RJ. Management of the major coagulopathy with onset during laparotomy. Ann Surg. 1983;197(5):532–5.
5. Rotondo MF, Schwab CW, Mcgonigal MD, Phillips GR, Fruchterman TM, Kauder DR, Latenser BA, Angood PA. "Damage Control": an approach for improved survival in exsanguinating penetrating abdominal injury. J Trauma. 1993;35:375–82; Discussion 82–3
6. Rotondo MF, Zonies DH. The damage control sequence and underlying logic. Surg Clin North Am. 1997;77:761–77.
7. Becker HP, Willms A, Schwab R. Small bowel fistulas and the open abdomen. Scand J Surg. 2007;96:263–71.
8. Richter S, Dold S, Doberauer JP, Mai P, Schuld J. Negative pressure wound therapy for the treatment of the open abdomen and incidence of enteral fistulas: a retrospective bicentre analysis. Gastroenterol Res Pract. 2013;2013:1–6.
9. Coccolini F, Biffl W, Catena F, Ceresoli M, Chiara O, Cimbanassi S, Fattori L, Leppäniemi A, Manfredi R, Montori G, Pesenti G, Sugrue M, Ansaloni L. The open abdomen, indications, management and definitive closure. World J Emerg Surg. 2015;10:32.
10. Schecter W, Ivatury R, Rotondo M, Hirshberg A. Open abdomen after trauma and abdominal sepsis: a strategy for management. J Am Coll Surg. 2006;203:390–6.
11. Chiara O, Cimbanassi S, Biffl W, Leppaniemi A, Henry S, Scalea TM, Catena F, Ansaloni L, Chieregato A, De Blasio E, Gambale G, Gordini G, Nardi G, Paldalino P, Gossetti F, Dionigi P, Noschese G, Tugnoli G, Ribaldi S, Sgardello S, Magnone S, Rausei S, Mariani A, Mengoli F, Di Saverio S, Castriconi M, Coccolini F, Negreanu J, Razzi S, Coniglio C, Morelli F, Buonanno M, Lippi M, Trotta L, Volpi A, Fattori L, Zago M, De Rai P, Sammartano F, Manfredi R, Cingolani E. International consensus conference on open abdomen in trauma. J Trauma Acute Care Surg. 2016;80:173–83.
12. Department Of Defense. Surface ship survivalility. Washington, DC: Naval War Pubblication; 1996. p. 20–31.
13. Mutschler M, Nienaber U, Brockamp T, Wafaisade A, Fabian T, Paffrath T, Bouillon B, Maegele M, Traumaregister DGU. Renaissance of base deficit for the initial assessment of trauma patients: a base deficit-based classification for hypovolemic shock developed on data from 16,305 patients derived from the Traumaregister Dgu(R). Crit Care. 2013;17:R42.
14. Mutschler M, Nienaber U, Nzberg MM, Lfl CW, Schoechl H, Paffrath T, Bouillon B, Maegele M. The Shock Index Revisited a fast guide to transfusion requirement? A retrospective analysis on 21,853 patients derived from the Traumaregister DGU. Crit Care. 2013;17(4):R172.
15. Burlew CC. The open abdomen: practical implications for the practicing surgeon. AJS. 2012:1–10.
16. MLNG M, Cheatham ML, Kirkpatrick A, Sugrue M, Parr M, De Waele J, Balogh Z, Leppäniemi A, Olvera C, Ivatury R, D'amours S, Wendon J, Hillman K, Johansson K, Kolkman K, Wilmer A. Results from the international conference of experts on intra-abdominal hypertension and abdominal compartment syndrome. I. Definitions. Intensive Care Med. 2006;32(11):1722–32.
17. Balogh ZJ, Van Wessem K, Yoshino O, Moore FA. Postinjury abdominal compartment syndrome: are we winning the battle? World J Surg. 2009;33:1134–41.
18. Balogh ZJ, Lumsdaine W, Moore EE, Moore FA. Postinjury abdominal compartment syndrome: from recognition to prevention. Lancet. 2014;384:1466–75.
19. Huang Q, Li J, Lau WY. Techniques for abdominal wall closure after damage control laparotomy: from temporary abdominal closure to early/delayed fascial closure-a review. Gastroenterol Res Pract. 2016;2016:2073260.
20. Quyn AJ, Johnston C, Hall D, Chambers A, Arapova N, Ogston S, Amin AI. The open abdomen and temporary abdominal closure systems - historical evolution and systematic review. Color Dis. 2012;14:E429–38.
21. Bruhin A, Ferreira F, Chariker M, Smith J, Runkel N. Systematic review and evidence based recommendations for the use of negative pressure wound therapy in the open abdomen. Int J Surg. 2014;12:1105–14.
22. Rasilainen SK, Mentula PJ, Leppaniemi AK. Vacuum and mesh-mediated fascial traction for primary closure of the open abdomen in critically ill surgical patients. Br J Surg. 2012;99:1725–32.
23. Fortelny RH, Hofmann A, Gruber-Blum S, Petter-Puchner AH, Glaser KS. Delayed closure of open abdomen in septic patients is facilitated by combined negative pressure wound therapy and dynamic fascial suture. Surg Endosc. 2014;28:735–40.
24. Willms A, Gusgen C, Schaaf S, Bieler D, Von Websky M, Schwab R. Management of the open abdomen using vacuum-assisted wound closure and mesh-mediated fascial traction. Langenbecks Arch Surg. 2015;400:91–9.
25. Smith PC, Tweddell JS, Bessey PQ. Alternative approaches to abdominal wound closure in severely injured patients with massive visceral edema. J Trauma. 1992;32:16–20.
26. Fernandez L, Norwood S, Roettger R, Wilkins HE. Temporary intravenous bag silo closure in severe abdominal trauma. J Trauma. 1996;40:258–60.
27. Friese RS. The open abdomen: definitions, management principles, and nutrition support considerations. Nutr Clin Pract. 2012;27:492–8.
28. Roberts DJ, Jenne CN, Ball CG, Tiruta C, Léger C, Xiao Z, Faris PD, Mcbeth PB, Doig CJ, Skinner CR, Ruddell SG, Kubes P, Kirkpatrick AW. Efficacy and safety of active negative pres-

sure peritoneal therapy for reducing the systemic inflammatory response after damage control laparotomy (the intra-peritoneal vacuum trial): study protocol for a randomized controlled trial. Trials. 2013;14:141.
29. Yin J, Wang J, Yao D, Zhang S, Mao Q, Kong W, Ren L, Li Y, Li J. Is it feasible to implement enteral nutrition in patients with enteroatmospheric fistulae? A single-center experience. Nutr Clin Pract. 2014;29:656–61.
30. Willcutts K, Mercer D, Ziegler J. Fistuloclysis: an interprofessional approach to nourishing the fistula patient. J Wound Ostomy Continence Nurs. 2015;42:549–53.
31. Moore FA, Feliciano DV, Andrassy RJ, Mcardle AH, Booth FV, Morgenstein-Wagner TB, Kellum JM, Welling RE, Moore EE. Early enteral feeding, compared with parenteral, reduces postoperative septic complications. the results of a meta-analysis. Ann Surg. 1992;216(2):172–83.
32. Kudsk KA, Croce MA, Fabian TC, Minard G, Tolley EA, Poret HA, Kuhl MR, Brown RO. Enteral versus parenteral feeding. Effects on septic morbidity after blunt and penetrating abdominal trauma. Ann Surg. 1992;215(5):503–11. Discussion 11–3
33. Byrnes MC, Reicks P, Irwin E. Early enteral nutrition can be successfully implemented in trauma patients with an "Open Abdomen". Am J Surg. 2010;199:359–62; Discussion 63
34. Yuan Y, Ren J, Gu G, Chen J, Li J. Early enteral nutrition improves outcomes of open abdomen in gastrointestinal fistula patients complicated with severe sepsis. Nutr Clin Pract. 2011;26(6):688–94.
35. Dissanaike S, Pham T, Shalhub S, Warner K, Hennessy L, Moore EE, Maier RV, O'keefe GE, Cuschieri J. Effect of immediate enteral feeding on trauma patients with an open abdomen: protection from nosocomial infections. J Am Coll Surg. 2008;207:690–7.
36. Tsuei BJ, Magnuson B, Swintosky M, Flynn J, Boulanger BR, Ochoa JB, Kearney PA. Enteral nutrition in patients with an open peritoneal cavity. Nutr Clin Pract. 2003;18(3):253–8.
37. Majercik S, Kinikini M, White T. Enteroatmospheric fistula: from soup to nuts. Nutr Clin Pract. 2012;27(4):507–12.
38. Polk TM, Schwab CW. Metabolic and nutritional support of the enterocutaneous fistula patient: a three-phase approach. World J Surg. 2012;36:524–33.
39. Cheatham ML, Safcsak K, Brzezinski SJ, Lube MW. Nitrogen balance, protein loss, and the open abdomen. Crit Care Med. 2007;35:127–31.
40. Weissenfluh GM, Brundage SI, Spain DA. Early enteral nutrition after abdominal trauma: effects on septic morbidity and practicality. Nutr Clin Pract. 2006;21(5):479–84.
41. Open Abdomen Advisory Panel, Campbell A, Chang M, Fabian T, Franz M, Kaplan M, Moore F, Reed RL, Scott B, Silverman R. Management of the open abdomen: from initial operation to definitive closure. Am Surg. 2009;75:S1–22.
42. Bruhin A, Ferreira F, Chariker M, Smith J, Runkel N. Systematic review and evidence based recommendations for the use of negative pressure wound therapy in the open abdomen. Int J Surg. 2014;12(10):1025–136.
43. Atema JJ, Gans SL, Boermeester MA. Systematic review and meta-analysis of the open abdomen and temporary abdominal closure techniques in non-trauma patients. World J Surg. 2014;39:912–25.
44. Kirshtein B, Mizrahi S. Vacuum-assisted management of enteroatmospheric fistula within the open abdomen. Am Surg. 2014;80:209–10.
45. Miller RS, Morris JA, Diaz JJ, Herring MB, May AK. Complications after 344 damage-control open celiotomies. J Trauma. 2005;59:1365–71; Discussion 71-4
46. Mintziras I, Miligkos M, Bartsch DK. High risk of fistula formation in vacuum-assisted closure therapy in patients with open abdomen due to secondary peritonitis-a retrospective analysis. Langenbeck's Arch Surg. 2016;401:619–25.
47. Schmelzle M, Alldinger I, Matthaei H, Aydin F, Wallert I, Eisenberger CF, Schulte Am Esch J 2nd, Dizdar L, Topp SA, Yang Q, Knoefel WT. Long-term vacuum-assisted closure in open abdomen due to secondary peritonitis: a retrospective evaluation of a selected group of patients. Dig Surg. 2010;27:272–8.
48. Bradley MJ, Dubose JJ, Scalea TM, Holcomb JB, Shrestha B, Okoye O, Inaba K, Bee TK, Fabian TC, Whelan JF, Ivatury RR, AAST Open Abdomen Study Group. Independent predictors of enteric fistula and abdominal sepsis after damage control laparotomy: results from the prospective AAST Open Abdomen registry. JAMA Surg. 2013;148:947–54.
49. Kaushal M, Carlson GL. Management of enterocutaneous fistulas. Clin Colon Rectal Surg. 2004;17(2):79–88.
50. Lloyd DA, Gabe SM, Windsor AC. Nutrition and management of enterocutaneous fistula. Br J Surg. 2006;93:1045–55.
51. Stevens P, Foulkes RE, Hartford-Beynon JS, Delicata RJ. Systematic review and meta-analysis of the role of somatostatin and its analogues in the treatment of enterocutaneous fistula. Eur J Gastroenterol Hepatol. 2011;23(10):912–22.
52. Ren J, Yuan Y, Zhao Y, Gu G, Wang G, Chen J, Fan C, Wang X, Li J. Open abdomen treatment for septic patients with gastrointestinal fistula: from fistula control to definitive closure. In: Am Surg, vol. 80; 2014. p. 339–47.
53. Cirocchi R, Birindelli A, Biffl WL, Mutafchiyski V, Popivanov G, Chiara O, Tugnoli G, Di Saverio S. What is the effectiveness of the negative pressure wound therapy (Npwt) in patients treated with open abdomen technique? A systematic review and meta-analysis. J Trauma Acute Care Surg. 2016;81:575–84.
54. Navsaria P, Nicol A, Hudson D, Cockwill J, Smith J. Negative pressure wound therapy management of the "Open Abdomen" following trauma: a prospective study and systematic review. World J Emerg Surg. 2013;8:4.
55. Navsaria PH, Bunting M, Omoshoro-Jones J, Nicol AJ, Kahn D. Temporary closure of open abdominal wounds by the modified sandwich-vacuum pack technique. Br J Surg. 2003;90:718–22.
56. Girard S, Sideman M, Spain DA. A novel approach to the problem of intestinal fistulization arising in patients managed with open peritoneal cavities. Am J Surg. 2002;184:166–7.
57. Jamshidi R, Schecter WP. Biological dressings for the management of enteric fistulas in the open abdomen: a preliminary report. Arch Surg. 2007;142:793–6.
58. Bhat YM, Banerjee S, Barth BA, Chauhan SS, Gottlieb KT, Konda V, Maple JT, Murad FM, Pfau PR, Pleskow DK, Siddiqui UD, Tokar JL, Wang A, Rodriguez SA, ASGE Technology Committee. Tissue adhesives: cyanoacrylate glue and fibrin sealant. Gastrointest Endosc. 2013;78:209–15.
59. Subramaniam MH, Liscum KR, Hirshberg A. The floating stoma: a new technique for controlling exposed fistulae in abdominal trauma. J Trauma. 2002;53:386–8.
60. Goverman J, Yelon JA, Platz JJ, Singson RC, Turcinovic M. The "Fistula Vac," a technique for management of enterocutaneous fistulae arising within the open abdomen: report of 5 cases. J Trauma. 2006;60:428–31.
61. D'hondt M, Devriendt D, Van Rooy F, Vansteenkiste F, D'hoore A, Penninckx F, Miserez M. Treatment of small-bowel fistulae in the open abdomen with topical negative-pressure therapy. Am J Surg. 2011;202:E20–E4.
62. Piazza R, Armstrong S, Vanderkolk W, Eriksson E, Ringler S. A modified "Fistula-Vac" technique: management of multiple enterocutaneous fistulas in the open abdomen. Plast Reconstr Surg. 2009;124:453e–5e.
63. Pang TC, Morton J, Pincott S. Novel technique for isolating and dressing enteroatmospheric fistulae. ANZ J Surg. 2012;82:747–9.
64. Timmons J, Russell F. The use of negative-pressure wound therapy to manage enteroatmospheric fistulae in two patients with large abdominal wounds. Int Wound J. 2013;11(6):723–9.

65. Al-Khoury G, Kaufman D, Hirshberg A. Improved control of exposed fistula in the open abdomen. J Am Coll Surg. 2008;206:397–8.
66. Pepe G, Magalini S, Callari C, Persiani R, Lodoli C, Gui D. Vacuum assisted closure (Vac) Therapy(Tm) as a swiss knife multi-tool for enteric fistula closure: tips and tricks: a pilot study. In: Eur Rev Med Pharmacol Sci; 2014 18(17):2527–2532.
67. Verhaalen A, Watkins B, Brasel K. Techniques and cost effectiveness of enteroatmospheric fistula isolation . In: Wounds; 2010 22(8):212–217.
68. Ramsay PT, Mejia VA. Management of enteroatmospheric fistulae in the open abdomen. In: Am Surg; 2010 76(6):637–639.
69. Layton B, Dubose J, Nichols S, Connaughton J, Jones T, Pratt J. Pacifying the open abdomen with concomitant intestinal fistula: a novel approach. Am J Surg. 2010;199:E48–50.
70. Di Saverio S, Villani S, Biscardi A, Giorgini E, Tugnoli G. Open abdomen with concomitant enteroatmospheric fistula: validation, refinements, and adjuncts to a novel approach. J Trauma. 2011;71:760–2.
71. Rekstad LC, Wasmuth HH, Ystgaard B, Stornes T, Seternes A. Topical negative-pressure therapy for small bowel leakage in a frozen abdomen. J Trauma Acute Care Surg. 2013;75:487–91.
72. Heineman JT, Garcia LJ, Obst MA, Chong HS, Langin JG, Humpal R, Pezzella PA, Dries DJ. Collapsible enteroatmospheric fistula isolation device: a novel, simple solution to a complex problem. J Am Coll Surg. 2015;221(2):e7–14.
73. Wang G, Ren J, Liu S, Wu X, Gu G, Li J. "Fistula patch": making the treatment of enteroatmospheric fistulae in the open abdomen easier. J Trauma Acute Care Surg. 2013;74:1175–7.
74. Ozer MT, Sinan H, Zeybek N, Peker Y. A simple novel technique for enteroatmospheric fistulae: silicone fistula plug. Int Wound J. 2014;11(Suppl 1):22–4.
75. Sriussadaporn S, Sriussadaporn S, Kritayakirana K, Pak-Art R. Operative management of small bowel fistulae associated with open abdomen. Asian J Surg. 2006;29:1–7.
76. Wind J, Van Koperen PJ, Slors JFM, Bemelman WA. Single-stage closure of enterocutaneous fistula and stomas in the presence of large abdominal wall defects using the components separation technique. Asian J Surg. 2009;197:24–9.
77. Stephensen B, Brown J, Lambrianides A. A novel method for managing enterocutaneous fistulae in the open abdomen using a pedicle flap. J Surg Case Rep. 2012;2012:5.
78. Al-Nahawi M. A rare approach to entero-atmospheric fistula. Am J Case Rep. 2013;14:476–80.
79. Gupta R, Singh H, Talukder S, Verma GR. A new technique of closing a gastroatmospheric fistula with a rectus abdominis muscle flap. BMJ Case Rep. 2015; https://doi.org/10.1136/bcr-2015-209309.
80. Lambe G, Russell C, West C, Kalaiselvan R, Slade DA, Anderson ID, Watson JS, Carlson GL. Autologous reconstruction of massive enteroatmospheric fistulation with a pedicled subtotal lateral thigh flap. Br J Surg. 2012;99(7):964–72.
81. Clark CE, Walker T, Bacon L, Mccoy J, Babaloa O. Staged suspension of an enteroatmospheric fistula: a novel surgical approach. Am Surg. 2013;79:E139–40.
82. Di Saverio S, Tarasconi A, Inaba K, Navsaria P, Coccolini F, Costa Navarro D, Mandrioli M, Vassiliu P, Jovine E, Catena F, Tugnoli G. Open abdomen with concomitant enteroatmospheric fistula: attempt to rationalize the approach to a surgical nightmare and proposal of a clinical algorithm. J Am Coll Surg. 2015;220:E23–33.
83. Di Saverio S, Tarasconi A, Walczak DA, Cirocchi R, Mandrioli M, Birindelli A, Tugnoli G. Classification, prevention and management of entero-atmospheric fistula: a state-of-the-art review. Langenbecks Arch Surg. 2016;401(1):1–13.
84. Björck M, Bruhin A, Cheatham M, Hinck D, Kaplan M, Manca G, Wild T, Windsor A. Classification--important step to improve management of patients with an open abdomen. World J Surg. 2009;33:1154–7.
85. Andrew W. Kirkpatrick, Derek J. Roberts, Jan De Waele, Roman Jaeschke, Manu L. N. G. Malbrain, Bart De Keulenaer, Juan Duchesne, Martin Bjorck, Ari Leppaniemi, Janeth C. Ejike, Michael Sugrue, Michael Cheatham, Rao Ivatury, Chad G. Ball, Annika Reintam Blaser, Adrian Regli, Zsolt J. Balogh, Scott D'Amours, Dieter Debergh, Mark Kaplan, Edward Kimball, Claudia Olvera, (2013) Intra-abdominal hypertension and the abdominal compartment syndrome: updated consensus definitions and clinical practice guidelines from the World Society of the Abdominal Compartment Syndrome. Intensive Care Medicine 39 (7):1190–1206
86. Rycerz AM, Slack P, Mcnulty AK. Distribution assessment comparing continuous and periodic wound instillation in conjunction with negative pressure wound therapy using an agar-based model. Int Wound J. 2013;10:214–20.
87. Lindstedt S, Malmsjö M, Hlebowicz J, Ingemansson R. Comparative study of the microvascular blood flow in the intestinal wall, wound contraction and fluid evacuation during negative pressure wound therapy in laparostomy using the V.A.C. abdominal dressing and the abthera open abdomen negative pressure therapy system. In: International Wound Journal: 12(1); 2015:83–88.
88. Hlebowicz J, Hansson J, Lindstedt S. Microvascular blood flow response in the intestinal wall and the omentum during negative wound pressure therapy of the open abdomen. Int J Color Dis. 2012;27:397–403.
89. Carlson GL, Patrick H, Amin AI, Mcpherson G, Maclennan G, Afolabi E, Mowatt G, Campbell B. Management of the open abdomen: a national study of clinical outcome and safety of negative pressure wound therapy. Ann Surg. 2013;257:1154–9.
90. Zosa BM, Como JJ, Kelly KB, He JC, Claridge JA. Planned ventral hernia following damage control laparotomy in trauma: an added year of recovery but equal long-term outcome. Hernia. 2016;20:231–8.
91. Marinis A, Gkiokas G, Argyra E, Fragulidis G, Polymeneas G, Voros D. "Enteroatmospheric fistulae" - gastrointestinal openings in the open abdomen: a review and recent proposal of a surgical technique. Scand J Surg. 2013;102:61–8.
92. Krpata DM, Stein SL, Eston M, Ermlich B, Blatnik JA, Novitsky YW, Rosen MJ. Outcomes of simultaneous large complex abdominal wall reconstruction and enterocutaneous fistula takedown. Am J Surg. 2013;205:354–9.
93. Dionigi G, Dionigi R, Rovera F, Boni L, Padalino P, Minoja G, Cuffari S, Carrafiello G. Treatment of high output entero-cutaneous fistulae associated with large abdominal wall defects: single center experience. Int J Surg. 2008;6:51–6.
94. Demetriades D. A technique of surgical closure of complex intestinal fistulae in the open abdomen. J Trauma. 2003;55:999–1001.
95. Latifi R, Joseph B, Kulvatunyou N, Wynne JL, O'keeffe T, Tang A, Friese R, Rhee PM. Enterocutaneous fistulas and a hostile abdomen: reoperative surgical approaches. World J Surg. 2012;36(3):516–23.
96. Chen Y, Ye J, Song W, Chen J, Yuan Y, Ren J. Comparison of outcomes between early fascial closure and delayed abdominal closure in patients with open abdomen: a systematic review and meta-analysis. Gastroenterol Res Pract. 2014;2014:784056.
97. Diaz JJ Jr, Dutton WD, Ott MM, Cullinane DC, Alouidor R, Armen SB, Bilanuik JW, Collier BR, Gunter OL, Jawa R, Jerome R, Kerwin AJ, Kirby JP, Lambert AL, Riordan WP, Wohltmann CD. Eastern association for the surgery of trauma: a review of the management of the open abdomen—Part 2 "Management Of The Open Abdomen". J Trauma. 2011;71:502–12.

Basic Operative Techniques in Abdominal Injury

24

Paolo Aseni, Antonino M. Grande, Federico Romani, Arianna Birindelli, and Salomone Di Saverio

Key Points

- Any patient who has persistent haemodynamic instability or signs of peritonitis following abdominal trauma requires emergent laparotomy.
- Lower thoracic and upper abdominal trauma should be considered as a unit, and any penetrating wound below the level of the nipple should be suspected as abdominal injury.
- Basic principles of abdominal techniques in abdominal injury include abbreviated surgery to control blood loss and contamination in the abdomen, simultaneous resuscitation of the patient's physiology and definitive surgical management at a later stage after the restoration of physiology.
- Up to 25% of patients with penetrating abdominal trauma will have major vascular injury, and inferior vena cava (IVC) and its branches are the most commonly injured vessel.
- Shock out of proportion to injury extent suggests major vascular injury.
- Supracoeliac aortic cross-clamping and cross-clamping of the thoracic aorta are important surgical manoeuvres to control massive intra-abdominal bleeding in patients with haemodynamic instability.
- Abdominal aorta and IVC and major branches are retroperitoneal and covered with viscera; they are difficult to expose in the presence of a large haematoma in patients with penetrating injury. Medial visceral rotations (Cattell-Braasch and Mattox manoeuvre) are paramount to expose retroperitoneal major midline vessels.
- In case of major abdominal vessel injury, the key procedural sequence is (a) expose, (b) achieve proximal control, (c) explore and evaluate the injury and (d) restore flow.
- Angiographic embolization has become an indispensable tool to control the bleeding source.
- Laparoscopy in abdominal trauma has demonstrated to be an extremely useful diagnostic and therapeutic tool, either immediate or interval, since it significantly reduces the rate of negative laparotomies up to almost 90% as well as decreases the rate of postoperative morbidity and allows a faster postoperative recovery.

P. Aseni (✉)
Dipartimento di Emergenza Urgenza, ASST Grande Ospedale Metropolitano Niguarda, Milan, Italy

A. M. Grande
Department of Cardiac Surgery, IRCCS Fondazione Policlinico San Matteo, Pavia, Italy

F. Romani
S.C. Chirurgia Vascolare, Dipartimento Cardiotoracovascolare, ASST Grande Ospedale Metropolitano Niguarda, Milan, Italy
e-mail: federico.romani@ospedaleniguarda.it

A. Birindelli
University of Bologna, Queen Elizabeth University Hospital Birmingham, Birmingham, UK

S. Di Saverio
Cambridge Colorectal Unit, Cambridge University Hospitals NHS Foundation Trust, Addenbrooke's Hospital, Cambridge, UK

P. Aseni et al. (eds.), *Operative Techniques and Recent Advances in Acute Care and Emergency Surgery*,
https://doi.org/10.1007/978-3-319-95114-0_24

24.1 General Principles

The abdomen is the third most common *injured* region; for this reason, diagnosis and management of abdominal trauma may present a great challenge even to best trauma surgeons who have to face a bunch of different injuries in patients where simultaneous multiple lesions may be present. Lower thoracic and upper abdominal trauma should be considered as a unit, and abdominal injury in any penetrating wound below the level of the nipple should be suspected. Thanks to many technological developments, the surgical management of significantly injured trauma patients has gone through a major change over the last decade, and the basic principles of the contemporary approach include different therapeutic strategies from **damage control** (DC) operations to damage control resuscitation and appropriate utilization of adjunctive bleeding control strategies. DC is not a surgical manoeuvre but an alternative treatment modality to offer primary surgical care. The principles of DC surgery in trauma care (discussed in a dedicated chapter) have become the standard of care in the treatment of injured patients with severe physiological compromise who require surgical intervention [1]. Basic principles include abbreviated surgery to control blood loss and contamination in the abdomen, simultaneous resuscitation of the patient's physiology, and definitive surgical management at a later stage after the restoration of physiology. In another term, damage control is a way to find a practical method, maybe not the optimal or the perfect solution but sufficiently advantageous for the immediate goal to guarantee a life-saving strategy [2–5]. A heuristic approach can help to find the algorithm throughout a common-sense clinical and anatomical information to decide which procedure to follow first for that specific injury considered as having the highest probability of death for exsanguination (Fig. 24.1).

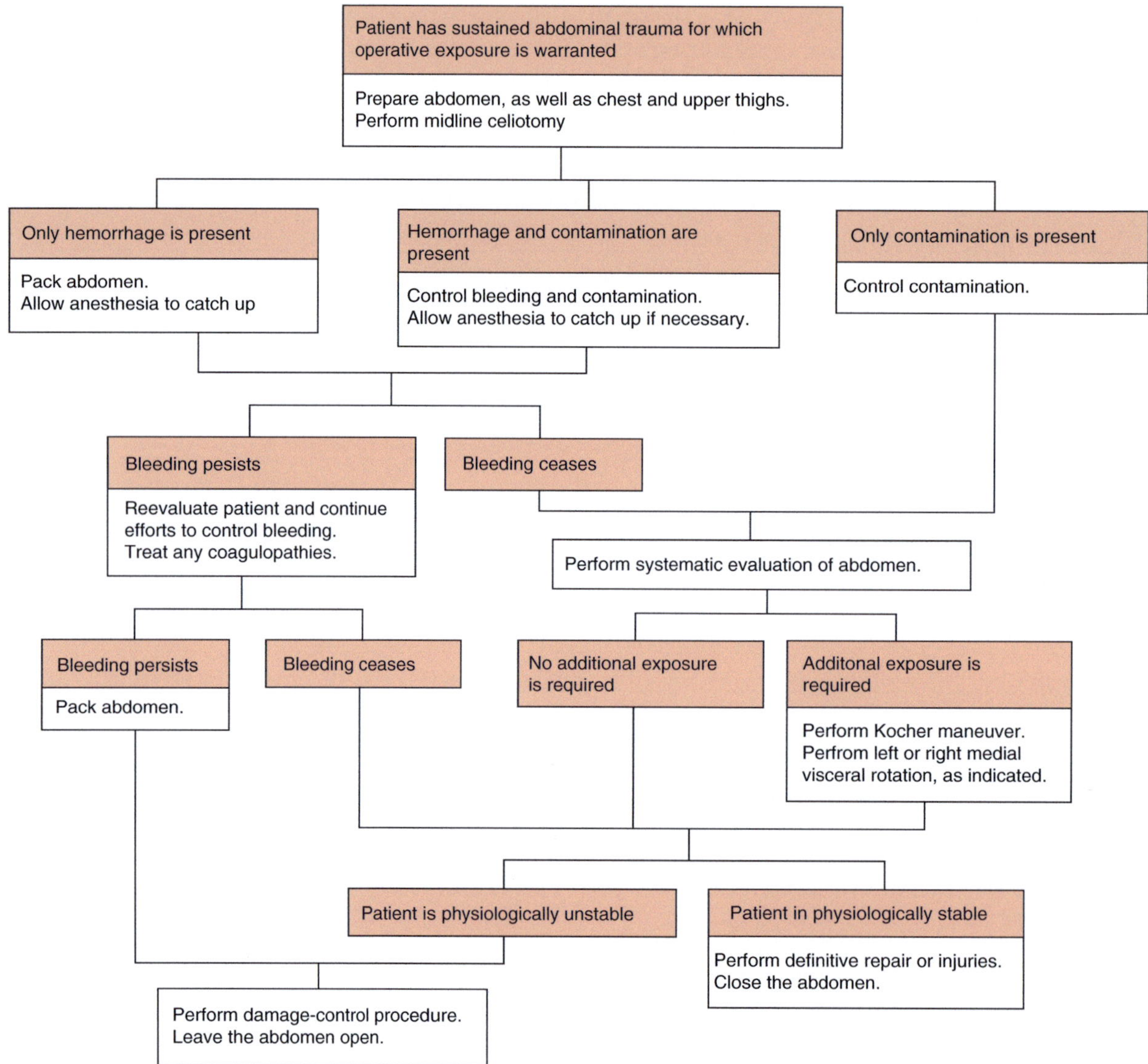

Fig. 24.1 Algorithm for exposure and control of abdominal trauma

The goal of the first phase of DC surgery is to perform an **abbreviated operation** focusing on both bleeding and contamination control, early recognition of surgically correctable bleeding points and avoidance of gastrointestinal soilage. Consequently, the majority of laparotomies in damage control surgery involve early laparotomy and pad packing of the surgical bed for haemostasis. The opening of the peritoneal cavity results in adverse effects on body core temperature as a function of time; therefore, damage control operations should be as rapid as possible, less than 90 min if possible. After rewarming and resuscitation, the patient is usually taken back in surgery for a second look, repacking or definitive care. All abdominal packs need to be removed before 48–72 h after the initial placement as a result of increased risk for infection after this period. Also, a **second look** can provide an opportunity to diagnose any missed injuries during the initial damage control procedure. When the clinical decision is made in order to perform a definitive operation, the bowel is anastomosed to preserve intestinal continuity; colostomies are refined, temporary vascular shunts are removed, necrotic parenchyma and devascularized tissues should be entirely removed, and biliary, pancreatic and gastroduodenal transit can be definitively restored. If the patient presents still a clinical coagulopathy, the operation may be turned into a simple second look with packs replaced, and the patient is returned to the intensive care unit (ICU). Unless the intraperitoneal contents are without any clinical evidence of tissue oedema, the abdominal fascia should be left open to allow further evacuation to minimize the risk of an increase of intra-abdominal pressure. In patients with ongoing haemorrhage or developing a secondary **acute compartment syndrome** (ACS), urgent relaparotomy should be performed. In the absence of strong indications for an early re-exploration, definitive treatment should be scheduled when the probability of achieving complete fascial closure is greatest. This can usually occur 3–4 days after the initial celiotomy when diuresis and negative fluid balance have occurred with evidence of decreasing abdominal girth and peripheral and abdominal wall oedema. However, often the abdominal wall cannot be closed resulting in the acceptance of a subsequent ventral hernia that generally requires a later planned repair.

24.2 Evolving Concepts in Nonoperative Management of Abdominal Emergencies

The last decade showed important improvements in medical technology in managing patients with abdominal trauma and acute care surgery, and probably the most significant improvement was in diagnostic and interventional radiology and **nonoperative management (NOM)** of abdominal injuries [6–9]. Selective nonoperative management of significant abdominal injuries has represented one of the most important changes in the trauma patient care over the last decades. **Angiographic embolization** has also become an indispensable tool to control the bleeding in various and less easily accessible anatomical areas such as in the head-face-neck regions as well as the pelvis. A novel trauma workflow, comprising immediate CT diagnosis and rapid bleeding control without patient transfer, as realized in the hybrid ER, may improve mortality in severe trauma [10]. Furthermore, embolization and surgical control are not mutually exclusive. Damage control embolization is a rapid procedure that can be performed in most of the institutions without the need for very advanced equipment. Critically bleeding patients are taken to the operating room for packing of major bleeding such as the liver or pelvis, and angioembolization can be usefully considered to consolidate the haemorrhage control and to obtain early and safe removal of the packs. The radiologist's main task is to rapidly and temporarily control the source of blood loss of the specific bleeding points. Pelvic embolization should routinely involve the injection of microcoils and gel-foam slurry inside both internal iliac arteries decreasing the pelvic perfusion and the bleeding, so allowing the clotting process to occur. Blood supply is usually present to ensure organ viability and to minimize significant ischaemic complications which are extremely rare. The sponge particles are reabsorbed within few days with the restoration of normal perfusion. Splenic haemorrhage can also be controlled by embolizing the main splenic artery although this should be avoided in all unstable patients in whom a prompt splenectomy is a much better option. Embolization of other organs, such as the liver or kidney, requires a higher degree of selectivity and is usually performed by placing coils in the bleeding branch. NOM in children with splenic injuries gained diffusion rapidly because of the significant incidence and seriousness of post-splenectomy sepsis. More recently, NOM has been extended to blunt hepatic injuries in children with similar success. Currently NOM of isolated blunt hepatic and splenic injuries is considered the standard of care for haemodynamically stable paediatric and adult patients. Although there is still no consensus on which parameters to use for definition of haemodynamic stability [11], physiologic stability is usually indicated by normal blood pressure, lack of tachycardia, no physical findings suggesting shock and absence of metabolic acidosis. NOM should be considered in patients who have no physiologic indicators of ongoing bleeding with a demonstrated haemodynamic stability without the need for intravascular volume support. During the past 10 years, we have assisted to growing evidence in favour of NOM in haemodynamically stable patients, in association to angiographic embolization which is a useful additional therapeutic tool with fewer intra-abdominal complications [6].

24.3 Surgical Management: Laparotomy, Damage Control, and Operative Exposure of the Abdominal Injuries

The surgeon's purpose in the preoperative phase is to plane early surgery in the bleeding patient when indicated. Patient selection is crucial as patients with relatively simple abdominal injuries should not undergo unnecessary surgical procedures. Haemodynamic instability manifestations include hypotension, tachycardia and tachypnoea; coagulopathy associated with hypothermia is an important hint for the damage control approach.

Trauma surgeon's primary task is to stop the bleeding; therefore, all unstable patients presenting in extremis with massive intra-abdominal haemorrhage should be immediately taken to the operating room for emergency surgery. The massive transfusion protocol should also be activated preferably by the attending trauma surgeon, trauma fellow or chief surgical resident, and the blood products must also be present in the operating room at the time of the patient's arrival. **Control of massive bleeding** from the vascular or parenchymal structures is dependent on whether the injury has resulted in tamponade (retroperitoneal haematoma) or free rupture into the peritoneal cavity. In the profoundly hypotensive trauma patient with massive abdominal distention, proximal vascular control with a left anterolateral thoracotomy for aortic cross-clamping may be considered; sudden decompression during laparotomy may result in cardiac arrest before the alternative supracoeliac aortic compression and clamping are established.

If the haematoma has ruptured, patients will likely present in a volume unresponsive haemorrhagic shock. However, if the injury remains contained in the retroperitoneum, the patient may remain stable or became a transient responder to fluid resuscitation. In the blunt trauma patient with associated significant traumatic brain injury, however, resuscitation to a systolic blood pressure above 90 mmHg is more important, in order to preserve cerebral blood flow and avoid the potential for secondary brain injury associated with hypotension [1, 3, 7–9].

Despite a surprising lack of evidence for temperature management in trauma patients, the majority of trauma centres have protocols for warming blankets, warming mattresses, heated intravenous fluids and adequately **rewarming** of the ambient room temperature. **Preparation of the operative field** must be undertaken quickly and should extend from the chin to the knees between the posterior axillary lines and with both arms fully abducted. The thoracic cavity should be easily accessible if a left anterolateral thoracotomy is required for aortic cross-clamping and open cardiopulmonary resuscitation. It is important to include the proximal thigh in the surgical field; this can ensure availability of an autogenous venous conduit such as great saphenous or femoral vein. Exploration of the abdomen begins with a midline abdominal incision extending from the xiphoid to pubis. If in this phase a cardiac arrest occurs before laparotomy, a left anterolateral thoracotomy in fifth intercostal space with aortic cross-clamping can be rapidly performed.

24.3.1 Control of Life-Threatening Haemorrhage

All the initial efforts should focus on the immediate control of life-threatening haemorrhage followed by containment of leaking of the gastrointestinal contents. A large Balfour retractor positioned above the abdomen facilitates the approach to the peritoneal cavity and optimizes exposure of intra-abdominal organs while the surgeon inserts the left hand into the abdomen to protect the organs using the right hand to evacuate the clots. Control of the massive haemorrhage requires systematic evaluation of the intra-abdominal cavity and retroperitoneal space which is divided into three anatomic zones (Fig. 24.2). Facing massive intra-abdominal bleeding, rapid packing of all four quadrants is the first manoeuvre and should be quickly performed. Packing of the liver and spleen in case of liver and spleen injuries should be performed both above and below the organs to create maxi-

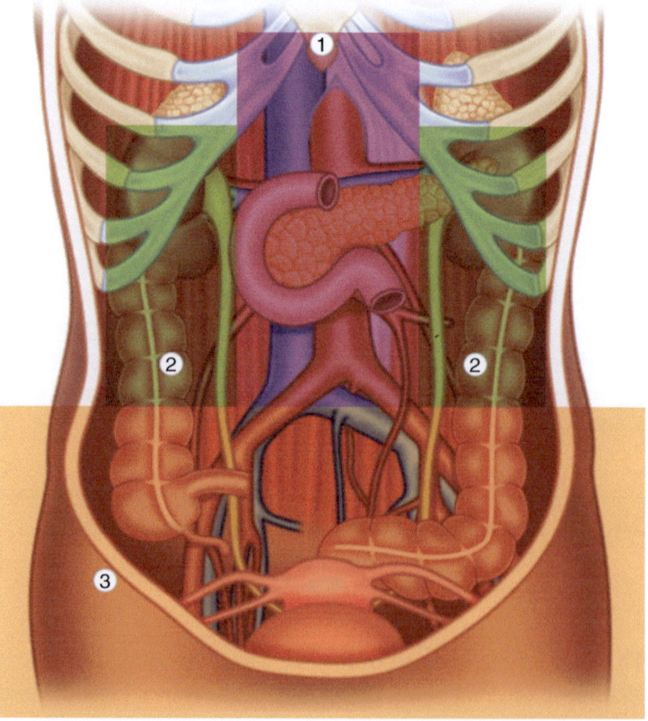

Fig. 24.2 The retroperitoneal space is divided into three anatomic Zones I, II and III

mal tamponade. Once haemorrhage is controlled with packing, resuscitation should be continued until stabilization of the patient has been obtained.

24.3.2 Supracoeliac Control of the Abdominal Aorta

If packing of all four quadrants fails to control blood loss or in case the patient is in cardiac arrest, supracoeliac control of the aorta is required. The hepatoduodenal and gastrohepatic ligaments should be opened and dissected as near as possible to the lesser gastric curvature, avoiding possible damage to an accessory or replaced left hepatic artery from the left gastric artery. Then, an assistant should retract the left lobe of the liver to the patient's right. To allow retraction of the left liver lobe, the left triangular ligament should be divided (Fig. 24.3). Opening the oesophageal hiatus with a wide incision on the right and left crura of the diaphragm facilitates the subsequent surgical steps (Fig. 24.4). The distal oesopha-

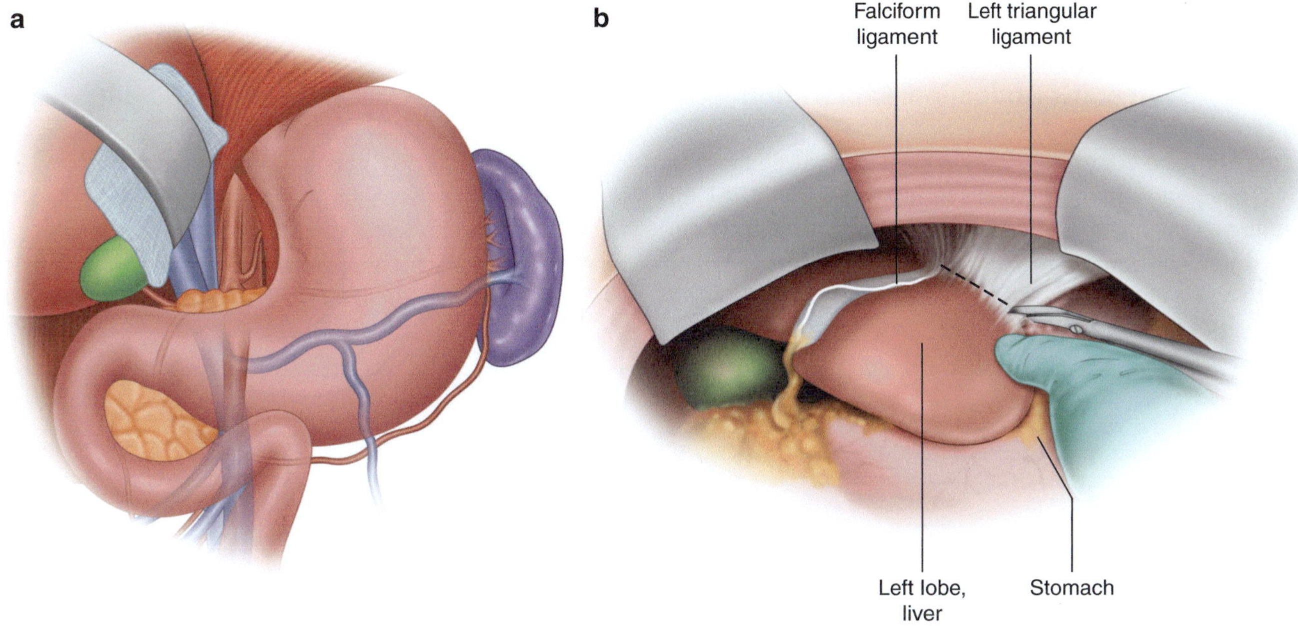

Fig. 24.3 Supracoeliac control of the abdominal aorta (**a**). Exposure of coeliac axis (**b**) is obtained by retraction of the left liver lobe and division of the left triangular ligament

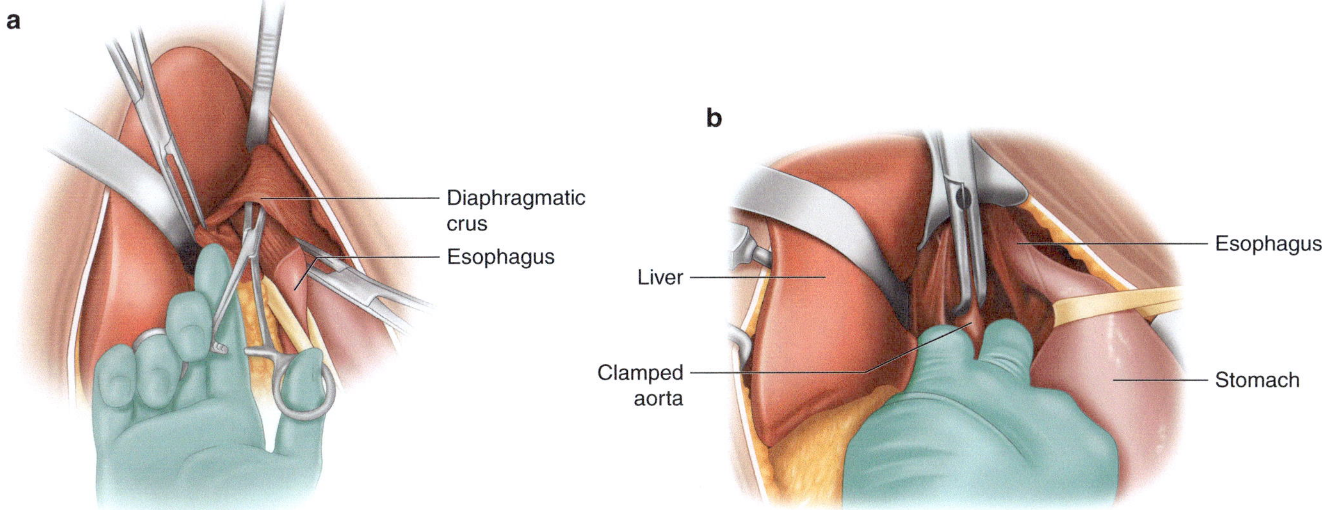

Fig. 24.4 Supracoeliac clamping of abdominal aorta: opening the oesophageal hiatus with a wide incision on the right and left crura of the diaphragm facilitates the subsequent surgical steps

gus and stomach are then retracted to the left. The aorta can then be manually compressed or occluded by an aortic clamp. To insert a vascular clamp on the supracoeliac aorta at the hiatus, the periaortic fat tissue should be cleared. Then the aortic adventitia is cut from either side by blunt dissection. This manoeuvre requires some minutes and can be challenging in emergency above all in patients with high body mass index. In this case, a left thoracotomy in the fifth intercostal space and cross-clamping of the thoracic aorta can offer the advantages to be a faster and more simple procedure in those markedly hypotensive patients with intra-abdominal massive bleeding and impending cardiac arrest.

24.3.3 Systematic Abdominal Exploration

Intraperitoneal control of haemorrhage using packing of all four quadrants should be done in less than 5 min. At this moment systematic abdominal exploration can be undertaken to identify injuries. After control of haemorrhage, the next step is the control of contamination. The intestine is inspected from the Treitz ligament to the rectum, and contamination is controlled initially with non-crushing bowel clamps and if required with simple sutures. Gastrointestinal staplers may be used to resect some devitalized areas. The packs are then removed, beginning in the quadrant farthest away from the greatest source of bleeding. If ongoing non-surgical bleeding continues, the packs are replaced and may be left in the abdomen. All surgical bleeding points should be controlled with suture. Vascular injuries may be treated with vascular shunts, ligation, or extra-anatomic bypass rather than with definitive repair. Ureter injuries may also be treated with temporary stenting during damage control.

All surgeons involved in the operative management of trauma patients must be familiar with the retroperitoneal anatomic zones and exposure techniques [12–18] for each of the following area:

Zone 1 (Fig. 24.5): It begins at the aortic hiatus and ends at the sacral promontory throughout the midline of the abdomen. Zone 1 is subdivided into **supramesocolic** and **inframesocolic**. The supramesocolic portion contains the suprarenal aorta and its major branches, the coeliac axis, the

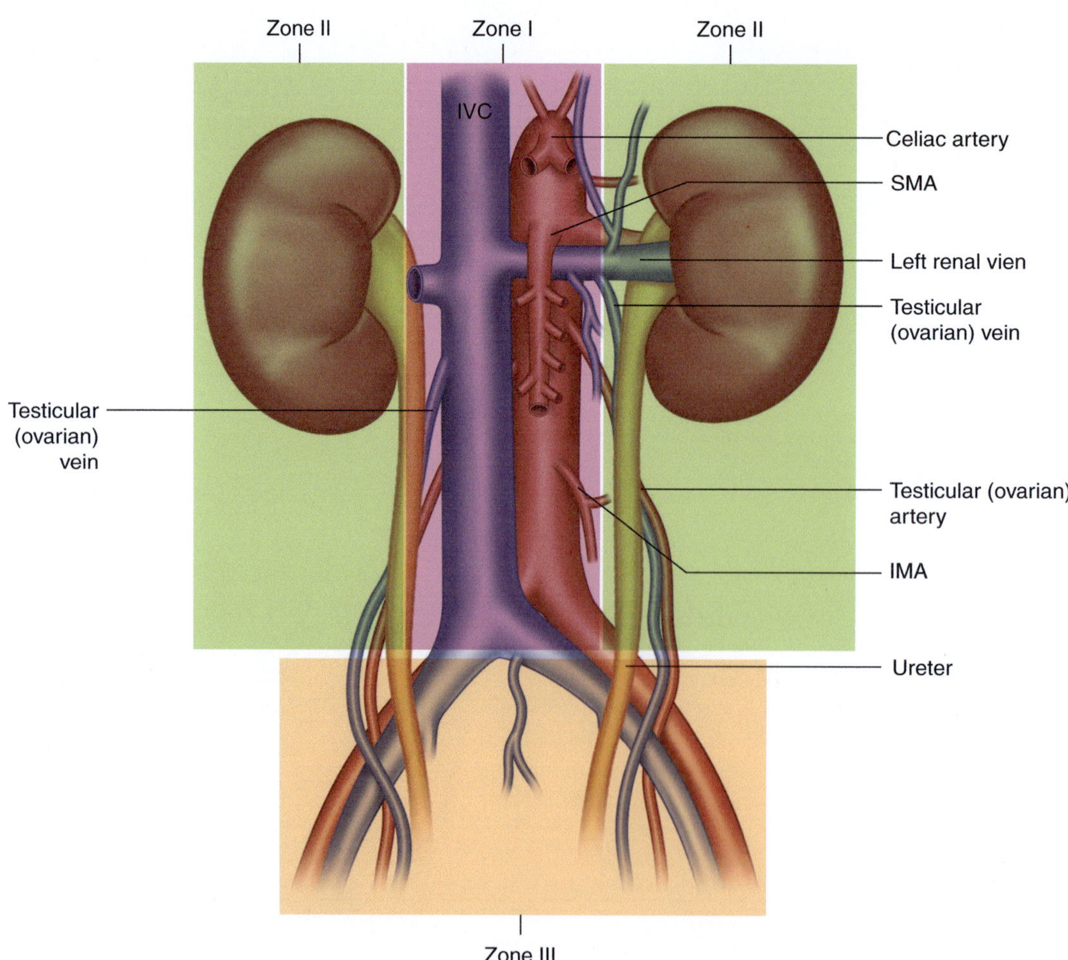

Fig. 24.5 Schematic representation of retroperitoneal Zones I, II and III

superior mesenteric artery (SMA), the renal arteries, the supramesocolic inferior vena cava (IVC) and the superior mesenteric vein (SMV). The infrarenal aorta and inferior vena cava belong to the inframesocolic portion of Zone 1.

Zone 2: The right and left Zone 2 areas each contains the kidneys, paracolic gutters and renal vessels.

Zone 3: It begins at the sacral promontory encompassing the pelvis, the iliac arteries and veins and the left and right ureters.

The retrohepatic region is occasionally referred to as Zone 4 and contains the retrohepatic vena cava and hepatic veins.

Retroperitoneal haematoma caused by a penetrating injury should be explored regardless of the zone, and the one possible exception to this rule is a stable and not expanding haematoma in Zone 4. Otherwise, retroperitoneal haematomas caused by blunt trauma do not require exploration with the exception of blunt injury to Zone 2 and Zone 3 in the presence of a pulsatile or expanding haematoma. The presence of bowel ischaemia necessitates exploration of the associated haematoma.

24.3.4 Mattox and Cattell–Braasch Manoeuvres

These two left side and right side medial visceral rotation manoeuvres provide rapid access to the great abdominal vessels (aorta and vena cava) and their major branches, as well as other retroperitoneal structures (such as the duodenum and kidneys). Both manoeuvres became part of trauma surgeons' common background of experience, and they are based on the same anatomical principle of lifting the intraperitoneal viscera off the posterior abdominal wall and rolling them medially in order to expose the midline retroperitoneal structures. The **Mattox manoeuvre** (Fig. 24.6) is used to gain access to the suprarenal aortic segment which is paramount in the presence of a central retroperitoneal haematoma. The **Cattell-Braasch manoeuvre** (Fig. 24.7) provides access to the entire inframesocolic (or infrarenal) retroperitoneum and has therefore much wider use for different purposes and in various operative situations.

The left-sided visceral rotation first requires mobilizing the lowermost descending colon and incising along the avascular line of Toldt in the left colon and the lieno-splenic ligament (Fig. 24.8). This enables the surgeon to make a blunt dissection behind the left colon and to rapidly mobilize the splenic flexure, left colon, spleen, tail and body of the pancreas and stomach. Note that all these structures are medially rotated: this allows to expose the entire abdominal aorta up to the diaphragmatic hiatus, the origin of the coeliac axis, SMA and left renal artery. In case of a large supramesocolic retroperitoneal haematoma, this manoeuvre facilitates the dissection by lifting the peritoneal organs upward, outside the posterior abdominal wall. The extended Mattox manoeuvre always includes the left kidney medial rotation (Fig. 24.8) which allows full control the abdominal aorta without division of the prerenal fascia with the risk of injury to the left renal vein and the left ureter. The surgeon can achieve

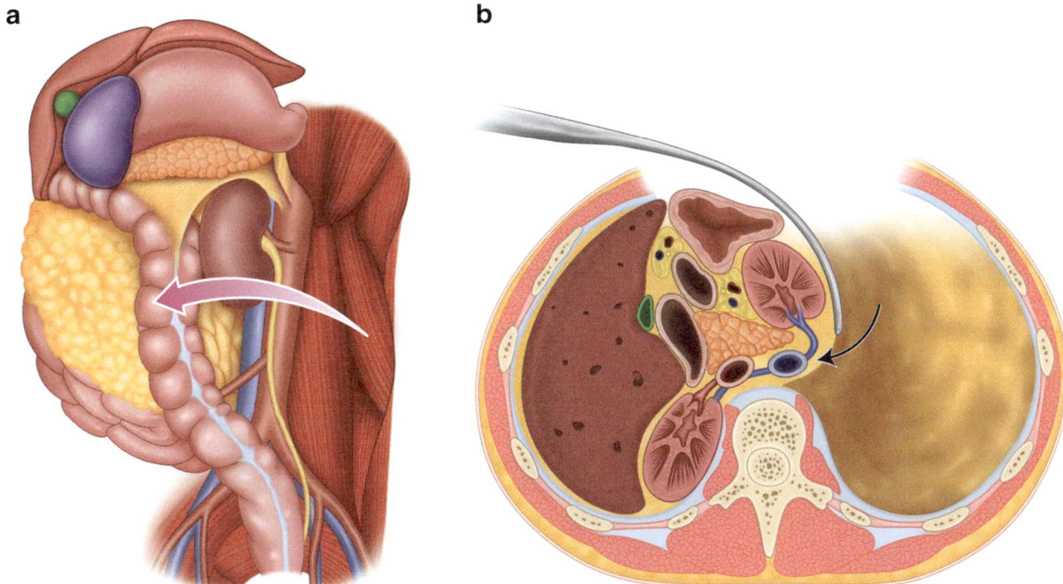

Fig. 24.6 The left-sided visceral rotation (Mattox manoeuvre) is obtained mobilizing the lowermost descending colon and incising along the avascular line of Toldt in the left colon and the lieno-splenic ligament

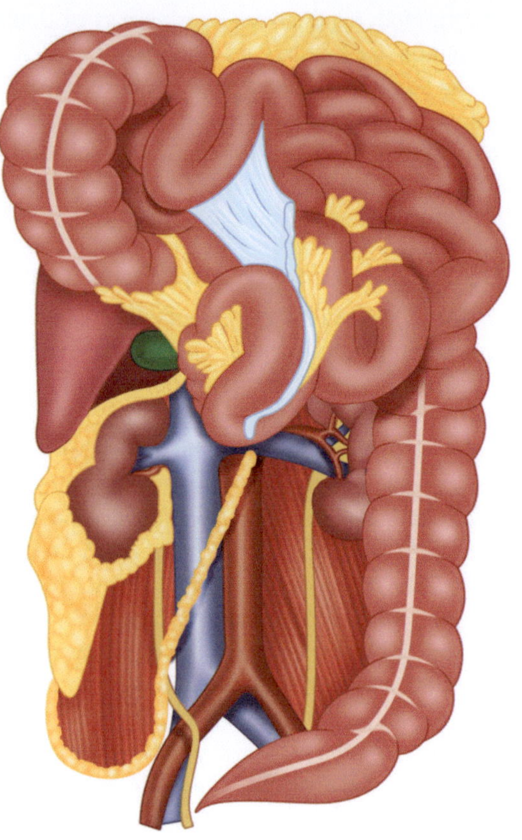

Fig. 24.7 Cattell-Braasch manoeuvre

proximal control of the supracoeliac aorta immediately below the diaphragm or incise the left diaphragmatic crus laterally, bluntly dissecting the periaortic tissue and adventitia and clamping it in the abdomen. The most common complication of the left-sided medial visceral rotation laparotomy is splenic injury, which is usually treated by removing the injured spleen. Other sources of bleeding are avulsion of the descending lumbar vein from the left renal vein and clamp injury causing an aortic wall tear during supracoeliac aortic clamping. Pancreatitis and gut ischaemia related to retraction are rare and late complications that emphasize the need for gentle handling and protection of the rotated viscera. On the right side, the Cattell-Braasch manoeuvre can be divided into three stages:

Stage I: It requires the complete mobilization of the duodenum starting with a Kocher manoeuvre (Fig. 24.9) with the mobilization of the entire right hemicolon including the duodenum from caudal to cranial via an incision of the peritoneum from parietal to visceral and slightly lateral to the reflection. The entire right hemicolon can then be lifted medially, the duodenum is identified and the posterior peritoneum is incised laterally allowing mobilization of the duodenum and the pancreas head. In this way, it is possible to obtain wide access to the right half of the retroperitoneum. Superiorly, the dissection is directed to the level of the *porta hepatis*. This manoeuvre allows access to infrahepatic IVC, distal common bile duct, duodenum, pancreatic head and the right renal hilum.

Stage II: The extended Kocher manoeuvre carries the classic Kocher incision caudally along white line of Toldt

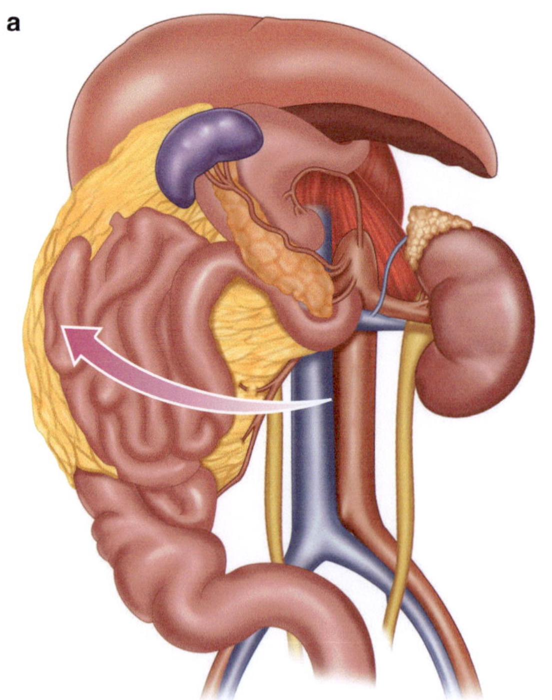

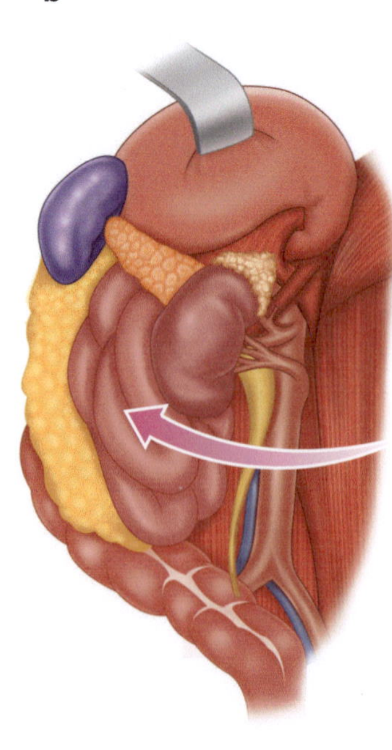

Fig. 24.8 Mattox (**a**) and extended Mattox manoeuvre [8] which includes the left kidney rotation and allows full control the abdominal aorta

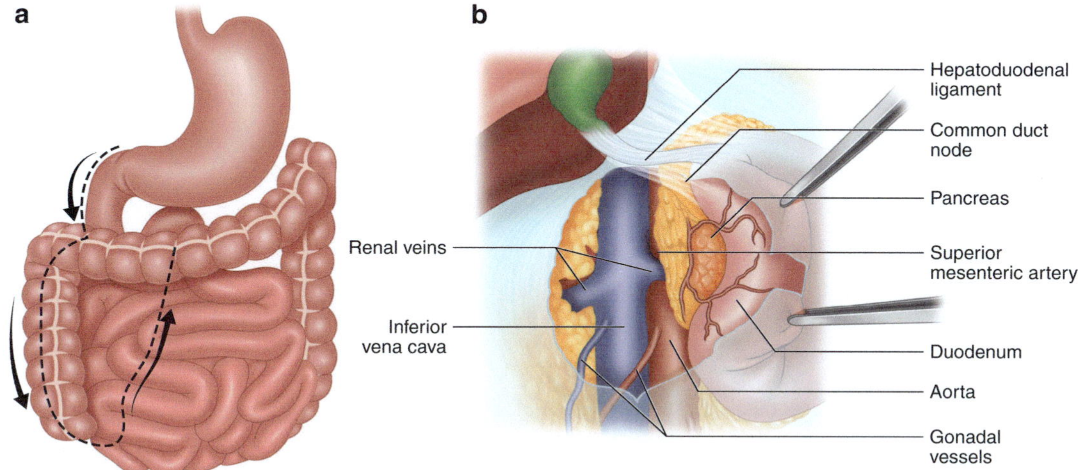

Fig. 24.9 Cattell-Braasch stage I requires complete mobilization of the duodenum starting with a Kocher manoeuvre with the mobilization of the entire right hemicolon including the duodenum. The Kocher manoeuvre reflects duodenum and the pancreatic head from the retroperitoneum, allowing access in the infrahepatic inferior vena cava as well as to the distal common bile duct and the pancreatic head

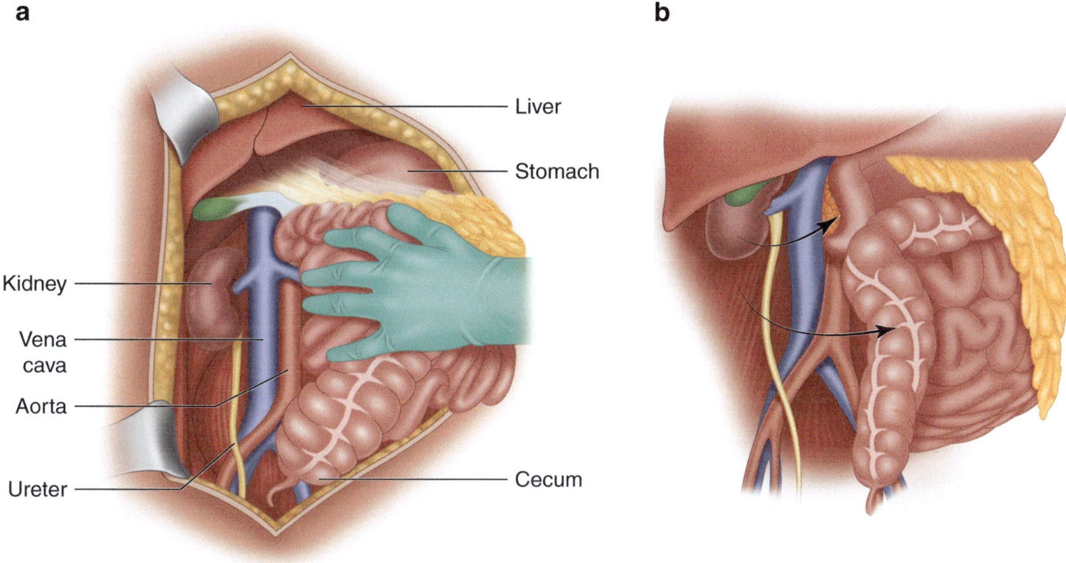

Fig. 24.10 Extended Kocher manoeuvre gives access to the entire infrahepatic IVC until iliac bifurcation, right kidney and hilum, right iliac vessels, right ureter, right iliac vessels

(Fig. 24.10) and gives access to the entire infrahepatic IVC until iliac bifurcation, right kidney and hilum, right ureter, and right iliac vessels.

Stage III: Super-extended Kocher (Cattell-Braasch) manoeuvre (Fig. 24.11)—after the extended Kocher, incise the line of fusion of small bowel mesentery to the posterior peritoneum swinging the small bowel and right colon out of the abdomen. Pitfalls of the Cattell-Braasch manoeuvre are represented by a possible injury to the SMV at the root of the mesentery.

24.3.5 Splenic Injuries

Many blunt splenic injuries may be managed without splenectomy if a careful selection of patients is applied. It is critical that only patients who are stable and have no evidence of ongoing blood loss should be considered for NOM. Splenic angiography and transarterial embolization represent the most recent advances in the evaluation and management of spleen injuries in trauma patients. The majority of trauma centres use angiography to evaluate and often to treat stable

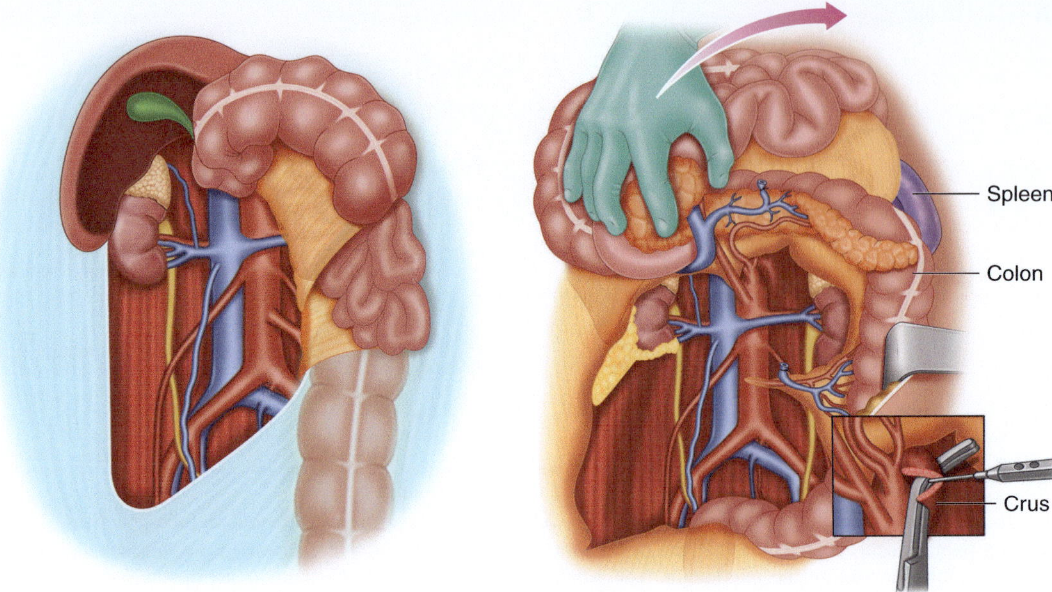

Fig. 24.11 Super-extended Kocher manoeuvre (Cattell-Braasch) after the extended Kocher; incise the line of fusion of small bowel mesentery to the posterior peritoneum swinging the small bowel and right colon out of the abdomen

patients who show active extravasation of contrast medium on CT imaging. Physiologic stability includes normal blood pressure, lack of tachycardia, no physical examination findings indicating shock and absence of metabolic acidosis. Many centres reserve NOM for stable grade I, II and III injuries, with the assistance of angioembolization when the bleeding risk is substantial. Operative management of splenic injuries may be required in the setting of instability at the time of admission, after failed NOM or in the case of rebleeding after a period of stability. A possible protective effect of immediate splenectomy versus NOM in haemodynamically stable patients with traumatic brain injury and coexisting grade III splenic injury has been suggested [19].

Despite the failure rate >25%, the definitive management of splenic bleeding for the majority of patients with grade ≥IV splenic injury remains splenectomy. This approach does not carry a significant operative risk, especially in comparison to the adverse outcomes related to ongoing haemorrhage. Therefore, no unstable bleeding patient should remain without splenectomy. Nevertheless, the majority of patients are no longer bleeding at presentation and do benefit from avoiding an unnecessary operation. Based on the patient's physiologic state, it is usually possible to identify those who have a haemostatic splenic injury and are appropriate candidates for NOM. A midline incision represents the best approach for splenectomy with or without the packing of all four quadrants, depending on whether the patient is unstable or not. An abdominal retractor can improve exposure, and the packs are removed to expose the injured spleen. The spleen is mobilized by dividing laterally the peritoneum along the white line of Toldt by retracting the spleen medially to expose the retroperitoneal attachments. This division of the peritoneum begins by dividing the splenocolic ligament and then continuing cranially until the short gastric vessels are encountered, divided and ligated. A working space by pulling the spleen gently in a medial direction should be created (Fig. 24.12). Then the splenorenal and splenophrenic ligaments are divided. The posterior plane of the peritoneum is now completely opened laterally, extending behind the tail of the pancreas. This manoeuvre mobilizes the entire spleen and the distal pancreas, allowing the spleen to be delivered from the abdomen (Fig. 24.13). While avoiding injury to the greater curvature of the stomach, the short gastric vessels are ligated and divided. The spleen can be removed after ligation and section of the hilar vessels, preventing pancreatic tail injuries.

24.3.6 Liver Injury

Patients with liver injuries who demonstrate haemodynamic stability benefit from a conservative approach. Similar to spleen injuries, most liver injuries may stop bleeding during the evaluation time and in this case do not require immediate operation but instead may benefit close surveillance for indicators of rebleeding and associated complications. NOM of liver injuries has been shown excellent results with a successful outcome achieved in more than 85% of patients. To avoid unnecessary operation in a significant number of patients, the application of a NOM approach for selected patients resulted in a decrease in mortality for liver injuries during the last decade.

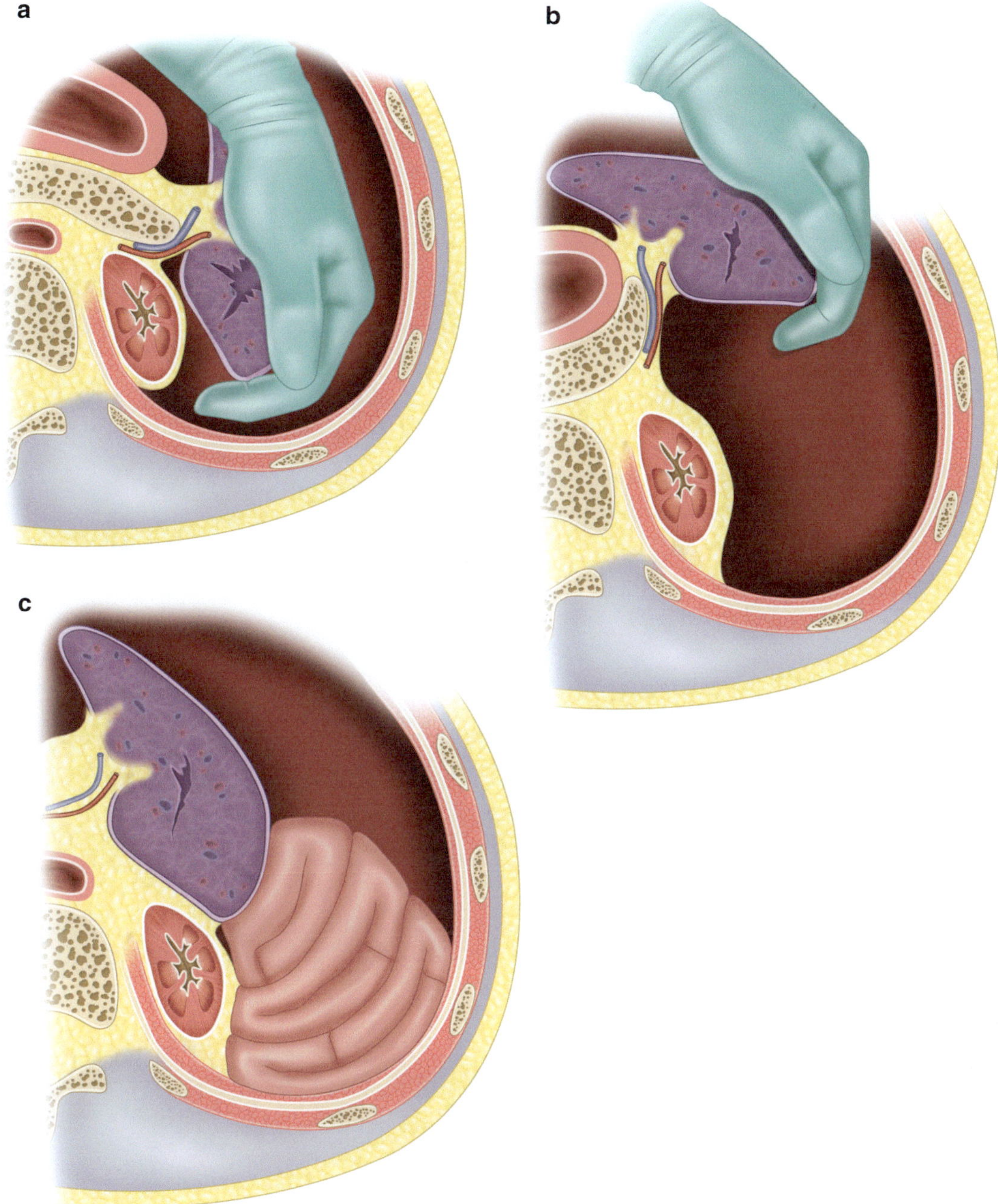

Fig. 24.12 Operative exposure for urgent splenectomy

Dealing with liver injury, two possible strategies are available:

- Option 1, NOM: This can be applied to more than 80% of patients and requires CT scan evaluation + angioembolization if needed + intensive care surveillance + delayed surgery if needed.
- Option 2, immediate surgery: Perihepatic packing + postoperative embolization if needed + scheduled reoperation, if needed.

The main indication for immediate surgery is haemodynamic instability, not the grading of the liver injury [20–23]. If surgical management is urgently required, a midline laparotomy is the most versatile approach. However, in the hypotensive trauma patients with impending cardiac arrest, proximal vascular control with a left anterolateral thoracotomy and thoracic aortic cross-clamping can be considered to avoid sudden abdominal decompression. In patients with massive bleeding from the hepatic dome of the liver or hepatic veins, the midline incision can be extended superi-

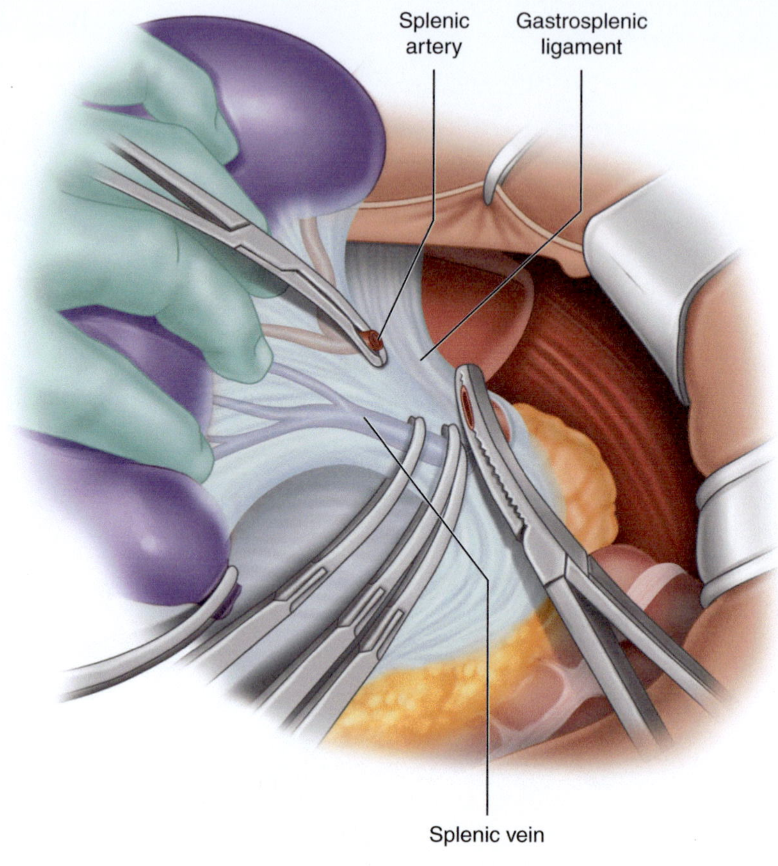

Fig. 24.13 The posterior plane of the peritoneum is completely opened laterally, extending behind the tail of the pancreas. This manoeuvre mobilizes the entire spleen and the distal pancreas, allowing the spleen to be delivered from the abdomen

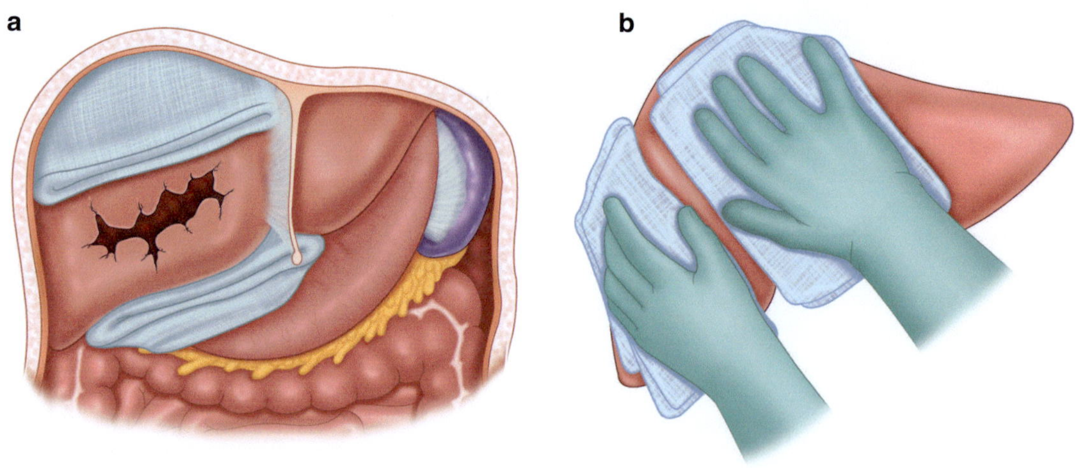

Fig. 24.14 Perihepatic packing and bimanual compression can reduce the bleeding from liver injury and provide extra time for resuscitation

orly with a median sternotomy to get better control of the suprahepatic vena cava. A perihepatic packing and manual sub-diaphragmatic aortic compression can also be useful for temporary control of massive liver bleeding. After laparotomy, the first important manoeuvre is the division of the falciform ligament to obtain a correct perihepatic packing with bimanual compression which can at least reduce the amount of bleeding and provide extra time for resuscitation (Fig. 24.14). In some penetrating injuries with long narrow wounds that bleed from deep within the tract, a Sengstaken-Blakemore or a Foley catheter can be introduced into the wound and inflated with saline until compression is obtained (Fig. 24.15). After perihepatic packing, the hepatic pedicle can be encircled with a tape to be ready for a Pringle manoeu-

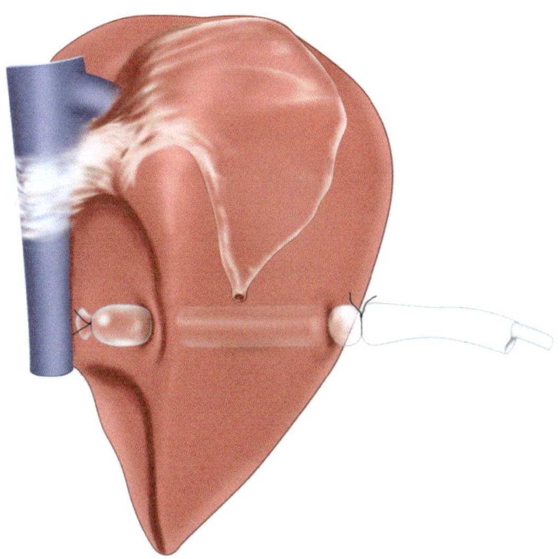

Fig. 24.15 In some penetrating liver injuries, a Sengstaken-Blakemore tube can be introduced into the wound and inflated with saline until compression is obtained

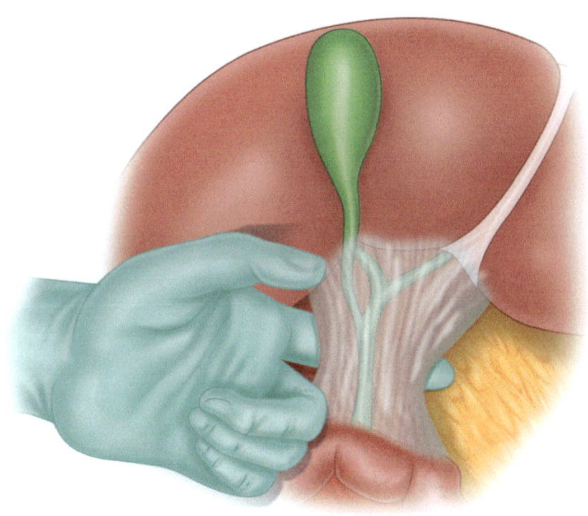

Fig. 24.16 Encircling the hepatic pedicle for clamping (Pringle manoeuvre)

vre (Fig. 24.16). When reasonable haemodynamic stability has been obtained and there is no need for manual sub-diaphragmatic aortic compression, the packs can be removed, and the injuries to the liver are evaluated. Small parenchymal injuries with minimal ongoing bleeding may be managed with topical haemostatic agents or suture hepatorrhaphy. Division of the triangular and coronary ligaments of the liver may offer better mobilization of the right or left hepatic lobes; this can allow visualization of the posterior liver segments. However, these manoeuvres should be carefully considered since the liver attachments can provide a life-saving natural tamponade in case of retrohepatic bleeding. Most liver injuries will require only superficial techniques for obtaining haemostasis. Consider superficial techniques when:

(a) Hepatic compression is effective.
(b) The hepatic bleeding site is anterior and easily visualized.
(c) The patient is not shocked and hypothermic, and he needed no more than five units of blood.

In these cases, direct exploration of the injury and haemostasis should be done. Hepatic pedicle clamping (Pringle manoeuvre) can be performed during haemostasis, and when effective, this slows bleeding. The edges of the hepatic wound can be then gently opened and haemostatic sutures directly placed usually using a 2–0 or 3–0 polypropylene. Closure with large mattress sutures should be avoided. In this case, duration of pedicle clamping should be short; if the clamping time exceeds 20 min, it is clear that the gesture is more complex than anticipated. If profuse bleeding appears, proceed again with bimanual compression and perihepatic packing. Sometimes, a nearly complete traumatic hepatectomy *à la demand* or non-anatomic hepatic debridement can be quickly completed. Anatomical hepatectomy is too dangerous and has virtually no place in emergency liver surgery. When haemostasis can be simply obtained, without haemodynamic derangement or prolonged pedicle clamping, parietal closure can be performed. The anatomic surgical area should be carefully inspected for major bile orifices and widely drained; postoperative bile leaks or biloma should be treated by multidisciplinary approach. Associated lesions conditioning intestinal oedema after hilum clamping or the presence of retroperitoneal haematoma, severe pelvic fractures or serious traumatic brain injury may be good indications for open abdomen or for vacuum-assisted laparostomy to prevent intra-abdominal hypertension and acute compartment syndrome. If hepatic pedicle clamping is ineffective in bleeding control, consider technical reasons for this failure such as the presence of a replaced left artery arising from the left gastric artery. If this is not the case, there is probably a leak from hepatic veins. Only seldom there is a manoeuvre that is feasible and simple for an obvious left hepatic vein tear. Although the hepatic hilum is too short, sometime portal vein injury requires a **double Pringle manoeuvre**, distal and proximal; this can allow a direct suture of the lesion, avoiding the backflow. Liver injuries in the proximity of the retrohepatic vena cava, the so-called big blue haematoma, which are not actively bleeding should be simply packed and not explored. There are many challenging techniques described in the literature that outline the repair of retrohepatic vena cava injuries, but in small injuries, the conservative approach has the greatest likelihood of success. Most often when the patient is bleeding copiously and the lethal triad is developing, the surgeon should remember that liver compression and a **perihepatic packing (PHP)** will control most of venous injuries, even when located high on the liver dome.

If PHP is ineffective and the Pringle manoeuvre does not decrease the bleeding, the surgeon must reinforce PHP by manually compressing the liver, adding more packs, wedged against the kidney posteriorly or against the stomach on the left side. Sometimes in patients with profound haemorrhagic shock who have other injuries, the inflow control via aortic occlusion (either by manual or aortic cross-clamping) can have some advantages. Aortic occlusion above the level of the coeliac axis can markedly decrease the liver flow.

Selective clamping of the right or left hepatic artery is better tolerated than proper hepatic artery clamping. However, selective clamping is rarely a real advantage in severely bleeding trauma patients. Prolonged hepatic arterial clamping implies a high risk of postoperative liver failure and should be considered only in case of arterial reconstruction for concomitant traumatic injury of the hepatic artery. A further option can be **aggressive PHP**, avoiding vena cava compression due to excessive retrohepatic packing, and immediate transfer to the radiology suite with ongoing maximal resuscitation for angiography and **distal hepatic artery embolization**.

In case both aggressive PHP and Pringle manoeuvre may not improve the situation and although the packing the continuous bleeding is too heavy to allow transfer to angiography, there are two procedural options:

(a) Aggressive PHP + closure + warming + maximal fluid resuscitation on the table and reoperation if the situation seems to be improving.
(b) **Supracoeliac aortic clamping** and **total hepatic vascular exclusion**. This is an aggressive but dangerous surgical approach. While one surgeon maintains compression on the liver pushing against the diaphragm, the first operator can achieve a wider exposure of the liver by extending the midline incision on the right side with a transverse incision (two finger's breadth above from the umbilicus) and placing a suitable retractor. **Total hepatic vascular exclusion** may then, theoretically, have a role in such exceptional conditions. Triple clamping without supracoeliac aortic clamping can result in a lethal collapse and should be avoided. The only possibility is a quadruple clamping (Fig. 24.17) as originally described by Heaney which includes concomitant clamping of the

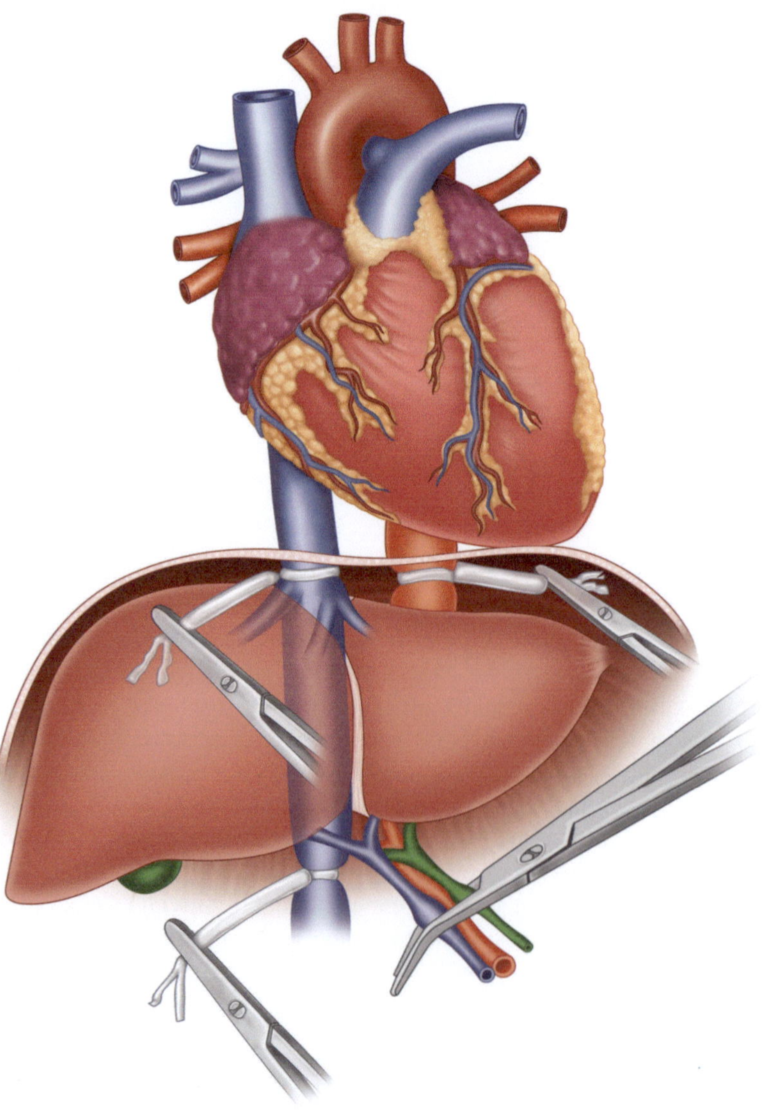

Fig. 24.17 Hepatic vascular exclusion with quadruple vascular clamping

supra-coeliac aorta, followed by clamping od the portal triad, suprarenal IVC, and suprahepatic IVC [24, 25]. The aortic cross-clamping (see Sect. 24.3.2) is essential as a first manoeuvre to avoid cardiac pump depression and consequent cardiac arrest. In the emergency setting, fast **control of the suprahepatic inferior vena cava (IVC)** can be only obtained by intrapericardial IVC isolation through a trans-diaphragmatic pericardial window or extending the midline incision with a median sternotomy. During laparotomy the fast way to control the IVC is by intrapericardial access (Fig. 24.18). The diaphragm is opened from the posterior aspect of the sternum. A small incision in the diaphragmatic pericardium is obtained with the aid of McKenzie forceps avoiding possible injury to the heart. With a clamp protecting the heart, obtain a larger incision on the diaphragm and on the pericardium paying attention to stay on the right side of the pericardium. With a Mayo scissor, free the IVC from pericardial attachments, and place an angled DeBakey vascular clamp on the IVC. To avoid the severe haemodynamic instability when IVC is clamped, there are two other strategic alternatives to supracoeliac aortic cross-clamping: the internal atriocaval shunt of Schrock (Fig. 24.19) and veno-venous bypass without systemic heparinization (Fig. 24.20), technique utilized sometimes in liver transplantation. However, atriocaval shunts and quadruple clamping techniques are reputed to have had more articles written on the subject than patients who have survived the procedure. These patients would probably have been better managed by aggressive PHP. Vascular exclusion with quadruple clamping or emergency percutaneous **veno-venous bypass** (better option with heat exchanger) might have a role in particular centres with experience in liver surgery and transplantation for those rare desperate cases of high-grade liver injury that fail to respond to correctly applied safer protocols of aggressive PHP, pedicle clamping, surgical haemostasis and embolization. **Total hepatectomy**

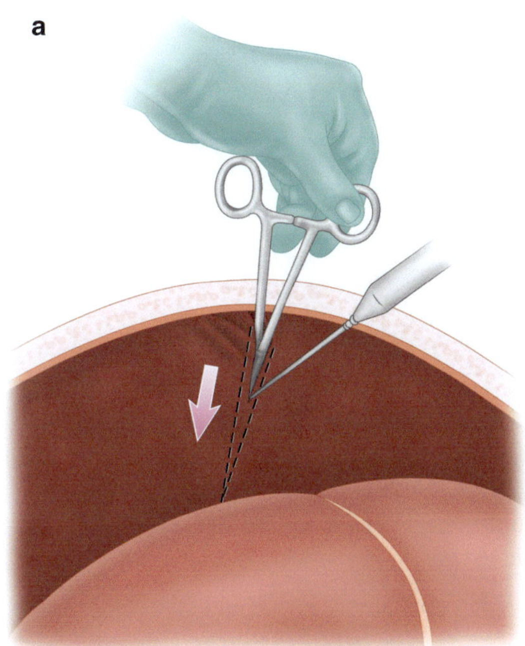

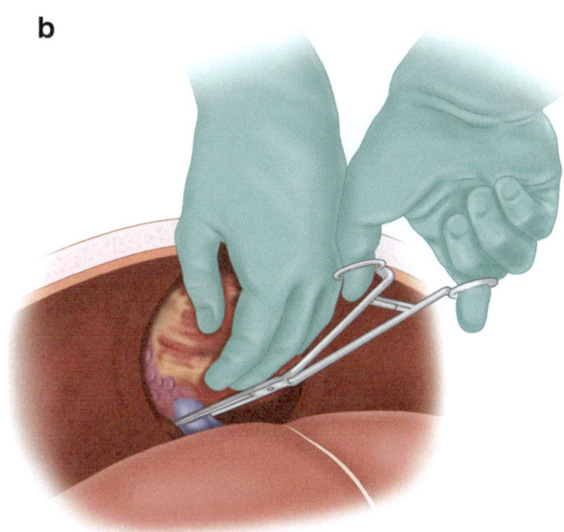

Fig. 24.18 Intrapericardial control of the inferior vena cava. (**a**) The pericardium is bluntly dissected from the posterior aspect of the sternum. A small hole is made in the diaphragmatic pericardium as superiorly as possible. With a clamp protecting the heart, the electrocautery or scissors is used to split the diaphragm and pericardium posteriorly. (**b**) The heart is lifted cephalad and anteriorly; a vascular clamp is placed on the suprahepatic IVC

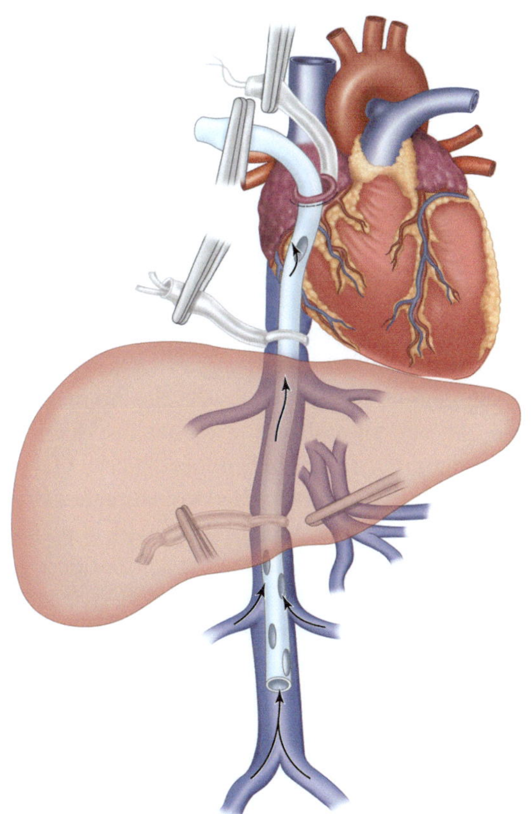

Fig. 24.19 Schrock atriocaval shunt

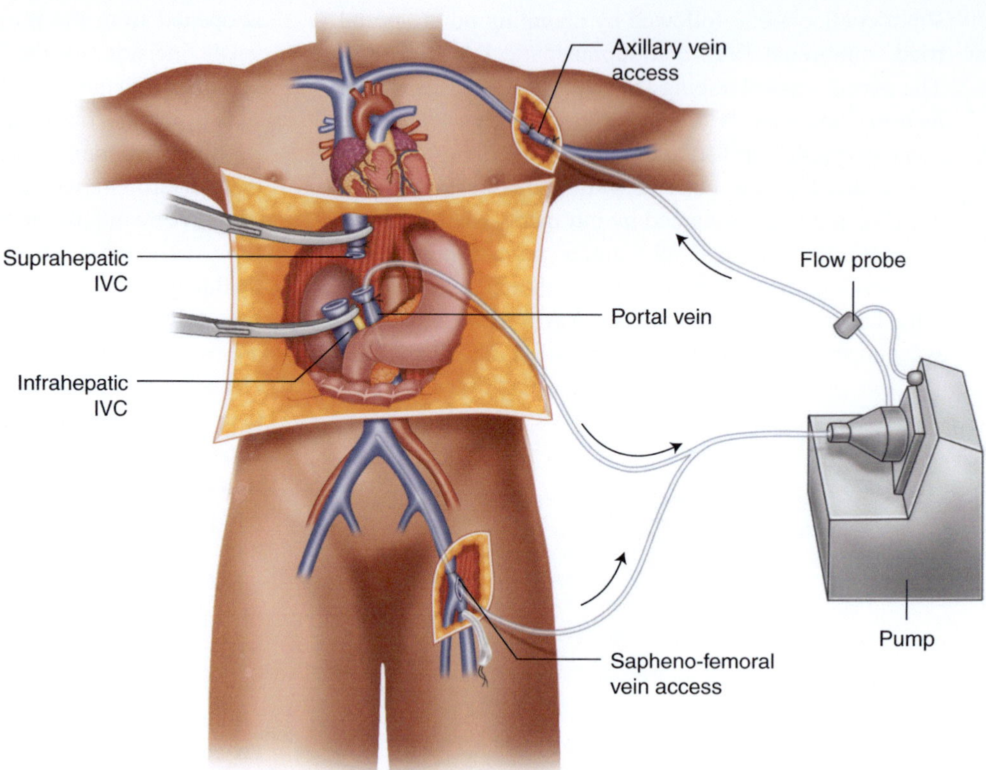

Fig. 24.20 Veno-venous bypass during anhepatic phase using a centrifugal pump

following veno-venous bypass **and liver transplantation** remain the last resort therapy limited to specialized centres. The European Liver Transplant Registry recently reported 73 patients who received a liver transplant procedure for hepatic trauma with a survival rate of less than 50% at 1 year [26].

24.3.7 Gastric Injury

Penetrating mechanisms are the most common cause of injuries to the stomach, and blunt gastric rupture is very rare, usually in relation to an acute increase in intraluminal gastric pressure. The surgical repair of gastric injuries is based on the amount of tissue loss and the injury location. Intramural haematomas should be evacuated with closure in one or two layers of the seromusculature with nonabsorbable suture during laparotomy for other indications. In case of a solitary gastric lesion, this can be controlled to ensure the absence of perforation and bleeding. When perforation is present, the most common approach is to close the perforation with continuous absorbable suture and then to apply a second layer with nonabsorbable seromuscular stitches. A stapler can also be used to close the perforation. Injuries involving the gastro-oesophageal junction, lesser curve, fundus and posterior wall may be more challenging to approach and require a larger exposure of the upper abdomen. Rarely, gastric injuries presenting with large portions of necrotic tissue of the stomach are secondary to acute necrotizing ischaemic injury complicating other surgical procedures; these types of lesions require partial or total gastrectomy with Billroth I or II gastroenterostomy or even a creation of a Roux-en-Y oesophagojejunostomy, depending on the extent of the gastric necrotic lesion.

24.3.8 Duodenal Injury

Duodenal injuries are uncommon after blunt trauma due to retroperitoneal location of the duodenum [27]. Penetrating injuries are prevalent making diagnostic and therapeutic challenges, are often diagnosed in about 90% of cases during laparotomy and are associated with a high mortality rate. The duodenum should be explored if free gas or fluid looking like bile with undetermined origin is found at laparotomy or in the presence of intestinal juice, oedema, haematoma, ecchymosis or crepitus in the periduodenal retroperitoneum or root of mesentery and mesocolon. It requires careful detection of an accompanying injury to the pancreas as well as the bile duct and the ampulla, especially when the second portion of duodenum is injured. The management of duodenal injuries depends on the injury location and the amount of tissue destruction. Haematomas of the duodenal wall will often resolve without intervention and can be managed only if they cause gastric outlet obstruction. Continuous gastric decompression by nasogastric tube and total parenteral nutrition can be the definitive care with a re-evaluation of gastric emptying after 8–10 days. If the duodenal obstruction persists or in the presence of an increase in bilirubin or amylase, endoscopic ultrasound can be considered with subsequent biliary and pancreatic stenting if needed. Operative exploration should be considered in the concern of duodenal ischaemic damage or associated pancreatic injury. Full surgical exploration of the duodenum involves the following steps:

- Perform a Kocher manoeuvre.
- Divide the gastrocolic ligament to allow entry into the lesser sac and inspection of the posterior aspect of the first, the second portion of the duodenum and the anterior surface of the pancreas.
- Divide the retroperitoneum inferior to the pancreas to inspect the posterior pancreas after mobilizing and lifting the inferior edge of the pancreas.
- Expose the third portion of the duodenum with a right medial visceral rotation.
- -Mobilize the ligament of Treitz to expose the fourth portion of the duodenum and pancreas.

Simple haematomas will frequently decompress spontaneously after a nonextended **mobilization of the duodenum**. Duodenal haematomas identified during a laparotomy performed for other causes should not be opened unless there is a concern for severe full-thickness injury or pancreatic-associated injury. Subtle full-thickness injuries can be identified by instilling methylene blue through the nasogastric tube and looking for small leak or duodenal subserosal staining. The majority of duodenal wall perforations can be repaired by **duodenorrhaphy** with a single- or double-layer approach. Complete mobilization of the duodenum with a wide Kocher manoeuvre is required to provide necessary exposure and to ensure a tension-free repair (Fig. 24.21). If the primary closure of the defect may narrow the lumen of the duodenum or result in undue tension and subsequent breakdown of the suture lines, segmental resection and primary **end-to-end duodenoduodenostomy** are advised, especially when the first, second or third part of duodenum is injured.

Duodenal disruption with large amounts of tissue loss should be managed as a pancreatic injury for the high

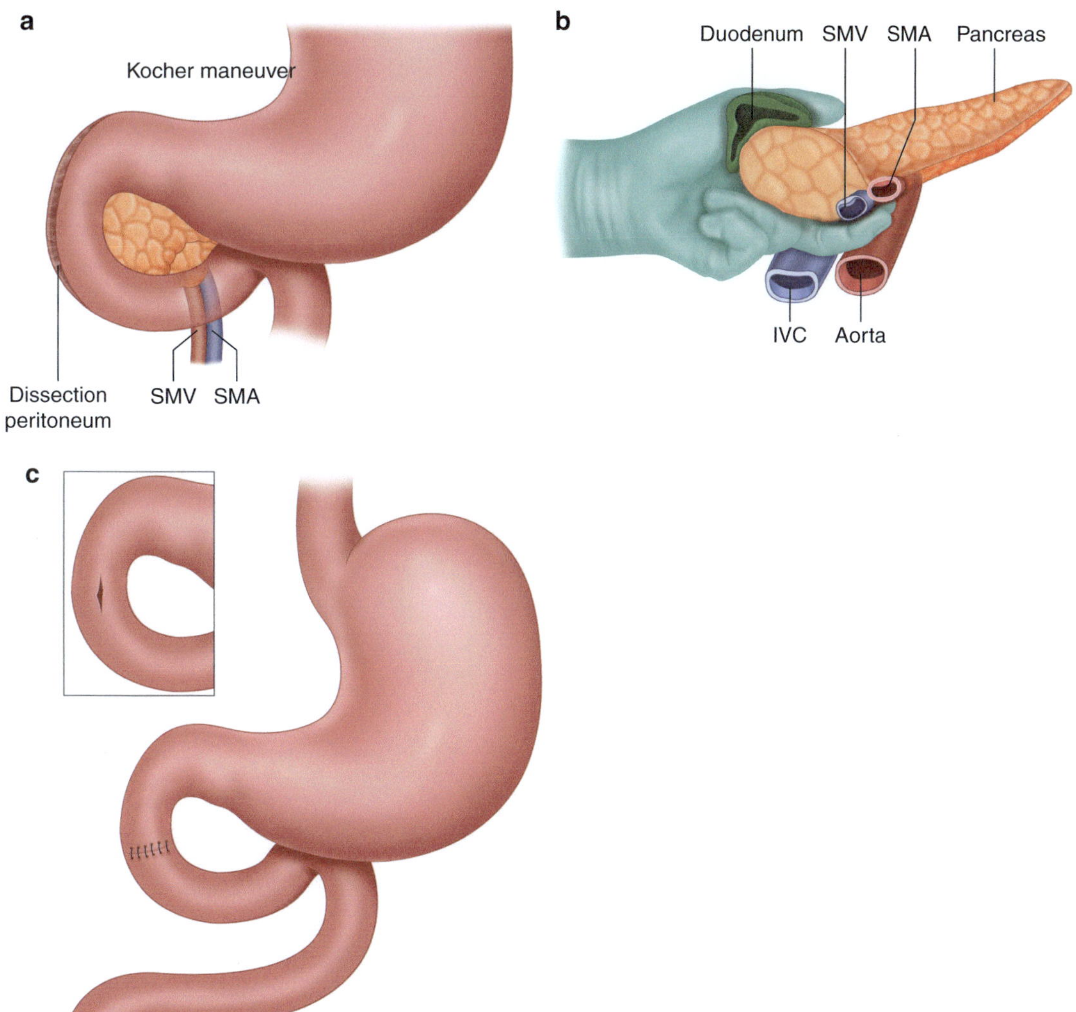

Fig. 24.21 Mobilization of the duodenum with a wide Kocher manoeuvre is required to provide necessary exposure and to ensure a tension-free repair

prevalence of the ampulla-associated lesion. If there is concern about possible stenosis of the ampulla, consider a cholecystectomy with passage of a probe through the cystic duct and the ampulla. Techniques for duodenal repair include simple suture repair, with or without intraluminal decompression, duodenorrhaphy with pyloric exclusion, (Fig. 24.22), duodenal diverticulization (Fig. 24.23) and pancreaticoduodenectomy for the most destructive injuries. In the damage control setting, simple duodenal repair with duodenal decompression with 1-, 2- or 3-tube system (Fig. 24.24) (gastrostomy, retrograde jejunostomy and antegrade jejunostomy for feeding) and pyloric exclusion

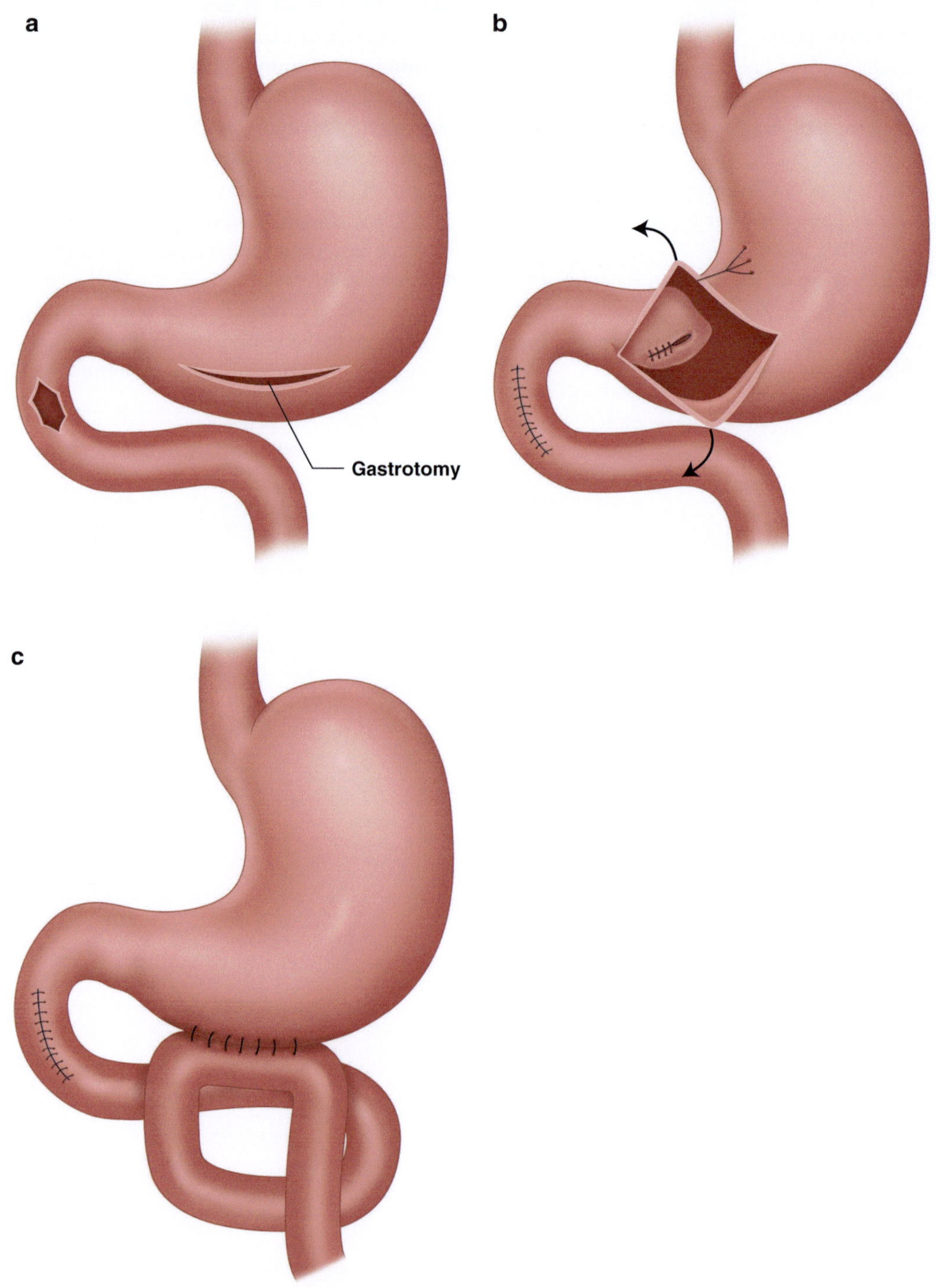

Fig. 24.22 Duodenorrhaphy and pyloric exclusion

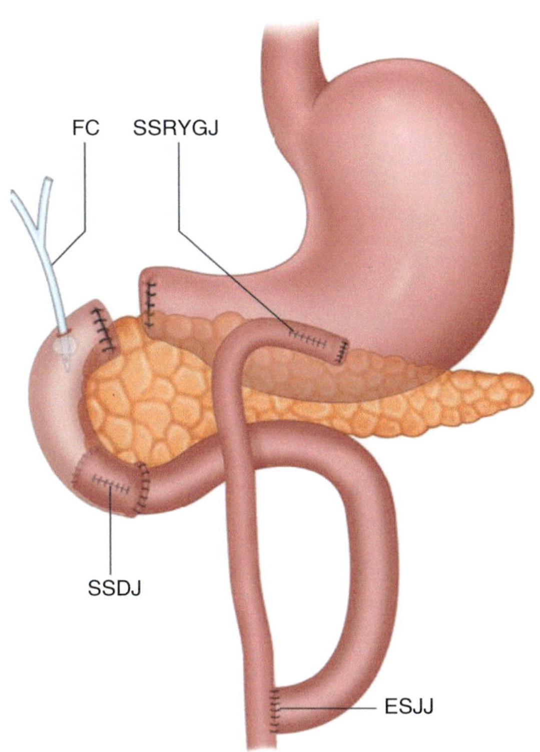

Fig. 24.23 For more destructive injuries of D4 a duodenal diverticulization can be performed with the duodenal resection of the first, third and fourth part of the duodenum. The procedure is completed by a side-to-side Roux-en-Y gastrojejunostomy (SSRYGJ) and end-to-side jejuno-jejunostomy (ESJJ), side-to-side or end-to-end duodenojejunostomy (ESDJ) using the afferent jejunal loop and duodenostomy with a Foley catheter (FC)

are the procedures of choice with comparable results in terms of morbidity and mortality. Duodenal diverticulization that involves the duodenal resection of the first, third and fourth parts of duodenum (Fig. 24.23) has been largely abandoned because of the procedural duration, the relative complexity and the need for healthy duodenal tissue removal. Definitive repair of large segments of duodenal injury requires pancreatoduodenectomy which should be planned as a second-stage procedure.

24.3.9 Pancreatic Injury

Pancreatic injury is seldom seen as a single isolated lesion [28]. Patients who sustain pancreatic trauma tend to have a high severity of illness on presentation with mortality rates reported from 15 to 30% for blunt and penetrating mechanisms, respectively. The identification of pancreatic injuries can be challenging, particularly because available imaging modalities are not highly effective, and in the presence of clinical suspicion, repeated CT imaging might suggest a pancreatic injury since its development is not immediate and radiographically evident following the mechanism of post-injury pancreatic inflammation. The integrity of the pancreatic duct or active pancreatic bleeding determines the course of treatment for pancreatic injuries.

NOM for blunt pancreatic injury should always be attempted if the main pancreatic duct is intact and in the absence of active bleeding. NOM has not been reported for penetrating mechanisms. In this way, patients with low-grade (I–II) blunt pancreatic injuries without disruption of the main pancreatic duct are best managed by conservative treatment. During laparotomy for associated lesions, pancreatic injuries not involving the pancreatic duct, including haematomas, parenchymal contusions and lacerations of the capsule, should be managed with simple external drainage. Operative management is recommended for patients with high-grade pancreatic injuries (grade ≥ III) and involvement of the main pancreatic duct. The use of endoscopic retrograde cholangiopancreatography (ERCP) in the damage control setting is a possible option as a diagnostic supplemental diagnosis and as a therapeutic procedure. Stenting the pancreatic duct, when a lesion at this level has been diagnosed, may be an attractive procedure in a damage control setting. However, ERCP has no indication in patients with multisystemic injuries and should be considered only in haemodynamically stable patients. Surgical management of pancreatic injuries requires exposure of the entire pancreas to evaluate the lesion and to plan the best surgical treatment. Pancreatic exposure includes mobilization of the hepatic flexure of the colon and division of the gastrocolic ligament to retract the transverse colon and mesocolon inferiorly. A Kocher manoeuvre will help to better mobilize the pancreatic head and facilitate visualization. A better and complete exploration of the pancreas requires that the retroperitoneum inferiorly to the pancreas should be divided lifting its posterior edge (Fig. 24.25). The third portion of the duodenum is accessed with a right medial visceral rotation and section of the Treitz ligament. Assessment of the pancreatic injury includes parenchymal involvement evaluation, injury site and presence of ductal involvement. Evaluation of the tail of the pancreas involves division of the peritoneum lateral to the spleen and colon with Aird's manoeuvre. Aird's manoeuvre, originally described in 1955 for adrenalectomy, involves division of the avascular splenic ligaments, splenorenal, splenocolic and splenophrenic, followed by mobilization of the body and tail of the pancreas from the patient's left to right (Fig. 24.26); this allows visualization of the anterior and posterior portion of the body and tail of the pancreas. The manoeuvre provides also exposure to

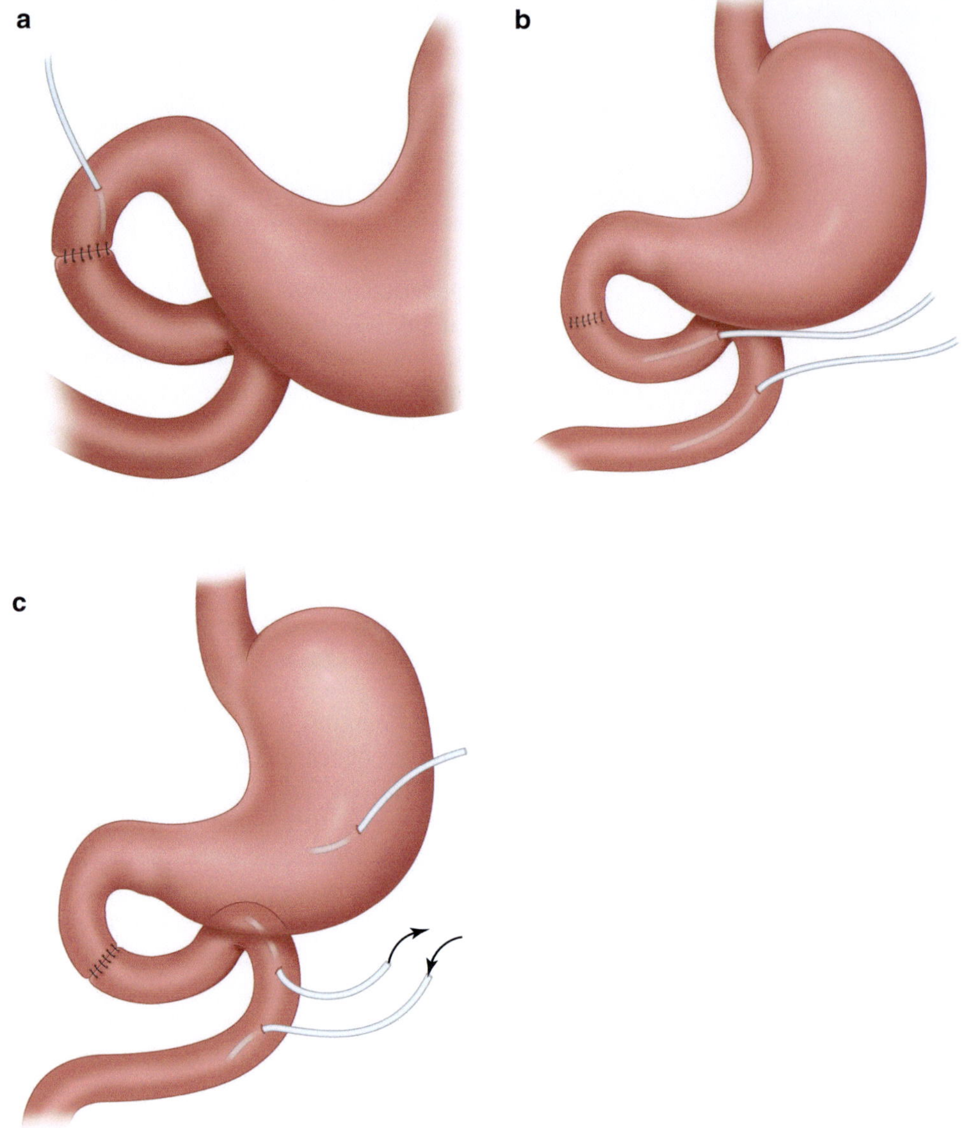

Fig. 24.24 Duodenal repair with duodenal decompression with 1-, 2- or 3-tube system: gastrostomy, retrograde jejunostomy and antegrade jejunostomy for feeding

Zones I and II of the retroperitoneum. Pancreatic ductal injuries to the left of the superior mesenteric vessels are managed with a distal pancreatectomy without splenectomy under favourable conditions. Grade ≥ III injuries of pancreatic body and tail required distal pancreatectomy. The proximal pancreatic stump can be treated by duct ligation and oversewing the parenchyma also with stapling device. Coverage of the suture with a piece of healthy omentum and a closed suction drain should be placed to manage possible pancreatic leaks. Managing injuries of the ductal system within the head of the pancreas can be really a challenging decision. When tissue injury is limited, a simple drainage alone often may divert externally the pancreatic fluid leakage, creating a **controlled fistula** that frequently with the help of endoscopic pancreatic duct stent placement will close in a variable range of time. Biliary and pancreatic stents have become one of the major advances in therapeutic endoscopy and the closure of a fistula may be facilitated by **biliary decompression** through the placement of pancreatic stents during ERCP. Most patients with pancreatic injury and bleeding from multiple associated lesions should undergo an **abbreviated damage control operation** with later reconstruction including control of all the bleeders, adequate external drainage and

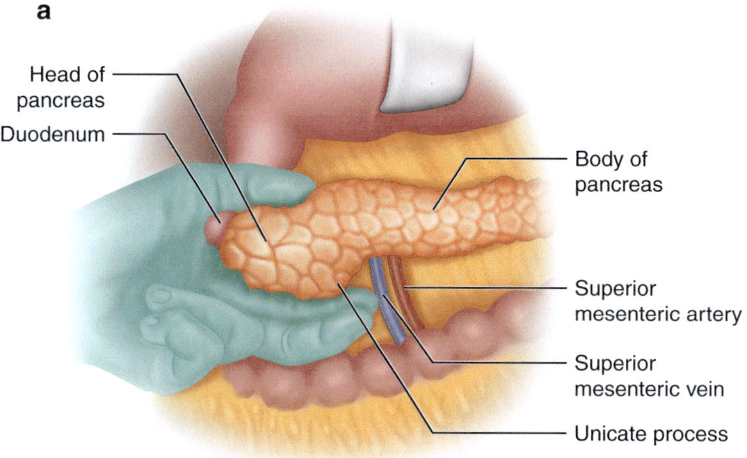

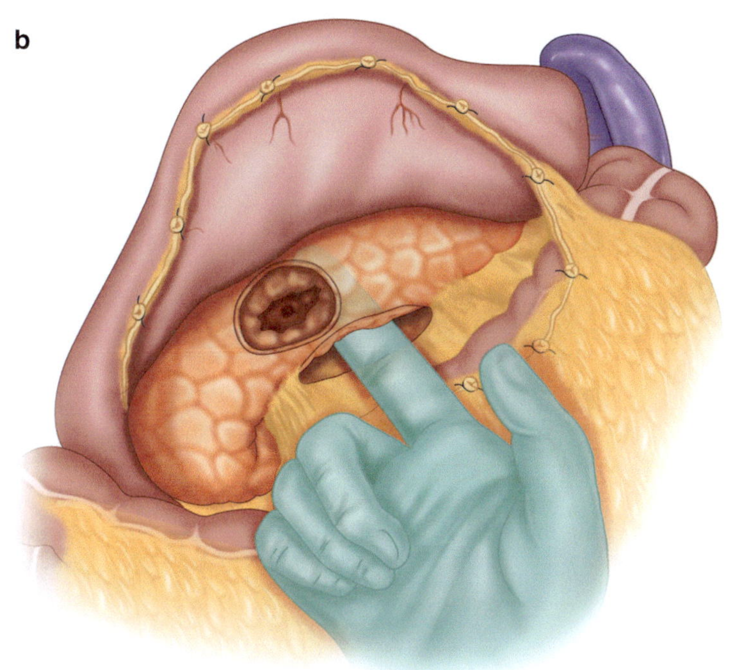

Fig. 24.25 After Kocher manoeuvre (**a**), the assessment of the pancreatic injury includes division of adhesive attachments between the posterior stomach and the pancreas and incision in peritoneum along the inferior margin of the pancreas. The finger is splitted behind to evaluate for parenchymal defects

temporary abdominal closure with a planned strategy for re-exploration. Destruction of the pancreatic head with a large amount of devitalized parenchyma (grade V injury) or combined pancreatic and duodenal injuries may require a **duodenopancreatectomy** which is associated with a high morbidity and mortality rate in the emergency setting and should be planned as a second-stage procedure. Only a few patients with favourable conditions and haemodynamic stability are considered candidates for first-stage duodenopancreatectomy. For complex duodenal and pancreatic head injury, duodenal suture repair protected by proximal tube gastrostomy, drainage of the biliary tree by a cholecystostomy, wide drainage of the region of the pancreatic head and a feeding jejunostomy may be the first-stage procedure, planning a later definitive duodenopancreatectomy. Effective external drainage is an important component in the management of pancreatic injuries. Depending on the patient's clinical conditions, distal enteral feeding access may help to provide early enteral nutrition.

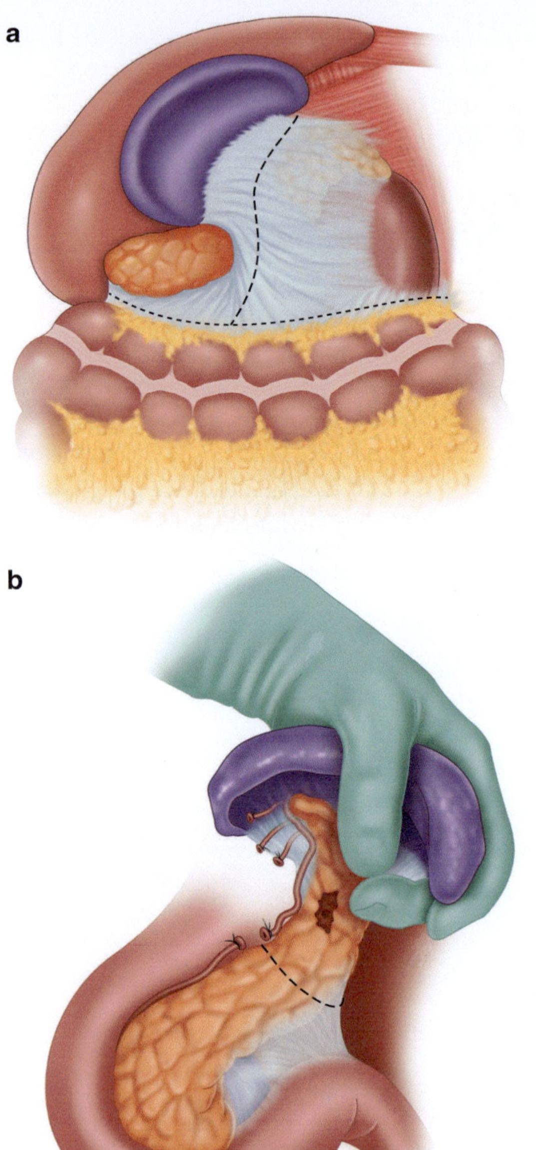

Fig. 24.26 Aird's manoeuvre for evaluation of the tail of the pancreas involves division of the avascular splenic ligaments, splenorenal, splenocolic and splenophrenic, followed by mobilization of the body and tail of the pancreas from the patient's left to right

24.3.10 Small Bowel and Mesenteric Injury (SBMI)

The small bowel is the most frequently involved hollow viscus in abdominal trauma. Injuries occur more often in penetrating than in blunt trauma. Small bowel injuries should be searched in all patients at risk since they are difficult to diagnose and treacherous when missed. The timing of surgery for isolated SBMI depends on the haemodynamic status of trauma victims and accuracy of diagnosis. However, in the setting of penetrating mechanisms, SBMI are often identified at the time of abdominal exploration. The repair of small bowel injuries depends on the amount of intestinal wall destruction in relation to the overall luminal circumference. Grade I injuries are treated by inversion with seromuscular sutures. Grade II injuries are treated by careful debridement and primary closure avoiding to compromise the size of the intestinal lumen. Grade III, IV and V injuries are usually treated by resection and anastomoses. In the setting of multiple perforations, primary repair can still be safely performed as long as the injuries are not at risk of narrowing of the bowel lumen. Many surgeons prefer to perform a resection with anastomosis also in the presence of multiple perforations. No difference in leak rates was clearly demonstrated between stapled and handsewn anastomoses following resection, and the latter is frequently constructed in two layers. Damage control for small bowel injuries includes the rapid closure of perforations to control contamination and resection when there are large injuries. Unstable patients with the need for an abbreviated operation may benefit from resection with stapled closure without immediate anastomosis because of a higher risk of anastomotic dehiscence, and the abdomen is temporarily closed. Only after complete resuscitation the patient returns to the operating room, and intestinal continuity can be re-established. Experienced and skilled surgeons in both **laparoscopy** and trauma surgery may obtain through a laparoscopic approach a correct diagnosis (especially after a stab wound) and treatment (see Sect. 24.3.14). **Mesenteric injuries** can be caused by blunt and penetrating mechanisms. If the blood supply is disrupted enough to lead to the possibility that the viability of a short or long segment of the small intestine is compromised, the affected segment should be resected. Treatment of isolated mesenteric injuries without bowel perforation is dependent on the viability of the bowel. The most critical issue in wide resection of the small bowel is the length of the remaining small bowel. Preserving as much of the ileum as clinically possible and the ileocecal valve may obviate the complications related to the short bowel syndrome.

24.3.11 Colorectal Injury

Colon and rectal injuries occur most commonly after penetrating abdominal injuries and rarely after blunt trauma. After penetrating abdominal trauma, colon injuries are second only to small bowel trauma. Depending on the involved colonic segment, the colon injury and perforation can occur into the retroperitoneum. Rectum injury can also occur in association of severe pelvic fractures with sharp bone fragments that cause a laceration. Colon injuries may first be identified at the time of laparotomy for other associated injuries. The approach to operative repair depends on the extent of the colonic wall injury and the patient's overall condition. Historically, the approach to all colon injuries included resection with the creation of a **colostomy** because anastomotic dehiscence was of great concern. Subsequent experience examined the need for proximal faecal diversion to manage colonic perforations. Several randomized prospective trials have concluded that primary repair or resection with anastomosis can be safe in selected patients, resulting in a leak rate that is not significantly greater than that observed in patients with colonic diversion. Therefore, injuries that involve less than 50% of the colonic wall circumference can be repaired with one or two layers, being sure to imbricate the mucosal edge. Destructive colon injuries that involve more than 50% of the colonic wall should be resected, and immediate anastomosis is possible in many cases. Injuries proximal to the middle colic artery are best managed with a right hemicolectomy and isoperistaltic ileocolic anastomosis. Distal injuries require segmental resection with end-to-end colo-colic anastomosis. In the setting of shock, in patients with multiple injuries, immediate anastomosis should be avoided because of an unacceptably high rate of anastomotic leaks [29].

Depending on the need to abbreviate the operation, colostomy can be created leaving the gastrointestinal tract in discontinuity until the patient has been adequately resuscitated. Delayed primary anastomosis or creation of a colostomy can be performed in a second-stage surgery. Leak rates after delayed primary anastomosis resulted equivalent to those with immediate anastomosis performed in the setting of patients with good haemodynamic stability. Associated significant injuries, underlying medical disease or delayed injury recognition with the possibility of a development of severe peritoneal inflammation may suggest primary repair and colostomy.

Rectal injuries that result in perforation can cause significant contamination, leading to pelvic sepsis. For this reason, surgical management is often required. Rectal injuries are predominantly managed **with faecal diversion** and **presacral drainage** until healing has occurred. After complete healing which can occur in a variable range of time, the colostomy can be reversed. An end colostomy or a loop configuration can be used as long as complete faecal diversion is achieved. **Drainage of the presacral space** by Jackson-Pratt drains has traditionally been a component for managing rectal perforations. Some authors have reported that presacral drainage can be unnecessary, especially in the setting of low-energy, non-military types of penetrating rectal trauma [18]. However, until more definitive studies emerge, one approach is to drain lower rectal injuries that occur posteriorly or laterally because these will likely enter the presacral space and are at greater risk of abscess formation. Rectal injuries that involve more than 50% of the luminal circumference may require resection of the rectum above the injury with the creation of an end colostomy leaving a distal stapled rectal stump as long as possible for further colorectal or recanalization.

24.3.12 Renal Injury

The most commonly injured genitourinary organ in trauma is the kidney with an incidence ranging from 1 to 3% of overall trauma cases. The most important predictor of genitourinary tract trauma is haematuria. CT scan protocol in trauma patients is paramount to include the nephrogenic, vascular or excretory renal injuries. Once the severity of renal injury is determined, the treatment algorithm includes open repair, endovascular intervention or nonoperative management. Low-grade injuries (grade 1–3 lacerations) from blunt abdominal trauma are not often associated with adjacent intra-abdominal organ damage and are best managed with conservative treatment.

Zone 2 retroperitoneal haematomas secondary to penetrating trauma require exploration. For renovascular injuries due to blunt trauma, the diagnosis is also made intraoperatively in the unstable patient. In this case, only expanding Zone 2 retroperitoneal haematomas warrant exploration.

The absolute indications for immediate surgical exploration is a life-threatening haemorrhage from a renal pedicle laceration (artery and vein) that may not be managed by the interventional radiological procedure in those patients with an expanding or pulsatile haematoma, haemodynamic instability and penetrating trauma. In cases of patients that require immediate laparotomy without prior imaging, a "one-shot" intravenous pyelogram may be crucial to evaluate presence of two renal units in case nephrectomy is needed. The midline laparotomy is recommended to allow complete exposure of all abdominal organs. The use of self-retaining retractors is often helpful. Renal vascular control may be performed by two distinct methods:

(a) Via an incision through the mesentery, just proximal to the inferior mesenteric artery identifying and isolating the renal vessels.
(b) By incision of the line of Toldt with rapid mobilization and medial rotation of the right or left colon.

Quick control of the renal vessels is obtained with anterior and posterior bimanual control. The method of choice will depend on surgeon's experience, and it remains controversial whether technique is superior to prevent total nephrectomy rates. Several studies evaluated selective angiography, stent placement and embolization in patients with high-grade renal lacerations who otherwise would not require a laparotomy. Penetrating injuries to the retroperitoneum identified during laparotomy for other associated lesions require exploration and repair. On the right side, mobilization of the right colon combined with extended and super extended Kocher manoeuvre provides excellent visualization of the right and left renal system (Fig. 24.11). Injuries to the renal veins are located anteriorly the renal arteries. The left renal vein passes below the origin of the SMA anterior to the aorta to reach the IVC slightly superiorly to the right renal vein. Exposure of the right renal vein involves medial rotation of the right colon with an extended Kocher manoeuvre, while the left kidney and left renal artery can be better visualized with a left-sided medial visceral rotation (Mattox manoeuvre) (Fig. 24.8). If renal pedicle or suprarenal aortic clamping is necessary for vascular repair, 6 h of warm ischaemia can be considered a safe limit of tolerance for renal salvage. Injuries of the genitourinary system are discussed in different dedicated chapters.

24.3.13 Abdominal Great Vessel Injuries

Major abdominal vascular injuries are usually secondary to penetrating mechanisms, and about 25% of patients with major abdominal penetrating injuries have significant vascular trauma [30]. For this reason, abdominal vascular injuries are often first recognized during a laparotomy performed for penetrating abdominal trauma. The major abdominal blood vessels are predominantly located within the retroperitoneum, with some larger vessels also in the intestinal mesenteries. Exposure of major blood vessels can be particularly challenging for retrohepatic IVC, suprarenal aorta, coeliac axis, proximal SMA, junction of superior mesenteric vein with the splenic and portal veins and iliac bifurcation of IVC. Because of massive associated blood loss, visualization of the vessels can be compromised, making management of these injuries challenging. These injuries are frequently associated with significant ongoing blood loss and haemodynamic instability. In patients with haemodynamic collapse or in cardiac arrest and PEA, **emergency left thoracotomy** with aortic cross-clamping is the only possible manoeuvre (Fig. 24.27). In short, perform a left anterolateral thoracotomy in the fifth intercostal space, retract the left lung anteriorly, feel concavity of ribs as they arch towards the thoracic spine, open the parietal pleura by blunt dissection and perform a blind cross-clamping of the first tubular structure. The technique has been reported more extensively in a dedicated chapter.

In stable patients, contrast-enhanced CT is used to identify the path of the injury and possible involvement of adjacent structures. In some patients the retroperitoneal vascular injury is identified during emergency laparotomy, although further identification of specific injuries depends on the location of the haematoma.

The **key sequence** is always the same: (a) expose, (b) achieve proximal control, (c) explore and evaluate the injury and (d) restore flow. A knowledge of the basic exposure of these structures is important. Haematomas of the infrarenal vasculature or the right renal hilum are exposed with a right medial visceral mobilization, also known as Cattell-Braasch manoeuvre (Fig. 24.7) with a wide Kocher manoeuvre followed by peritoneal dissection and mobilization of the right colon. The dissection is then continued below the caecum and superiorly up the mesenteric root. Retraction of the abdominal viscera superior and to the left will expose the lower midline vascular structures. Basic principles of vascular repair including proximal and distal control of the injured vessel have been discussed in a dedicated chapter. Injuries to the left suprarenal great vessels or the left renal hilum are exposed by performing a left medial visceral mobilization also known as the Mattox manoeuvre (Fig. 24.8). This is achieved by dividing the peritoneum along the entire left side of the abdomen, from above the spleen down to the distal left colon. The plane posterior to the colonic mesentery and to the pancreas is developed, and the abdominal viscera are retracted to the right to expose the superior retroperitoneal vasculature. At this point, three layers can be controlled: (a) the superficial layer with the pancreaticoduodenal complex; (b) the middle layer with the retropancreatic vessels, SMA/SMV and portal vein; and (c) the deep layer with IVC and renal pedicle (Fig. 24.28).

All retroperitoneal haematomas from penetrating trauma should be explored. Haematomas from blunt abdominal vascular injuries which are not actively bleeding may require operative repair or may be considered for endovascular treatment, depending on the nature of the vascular lesion. During laparotomy, the site of retroperitoneal haematoma guides surgical decision making. Zone 1 haematomas require exploration since these frequently involve the aorta or inferior vena cava. An exception may be a haematoma behind the

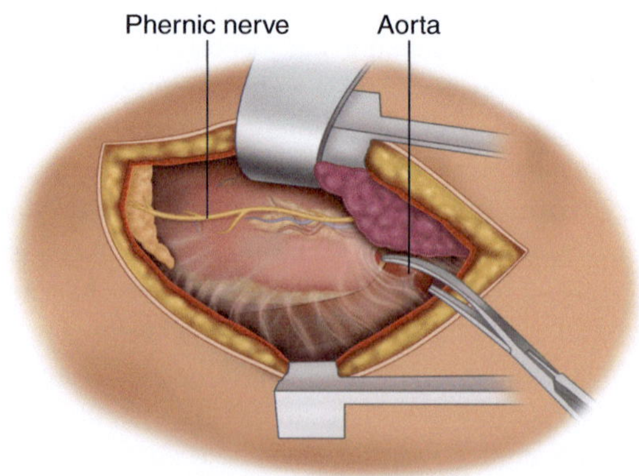

Fig. 24.27 Left anterolateral thoracotomy in the fifth intercostal space and thoracic aortic cross-clamping

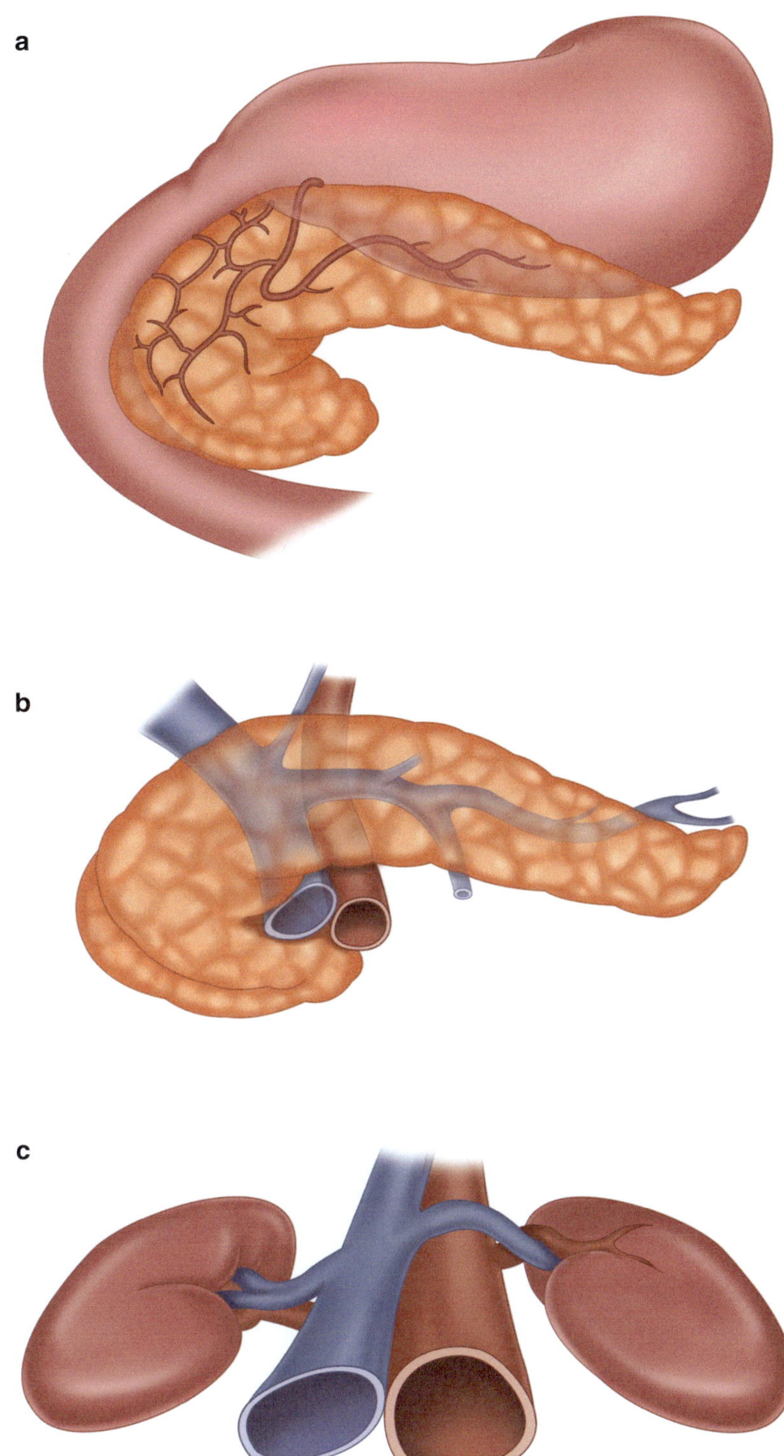

Fig. 24.28 (**a**) The superficial layer with the pancreaticoduodenal complex; (**b**) the middle layer with the retropancreatic vessels, SMA/SMV and portal vein; and (**c**) deep layer with IVC and renal pedicle

liver (Zone 4), which suggests a retrohepatic vena cava injury. Injuries to the retrohepatic vena cava are best treated by gently packing the surrounding area. A haematoma following blunt injury in the Zone 2, which predominantly encompasses the right and left kidneys, should be explored only if expanding. Finally, a haematoma due to blunt trauma in Zone 3 with ongoing instability is usually secondary to pelvic fracture. Bleeding in this zone should not be explored unless there is haemodynamic collapse; in this case a coordinated approach by a multimodal treatment with extraperitoneal pelvic packing, stabilization of the pelvic ring and angiography with embolization may be required. In patients with important haemodynamic instability and in the presence of bilateral iliac injuries, the only way to achieve bleeding control is the total pelvic vascular exclusion: proximal cross-clamping of the infrarenal aorta and vena cava, above their bifurcation, and a distal cross-clamping of the external iliac arteries and veins on both sides.

24.3.14 The Role of Laparoscopy in Abdominal Trauma

Although the level of evidence on the use of laparoscopy in trauma patients is overall poor, this technique has demonstrated to be an extremely useful diagnostic and therapeutic tool, either immediate or interval, since it significantly reduces the rate of negative laparotomies up to almost 90% [31], as well as decreases the rate of postoperative morbidity and allows a faster postoperative recovery with consequent better cost-effectiveness [32, 33]. However, patient selection is of paramount importance in order to safely use laparoscopy in trauma patients. First of all, patients must be haemodynamically stable (ATLS class I–II fully responders to initial small-volume fluid bolus administration) [34]. **Severe brain traumatic injury** [35] and **cardiorespiratory impairment are absolute contraindications** to laparoscopy. Moreover, we do not recommend laparoscopic exploration and opening of the retroperitoneum in trauma patients. Non-expanding retroperitoneal or pelvic haematomas in stable patients should never be explored or the retroperitoneum opened neither laparoscopically nor in open surgery. Haemodynamically stable patients with expanding or pulsating retroperitoneal or pelvic haematomas should be immediately converted to open surgery. Overall, a low threshold for open conversion should be maintained if the surgeon is not confident, in case if uncontrolled bleeding or if missing injuries are suspected [36]. Diagnostic laparoscopy has revealed to be particularly useful in trauma patients with equivocal CT scan findings or discrepancy between the clinical examination and the imaging, the so-called unclear abdomen [37]. Other important indications to diagnostic laparoscopy in trauma patients are:

- Unexplained free fluid with no parenchymal injuries to rule out mesenteric tears and bowel ischaemia [38].
- Penetrating injuries with uncertain peritoneal violation [39].
- Suspected diaphragmatic injury (penetrating or blunt) [40].
- Penetrating trauma to exclude intra-abdominal injuries [41].
- Penetrating injuries with evisceration to rule out visceral injuries [42].

Either in case of CT-diagnosed abdominal injuries or positive diagnostic laparoscopy, in the presence of a highly skilled and experienced laparoscopic trauma surgeon, most of the intraperitoneal traumatic lesions can be treated laparoscopically [33, 43]. In case of hollow viscus injuries, according to the extent of the disruption, a primary intracorporeal suture or resection and anastomosis can be performed. Diaphragmatic tears can be intracorporeally sutured and in case of gallbladder tear or avulsion laparoscopic cholecystectomy can be performed. Some complex pelvic trauma with perineal injuries and/or rectal perforation may benefit from a laparoscopic stoma formation to divert the transit and allow better healing.

The main indications to laparoscopic splenectomy for trauma include [44]:

- **High-grade splenic injury** in >40-year-old patients.
- Unavailable, failed or contraindicated angioembolization, such as in socially or mentally impaired or nephropathic patients, or in case of urgent orthopaedic surgery required.

The main risk related to the use of laparoscopy in trauma is the rate of missed injuries and delayed surgical treatment. However, this rate is significantly lower if the surgeon is experienced and skilled [45].

References

1. American College of Surgeons Committee on Trauma. Resources for the optimal care of the injured patient. 6th ed. Chicago: American College of Surgeons; 2014.
2. Jensen SD, Cotton BA. Damage control laparotomy in trauma. Br J Surg. 2017;104:959–61.
3. Peitzman A, Schwab CW, Fabian TC, Rhodes M, Yealy DM. The trauma manual: trauma and acute care surgery. Philadelphia: Lippincott Williams & Wilkins; 2013.
4. Scalea Thomas M. Resuscitation maneuvers for "extremis". In: Ivatury RR, editor. Operative techniques for severe liver injury. New York: Springer; 2015. p. 29–34.
5. Germanos S, Gourgiotis S, Villias C, Bertucci M, Dimopoulos N, Salemis N. Damage control surgery in the abdomen: an approach for the management of severe injured patients. Int J Surg. 2008;6(3):246–52.
6. Cimbanassi S, Chiara O, Leppaniemi A, et al. Non-operative management of abdominal solid organ injuries following blunt trauma in adults: results from an international consensus conference. J Trauma Acute Care Surg. 2018;84(3):517–31.
7. Di Saverio S, Tugnoli G, Catena F, Ansaloni L, Naidoo N, editors. Trauma surgery, thoracic and abdominal trauma, vol. 2. Milan: Springer; 2014.
8. Scalea TM, editor. The shock trauma manual of operative techniques. New York: Springer; 2015.
9. Mattox KL, Feliciano DV, Moore EE. Trauma. 7th ed. New York: McGraw-Hill; 2012.
10. Kinoshita T, Yamakawa K, Matsuda H, et al. The survival benefit of a novel trauma workflow that includes immediate whole-body computed tomography, surgery, and interventional radiology, all in one

trauma resuscitation room: a retrospective historical control study. Ann Surg. 2017. https://doi.org/10.1097/SLA.0000000000002527.
11. Loggers SAI, Koedam TWA, Giannakopoulos GF, Vandewalle E, Erwteman M, Zuidema WP. Definition of hemodynamic stability in blunt trauma patients: a systematic review and assessment amongst Dutch trauma team members. Eur J Trauma Emerg Surg. 2017;43(6):823–33. https://doi.org/10.1007/s00068-016-0744-8. Epub 2016 Nov 30.
12. Velmahos GC, Degiannis E, Doll D, editors. Penetrating trauma a practical guide on operative technique and peri-operative management. 2nd ed. Berlin: Springer; 2017.
13. Cioffi W, Asensio JA, editors. Atlas of trauma/emergency surgical techniques. Philadelphia: Elsevier; 2014.
14. Britt LD, Barie PS, Peitzman AB, Jurkovich G, editors. Acute care surgery. Philadelphia: Lippincott Williams & Wilkins; 2012.
15. Kozar RA, Feliciano DV, Moore EE, et al. Western Trauma Association/critical decisions in trauma: operative management of adult blunt hepatic trauma. J Trauma. 2011;71:1–5.
16. Brenner M, Hicks C. Major Abdominal Trauma. Emerg Med Clin North Am. 2018;36:149–60.
17. Brenner M, Hoehn M, Pasley J, et al. Basic endovascular skills for trauma course: bridging the gap between endovascular techniques and the acute care surgeon. J Trauma Acute Care Surg. 2014;77:286–91.
18. Johnsen NV, Betzold RD, Guillamondegui OD, Dennis BM, Stassen NA, Bhullar I, Ibrahim JA. Surgical management of solid organ injuries. Surg Clin N Am. 2017;97:1077–105.
19. Alabbasi T, Nathens AB, Tien H. Blunt splenic injury and severe brain injury: a decision analysis and implications for care. Can J Surg. 2015;58(Suppl 3):S108–17.
20. Ivatury RR. Operative techniques for severe liver injury. New York: Springer; 2014.
21. Peitzman AB, Marsh JW. Advanced operative techniques in the management of complex liver injury. J Trauma Acute Care Surg. 2012;73:765–70.
22. Asensio JA, Roldan G, Petrone P, et al. Operative management and outcomes in 103 AAST-OIS grades IV and V complex hepatic injuries: trauma surgeons still need to operate, but angioembolization helps. J Trauma. 2003;54:647–53, discussion 653–654.
23. Demetriades D, Gomez H, Chahwan S, et al. Gunshot injuries to the liver: the role of selective nonoperative management. J Am Coll Surg. 1998;188:343.
24. Burch JM, Feliciano DV, Mattox KL. The atriocaval shunt. Facts and fiction. Ann Surg. 1988;207:555–68.
25. Hansen CJ, Bernadas C, West MA, et al. Abdominal vena caval injuries: outcomes remain dismal. Surgery. 2000;128:572.
26. Letoublon C, Amariutei A, Taton N, Lacaze L, Abba J, Risse O, Arvieux C. Management of blunt hepatic trauma. J Visc Surg. 2016;153:33–43.
27. García Santos E, Soto Sánchez A, Verde JM, Marini CP, Asensio JA, Petrone P. Duodenal injuries due to trauma: review of the literature. Cir Esp. 2015;93:68–74.
28. Lahiri R, Bhattacharya S. Pancreatic trauma. Ann R Coll Surg Engl. 2013;95:241–5.
29. Gonzalez RP, Falimirski ME, Holevar MR. The role of presacral drainage in the management of penetrating rectal injuries. J Trauma. 1998;45:656–61.
30. Kobayashi LM, Costantini TW, Hamel MG, et al. Abdominal vascular trauma. Trauma Surg Acute Care Open. 2016;1:e000015. https://doi.org/10.1136/tsaco-2016-000015.
31. Johnson JJ, Garwe T, Raines AR, et al. The use of laparoscopy in the diagnosis and treatment of blunt and penetrating abdominal injuries: 10-year experience at a level 1 trauma center. Am J Surg. 2013;205:317–20.
32. Lim KH, Chung BS, Kim JY, Kim SS. Laparoscopic surgery in abdominal trauma: a single center review of a 7-year experience. World J Emerg Surg. 2015;10:16.
33. Chakravartty S, Sarma DR, Noor M, Panagiotopoulos S, Patel AG. Laparoscopy has a therapeutic role in the management of abdominal trauma: a matched-pair analysis. Int J Surg. 2017;44:21–5.
34. Khubutiya MS, Yartsev PA, Guliaev AA, Levitsky VD, Tlibekova MA. Laparoscopy in blunt and penetrating abdominal trauma. Surg Laparosc Endosc Percutan Tech. 2013;23(6):507–12.
35. Marks JM, Youngelman DF, Berk T. Cost analysis of diagnostic laparoscopy vs laparotomy in the evaluation of penetrating abdominal trauma. Surg Endosc. 1997;11:272–6.
36. Taner AS, Topgul K, Kucukel F, et al. Diagnostic laparoscopy de- creases the rate of unnecessary laparotomies and reduces hospital costs in trauma patients. J Laparoendosc Adv Surg Tech. 2001;11:207–11.
37. Uranues S, Dorr K. Laparoscopy in abdominal trauma. Eur J Trauma Emerg Surg. 2010;36:19–24.
38. Kamine TH, Elmadhun NY, Kasper EM, Papavassiliou E, Schneider BE. Abdominal insufflation for laparoscopy increases intracranial and intrathoracic pressure in human subjects. Surg Endoscopy. 2016;30:4029–32.
39. Matsevych O, Koto M, Balabyeki M, Aldous C. Trauma laparoscopy: when to start and when to convert? Am J Surg. 2015;210:326–33.
40. Lin H, Chen Y, Lin K, et al. Laparoscopy decreases the laparotomy rate for hemodynamically stable patients with blunt hollow viscus and mesenteric injuries. Am J Surg. 2015;210:326–33.
41. Miles EJ, Dunn E, Howard D, Mangram A. The role of laparoscopy in penetrating abdominal trauma. JSLS. 2004;8:304–9.
42. Stefanidis D, Richardson WS, Chang L, Earle DB, Fanelli RD. The role of diagnostic laparoscopy for acute abdominal conditions: an evidence based review. Surg Endosc. 2009;23:16–23.
43. Matsevych OY, Koto MZ, Motilall SR, Kumar N. The role of laparoscopy in management of stable patients with penetrating abdominal trauma and organ evisceration. J Trauma Acute Care Surg. 2016;81:307–11.
44. Zafar SN, Onwugbufor MT, Hughes K, et al. Laparoscopic surgery for trauma: the realm of therapeutic management. Am J Surg. 2015;209:627–32.
45. O'Malley E, Boyle E, O'Callaghan A, et al. Role of laparoscopy in penetrating abdominal trauma: a systematic review. World J Surg. 2013;37:113–22.

25 Current Management of Urinary Tract Injuries

Nicolaas Lumen and Florence Desmidt

Key Points

- Hematuria is a predominant clinical sign of injury to the urinary tract.
- Except for high-grade renal injury, injury to the urinary tract is seldom directly life-threatening.
- Conservative management is safe for stable renal injuries.
- Diagnosis of ureteral injury is often delayed.
- Urinary diversion (transurethral catheter or suprapubic catheter) is the cornerstone in the management of extraperitoneal bladder injuries and urethral injuries.
- Intraperitoneal bladder injuries require surgical repair of the bladder rupture.
- Testicular ruptures require surgical repair.

25.1 Renal Trauma

25.1.1 Etiology and Epidemiology

The kidney(s) are involved in 1–5% of all trauma cases [1] and account for 24% of traumatic abdominal solid organ injuries [2].

Blunt renal injury is most commonly due to traffic road accidents, followed by falls and sports injuries [1]. Gunshot and stab wounds represent the most common causes of **penetrating** injuries and are usually more severe. In urban settings, where more violence prevails, the percentage of penetrating injuries may be as high as 20% or more [3, 4]. Bullets have the potential for more parenchymal damage and are frequently associated with other organ injuries [5].

The classification system of the American Association for the Surgery of Trauma (AAST) [6] (Table 25.1) is important as it guides further management.

Table 25.1 AAST renal injury grading scale

Grade[a]	Description of injury
1	Contusion or non-expanding subcapsular hematoma
	No laceration
2	Non-expanding perirenal hematoma
	Cortical laceration <1 cm deep without extravasation
3	Cortical laceration >1 cm without urinary extravasation
4	Laceration: through corticomedullary junction into collecting system *or* Vascular: segmental renal artery or vein injury with contained hematoma, or partial vessel laceration, or vessel thrombosis
5	Laceration: shattered kidney *or* Vascular: renal pedicle or avulsion

[a]Advance one grade for bilateral injuries up to grade III

25.1.2 Diagnosis

25.1.2.1 Clinical Features and Examination

A stab wound or bullet entrance/exit wound in the lower thoracic back, flank, or upper abdomen should raise suspicion for a penetrating injury. Blunt trauma with flank pain, ecchymosis, and/or fractured floating ribs suggests kidney involvement [1]. **Hematuria** is often present but does not predict the severity of the injury and is not specific as other injuries at the urogenital tract may also cause hematuria [7]. **Hemodynamic status** must be checked by measuring blood pressure and heart frequency.

N. Lumen (✉)
Department of Urology, Ghent University Hospital, Ghent, Belgium
e-mail: nicolaas.lumen@uzgent.be

F. Desmidt
Department of Urology, Gronau St. Antonius Hospital, Gronau, Germany

P. Aseni et al. (eds.), *Operative Techniques and Recent Advances in Acute Care and Emergency Surgery*,
https://doi.org/10.1007/978-3-319-95114-0_25

25.1.2.2 Further Diagnostics

Laboratory Findings

Perform **urinalysis**, **hematocrit,** and **baseline creatinine** measurement. To diagnose microscopic hematuria, urine dipstick is a very rapid test, but up to 10% is false negative. Serial blood tests with hematocrit determination are important to evaluate the rate of blood loss. Continuous decrease in hematocrit can also be due to associated injuries. Baseline creatinine is used to screen for preexisting renal pathology and renal insufficiency [1].

Imaging

Although abdominal ultrasonography is widely used to screen for the presence of hemoperitoneum, it is not an appropriate tool in the diagnosis of renal trauma. In unstable patients not able to undergo preoperative imaging, an intraoperative single-shot intravenous urography (plain X-ray 10 min after 2 mg/kg of intravenous contrast injection) remains a useful technique to confirm the presence of a functioning contralateral kidney [8]. In stable patients, multiphase contrast-enhanced **computed tomography (CT)** is the preferred imaging modality. Grade of renal injury, presence of a functional contralateral kidney, and concomitant injuries can be adequately assessed [9] (Fig. 25.1). The arterial phase assesses vascular injury and presence of active contrast extravasation. The venous phase reveals parenchymal contusions and lacerations. The delayed phase is used to screen for injury to the collecting system (and ureter) [10]. However, multiphase imaging in the multitrauma patient is not routinely performed. If the renal injury cannot be adequately diagnosed, repeat imaging should be performed if the condition of the patient allows for it.

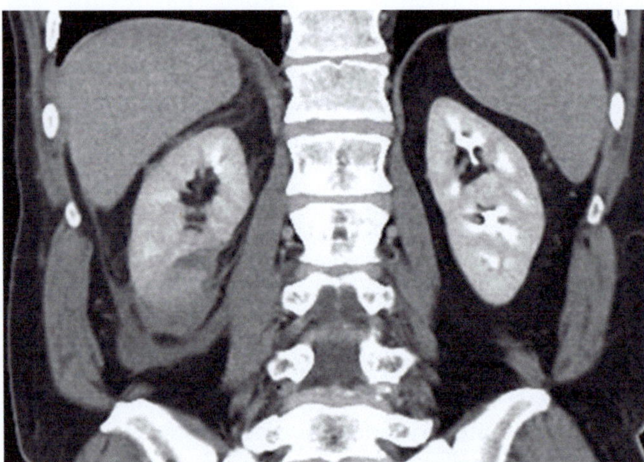

Fig. 25.1 CT image of grade 3 renal injury at the lower pole of the right kidney

25.1.3 Management

The management of renal injuries is primarily dictated by the hemodynamic status of the patient. The presence or absence of a functional contralateral kidney and any preexisting renal insufficiency are also important in the decision-making. The main goal of management is to preserve a maximum of functioning renal units.

25.1.3.1 Conservative Management

This means supportive care (with or without blood transfusion), bed rest, and observation (serial hematocrit measurement and imaging). It is the standard treatment for renal injuries in the hemodynamic stable patient, regardless of the grade of injury (except vascular grade 5). Conservative management is associated with a lower nephrectomy rate, without any rise in the immediate or long-term morbidity [11]. Unilateral main arterial injuries are managed conservatively in the hemodynamic stable patient; however bilateral artery injuries or arterial injury in a solitary kidney should be managed by surgical intervention. Conservative management is also recommended in the treatment of unilateral complete blunt arterial thrombosis. Selective nonoperative management of stab wounds and low-velocity gunshot wounds is generally accepted following complete staging in stable patients [12–14]. Grade 4–5 injuries with urinary extravasation must undergo repeated imaging after 2–3 days. In case of persistent extravasation, a double-J stent must be placed. An infected perirenal hematoma or urinoma is treated by percutaneous drainage [7].

25.1.3.2 Interventional Radiology

Angiography and angioembolization are increasingly used as an adjunct to the nonoperative management of blunt renal trauma in hemodynamically stable patients [15–17]. Active extravasation of contrast, arteriovenous fistula, and pseudoaneurysm are generally accepted indications for angioembolization [18].

25.1.3.3 Surgical Management

Persistent hemodynamic instability, unresponsive to aggressive resuscitation, is an absolute indication for renal exploration [19, 20]. Renal exploration must also be performed in case of an expanding or pulsatile perirenal hematoma identified at laparotomy performed for other injuries. During exploration, control of the bleeding and renal salvage is the main goal. A transperitoneal approach by midline abdominal incision is preferred. The renal pedicle is approached through the posterior parietal peritoneum, which is incised over the aorta, just medial to the inferior mesenteric vein. An alternative approach is achieved by blunt dissection along the plane of the psoas muscle fascia, adjacent to the great vessels, and directly placing a vascular clamp on the hilum [21]. After vascular control, renal reconstruction is possible in most cases of parenchymal injury. Renorrhaphy with closure of the collecting system (if open) and partial nephrectomy in case of a clearly devascularized segment are possible options [1]. Hemostatic agents and/or sealants are helpful in control of venous/parenchymal bleeding. Persistent major bleeding after renal reconstruction and release of the vascular clamp must be followed by nephrectomy. Repair of vascular grade 5 injuries is usually not possible, and nephrectomy is recommended. However, vascular repair should be attempted in case of a solitary kidney or bilateral injuries.

25.2 Ureteral Trauma

25.2.1 Etiology and Epidemiology

Trauma to the ureters is **rare**, accounting for 1–2.5% of all urologic traumas [22, 23]. This is explained by their small size, their mobility, and their protection by the vertebral bodies, pelvic bones, and adjacent muscles [1, 24]. Penetrating injuries are more common compared to blunt injuries, and the upper part of the ureter is the most affected portion [22, 23]. Ureteric injuries are almost always (90.4%) **associated with other injuries** [22]. Trauma to the ureter frequently results in severe complications [22, 24].

25.2.2 Diagnosis

25.2.2.1 Clinical Features and Examination

The diagnosis is difficult and **often delayed** as the clinical features of associated injuries are more prominent [1, 24]. Any penetrating injury close to the course of the ureter should raise suspicion for a ureteric injury. Vascular and intestinal injuries are mostly associated [25]. Blunt trauma with fractures of the pelvic bones, sacrum, or lumbar vertebrae should also raise suspicion for ureteric injury [1]. **Hematuria** is a nonspecific sign and only present in 40–75% of the cases [22, 24, 26]. Delayed signs in case of missed diagnosis are caused by urinary extravasation: prolonged ileus, flank pain, fever, sepsis, and urinary leakage through drains [1, 24]. Biochemical analysis might reveal elevated creatinine and urea-nitrogen levels [24].

25.2.2.2 Further Diagnostics

In case of immediate laparotomy for other injuries, the ureter(s) must be inspected for its integrity in case a ureteric injury is suspected [24, 27]. Intravenous injection of methylene blue can be helpful. **Direct recognition during laparotomy** facilitates the repair and reduces late complications [24]. Single-shot intravenous urography during laparotomy is unreliable, as negative findings cannot rule out a ureteric injury [24, 26, 27].

In stable patients, **abdominopelvic CT with excretory phase** is the preferred modality. Extravasation of contrast medium along the course of the ureter is pathognomonic for a ureteric injury. However, sometimes only minor signs are visible such as hydronephrosis, mild ureteric dilation, ascites, or urinoma [1]. In case of any doubt, **retrograde ureterography** should be performed, but this is often difficult in the acute trauma setting [1, 24, 27].

25.2.3 Management

25.2.3.1 Immediate Recognition

In case of a persistent unstable patient during laparotomy, "damage control" of the ureteric injury must be performed [1, 28]. Urinary diversion is essential here with the least damage to the ureter. An options is insertion of a single-J stent at the lesion in the proximal ureter and externalization of this stent through a small skin incision. The distal part is left unaffected. If this is not possible, proximal ureteric ligation and placement of a nephrostomy tube are an alternative. Further ureteric reconstruction is performed once the patient's condition allows it [28]. In other cases, immediate repair is performed. Ureteric contusions and gunshot wounds very close to the ureter are treated by a ureteric stent or by nephrostomy as delayed necrosis can cause fistulation [24]. Partial injuries are repaired primarily with resorbable 5.0 sutures and with placement of a ureteric stent or nephrostomy [1, 24]. However, stenting must be done very carefully as it might aggravate the ureteric injury [1]. In case of a complete lesion in the upper and middle part of the ureter, the ureteric ends are inspected and debrided if necessary. The ureteric ends are spatulated and thereafter mobilized sufficiently to allow for a tension-free anastomotic repair over a ureteric stent with absorbable 5.0 sutures [27]. An external drain is placed close to the lesion. A complete injury at the lower third (below the crossing with the iliac vessels) is treated by ureteric reimplantation in the bladder, if necessary in combination with a psoas hitch of the bladder to diminish tension [24]. As the lesion is usually short, other techniques such as transureteroureterostomy and ureteric reimplantation into the bladder with the use of a Boari flap are seldom needed [27].

25.2.3.2 Delayed Recognition

First, urinary diversion must be accomplished. Usually, this is performed by insertion of a nephrostomy tube as retrograde stenting is seldom successful in this setting [24]. Large urinomas must be drained as well (percutaneous or open) [24]. Definitive reconstruction is performed once the acute inflammatory phase has ended and the local tissues are healed. This usually takes at least 6 weeks. Definitive reconstruction depends on the site and extent of the final lesion [1].

Short lesion at the upper and middle part of the ureter can be treated by excision and primary anastomosis (as described above). Longer lesions can be treated by transureteroureterostomy. A window is made through the mesentery of the sigmoid, and an end-to-side anastomosis with the other ureter is made. The injured ureter is stented. For longer lesion at the upper part, renal mobilization and ureteropyelostomy are an alternative. For longer lesions at the middle part, ureteric reimplanation with a Boari flap can be performed, especially in case of contraindication for transureteroureterostomy (e.g., nephrolithiasis) [1, 24, 27]. In case of extensive ureteric tissue loss, ileal interposition is an option. Patients might develop hyperchloremic metabolic acidosis [29]. In case of contraindication (impaired renal function, intestinal disease) or failure of ileal interposition (or other reconstructive techniques), renal autotransplantation is feasible but requires a high level of expertise. The kidney is relocated in the pelvis, the renal vessels are anastomosed end to side to the iliac vessels, and a ureteric reimplantation is performed in the bladder [30].

25.3 Bladder Trauma

Bladder injury is herein defined as full-thickness laceration of the bladder wall. For therapeutic reasons, it is important to distinguish between extraperitoneal, intraperitoneal, and combined extra-and intraperitoneal perforations [31].

25.3.1 Etiology and Epidemiology

The majority of bladder traumata are blunt and related to motor vehicle collisions [23]. Extraperitoneal ruptures are almost always associated with **pelvic fractures**. Intraperitoneal ruptures are caused by a sudden rise in intravesical pressure, secondary to a **blow** to the pelvis or lower abdomen. Because the bladder dome is the weakest and most mobile point of the bladder, ruptures will usually occur at that site [32]. Penetrating injuries, mainly gunshot wounds, are rare except in war zones and some violent urban settings [33, 34]. Patients with bladder injuries are likely to have at least one other intra-abdominal injury [35]. Furthermore, a combination of bladder and urethral injury is reported in 10–20% of cases [32, 35].

25.3.2 Diagnosis

25.3.2.1 Clinical Features and Examination

The cardinal sign of bladder injury is **macroscopic (visible) hematuria** [31, 32]. The combination of macroscopic hematuria and pelvic fracture is highly suggestive of bladder injury. Inability to void and abdominal tenderness are nonspecific signs. Abdominal distension is possible in case of urinary ascites due to an intraperitoneal rupture. Due to reabsorption of urea nitrogen and creatinine, intraperitoneal ruptures might be associated with uremia and elevated creatinine. Severe blast injuries to the pelvis and entrance/exit wounds at the lower abdomen, perineum, or buttocks must raise suspicion for a penetrating bladder injury [31, 32]. During surgical exploration for other injuries, signs of bladder injury are visible laceration, urine (clear fluid) in the surgical field, appearance of the bladder catheter, and/or blood in the urine bag during laparoscopy. Intravesical instillation of methylene blue may be helpful.

25.3.2.2 Further Diagnostics

Cystography is the standard diagnostic modality [31]. Both plain (conventional) cystography and CT cystography are appropriate as these modalities have a comparable sensitivity (90–95%) and specificity (100%) [36]. CT cystography has the advantage of the possibility of diagnosing bony fragments in the bladder, bladder neck injuries, and other abdominal injuries [32, 35]. Conventional or CT cystography must be performed using slow retrograde filling of the bladder by the transurethral or suprapubic catheter with a minimum of 350 mL of dilute contrast material. A plain film, a complete filling film, and a post-drainage film are the absolute minimum during conventional cystography, while 3D reconstruction during CT cystography makes a post-drainage series unnecessary. Passive bladder filling by clamping the urinary catheter during the excretory phase of CT or IVP is not sufficient to exclude bladder injury [32]. Contrast extravasation outside the boundaries of the bladder is pathognomonic for bladder injury. With intraperitoneal extravasation, free contrast medium will surround and highlight bowel loops and other abdominal viscera (Fig. 25.2). Extraperitoneal bladder injury is associated with irregular flame-shaped areas of contrast extravasation in the perivesical area (Fig. 25.3).

Cystoscopy is the preferred method for detection when the patient is already on the operation table and a bladder injury is suspected (e.g., blood in de urine bag) but not directly visualized. Cystoscopy will directly visualize the laceration and localize it in relation to the position of the trigone and ureteral orifices of which the integrity must be checked. A lack of bladder distension during cystoscopy suggests a large perforation. Bowel loops can be visible in case of an intraperitoneal rupture.

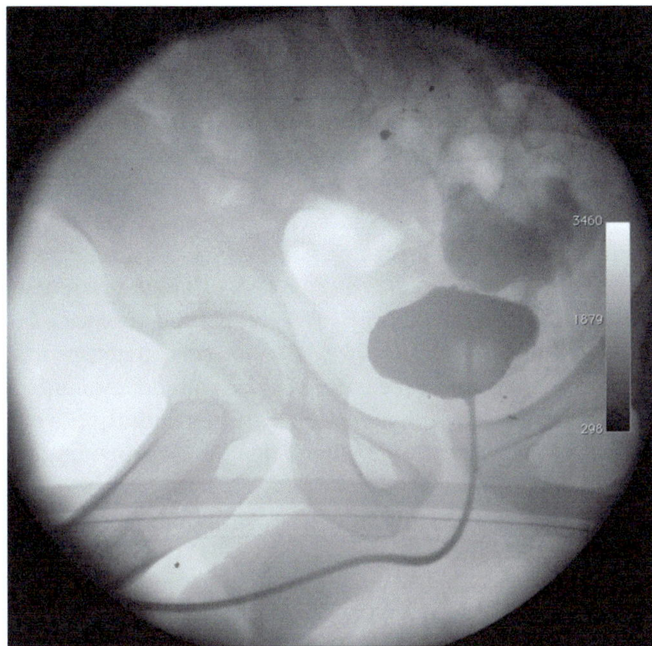

Fig. 25.2 Conventional cystography after a blunt trauma in the lower abdomen highlighting an intraperitoneal rupture

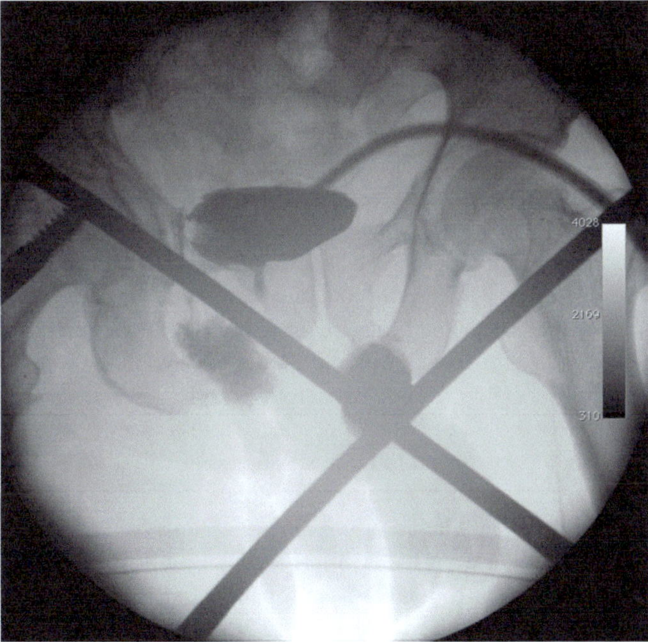

Fig. 25.3 Conventional cystography in a male with a pelvic fracture injury. At the right lateral side of the bladder, contrast extravasation is seen into the extraperitoneal (retropubic) space

25.3.3 Initial Management

Uncomplicated blunt extraperitoneal bladder injuries can be safely managed by catheter drainage (urethral or suprapubic) combined with antibiotic treatment [31, 32, 35]. On the contrary, the following conditions require surgical intervention [31, 32]:

- Penetrating bladder injury
- Blunt intraperitoneal injury
- Blunt extraperitoneal injury with concomitant rectum injury, bladder neck injury, or bony fragment in the bladder
- Blunt extraperitoneal injury in which the pelvic fracture will be treated by open stabilization and internal fixation with osteosynthetic material

If open surgery is performed, a midline lower abdominal incision is made and the prevesical ("Retzius") space is developed. In case of suspicion of intra-abdominal lesions and/or in case of an intraperitoneal injury, the peritoneal cavity is opened as well. A midline exploratory cystotomy is advised to have a good exposure to the entire bladder wall. In case of gunshot wounds, always search for an entrance and exit wound at the bladder wall [33]. Remaining bullet fragments or shrapnels are removed. The integrity of the ureteric orifices and the distal ureters are checked. In case the injury extends into the ureteric orifice or in case of concomitant trauma to the distal ureter, ureteric reimplantation must be performed. At the site of injury, debridement of any devitalized bladder muscle must be performed. However, this debridement should be done minimally because of the excellent vascularization of the bladder. Thereafter, a two-layer repair (detrusor muscle and mucosa) is performed with absorbable sutures. However, a watertight single-layer closure might be as good [31, 35]. A drain is left in space in the retropubic space or in the perineal cavity in case of respectively an extraperitoneal and intraperitoneal bladder injury.

In the absence of other intra-abdominal injuries, laparoscopic suturing of an uncomplicated intraperitoneal rupture is an option [37]. The camera trocar is placed at the umbilicus with two trocars for instruments at the left and right iliac fossa.

In some cases of major injury with extensive bladder tissue loss and/or avulsion of the lower abdominal wall or perineum, direct closure of the traumatized bladder wall will lead to excessive tension and eventual breakdown of the repair. Therefore, a bladder wall substitute is needed for the repair of bladder defect as well as a substitute to restore the lower abdominal wall or perineum. Use of a pedicled vastus lateralis myocutaneous flap has been reported for this [38].

25.3.4 Further Management

Infective complications are possible after surgical repair or in case of a conservative approach. Perivesical abcedation requires drainage and surgical repair of the bladder (if an initial conservative approach was chosen). Postoperative continuous bladder drainage is required in case of conservative treatment but also after surgical repair as it prevents elevated intravesical pressure and subsequent risk of disruption of the suture line [32].

Bladder healing is assessed by cystography which is first planned after 7–14 days, depending on the extent of the laceration. The catheter can be removed in the absence of contrast extravasation. However, persistent extravasation must raise suspicion for bony fragments in the bladder, especially after conservative treatment. To rule this out, cystoscopy must be performed. In the absence of bony fragments, cystography is repeated after 1 week [32]. Only after operative repair of a noncomplicated injury in a healthy patient, the catheter can be removed without control cystography after 7–10 days [39].

25.4 Urethral Trauma

25.4.1 Etiology and Epidemiology

25.4.1.1 Posterior Urethra

A **pelvic fracture** is complicated by a urethral injury in 1.54% of cases [40]. This urethral injury is a stretch injury in about 25%, a partial rupture in another 25%, and a complete rupture in 50% of cases. Especially the straddle fracture (fracture of the four rami of the pubic bone) and the Malgaigne fracture (fracture of two pubic rami with a diastasis of the sacroiliac joint) have a high likelihood of being associated with a urethral lesion [41]. In women, a urethral lesion is rare [42]. In children, the prostate is only rudimentary developed, and here, a pelvic fracture can cause damage to the bladder neck and the prostatic urethra, rather than a rupture at the membranous urethra. **Penetrating injuries** at the perineum can be caused by gunshot or stab wound injuries or by explosive devices [33]. These injuries are rare in the civilian setting but not uncommon in war circumstances [43].

25.4.1.2 Anterior Urethra

Fall-astride injuries, in which the bulb is compressed against the inferior surface of the pubic symphysis, can lead to rupture of the bulbar urethra [44]. **Penetrating injuries** such as gunshot and stab wounds can affect the penile and bulbar urethra, while dog bites will usually cause trauma to the penile urethra [45, 46]. **A penile fracture** is complicated by a urethral injury, usually at the penoscrotal angle in up to one third of cases [47, 48].

25.4.2 Diagnosis

Adequate diagnosis and management of urethral injuries are important because the urological incapacity of urethral injuries might be very important (urethral stricture, urinary incontinence, impotence), often in young men.

25.4.2.1 Clinical Features and Examination

A urethral injury must be considered in case of an unstable pelvic fracture, severe fall-astride injury, and penetrating penile or perineal injury and after every severe perineal or genital trauma.

Meatal blood loss, the cardinal sign of urethral injury, is present in the large majority of cases, but the absence of it does not rule out an injury [42]. **Hematuria** is a nonspecific sign of urethral injury because bladder and kidney injuries are also associated with hematuria [1, 31]. **Inability to void** suggests a complete urethral disruption [32]. **Perineal, scrotal, or penile swelling/hematoma** also suggests urethral trauma but is a delayed sign (>1 h after initial trauma) [31]. In females, labial swelling and blood at the vaginal introitus must raise suspicion for a urethral injury [31].

Clinical examination must include a **digital rectal examination**. A high-riding prostate is suggestive for posterior urethral disruption but is difficult to assess in the acute phase. Rectal examination is of utmost importance to screen for rectal injuries. Although rare, this injury is life-threatening if unrecognized [32, 42, 49].

25.4.2.2 Further Diagnostics

Retrograde urethrography (RUG) is the standard to diagnose a urethral injury [31]. This examination can be done, while the patient is on the X-ray table for other radiographic examinations (e.g., X-ray thorax, pelvis, extremities), but should be postponed in the unstable patient [42, 49]. The tip of a Foley catheter is introduced at the urethral meatus, and contrast is injected, while films are made in a slight oblique position (if possible). Extravasation of contrast is pathognomonic for urethral injury. Retrograde urethrography provides information on the site of the injury and is able to differentiate between a partial rupture (extravasation, but still bladder filling; Fig. 25.4) and a complete rupture (massive urethral extravasation, no bladder filling; Fig. 25.5), although this difference is not always clear [50]. Flexible **cystourethroscopy** is an alternative to diagnose (and manage) an acute urethral injury and is preferred above RUG in case of suspicion of penile fracture-related urethral injuries and in case of female urethral injuries [42, 49, 51]. In females, concomitant vaginoscopy must be performed to rule out a vaginal laceration [31].

25.4.3 Initial Management

Urethral injuries itself are **not life-threatening**, but they mostly occur in the context of a poly-traumatized patient with associated injuries [40]. Treatment of these patients requires a multidisciplinary approach. The initial management, therefore, consists of stabilization of the patient and

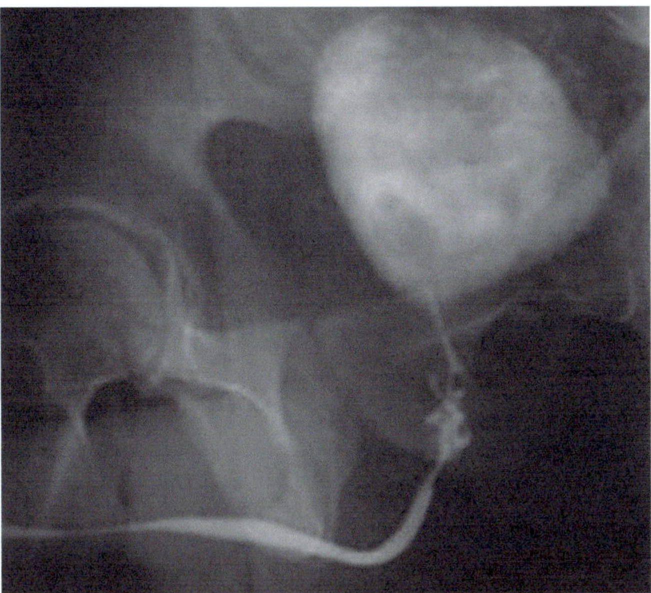

Fig. 25.4 RUG of partial posterior urethral injury: contrast extravasation but still bladder filling

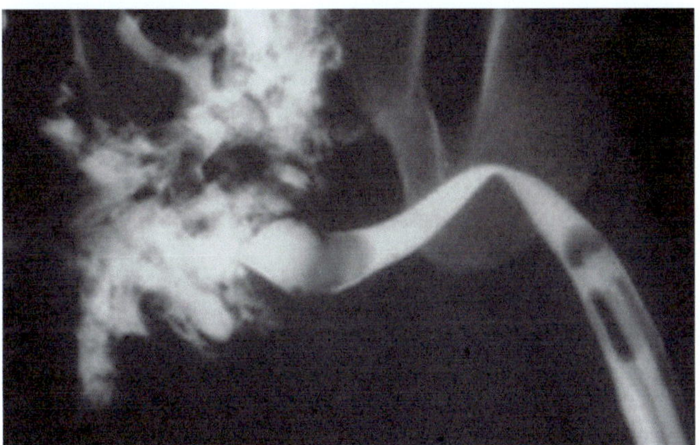

Fig. 25.5 RUG of complete posterior urethral injury: contrast extravasation without bladder filling

treatment of life-threatening problems according to the principle "treat first what kills first." Initial management of urethral injury comprises of **urinary diversion** (urethral catheter or suprapubic diversion), and even this is not essential on the first hours after trauma [31]. In case of severe urethral blood loss, perineal compression or a penile circumferential dressing can be applied.

25.4.3.1 Penetrating Urethral Injuries and Urethral Injuries Related to Penile Fracture

If the patient is stable, **immediate exploration** is warranted [31]. Simple tears are closed primarily, whereas short complete injuries can be treated with anastomotic repair. In case of longer defects, extensive tissue loss, or infection (esp. bite wounds), a primary repair must be aborted. In this case, the urethral mucosa is marsupialized, and a definitive repair is performed at least 3 months later (two-stage repair). Because of the risk of infection and the uncertain blood supply, grafts or flaps have no place in penetrating injuries [52].

In case the patient is unstable, a suprapubic catheter is placed and a delayed repair is performed.

25.4.3.2 Blunt Injuries

Stretch Injury

In case no extravasation is seen on urethrography and thus only a stretch injury is diagnosed, placement of a urethral catheter is not a problem. In fact, a urethral catheter is not needed in case spontaneous voiding is possible. This avoids further urethral manipulation.

Partial Rupture

A urinary diversion is needed because extravasation of urine can lead to periurethral inflammation, abcedation, and stricture formation [31]. One attempt of **skilled urethral catheterization** is allowed. One must always check whether the urethral catheter is in the bladder (and not in the pelvic hematoma). In case of any problems, the attempt is stopped, and a **suprapubic catheter** must be placed. The advantage of a urethral catheter is that a possible hazardous suprapubic puncture is avoided. A urethral catheter can also be placed after insertion of a guidewire in the bladder with the aid of cystoscopy (early urethral realignment, see later).

Complete Rupture

Insertion of a **suprapubic catheter** is the standard treatment [31]. However, if associated with pelvic fractures, the bladder is usually displaced by the pelvic hematoma, and insertion is not always easy. Placement under echographic vision is necessary to safely insert the catheter. If the patient undergoes lower abdominal surgery, the suprapubic catheter can be placed under "direct vision."

25.4.4 Further Management

25.4.4.1 Partial Ruptures

The urinary diversion (urethral or suprapubic catheter) is usually maintained for 2–4 weeks and removed if voiding cystourethrography shows no longer extravasation [53, 54]. These patients must be followed regularly because stricture formation can develop.

25.4.4.2 Complete Ruptures

Early Urethral Realignment (EUR)

This can only be performed when the patient is **stable within 14 days** after the trauma. EUR can be performed when the patient is under anesthesia for other surgery, or it can be as a stand-alone procedure. **Endoscopic** realignment is the preferred modality. The aim is rather to correct severe distraction than preventing urethral stricture formation [55]. Unlike partial injuries, complete injuries are not likely to heal with EUR. If subsequent stricture formation occurs, the stricture is usually shorter and easier to treat (endoscopic incision or simple perineal urethroplasty) [56, 57]. However, repetitive endoscopic incisions after EUR delay definitive cure and might make the final urethroplasty more complex [58].

Delayed Formal Urethroplasty

This is the standard modality [31]. The suprapubic catheter is maintained for at least 3 months after which the repair can be done. The standard technique is the elaborated anastomotic repair by perineal route except in the presence of a rectourethral fistula, periurethral cavities, and/or bladder neck abnormalities. The recurrence rate is ca.10% with no additional risk of impotence caused by the urethroplasty [31, 59].

A first crucial step during the procedure is the correct identification of the urethral ends. The distal end is easily identified by inserting a catheter or a metal sound through the meatal orifice, and the urethra is transected at the site of obstruction. The proximal end is harder to identify, and in case of any difficulty, it is strongly advised to use the suprapubic tract for suprapubic cystoscopy (Fig. 25.6). A second crucial step is resection of the fibrotic tissue. An anastomosis of fibrotic urethral ends will lead to failure. Therefore, resect until healthy mucosa is visible, and thereafter spatulate for about 1.5 cm [60]. In order to bridge the distraction defect, four consecutive maneuvers can be used, and the procedure is stopped at the moment where a tension-free anastomosis can be performed [61]. These maneuvers consist of:

1. Mobilization of the bulbar urethra (up to the penoscrotal angle)
2. Separation of the cavernosal bodies
3. Inferior pubectomy
4. Supracrural rerouting (Fig. 25.7)

For longer defects (>8 cm) or in case of redo, a transverse island flap from the prepuce can be used and tubularized.

25.4.4.3 Female Urethral Injuries

The level of the disruption is crucial for the approach and treatment [31]. Distal injuries can be left unrepaired or are closed primarily by vaginal approach. Midurethral and proximal injuries require primary repair as they involve the sphincteric mechanism. Midurethral injuries can be treated by transvaginal route, whereas proximal injuries require a retropubic approach. Concomitant vaginal injuries are repaired at the same time by the vaginal approach, and the use of an interposition flap (e.g., Martius flap) is advised to avoid urethrovaginal fistulation [62].

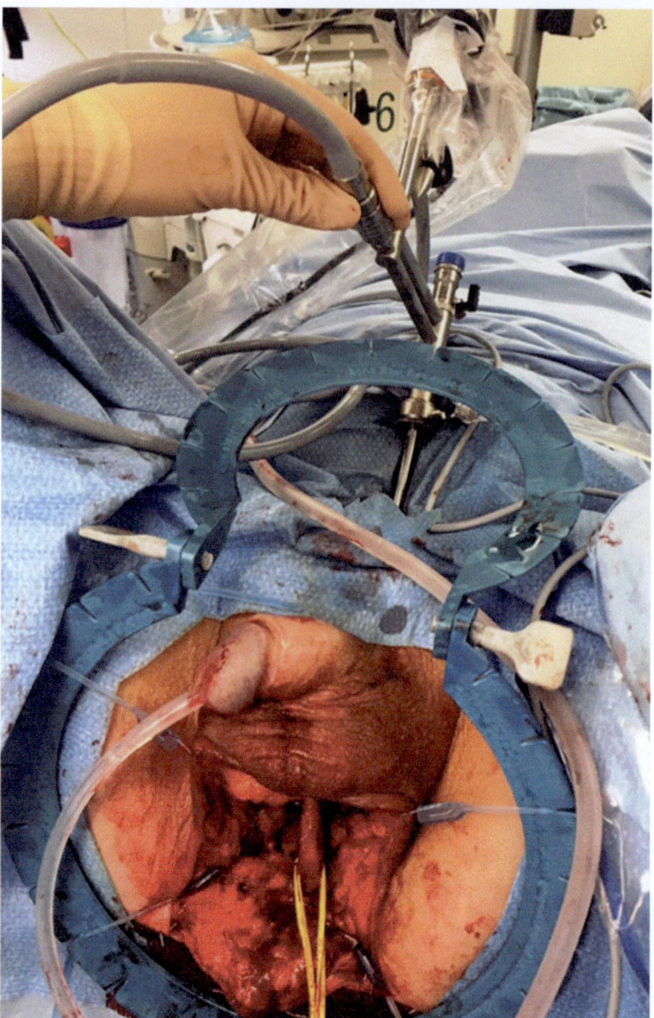

Fig. 25.6 Rigid suprapubic cystoscopy to identify the proximal end of the urethral obliteration. The distal end is identified by a transurethral catheter

25.5 Scrotal Trauma

25.5.1 Etiology and Epidemiology

The majority is caused by blunt trauma [7, 63]. Possible subtypes are testicular dislocation (ectopic posttraumatic position), testicular hematocele (blood in tunica vaginalis), or testicular rupture (tear of tunica albuginea). Testicular rupture requires a force of approximately 50 kg [64]. **Sports trauma**, especially contact sports, is the main cause of blunt trauma [63]. Penetrating trauma is less frequent. In conflict areas, improvised explosive devices are an important cause [65], whereas, in the civilian setting, gunshot wounds are predominant [66, 67].

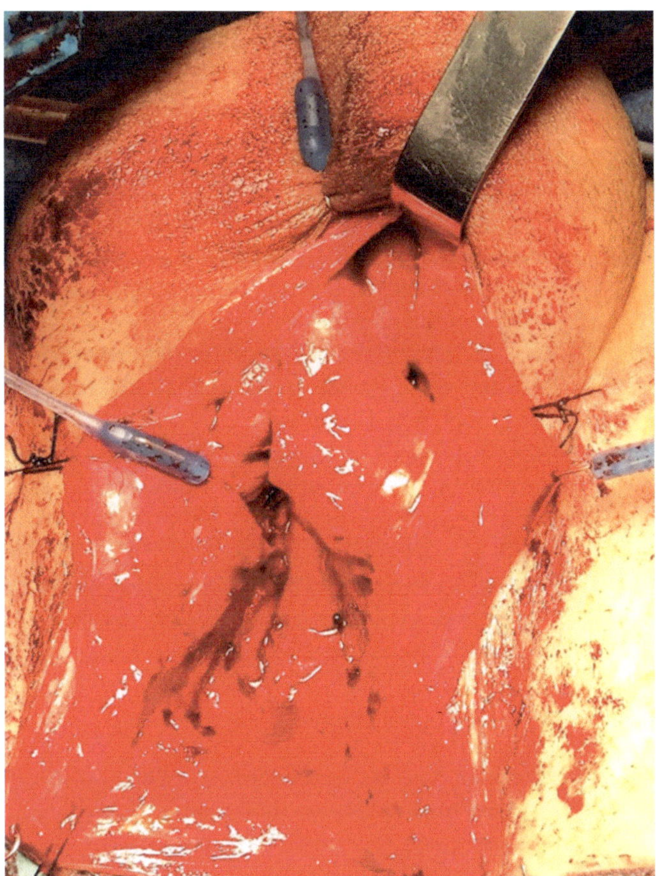

Fig. 25.7 Bulboprostatic anastomosis after full bulbar urethral mobilization, splitting of the corporal bodies, inferior pubectomy, and supracrural rerouting

25.5.2 Diagnosis

25.5.2.1 Clinical Features and Examination

Symptoms are **localized pain** and **swelling** [7, 63]. The pain can be such intense that vagal symptoms (nausea, vomiting, fainting) occur [63]. Direct inspection and physical examination are of utmost importance. However, scrotal examination is often not possible because of patient's discomfort and agitation [63]. Testicular dislocation can be subcutaneous in case of epifascial displacement. In case of internal dislocation, the testis is displaced at the external inguinal ring, inguinal canal, or abdominal cavity [68]. In case of hematocele or testicular rupture, local swelling is evident but makes it difficult to palpate the testis. Meatal blood loss suggests a concomitant urethral injury [31].

25.5.2.2 Further Diagnostics

Scrotal **ultrasound** ($\geq$7.5 MHz) is advised as to discriminate between hematocele, testicular contusion, and rupture, although differentiation between testicular rupture and hematocele is not evident. Signs of testicular rupture are heterogeneous parenchyma, testicular contour irregularity, and direct tunica albuginea breach [7, 63, 69]. Addition of color Doppler duplex is helpful to evaluate testicular perfusion. In case of equivocal findings on ultrasound, MRI is helpful in further diagnostics but however often limited by its availability [63].

25.5.3 Management

In case of traumatic **dislocation**, manual replacement is advised with secondary orchidopexy at a later time. If this fails, immediate orchidopexy should be performed [68].

Small **hematoceles** (<3× size of contralateral testis) are managed conservatively with relative rest and analgesics. In order to reduce the rate of delayed surgery and orchiectomy, larger hematoceles should be explored as soon as possible with evacuation of the blood from the tunica vaginalis [70].

In case of **testicular rupture**, or in case clinical examination and ultrasound cannot rule it out, early surgical exploration should be performed. During this exploration, blood clots are evacuated, necrotic testicular tissue is excised, and the tunica albuginea is closed with an absorbable running suture [7, 63].

Penetrating injuries require surgical exploration [67, 69]. Primary reconstruction of the testis and closure of the scrotum can usually be performed, especially in case of low-velocity injuries. In case of injury to the vas deferens, vasovasostomy can be performed if the clinical condition allows for this. In case of blast injuries or high-velocity injuries, the trauma is extensive, and mobilization of a tunica vaginalis flap might be required to replace the tunica albuginea for testicular closure [7]. In the unstable patient, or if reconstruction is not possible, orchiectomy has to be performed [67]. Extensive scrotal skin loss is treated by delayed scrotal reconstruction. The testicles (if preserved) are placed at the groin or thigh in this case.

Case Scenario: Combined Bladder and Urethral Injury

A 57-year-old man went through a serious car accident and was admitted to the nearest hospital with signs of hemodynamic instability. He complained about lower abdominal discomfort and the inability to void. During clinical examination, urethral blood loss was seen and pelvic instability was affirmed. After starting resuscitation, a contrast-enhanced full-body CT scan (no excretory phase) was performed. This exam revealed small liver damage as well as unstable pelvic fracture and an empty bladder, although the kidneys were not injured. After external fixation of the pelvis, the patient went to the intensive care unit for further careful observation and resuscitation. Abdominal echography showed free intraperitoneal fluid and no bladder filling and therefore no possibility for insertion of a suprapubic catheter. The decision to perform an excretory phase CT scan was made: an upward displaced empty bladder was discovered together with intraperitoneal contrast leakage. Therefore a percutaneous intraperitoneal drain was placed. On the second day after the accident, the patient developed increased temperature with leukocytosis and increased CRP. After sampling urine and taking blood culture, broad-spectrum antibiotics were given. One day later (third day after the accident), signs of hemodynamic instability with tachycardia, hypotension, tachypnea, and increased abdominal pain were observed. The patient was transferred to an academic hospital. Blood test revealed acute renal insufficiency, low hemoglobin, and unmistakable electrolyte changes, so urgent dialysis was performed followed by laparotomy (after detachment of the external fixation). Immediately after opening of the abdominal cavity, a large amount of urine was evacuated, and a clear rupture at the bladder dome, extending toward the anterior bladder wall, was noticed. The ruptured bladder allowed us to detect the intact ureteric orifices and bladder neck. Separated bone fragments were removed, and the pelvic hematoma was drained. A suprapubic catheter was inserted and the bladder was closed in two layers. Moreover, a second drain was placed extraperitoneal. Before finishing the theater, the external fixation was reattached. Two days later, a normalization of laboratory parameters was seen with disappearance of the abdominal pain. Revalidation program was started 1 day later (sixth day after the accident) with his suprapubic catheter on continuous drainage to give the bladder a chance to heal. Ten days postoperative, cystography demonstrated integrity of the bladder wall. Flexible cystoscopy showed a completed urethral injury. The suprapubic catheter was maintained on continuous drainage for 3 months more. Later, a combination of retrograde and antegrade cystourethrography was performed which showed a complete obliteration of the membranous urethra. Three weeks later, a urethroplasty was performed. A midline perineal incision was made, fibrotic tissue was excised, both urethral ends were spatulated, the corporal bodies were separated, and an inferior pubectomy was performed in order to bridge the distraction defect. Two weeks later, a voiding cystourethrography was performed which showed no urethral extravasation, and the urinary catheter was removed. At present, patient is voiding without any difficulties and is continent. Erectile dysfunction is treated by medication (PDE-5 inhibitor).

Questions

1. Did the emergency team act well (according to the EAU guidelines) to admit the patient after the severe car accident to the nearest local hospital?
   A. Yes, the faster the patient reaches the hospital, the lower the mortality.
   B. **No, the patient should be admitted to a major trauma center because the risk of mortality and morbidity is reduced.**
   C. Yes, the initial resuscitation should be performed in the nearest hospital; afterward, the patient can be transported to a more specialized trauma center.
   D. No, the patient should be admitted directly to a major trauma center with possible inputs from all major surgical specialties and trauma teams which reduce mortality by 25% but without influence on the length of stay.

2. Did the urologists act well to postpone the diagnostics and treatment of the urethral injury?
   A. Yes, because urethral injury has no serious long-term consequences.
   B. Yes, because urethral injury is not life-threatening in most cases and doesn't have long-term consequences.
   C. **Yes, because it has low priority in the management of severely injured trauma patients.**
   D. No, the urologist should have performed an immediate retrograde urethrography after the first laparotomy: the faster the suturing of the urethral ends, the easier the surgery without enhancing the complications.

3. The standard to rule out bladder injury is:
   A. **Cystography with filling of the bladder with a minimum of 350 ml**
   B. Three-phase CT
   C. Four-phase CT
   D. Cystoscopy

4. After discovering contrast extravasation intraperitoneal, did the urologist act well to perform a percutaneous intraperitoneal drain without following a laparotomy and vesicorraphy?
   A. **No, there is a strong recommendation to perform a direct surgical exploration and bladder repair in case of intraperitoneal or combined intra- and extraperitoneal bladder injury.**

B. Yes, intraperitoneal injuries can be solved with a bladder drainage only. Extraperitoneal injuries need a direct laparotomy.
C. Yes, a laparotomy should be postponed for at least 2 weeks after intraperitoneal drain insertion to reduce the mortality.
D. No, because insertion of a drain is waste of time and can't be seen as a part of damage control strategy.

5. What is wrong about immediate realignment in this case?
A. Because the patient was unstable, we decided not to perform it.
B. It would be justified because there is a lower stricture rate than with suprapubic catheter placement alone.
C. **It would be justified because treatment might be easier if a stricture occurs without lowering the stricture rate than with suprapubic catheter placement alone.**
D. It would be justified, but in case of a complete posterior urethral rupture, an initial suprapubic diversion and delayed urethroplasty >3 months after trauma remain strongly recommended.

Please see Chap. 58 for the correct answer

References

1. Serafetinides E, Kitrey ND, Djakovic N, Kuehhas FE, Lumen N, Sharma DM, et al. Review of the current management of upper urinary tract injuries by the EAU Trauma Guidelines Panel. Eur Urol. 2015;67(5):930–6.
2. Smith J, Caldwell E, D'Amours S, Jalaludin B, Sugrue M. Abdominal trauma: a disease in evolution. ANZ J Surg. 2005;75(9):790–4.
3. Sangthong B, Demetriades D, Martin M, Salim A, Brown C, Inaba K, et al. Management and hospital outcomes of blunt renal artery injuries: analysis of 517 patients from the National Trauma Data Bank. J Am Coll Surg. 2006;203(5):612–7.
4. Kansas BT, Eddy MJ, Mydlo JH, Uzzo RG. Incidence and management of penetrating renal trauma in patients with multiorgan injury: extended experience at an inner city trauma center. J Urol. 2004;172(4 Pt 1):1355–60.
5. Najibi S, Tannast M, Latini JM. Civilian gunshot wounds to the genitourinary tract: incidence, anatomic distribution, associated injuries, and outcomes. Urology. 2010;76(4):977–81; discussion 81
6. Moore EE, Shackford SR, Pachter HL, McAninch JW, Browner BD, Champion HR, et al. Organ injury scaling: spleen, liver, and kidney. J Trauma. 1989;29(12):1664–6.
7. Zinman LN, Vanni AJ. Surgical management of urologic trauma and iatrogenic injuries. Surg Clin North Am. 2016;96(3):425–39.
8. Morey AF, McAninch JW, Tiller BK, Duckett CP, Carroll PR. Single shot intraoperative excretory urography for the immediate evaluation of renal trauma. J Urol. 1999;161(4):1088–92.
9. Heller MT, Schnor N. MDCT of renal trauma: correlation to AAST organ injury scale. Clin Imaging. 2014;38(4):410–7.
10. Fischer W, Wanaselja A, Steenburg SD. JOURNAL CLUB: incidence of urinary leak and diagnostic yield of excretory phase CT in the setting of renal trauma. AJR Am J Roentgenol. 2015;204(6):1168–72; quiz 73
11. Schmidlin FR, Rohner S, Hadaya K, Iselin CE, Vermeulen B, Khan H, et al. The conservative treatment of major kidney injuries. Ann Urol. 1997;31(5):246–52.
12. Buckley JC, McAninch JW. Selective management of isolated and nonisolated grade IV renal injuries. J Urol. 2006;176(6 Pt 1):2498–502; discussion 502
13. Jansen JO, Inaba K, Resnick S, Fraga GP, Starling SV, Rizoli SB, et al. Selective non-operative management of abdominal gunshot wounds: survey of practise. Injury. 2013;44(5):639–44.
14. Baniel J, Schein M. The management of penetrating trauma to the urinary tract. J Am Coll Surg. 1994;178(4):417–25.
15. Lanchon C, Fiard G, Arnoux V, Descotes JL, Rambeaud JJ, Terrier N, et al. High grade blunt renal trauma: predictors of surgery and long-term outcomes of conservative management. A prospective single center study. J Urol. 2016;195(1):106–11.
16. Shoobridge JJ, Bultitude MF, Koukounaras J, Martin KE, Royce PL, Corcoran NM. A 9-year experience of renal injury at an Australian level 1 trauma centre. BJU Int. 2013;112(Suppl 2):53–60.
17. van der Wilden GM, Velmahos GC, Joseph DK, Jacobs L, Debusk MG, Adams CA, et al. Successful nonoperative management of the most severe blunt renal injuries: a multicenter study of the research consortium of New England Centers for Trauma. JAMA Surg. 2013;148(10):924–31.
18. Charbit J, Manzanera J, Millet I, Roustan JP, Chardon P, Taourel P, et al. What are the specific computed tomography scan criteria that can predict or exclude the need for renal angioembolization after high-grade renal trauma in a conservative management strategy? J Trauma. 2011;70(5):1219–27; discussion 27–8
19. Armenakas NA, Duckett CP, McAninch JW. Indications for nonoperative management of renal stab wounds. J Urol. 1999;161(3):768–71.
20. McAninch JW, Carroll PR, Klosterman PW, Dixon CM, Greenblatt MN. Renal reconstruction after injury. J Urol. 1991;145(5):932–7.
21. Gonzalez RP, Falimirski M, Holevar MR, Evankovich C. Surgical management of renal trauma: is vascular control necessary? J Trauma. 1999;47(6):1039–42; discussion 42–4
22. Pereira BM, Ogilvie MP, Gomez-Rodriguez JC, Ryan ML, Pena D, Marttos AC, et al. A review of ureteral injuries after external trauma. Scand J Trauma Resusc Emerg Med. 2010;18:6.
23. McGeady JB, Breyer BN. Current epidemiology of genitourinary trauma. Urol Clin North Am. 2013;40(3):323–34.
24. Brandes S, Coburn M, Armenakas N, McAninch J. Diagnosis and management of ureteric injury: an evidence-based analysis. BJU Int. 2004;94(3):277–89.
25. Siram SM, Gerald SZ, Greene WR, Hughes K, Oyetunji TA, Chrouser K, et al. Ureteral trauma: patterns and mechanisms of injury of an uncommon condition. Am J Surg. 2010;199(4):566–70.
26. Elliott SP, McAninch JW. Ureteral injuries from external violence: the 25-year experience at San Francisco General Hospital. J Urol. 2003;170(4 Pt 1):1213–6.
27. Elliott SP, McAninch JW. Ureteral injuries: external and iatrogenic. Urol Clin North Am. 2006;33(1):55–66, vi
28. Smith TG 3rd, Coburn M. Damage control maneuvers for urologic trauma. Urol Clin North Am. 2013;40(3):343–50.
29. Chung BI, Hamawy KJ, Zinman LN, Libertino JA. The use of bowel for ureteral replacement for complex ureteral reconstruction: long-term results. J Urol. 2006;175(1):179–83; discussion 83-4
30. Meng MV, Freise CE, Stoller ML. Expanded experience with laparoscopic nephrectomy and autotransplantation for severe ureteral injury. J Urol. 2003;169(4):1363–7.

31. Lumen N, Kuehhas FE, Djakovic N, Kitrey ND, Serafetinidis E, Sharma DM, et al. Review of the current management of lower urinary tract injuries by the EAU Trauma Guidelines Panel. Eur Urol. 2015;67(5):925–9.
32. Figler BD, Hoffler CE, Reisman W, Carney KJ, Moore T, Feliciano D, et al. Multi-disciplinary update on pelvic fracture associated bladder and urethral injuries. Injury. 2012;43(8):1242–9.
33. Cinman NM, McAninch JW, Porten SP, Myers JB, Blaschko SD, Bagga HS, et al. Gunshot wounds to the lower urinary tract: a single-institution experience. J Trauma Acute Care Surg. 2013;74(3):725–30; discussion 30–1
34. Pereira BM, de Campos CC, Calderan TR, Reis LO, Fraga GP. Bladder injuries after external trauma: 20 years experience report in a population-based cross-sectional view. World J Urol. 2013;31(4):913–7.
35. Matlock KA, Tyroch AH, Kronfol ZN, McLean SF, Pirela-Cruz MA. Blunt traumatic bladder rupture: a 10-year perspective. Am Surg. 2013;79(6):589–93.
36. Quagliano PV, Delair SM, Malhotra AK. Diagnosis of blunt bladder injury: a prospective comparative study of computed tomography cystography and conventional retrograde cystography. J Trauma. 2006;61(2):410–21; discussion 21–2
37. Wirth GJ, Peter R, Poletti PA, Iselin CE. Advances in the management of blunt traumatic bladder rupture: experience with 36 cases. BJU Int. 2010;106(9):1344–9.
38. Wu CW, Lin CH, Lin CH. One-stage posttraumatic bladder reconstruction and soft-tissue coverage of the lower abdomen or perineum. Ann Plast Surg. 2010;64(1):65–8.
39. Inaba K, Okoye OT, Browder T, Best C, Branco BC, Teixeira PG, et al. Prospective evaluation of the utility of routine postoperative cystogram after traumatic bladder injury. J Trauma Acute Care Surg. 2013;75(6):1019–23.
40. Bjurlin MA, Fantus RJ, Mellett MM, Goble SM. Genitourinary injuries in pelvic fracture morbidity and mortality using the National Trauma Data Bank. J Trauma. 2009;67(5):1033–9.
41. Koraitim MM, Marzouk ME, Atta MA, Orabi SS. Risk factors and mechanism of urethral injury in pelvic fractures. Br J Urol. 1996;77(6):876–80.
42. Brandes S. Initial management of anterior and posterior urethral injuries. Urol Clin North Am. 2006;33(1):87–95, vii
43. Tausch TJ, Cavalcanti AG, Soderdahl DW, Favorito L, Rabelo P, Morey AF. Gunshot wound injuries of the prostate and posterior urethra: reconstructive armamentarium. J Urol. 2007;178(4 Pt 1):1346–8.
44. Elgammal MA. Straddle injuries to the bulbar urethra: management and outcome in 53 patients. Int Braz J Urol. 2009;35(4):450–8.
45. Bjurlin MA, Kim DY, Zhao LC, Palmer CJ, Cohn MR, Vidal PP, et al. Clinical characteristics and surgical outcomes of penetrating external genital injuries. J Trauma Acute Care Surg. 2013;74(3):839–44.
46. Kommu SS, Illahi I, Mumtaz F. Patterns of urethral injury and immediate management. Curr Opin Urol. 2007;17(6):383–9.
47. Amit A, Arun K, Bharat B, Navin R, Sameer T, Shankar DU. Penile fracture and associated urethral injury: experience at a tertiary care hospital. Can Urol Assoc J. 2013;7(3–4):E168–70.
48. Cavalcanti AG, Krambeck R, Araujo A, Rabelo PH, Carvalho JP, Favorito LA. Management of urethral lesions in penile blunt trauma. Int J Urol. 2006;13(9):1218–20.
49. Rosenstein DI, Alsikafi NF. Diagnosis and classification of urethral injuries. Urol Clin North Am. 2006;33(1):73–85, vi–vii
50. Mundy AR, Andrich DE. Urethral trauma. Part I: introduction, history, anatomy, pathology, assessment and emergency management. BJU Int. 2011;108(3):310–27.
51. Kamdar C, Mooppan UM, Kim H, Gulmi FA. Penile fracture: preoperative evaluation and surgical technique for optimal patient outcome. BJU Int. 2008;102(11):1640–4; discussion 4
52. Chapple C, Barbagli G, Jordan G, Mundy AR, Rodrigues-Netto N, Pansadoro V, et al. Consensus statement on urethral trauma. BJU Int. 2004;93(9):1195–202.
53. Koraitim MM. Pelvic fracture urethral injuries: the unresolved controversy. J Urol. 1999;161(5):1433–41.
54. Koraitim MM. Pelvic fracture urethral injuries: evaluation of various methods of management. J Urol. 1996;156(4):1288–91.
55. Mundy AR, Andrich DE. Urethral trauma. Part II: types of injury and their management. BJU Int. 2011;108(5):630–50.
56. Koraitim MM. Effect of early realignment on length and delayed repair of postpelvic fracture urethral injury. Urology. 2012;79(4):912–5.
57. Kizer WS, Armenakas NA, Brandes SB, Cavalcanti AG, Santucci RA, Morey AF. Simplified reconstruction of posterior urethral disruption defects: limited role of supracrural rerouting. J Urol. 2007;177(4):1378–81; discussion 81–2
58. Tausch TJ, Morey AF, Scott JF, Simhan J. Unintended negative consequences of primary endoscopic realignment for men with pelvic fracture urethral injuries. J Urol. 2014;192(6):1720–4.
59. Feng C, Xu YM, Barbagli G, Lazzeri M, Tang CY, Fu Q, et al. The relationship between erectile dysfunction and open urethroplasty: a systematic review and meta-analysis. J Sex Med. 2013;10(8):2060–8.
60. Lumen N, Hoebeke P, Troyer BD, Ysebaert B, Oosterlinck W. Perineal anastomotic urethroplasty for posttraumatic urethral stricture with or without previous urethral manipulations: a review of 61 cases with long-term followup. J Urol. 2009;181(3):1196–200.
61. Webster GD, Ramon J. Repair of pelvic fracture posterior urethral defects using an elaborated perineal approach: experience with 74 cases. J Urol. 1991;145(4):744–8.
62. Singh O, Gupta SS, Mathur RK. Urogenital fistulas in women: 5-year experience at a single center. Urol J. 2010;7(1):35–9.
63. Wang Z, Yang JR, Huang YM, Wang L, Liu LF, Wei YB, et al. Diagnosis and management of testicular rupture after blunt scrotal trauma: a literature review. Int Urol Nephrol. 2016;48(12):1967–76.
64. Wasko R, Goldstein AG. Traumatic rupture of the testicle. J Urol. 1966;95(5):721–3.
65. Hudak SJ, Hakim S. Operative management of wartime genitourinary injuries at Balad Air Force Theater Hospital, 2005 to 2008. J Urol. 2009;182(1):180–3.
66. Phonsombat S, Master VA, McAninch JW. Penetrating external genital trauma: a 30-year single institution experience. J Urol. 2008;180(1):192–5; discussion 5–6
67. Simhan J, Rothman J, Canter D, Reyes JM, Jaffe WI, Pontari MA, et al. Gunshot wounds to the scrotum: a large single-institutional 20-year experience. BJU Int. 2012;109(11):1704–7.
68. Shefi S, Mor Y, Dotan ZA, Ramon J. Traumatic testicular dislocation: a case report and review of published reports. Urology. 1999;54(4):744.
69. Morey AF, Brandes S, Dugi DD 3rd, Armstrong JH, Breyer BN, Broghammer JA, et al. Urotrauma: AUA guideline. J Urol. 2014;192(2):327–35.
70. Altarac S. Management of 53 cases of testicular trauma. Eur Urol. 1994;25(2):119–23.

Operative Techniques in Vascular Injuries of Extremities

26

A. Lista, F. Riolo, A. G. Rampoldi, P. A. Rimoldi, I. D'Alessio, and F. Romani

Key Points

- Precocity of diagnosis is critical in vascular injuries of extremities.
- Every injured limb must undergo a deep vascular clinical examination followed by strict surveillance.
- In the absence of palpable peripheral pulse, arterial injury must be suspected.
- Palpable pulse means patency of the vessel at that moment but does not mean the absence of arterial injury, which could be evident later.
- Every blunt trauma must be monitored, and, if in doubt, a diagnostic test must be performed (Doppler ultrasound scan, arteriography, or CT angiogram).
- Different etiology is considerable in vascular trauma.
- Tissue contusion, severity of ischemia, and infection are most responsible for revascularization procedure failure.
- The quality of arterial surgery and tissue covering affect therapeutic result; surveillance and treatment of muscular necrosis allow limiting secondary amputation rate.
- Functional prognosis of the revascularized limb is often better than amputation, despite sequelae.
- The adoption of different prognostic scoring systems cannot replace multidisciplinary discussion among orthopedic, vascular, and plastic surgeons.

26.1 Introduction

The majority of arterial trauma (90% in most records) involves limb arteries, and vascular trauma of the limbs is associated with injury to other organs. Furthermore, in recent years, due to the increasing numbers of endovascular procedures, there is a growth in iatrogenic injuries, and drug addiction injuries are also considered as classic vascular trauma.

A. Lista (✉) · F. Riolo · P. A. Rimoldi · F. Romani
S.C. Chirurgia Vascolare, Dipartimento Cardiotoracovascolare, ASST Grande Ospedale Metropolitano Niguarda, Milan, Italy
e-mail: alfredo.lista@ospedaleniguarda.it; franco.riolo@ospedaleniguarda.it; pierantonio.rimoldi@ospedaleniguarda.it; federico.romani@ospedaleniguarda.it

A. G. Rampoldi
S.C. Radiologia Interventistica, Dipartimento Tecnologie Avanzate Diagnostico-Terapeutiche, ASST Grande Ospedale Metropolitano Niguarda, Milan, Italy
e-mail: antoniogaetano.rampoldi@ospedaleniguarda.it

I. D'Alessio
Università di Milano-Bicocca, Milan, Italy

26.2 Classification and Pathology

Typical classification of vascular trauma is divided in penetrating and blunt injuries. In penetrating trauma, the vascular lesion consists of a partial or complete section of the vessel, independently from the agent. In blunt trauma, instead, the mechanism is an indirect compression, deceleration, or stretching of the vessel often associated with osteoarticular injuries. Gunshot wounds have different mechanisms. The bullet forms a *temporary* cavity along its trajectory and a *permanent* cavity filled by tissue debris, causing a sudden shift of tissues.

Complete transections of the artery consist of adventitia, media, and intima laceration; such injuries are circumferential, causing a retraction of arterial extremities, followed by obstruction of the arterial lumen with temporary hemostasis. Partial lesions, instead, lead to a pulsating hematoma formation and a pseudoaneurysm thereafter as often happens in the iatrogenic trauma due to arterial catheterization. Arteriovenous fistula could form when a lateral arterial lesion involves the nearby vein.

P. Aseni et al. (eds.), *Operative Techniques and Recent Advances in Acute Care and Emergency Surgery*,
https://doi.org/10.1007/978-3-319-95114-0_26

Arterial contusions are often met in blunt trauma due to stretching, deceleration, or cavitation. A broken intima or media can occur.

The intimal layer is by far less extensible compared to media or adventitia. Therefore it could be torn along with the formation of dissecting flap leading to secondary thrombosis. Exposition of medial layer, after intimal rupture, has a thrombogenic effect. Adventitial layer, instead, is more resistant and can often stop blood spilling. The mechanism of iatrogenic complications due to percutaneous sealing systems in endovascular procedures is different: in these cases, thrombosis is due to posterior intimal detachment, associated to the presence of an intra-arterial component of the percutaneous sealing system.

In the most critical arterial trauma, rupture of three layers is observed with the formation of pseudoaneurysm (PSA). Arterial spasms determine a reduction in caliber of the vessel: they are typical in small caliber arteries and more frequent in young people with normal vessels.

26.3 Diagnosis, Signs, and Symptoms

We can distinguish between "hard" signs, in which arterial injury is almost always present, thus leading to mandatory surgical exploration, and "soft" signs, in which arterial lesion is suspected, leading, at least initially, to noninvasive diagnostic tests:

Hard Signs

- Active hemorrhage
- Pulsatile or expanding hematoma
- Bruit or thrill
- Absent or diminished pulses
- Distal ischemia

Soft Signs

- Stable hematoma
- Trauma close to major nervous or vascular structures
- Bone fractures
- Unexplained hypotension
- Limb paresis or paresthesias

Clinical signs of arterial injury can be furtherly distinguished as hemorrhagic or ischemic.

26.3.1 Hemorrhagic Signs

The most commonly encountered sign of arterial injury is hematoma.

It can be compressive or expanding, rarely pulsating. If it is localized in a close space, it can worsen ischemic and neurologic complications.

External pulsating hemorrhage allows determining the location of the arterial injury. Most of the times, it is a self-limiting blood loss due to arterial stump spasm. A thrombus is evident in the lumen.

26.3.2 Ischemic Signs

- The classical description of patients with acute limb ischemia is represented by the "six Ps": pain, pallor, paralysis, pulse deficit, paresthesia, and poikilothermia. Pain may be either constant or elicited by passive movement of the involved extremity. History should include relation to trauma, duration, location, intensity, and suddenness of the onset of pain and changes over time.
- More frequently, however, subacute ischemia is encountered. The extremity is cold and pale; pulses are absent, and neurological examination is normal.
- Compartment syndrome appears most of the times after revascularization: absence of a peripheral palpable pulse is first noticed, followed by painful muscular swelling causing progressive neurological sensory deficit first and, ultimately, also motor.
- Muscular ischemia is due to revascularization edema.
- Diagnosis is easier if edema is localized in anterior, lateral, or superficial posterior compartment of the foreleg, more difficult if in the deep posterior lower limb.
- Compartment syndrome requires urgent fasciotomies: different studies limit the pressure in 45 mmHg. Fasciotomies in forearms can be performed anteriorly and posteriorly.
- Arteriovenous fistula is characterized by the presence of continuous systolic-diastolic bruit and palpable thrill, although its formation in trauma is rare.

26.3.3 Hidden and in Development Clinical Pictures

Hidden clinical pictures are common in polytrauma with multilevel bone injury leading to swelling for tissue ischemia and contusion.

In-development clinical pictures are sneaky: pulses, initially palpable, can later disappear due to intimal tear leading to thrombus formation. Hence it is necessary to check pulses after reduction of fracture or dislocation in any major joint (shoulder, elbow, hip, knee, etc.).

26.4 Instrumental Diagnosis

Emergency treatment of vascular trauma, in the presence of massive hemorrhage or compressive hematoma, can lead to leaving out any further diagnostic investigation in order to transfer the patient in the operating room, as rapidly as possible.

In the majority of cases, however, there is time to perform a deep diagnostic investigation.

26.4.1 Doppler Ultrasound Scan

Advantages of Doppler ultrasound scan are:

- Point of care at patient's bedside
- Noninvasive procedure
- Easily repeatable, allowing to detect evolution of the injury
- Screening methods in asymptomatic lesions

Disadvantages of Doppler ultrasound scan are:

- Operator dependent
- Lack of detection of injuries to side branches and isolated intimal tears
- Troublesome performance in painful limb

Different authors studied the diagnostic value of ankle-brachial index (ABI), showing that a value <0.9 has a 95% sensibility and 97% specificity in diagnosing traumatic arterial injuries.

ABI could have a predictive value in screening arterial injuries after knee dislocation: in different studies, patients with a value <0.9 showed, after the angiogram, injuries needing operating treatment; in patients with a value >0.9, no significant arterial injury has been detected.

ABI could, therefore, replace angiogram; there is a consensus in trauma patients with ABI $\geq$ 1, on performing only noninvasive vascular studies followed by clinical surveillance and US Doppler scan after 48 h. ABI cannot be trusted in patients with PAOD (peripheral artery occlusive disease).

26.4.2 CT Angiogram

Ultrasound scan limits (massive musculocutaneous injuries and low sensitivity in traumatic injuries of the base of neck) have made CT angiogram the gold standard in the vascular trauma of the extremities.

Total body CT scan is part of the initial step in polytrauma patient with suspected vascular injuries.

A recent meta-analysis showed CT angiogram as the first choice diagnostic tool in vascular trauma in which therapeutic needs could differ.

In blunt cervical trauma, sensitivity varies from 82 to 100% and specificity from 90 to 99%. In penetrating cervical trauma, CT angiogram allows, in the majority of cases, to detect the route of injurious agent, thus identifying all injuries, excluding at the same time any damage to the digestive and respiratory tract.

The highly predictive value of CT angiogram (97–100%) has led in many centers to a decrease of surgical cervical exploration for 68–0%.

CT angiogram is fundamental in blunt traumatic aortic injuries, either for direct diagnosis (simple intimal tear, PSA, intramural hematoma, dissections, blood spills) or indirect (hemo-mediastinum) or for planning endovascular treatment. In limbs trauma, in particular, CT angiogram has a sensitivity of 95–100% and specificity of 86–100% in the femoropopliteal region. It loses reliability in more distal injuries.

26.4.3 Arteriography

Before CT angiogram era, arteriography was frequently utilized in case of Doppler ultrasound scan anomalies, also in particular cases like a patient with PAOD or in the case of multiple wounds with large loss of tissues.

Angiogram can be used intraoperatively in case of hemodynamic instability or active hemorrhage, once obtained hemostatic control.

Arteriography with the mobile digital tool is simple to perform. It allows checking distal segment of the artery, before a revascularization, to ensure the absence of peripheral emboli and to control final revascularization. Arteriography is again fundamental in the endovascular procedures, associated with classic open procedures, allowing, for example, a temporary hemostasis with a balloon catheter or to place covered stent or hemostasis by embolization.

Five kinds of images can be seen in trauma:

- Complete interruption of the vessel indicates either complete rupture or subintimal flap associated with thrombosis; distal artery flow is present in case of an elevate number of collateral vessels.
- Spill of contrast medium is a sign of lateral laceration, with possible formation of PSA.
- Early venous opacification is a sign of arteriovenous fistula, typical of lateral laceration.
- Evidence of fusiform arterial stenosis is seen in the arterial spasm; in such case, a possible intimal tear causing secondary thrombosis must be ruled out.
- Minimal intimal injury usually determines patency of the vessel.

26.5 Surgical Technique

In polytrauma, patient treatment priority is survival, followed by salvage of the limb.

26.5.1 Minor Arterial Trauma

In minimal arterial lesion, without hemorrhage and/or ischemia, the patient must be evaluated with complete physical examination, associated with a Doppler ultrasound scan, and monitored with periodic checking of pulses and ABI. Invasive tools should be used only if there are significant clinical variations (absence of pulses or ischemia).

Different studies confirmed the efficacy of surveillance of patients with silent arterial injury, due to low-velocity agents, determining non-occluding intimal lesions or PSA without external hemorrhage.

26.5.2 Major Arterial Trauma

In case of major arterial trauma, with frank hemorrhage or ischemia, the patient is treated in shock room. Initial steps are intensive care with effective compression, associated to correction of hypovolemia. Clinical examination must precisely localize arterial lesion, regarding location and gravity. Temporary hemostasis must be done with manual compression; trying to place clamp blindly is generally ineffective and associated with injury to the nearby anatomic structures. Compression must be maintained until complete artery control is possible in the operating room (OR).

Use of balloon or Foley catheter can ease initial control of an external hemorrhage, especially in the supraclavicular or axillary region, where manual compression is particularly difficult.

Use of tourniquet, although often used, should be avoided because it can worsen ischemia for simultaneous interruption of venous return and arterial collateral flow.

In case of ischemia, alkalinization of blood must be taken as soon as possible, to grant a correct electrolytic balance, and must be associated to a correct diuresis. Systemic broad spectrum antibiotic must be administered in case of a contaminated wound. Operative asepsis in an emergency is not granted; it is, therefore, important to remove tissue debris and to perform intraoperative bacteriological tests.

If other major injuries are present and revascularization of the limb is delayed, it's essential to place a temporary arterial shunt to limit ischemic time: it is usually used a 3–3.5 mm shunt in diameter, thus allowing a 300 mL/min flow with a mean pressure of 75 mmHg.

Operating field must include both complete legs, for the collection of saphenous vein of both lower limbs.

Access route to expose vascular stump anatomically, if possible, must be through the classic elective incision avoiding to use the trauma wounds. Associated osteoarticular injuries are particularly frequent at brachial and popliteal level.

Most of the authors prefer to perform reduction and stabilization of bones with external fixation first, to avoid secondary mobilization that could threaten arterial revascularization. Timing of reduction and fixation of fractures, with external fixation, do not delay significantly revascularization.

Simple aligning of fracture or dislocation reduction without specific orthopedic procedure results in a risk of secondary failure of revascularization itself. It's, anyway, important that vascular surgeon attends orthopedic procedure, to check the correct performance of revascularization at the end of osteosynthesis. In case of particularly serious trauma with important muscular involvement, crushing, and necrosis, primary amputation *quoad vitam* must be performed.

A prosthetic leg is far better than a paralyzed limb. In the upper limb, primary amputation is a more difficult decision, because the prosthetic outcome is less beneficial. Contraindications to lower limb revascularization, universally accepted, are:

- Loss of tibial bone substance greater than 8 cm
- Duration of ischemia greater than 6 h
- Posterior tibial nerve injury

Mangled extremity severity score (MESS) has an important prognostic value: a score greater than 7 has a positive predictive value of amputation of 100%, for both upper and lower limb trauma.

This score, however, does not take in account seriousness of nerve injury, very important for the ultimate functional prognosis.

Other scoring systems fill this gap, but they cannot replace multidisciplinary consultation among orthopedic, vascular, and plastic surgeons.

26.5.3 Methods of Arterial Repair

Arterial suture must be made on healthy arterial tissue, resecting arterial stump with no tension. Isolation of the injured artery, for few centimeters, proximally and distally, allows to gain a proper length for direct suture, but it is necessary to avoid, with such maneuver, damage of side branches. Arterial suture, either direct or made with bypass, must be covered with vital tissues: such procedure is more comfortable in blunt trauma than penetrating one where pedunculated or free muscular grafts must be used. If loss of

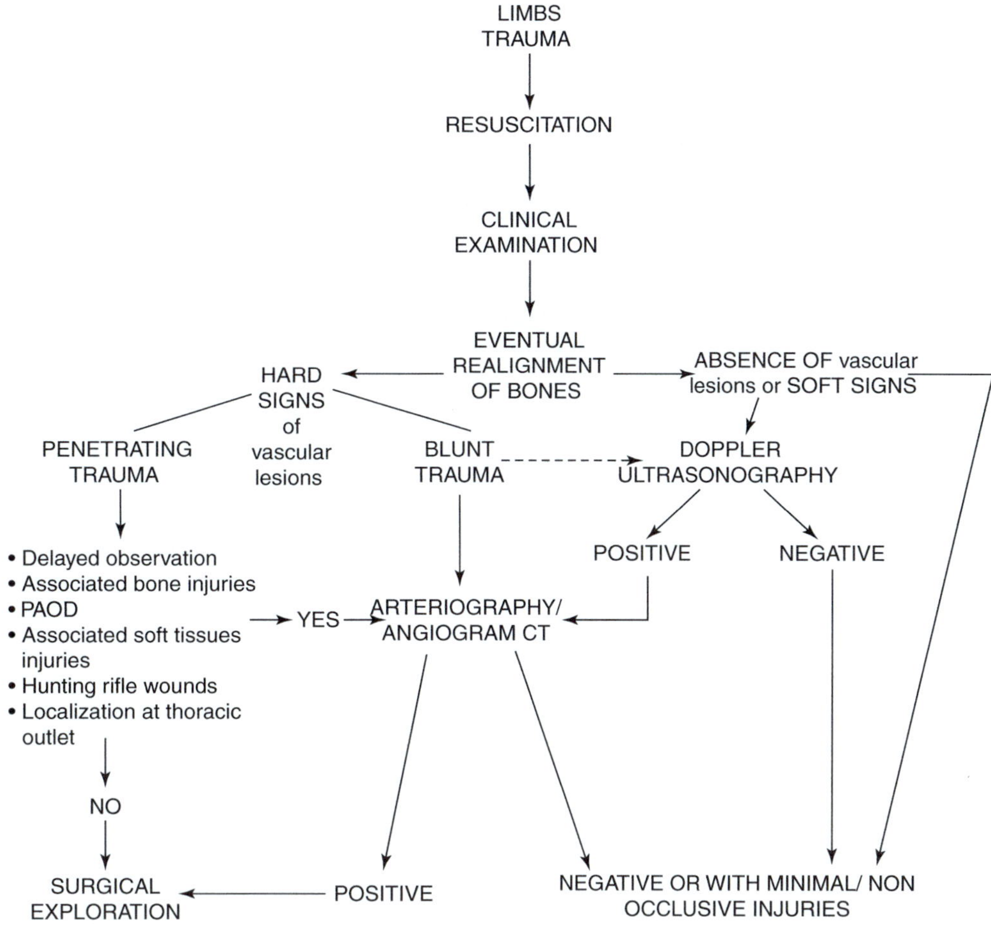

Fig. 26.1 Algorithm for limb trauma

tissue or necrosis, factors of elevated septic risk, is widespread, an extra anatomical revascularization is mandatory. Direct suture is possible inside lacerations, with appropriate control of intimal layer: direct longitudinal suture always causes a relative stenosis, acceptable for arterial calibers >10 mm and dangerous if <10 mm diameters, where a patch, better if biological (vein), is requested.

Termino-terminal suture, better if beveled anastomosis, is ideal in complete traumatic transections, as long as the approach is without tension: approved limits are 25 mm for brachial or superficial femoral artery and 10 mm for arteries in forearms and forelegs.

Bypass, using an inverted saphenous vein, is the best revascularization technique in case of extensive arterial injury.

Extra-anatomical bypass is wise in case of diffuse soft tissue trauma, to prevent infection of the graft.

Distal stump is catheterized with Fogarty, to remove thrombi and perfused with local heparin.

The graft of choice is contralateral saphenous vein (especially in lower limbs), for its infection resistance.

If the vein is not available, PTFE seems to grant better infection resistance than Dacron.

Associated venous injuries are present in 40% of cases, mainly at popliteal level. They could not be evident initially, but overt after arterial reperfusion. It is necessary to preserve blood return in at least one main venous vessel and to repair vein with the same surgical principles as arteries (Fig. 26.1).

26.6 Surgical Technique Notes (Based on Anatomic Site)

Ninety percent of vascular trauma belongs to the lower limb (60%) or upper limb (30%). Popliteal, brachial, and superficial femoral arteries are the most involved.

The most dangerous areas of vascular trauma are those in which collateral circulation is poor. Common femoral, supra-articular popliteal, and proximal brachial arteries have very few collaterals. As a consequence, traumatic occlusion of the flow often causes severe ischemia, leading to irreversibility if not corrected. Subclavian and distal brachial artery better tolerate an obstruction, due to greater collateral.

26.6.1 Subclavian Artery

Subclavian artery (SA) is divided into three segments: pre-scalenic, retro-scalenic, and post-scalenic. Due to sterno-costo-clavicular bone protection, injuries of SA are rare but particularly serious: different authors report a mortality up to 40%. In patients with unstable conditions, with or without acute hemorrhage, hemostasis has its gold standard in a mini-invasive endovascular solution, increasingly common today. Endoluminal control is reached through common femoral artery catheterization with long (90 cm) introducers, supra-aortic probe, and angioplasty balloons.

Endovascular approach reduces morbidity because of avoiding iatrogenic injuries of brachial plexus and subclavian vein, quite frequent in case of open emergency surgery. Covered stents well fit in the treatment of iatrogenic injuries, arteriovenous fistulas, avulsions of side branches, and intimal tears. Short-term graft patency is between 86 and 100%. Most frequent contraindications to endovascular treatment are unstable arterial pressure, bulky hematoma compressing brachial plexus, complete transection of the vessel, or long occlusion.

If the endovascular approach is not feasible, massive hemorrhage can be controlled through anterolateral thoracotomy on third intercostal space for left SA and median sternotomy for right SA.

In the absence of acute hemorrhage, SA exploration can be made through a supraclavicular incision (Fig. 26.2), with section of the clavicular head of sternocleidomastoid muscle and of anterior scalene muscle, paying particular attention to the phrenic nerve.

Rarely a direct suture can be performed. More often a SA transposition on common carotid or bypass between SA and carotid is requested.

The majority of authors prefer, in case of plexus injury, to mark nerves for a subsequent repair.

26.6.2 Axillary Artery (Fig. 26.3)

Axillary trauma is relatively rare, either in civilian or military settings. The majority of them is due to penetrating trauma. In case of short segmental lesion without important hematoma, surgical access is made through deltoid-pectoral sulcus with section of pectoralis minor muscle.

In case of more severe trauma, section of pectoralis major is also performed, thus obtaining sub-clavicular control.

Arterial reconstruction is made with termino-terminal direct suture, after resection of damaged arterial stumps in case of minimal tissue loss, or with saphenous vein graft, preferred to synthetic grafts, because it better tolerates mechanical stress and is more resistant to infections.

Treatment of injury to axillo-subclavian junction after shoulder dislocation, typical of motor bike accident, is more difficult. In this case, lesions to veins and brachial plexus are frequently associated. Extra-anatomical bypass between carotid and the brachial artery is the treatment of choice, thus avoiding access through traumatized area.

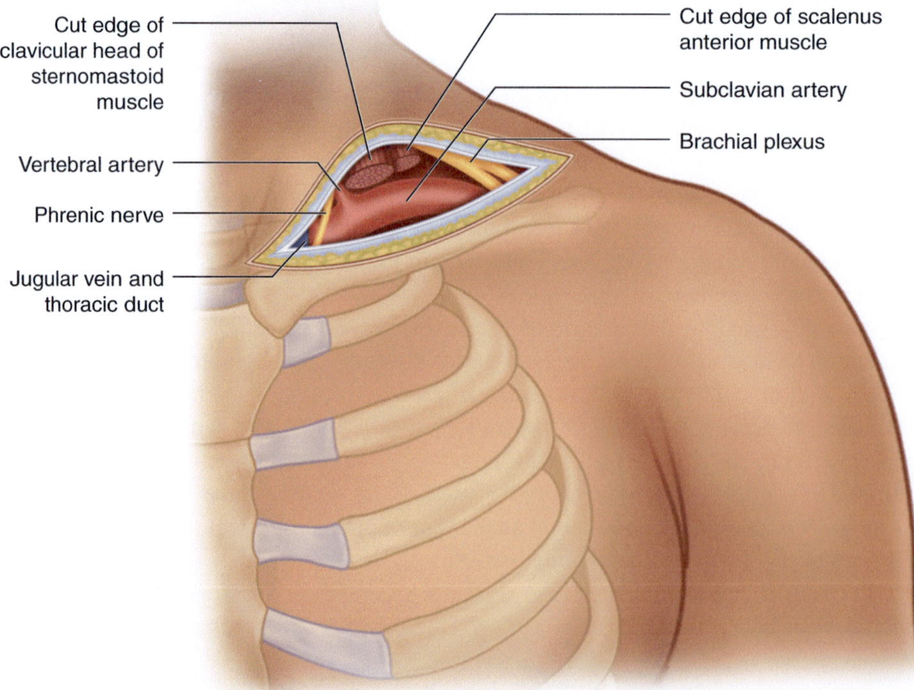

Fig. 26.2 Subclavian artery

26.6.3 Brachial Artery (Fig. 26.4)

Superficial route of brachial artery explains the frequent damage to this vessel. Access to the brachial artery is relatively simple. It is made in the internal biceps groove and is sometimes associated with section of biceps aponeurosis, to reach the vessel bifurcation. If tissue loss is poor, termino-terminal anastomosis is performed; otherwise saphenous vein grafting is mandatory. Associated venous injuries require ligation, due to large collateral venous circulation. It

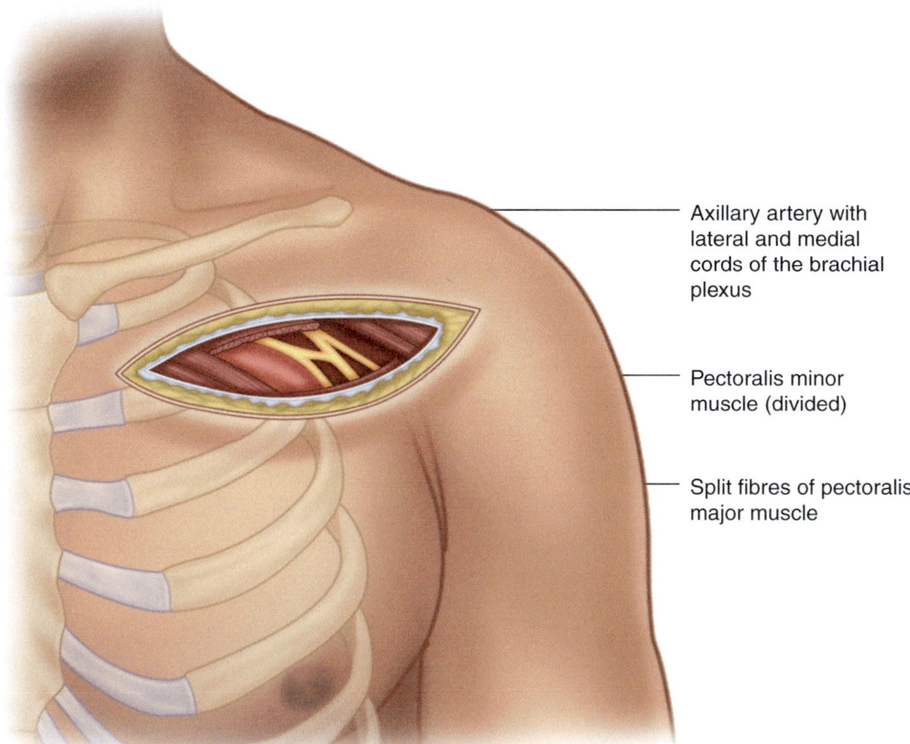

Fig. 26.3 Axillary artery

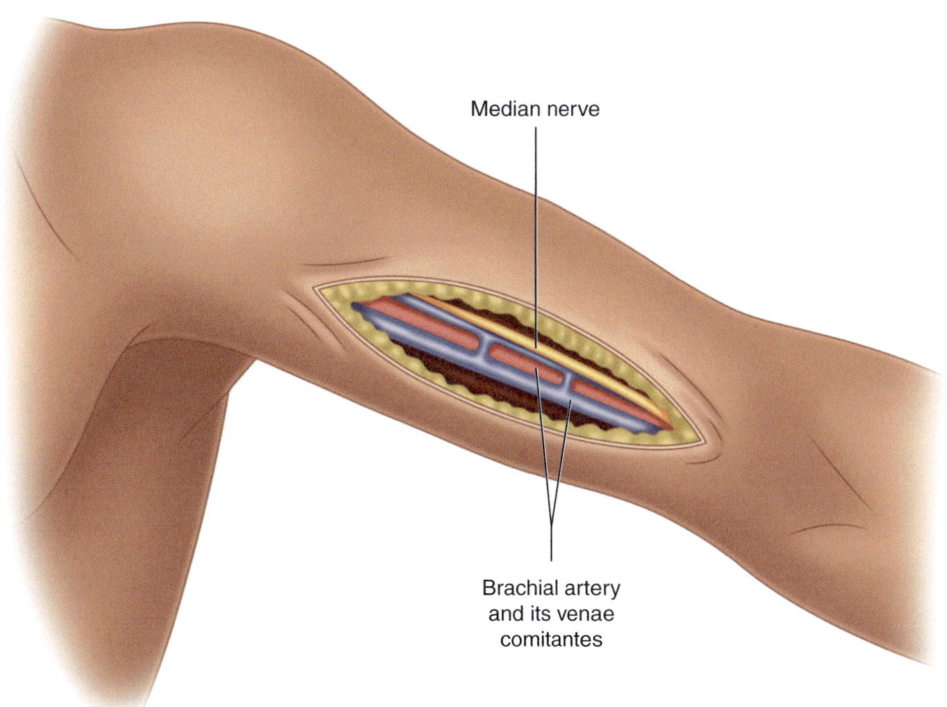

Fig. 26.4 Brachial artery

is always recommended to cover arterial reconstruction, difficult in case of loss of tissue of anterior area of elbow. In this case, extra-anatomical saphenous graft on the interior or exterior aspect of the arm must be made.

26.6.4 Forearm Arteries

Revascularization techniques of radial or ulnar arteries do not raise particular problems of surgical access. Direct reconstruction, venous patch, and grafting are the treatment of choice.

26.6.5 Femoral Artery

Femoral vessels are often affected by stab injuries. Access route to femoral artery tripod is a longitudinal crural incision (Fig. 26.5), sometimes associated with a supracrural extraperitoneal access to control external iliac vessel, in case of large hematoma in Scarpa's triangle. Superficial femoral artery is reached through an internal middle third thigh incision (Fig. 26.6). In case of large tissue loss, mobilized and rotated sartorius or internal rectus femoris muscle can be used to cover arterial reconstruction.

26.6.6 Popliteal Artery

Popliteal artery (PA) is the most frequently involved segment in trauma for the concomitant osteoarticular knee injury. The seriousness of popliteal trauma is well known since the Second World War, where PA ligation after trauma led to 73% of amputations. The risk of loss of limb, in knee trauma with vascular and osteoarticular lesions, depends on the delay of treatment, severity of bone and muscular injuries, and lesion of skin coverage. Diagnosis is relatively easy; in 75% of patients, there is the absence of distal pulses and presence of typical signs of ischemia.

Access to supra-articular popliteal artery is medial, through the anterior edge of sartorius muscle; section of adductor magnus tendon allows to find distal segment of the superficial femoral artery.

The distal part of popliteal artery is reached through a medial route, 2 cm posteriorly to the posterior edge of tibia (Fig. 26.7); section of medial gastrocnemius, semitendino-

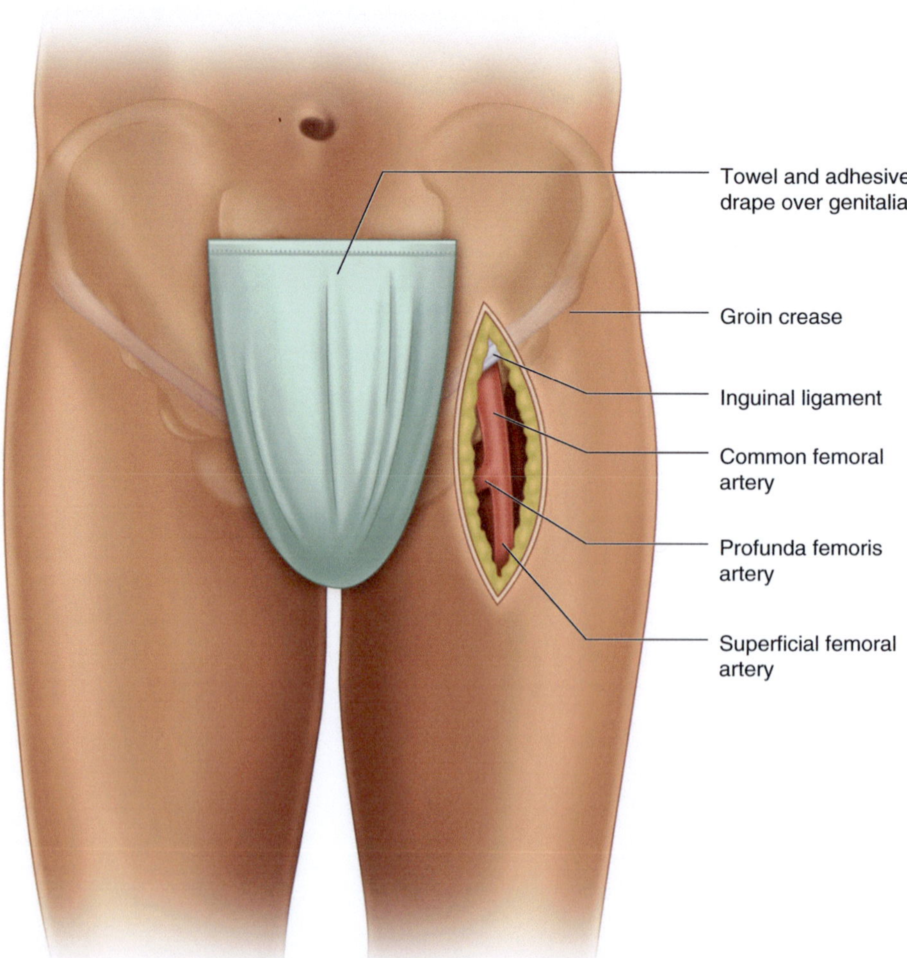

Fig. 26.5 Profunda femoris artery

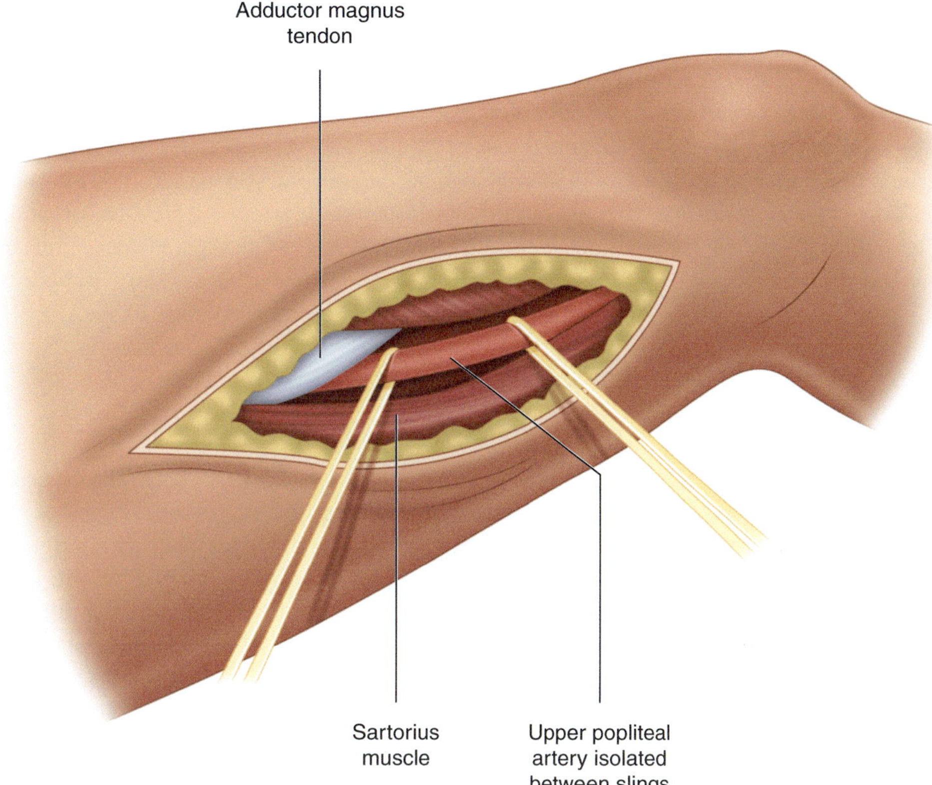

Fig. 26.6 Upper popliteal artery

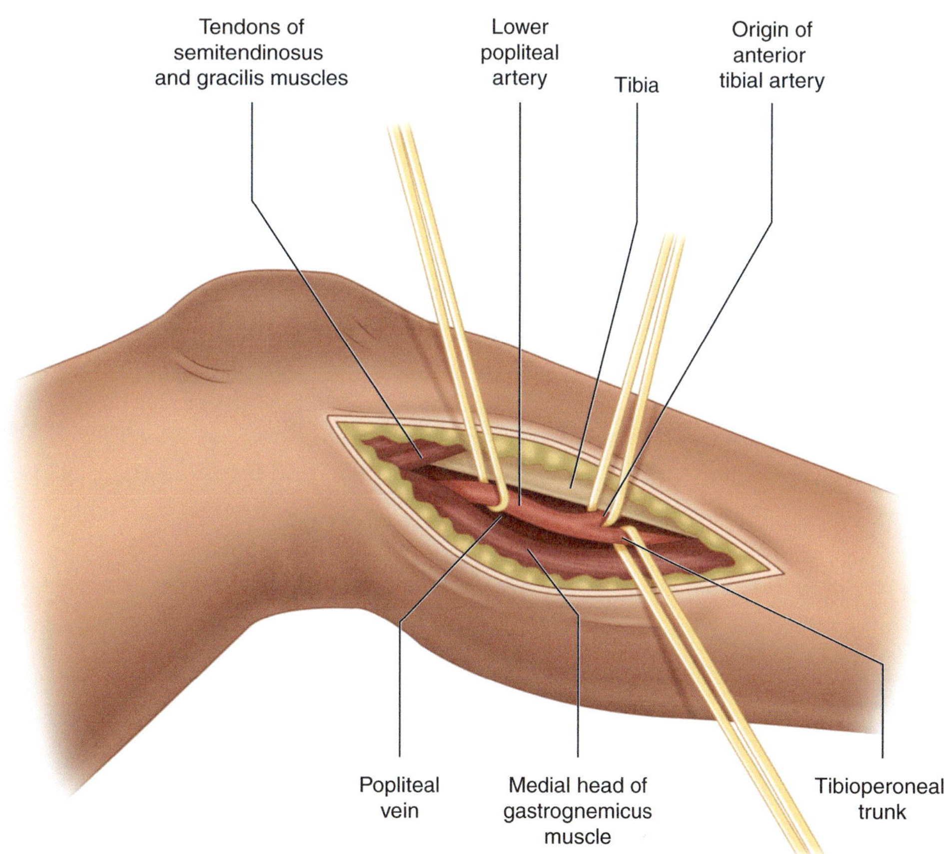

Fig. 26.7 Lower popliteal artery

sus, and semimembranosus muscles allows to reach popliteal artery deeply. In this access it is necessary to preserve saphenous vein. Posterior access route is seldom used in vascular trauma because of prone decubitus and difficult harvesting of the saphenous vein. Bypass is the treatment of choice for arterial repair, with the harvesting of the vein in contralateral limb if feasible. Endovascular treatment with covered stent rarely applies to this site for possible stenting fracture risk at the articular knee fold.

26.6.7 Arteries of Forelegs

At this level, surgical repair is mandatory if two out of the three vessels or tibio-peroneal trunk are involved.

Posterior tibial artery and tibio-peroneal trunk are accessed through a prolongation of already discussed popliteal incision, with section of soleus arch. Posterior tibial is reached through intern retromalleolar space (Fig. 26.8). Proximal *anterior tibialis* is anteriorly and laterally approached between anterior tibial muscle and *extensor longus* of toe (Fig. 26.9), halfway distally of intermalleolar line. In the foreleg, covering of arterial reconstruction is often difficult, consequently leading to primary amputation.

26.7 Particular Cases

26.7.1 Iatrogenic Pseudoaneurysm (PSA)

Surgical treatment of PSA consists of proximal and distal control of the injured vessel and direct suture of arterial breach. If a stenosis is expected, a venous patch must be placed; rarely a terminal suture is requested. Since the 1980s, mini-invasive methods are increasingly used. Thrombin injection in the PSA, along with eco-guided compression, give excellent results, with primary thrombosis of PSA > 97%. Other authors prefer percutaneous embolization with coils during the angiogram, with a success rate close to 90%. Another largely used method is positioning covered stents, easily feasible in a straight tract of injured vessel. Traditional surgical treatment in case of injury near artery bifurcation or in large PSA (absolute indication if >8 cm) is, instead, preferred, especially if infected or with neurologic or ischemic signs due to compression. Surveillance of PSA < 3 cm with Doppler US scan is suggested, considering that small PSAs very often thrombose spontaneously.

26.7.2 Arteriovenous Fistula

The presence of contiguous penetrating arterial and venous injury can lead to arteriovenous fistula formation, clinically manifested with a bruit and a thrill.

If communication is wide, hemodynamic steal occurs, leading to chronic arterial ischemia associated with venous hypertension and to cardiac overload. Iatrogenic fistulas after catheterization often have low output and thrombose either spontaneously or by eco-guided compression. It is hence accepted an observational attitude: after 6 months, however, it is preferred to close the fistula, in order to avoid hemodynamic overload. Diagnosis is usually made by ultrasonography. Gold standard treatment consists of placing a covered stent, if anatomically feasible away from bifurcations. Open surgery, instead, consists of simple suture of the artery, adding a venous patch in case of wider lesion.

Embolization of fistulous conduit is rarely possible on large caliber arteries because of greater output.

It grants better results in smaller vessels, such as in the foreleg where traditional surgical access is more difficult. The disappearance of bruit and thrill is a sign of success.

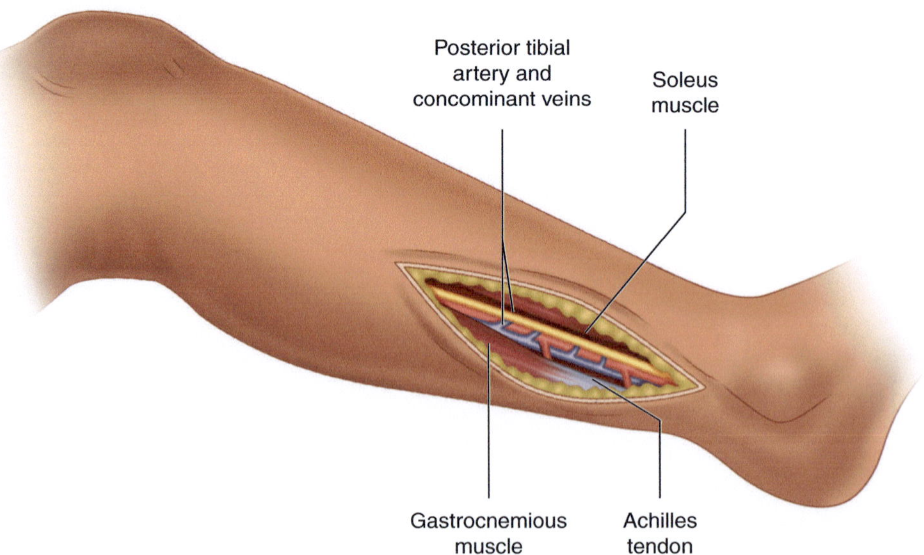

Fig. 26.8 Posterior tibial artery

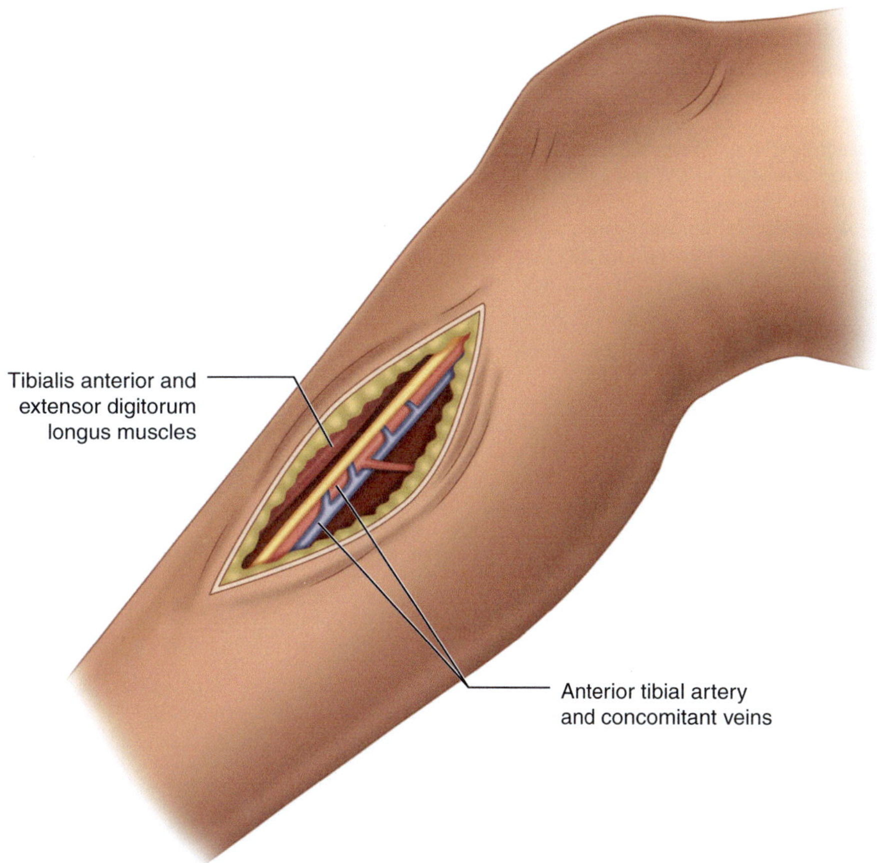

Fig. 26.9 Anterior tibial artery

Case Scenario

A 35-year-old white male was admitted to the emergency room after a motorbike accident. History of patient was uneventful; vitals were abnormal (blood pressure 75/50 mmHg, heart rate 110 bpm); clinical examination revealed GCS 15; absence of brain, thoracic, and abdominal injuries after CT scan; ischemia of left leg (pallor, pain, poikilothermia, paresthesia, absence of popliteal and tibial pulses); rapidly expanding left groin hematoma; exposed fracture of upper third of left femur; lacerations to quadriceps and biceps muscles. Correction of shock was started. Worsening in volume hematoma and deteriorating blood pressure led the patient directly in the operating room around 6 h after accident. Surgical exploration of left groin revealed complete transection of superficial femoral artery 2 cm after its origin, complete transection of *profunda femoris* vein and complete transection of femoral nerve. Proximal and distal stumps of artery were found. Harvesting of contralateral greater saphenous vein and bypass to restore arterial flow was made. *Profunda femoris* vein was ligated. Primary fasciotomies of the foreleg were performed. Venous bleeding difficult to control in the mangled muscles caused in the following hours hemodynamic instability. Irreversible ischemia of the foreleg has also developed, leading to secondary amputation of the thigh.

Questionnaire

1. In penetrating trauma with active bleeding, suggested is:
   A. Immediate surgical exploration X
   B. Doppler Ultrasound scan
   C. Angiography
   D. CT angiogram
2. Immediate action for injuries in penetrating trauma of limbs involving bones is:
   A. Immediate surgical exploration
   B. Arteriography X
   C. Doppler ultrasound scan
   D. Clinical observation
3. In arterial reconstruction with prosthetic interposition, if autologous vein is unavailable, the first choice graft is:
   A. Dacron
   B. Homograft
   C. PTFE X
   D. Others

Please see Chap. 58 for the correct answer.

Suggested Reading

Feliciano DV, et al. Evaluation and management of peripheral vascular injury: part I. Western Trauma Association/Critical decisions in trauma. J Trauma. 2011;70:1551–6.

Feliciano DV, et al. Western Trauma Association critical decisions in trauma: evaluation and management of peripheral vascular injury: part II. J Trauma Acute Care Surg. 2013;75:391–7.

Fox N, et al. Evaluation and management of penetrating lower extremity arterial trauma: an Eastern Association for the Surgery of Trauma practice management guideline. J Trauma Acute Care Surg. 2012;73(5 Suppl 4):S315–20.

Percival TJ, et al. Reperfusion strategies in the management of extremity vascular injury with ischaemia. Br J Surg. 2012;99(Suppl 1): 66–74.

Perkins ZB, et al. Meta-analysis of prognostic factors for amputation following surgical repair of lower extremity vascular trauma. Br J Surg. 2015;102(5):436–50.

Wahlgren CM, et al. Penetrating vascular trauma of the upper and lower limbs. Curr Trauma Rep. 2016;2:11–20.

Part III

Non-traumatic Emergency Surgery

Point-of-Care Ultrasound in the Diagnosis of Acute Abdominal Pain

27

Francesca Cortellaro, Cristiano Perani, Linda Guarnieri, Laura Ferrari, Michela Cazzaniga, Giovanni Maconi, Maddalena Alessandra Wu, and Paolo Aseni

Key Points

- In the emergency department, the use of point-of-care ultrasound has greatly improved the ability of physicians to diagnose emergent conditions rapidly, but a related area of concern is the operator dependence of this technology.
- The lower cost of ultrasounds and the lack of radiation exposure and side effects secondary to contrast medium make point-of-care sonography the first diagnostic choice in many clinical conditions characterized by acute abdominal pain such as ruptured abdominal aortic aneurysm, biliary tract disease including cholecystitis and cholangitis, complications of acute pancreatitis, acute appendicitis, diverticulitis, Crohn's disease, and bowel obstruction and perforation and in gynecological emergencies.
- Transabdominal ultrasound is the preferred imaging examination for the diagnosis of acute cholecystitis and should be considered the first diagnostic tool when the clinical presentation is suggestive of acute biliary pathology.
- Transabdominal sonography should be performed with a full bladder that acts as an acoustic window.
- In patients with bowel obstruction, it is important to search with US the transit point, i.e., the point between the dilated proximal and collapsed distal bowel loops; serial US examinations are safe and can be used to evaluate the progress of bowel obstruction in patients who are treated conservatively.
- Clinic-based point-of-care intestinal ultrasound has been proved to play a significant role in guiding therapeutic management of patients with Crohn's disease where sonographic detection of bowel wall thickening >3 mm is considered the most important parameter to suspect the active inflammatory phase of the disease.
- In patients with pneumoperitoneum, free abdominal air produces a sonographic appearance of linear enhancement of the peritoneal stripe from which start distinct posterior hyperechoic reverberation and shadowing artifacts. Sonography for pneumoperitoneum has been proved to have high accuracy and shows superior sensitivity to diagnose free peritoneal air compared with abdominal radiography.
- The site of the ectopic pregnancy can be determined with the transvaginal sonography: ultrasonographic findings of an empty uterus, a pseudosac, an adnexal mass, and/or a free fluid have good specificity, especially when found in combination, and they are useful for "ruling in" an ectopic pregnancy.

F. Cortellaro (✉)
ASST Santi Paolo e Carlo, Milan, Italy

C. Perani
ASST degli Spedali Civili di Brescia, Brescia, Italy

L. Guarnieri · L. Ferrari · M. Cazzaniga · P. Aseni
ASST Dipartimento di Emergenza-Urgenza, ASST Grande Ospedale Metropolitano Niguarda, Milan, Italy

G. Maconi
Gastroenterology Unit, Department of Biomedical and Clinical Sciences, Luigi Sacco University Hospital, University of Milan, Milan, Italy

M. A. Wu
Department of Biomedical and Clinical Sciences "Luigi Sacco", University of Milan, ASST Fatebenefratelli Sacco, Luigi Sacco Hospital, Milan, Italy

P. Aseni et al. (eds.), *Operative Techniques and Recent Advances in Acute Care and Emergency Surgery*,
https://doi.org/10.1007/978-3-319-95114-0_27

27.1 Introduction

The term "acute abdomen" can be defined as a possible medical emergency in a patient with recent onset of sudden abdominal pain with accompanying signs and symptoms that focus on abdominal organ involvement. Abdominal pain can be classified as visceral, somatoparietal, or referred pain and can be a manifestation of a broad group of systemic and local causes.

Acute abdominal pain (AAP) is a common complaint of patients presenting to the emergency department. Approximately 10% of patients presenting to the emergency department complain AAP, and approximately half of these patients have nonspecific findings [1]. The other half have a more serious disorder, life-threatening in a small number, which warrants further evaluation and treatment. Nearly 90% of most presentations of AAP fall into one of the following eight diagnoses: appendicitis, cholecystitis, bowel obstruction, renal colic, peptic ulcer disease, pancreatitis, diverticular disease, and nonspecific abdominal pain. Causes of acute abdominal pain can be classified as urgent or non-urgent [2]. Urgent conditions require immediate treatment (within 24 h) to prevent complications. Most common urgent causes are cholecystitis-cholangitis, acute appendicitis, acute diverticulitis, and bowel obstruction. Less common are abdominal aortic aneurysm rupture, visceral perforation, mesenteric ischemia, and complicated inflammatory bowel diseases. Most common non-urgent causes are the nonspecific abdominal pain (NSAP) and non-complicated gastrointestinal diseases.

Only about one-quarter of patients who have previously been classified with an acute abdomen will receive surgical treatment; so the clinical dilemma is to decide if the patient needs a surgical treatment or not and in which patients a surgical option needs to be urgently adopted [3, 4]. Therefore, a thorough and heuristic approach to the diagnosis of abdominal pain is necessary.

Associate symptoms, medical history, or drug therapy often allow the physician to further focus on the differential diagnosis. However, an accurate diagnosis by medical history, physical examination, and laboratory test findings is possible in only a small proportion of patients (in 20–40% of patients with abdominal pain) so that imaging by different radiological techniques plays a pivotal role [4, 5]. CRP and WBC count alone are usually insufficient to differentiate urgent from non-urgent conditions; however, when their count is elevated, the suspicion of an urgent condition rises, and additional imaging is necessary [6]. Conventional radiography correctly can diagnose the presence of a cause in 47% of patients [7], but it cannot accurately discriminate between urgent and non-urgent conditions [5]. For bowel obstruction, the conventional radiology with a simple plain abdominal X-ray has a higher sensitivity than clinical evaluation (74 vs. 57%). However, since it is impossible to diagnose the underlying cause of the bowel obstruction with conventional radiography only, a computed tomography scan is usually mandatory. The value of plain abdominal X-rays has been questioned by many authors in the workup of patients with AAP due to the lack of added benefit on top of clinical assessment. However, in patients with clinical suspicion of perforation of hollow viscus by foreign bodies [5–8] and bowel obstruction, a conventional X-ray can be still considered the useful first approach as a triage test to distinguish between patients who need further investigations and those who can be safely observed without additional urgent examination.

CT leads to the highest sensitivity and specificity in patients with acute abdominal pain, and it is still the gold standard. The use of multidetector computed tomography has completely changed the clinical approach to patients with AAP, simplifying the diagnosis but burdening the patients with radiation exposure.

The use of a sequential strategy that performs a CT scan after negative or inconclusive ultrasonography (US) reduces the use of CT scan. The CT strategy has a sensitivity of 94% and a specificity of 68% [9]. Some authors concluded that in nonpregnant women with acute abdominal pain, the sequential strategy using CT after US could reduce the use of CT to about a half [5].

The location of pain is a useful starting point and will guide a further evaluation. The American College of Radiology has recommended the use of different imaging studies to assess AAP based on pain location: the US is recommended to evaluate the right upper-quadrant pain, and CT is recommended for the right and left lower-quadrant pain (Table 27.1) [10]. However, the sensitivity of US in identifying patients with appendicitis and diverticulitis in the presence of clinical suspicion ranges from 80% to 90%. For this reason, US remains the primary imaging technique in the majority of cases, especially in young or female patients, when the limitation of the radiation exposure should be mandatory. The use of CT should be limited to patients with the nondiagnostic US and patients showing a discrepancy between clinical symptoms and negative imaging obtained by the US.

Moreover, if the US is performed by the emergency physician, the accuracy is high in most common conditions and can give real-time answers in unstable or septic patients where the choice of antibiotic therapy, need of early surgical operation, and immediate control of septic source by the interventional radiologist or endoscopist can be lifesaving [11]. In the next paragraph, we will focus on the role of POCUS in the different clinical situations and its respective values of sensibility and specificity.

Table 27.1 Pain location and possible diagnosis in patients with acute abdominal pain

Pain location	Possible diagnosis
Right upper quadrant	Biliary: cholecystitis, cholelithiasis, cholangitis
	Colonic: colitis, diverticulitis
	Hepatic: abscess, hepatitis, mass
	Pulmonary: pneumonia, embolus
	Renal: nephrolithiasis, pyelonephritis
Epigastric	Biliary: cholecystitis, cholelithiasis, cholangitis
	Cardiac: myocardial infarction, pericarditis
	Gastric: esophagitis, gastritis, peptic ulcer
	Pancreatic: mass, pancreatitis
	Vascular: aortic dissection, mesenteric ischemia
Left upper quadrant	Cardiac: angina, myocardial infarction, pericarditis
	Gastric: esophagitis, gastritis, peptic ulcer
	Pancreatic: mass, pancreatitis
	Renal: nephrolithiasis, pyelonephritis
	Vascular: aortic dissection, mesenteric ischemia
Periumbilical	Colonic: early appendicitis
	Gastric: esophagitis, gastritis, peptic ulcer, small bowel mass or obstruction
	Vascular: aortic dissection, mesenteric ischemia
Right lower quadrant	Colonic: appendicitis, colitis, diverticulitis, IBD, IBS
	Gynecologic: ectopic pregnancy, fibroids, ovarian mass, torsion, PID
	Renal: nephrolithiasis, pyelonephritis
Suprapubic	Colonic: appendicitis, colitis, diverticulitis, IBD, IBS
	Gynecologic: ectopic pregnancy, fibroids, ovarian mass, torsion, PID
	Renal: cystitis, nephrolithiasis, pyelonephritis
Left lower quadrant	Colonic: colitis, diverticulitis, IBD, IBS
	Gynecologic: ectopic pregnancy, fibroids, ovarian mass, torsion, PID
	Renal: nephrolithiasis, pyelonephritis
Any location	Abdominal wall: herpes zoster, muscle strain, hernia
	Other: bowel obstruction, mesenteric ischemia, peritonitis, narcotic withdrawal, sickle-cell crisis, porphyria, IBD, heavy metal poisoning

From: Cartwright SL, Knudson MP: Evaluation of acute abdominal pain in adults. Am Fam Physician 2008, 77:971–8

IBD inflammatory bowel disease, *IBS* irritable bowel syndrome, *PID* pelvic inflammatory disease

27.2 Abdominal Aortic Aneurysm

A dilation of the infrarenal aorta, due to a chronic weakening of the arterial wall, has an increased risk of fatal rupture [12–14]. It is estimated that abdominal aortic aneurysm (AAA) affects up to 8% of men over 65 years of age [14–16]. Data from CDC's National Center for Health Statistics showed that abdominal aortic aneurysms (AAAs) and acute aortic syndrome are among the 15 leading causes of death for people aged 60–84 years in the USA, accounting for up to 0.7% of total deaths for that age group [17]. AAAs are usually asymptomatic, and diagnosis is an incidental finding during evaluation of routine screening or other health complaints. AAA size is considered the main predictive factor of rupture, and when the diameter is evaluated less than 50 mm, the risk of rupture is evaluated at a rate of <1% per year, while for those with a diameter larger than 60 mm the associated rupture risk is about 10% per year. Mortality of AAA rupture is still very high among 75–80%, and half of these patients die before coming into the hospital [18]. Once patients present to the emergency department (ED), early diagnosis significantly decreases mortality from 75% to 35% [19].

Less than half of the patients with a ruptured AAA will present with the classic triad of abdominal pain, hypotension, and a pulsatile abdominal mass [20]. For these reasons, it is essential to have a rapid and accurate diagnostic test for patients at risk for AAA presenting with symptoms suggestive of this disease.

US-based assessments can quantify the maximal anterior-posterior and transverse diameter of the aorta and are the method of choice for AAA screening and follow-up. The reported sensitivity and specificity of US for AAA diagnosis are 87.4–98.9% and 99.9%, respectively [21]; for this reason, it is considered very useful in the emergency setting.

In particular, the US performed by emergency medicine residents with appropriate training had a sensitivity of 0.94 (95% CI 0.86–1.0) for AAA. Specificity was 1.0 (95% CI 0.984–1.0). These data don't differ from those obtained by conventional radiology (US, CT, RMN) [22].

The other main modality used to diagnose and assess AAA is CT or computed tomography angiography (CTA) with intravenous contrast. CTA, however, has the advantage to provide a much more accurate assessment of the morphology and surgical anatomy of the AAA which is a prerequisite for decisions regarding the appropriate surgical repair [23].

27.3 Biliary Tract Disease

Epigastric and right hypochondrium pain is one of the most common complaints in patients presenting to an emergency department (ED) in about 2–4% and accounts for approximately 20–25% of all patients with non-traumatic abdominal pain [24]. The differential diagnoses of isolated acute non-traumatic epigastric pain include a broad spectrum of diseases ranging from benign, self-limited conditions to diseases with high morbidity and mortality. Isolated acute epigastric pain is one of the presenting symptoms of cholelithiasis and cholecystitis [25, 26]. Abdominal ultrasound is noninvasive, does not use ionizing radiation, and is relatively inexpensive, so it may be the imaging modality of choice for these patients [27].

In this paragraph for brevity, we will only deal with the two most commonly encountered pathologies that share the same etiology and the role of US in their management: acute calculous cholecystitis and acute biliary pancreatitis (ABP).

27.3.1 Acute Calculous Cholecystitis

Acute cholecystitis is defined as an acute inflammation of the gallbladder, regardless of the cause. In the many of cases, the underlying etiology is the obstruction of the cystic duct due to an impacted stone in either the neck of the gallbladder or the cystic duct (acute calculous cholecystitis). Acute cholecystitis can also develop without associated cholelithiasis (acute acalculous cholecystitis) [28].

US is the preferred imaging examination for the diagnosis of acute cholecystitis and should be considered the first diagnostic tool when the clinical presentation is suggestive of biliary pathology. Acute calculous cholecystitis is diagnosed radiologically by the concomitant presence of gallstones, thickening of the gallbladder wall (5 mm or greater), pericholecystic fluid, or direct tenderness when the probe is pushed against the gallbladder (ultrasonographic Murphy's sign) [29] (Figs. 27.1 and 27.2).

A meta-analysis of the diagnostic performance of US in detecting acute cholecystitis indicated an unadjusted sensitivity and specificity of 94% and 78%, respectively [30]. Some investigators included in their analysis some appropriate adjustments for verification bias (workup bias) [31], to be as close as possible to the "real life," and they found that US detects acute cholecystitis with sensitivity of 88% (95% confidence interval [CI], 74–100%) and specificity of 80% (95% CI, 62–98%). Sensitivity for the detection of cholelithiasis was comparable, but specificity was higher at approximately 99% [32]. CT of the abdomen, though useful for the evaluation of suspected complications and concurrent intra-abdominal conditions, is inferior to US in the assessment of acute biliary disease [33].

Some US findings are more strongly associated with acute cholecystitis than others: a positive Murphy's sign (pain can be provoked by either the transducer or the sonographer's palpation under guidance, in the exact area of the gallbladder) is reported to have sensitivity as high as 88% [34]. Ultrasonographic Murphy's sign shows a better performance than clinical Murphy's sign, which seems to have lower sensitivity and specificity (respectively, 65% and 87%) to detect acute cholecystitis, with a positive likelihood ratio of 2.8 (95% CI 0.8–8.6) [32].

In a study involving 497 patients with suspected acute cholecystitis, the positive predictive value of the presence of stones and a positive ultrasonographic Murphy's sign was

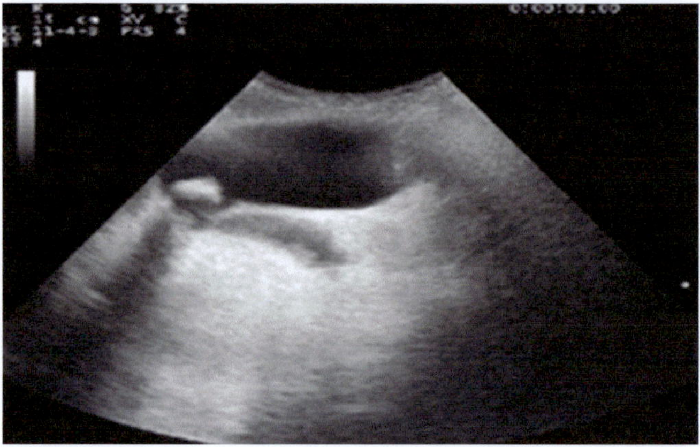

Fig. 27.2 Gallbladder hydrops with big gallstone and cone-shaped shadow

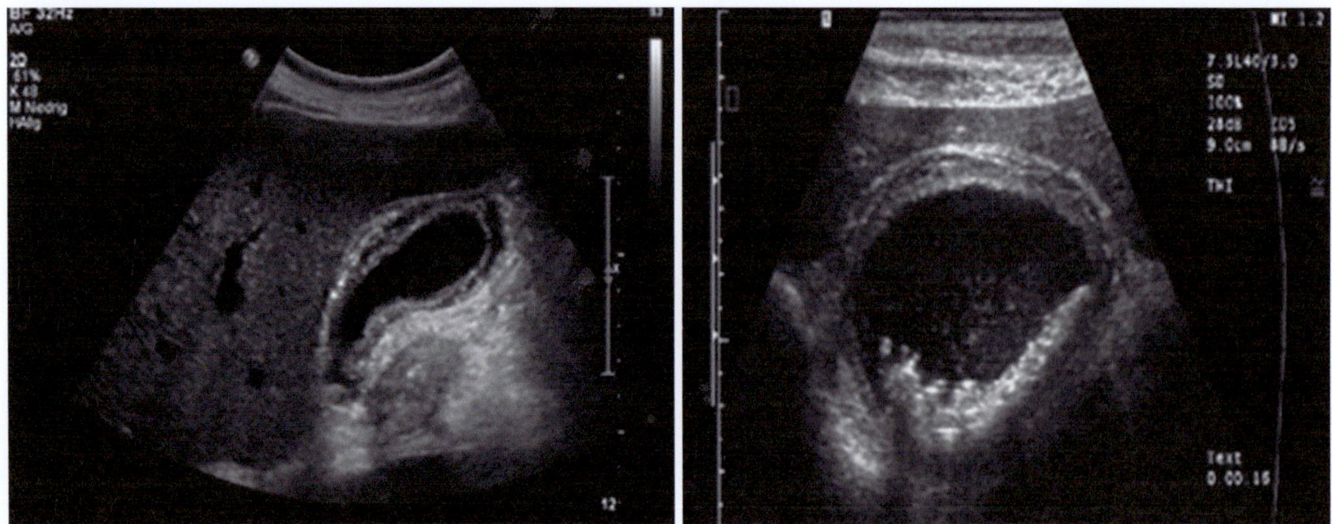

Fig. 27.1 US image of acute cholecystitis showing the concomitant presence of thickening of the gallbladder wall and a pericholecystic fluid

92%, and that of stones and thickening of the gallbladder wall was 95%. The negative predictive value of the absence of stones combined with either a normal gallbladder wall or a negative Murphy's sign was 95% [35]. It should be remembered that thickening of the gallbladder wall in the absence of cholecystitis may be observed in systemic conditions, such as liver, renal, and heart failure, possibly due to the elevated portal and systemic venous pressures [36]. No differences are shown in sensitivity and specificity for acute calculous cholecystitis when US is performed by a radiologist or by a trained emergency physician [37].

However, due to differences among reports in the frequency of the occurrence of individual findings, sensitivity, and specificity, the diagnosis should be made after a comprehensive judgment of the individual clinical evaluation [37, 38].

27.3.2 Acute Biliary Pancreatitis

Gallstones represent the most frequent etiology of acute pancreatitis. The proportion of the total number of cases of acute pancreatitis associated to biliary lithiasis can be estimated between 40% and 60%. An accurate diagnosis of acute biliary pancreatitis (ABP) is of utmost importance since the clearance of lithiasis from the gallbladder, and common bile duct can rule out recurrences, very frequent otherwise, with 30% to 50% of the patients developing recurrent acute pancreatitis relatively soon after discharge. Over 90% of the CBD stones come from the gallbladder through the cystic duct [39], (Fig. 27.2). The US is the first and the most available and commonly performed imaging method. It seeks for lithiasis in the gallbladder and in the common bile duct (CBD) or indirect signs of biliary obstruction (dilation of the CBD). The sensitivity of the US in the detection of gallstones is over 95% in uncomplicated cases, [40] but in ABP, the sensitivity for gallstone detection is lower, being only 67–78% due to the ileus and bowel distension [41]. The sensitivity of US for choledocholithiasis varies between 50% and 80% from different studies, but the specificity is high, reaching 95% [42]. Although ultrasound is very useful in the first phase to identify the etiology of ABP, contrast-enhancement CT remains the gold standard for the management to identify the severity of the disease and any complications [43].

27.4 Acute Appendicitis

Acute appendicitis (AA) is one of the most common causes of abdominal-related emergency seen in the ED, as well as the most common reason for urgent surgery in pediatric population. Among ED accesses for abdominal pain, AA represents the first diagnosis for 5–15% of patients above 50 years and 15–30% of youngers. Acute appendicitis can progress to perforation and peritonitis. It has been estimated that the perforation rate of above 30% [44] is associated with significant morbidity. A delay in diagnosis later than 24 h increases the risk of perforation [45].

The diagnosis of AA can sometimes be clinically challenging. The classic presentation of periumbilical pain followed by nausea and vomiting with migration of pain to the right lower quadrant may be absent in more than one-third of patients, and the diagnosis can sometimes be clinically challenging. Moreover, when typical symptoms are present, they can be similar to other conditions, especially in the early stage [46, 47]; the diagnosis can be particularly difficult in children, elderly patients, pregnant, and childbearing age women.

Differential diagnosis of AA includes in women gynecological emergencies and pelvic inflammatory disease (PID) and, in both sexes, right-sided diverticula (that occur more often in younger patients than do left-sided ones), left-sided diverticula with a redundant sigmoid colon, torsion of epiploic appendix, complicated IBD, and perforation of colonic neoplasia. Laboratory examinations alone have weak discriminatory and predictive capacity. When the laboratory values of two or more inflammatory variables are normal, the diagnosis of appendicitis is unlikely. Conversely, appendicitis is very likely when the values of two or more inflammatory variables are increased [48]. A variable combination of clinical signs and symptoms has been used together with laboratory findings in several scoring systems proposed for suggesting the probability of AA and the possible subsequent management pathway. Laboratory tests of inflammatory response and clinical descriptors of peritoneal irritation and migration of pain are the strongest discriminators and have been included in all diagnostic scores; the Alvarado score (Table 27.2) is the most extensively studied. Its validity has

Table 27.2 Alvarado score for acute appendicitis

		Value
Symptoms	Abdominal pain that migrates to the right iliac fossa	1
	Anorexia or ketones in the urine	1
	Nausea or vomiting	1
	Tenderness in the right iliac fossa	2
Signs	Rebound tenderness (Blumberg)	1
	Fever of 37.3 °C or more	1
Laboratory	Leukocytosis >10,000	2
	Neutrophilia >70%	1
Total score		10
Score		
1–4	Appendicitis unlikely	
5–6	Appendicitis possible	
7–8	Appendicitis probable	
9–10	Appendicitis very probable	

From Alvarado A. A practical score for the early diagnosis of acute appendicitis. Ann. Emerg. Med 1986

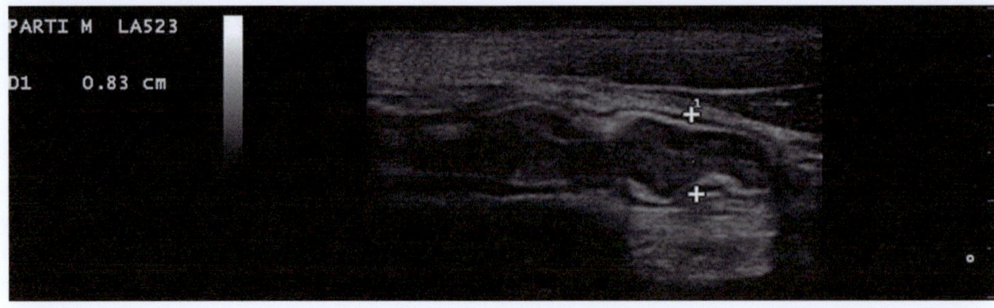

Fig. 27.3 US of the appendix with increased diameter

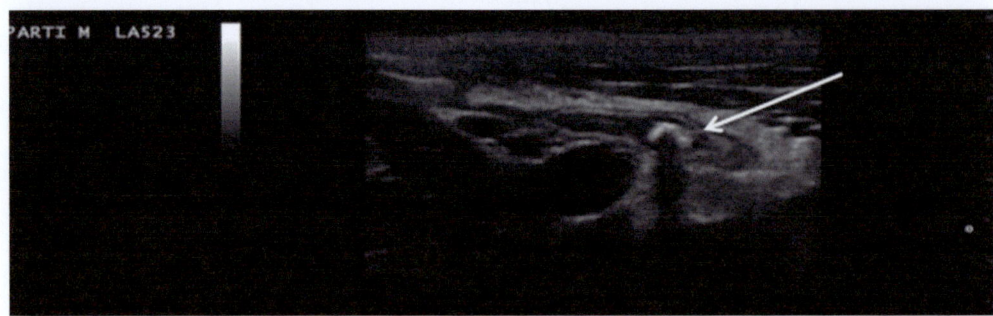

Fig. 27.4 US image of intraluminal appendicolith (arrow) with posterior acoustic shadowing

been summarized in a meta-analysis including 5.960 patients in 29 studies [49]. A clinical cutoff score of less than 5 can be applied to "rule out" appendicitis with a sensitivity of 99% (95% CI 97–99%) and a specificity of 43% (36–51%), while a cutoff score of fewer than 7 results in a sensitivity of 82% (76–86%) and a specificity of 81% (76–85%), suggesting it is not sufficiently accurate to rule in or rule out surgery.

The role of imaging in the diagnosis of AA is still debated, with variable use of US, CT, and MRI in different clinical settings. A diagnostic scoring system that incorporates imaging to the primary clinical diagnosis of acute appendicitis has not yet been developed [50]. CT scan has more sensitivity and specificity than US: overall sensitivity and specificity of US and CT are 58–76 and 95 and 99 and 84%, respectively [51, 52]. On the other hand, it has been estimated that the benefit of universal imaging in avoiding 12 unnecessary appendectomies could result in one additional cancer death [53]. MRI is much less affordable than US but, in settings having availability of such resource, can be considered for the young population and in pregnant women, being a non-radiative imaging modality, potentially valuable in the setting of negative US.

The US diagnosis of AA is made using a linear high-frequency probe (7–10 MHz) or a convex-medium frequency probe (3–5 MHz). Scanning starts using the highest-frequency transducer providing penetration adequate to visualize the right psoas muscle and the iliac vessels, and then transverse and longitudinal images of the cecal region are obtained. The technique used is known as graded compression of the right lower quadrant, with patient in supine position and gradual increasing pressure exerted to displace normal overlying bowel gas. The potential adverse effect of high BMI on US accuracy is almost unclear [54].

During US examination, a digitiform dead-end image should be visualized with these characteristics: diameter greater than 6 mm, thickened wall >3 mm, non-compressible lumen, hypo-aperistalsis, and McBurney echographic sign.

Other findings include the absence of gas in the lumen, appendicoliths, hyperechogenic peri-appendicular fat thickening, or fluid collection consistent with an abscess, free fluid, and lymphadenopathy (Figs. 27.3 and 27.4). The most sensitive sign seems to be a non-compressible appendix that exceeds 6 mm in diameter (up to 98% sensitive). A method of self-localization added to graded compression US of the right lower quadrant reduces the time of the examination and has been a valuable addition to the diagnostic evaluation of acute appendicitis [55]. A three-step sequential positioning has been suggested to optimize sensitivity and specificity. Since the appendix lies in retrocecal position in 25–65% of patients, an additional use of scanning with the patient lying in a 45° left posterior oblique (LPO) position and then rescanning in the supine position significantly improves the appendiceal visualization rate, with a decreasing need of CT scan [52].

In the emergency department, the use of POCUS has greatly improved the ability of physicians to diagnose emergent conditions rapidly, but a related area of concern is the operator dependence of this technology. A recent systematic review [56] of the literature on diagnostic accuracy of POCUS for AA when performed by non-radiologist physicians shows that it is as specific as the US performed by radiologists but less sensitive (80% vs. 90%). Nonetheless, it should be considered that the level of training and experience in the different considered studies varied from novice to expert. US of the appendix may be more difficult to learn than other modalities because the normal appendix is typically air-filled making it more difficult to localize than the pathologic appendix, which is usually enlarged and fluid-filled.

This review concludes that POCUS has a reasonable diagnostic accuracy in the hands of trained operators and could be considered in the routine workup of acute appendicitis.

The controversies in diagnosis and management of AA lead the World Society of Emergency Surgery (WSES) to convene a consensus conference (CC) in 2016 to study the topic and define its guidelines [57].

These guidelines state that using a scoring system (such as Alvarado score) is important in tailoring management:

- Low-risk patients could be discharged with appropriate short outpatient-department follow-up or admitted for observation if strongly symptomatic.
- Intermediate-risk patients benefit from observation and systematic diagnostic imaging. In this kind of patients, an abdominal US would be the first line in diagnostic imaging. Patients with the positive US would receive appendectomy, and those with negative test should be submitted to either CT or further clinical observation, followed by serial US.
- High-risk patients (younger than 60 years old) may not always require CT; in specific clinical settings when the US is negative or uncertain, CT before surgery is routinely performed in Western countries.

27.5 Crohn's Disease (CD)

CD is a chronic inflammatory bowel disease (IBD) that may involve any part of the gastrointestinal tract. It is characterized by a relapsing behavior or variable severity and clinical activity and by intestinal complications such as strictures, fistulas, or abscesses. For this reason, CD patients need clinical, endoscopic, radiological, and sonographic assessment. Although endoscopy is the main diagnostic procedure in the management of patients, intestinal ultrasound (IUS) is well known as an accurate, useful, and practical tool for prompt assessment of extension and activity of the disease and for detecting abdominal complications of CD [58, 59]. Several European guidelines, namely, the European Crohn's and Colitis Organization (ECCO), European Society of Gastrointestinal Radiology (ESGAR), and European Federation of Societies of Ultrasound in Medicine and Biology (EFSUMB), recommend IUS as a useful technique to detect small bowel CD at its first presentation, to assess disease activity, to diagnose stenoses of the small bowel, and to assess penetrating complications such as fistulas and abscesses [60]. More importantly, thanks to the advantage to be well-tolerated, radiation-free, repeatable, and cheap, the bedside and ambulatory use of IUS is considered as the main tool to monitor the course of the disease. Clinic-based point-of-care IUS has been proved to play a significant role in guiding therapeutic management of IBD patients and an important adjunct to routine clinical and laboratory assessment [61].

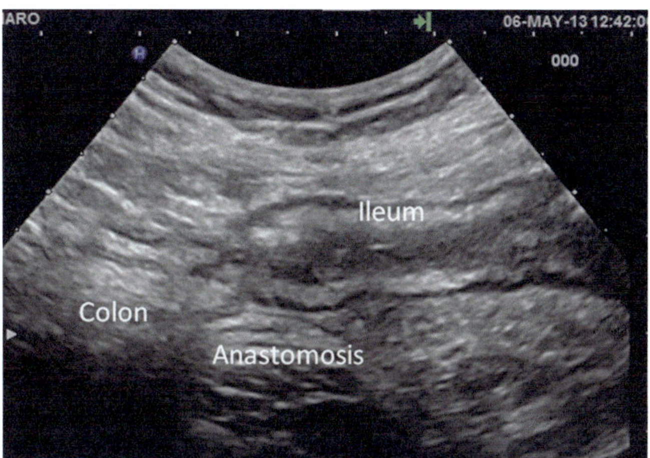

Fig. 27.5 Sonographic detection of bowel wall thickening >3 mm is the most important parameter to suspect CD

Sonographic detection of bowel wall thickening (BWT) >3 mm is considered the most important parameter to suspect CD (Fig. 27.5). Although it is not specific for the diagnosis of CD, systematic review and meta-analyses showed that this parameter is the most accurate in detecting CD with a sensitivity and specificity of 89% and 96%. This is also the main sonographic parameter to detect CD recurrence after surgery. The assessment of specific features of BWT such as echo pattern and vascularization, the latter using echo-Doppler or contrast-enhanced ultrasound (CEUS), is useful to evaluate CD activity, to monitor the disease after treatment, and to predict its behavior. One of the main indications for IUS is the detection of abdominal complications of CD. These are a frequent reason for surgery, an event occurring in the natural history of approximately 70% of CD patients. Stenoses represent the most frequent complication and the main reason for surgical intervention (up to 90%). It can be detected by IUS as a thickened and stiff bowel wall, coupled with narrowing of the lumen (diameter less than 1 cm), proximal dilatation (> 25–30 mm), and hyperperistalsis of the pre-stenotic gut (Fig. 27.6). Depending on the severity of the stricture, the accuracy of IUS for the diagnosis ranges from 74% to 100% in sensitivity and from 89% to 93% in specificity [60]. Intestinal fistulas, sinus tracts, and fissures originating from deep ulcers in CD are frequent complications of CD. Fistulas may be classified as internal

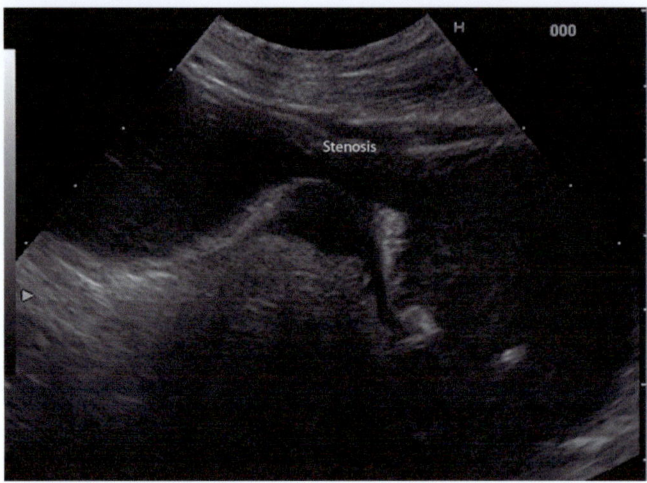

Fig. 27.6 Sonographic appearance of enteric stenosis

(e.g., entero-enteric) and external and are detected as hypoechoic areas or tracts between ileal loops with or without internal gaseous artifacts. The sensitivity of IUS for the diagnosis of these lesions ranges from 67% to 87%, with specificity of 90% to 100%, similar to CT and MRI [62]. Abdominal abscesses in CD are usually the results of internal fistula or surgical interventions. These lesions appear at IUS as hypo-anechoic lesions containing fluid and gaseous artifacts with posterior enhancement and irregular margins, sometimes within hypertrophic mesentery. IUS can detect this complication with a sensitivity of 81–100% and a specificity of 92–94%, similar to CT and MR (5). The use of CEUS accurately discriminates abscesses from phlegmons. For these reasons, absence of radiation and low cost, IUS should be preferred over CT to monitor CD patients with abscess under conservative treatment and patients under treatment with biologic agents, which are contraindicated in the presence of intra-abdominal abscesses.

27.6 Acute Diverticulitis

Acute diverticulitis results from inflammation of a colonic diverticulum, which is a herniation of mucosa and submucosa, corresponding to a weak point of the colonic wall, in particular in the sigmoid colon, because of its highest intraluminal pressure [34, 63, 64]. It represents the most common cause of acute left lower-quadrant pain in adults who require acute hospitalization. The incidence of diverticular disease has increased over the past century affecting over half of the people over 65 years with a prevalence that increases with age. About 10–25% of patients with diverticulosis will develop an acute episode of diverticulitis in their life [65, 66]. From a clinical point of view, patients with diverticulitis are more likely to have a non-complicated pain in the left lower abdominal quadrant, with or without nausea or vomiting or fever, and although 85% of colonic diverticulitis will recover with a nonoperative treatment, some patients may have complications such as abscesses, fistulas, obstruction, and/or perforation at presentation [67, 68].

Modified Hinchey classification (1997) and others based on clinical severity and presentation of the disease have been made to guide the clinical management and treatment. Clinical differentiation from other causes of abdominopelvic pain is often difficult, so imaging is used in most cases both to realize a differential diagnosis and to guide the therapeutic management [69, 70].

Currently, conventional contrast-enhanced CT of the abdomen is the diagnostic test of choice, especially in the ED, with sensitivity, specificity, and positive and negative predictive values as well greater than 95%, allowing the identification of both colonic abnormalities (particularly segmental wall thickening, submucosal edema, vascular engorgement, and diverticula) and inflammatory changes in the pericolic fat planes plus fascial, mesenteric, and/or peritoneal fluid, grading its severity and identifying most usual complications, excluding an underlying carcinoma [70, 71].

Some authors claim that CT sensitivity is higher than that of US in detecting diverticulitis (81% versus 61%, $p = 0.048$) in unselected patients presenting with acute abdominal pain, but the positive predictive values are comparable, whereas in the presence of clinical suspicion of diverticulitis, the sensitivity of US reaches 92% [72–74].

CT may be more likely to recognize alternative causes of abdominal pain, and it is essential for investigating complicated diverticular disease especially where there are signs and clinical suspicion of secondary peritonitis. However, in most of the uncomplicated cases, the experienced sonographer may quickly confirm a diagnosis guided by clinical symptoms [75–79]. Moreover, the lower cost and the lack of radiation exposure and side effects secondary to contrast, in particular in pregnancy, young, and premenopausal women on one side and patients with kidney failure or nephropathy on the other, are strong advantages of US compared to CT. Furthermore, US is a real-time, always available, dynamic examination, and this characteristic conveys dynamic information about bowel motility and changes in position and can also depict visceral blood flow [75]. Another important advantage of US is the possibility to correlate the US finding with the point of maximal tenderness. Bedside, in not too obese patients, US may be superior to CT, and it is most useful in early, uncomplicated diverticulitis, with a high sensitivity and specificity for the primary complication of pericolic abscess, too [79]. From a technical point of view, both curved (3.5–5 MHz) and linear (5–12 MHz) transducers can be used; the higher-frequency probes are useful for detailed investigation of the large bowel wall, identifying its typical haustral pattern or changes in the layers of the bowel wall. Focal bowel masses or segments of wall thickening or dilated loops may be evident even at lower frequencies. The diagnostic criteria for diverticulitis that have been used in US and CT are the same [80, 81]. The presence of the following three criteria at the point of maximum tenderness allows a specific sonographic diagnosis of diverticulitis:

- Demonstration of at least one inflamed diverticulum: in contrast to normal, inflamed diverticula are hypoechoic or hyperechoic with a hypoechoic rim, and they are surrounded by hyperechoic fatty tissue.
- Signs of inflammation of pericolic fat ranging from hyperechoic non-compressible fat to hypoechoic phlegmonous inflammation with fibrinopurulent exudate.
- Short segmental bowel wall thickening >4–5 mm, in particular, if graded compression causes pain; the bowel wall layers are usually preserved; hypertrophy of the muscular layer is frequently seen (Figs. 27.7, 27.8, and 27.9).

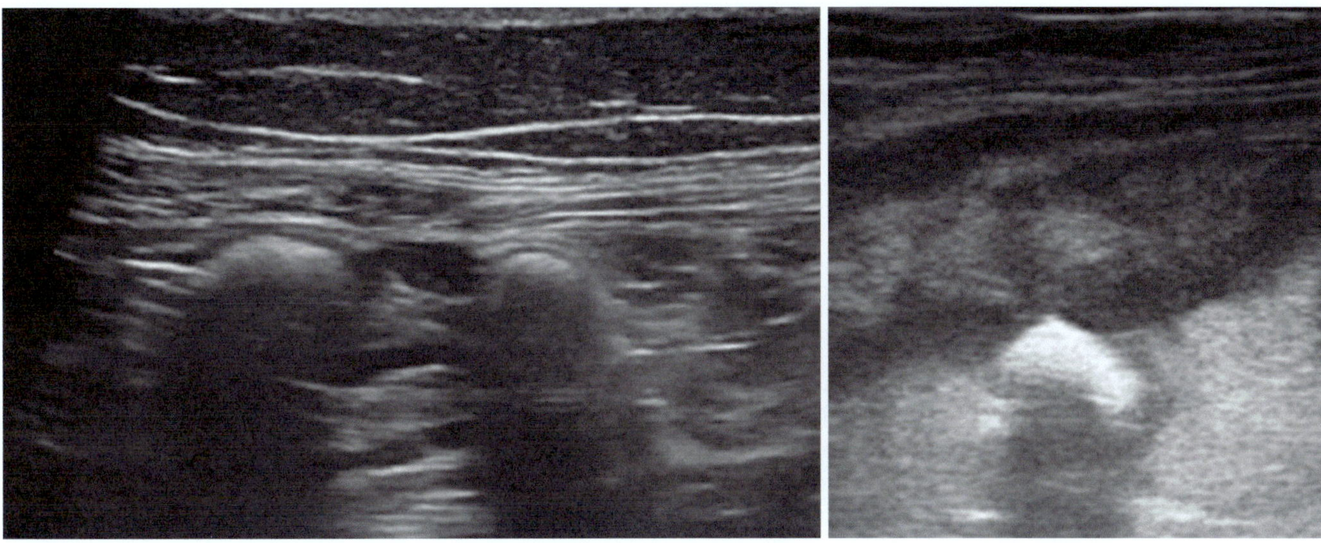

Fig. 27.7 Sonographic features of uncomplicated diverticulitis. Diverticula appear as bright "ear" out of the bowel wall, often hyperechoic because of the air inside. A central acoustic shadowing echogenicity may indicate the presence of fecalith. The neck of diverticulum may be identified as an echogenic band traversing hypoechoic muscularis propria, which is often thickened. A thinned diverticular wall may be demonstrated at higher probe frequencies with a reduced gut signature due to the absence of muscularis propria

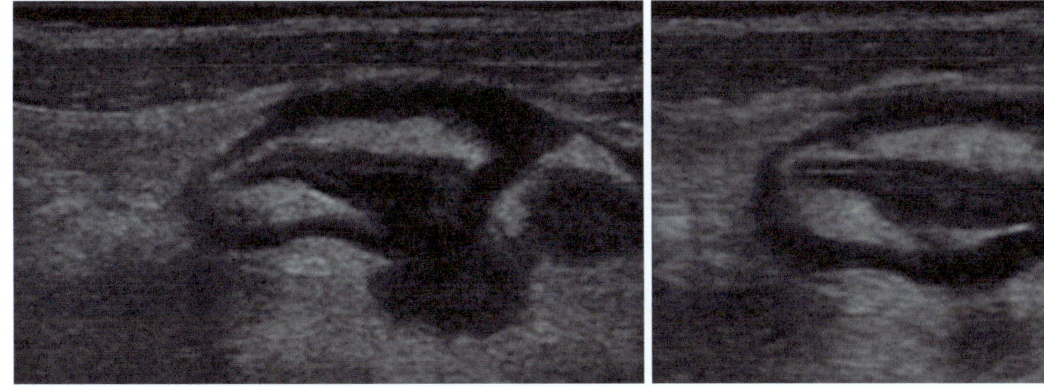

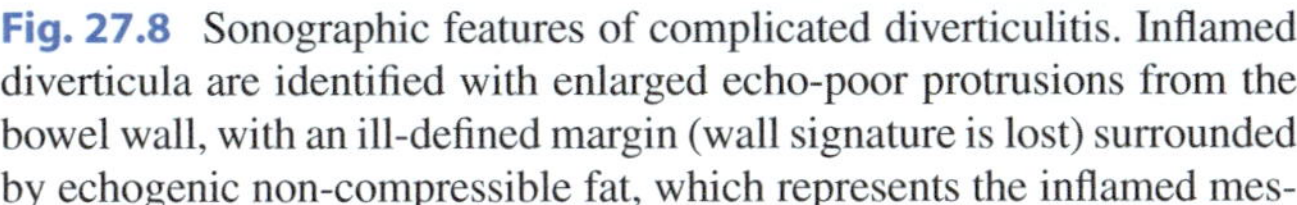

Fig. 27.8 Sonographic features of complicated diverticulitis. Inflamed diverticula are identified with enlarged echo-poor protrusions from the bowel wall, with an ill-defined margin (wall signature is lost) surrounded by echogenic non-compressible fat, which represents the inflamed mesentery and omentum sealing off the imminent perforation and may contain pockets of air and pericolic anechoic fluid. Often the inflammation extends into the bowel producing asymmetrical hypoechoic mural thickening that may demonstrate hyperemia on Doppler scanning

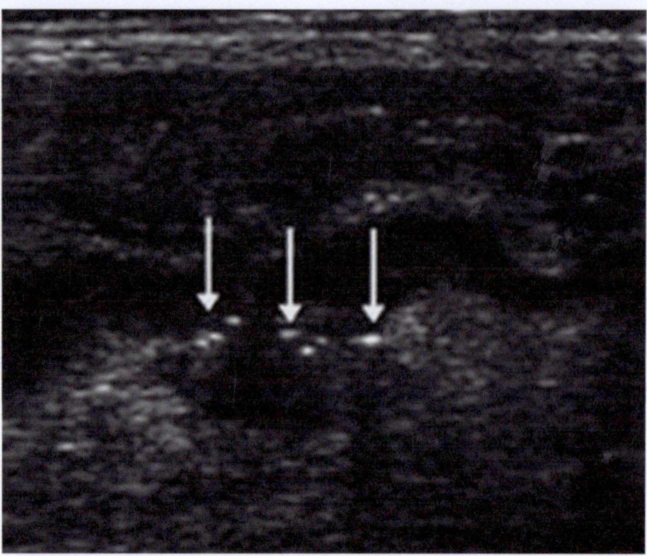

Fig. 27.9 Sonographic features of complicated diverticulitis with micro-perforation of the bowel wall showing the presence of small pockets of air (arrows) in the pericolic inflamed fat

27.7 Bowel Obstruction

Intestinal obstruction is a common cause of acute abdominal pain. Effective treatment depends on rapid and accurate diagnosis especially for patients who need early surgery. Diagnosis is usually based on clinical history, physical examination, and plain abdominal radiographs; recently multidetector CT scanning is becoming the first-line diagnostic imaging method for bowel obstruction, particularly useful in revealing the site and cause of obstruction [82].

The increased use of sonography in the initial assessment of patients with abdominal pain has made the point-of-care US a valuable adjunctive tool for the diagnosis of bowel obstruction. US is cheap, readily available, and noninvasive, does not use ionizing radiation, and is easy and safe to perform in critically ill patients. In expert hands, it is relatively quick to perform and accurate and may offer specific information about the etiology and level of obstruction. It has been demonstrated that non-radiology residents after a short training can diagnose the presence of small bowel obstruction (SBO) using POCUS with a high degree of accuracy, comparable with that of radiology residents [83].

US bowel examination usually starts with abdominal curvilinear (convex, 3.5–5.0 MHz) probe but should be completed with high-frequency (5.0–12.0 MHz) linear probe. The latter transducer allows an accurate evaluation of histologic bowel wall layers: inner hyperechoic lumen-mucosal interface, hypoechoic mucosa (or muscularis mucosae for other authors), hyperechoic submucosa, hypoechoic muscularis layer, and peripheral hyperechoic serosa [84, 85].

The different anatomical segments of the gut can be identified by their topographical position and specific morphological criteria. The duodenum can be identified by its "C-shaped" course around the pancreatic head and by the location of the third part of the duodenum, which lies between the aorta and the superior mesenteric vessels. The small bowel cannot be evaluated continuously, and a systematic examination can be performed by making vertical, parallel, and overlapping lanes with the transducer. The jejunum is usually located in the left upper and mid-abdomen and the ileum in the right mid- and lower abdomen. Fluid-filled loops allow optimal visualization of the *valvulae conniventes*, typical of the small intestine; they may help differentiate the *jejunum* (where they are numerous and widespread) and the *ileum* (where they are rare and smaller). The colon is characterized by its haustration, best visible with US on the anterior wall at the ascending and transverse colon. The left hemicolon is seen more often in a contracted condition. The sigmoid colon takes a variable course over the left iliac vessels to the small pelvis, and the rectum can be scanned using a filled bladder as the sonic window [86, 87].

Approaching the US in bowel obstruction may be difficult in the very gassy or obese patient, but the use of technical tricks, as graded compression or examination in the coronal plane and lateral decubitus positions, may help to overcome bowel gas. Contrarily, if the lumen of the bowel is filled with fluid, mucus, or food, evaluation of the walls is improved, and fluid-filled bowel loop may act as a sonic window [88].

The main characteristic findings that suggest the diagnosis of small bowel obstruction are fluid-filled small bowel loops with lumen >3 cm. Those dilated loops may show thickened wall (normally up to 3 mm) and lack of normal compressibility under direct pressure with the probe. In the early stage of obstruction, there is increased peristalsis of the dilated segment; later on, the peristalsis is reduced with a just "to-and-fro motion" of the bowel contents. Distal to the stenosis, typically there are just collapsed bowel loops [89], (Fig. 27.10).

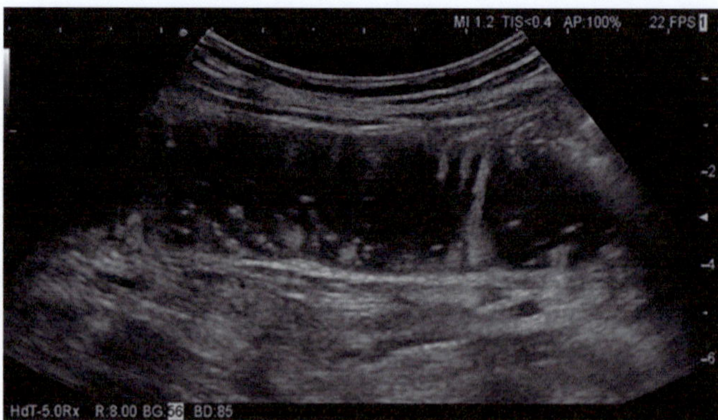

Fig. 27.10 Small bowel occlusion. Dilated aperistaltic loop of jejunum with valvulae conniventes and some hyperechoic spot in the lumen (*gas bubbles and debris*)

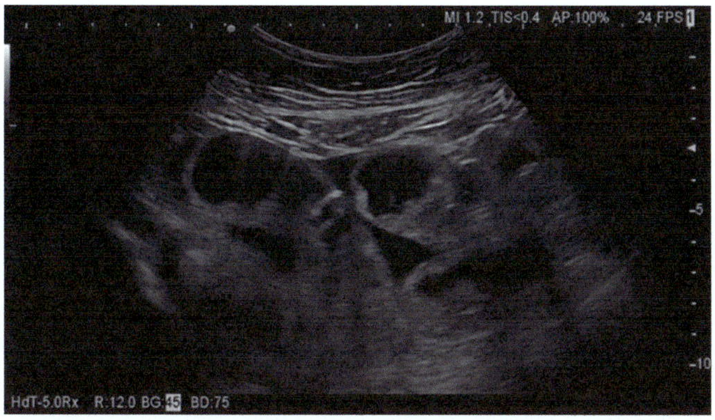

Fig. 27.11 Sonographic appearance of small bowel occlusion. Free fluid between fluid-filled loops; triangular-shaped "tanga sign"

The severity of the obstruction can also be assessed. Free peritoneal fluid associated with aperistalsis and wall thickening (>3 mm) in a fluid-filled distended bowel segment suggests a high-grade obstruction. The presence of free peritoneal fluid in SBO is due to the elevated intraluminal pressure that exceeds capillary pressure, resulting in impaired parietal permeability, and may be followed by ischemia. The free fluid can be seen in the recess between dilated small bowel loops and assumes a typical triangular shape ("tanga sign") [89], (Fig. 27.11).

Even the characteristics of the free fluid are relevant. The fluid can eventually be aspirated under US guidance, and the findings of bloody intraperitoneal fluid may indicate bowel gangrene that needs immediate surgical exploration and treatment [90].

The level of obstruction can be determined by the anatomical position and specific structure of the latest dilated proximal bowel loop before collapsed bowel segments (transit point).

Paralytic ileus can be diagnosed by US by demonstrating very reduced or absence of peristalsis in dilated loops, usually affecting the entire bowel. When pressure is applied to the transducer, the bowel compresses and appears pliable.

Even if scanning could be impaired by extensive intraluminal gas and associated shadowing, it is possible to see debris in the dependent part of fluid-filled dilated loops, confirming the absence of propulsive movements.

It is important to remember that also in the late stage of mechanical obstruction, the obstructed segment becomes paralytic. This situation should not be mistaken for paralytic ileus. Contracted bowel loops distal to the stenosis still allow correct diagnosis [91].

Large bowel obstruction (LBO) is rarer than paralytic ileus, and US diagnosis could be relatively more difficult because of its contents (feces and air, rather than fluids like in the small abdomen). However, thanks to its fixed position, it is easier to identify each segment during the scan and the anatomical level of obstruction.

To make a diagnosis of obstruction, the colon has to be dilated with usually hyperechoic content (air artifacts). Normal colonic caliber ranges from 3 to 8 cm, with the largest diameter in the cecum; the colon is deemed to be dilated when its diameter in the transverse scan is greater than 6 cm, or at the cecum level, it is larger than 9 cm. This dilated tract ends abruptly at the level of the lesion, with or without the presence of a mass lesion, and the colon distal to it has paucity or absence of gas [92].

Taylor et al. with a systematic review and meta-analysis [93] have proven that plain radiology has just moderate accuracy for small bowel obstruction, with sensitivity of 75% (95% CI 68–80) and specificity of 66% (55–76), with positive and negative likelihood ratio of 1.6 (1.1–2.5) and 0.43 (0.24–0.79). US performed better, with these formal radiological US results: sensitivity 87% (95% CI 83–90) and specificity 81% (74–87), with +LR 14.1 (3.57–55.66) and –LR 0.13 (0.08–0.20). For bedside US performed by non-radiologists, the sensitivity was 92% (80–98), and specificity 89% (65–99), with +LR of 9.55 (2.16–42.21) and –LR 0.04 (0.1–0.13).

Sonography has particular advantage for the diagnosis of proximal (duodenal or proximal jejunal) obstruction. In these pathologies, plain abdominal radiographs are often normal because frequent vomiting causes lack of air in the obstructed tract [94]. Even if US has lower accuracy than CT providing the surgeon some relevant information (the specific cause for SBO), POCUS may be very useful to detect it, allowing to initiate immediate treatment with nasogastric suction, which can hasten symptom relief, and refer promptly to another imaging study. On the other side, a normal sonography in the emergency department may serve as a diagnostic end point to exclude SBO [95].

It is important to search always for the cause of obstruction at the transit point (the point between the dilated proximal and collapsed distal bowel loop). The most frequent cause of SBO, adhesion, is suggested by the identification of obstruction pattern, in the absence of obstructing masses, in patients with a previous history of surgery. This may prompt a trial of conservative therapy in the absence of signs of vascular compromise. Obviously, serial US examinations are safe and can be used to evaluate the progress of bowel obstruction in patients who are treated conservatively [96].

Tumors are the leading cause of large bowel obstruction and may be identified by US. The sonographic aspect reflects the pathology: it is possible to find bulky eccentric mass, small or relatively large, at the end of the dilated intestinal tract. Another possible appearance is the presence of a segmental, eccentric or circumferential, irregular wall thickening, with narrow lumen. Typically, the normal colonic wall multilayered pattern is disrupted [94, 97].

27.8 Intussusception

US is well established as the first-line imaging modality for diagnosing intussusception in children. For these patients, ultrasound accuracy is very high (sensibility 98–100%, specificity 88–89%) [98]. Adult intussusception represents 5% of all cases of intestinal intussusception and accounts for only 1–5% of intestinal obstructions in adults. But even in the adult population, bowel sonography can be very useful [99], above all when the patient constitution and intestinal gas allow a good-quality bowel scan [100]. Features of US include in transverse sections a swirled pattern of alternating hyperechogenicity and hypoechogenicity, representing alternating layers of the mucosa, muscularis, and serosa: the "doughnut" or "bull's eye" sign [101].

On longitudinal or oblique sections, alternating loops of bowel and a loop-within-loop have a sandwich-like appearance ("pseudokidney" sign or "hay-fork" sign) [101, 102].

27.9 Abdominal Wall Hernias

US can confirm clinical suspect of abdominal wall hernia. It can show the protrusion of organs or tissue (even in real time during a Valsalva maneuver) and can be appreciated the dimension of the defect in the surrounding fascia. US has been shown to be quite accurate in identifying the presence of an inguinal hernia (>90% accuracy) [103]. When the bowel is contained within the hernial sac, US will easily demonstrate distinctive bright artifacts from the intestinal gas and active peristalsis [104].

In small bowel obstruction due to a hernia, it is possible to see sign of complication: irreducibility of the hernial sac, dilated bowel loop in the sac, bowel wall thickening, absence of peristalsis, and free fluid inside the sac (Fig. 27.12).

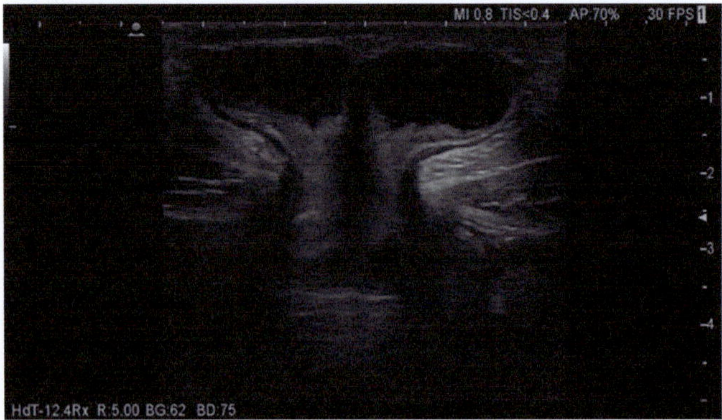

Fig. 27.12 Sonography of complicated umbilical hernia. Incarcerated bowel loop penetrating through peritoneal defect. No peristalsis and free fluid surrounding the loop

US may also detect other frequent causes of intestinal obstruction (as seen for diverticulitis and appendicitis) and rarer causes with specific sonographic findings such as volvulus, ascariasis, superior mesenteric artery syndrome, gallstone ileus, bezoars, afferent loop syndrome, foreign bodies, and Crohn's disease [87, 105–111].

27.10 Ischemic Bowel Disease

In acute ischemia, during the first hour, little or no signal from color Doppler or echo-enhancing contrast US can be observed. This sign is suggestive of ischemia but has a low sensitivity. If the ischemia has lasted a few hours, dilated bowel loops and a thickened bowel wall with the absence of stratification can be observed, with often free peritoneal fluid. But all these signs are nonspecific, and the examination is often made difficult by increasing amounts of intraluminal air [112–114].

Ultrasound can be used to identify complications of ischemic bowel disease, such as pneumatosis intestinalis [115], portal venous gas [116], and pneumoperitoneum.

In chronic ischemia of the small bowel, stenotic or occlusive lesions are found in the coeliac and/or mesenteric arteries. However, Doppler scanning is not the method of choice for diagnosing acute ischemia of the small bowel because it does not permit the evaluation of the compensatory collateral circulation and distal embolization. Thus, CT angiography must be performed for a definite diagnosis and evaluation of the possible best treatment [117–119].

27.11 Perforation/Pneumoperitoneum

Detection of pneumoperitoneum is of extreme importance as it often indicates an acute underlying abdominal emergency and is the clue to the diagnosis of perforation of the gastrointestinal tract. Clinical signs and symptoms have low diagnostic accuracy, and abdominal radiography is positive in 55–85% of cases [120]. Computed tomography is considered the "gold standard" for the recognition of pneumoperitoneum owing to its high spatial resolution and capability to detect even the smallest amount of free intraperitoneal air. US displays normal air within the lumen of the gastrointestinal tract by its association with bowel and peristaltic movements. The normal peritoneal stripe is identified as a single or double echogenic line posterior to the anterior abdominal wall. US ability to identify free peritoneal air is known since more than three decades [121]. In pneumoperitoneum, free abdominal air produces a sonographic appearance of linear enhancement of the peritoneal stripe from which start distinct posterior hyperechoic reverberation and shadowing

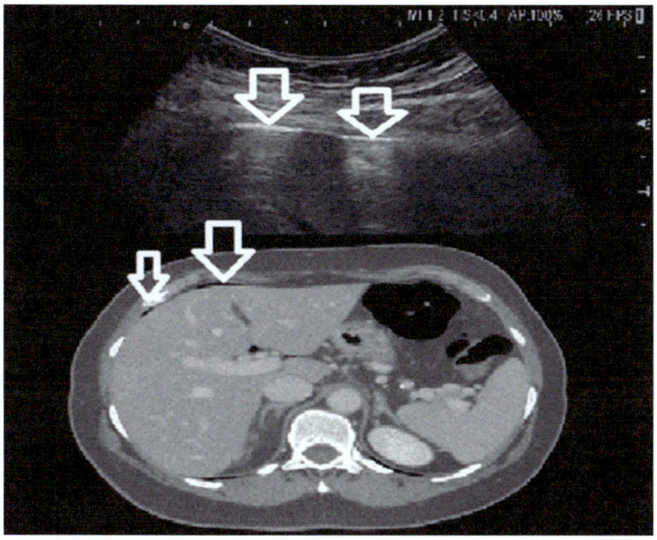

Fig. 27.13 Sonography of perforated diverticulitis. Small amount of free air is detected in supine position under anterior to abdominal wall before the right liver lobe. In the figure, two air sacs (*arrows*) identified by the enhancement of peritoneal stripe of pneumoperitoneum (EPPS) and posterior typical bright air artifacts. CT scan confirms small amount of free peritoneal air, on plain abdominal radiographs missed

artifacts. This is best visible anterior to the liver surface or immediately below the anterior abdominal wall in the supine position with the thorax slightly elevated. In supine position, the enhancement of peritoneal stripe of pneumoperitoneum (EPPS) [122] disappears when pressure is increasingly applied on the abdomen, leading to a migration of the free peritoneal air. This sign, called the "scissor's phenomenon" [123], helps to differentiate free air from gas inside the bowel lumen (Fig. 27.13).

To complete the scan, the patient should also turn on the left semi-lateral decubitus position. Extra-luminal gas moves by changing the patient's position, with "shifting" of free air to the highest point of peritoneal cavity, the ventral hepato-peritoneal space, where it can be easily detected. Several large prospective trials have proved high accuracy of sonography for pneumoperitoneum demonstrating that US has a superior sensitivity to diagnose free peritoneal air compared with abdominal radiography [121]. Seitz and Reising evaluating 4000 consecutive patients with non-traumatic acute abdominal pain described a sensitivity of 90% and a specificity of 100% for the detection of pneumoperitoneum. Moriwaki et al. [124] found a sensitivity and specificity of 85 and 100%, respectively, on 487 consecutive patients with blunt trauma and abdominal pain. Although a large amount of free peritoneal air may be easily detected, some specific cases need adjunctive attention. That is the case of contained gastric or duodenal perforation when gas could be found only in the fissure for *ligamentum teres*. Retroperitoneal perforation with retroperitoneum may be difficult to detect; in these rare cases, air reverberations obscure retroperitoneal vessels and organs, and the air shifting phenomenon is not observed [125].

27.12 Female Pelvis in Acute Abdominal Pain

POCUS is the first imaging tool to evaluate women with acute pelvic pain. It has good accuracy to detect or rule out gynecologic disorders and can evaluate other causes of acute abdominal pain that may require surgical repair. Ectopic pregnancy, pelvic inflammatory disease, and hemorrhagic ovarian cysts are the most commonly diagnosed gynecologic conditions presenting with acute pelvic pain. Ovarian torsion occurs less frequently, but a quick diagnosis is required to save the adnexal structures from infarction. If a gynecologic disorder is confirmed, the following workup expedites [126, 127]; other imaging studies might be unnecessary, thereby reducing cost, length of hospitalization, and adverse complications of CT [128].

Point-of-care female pelvis US can be performed by two complementary ways: transabdominal and transvaginal approach. Each technique has its advantages. The transabdominal approach shows the spatial orientation of the pelvis and defines the relationship of the uterus with adjacent pelvic and abdominal structures. It may detect large masses, free fluid, and other pathologies extending outside of the pelvis. The transvaginal approach offers a better imaging of intrauterine contents and adnexal abnormalities, because of probe proximity to the pelvic organs and higher frequencies. The transabdominal examination should be performed with a full bladder that acts as an acoustic window and displaces bowel loops. On the other side, transvaginal scan always needs an empty bladder.

Emergency physicians (non-radiologist and non-gynecologist) who performe transvaginal sonography are not always available and uniformely distributed in different Hospitals and Institution. Anyway, even the use of just trans-abdominal approach may be useful in women with acute pelvic pain of suspected genital origin [129].

27.12.1 Ectopic Pregnancy

Ectopic pregnancy is still the leading cause of pregnancy-related morbidity and mortality. US, together with quantitative measurements of β-hCG levels, can be considered the best imaging procedure to guide the diagnosis and may confirm the presence of intraperitoneal bleeding, which in turn helps guide treatment decisions. When an ectopic pregnancy is suspected, the goal of POCUS is to diagnose an intrauterine pregnancy (IUP). Ectopic pregnancy can be reliably excluded in women when IUP is found. Heterotopic pregnancies (when an IUP and ectopic pregnancy occur simultaneously) are very rare, as low as 1 in 30,000 pregnancies. It is important to remember anyway that the incidence increases to as high as 1 in 100 in women undergoing fertility stimulation or in vitro fertilization procedures [130]. The first sign of an early intrauterine pregnancy is the gestational sac, which can be visualized with transvaginal ultrasound at approximately 4–5 weeks of gestation (menstrual age) when it would measure 2–3 mm in diameter (or about 1 week later by transabdominal approach). Usually, the sac can be detected transvaginal when the serum level of beta human chorionic gonadotropin (β-hCG) is higher than 1500 mIU/ml and transabdominal when it is approximately higher than 6500 mIU/ml. The gestational sac appears as a small round or oval intrauterine fluid collection with an echogenic rim (Fig. 27.14). Unfortunately, also in up to 20% of cases of ectopic pregnancy, a collection of fluid (without any border) may be seen within the uterine cavity. It is referred as a "pseudosac" and must not be confused with a gestational sac [131, 132]. Early intrauterine pregnancy is definitively identified if a yolk sac (fifth week) and/or a fetal pole (sixth week) is visualized in the uterus. A small amount of free peritoneal anechoic fluid in the pouch of Douglas may be found in both intrauterine and ectopic pregnancies [133]. A small quantity is not diagnostic by itself, but a larger amount, or the presence of echogenic fluid in the Douglas pouch, suggests tubal rupture [134, 135]. The site of the ectopic pregnancy is determined just with transvaginal US. An extra-ovarian complex adnexal mass is the most common ultrasound finding in ectopic pregnancy and is present in 89% or more of cases [136]. Stein et al. meta-analysis revealed that emergency physician POCUS accuracy to detect intrauterine pregnancy had a sensitivity of 99.3% and

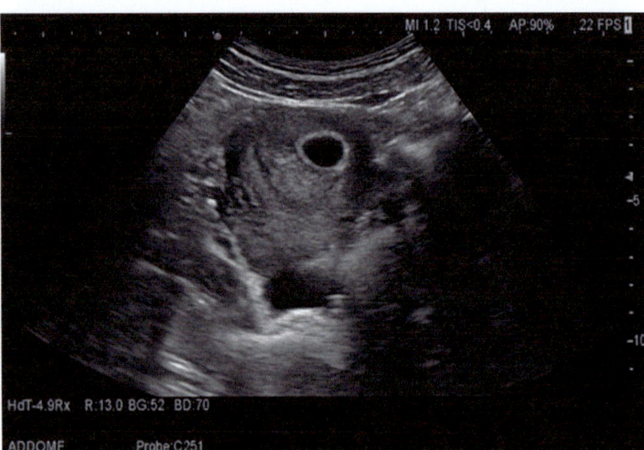

Fig. 27.14 Sonogram of a 5-week intrauterine pregnancy. Transabdominal pelvic ultrasonography demonstrating a hypoechoic rounded gestational sac with hyperechoic border inside the uterus

a negative predictive value of 99.96% [137]. Another systematic review of US features for diagnosis of ectopic pregnancy indicated that an empty uterus predicts an ectopic pregnancy with a sensitivity of 32.4% and a specificity of 93.3% [138]. These studies confirm that the ultrasonographic findings of an empty uterus, a pseudosac, an adnexal mass, and/or a free fluid have a good specificity, especially when found in combination, and they are useful for "ruling in" an ectopic pregnancy. Many different gynecologic other causes of acute pelvic pain can be detected by bedside ultrasonography. For most of them, endocavitary ultrasonography is recommended, although if the finding is large enough, it may be appreciated on transabdominal ultrasonography as well.

27.12.2 Pelvic Inflammatory Disease (PID)

PID can produce acute symptoms and may result in infertility, raising the risk for ectopic pregnancy and chronic pelvic pain. Hydrosalpinx is diagnosed by the US when the fallopian tubes (one or both) appear elongated or folded, tubular, C-shaped or S-shaped, dilated, and filled with hypoechoic fluid, measuring more than 5 mm in diameter. In pyosalpinx, the tube content appears heterogeneous and hyperechoic, and the tube walls appear thicker in diameter than in hydrosalpinx. A tubo-ovarian abscess is usually easily identified also by transabdominal scan; it appears as heterogeneous and tender adnexal mass, often multiloculated, with septations and irregular thick walls with increased color Doppler blood flow in the periphery, due to acute inflammation [139].

27.12.3 Ruptured or Hemorrhagic Ovarian Cyst

A hemorrhagic ovarian cyst (HOC) is an adnexal mass formed because of the occurrence of bleeding into a follicular or *corpus luteum* cyst. It is the most common cause of acute pelvic pain in an afebrile, premenopausal woman with acute pelvic pain. The sonographic appearance depends on whether a simple functional or hemorrhagic ovarian cyst ruptures and whether the cyst has completely collapsed. The simple cysts have smooth avascular capsule with thin walls, anechoic content, and posterior enhancement (Fig. 27.15). The ruptured cyst may have a deflated or angular appearance with adjacent free fluid. Since the hemorrhagic cysts typically develop because of bleeding within a *corpus luteum*, its sonographic aspects are dependent on the stage of evolution (bleeding, clot formation inside the cyst, clot lysis, clot retraction, and resolution). In the early stage, US show diffuse low-level internal echoes, and it may resemble a homogeneous solid adnexal mass. A fluid/

Fig. 27.15 Ovarian cyst. Abdominal ultrasonography demonstrating a simple cyst, with anechoic fluid content, with smooth and thin walls

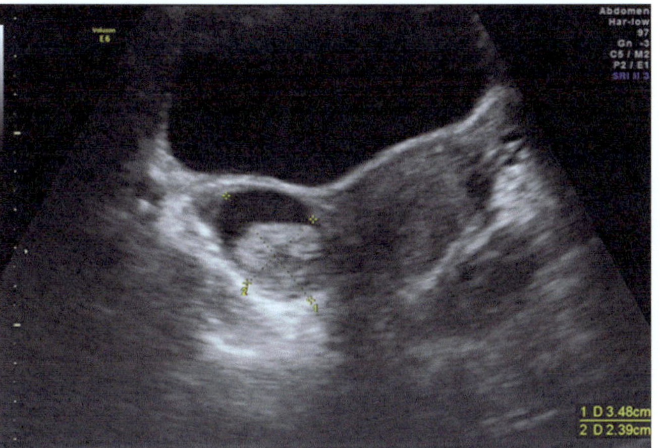

Fig. 27.16 Hemorrhagic luteal body. Transabdominal pelvic ultrasonography showing a small adnexal complex mass in a patient with severe lower-quadrant abdominal pain. A corpus luteum is evident with US showing signs of recent hemorrhage in its interior (it is possible to identify the retracting clot). Color Doppler US must rule out the presence of vascularization within the interior echogenic mass, supporting the characterization of the clot and excluding neoplasia

fluid level due to layering of the dependent red blood cells and/or debris may be observed later and may be possible to identify a "fishnet weave" pattern due to fibrin strands or a retracting clot inside the anechoic cyst. Color Doppler may exhibit low resistance blood flow around the cyst also known as hypervascular "ring of fire" and no vascularity within [140, 141] (Fig. 27.16).

27.12.4 Ovarian Torsion

The rotation of the ovary and portion of the fallopian tube on the supplying vascular pedicle causes venous, arterial, and lymphatic stasis. A quick point POCUS diagnosis may help to expedite surgery and preserve ovarian function avoiding adnexal necrosis. In reproductive-aged women, torsion occurs because of the presence of an ovarian mass, such as large functional or dermoid cysts, which can be seen by transabdominal approach too. The ovary is usually enlarged because of venous and lymphatic congestion, with peripherally displaced follicles and hyperechoic central stroma. It is painful when pressure is applied to the probe and is pulled toward the midline of the pelvis. Ovarian torsion is often associated with a small amount of free fluid in the pelvis. Even if little or no intra-ovarian venous flow is common, color Doppler findings can be widely variable and do not confirm or rule out the diagnosis [142].

Case Scenario

A 27-year-old Caucasian woman presented to the emergency department complaining of intermittent abdominal pain-associated with nausea, abdominal distention and mild dyspnea during the last 24 h. She reported similar recurrent episodes of abdominal pain (sometimes associated with nausea, vomiting, and diarrhea), which had led to previous extensive diagnostic workup including a CT scan, with two hospitalizations without a clear diagnosis. Her past medical history also revealed a hiatal hernia and lactose intolerance, while the diagnostic workup for celiac disease reported inconclusive results. A detailed reiterated evaluation of her medical history revealed that the patient had suffered from several episodes of posttraumatic edema involving the skin and submucosal tissues since childhood. Her physical examination revealed tenderness in the central and right upper quadrant upon light palpation without guarding or rebound tenderness. Laboratory workup revealed a normal complete blood count, C-reactive peptide, and metabolic panel. An abdominal US showed an abundant ascitic fluid and edematous jejunal loop thickening, without hepatosplenomegaly; no intra- and extra-hepatic biliary duct dilation and no focal lesions were found. The patient was admitted to the internal medicine department.

Question no. 1: Which is the most likely diagnosis in this young woman with abdominal pain and nausea and US showing jejunal thickening and ascites?

A. Inflammatory bowel disease
B. *Campylobacter jejuni* infection
C. Small bowel intussusception
D. Endometriosis

E. Pelvic inflammatory disease
F. Hereditary angioedema due to C1 inhibitor deficiency (HAE)

Question no. 2: What is the best diagnostic workup after POCUS?

A. Endoscopy with biopsies (esophagogastroduodenoscopy and/or colonoscopy)
B. Laparoscopy
C. Video capsule endoscopy imaging
D. Abdominal CT scan
E. Paracentesis with analysis of abdominal free fluid
F. Blood tests including C4 and C1 inhibitor antigenic and functional levels
G. All the above-mentioned tests

Question no.3: Which of the following can be the best treatment(s)?

A. Anti-inflammatory drugs
B. Antibiotics
C. Intravenous steroids
D. Antihistamines
E. C1 inhibitor concentrates
F. Antagonist of the bradykinin B2 receptor

Please see Chap. 58 for the correct answer.

Clinical Commentary [143]

This case scenario in a patient with HAE underlines that:

1. Differential diagnosis of abdominal pain and ascites in a patient with HAR can be challenging, even with advanced diagnostic tools like CT.
2. Gastrointestinal symptoms can be the only manifestation of angioedema (up to 50% of reported cases), and they may mimic an acute abdomen sometime with various degrees of small bowel obstruction. The condition usually involves a complex diagnostic workup with useless invasive procedures and sometime unnecessary surgical intervention.
3. Ultrasonography is the first valuable reproducible noninvasive tool and may show signs which are nonspecific but useful clues when associated with a thorough medical history for the diagnosis of abdominal pain related to hereditary angioedema due to C1 inhibitor deficiency.
4. Free peritoneal and retroperitoneal fluid and various degrees of small bowel or colonic wall thickening may be detected by US or CT scan during abdominal angioedema attacks. The intraperitoneal fluid may vary from small volumes identifiable only in the Douglas cul-de-sac to large volume ascites, with the intestinal loops floating in the peritoneal fluid. The wall thickening is usually mild but rarely can lead to small bowel or colonic intussusception.
5. The diagnostic value of C4 test in patients with HAE should not be underestimated because it has high sensitivity and specificity in patients with C1-INH-HAE.

References

1. McCaig LG, Stussamm BJ. National Hospital Ambulatory Medical Care Survey: 1996 Emergency Department Summary. Adv Data. 1997; (293):1–20.
2. Tintinalli JE. Emergency medicine. New York: McGraw-Hill Education; 2016.
3. Cartwright SL, Knudson MP. Evaluation of acute abdominal pain in adults. Am Fam Physician. 2008;77:971–8. Review
4. Scaglione M. Imaging features and differential diagnosis for a timely management approach. Emergency radiology of the abdomen. 1st ed. Heidelberg: Springer; 2012. p. 133–64.
5. Lameris W, van Randen A, van Es HW, van Heesewijk JP, van Ramshorst B, Bouma WH, et al. Imaging strategies for detection of urgent conditions in patients with acute abdominal pain: diagnostic accuracy study. BMJ. 2009;338:b2431.
6. Laurell H, Hansson LE, Gunnarsson U. Diagnostic pitfalls and accuracy of diagnosis in acute abdominal pain. Scand J Gastroenterol. 2006;41:1126–35.
7. Prasannan S, Zhueng TJ, Gul YA. Diagnostic value of plain abdominal radiographs in patients with acute abdominal pain. Asian J Surg. 2005;28:246–51.
8. MacKersie AB, Lane MJ, Gerhardt RT, Claypool HA, Keenan S, Katz DS, et al. Nontraumatic acute abdominal pain: unenhanced helical CT compared with three-view acute abdominal series. Radiology. 2005;237:114–22.
9. Gans SL, Pols MA, et al. Guideline for the diagnostic pathway in patients with acute abdominal pain. Dig Surg. 2015;32:23–31. https://doi.org/10.1159/00037158.
10. Rosen MP, Ding A, Blake MA, Baker ME, Cash BD, Fidler JL, Grant TH, Greene FL, Jones B, Katz DS, Lalani T, Miller FH, Small WC, Spottswood S, Sudakoff GS, Tulchinsky M, Warshauer DM, Yee J, Coley BD. ACR Appropriateness Criteria® right lower quadrant pain–suspected appendicitis. J Am Coll Radiol. 2011;8:749–55. Review
11. Cortellaro F, Ferrari L, et al. Accuracy of point of care ultrasound to identify the source of infection in septic patients: a prospective study. Intern Emerg Med. 2016;12(3):371–8.
12. Lederle FA, Johnson GR, Wilson SE, Chute EP, Littooy FN, Bandyk D, et al. Prevalence and associations of abdominal aortic aneurysm detected through screening. Aneurysm Detection and Management (ADAM) Veterans Affairs Cooperative Study Group. Ann Intern Med. 1997;126:441–9.
13. Sakalihasan N, Limet R, Defawe OD. Abdominal aortic aneurysm. Lancet. 2005;365:1577–89.

14. Thompson MM. Controlling the expansion of abdominal aortic aneurysms. Br J Surg. 2003;98:897–8.
15. Chichester Aneurysm Screening Group. Viborg Aneurysm Screening Study, Western Australian Abdominal Aortic Aneurysm Program, Multicentre Aneurysm Screening Study. A comparative study of the prevalence of abdominal aortic aneurysms in the United Kingdom, Denmark, and Australia. J Med Screen. 2001;8:46–50.
16. Norman PE, Powell JT. Abdominal aortic aneurysm: the prognosis in women is worse than in men. Circulation. 2007;115:2865–9.
17. U.S. Department of Health and Human Services Centers for Disease Control and Prevention National Center for Health Statistics. MD LCWK1. Deaths, percent of total deaths, and death rates for the 15 leading causes of death in 5-year age groups, by race and sex: United States, 2006. 2009. [10/11/09]. pp. 7–9.
18. Lederle FA, Johnson GR, Wilson SE, Ballard DJ, Jordan WDJ, Blebea J, et al. Rupture rate of large abdominal aortic aneurysms in patients refusing or unfit for elective repair. JAMA. 2002;287:2968–72.
19. Hoffman M, Avellone JC, Pleecha GR, et al. Operation for ruptured abdominal aortic aneurysm: a community-wide experience. Surgery. 1982;91:597.
20. Kiell CS, Ernst CB. Advances in management of abdominal aortic aneurysm. Adv Surg. 1993;26:73–98.
21. Lindholt JS, Vammen S, Juul S, Henneberg EW, Fasting H. The validity of ultrasonographic scanning as screening method for abdominal aortic aneurysm. Eur J Vasc Endovasc Surg. 1999;17:472–5.
22. Costantino TG, Bruno EC, Handly N, Den AJ. Accuracy of emergency medicine ultrasound in the evaluation of abdominal aortic aneurysm. J Emerg Med. 2005;29(4):455–60.
23. Lederle FA, Wilson SE, Johnson GR, Reinke DB, Littooy FN, Acher CW, et al. Variability in measurement of abdominal aortic aneurysms. Abdominal Aortic Aneurysm Detection and Management Veterans Administration Cooperative Study Group. J Vasc Surg. 1995;21:945–52.
24. Testa A, Lauritano EC, Giannuzzi R, Pignataro G, Casagranda I, Gentiloni Silveri N. The role of emergency ultrasound in the diagnosis of acute non-traumatic epigastric pain. Intern Emerg Med. 2010;5(5):401–9.
25. Johnson CD. ABC of the upper gastrointestinal tract. Upper abdominal pain: gall bladder. BMJ. 2001;323(7322):1170–3.
26. Grimpen F, Pavli P. Rational investigation of upper abdominal pain. Aust Fam Physician. 2008;37(8):602–7.
27. Rubens DJ. Ultrasound imaging of the biliary tract. Ultrasound Clin. 2007;2:391–413.
28. Menu Y, Vuillerme M-P. Non-traumatic abdominal emergencies: Imaging and intervention in acute biliary conditions. In: Marincek B, Dondelinger RF, editors. Emergency radiology. Berlin: Springer; 2007. p. 481–91.
29. Steven M, Strasberg MD. Acute calculous cholecystitis. N Engl J Med. 2008;358:2804–11.
30. Shea JA, Berlin JA, Escarce JJ, et al. Revised estimates of diagnostic test sensitivity and specificity in suspected biliary tract disease. Arch Intern Med. 1994;154:2573–81.
31. Guyatt G, Rennie D, for the Evidence-Based Medicine Working Group, American Medical Association. Users' guides to the medical literature: a manual for evidence-based clinical practice. Chicago, IL: AMA Press; 2002.
32. Trowbridge RL, Rutkowski NK, Shojania KG. Does this patient have acute cholecystitis. JAMA. 2009;289:80–6.
33. Harvey RT, Miller WT Jr. Acute biliary disease. Radiology. 1999;213:831–6.
34. Reginelli A, Pezzullo MG, Scaglione M, Scialpi M, Brunese L, Grassi R. Gastrointestinal disorders in elderly patients. Radiol Clin N Am. 2008;46(4):755–71.
35. Ralls PW, Colletti PM, Lapin SA, et al. Real-time sonography in suspected acute cholecystitis: prospective evaluation of primary and secondary signs. Radiology. 1985;155:767–71.
36. Van Breda Vriesman AC, Engelbrecht MR, Smithuis RH, Puylaert JB. Diffuse gallbladder wall thickening: differential diagnosis. Am J Roentgenol. 2007;188:495–501.
37. Takada T, Strasberg SM, Solomkin JS, Pitt HA, et al. Tokyo Guidelines Revision Committee. TG13:Updated Tokyo Guidelines for the management of acute cholangitis and cholecystitis. J Hepatobiliary Pancreat Sci. 2013;20(1):1–7.
38. Ansaloni L, Pisano M, Coccolini F, Peitzmann AB, et al. WSES guidelines on acute calculous cholecystitis. World J Emerg Surg. 2016;11:25.
39. Larson SD, Nealon WH, Evers BM. Management of gallstone pancreatitis. Adv Surg. 2006;40:265–84.
40. Vilgrain V, Palazzo L. Choledocholithiasis: role of US and endoscopic ultrasound. Abdom Imaging. 2001;26:7–14.
41. Neoptolemos JP, Hall AW, Finlay DF, Berry JM, CarrLocke DL, Fossard DP. The urgent diagnosis of gallstones in acute pancreatitis: a prospective study of three methods. Br J Surg. 1984;71:230–3.
42. Şurlin V, Săftoiu A, Dumitrescu D. Imaging tests for accurate diagnosis of acute biliary Pancreatitis. World J Gastroenterol. 2014;20(44):16544–9.
43. Koo BC, Chinogureyi A, Shaw AS. Imaging acute pancreatitis. Br J Radiol. 2010;83(986):104–12.
44. Barrett ML, Hines AL, Andrews RM. Trends in rates of perforated appendix, 2001–2010. HCUP Statistical Brief #159. July 2013.
45. United Kingdom National Surgical Research Collaborative, Bhangu A. Safety of short, in-hospital delays before surgery for acute appendicitis: multicentre cohort study, systematic review, and meta-analysis. Ann Surg. 2014;259(5):894–903.
46. Velanovich V, Satava R. Balancing the normal appendectomy rate with the perforated appendicitis rate: implications for quality assurance. Am Surg. 1992;58(4):264–9.
47. Kirkil C, et al. Appendicitis scores may be useful in reducing the costs of treatment for right lower quadrant pain. Ulus Travma Acil Cerrahi Derg. 2013;19(1):13–9.
48. Hallan S, Asberg A. The accuracy of C-reactive protein in diagnosing acute appendicitis–a meta-analysis. Scand J Clin Lab Invest. 1997;57(5):373–80.
49. Ohle R, et al. The Alvarado score for predicting acute appendicitis: a systematic review. BMC Med. 2011;9:139.
50. Debnath J, et al. Alvarado score: is it time to develop a clinical-pathological- radiological scoring system for diagnosing acute appendicitis? Am J Emerg Med. 2015;33(6):839–40.
51. Atema JJ, et al. Scoring system to distinguish uncomplicated from complicated acute appendicitis. Br J Surg. 2015;102(8):979–90.
52. Chang ST, Jeffrey RB, Olcott EW. Three-step sequential positioning algorithm during sonographic evaluation for appendicitis increases appendiceal visualization rate and reduces CT use. AJR Am J Roentgenol. 2014;203(5):1006–12.
53. Nielsen JW, et al. Reducing computed tomography scans for appendicitis by introduction of a standardized and validated ultrasonography report template. J Pediatr Surg. 2015;50(1):144–8.
54. Koseekriniramol V, et al. Abdominal wall thickness is not useful to predict appendix visualization on sonography in adult patients with suspected appendicitis. J Clin Ultrasound. 2015;43(5):269–76.
55. Chesbrough RM, et al. Self-localization in US of appendicitis: an addition to grades compression. Radiology. 1993;187:349–51.
56. Fields MJ, et al. Accuracy of point of care ultrasonography for diagnosing acute appendicitis: a systematic review and meta-analysis. Acad Emerg Med. 2017;24(9):1124–36.
57. Saverio D, et al. WSES Jerusalem guidelines for diagnosis and treatment of acute appendicitis. World J Emerg Surg. 2016;11:34.
58. Maconi G, Sampietro GM, Sartani A, Bianchi Porro G. Bowel ultrasound in Crohn's disease: surgical perspective. Int J Color Dis. 2008;23:339–47.

59. Maconi G, Radice E, Greco S, Bianchi Porro G. Bowel ultrasound in Crohn's disease. Best Pract Res Clin Gastroenterol. 2006;20:93–112.
60. Panes J, Bouhnik Y, Reinisch W, Stoker J, Taylor SA, Baumgart DC, et al. Imaging techniques for assessment of inflammatory bowel disease: joint ECCO and ESGAR evidence-based consensus guidelines. J Crohns Colitis. 2013;7:556–85.
61. Novak K, Tanyingoh D, Petersen F, Kucharzik T, Panaccione R, Ghosh S, et al. Clinic-based point of care transabdominal ultrasound for monitoring Crohn's disease: impact on clinical decision making. J Crohns Colitis. 2015;9:795–801.
62. Panés J, Bouzas R, Chaparro M, García-Sánchez V, Gisbert JP, Martínez de Guereñu B, et al. Systematic review: the use of ultrasonography, computed tomography and magnetic resonance imaging for the diagnosis, assessment of activity and abdominal complications of Crohn's disease. Alim Pharmacol Ther. 2011;34:125–45.
63. Hammond NA, Nikolaidis P, Miller FH. Left lower-quadrant pain: guidelines from the American College of Radiology appropriateness criteria. Am Fam Physician. 2010;82:766–70. Review
64. Jacobs DO. Clinical practice. Diverticulitis. N Engl J Med. 2007;357:2057–66. Review
65. Hollerweger A, Macheiner P, Rettenbacher T, Brunner W, Gritzmann N. Colonic diverticulitis: diagnostic value and appearance of inflamed diverticula-sonographic evaluation. Eur Radiol. 2001;11:1956–63.
66. Cuccurullo V, Cioce F, Sica A, Iasiello F, Capasso R, Gatta G, Rubini G. Gastroenteric diseases in the third millennium: a rational approach to optimal imaging technique and patient selection. Recenti Prog Med. 2012;103(11):426–30.
67. Tack D, Bohy P, Perlot I, De Maertelaer V, Alkeilani O, Sourtzis S, Gevenois PA. Suspected acute colon diverticulitis: imaging with low-dose unenhanced multi-detector row CT. Radiology. 2005;237:189–96.
68. van Randen A, Laméris W, van Es HW, van Heesewijk HP, van Ramshorst B, Ten Hove W, Bouma WH, van Leeuwen MS, van Keulen EM, Bossuyt PM, Stoker J, Boermeester MA, OPTIMA Study Group. A comparison of the accuracy of ultrasound and computed tomography in common diagnoses causing acute abdominal pain. Eur Radiol. 2011;21:1535–45.
69. Klarenbeek BR, de Korte N, van der Peet DL, Cuesta MA. Review of current classifications for diverticular disease and a translation into clinical practice. Int J Color Dis. 2012;27:207–14. Review
70. Jang HJ, Lim HK, Lee SJ, Lee WJ, Kim EY, Kim SH. Acute diverticulitis of the cecum and ascending colon: the value of thin-section helical CT findings in excluding colonic carcinoma. Am J Roentgenol. 2000;174:1397–402.
71. Sai VF, Velayos F, Neuhaus J, Westphalen AC. Colonoscopy after CT diagnosis of diverticulitis to exclude colon cancer: a systematic literature review. Radiology. 2012;263:383–90. Review, Erratum in: Radiology 2012, 264:306
72. Andeweg CS, et al. Toward an evidence-based step-up approach in diagnosing diverticulitis. Scand J Gastroenterol. 2014;49:775–84.
73. Baker JB, et al. Diagnosis of diverticulitis by bedside ultrasound in the Emergency department. J Emerg Med. 2006;30(3):327–9.
74. Helou N, et al. Sonography: first-line modality in the diagnosis of acute colonic diverticulitis? J Ultrasound Med. 2013;32:1689–94.
75. Talabani AJ, et al. Clinical diagnostic accuracy of acute colonic diverticulitis in patients admitted with acute abdominal pain, a receiver operating characteristic curve analysis. Int J Color Dis. 2017;32:41–7.
76. Sartelli M, Catena F, et al. WSES Guidelines for the management of acute left sided colonic diverticulitis in the emergency setting. World J Emerg Surg. 2016;11:37.
77. Salem TA, Molloy RG, O'Dwyer PJ. Prospective, five-year follow-up study of patients with symptomatic uncomplicated diverticular disease. Dis Colon Rectum. 2007;50:1460–4.
78. Ambrosetti P. Acute diverticulitis of the left colon: value of the initial CT and timing of elective colectomy. J Gastrointest Surg. 2008;12:1318–20. Review
79. Lameris W, van Randen A, et al. Graded compression ultrasonography and computed tomography in acute colonic diverticulitis: meta-analysis of test accuracy. Eur Radiol. 2008;18:2498–511.
80. Mazzei MA, et al. Sigmoid diverticulitis: US findings. Crit Ultrasound J. 2013;5:S1/S5.
81. Liljegren G, Chabok A, Wickbom M, et al. Acute colonic diverticulitis: a systematic review of diagnostic accuracy. Color Dis. 2007;9:480–8.
82. Patak MA, Mortele KJ, Ros PR. Multidetector row CT of the small bowel. Radiol Clin N Am. 2005;43:1063–77.
83. Unluer EE, Yavasi O, Eroglu O, Yilmaz C, Akarca FK. Ultrasonography by emergency medicine and radiology residents for the diagnosis of small bowel obstruction. Eur J Emerg Med. 2010;17:260–4.
84. Muradali D, Goldberg DR. US of gastrointestinal tract disease. Radiographics. 2015;35(1):50–68.
85. Ødegaard S, Nesje LB, Lærum OD, Kimmey MB. High-frequency ultrasonographic imaging of the gastrointestinal wall. Expert Rev Med Devices. 2012;9(3):263–73.
86. Maconi G, Porro GB. Ultrasound of the gastrointestinal tract. Berlin: Springer; 2007. p. 27–34.
87. Silva AC, Pimenta M, Guimarães LS. Small bowel obstruction: what to look for. Radiographics. 2009;29:423–39.
88. Scheible W, Goldberger LE. Diagnosis of small bowel obstruction: the contribution of diagnostic ultrasound. AJR Am J Roentgenol. 1979;133:685–8.
89. Guttman J, Stone MB, Kimberly HH, Rempell JS. Point-of-care ultrasonography for the diagnosis of small bowel obstruction in the emergency department. CJEM. 2015;17(2):206–9.
90. Grassi R, Romano S, D'amario F, et al. The relevance of free fluid between intestinal loops detected by sonography in the clinical assessment of small bowel obstruction in adults. Eur J Radiol. 2004;50(1):5–14.
91. Wilson SR. The acute abdomen of gastrointestinal tract origin: sonographic evaluation. In: Margulis AR, Burhenne HJ, editors. Alimentary tract radiology. 5th ed. St. Louis: Mosby; 1994. p. 2099–117.
92. Jaffe T, Thompson WM. Large-bowel obstruction in the adult: classic radiographic and CT findings, etiology, and mimics. Radiology. 2015;275(3):651–63.
93. Taylor M. Adult small bowel obstruction. Acad Emerg Med. 2013;20:528–44.
94. Jae Hoon Lim. Ultrasound examination of gastrointestinal tract disease. J Korean Med Sci. 2000;15:371–9.
95. Carpenter CR, Pines JM. The end of x-rays for suspected small bowel obstruction? Using evidence based diagnostics to inform best practices in emergency medicine. Acad Emerg Med. 2013;20:618–20.
96. Ogata M, Mateer JR, Condon RE. Prospective evaluation of abdominal sonography for the diagnosis of bowel obstruction. Ann Surg. 1996;223:237–41.
97. Ko YT, Lim JH, Lee DH, Lee HW, Lim JW. Small bowel obstruction: sonographic evaluation. Radiology. 1993;188(3):649–53.
98. Akbulut S. Intussusception due to inflammatory fibroid polyp: a case report and comprehensive literature review. World J Gastroenterol. 2012;18:5745–52.
99. Marinis A, Yiallourou A, Samanides L, et al. Intussusception of the bowel in adults: a review. World J Gastroenterol. 2009;15:407–11.
100. Rafailidis V, Phillips C, Yusuf G, Sidhu P. A case of adult intussusception with greyscale, contrast-enhanced ultrasound and computerised tomography correlation. Ultrasound. 2017;25(2):120–5.
101. Weissberg DL, Scheible W, Leopold GR. Ultrasonographic appearance of adult intussusception. Radiology. 1977;124:791–2.
102. Boyle MJ, Arkell LJ, Williams JT. Ultrasonic diagnosis of adult intussusception. Am J Gastroenterol. 1993;88:617–8.

103. Light D, Ratnasingham K, Banerjee A, Cadwallader R, Uzzaman MM, Gopinath B. The role of ultrasound scan in the diagnosis of occult inguinal hernias. Int J Surg. 2011;9(2):169–72.
104. Jain N, Goyal N, Mukherjee K, Kamath S. Ultrasound of the abdominal wall: what lies beneath? Clin Radiol. 2013;68:85–93.
105. Lim JH. Ultrasound examination of gastrointestinal tract diseases. J Korean Med Sci. 2000;15:371–9.
106. Santín-Rivero J, Núñez-García E, Aguirre-García M, Hagerman-Ruiz-Galindo G, de la Vega-González F, Moctezuma-Velasco CR. Intestinal volvulus. Case report and a literature review. Cir Cir. 2015;83(6):522–6.
107. Abu-Zidan FM, Hefny AF, Saadeldinn YA, El-Ashaal YI. Sonographic findings of superior mesenteric artery syndrome causing massive gastric dilatation in a young healthy girl. Singap Med J. 2010;51:e184–6.
108. Nuño-Guzmán CM, Marín-Contreras ME, Figueroa-Sánchez M, Corona JL. Gallstone ileus, clinical presentation, diagnostic and treatment approach. World J Gastrointest Surg. 2016;8(1):65–76.
109. Ko YT, Lim JH, Lee DH, Yoon Y. Small bowel phytobezoars: sonographic detection. Abdom Imaging. 1993;18:271–3.
110. Hosokawa T, Yamada Y, Sato Y, Tanami Y, Nanbu R, Hagiwara SI, Oguma E. Role of sonography for evaluation of gastrointestinal foreign bodies. J Ultrasound Med. 2016;35(12):2723–32.
111. Lee DH, Lim JH, Ko YT. Afferent loop syndrome: sonographic findings in seven cases. AJR Am J Roentgenol. 1991;157:41–3.
112. Danse E, Jamart J, Hoang P, et al. Focal bowel wall changes detected with colour Doppler ultrasound: diagnostic value in acute non-diverticular diseases of the colon. Br J Radiol. 2004;77:917–21.
113. Danse EM, Van Beers BE, Jamart J, et al. Prognosis of ischemic colitis: comparison of color Doppler sonography with early clinical and laboratory findings. AJR Am J Roentgenol. 2000;175:1151–4.
114. Ripolles T, Simo L, Martinez-Perez MJ, et al. Sonographic findings in ischemic colitis in 58 patients. AJR Am J Roentgenol. 2005;184:777–85.
115. James V, Warier A, Lee KP, Ong GY-K. Point-of-care ultrasound identification of pneumatosis intestinalis in paediatric abdominal pain: a case report. Crit Ultrasound J. 2017;9:2.
116. Pan HB, Huang JS, Yang TL, Liang HL. Hepatic portal venous gas in ultrasonogram - Benign or noxious. Ultrasound Med Biol. 2007;33(8):1179–83.
117. Roccarina D, Garcovich M, Ainora ME, Caracciolo G, Ponziani F, Gasbarrini A, Zocco MA. Diagnosis of bowel diseases: the role of imaging and ultrasonography. World J Gastroenterol. 2013;19(14):2144–53.
118. Dietrich CF, Jedrzejczyk M, Ignee A. Sonographic assessment of splanchnic arteries and the bowel wall. Eur J Radiol. 2007;64:202–12.
119. Gebel M. Ultrasound in gastroenterology and hepatology. Berlin: Blackwell; 1999. p. 159–230.
120. Nazerian P, Tozzetti C, Vanni S, Bartolucci M, Gualtieri S, Trausi F, Vittorini M, Catini E, Cibinel GA, Grifoni S. Accuracy of abdominal ultrasound for the diagnosis of pneumoperitoneum in patients with acute abdominal pain: a pilot study. Crit Ultrasound J. 2015;7:15.
121. Seitz K, Reising KD. Ultrasound detection of free air in the abdominal cavity. Ultraschall Med. 1982;3:4–6.
122. Muradali D, Wilson S, Burns PN, Shapiro H, Hope-Simpson D. A specific sign of pneumoperitoneum on sonography: enhancement of the peritoneal stripe. Am J Roentgenol. 1999;173:1257–62.
123. Karahan OI, Kurt A, Yikilmaz A, Kahriman G. New method for the detection of intraperitoneal free air by sonography: scissors maneuver. J Clin Ultrasound. 2004;32:381–5.
124. Moriwaki Y, Sugiyama M, Toyoda H, Kosuge T, Arata S, Iwashita M, et al. Ultrasonography for the diagnosis of intraperitoneal free air in chest- abdominal- pelvic blunt trauma and critical acute abdominal pain. Arch Surg. 2009;144:137–41. discussion 42
125. Numberg D, Mauch M, Spengler J, Holle A, Pannwitz H, Seitz K. Sonographical diagnosis of pneumoretroperitoneum as a result of retroperitoneal perforation. [in German. Ultraschall Med. 2007;28:612–21.
126. Wilson SP, Connolly K, Lahham S, et al. Point-of-care ultrasound versus radiology department pelvic ultrasound on emergency department length of stay. World J Emerg Med. 2016;7(3):178–82.
127. Thamburaj R, Sivitz A. Does the use of bedside pelvic ultrasound decrease length of stay in the emergency department? Pediatr Emerg Care. 2013;29(1):67–70.
128. Mazzei MA, et al. The role of US examination in the management of acute abdomen. Crit Ultrasound J. 2013;5(Suppl 1):S6.
129. Kameda T, Kawai F, Taniguchi N, Kobori Y. Usefulness of transabdominal ultrasonography in excluding adnexal disease. J Med Ultrason. 2016;43(1):63–70.
130. Li XH, Ouyang Y, Lu GXT. value of transvaginal sonography in diagnosing heterotopic pregnancy after in-vitro fertilization with embryo transfer. Ultrasound Obstet Gynecol. 2013;41:563.
131. Marks WM, Filly RA, Callen PW, Laing FC. The decidual cast of ectopic pregnancy: a confusing ultrasonographic appearance. Radiology. 1979;133:451–4.
132. Benson CB, Doubilet PM, Peters HE, Frates MC. Intrauterine fluid with ectopic pregnancy: a reappraisal. J Ultrasound Med. 2013;32:389–93.
133. Elson CJ, Salim R, Potdar N, Chetty M, Ross JA, Kirk EJ on behalf of the Royal College of Obstetricians and Gynaecologists. Diagnosis and management of ectopic pregnancy. BJOG 2016 123(13):e15-e55.
134. Nyberg DA, Hughes MP, Mack LA, Wang KY. Extrauterine findings of ectopic pregnancy of transvaginal US: importance of echogenic fluid. Radiology. 1991;178:823–6.
135. Fleischer AC, Pennell RG, McKee MS, Worrell JA, Keefe B, Herbert CM, et al. Ectopic pregnancy: features at transvaginal sonography. Radiology. 1990;174:375–8.
136. Dialani V, Levine D. Ectopic pregnancy: a review. Ultrasound Q. 2004;20(3):105.
137. Stein JC, Wang R, Adler N, Boscardin J, Jacoby VL, Won G, et al. Emergency physician ultrasonography for evaluating patients at risk for ectopic pregnancy: a meta-analysis. Ann Emerg Med. 2010;56(6):674–83.
138. Richardson A, Gallos I, Dobson S, Campbell BK, Coomarasamy A, Raine-Fenning N. Accuracy of first trimester ultrasound features for diagnosis of tubal ectopic pregnancy in the absence of an obvious extra-uterine embryo: a systematic review and meta-analysis. Ultrasound Obstet Gynecol. 2015;47(1):28–37.
139. Sohoni A, Bosley J, Miss JC. Bedside ultrasonography for obstetric and gynecologic emergencies. Crit Care Clin. 2014;30:207–26.
140. Jain KA. Sonographic spectrum of hemorrhagic ovarian cysts. J Ultrasound Med. 2002;21:v879–86.
141. Amirbekian S, Hooley RJ. Ultrasound evaluation of pelvic pain. Radiol Clin N Am. 2014;52(6):1215–35.
142. Lee EJ, Kwon HC, Joo HJ, et al. Diagnosis of ovarian torsion with color Doppler sonography: depiction of twisted vascular pedicle. J Ultrasound Med. 1998;17(2):83–9.
143. Cicardi M, Aberer W, Banerji A, et al. Classification, diagnosis, and approach to treatment for angioedema: consensus report from the Hereditary Angioedema International Working Group. Allergy. 2014;69:602–16.

Updates in Diagnosis and Management of Acute Gastrointestinal Hemorrhage

28

Alberto Tringali and Silvia Gheda

Key Points

- Acute gastrointestinal hemorrhage still represents a cause of death despite the improvement of medical and endoscopic treatment.
- Risk stratification is an essential part of patient assessment because it allows identifying patients who need treatment and those at high risk of rebleeding and mortality.
- Endoscopy is an essential tool for diagnosis and treatment of acute gastrointestinal hemorrhage and should be performed after hemodynamic resuscitation and in any case within 12 h for variceal bleeding and 24 h for non-variceal bleeding and lower GI bleeding.
- The best treatment should be based on different specialist skill ("bleeding team") including ER physicians, anesthesiologist, endoscopist, interventional radiologist, surgeons, and cardiologist. The team-based approach has been shown to be associated with better outcome.
- Endoscopic treatment is based on combined injection, thermal, and mechanical modalities using different devices that need to know how to use it.
- In case of medical and endoscopic treatment failure, radiological or surgical approach should be used.

28.1 Introduction

Gastrointestinal bleeding (GIB) is a common problem encountered in the emergency department and the primary care setting. Acute gastrointestinal bleeding is visible in the form of hematemesis, melena, or hematochezia. GIB is historically divided into two main types: upper gastrointestinal bleeding (UGIB) and lower GI bleeding (LGIB).

28.2 Upper Gastrointestinal Bleeding

UGIB includes hemorrhage originating from the esophagus to the ligament of Treitz, at the duodenojejunal flexure. UGIB is broadly divided into two main groups: non-variceal and variceal UGIB. Acute UGIB is a common cause of hospitalization, with incidences ranging from 48 to 160 cases per 100,000 adults per year [1]. For the past 20 years, epidemiology of UGIB is changed being increased the median age of patients, comorbidity, episodes of UGIB in patients admitted for other reason and UGIB related to NSAID, antiplatelet an anticoagulant users. Recent data suggest a decrease in the incidence and mortality of UGIB by 22.7% and 16.9%, respectively [2], most likely because of advances in both medical and endoscopic therapies. Despite the introduction of PPI, HP eradication, and efficacy of endoscopic treatment, mortality still remains unchanged around 5–10% [3]. A large prospective cohort study by Sung et al. analyzed the cause of mortality in patients with UGIB explaining that the reasons for the high mortality in these patients were determined by the fact that patients died of nonbleeding-related causes in about 80% of cases mostly due to MOF and cardiopulmonary conditions [3].

Electronic Supplementary Material The online version of this chapter (https://doi.org/10.1007/978-3-319-95114-0_28) contains supplementary material, which is available to authorized users.

A. Tringali (✉)
Endoscopy Unit, ASST GOM NIGUARDA, Milan, Italy
e-mail: alberto.tringali@ospedaleniguarda.it

S. Gheda
Department of Emergency Medicine, ASST GOM NIGUARDA, Milan, Italy

P. Aseni et al. (eds.), *Operative Techniques and Recent Advances in Acute Care and Emergency Surgery*,
https://doi.org/10.1007/978-3-319-95114-0_28

28.3 Non-variceal Upper Gastrointestinal Bleeding (NVUGB)

The most common causes of acute UGIB are non-variceal. This includes peptic ulcers, 28–59% (duodenal ulcer 17–37% and gastric ulcer 11–24%); mucosal erosive disease of the esophagus/stomach/duodenum, 1–47%; Mallory-Weiss syndrome, 4–7%; upper GI tract malignancy, 2–4%; other diagnosis, 2–7%; or not exact cause identified, 7–25% [4, 5].

28.3.1 NVUGB: Initial Assessment

The assessment of patients with acute UGIB should start with evaluation of their hemodynamic status. This directs resuscitation and allows prompt risk stratification. The first step in the management of UGIB is fluid resuscitation with isotonic intravenous fluid (e.g., normal saline solutions) administered to restore a normal circulating blood volume. In patients with hemodynamic instability (heart rate >100 bpm; systolic blood pressure <100 mmHg, or orthostatic hypotension), a bolus of 500 mL of normal saline should be given and repeated as necessary to achieve hemodynamic stability. Furthermore, a vasopressor therapy could be necessary to maintain adequate end-organ perfusion if a patient remains hypotensive despite aggressive fluid resuscitation. Stevens P et al. have shown that the management of patients with UGIB by a dedicated team (e.g., bleeding team) significantly reduced rebleeding rate, surgery rate, and length of hospital stay [6]. Furthermore, in a small trial, Baradarian et al. showed that early intensive resuscitation in patients with UGIB reduced mortality [7].

ESGE guideline recommends immediate assessment of hemodynamic status in patients with UGIB with prompt intravascular volume replacement using crystalloid fluid in case of hemodynamic instability [8].

28.3.2 Blood Transfusion

Blood transfusions should be administered to patients with a hemoglobin <7 g/dL [1], along with intravenous fluids.

A randomized controlled trial conducted by Villanueva et al. [10] that included 921 patients with acute UGIB, patients were assigned to a restrictive (transfusion for hemoglobin <7 g/dL) or a liberal (transfusion for hemoglobin <9 g/dL) strategy.

A restrictive target is associated with improved outcomes: notably decreased in-hospital mortality in critically ill patients [9], as well as higher 6-week survival, and decreased rebleeding in patients with UGIB [10] compared to a more liberal approach targeting hemoglobin levels above 10 g/dL and 9 g/dL, respectively. Mortality, rebleeding, and adverse event rates were all lower with the restrictive transfusion strategy compared with the liberal transfusion strategy.

A Cochrane review on transfusion in UGIB reports a non-significant trend toward increased rebleeding and mortality with transfusions [11].

Early transfusions within 12 h led to a twofold increase in rebleeding (odds ratio (OR) 2.26, 95% CI 1.76–2.90) [11]. Similar trends in rebleeding (OR 1.8, 95% CI 1.2–2.8) were seen with transfusion within 24 h [12, 13].

However, the applicability of a restrictive strategy should be individualized to each patient and may not apply to those, for instance, with severe bleeding or if the patient has significant cardiovascular comorbidities (e.g., unstable coronary artery disease) [14].

ESGE guideline recommends a restrictive strategy maintaining hemoglobin between 7 and 9 g/dL considering different target for patients with significant comorbidity [8].

28.3.3 NVUGB: Risk Stratification

Along with resuscitation, risk-stratifying patients into high- and low-risk categories can aid clinical decision-making regarding the timing of endoscopy and hospital discharge [15]. Some scoring tools have been developed for predicting outcomes following acute UGIB, with the Glasgow-Blatchford score (GBS) and Rockall score being the most widely evaluated and adopted. However, no single scoring tool has been shown to be superior at predicting all relevant outcomes in acute UGIB (e.g., rebleeding, need for intervention, mortality) [18]. This is not surprising as the most validated risk scores were derived to assess a specific UGIB outcome: that for the Rockall score being mortality and for the GBS being the need for intervention [16, 17].

Rockall score can be calculated using both pre-endoscopic (total = 7) and postendoscopic (total = 11) data. It predicts risk for further bleeding and mortality using clinical data and endoscopic findings. Glasgow-Blatchford risk score (GBS) (total = 23) was conceived to predict the need for interventions (i.e., transfusions, surgical and endoscopic treatment). The advantage of GBS is based on the fact that it incorporates only pre-endoscopic variables [17]. A GBS of 0 predicts a 0.5% risk for needing subsequent intervention. Stanley et al. used this cutoff to safely direct early discharge and outpatient endoscopy [18].

Comparing Rockall and GBS scores, the GBS's area under the ROC curve (0.90, 95% CI 0.88–0.93) outperformed the full Rockall score and pre-endoscopic Rockall score in predicting the need for reintervention or death [18].

International consensus recommends early discharge of low-risk patients after endoscopy [1] according to a set of criteria previously summarized [19] while American College of Gastroenterology guidelines for peptic ulcers bleeding even consider discharge before endoscopy for selected population [20]. High-risk patients should be hospitalized and monitored for 72 h [19]. ESGE recommends the use of GBS for pre-endoscopy risk stratification. Patients with GBS of 0–1 do not require early endoscopy or hospital admission [8].

28.3.4 NVUGIB: Management of Patients Receiving Antiplatelet or Anticoagulant Drugs

28.3.4.1 Antiplatelet Drugs

The most common antiplatelet agents in patients presenting with UGIB are aspirin and thienopyridines. These medications should be held at the time of presentation, and platelet transfusion can be considered for severe bleeding.

In a randomized controlled trial of patients presenting with acute peptic ulcer bleeding on daily aspirin for secondary prophylaxis of established cardiovascular or cerebrovascular diseases that required regular antiplatelet therapy, patients who resumed aspirin after successful hemostasis had a nonsignificant trend toward recurrent bleeding but a lower 30-day mortality compared with patients whose aspirin was held [21].

Current guidelines recommend restarting antiplatelet agents once patients are deemed stable after the UGIB [22].

28.3.4.2 Anticoagulants

For patients presenting with UGIB, an elevated international normalized ratio (INR) >1.5 has been associated with an increase in mortality [23, 24].

Warfarin: Warfarin should be stopped at the time of presentation. However, for patients at high risk of thromboembolic events, the benefits of stopping anticoagulation need to be weighed against the risks. Endoscopy does not need to be delayed for patients with mildly to moderately elevated INRs. Retrospective studies have shown that therapeutic upper endoscopy can be safely and effectively performed in such patients [25, 26, 27].

Current consensus guidelines advise that correction of a moderate coagulopathy (INR up to 2.5) should not delay endoscopy [28].

Direct-acting oral anticoagulants: This group of drugs currently includes the direct thrombin inhibitor dabigatran etexilate (Pradaxa) and the direct oral factor Xa inhibitors rivaroxaban (Xarelto), apixaban (Eliquis), and edoxaban (Lixiana) [29, 30].

Because of a fixed oral dosing schedule without the need for drug monitoring, direct-acting oral anticoagulants have become a popular anticoagulation alternative to warfarin therapy.

Also, new direct oral anticoagulants (DOAC) should be temporarily withheld. Given their relatively short half-life, time is the most important antidote against DOACs.

Anyway, if bleeding is severe and persistent, there is a potential role for transfusion of clotting factors such as fresh frozen plasma, activated factor VII, or prothrombin complex concentrate (which contains factors II, VII, IX, and X). Activated prothrombin complex concentrate is particularly effective for patients on dabigatran, although it may be replaced by the newly US FDA-approved reversal agent, idarucizumab (Praxibind), a monoclonal antibody against dabigatran that reverses the anticoagulant effect within minutes [31].

For patients on factor Xa inhibitors who have persistent, severe bleeding, non-activated prothrombin complex concentrate is the most effective product currently available [32].

28.3.5 NVUGIB: Pharmacological Therapy

28.3.5.1 PPI Prior to Endoscopy

A key element in the initial management of UGIB is initiation of proton pump inhibitor (PPI). By elevating the gastric pH, PPI facilitates clot stabilization within the stomach and have been shown to improve outcomes such as rebleeding and the need for surgery. In a Cochrane review, pre-endoscopic PPI led to a decreased proportion of patients with high-risk stigmata, as well as the need for endoscopic intervention [33, 34], but does not reduce rebleeding, surgery, or mortality. Nevertheless, the initiation of PPI while awaiting endoscopy should be considered, preferably using an 80 mg intravenous bolus followed by an 8 mg/h infusion. The decision to use PPI before endoscopy should be individualized, as additional data are still needed to define their optimal use in this setting.

ESGE guideline recommends initiating high-dose intravenous PPI (bolus followed by continuous infusion) awaiting endoscopy although should not delay the performance of early endoscopy [8].

28.3.5.2 Prokinetics Prior to Endoscopy

The use of prokinetics before endoscopy should be considered in selected patients. Erythromycin, a macrolide antibiotic with motilin-like properties, increases gastric emptying and thereby allows for improved views of the gastric mucosa [35].

ESGE recommends intravenous erythromycin (single dose, 250 mg given 30–120 min before endoscopy) in patients with severe UGIB because of significantly improved endoscopy visualization, reduces the need for second-look endoscopy, and decreases the number of unit of blood transfuses and length of hospital stay [8].

28.3.5.3 Nasogastric Tube

Nasogastric tube lavage is not necessary but can be considered prior to endoscopy. A bloody aspirate is linked to increased risk of finding a high-risk lesion, though a clear or bilious aspirate cannot rule it out [36].

ESGE do not recommend the routine use of nasogastric tube in patients with acute UGIB.

28.3.5.4 Orotracheal Intubation Prior to Endoscopy

Endotracheal intubation has been widely adopted as the preferred method for protection of the airway and prevention of aspiration during EGD for severe UGIB, although its utilization varies widely, even among experts. Between those patients who were prophylactically intubated prior to upper GI endoscopy as compared to those patients not intubated, published data show no significant difference in patient outcomes (e.g., pulmonary aspiration, in-hospital mortality) [37–40]. When performing emergency endoscopy, the sedation plan should be considered on case by case basis.

Unfortunately, there are few data and no prospective, randomized, or other comparative trial concerning the safety or efficacy of endotracheal intubation for UGIB.

A study published this year by Hayat et al. [42] showed that prophylactic endotracheal intubation before an EGD for brisk UGIB in critically ill patients is associated with an increased risk of unplanned cardiopulmonary events. The benefits and risks of intubation should be carefully weighted when considering airway protection before an EGD in this group of patients.

ESGE suggested endotracheal intubation prior to endoscopy in patients with ongoing active hematemesis, encephalopathy, or agitation, in an effort to protect the patient's airway from potential aspiration of gastric contents [8].

28.3.6 NVUGIB: Timing of Endoscopy

Early endoscopy within 24 h of presentation is recommended for most patients with UGIB. It allows for safe early discharge of low-risk patients [43, 44]. Very early endoscopy (<12 h) may be associated with increased findings of advanced stigmata but does not impact on rebleeding or mortality [44].

While some suggest very early endoscopy in selected high-risk patients [45, 46] such as those with bloody nasogastric aspirate [44] or high Blatchford risk score [47], the body of evidence that supports such practice changes outcomes is limited [46].

Current international guidelines do not advocate for routine endoscopy in less than 12 h in patients with suspected non-variceal UGIB [1], as opposed to variceal bleeding where endoscopy should be performed within 12 h [48].

Additional evidence for the availability of out-of-hours endoscopy just failed to reach significance with regard to mortality [49]; on the other hand, mortality has been reported to be increased in some high-risk patients undergoing early endoscopy [50].

Nine studies [44, 51–58] of patients with acute UGIB have evaluated the effect of endoscopy timing on clinical outcomes and/or healthcare resource use, although the studies differed significantly in their designs, which complicates the interpretation of the results as a whole. Three studies were randomized controlled trials, five were retrospective cohort trials, and one was a prospective cohort trial.

These studies defined differently timing of endoscopy. We divided, in attempt to homogenize the result, into three groups based on reported timing of endoscopy. A first group was called immediate endoscopy (within 2 h), a second group was defined as very early endoscopy (within 12 h), while a third group was named as early endoscopy (within 24 h).

The authors concluded that patients with high-risk bleeding prognostic scores benefit from earlier endoscopy, although it is also possible that clinical judgment underestimated the severity of bleeding or that high-risk patients with delayed endoscopy required more prolonged resuscitative efforts and thus were more likely to die.

Laursen et al. have analyzed the relationship between timing of endoscopy and mortality in patients with peptic ulcer bleeding in a nationwide cohort study. They showed no association between timing of endoscopy and mortality in hemodynamically stable patients with an ASA score of 1–2. In hemodynamically stable patients with ASA score of 3–5, endoscopy performed 12–36 h after admission was associated with lower in-hospital mortality (OR 0.48, 95%CI 0.34–0.67) compared with endoscopy outside this time frame. Finally in patients with hemodynamic instability, endoscopy 6–24 h after admission was associated with lower in-hospital mortality (OR 0.73, 95%CI 0.54–0.98) compared with endoscopy outside this time frame [59].

ESGE recommends early (<24 h) endoscopy following hemodynamic resuscitation. Very early (<12 h) upper GI endoscopy may be considered in patients with high-risk clinical features, namely, hemodynamic instability (tachycardia, hypotension) that persists despite ongoing attempts at volume resuscitation, in-hospital bloody emesis/nasogastric aspirate, or contraindication to the interruption of anticoagulation.

28.3.7 NVUGIB: Endoscopic Diagnosis and Management

Forrest classification should be used in all patient with peptic ulcer hemorrhage in order to differentiate low- and high-risk endoscopic stigmata.

28.3.7.1 Indication for Endoscopic Treatment

According to ESGE guidelines, peptic ulcers Ia and Ib or IIa receive endoscopic hemostasis because these lesions are at high risk for persistent bleeding or rebleeding and endoscopic treatment improved outcomes [8, 60, 68].

Peptic ulcers IIb should be considered for endoscopic clot removal. Once the clot is removed, any identified underlying active bleeding (Forrest classification Ia or Ib) or nonbleeding visible vessel (Forrest classification IIa) should receive endoscopic hemostasis.

In patients with peptic ulcers IIc or III, endoscopic hemostasis is not recommended as these stigmata present a low risk of recurrent bleeding. In selected clinical settings, these patients may be discharged to home on standard PPI therapy, e.g., oral PPI once daily.

Endoscopic treatment of peptic ulcer bleeding with adherent clot (F IIb) has been a matter of debate and controversy issue. A meta-analysis examining this issue suggested significant improvement in outcome attributable to endoscopic treatment in this patient population [61] that was criticized because of statistical shortcomings [62].

28.3.7.2 Endoscopic Treatment Modalities

Endoscopic modalities used in the management of acute UGIB are classified into injection, thermal, and mechanical therapies and shown in Fig. 28.1.

Any endoscopic therapy is superior to pharmacotherapy in patients with FIa, FIb and FIIa ulcers [48, 49].

Injection therapy includes epinephrine, hypertonic saline, sclerosants, (polidocanol, ethanolamine), and tissue adhesives (cyanoacrylate, thrombin, and fibrin glue). All injection therapies achieve hemostasis through local tissue and vascular tamponade [63]. Furthermore, thrombin and fibrin injection may create a tissue seal at the site of bleeding, whereas sclerosant causes direct tissue injury and induces thrombosis. Sclerosant is associated with more tissue necrosis, limiting use to less than 1 mL [63].

Thermal therapy**:** thermal devices are classified in contact and no contact methods. Heater probe and electrocautery probe are contact modalities whereas argon plasma coagulation (APC) is a contact modality. The most frequently used in UGIB are electrocautery probe which achieves hemostasis through coaptive coagulation which provides local tamponade and vessel occlusion through the application of pressure using the probe tip followed by heat to coagulate the vessel. APC uses argon to conduct electricity to treat superficial lesions (<1–2 mm deep).

Mechanical therapy**:** mechanical devices cause local tamponade of vessels via direct approximation of the submucosa surrounding the bleeding site without tissue injury. The most common devices used are clip, band ligation especially used for Dieulafoy lesion [64], and OVESCO clip.

To date, five meta-analyses assessed the optimal endoscopic therapy in peptic ulcer bleeding with high-risk stigmata [65, 66, 67, 69, 73].

A meta-analyses showed that thermal devices (contact and noncontact), injectable agents other than epinephrine (i.e., sclerosing agents, thrombin/fibrin glue), and clips are all effective methods for achieving hemostasis, with no single modality being superior [68, 69, 70–74].

ESGE recommends that epinephrine injection therapy not be used as endoscopic monotherapy. If used, it should be combined with a second endoscopic hemostasis modality. For patients with active NVUGIB not controlled by standard endoscopic hemostasis therapies, ESGE suggests the use of a topical hemostatic spray or over-the-scope clip as salvage endoscopic therapy.

28.3.8 NVUGIB: Novel Therapy

New endoscopic hemostasis modalities (topical hemostatic sprays and over-the-scope clips) are emerging as possible alternative endotherapies for primary hemostasis when bleeding is refractory or not amenable to standard endoscopic hemostasis therapies [75, 76]. Moreover, several small retrospective studies have reported that an over-the-scope clip (OVESCO) may have a role as rescue hemostasis therapy for severe NVUGIB when conventional endoscopic treatment modalities fail [77–79]. An inert nanopowder (Hemospray) that causes immediate hemostasis when sprayed onto active bleeding [75, 80] has recently been used as a primary hemostasis agent or as a second-line salvage therapy. Several prospective uncontrolled studies, a large European registry [81–86], and a systematic review of the currently limited data suggest that Hemospray is safe and effective and may be best used in high-risk cases as a temporizing measure or a bridge toward more definitive treatment [75]. However, RCTs directly comparing topical agents with traditional hemostasis methods are required to better define their optimal role and safety in the endoscopic management of NVUGIB. Endoscopic Doppler ultrasound is an

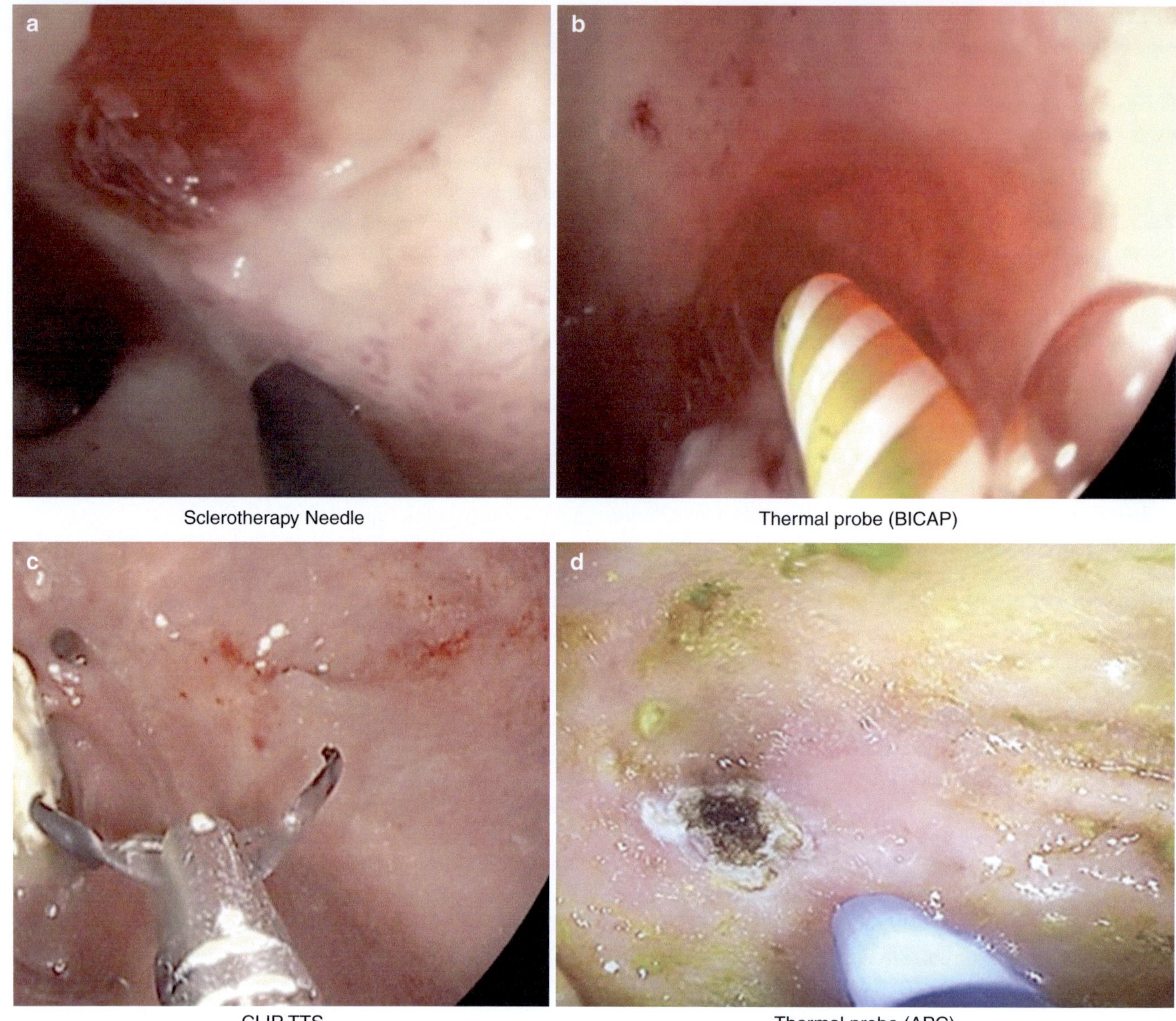

Fig. 28.1 Endoscopic treatment modalities of acute NVUGIB. (**a**) Sclerotherapy needle, (**b**) thermal probe (BICAP), (**c**) CLIP TTS, (**d**) thermal probe (APC)

adjunct method that can guide endoscopic therapy by identifying underlying vasculature before proceeding to focal injection of vessels [82, 84]. Endoscopic sutures and expandable stents have yet to be tested for acute NVUGIB at the time of writing of this chapter [75]. A hemostatic forceps is usually used in the ESD procedures to coagulate effectively and safely active bleeding vessel or visible vessels. In a small study, hemostatic forceps was used for ulcer bleeding as second-line approach during the same procedure or as rescue [87].

28.3.9 NVUGIB: Management Following Endoscopic Hemostasis

28.3.9.1 PPI Postendoscopic Treatment

The administration of a continuous-infusion, high-dose, intravenous PPI for 72 h has been demonstrated to be effective in reducing rebleeding rates to approximately 10% and mortality after endoscopic therapy of ulcers with high-risk stigmata [33, 68, 88, 89].

In a study designed to identify the lowest effective dose of PPI, rather than using a high (or low) dose, continuous infusion was the key to maintaining an intragastric pH greater than 6 [90].

Two meta-analyses have confirmed that an intravenous PPI bolus followed by continuous PPI infusion over 72 h reduces the rates of mortality (RR, 0.40, 0.28–0.59; NNT, 12), rebleeding (RR, 0.40, 0.28–0.59; NNT, 12), and surgery (RR, 0.43, 0.24–0.76; NNT, 28). Mortality was only reduced in patients who had previously undergone successful endoscopic hemostasis [33, 68].

More recently, a systematic review and meta-analysis compared intermittent versus continuous PPI therapy for the treatment of high-risk bleeding ulcers after endoscopic therapy [91]. This study revealed that intermittent PPI therapy might be as effective as continuous-infusion high-dose therapy in these high-risk patients.

However, overall, current guidelines remain ambivalent toward optimal postendoscopy PPI dosing because of an overall low quality of evidence secondary to a high risk of bias and imprecision in the aforementioned systematic review [92].

High-dose oral PPI treatment after endoscopy was efficacious in early trials conducted in India and Iran [33].

Accordingly, the evidence is currently insufficient to support the use of oral PPI therapy immediately after endoscopy in high-risk patients.

However, current recommendations do recommend oral PPI therapy in patients with lower-risk stigmata on endoscopy, such as a clean-based ulcer or a flat pigmented spot. In these lower-risk patients, the rates of significant rebleeding remain low [65].

Anyway our recent meta-analysis comparing oral vs. intravenous PPI after endoscopic treatment in patients with acute UGIB showed that there was no difference in primary and secondary outcomes [93].

28.3.9.2 Predictors of Rebleeding

Rebleeding after initial hemostasis occurs in 10–20% [49, 94, 95] of patients and is in itself a predictor of mortality [96]. Data from trials featuring sequential endoscopic evaluations of bleeding stigmata depict an evolution from high-risk stigmata to low-risk stigmata, where the majority of rebleeding occurs within the first 72 h [26]. Both clinical and endoscopic variables can help in predicting the risk of rebleeding. Several independent prognostic factors have been identified and include comorbid illness, the presence of hemodynamic instability, active bleeding at endoscopy, large ulcer size (most commonly >2 cm), ulcer location (posterior duodenal wall and lesser gastric curvature), hemoglobin value (most commonly <10 g/L), and the need for transfusion [95, 96]. The presence of such factors may help identify and manage patients at an especially high risk of rebleeding.

28.3.9.3 Second-Look Endoscopy

Second-look endoscopy is a pre-planned repeat endoscopy at 16–48 h after achieving initial endoscopic hemostasis. Moreover, the benefits of second-look endoscopy were not robust when very high-risk patients were excluded [97]. The added cost also needs to be considered [98]. Hence, second-look endoscopy is not recommended in all UGIB patients, but should be reserved for those at an especially high risk for rebleeding.

28.3.9.4 Endoscopy in Rebleeding

Repeat endoscopy is recommended in the setting of clinically evident rebleeding after successful hemostasis [1, 45].

A RCT showed that at a second attempt an endoscopic control of bleeding was achieved in 73% of patients [99]. Compared to surgery, it is associated with lower complications without increased mortality [99]. After the second episode of rebleeding, surgical and radiological options should be considered and are being increasingly used in contemporary practice for cases refractory to endoscopic treatment.

A national UK audit on NVUGIB revealed that surgery and transarterial embolization (TAE) was required in 2.3% and 1.3% of all patients, respectively [100]. Mortality was noted to be higher after surgery than after TAE, with rates of 29% (28/97 patients) versus 10% (6/60 patients), suggesting TAE may be an alternative for surgery in rebleeding [100]. Several retrospective studies support TAE after failed endoscopic treatment as being at least comparable to surgery with regard to complications, without adversely affecting mortality in retrospective studies [101].

28.3.9.5 Secondary Prophylaxis to Prevent Recurrent Bleeding

In patients with *Helicobacter pylori*-associated bleeding ulcers, continuing PPI therapy after *H. pylori* eradication is not required unless there are other ongoing risk factors, including NSAID use or antithrombotic therapy.

Similarly, in patients with low-dose aspirin-related ulcers, long-term PPI therapy is required if acetylsalicylic acid (ASA) must be continued (e.g., secondary prevention of cardiovascular disease) [102, 103].

Pooled results of two randomized trials have shown that ASA with PPI has significantly less risk of rebleeding than clopidogrel alone (OR, 0.06; 95% CI, 0.01–0.32) [104, 105].

28.3.9.6 *Helicobacter pylori* Eradication

All patients should be tested for infection with *H. pylori*, which is one of the principal causes of bleeding ulcers. The low prevalence reported for *H. pylori* infection in patients with UGIB might be related to delay in testing, which is often not performed until 4 weeks after the bleeding episode [106].

A second test should be performed if a negative index result is obtained at the time of acute UGIB because false-negative rates in the acute setting reach 55% and are increased for all diagnostic modalities [1].

After the completion of antibiotic and PPI treatment, a urea breath test might be the most convenient approach to assess the effectiveness of *H. pylori* eradication treatment, unless repeat endoscopy is indicated, at which time gastric biopsies can be performed.

28.4 Variceal Upper Gastrointestinal Bleeding

One of the most important complications of portal hypertension, in the setting of liver cirrhosis or of non-cirrhotic portal hypertension, is upper gastrointestinal bleeding from ruptured gastroesophageal varices and portal hypertensive gastropathy. The prevalence of varices in cirrhotic patients ranges from 30 to 60%, according to the presence of decompensation [107], and prospective studies have shown that more than 90% of patients will develop esophageal varices during their lifetime. The main prognostic factors associated with progression of small to large varices are decompensated cirrhosis (Child B/C), alcoholic etiology of cirrhosis, elevated hepatic venous pressure gradient (HVPG), and the presence of red wale markings on the esophageal varices at the time of baseline endoscopy [108, 109, 110].

Acute variceal bleeding in patients with cirrhosis indicates decompensation and a high risk of death [107]. The annual rate of bleeding, in the absence of treatment, is 10–15% [111, 112].

In patients with cirrhosis, ruptured esophageal varices cause approximately 70% of all upper digestive bleeding [113] and are the second most common cause of mortality for cirrhotic patients [114]. Mortality from variceal bleeding has greatly decreased during the last decades to the current rates of 6–12% [107, 115, 116–118].

The management of the acute variceal bleeding is a multidisciplinary process [94] that includes the initial assessment of the patient, effective resuscitation, timely diagnosis, control of bleeding, and prevention of early rebleeding and complications such as infection, hepatorenal syndrome, or hepatic encephalopathy.

28.4.1 VUGIB: Primary Prophylaxis

Since 30–50% of patients with portal hypertension will bleed from varices and about 20% will die from the effects of the first bleed, it seems rational to develop prophylactic regimens to prevent the development of, and bleeding from, these varices. Based on the expected bleeding and death rates in this group of patients, guidelines propose an algorithm for surveillance and primary prophylaxis of varices.

The mainstay of the pharmacological approach to the primary prophylaxis of variceal hemorrhage has been based on non-cardioselective beta-blockers (NSBB). According to international guidelines, NSBB treatment is only recommended in patients with medium to large varices as well as high-risk small varices. Propranolol has been shown to reduce the portal pressure gradient, azygos blood flow, and also variceal pressure. It achieves this by causing splanchnic vasoconstriction and reducing cardiac output. Nadolol exerts similar effects on portal hemodynamics, although the effect on blood pressure may not be as pronounced. Carvedilol is a NSBB like propranolol and a vasodilator due to $\alpha 1$ receptor blockade. The latter reduces porto-collateral resistance and by actions on hepatic stellate cells leads to a reduction in intrahepatic resistance. Hemodynamic studies demonstrate a greater reduction in portal pressure with carvedilol than with propranolol, although blood pressure is reduced. However, carvedilol has not been adequately compared head to head to traditional NSBB in clinical trials.

In case of contraindications or intolerance to NSBB, international guidelines recommend variceal band ligation. Beta-blockade should not be started in the acute setting, and those already taking NSBB as prophylaxis should probably stop taking them for 48–72 h so that patient's physiological response to blood loss can be allowed to manifest. Finally band ligation should be considered in patient on beta-blockers with refractory ascites who develop hypotension (SBP <90 mmHg), hyponatremia (<130 mEq/l), or acute kidney injury.

28.4.2 VUGIB: Initial Assessment

The most important step in the management of acute variceal hemorrhage is the initial resuscitation assessed according to standard "ABC" practice, together with protection of the airway to prevent aspiration. Although early endoscopy allows for accurate diagnosis of the bleeding site and decisions about management, therapeutic intervention in acute variceal bleeding can be initiated, safely in most cases, before diagnostic endoscopy.

The majority of patients with a variceal bleed will be sufficiently stable to enable a full history and examination to take place. Comorbidity is important when estimating risk and deciding on use of vasopressors. Intravenous access (two 16–18G cannulae) should have been secured on admission with a reported GI bleed. Intravenous fluid resuscitation should be initiated with plasma expanders aiming to maintain a systolic blood pressure of 100 mmHg. Overtransfusion has been shown to have a deleterious effect on outcome. A recent single-center RCT, a restrictive transfusion policy of maintaining hemoglobin between 7 and 8 g/dL, improved the control of variceal bleeding (11% vs. 22%, $p = 0.05$) and lowered HVPG compared with a liberal transfusion policy without effect on 45-day survival [10]. Interpretation and management of clotting profile are challenging in liver disease, where there is usually a balanced deficiency of both procoagulant and anticoagulant factors [160]. The NICE guidelines recommend activation of a hospital's massive transfusion policy when there is major hemorrhage, platelet support when the value is <50.000, and clotting factor support when the international normalized ratio (INR) is <1.5 times normal.

28.4.3 VUGIB: Pharmacological Therapy

Antibiotics that provide Gram-negative cover are one of the interventions which positively influence survival in variceal hemorrhage as shown in a Cochrane meta-analysis of 12 placebo-controlled trials (RR = 0.79, 95% CI 0.63–0.98). Antibiotics were also shown to reduce bacterial infections (RR = 0.43, 95% CI 0.19–0.97) and early rebleeding (RR = 0.53, 95% CI 0.38–0.74) [127].

Therefore, antibiotic prophylaxis should be instituted from admission in all cirrhotic patients who have a variceal bleed, irrespective of the presence of confirmed infection. It should consist of oral quinolones for most patients considering intravenous ceftriaxone in patients with advanced cirrhosis, in hospital settings with high prevalence of quinolone-resistant bacterial infections and patients on previous quinolone prophylaxis [119, 120, 121].

Vasoactive drugs (terlipressin, somatostatin, octreotide, vapreotide) should be started as soon as possible, even before endoscopy [122]. Vasoactive drugs used in combination with endoscopic therapy allow a better control of hemorrhage than drug therapy or endoscopy alone [123]. No significant differences have been found in several studies between different vasoactive drugs in the control of the index bleeding and the prevention of recurrence. Terlipressin is the only vasoactive drug that has a positive effect on survival [111]. It is a synthetic analog of vasopressin, which has an immediate systemic vasoconstrictor action followed by portal hemodynamic effects due to slow conversion to vasopressin. The recommended dose of terlipressin is 2 mg IV every 4 h, although many units reduce the dose to 6 hourly as it may cause peripheral vasoconstriction which manifests as painful hands and feet.

In clinical practice, the choice of the vasoactive drug is based on its availability and its cost. Vasoactive drug therapy should be prolonged for 2–5 days according to control of bleeding and can be stopped after 24 h free from bleeding.

Endotracheal intubation may be needed in selected cases [122]. If a patient is vomiting blood or there is a perceived risk of a hemodynamically unstable patient having blood in the stomach, then the patient must be intubated before endoscopy and return to an intensive care or high dependency unit will be necessary until extubation.

Balloon tamponade can also be used as a bridge therapy to obtain temporary hemostasis (maximum 24 h) [124]. An appropriately placed Sengstaken-Blakemore tube allows for resuscitation, safe transportation, and either repeat endoscopy or radiological shunting in a patient with a stable cardiovascular system. It is however associated with serious complications such as esophageal ulceration and aspiration pneumonia in up to 15–20% of patients.

28.4.4 VUGIB: Endoscopic Therapy

Emergency EGD may be at the same time diagnostic and therapeutic. When it is performed early, 39–44% of patients present with active bleeding, 33–44% are with signs of recent bleeding (clots or "white nipple" on varices) [125], and 12–28% have no sign of active or recent hemorrhage [126].

Endoscopy should take place within 24 h of admission and earlier if there is excessive bleeding, based on low-level evidence [128]. While many guidelines and reviews suggest that endoscopy should be carried out within 12 h, the only study that examined the influence of timing on outcome failed to demonstrate any advantage of endoscopy before 12 h [129]. The optimal time is after sufficient resuscitation, and pharmacological treatment, with the endoscopy performed by a skilled endoscopy team, in a suitably equipped environment and with airway protection.

Airway protection is essential where risk of aspiration is high and affords the endoscopist time for thorough evaluation, including complete clot aspiration and controlled application of treatment, including tamponade if required.

Endoscopic treatment of esophageal varices may be performed by endoscopic sclerotherapy (ES) and endoscopic variceal ligation (EVL). ES is currently performed using flexible catheters with a short needle tip (23 or 25 gauge). Different sclerosant agents (e.g., sodium morrhuate, polidocanol, ethanolamine, alcohol, and sodium tetradecyl sulfate) have been used in controlled trials [130], and nowadays the most commonly used agents are ethanolamine oleate (5%) or polidocanol (1–2%) in Europe and sodium morrhuate (5%) in the United States [131, 132]. The injection of the sclerosant agent may be performed into the variceal lumen (intravariceal) or adjacent to it (paravariceal) inducing thrombosis of the vessel and inflammation of the surrounding tissues [133, 134] leading to fibrosis and resulting in variceal obliteration [135]. Injection of sclerosant should be first made immediately below the bleeding point (1–3 mL) and then in the remaining varices near the bleeding one (2–3 mL injections). The total amount of sclerosant per session is usually 10–15 mL. Both intravariceal and paravariceal injections have been associated with good outcomes [136], and no differences have been found with different sclerosants [137], the volume injected, or frequency of sessions [135]. Compared to EVL, ES is easier to use since it does not require to withdraw and reinsert the endoscope.

Complications of ES are more frequent than those of EVL [130, 138–145]. The complications can be classified as local (esophageal ulcers, ulcer bleeding, and esophageal stricture), cardiovascular and respiratory (pleural effusion, acute respiratory distress syndrome, and pericarditis), and systemic (fever, bacteremia, spontaneous bacterial peritonitis, distant embolism, or abscess) [146]. Frequent minor complications that do not require treatment occur within the first 24–48 h: retrosternal chest pain, low-grade fever, dysphagia, asymptomatic pleural effusions, and nonspecific chest radiographic changes [133].

In a Cochrane meta-analysis, ES was not shown to be superior to the vasoactive drug therapy for the control of bleeding, rebleeding, and mortality [147].

While ES used chemical action to obliterate varices, EVL causes a mechanical strangulation with rubber bands that induces thrombosis with ischemic necrosis of the mucosa. EVL consists in placing rubber rings on esophageal varices after sucking them into a plastic cylinder attached to the tip of the endoscope [148, 149]. During an emergency EGD, the bleeding varix is identified; the endoscope is then removed from the patient and the banding device is loaded. The endoscope is then reinserted into the esophagus up to the gastroesophageal junction to identify the varices. Then the tip of the endoscope is oriented toward the varix and a continuous suction is applied until the varix fills the cap. At this moment, the band can be "fired" [146]. The bands should be placed on the varix at the point of bleeding or starting from the gastroesophageal junction in a helical fashion [133] for 6–8 cm within the palisade and perforating zones [146]. The rubber bands on the ligated varix detach in 1–10 days, leaving shallow esophageal ulcers and smaller esophageal varices. The ulcers generated by EVL are bigger and shallower than those of ES and heal more rapidly [146, 150]. After band ligation, patients should start with liquids at room temperature for the first 12 h and then take soft foods gradually. Varices are considered eradicated when they have either disappeared or cannot be sucked and banded by the ligator [131]. Variceal eradication is obtained in about 90% of patients with up to four banding sessions [131], but recurrence is not uncommon [151].

A meta-analysis of seven randomized controlled trials (RCTs) showed that there is a tendency toward benefit of EVL compared to ES in terms of control of bleeding, recurrent bleeding, side effects, need for fewer endoscopic treatments, and survival [145]. Therefore, EVL has become the treatment of choice for variceal bleeding, but ES can be used when EVL is technically difficult [149]. Compared to ES, EVL has a higher frequency of recurrent varices [152–154], but they can be treated with repeated EVL [154].

Minor complications of EVL, which respond well to oral analgesia and antacids, include chest pain and transient dysphagia. Serious, but rare, complications include massive bleeding from untimely sloughing of bands, esophageal perforation (mostly for the use of overtube), esophageal strictures [155], and bacteremia [156] even if with a lower frequency than with ES [157].

Combination of vasoactive drugs plus EVL/ES is the standard of care for variceal bleeding [122]. In fact, a meta-analysis of eight trials demonstrated that combined therapy (endoscopic plus vasoactive drugs) compared to endoscopic therapy alone (ES or EVL) improved control of bleeding and 5-day hemostasis without differences in severe side effects or mortality [123].

Current guidelines define treatment failure a failure to control acute variceal bleeding within 24 h or failure to prevent clinically significant rebleeding or death within 5 days of treatment.

Approximately 10–15% of patients have a risk of treatment failure [122, 126]. Child-Pugh class, shock at admission, presence of portal vein thrombosis, active bleeding at endoscopy, and elevated hepatic venous pressure gradient >20 mmHg have been shown to be predictive of treatment failure [122]. A second attempt at endoscopic therapy can be tried, possibly changing the endoscopic technique, but if this is unsuccessful, a more aggressive approach by shunt therapy (TIPS or surgical) may be needed [122].

An early TIPS with PTFE-covered stents within 72 h (ideally <24 h) must be considered in patients bleeding from EV at high risk of treatment failure (e.g., Child-Pugh class C or Child-Pugh class B with active bleeding) after initial pharmacological and endoscopic therapy.

28.4.5 VUGIB: Novel Therapy

Hemostatic powder (TC-325, Hemospray, Cook Medical, USA) has been described in small studies of few patients who receive endoscopic spray treatment for acute variceal bleeding. A study by Ibrahim et al. reported no rebleeding within 24 h and no mortality at 15 days in nine patients [158]. Hemospray is currently not approved for routine management of AVB since a theoretical concern is that its application with a CO2 cartridge delivers the powder at the end of the catheter with an outflow pressure of 15 mmHg that might be associated with a risk, never observed in the current and previous studies, of venous thromboembolization. This is, however, highly improbable since, by definition, Hemospray is a noncontact method, and, in the case of esophageal or esogastric variceal bleeding, it is delivered with the catheter positioned in the center of the lumen and pulled backward, making the risk of impact with a millimeter-sized bleeding site almost null. Anecdotal experience suggests that the covered SEMSs may be useful in controlling esophageal variceal bleeding. A meta-analysis including four observational studies and one RCT for a total of 80 patients showed that the complete response to esophageal stenting was 93.9% with a rebleeding rate of 13.2% and the overall mortality was 34.5% mostly due to hepatic or multiple organ failure, and only 12.6% of patients died from uncontrolled bleeding. There was no stent-related complication reported, and the incidence of stent migration was 21.6% In conclusion, esophageal stent might be considered in patients with variceal bleeding refractory to conventional therapy.

28.4.6 VUGIB: Secondary Prophylaxis

Patients who survive an episode of acute variceal hemorrhage have a very high risk of rebleeding and death. The median rebleeding rate in untreated individuals is around 60% within 1–2 years of the index hemorrhage, with a mortality of 33% [151]. It is, therefore, essential that patients who have recovered from an episode of variceal hemorrhage and have had no evidence of hemorrhage for at least 24 h be started on therapy to prevent recurrence prior to discharge from the hospital.

A meta-analysis of 23 trials assessing sclerotherapy or EVL combined with NSBB reported that combination therapy reduced rebleeding more than either endoscopic therapy or NSBB alone (pooled RR = 0.68, 95% CI 0.52–0.89), although no difference in mortality was detected [159]. EVL should not be used as monotherapy unless there is intolerance or contraindications to NSBB. NSBB should be used as monotherapy in patients with cirrhosis who are unable or unwilling to be treated with EVL.

28.4.7 VUGIB: Gastric Variceal Bleeding

Bleeding from gastric varices (GV) is less frequent but more severe than bleeding from esophageal varices [113]. The treatment of GV is more difficult because of the torrential blood outflow and their treatment modality depends on their type. Gastric varices can be classified on the basis of their location in the stomach and the relationship with esophageal varices. The commonly used Sarin classification divides them into gastroesophageal varices (GOV) which are associated with esophageal varices and isolated gastric varices (IGV) which occur independently of esophageal varices. Type 1 GOV are an extension of esophageal varices along the lesser curvature of the stomach. Type 2 GOV extend beyond the gastroesophageal junction into the fundus of the stomach. Type 1 IGV refers to varices that occur in the fundus of the stomach, and type 2 IGV describes varices anywhere else in the stomach. Patients who bleed from IGV are at a significantly higher risk of dying from an episode of variceal bleeding than patients bleeding from GOV [160].

Although no studies have reported the use of vasopressors and antibiotics specifically for the initial management of gastric variceal hemorrhage, any patient with suspected variceal bleeding should be managed as described above for esophageal varices.

Once endoscopy has identified the source of bleeding as gastric varices, therapeutic options include endoscopic methods, TIPSS, other radiological procedures, surgery, and long-term NSBB. Sclerotherapy has been largely replaced by EVL and tissue adhesives or thrombin when appropriate for gastric varices, owing to the lower complication and rebleeding rates.

As GOV-1 are generally considered extensions of esophageal varices, EVL is often used to treat bleeding from here. However, given the larger diameter and the anatomy of other types of gastric varices, and the limited data on use of EVL in this situation, this technique is generally not recommended for these.

Gastric variceal obliteration consists in the injection of a tissue adhesive (polymers of cyanoacrylate) into a varix; the tissue adhesive upon contact with blood immediately polymerizes obliterating the varix. Gastric variceal obliteration is effective for acute fundal GV bleeding as it allows a better control of bleeding and reduces the rate of rebleeding in comparison with other treatments [161].

Intravariceal thrombin injection was useful in achieving initial hemostasis in GV bleeding without significant side effects in preliminary studies [161–164], but further evidence is needed before its use could be recommended in clinical practice.

In case of treatment failure of pharmacological and endoscopic therapy, TIPS should be considered, sometimes associated with coil embolization of GV [122].

28.5 LGIB

Acute lower gastrointestinal bleeding (LGIB) refers to blood loss from the gastrointestinal tract of recent onset emanating from a location distal to the ligament of Treitz and resulting in instability of vital signs, anemia, and/or need for blood transfusion [165].

The most common causes of lower gastrointestinal bleeding are diverticulosis (5–42%), angiodysplasia (1–4%), ischemic colitis (7–18%), IBD, colon adenocarcinoma (2–19%), and post-polypectomy bleeding (0–12.8%).

LGIB tends to be less severe in presentation than UGIB, and 80–85% of patients with LGIB will stop spontaneously. LGIB encompasses a wide clinical spectrum ranging from occult bleeding to overt hematochezia until massive hemorrhage with shock requiring emerging hospitalization. A mild-moderate LGIB occur in about 85–90% of cases; 10–15% of cases had a severe presentation with persistent or recurrent bleeding with hemodynamic effect (tachycardia, hypotension), drop in Hb levels (>2 g/dL), and need hospital admission.

28.5.1 Initial Assessment

Initial assessment of the patient presenting with presumed acute LGIB should include a focused history, physical examination, and laboratory testing with the goal of determining the severity of bleeding. Hematochezia associated with hemodynamic instability should lead to consideration of a brisk UGIB source. Patients with hemodynamic instability and/or suspected ongoing bleeding should receive intravenous fluid resuscitation with the goal of normalization of blood pressure and heart rate before endoscopic evaluation/intervention.

In contrast to UGIB, predictive factors of poor outcome in LGIB are not well defined. Most episodes of LGIB will stop spontaneously, the early identification of high-risk patients would allow the selection of those patients most likely to benefit from urgent therapeutic interventions. Several tools have been developed to assess risk in acute LGIB [166–171], although the number of available studies is modest in comparison with UGIB. Risk factors identified for poor outcome in LGIB include markers of hemodynamic instability at presentation (tachycardia, hypotension, and syncope), ongoing bleeding (gross blood on initial digital rectal examination and recurrent hematochezia), comorbid illnesses, age > 60 years, a history of diverticulosis or angioectasia, an elevated creatinine, and anemia (initial hematocrit ≤35%). In general, the likelihood of an adverse outcome increases with the number of risk factors present [169]. Monitoring in an intensive care setting should be considered in patients with high-risk features. These patients may also benefit from colonoscopy after a rapid bowel preparation or radiographic interventions.

Colonoscopy should be the initial diagnostic procedure for nearly all patients presenting with acute LGIB. The goal of colonoscopy in LGIB is to identify the site of bleeding and perform hemostasis, if indicated.

ACG guideline recommended that a focused history, physical examination, and laboratory evaluation should be obtained at the time of patients' presentation to assess the severity of bleeding and its possible localization and etiology. Initial patient assessment and hemodynamic resuscitation should be performed simultaneously (strong recommendation, very-low-quality evidence) [170].

Furthermore, hematochezia associated with hemodynamic instability may be indicative of an UGIB source, and an upper endoscopy should be performed. A nasogastric lavage/aspirate may be used to assess a possible upper GI source if suspicion of UGIB is moderate (strong recommendation, low-quality evidence).

Finally, risk assessment and stratification should be performed to help distinguish patients at high and low risks of adverse outcomes and assist in patient triage including the timing of colonoscopy and the level of care (conditional recommendation, low-quality evidence) [170].

28.5.2 Hemodynamic Resuscitation

Patients with hemodynamic instability and/or suspected ongoing bleeding should receive intravenous fluid resuscitation with the goal of normalization of blood pressure and heart rate prior to endoscopic evaluation/intervention (strong recommendation, very-low-quality evidence).

Packed red blood cells should be transfused to maintain the hemoglobin above 7 g/dl. A threshold of 9 g/dl should be considered in patients with massive bleeding, significant comorbid illness (especially cardiovascular ischemia), or a possible delay in receiving therapeutic interventions (conditional recommendations, low-quality evidence) [170].

28.5.3 Management of Anticoagulant Medications

Endoscopic hemostasis may be considered in patients with an INR of 1.5–2.5 before or concomitant with the administration of reversal agents. Reversal agents should be considered before endoscopy in patients with an INR >2.5 (conditional recommendation, very-low-quality evidence).

Platelet transfusion should be considered to maintain a platelet count of 50 × 10/l in patients with severe bleeding and those requiring endoscopic hemostasis (conditional recommendation, very-low-quality evidence).

Platelet and plasma transfusions should be considered in patients who receive massive red blood cell transfusions (conditional recommendation, very-low-quality evidence).

In patients on anticoagulant agents, a multidisciplinary approach (e.g., hematology, cardiology, neurology, and gastroenterology) should be used when deciding whether to discontinue medications or use reversal agents to balance the risk of ongoing bleeding with the risk of thromboembolic events (strong recommendation, very-low-quality evidence).

28.5.4 Timing of Endoscopy

28.5.4.1 Colonoscopy as a Diagnostic Tool

Colonoscopy should be the initial diagnostic procedure for nearly all patients presenting with acute LGIB (strong recommendation, low-quality evidence).

The colonic mucosa should be carefully inspected during both colonoscope insertion and withdrawal, with aggressive attempts made to wash residual stool and blood to identify the bleeding site. The endoscopist should also intubate the terminal ileum to rule out proximal blood suggestive of a small bowel lesion (conditional recommendation, very-low-quality evidence).

28.5.4.2 Bowel Preparation

Once the patient is hemodynamically stable, colonoscopy should be performed after adequate colon cleansing [173–176]. Four to six liters of a polyethylene glycol (PEG)-based solution or the equivalent should be administered over 3–4 h until the rectal effluent is clear of blood and stool. Unprepped colonoscopy/sigmoidoscopy is not recommended (strong recommendation, low-quality evidence).

A nasogastric tube can be considered to facilitate colon preparation in high-risk patients with ongoing bleeding who are intolerant to oral intake and are at low risk of aspiration (conditional recommendation, low-quality evidence).

Preparation of the colon facilitates endoscopic visualization and diagnosis and may reduce the risk of bowel perforation.

Nonetheless, there is a great controversy about the timing of colonoscopy [172, 177].

A systematic review and meta-analysis comparing urgent to elective colonoscopy in patients with LGIB showed that urgent colonoscopy was associated with increased use of endoscopic therapeutic intervention (RR 1.70, 95% CI 1.08–2.67), but there were no significant differences in bleeding source localization (RR 1.08; 95% CI, 0.92–1.25), adverse event rates (RR 1.05, 95%CI 0.65–1.71), rebleeding rates (RR 1.14, 95%CI 0.74–1.78), transfusion requirements (RR 1.02, 95%CI 0.73–1.41), or mortality (RR 1.17, 95% CI 0.45–3.02) [177, 178].

According to ASGE guideline, in patients with high-risk clinical features and signs or symptoms of ongoing bleeding, a rapid bowel purge should be initiated following hemodynamic resuscitation and a colonoscopy performed within 24 h of patient presentation after adequate colon preparation to potentially improve diagnostic and therapeutic yield (conditional recommendation, low-quality evidence).

In patients without high-risk clinical features or serious comorbid disease or those with high-risk clinical features without signs or symptoms of ongoing bleeding, colonoscopy should be performed next available after a colon purge (conditional recommendation, low-quality evidence) [179].

28.5.5 Endoscopic Treatment

Usually, a standard colonoscope is used because the larger (3.7 mm) working channel facilitates clearing of blood, clots, and residual stool material and enables passage of larger-diameter hemostatic devices. The goal of the procedure is to identify a bleeding site more than perform a cecal intubation. Meticulous examination is performed both during insertion and withdrawal of the scope because of intermittently bleeding lesion.

Areas containing or accumulating fresh blood or clots are vigorously washed and investigated as they are a potential bleeding site. Maximum dexterity is required when performing colonoscopy in patients with acute severe LGIB to negotiate the scope through the blood, clots, and diverticular segments to avoid perforation.

Endoscopic treatment modalities include injection, contact thermal coagulation, argon plasma coagulation, clipping, and band ligation. The use of one or a combination of these techniques depends on the site and features of the bleeding lesions, operator choice and familiarity with the device, and type of access to the bleeding site.

ASGE guidelines recommend that endoscopic therapy should be provided to patients with high-risk endoscopic stigmata of bleeding: active bleeding (spurting and oozing), nonbleeding visible vessel, or adherent clot (strong recommendation, low-quality evidence) [179].

28.5.6 Diverticular Bleeding

Endoscopic treatment of diverticular bleeding with active bleeding, nonbleeding visible vessel, and an adherent clot is treated with paradiverticular injection of a 1:10,000 dilution of epinephrine in 0.5 aliquots.

A submucosal injection of 1–2 mL in 2–4 sites around the diverticulum is often sufficient [180–183]. If the bleeding vessel is identified, it should be cauterized with bipolar probe (large probe 10–15 W, 1–2 s pulse) with light-to-moderate tamponade pressure avoiding the risk of perforation which is substantially higher when the vessel is located at the base of the diverticulum. In this circumstance, clipping of the visible vessel or entire diverticulum might be a safer alternative [185, 194].

It is useful to tattoo the site of the diverticular bleeding for future localization in case of rebleeding or in case of reinsertion of the scope to perform band ligation which could be useful in case of narrowed lumen associated to diverticular disease that may impair use of clipping and thermal coagulation probe.

According to ASGE guideline, in case of diverticular bleeding, through-the-scope endoscopic clips are recommended as clips may be safer in the colon than contact thermal therapy and are generally easier to perform than band ligation, particularly for right-sided colon lesions (conditional recommendation, low-quality evidence) [179].

28.5.7 Angiodysplasia

Typically, the bleeding caused by angiodysplasia is chronic, slow, and intermittent. The bleeding stops spontaneously in 85–90% of cases, but it recurs in 25–85% [185]. The characteristic endoscopic appearance is a red, flat lesion (2–10 mm diameter) with dilated blood vessels radiating from a central feeding vessel. The use of narcotics during colonoscopy may mask the detection of these lesions by reducing mucosal blood flow [186, 187].

Endoscopic management of actively bleeding angiodysplasia is straightforward; decision-making may be more difficult in patients who have stopped bleeding and are found to have nonbleeding angiodysplasia. In this case, it seems to be reasonable to ablate angiodysplasia in the absence of another definitive bleeding site. Contact and noncontact thermal techniques are effective at treating vascular ectasias.

ASGE guidelines recommend noncontact thermal therapy using argon plasma coagulation for angioectasia bleeding (conditional recommendation, low-quality evidence) [179].

28.5.8 Post-polypectomy Bleeding

Post-polypectomy bleeding can occur immediately or days to weeks following polyp removal [188]. Risk factors for post-polypectomy bleeding include large polyp size (>2 cm), thick stalk, right colon location, and resumption of antithrombotic therapy. Endoscopic hemostasis treatments for post-polypectomy bleeding include endoscopic clipping; thermal contact, with or without the combined use of dilute epinephrine injection; and band ligation. Use of through-the-scope clipping, with or without epinephrine injection, may be preferred to limit additional tissue injury that occurs with contact thermal coagulation therapy [188].

ASGE guidelines recommend mechanical (clip) or contact thermal endotherapy, with or without the combined use of dilute epinephrine injection in post-polypectomy bleeding (strong recommendation, low-quality evidence) [179].

Acute LGIB etiologies such as ischemic colitis, colitis due to inflammatory bowel disease, and colorectal neoplasms are generally not amenable to durable endoscopic hemostasis and are treated with supportive medical and/or surgical care of the underlying etiology.

28.5.9 Novel Therapy

Hemostatic topical powders/sprays have recently been reported as an endotherapy options for acute LGIB [189]. These powders/sprays (hemostatic agent TC-325 (Hemospray, Cook Medical, Winston-Salem, NC), EndoClot polysaccharide hemostatic system (EndoClot Plus Inc., Santa Clara, CA), and Ankaferd BloodStopper (Ankaferd ilac kozmetik A.S., Istanbul, Turkey) are delivered through the working channel of the endoscope and are intended to control "actively" bleeding lesions [190]. There are a limited number of case reports and small case series reporting on these modalities as primary or salvage therapy in post-polypectomy bleeding, colonic ulcerations including solitary rectal ulcer, radiation proctitis, colorectal neoplasia, and portal hypertensive colopathy [192–195].

In addition, an over-the-scope clip (OTSC, Ovesco Endoscopy, Tubingen, Germany), made from a nitinol alloy, has been applied as salvage therapy in post-polypectomy bleeding [195]. This clipping device is loaded onto an endoscope and deployed in a similar manner as a band-ligating device.

28.5.10 Role of Repeat Colonoscopy in the Setting of Early Recurrent Bleeding

In two randomized controlled studies, early rebleeding (defined as rebleeding prior to hospital discharge) following urgent colonoscopy is reported to be 22% and late rebleeding (defined as rebleeding after hospital discharge) is 16% [173, 177]. Factors that may contribute to early or late rebleeding include underlying comorbid conditions, concurrent medication use (e.g., NSAIDs, antiplatelet agents, anticoagulants), source of index bleeding, and initial hemostasis modality [196]. There are no published studies that directly evaluate the role of repeat colonoscopy in patients with early or late recurrent LGIB. However, small case series indicate that the yield of repeat colonoscopy for early rebleeding from a diverticular source is fairly high (20%) [128]. According to ASGE guideline, repeat colonoscopy, with endoscopic hemostasis if indicated, should be considered for patients with evidence of recurrent bleeding (strong recommendation, very-low-quality evidence) [179].

28.5.11 Non-endoscopic Treatments

Mesenteric angiography with or without a preceding nuclear red blood cell scan is reserved for patients with severe bleeding who cannot be stabilized or prepped for a colonoscopy and for those who have failed endoscopic management. The multidetector row CT scan may be superior to the nuclear red blood cell scan for evaluation of LGIB. It decreases scan time, allows accurate acquisition of arterial images, and demonstrates contrast material extravasation into any portion of the GI tract [197]. The multidetector row CT scan has therefore replaced the nuclear red blood cell scan at several centers [198].

Superselective embolization with microcoils, polyvinyl alcohol particles, or water-insoluble gelatin (gel foam) has improved the success rate of this technique and decreased the occurrence of the adverse event of bowel infarction. A meta-analysis of angiography and embolization as first-line therapy for LGIB found embolization to be an effective treatment for diverticular bleeding, with successful hemostasis in 85% of patients as compared with 50% of those with bleeding from other sources at 30-day follow-up [199]. However, in contrast to effective endoscopic treatment, early rebleeding after embolization has been reported in 22% of patients with LGIB [193]. Studies that have compared angiography (with the older technique of vasopressin infusion) to colonoscopy have found a significantly higher diagnostic yield and therapeutic success with endoscopic management [173, 200, 201].

Surgery is rarely required and should be reserved for the minority of patients who have persistent or refractory diverticular bleeding.

It is important to attempt localization of the bleeding site for a segmental colectomy as opposed to proceeding with a subtotal colectomy, which has a significantly higher mortality rate [202]. Preferentially, surgery should be performed on an elective basis, because there is a high mortality rate with emergent surgical intervention [203].

According to ASGE guideline, a surgical consultation should be requested in patients with high-risk clinical features and ongoing bleeding. In general, surgery for acute LGIB should be considered after other therapeutic options have failed and should take into consideration the extent and success of prior bleeding control measures, severity and source of bleeding, and the level of comorbid disease. It is important to very carefully localize the source of bleeding whenever possible before surgical resection to avoid continued or recurrent bleeding from an unresected culprit lesion (conditional recommendation, very-low-quality evidence).

Radiographic interventions should be considered in patients with high-risk clinical features and ongoing bleeding who have a negative upper endoscopy and do not respond adequately to hemodynamic resuscitation efforts and are therefore unlikely to tolerate bowel preparation and urgent colonoscopy (strong recommendation, very-low-quality evidence).

If a diagnostic test is desired for localization of the bleeding site before angiography, CT angiography should be considered (conditional recommendation, very-low-quality evidence).

28.5.12 Prevention of Recurrent LGIB

Non-aspirin NSAID use should be avoided in patients with a history of acute LGIB, particularly if secondary to diverticulosis or angioectasia (strong recommendation, low-quality evidence).

In patients with established high-risk cardiovascular disease and a history of LGIB, aspirin used for secondary prevention should not be discontinued. Aspirin for primary prevention of cardiovascular events should be avoided in most patients with LGIB (strong recommendation, low-quality evidence).

In patients on dual antiplatelet therapy or monotherapy with non-aspirin antiplatelet agents (thienopyridine), non-aspirin antiplatelet therapy should be resumed as soon as possible and at least within 7 days based on a multidisciplinary assessment of cardiovascular and GI risk and the adequacy of endoscopic therapy (as above, aspirin use should not be discontinued). However, dual antiplatelet therapy should not be discontinued in patients with an acute coronary syndrome within the past 90 days or coronary stenting within the past 30 days (strong recommendation, low-quality evidence) [179].

Case Scenario

A 44-year-old man in health conditions and without comorbidity was admitted to ER for significant and continuous rectal bleeding. The day before, he underwent to a colonoscopy removing two polyps at different colon segments, ascending colon (Fig. 28.2) and sigmoid colon (Fig. 28.3). He had a normal blood pressure and heart rate. FBC was normal. Chest and abdominal X-rays were normal (Video 28.1).

1. What is your diagnostic hypothesis?
   A. **Post-polypectomy bleeding**
   B. Hemorrhoid
   C. Ischemic colitis
   D. Other
2. What would you do?
   A. Clinical observation
   B. Check BP, HR, and FBC

   C. **Colonoscopy**
   D. Surgical consultation
3. What is your diagnosis?
   A. Post-polypectomy bleeding
   B. Hemorrhoid
   C. Rectal ulcer bleeding
   D. **Dieulafoy lesion**
4. What is your treatment?
   A. Adrenaline sclerotherapy
   B. **Clip**
   C. Thermal therapy (BICAP, APC)
   D. **Band ligation**

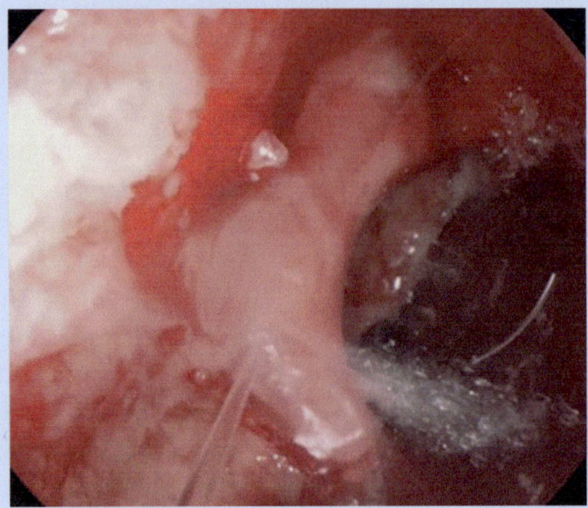

Fig. 28.2 Diulafoy lesion in the rectum

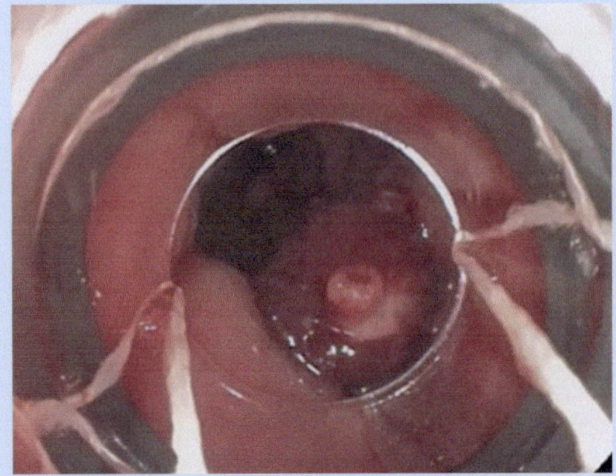

Fig. 28.3 Band ligation of rectal Dieulafoy

References

1. Barkun AN, Bardou M, Kuipers EJ, Sung J, Hunt RH, Martel M, Sinclair P. International consensus recommendations on the management of patients with nonvariceal upper gastrointestinal bleeding. Ann Intern Med. 2010;152(2):101–13.
2. Laine L, Yang H, Chang SC, Datto C. Trends for incidence of hospitalization and death due to GI complications in the United States from 2001 to 2009. Am J Gastroenterol. 2012;107(8):1190–5.
3. Sung JJ, Tsoi KK, Ma TK, et al. Causes of mortality in patients with peptic ulcer bleeding: a prospective cohort study of 10,428 cases. Am J Gastroenterol. 2010;105:84–9.
4. van Leerdam ME. Epidemiology of acute upper gastrointestinal bleeding. Best Pract Res Clin Gastroenterol. 2008;22:209–24.
5. Hearnshaw SA, Logan RF, Lowe D, et al. Acute upper gastrointestinal bleeding in the UK: patient characteristics, diagnoses and outcomes in the 2007 UK audit. Gut. 2011;60:1327–35.
6. Stevens PD, Finegold J, Garcia-Carrasquillo RJ, et al. Effectiveness of a protocol-based team approach to gastrointestinal hemorrhage. Gastrointest Endosc. 1997;45(4):AB 102 n 309.
7. Baradarian R, Ramdhaney S, Chapalamadugu R, Skoczylas L, Wang K, Rivilis S, et al. Early intensive resuscitation of patients with upper gastrointestinal bleeding decreases mortality. Am J Gastroenterol. 2004;99(4):619–22.
8. Gralnek IM, Dumonceau JM, Kuipers EJ, Lanas A, Sanders DS, Kurien M, et al. Diagnosis and management of nonvariceal upper gastrointestinal hemorrhage: European Society of Gastrointestinal Endoscopy (ESGE) Guideline. Endoscopy. 2015;47:a1–a46.
9. Hebert PC, Wells G, Blajchman MA, Marshall J, Martin C, Pagliarello G, Tweeddale M, Schweitzer I, Yetisir E. A multicenter, randomized, controlled clinical trial of transfusion requirements in critical care. Transfusion Requirements in Critical Care Investigators, Canadian Critical Care Trials Group. N Engl J Med. 1999;340(6):409–17.
10. Villanueva C, Colomo A, Bosch A, Concepcion M, Hernandez-Gea V, Aracil C, Graupera I, Poca M, Alvarez-Urturi C, Gordillo J, Guarner-Argente C, Santalo M, Muniz E, Guarner C. Transfusion strategies for acute upper gastrointestinal bleeding. N Engl J Med. 2013;368(1):11–21.
11. Jairath V, Hearnshaw S, Brunskill SJ, Doree C, Hopewell S, Hyde C, Travis S, Murphy MF. Red cell transfusion for the management of upper gastrointestinal haemorrhage. Cochrane Database Syst Rev. 2010;9:CD006613.
12. Hearnshaw SA, Logan RF, Palmer KR, Card TR, Travis SP, Murphy MF. Outcomes following early red blood cell transfusion in acute upper gastrointestinal bleeding. Aliment Pharmacol Ther. 2010;32(2):215–24.
13. Restellini S, Kherad O, Jairath V, Martel M, Barkun AN. Red blood cell transfusion is associated with increased rebleeding in patients with nonvariceal upper gastrointestinal bleeding. Aliment Pharmacol Ther. 2013;37(3):316–22.
14. Laine L. Blood transfusion for gastrointestinal bleeding. N Engl J Med. 2013;368(1):75–6.
15. de Groot NL, Bosman JH, Siersema PD, et al. Prediction scores in gastro intestinal bleeding: a systematic review and quantitative appraisal. Endoscopy. 2012;44:731–9.
16. Rockall TA, Logan RF, Devlin HB, et al. Risk assessment after acute upper gastrointestinal haemorrhage. Gut. 1996;38:316–21.

17. Blatchford O, Murray WR, Blatchford M. A risk score to predict need for treatment for upper-gastrointestinal haemorrhage. Lancet. 2000;356:1318–21.
18. Stanley AJ, Ashley D, Dalton HR, Mowat C, Gaya DR, Thompson E, et al. Outpatient management of patients with low-risk upper-gastrointestinal haemorrhage: multicentre validation and prospective evaluation. Lancet. 2009;373(9657):42–7.
19. Gralnek IM, Barkun AN, Bardou M. Management of acute bleeding from a peptic ulcer. N Engl J Med. 2008;359(9):928–37.
20. Hwang JH, et al. The role of endoscopy in the management of variceal hemorrhage. Gastrointest Endosc. 2014;80(2):221–7.
21. Sung JJ, Lau JY, Ching JY, et al. Continuation of low-dose aspirin therapy in peptic ulcer bleeding: a randomized trial. Ann Intern Med. 2010;152:1–9.
22. ASGE Standards of Practice Committee, Acosta RD, Abraham NS, Chandrasekhara V, et al. The management of antithrombotic agents for patients undergoing GI endoscopy. Gastrointest Endosc. 2016;83:3–16.
23. Shingina A, Barkun AN, Razzaghi A, et al. Systematic review: the presenting international normalised ratio (INR) as a predictor of outcome in patients with upper nonvariceal gastrointestinal bleeding. Aliment Pharmacol Ther. 2011;33:1010–8.
24. Saltzman JR, Tabak YP, Hyett BH, et al. A simple risk score accurately predicts in-hospital mortality, length of stay, and cost in acute upper GI bleeding. Gastrointest Endosc. 2011;74:1215–24.
25. Choudari CP, Rajgopal C, Palmer KR. Acute gastrointestinal haemorrhage in anticoagulated patients: diagnoses and response to endoscopic treatment. Gut. 1994;35:464–6.
26. Barkun A, Sabbah S, Enns R, et al. The Canadian Registry on Nonvariceal Upper Gastrointestinal Bleeding and Endoscopy (RUGBE): endoscopic hemostasis and proton pump inhibition are associated with improved outcomes in a real-life setting. Am J Gastroenterol. 2004;99:1238–46.
27. Wolf AT, Wasan SK, Saltzman JR. Impact of anticoagulation on rebleeding following endoscopic therapy for nonvariceal upper gastrointestinal hemorrhage. Am J Gastroenterol. 2007;102: 290–6.
28. Barkun AN, Bardou M, Kuipers EJ, Sung J, Hunt RH, Martel M, Sinclair P. International Consensus Upper Gastrointestinal Bleeding Conference Group International consensus recommendations on the management of patients with nonvariceal upper gastrointestinal bleeding. Ann Intern Med. 2010;152(2):101–13.
29. Abraham NS. Management of antiplatelet agents and anticoagulants in patients with gastrointestinal bleeding. Gastrointest Endosc Clin North Am. 2015;25:449–62.
30. Ruff CT, Giugliano RP, Braunwald E, et al. Comparison of the efficacy and safety of new oral anticoagulants with warfarin in patients with atrial fibrillation: a meta-analysis of randomised trials. Lancet. 2014;383:955–62.
31. Pollack CV Jr, Reilly PA, Eikelboom J, et al. Idarucizumab for dabigatran reversal. N Engl J Med 2015;373:511–520.
32. Majeed A, Schulman S. Bleeding and antidotes in new oral anticoagulants. Best Pract Res Clin Haematol. 2013;26:191–202.
33. Leontiadis GI, Sharma VK, Howden CW. Proton pump inhibitor therapy for peptic ulcer bleeding: Cochrane collaboration meta- analysis of randomized controlled trials. Mayo Clin Proc. 2007;82(3):286–96.
34. Sreedharan A, Martin J, Leontiadis GI, Dorward S, Howden CW, Forman D, Moayyedi P. Proton pump inhibitor treatment initiated prior to endoscopic diagnosis in upper gastrointestinal bleeding. Cochrane Database Syst Rev. 2010;7:CD005415.
35. Theivanayagam S, Lim RG, Cobell WJ, et al. Administration of erythromycin before endoscopy in upper gastrointestinal bleeding: a metaanalysis of randomized controlled trials. Saudi J Gastroenterol. 2013;19:205–10.
36. Aljebreen AM, Fallone CA, Barkun AN. Nasogastric aspirate predicts high-risk endoscopic lesions in patients with acute upper-GI bleeding. Gastrointest Endosc. 2004;59(2):172–8.
37. Koch DG, Arguedas MR, Fallon MB. Risk of aspiration pneumonia in suspected variceal hemorrhage: the value of prophylactic endotracheal intubation prior to endoscopy. Dig Dis Sci. 2007;52:2225–8.
38. Rehman A, Iscimen R, Yilmaz M, et al. Prophylactic endotracheal intubation in critically ill patients undergoing endoscopy for upper GI hemorrhage. Gastrointest Endosc. 2009;69:55–9.
39. Rudolph SJ, Landsverk BK, Freeman ML. Endotracheal intubation for airway protection during endoscopy for severe upper GI hemorrhage. Gastrointest Endosc. 2003;57:58–61.
40. Waye JD. Intubation and sedation in patients who have emergency upper GI endoscopy for GI bleeding. Gastrointest Endosc. 2000;51(6):768–71.
41. Rajala MW. Trips and tricks on How to Optimally Manage Patients with Upper Gastrointestinal Bleeding. Gastrointest Endosc Clin N Am. 2015;25:607–17.
42. Hayat U, et al. Association of prophylactic endotracheal intubation in critically ill patients with upper GI bleeding and cardiopulmonary unplanned events. Gastrointest Endosc. 2017;86(3):500–509.e1.
43. Barkun AN, Bardou M, Kuipers EJ, Sung J. How early should endoscopy be performed in suspected upper gastrointestinal bleeding? Am J Gastroenterol. 2012;107(2):328–9.
44. Lim LG, Ho KY, Chan YH, Teoh PL, Khor CJ, Lim LL, Rajnakova A, Ong TZ, Yeoh KG. Urgent endoscopy is associated with lower mortality in high-risk but not low-risk nonvariceal upper gastrointestinal bleeding. Endoscopy. 2011;43(4):300–6.
45. Laine L, Jensen DM. Management of patients with ulcer bleeding. Am J Gastroenterol. 2012;107(3):345–60.
46. Garcia-Tsao G, Sanyal AJ, Grace ND, Carey W. Prevention and management of gastroesophageal varices and variceal hemorrhage in cirrhosis. Hepatology. 2007;46(3):922–38.
47. Hearnshaw SA, Logan RF, Lowe D, Travis SP, Murphy MF, Palmer KR. Use of endoscopy for management of acute upper gastrointestinal bleeding in the UK: results of a nationwide audit. Gut. 2010;59(8):1022–9.
48. Marmo R, Del Piano M, Rotondano G, et al. Mortality from nonvariceal upper gastrointestinal bleeding: is it time to differentiate the timing of endoscopy? Digestive Disease Week, May 7–10 McCormick Place Convention Center, Chicago, IL, 2011.
49. Cook DJ, Guyatt GH, Salena BJ, Laine LA. Endoscopic therapy for acute nonvariceal upper gastrointestinal hemorrhage: a meta-analysis. Gastroenterology. 1992;102(1):139–48.
50. Sacks HS, Chalmers TC, Blum AL, Berrier J, Pagano D. Endoscopic hemostasis. An effective therapy for bleeding peptic ulcers. JAMA. 1990;264(4):494–9.
51. Lee JG, Turnipseed S, Romano PS, et al. Endoscopy-based triage significantly reduces hospitalization rates and costs of treating upper GI bleeding: a randomized controlled trial. Gastrointest Endosc. 1999;50:755–61.
52. Schacher GM, Lesbros-Pantoflickova D, Ortner MA, et al. Is early endoscopy in the emergency room beneficial in patients with bleed-

ing peptic ulcer? A "fortuitously controlled" study. Endoscopy. 2005;37:324–8.
53. Bjorkman DJ, Zaman A, Fennerty MB, et al. Urgent vs. elective endoscopy for acute non-variceal upper-GI bleeding: an effectiveness study. Gastrointest Endosc. 2004;60:1–8.
54. Targownik LE, Murthy S, Keyvani L, et al. The role of rapid endoscopy for high-risk patients with acute nonvariceal upper gastrointestinal bleeding. Can J Gastroenterol. 2007;21:425–9.
55. Tai CM, Huang SP, Wang HP, et al. High-risk ED patients with nonvariceal upper gastrointestinal hemorrhage undergoing emergency or urgent endoscopy: a retrospective analysis. Am J Emerg Med. 2007;25:273–8.
56. Lin HJ, Wang K, Perng CL, et al. Early or delayed endoscopy for patients with peptic ulcer bleeding. A prospective randomized study. J Clin Gastroenterol. 1996;22:267–71.
57. Cooper GS, Chak A, Way LE, et al. Early endoscopy in upper gastrointestinal hemorrhage: associations with recurrent bleeding, surgery, and length of hospital stay. Gastrointest Endosc. 1999;49:145–52.
58. Cooper GS, Kou TD, Wong RC. Use and impact of early endoscopy in elderly patients with peptic ulcer hemorrhage: a population-based analysis. Gastrointest Endosc. 2009;70:229–35.
59. Laursen SB, et al. Relationship between timing of endoscopy and mortality in patients with peptic ulcer bleeding: a nationwide cohort study. Gastrointest Endosc. 85(5):936–944.e3.
60. Lau JY, Chung SC, Leung JW, Lo KK, Yung MY, Li AK. The evolution of stigmata of hemorrhage in bleeding peptic ulcers: a sequential endoscopic study. Endoscopy. 1998;30(6):513–8.
61. Leung Ki EL, Lau JY. New endoscopic hemostasis methods. Clin Endosc. 2012;45(3):224–9.
62. Wong Kee Song L-M, et al. Emerging technologies for endoscopic hemostasis. Gastrointest Endosc. 75(5):933–93.
63. Lin HJ, Hsieh YH, Tseng GY, et al. A prospective, randomized trial of large versus small injection of epinephrine for peptic ulcer bleeding. Gastrointest Endosc. 2002;55(6):615–9.
64. Alis H, Oner OZ, Kalayci MU, et al. Is endoscopic band ligation superior to injection therapy for Dieulafoy lesion? Surg Endosc. 2009;23:1465–9.
65. Laine L, Peterson WL. Bleeding peptic ulcer. N Engl J Med. 1994;331:717–27.
66. Laine, Loren et al A prospective outcome study of patients with clot in an ulcer and the effect of irrigation . Gastrointest Endosc , Volume 43 , Issue 2 , 107–110.
67. Lin HJ, Wang K, Perng CL, et al. Natural history of bleeding peptic ulcers with a tightly adherent blood clot: a prospective observation. Gastrointest Endosc. 1996;43(5):470–3.
68. Laine L, McQuaid KR. Endoscopic therapy for bleeding ulcers: an evidence-based approach based on meta-analyses of randomized controlled trials. Clin Gastroenterol Hepatol. 2009;7:33–47.
69. Barkun AN, Martel M, Toubouti Y, et al. Endoscopic hemostasis in peptic ulcer bleeding for patients with high-risk lesions: a series of meta-analyses. Gastrointest Endosc. 2009;69:786–99.
70. Sung JJ, Tsoi KK, Lai LH, et al. Endoscopic clipping versus injection and thermo-coagulation in the treatment of non-variceal upper gastrointestinal bleeding: a meta-analysis. Gut. 2007;56:1364–1373 138.
71. Calvet X, Vergara M, Brullet E, et al. Addition of a second endoscopic treatment following epinephrine injection improves outcome in high-risk bleeding ulcers. Gastroenterology. 2004;126:441–450 139.
72. Marmo R, Rotondano G, Piscopo R, et al. Dual therapy versus mono-therapy in the endoscopic treatment of high-risk bleeding ulcers: a meta-analysis of controlled trials. Am J Gastroenterol. 2007;102:279–89.
73. Vergara M, Bennett C, Calvet X, et al. **Epinephrine injection versus epinephrine injection and a second endoscopic method in high risk bleeding ulcers. Cochrane Database Syst Rev. 2014;10:CD005584.
74. Hwang JH, Fisher DA, Ben-Menachem T, et al. Standards of Practice Committee of the American Society for Gastrointestinal Endoscopy. The role of endoscopy in the management of acute non-variceal upper GI bleeding. Gastrointest Endosc. 2012;75:1132–8.
75. Barkun AN, Moosavi S, Martel M. Topical hemostatic agents: a systematic review with particular emphasis on endoscopic application in GI bleeding. Gastrointest Endosc. 2013;77:692–700.
76. Wong Kee Song LM, Banerjee S, Barth BA, et al. Emerging technologies for endoscopic hemostasis. Gastrointest Endosc. 2012;75:933–7.
77. Kirschniak A, Kratt T, Stüker D, et al. A new endoscopic over-the-scope clip system for treatment of lesions and bleeding in the GI tract: first clinical experiences. Gastrointest Endosc. 2007;66:162–7.
78. Kirschniak A, Subotova N, Zieker D, et al. The over-the-scope clip (OTSC) for the treatment of gastrointestinal bleeding, perforations, and fistulas. Surg Endosc. 2011;25:2901–5.
79. Manta R, Galloro G, Mangiavillano B, et al. Over-the-scope clip (OTSC) represents an effective endoscopic treatment for acute GI bleeding after failure of conventional techniques. Surg Endosc. 2013;27:3162–4.
80. Giday SA, Kim Y, Krishnamurty DM, et al. Long-term randomized controlled trial of a novel nanopowder hemostatic agent (TC-325) for control of severe arterial upper gastrointestinal bleeding in a porcine model. Endoscopy. 2011;43:296–9.
81. Chen YI, Barkun AN, Soulellis C, et al. Use of the endoscopically applied hemostatic powder TC-325 in cancer-related upper GI hemorrhage: preliminary experience. Gastrointest Endosc. 2012;75:1278–81.
82. Leblanc S, Vienne A, Dhooge M, et al. Early experience with a novel hemostatic powder used to treat upper GI bleeding related to malignancies or after therapeutic interventions. Gastrointest Endosc. 2013;78:169–75.
83. Holster IL, Kuipers EJ, Tjwa ET. Hemospray in the treatment of upper gastrointestinal hemorrhage in patients on antithrombotic therapy. Endoscopy. 2013;45:63–6.
84. Yau AH, Ou G, Galorport C, et al. Safety and efficacy of Hemospray in upper gastrointestinal bleeding. Can J Gastroenterol Hepatol. 2014;28:72–6.
85. Sung JJ, Luo D, Wu JC, et al. Early clinical experience of the safety and effectiveness of Hemospray in achieving hemostasis in patients with acute peptic ulcer bleeding. Endoscopy. 2011;43:291–5.
86. Smith LA, Stanley AJ, Bergman JJ, et al. Hemospray application in non-variceal upper gastrointestinal bleeding: results of the survey to evaluate the application of hemospray in the luminal tract. J Clin Gastroenterol. 2014;48:89–92.
87. Coumaros D, Tsesmeli N. Active gastrointestinal bleeding: use of hemostatic forceps beyond endoscopic submucosal dissection. Word J Gastroenterol. 2010;16(16):2061–4.
88. Lau JY, Sung JJ, Lee KK, et al. Effect of intravenous omeprazole on recurrent bleeding after endoscopic treatment of bleeding peptic ulcers. N Engl J Med. 2000;343:310–6.
89. Sung JJ, Barkun A, Kuipers EJ, et al. Intravenous esomeprazole for prevention of recurrent peptic ulcer bleeding: a randomized trial. Ann Intern Med. 2009;150:455–64.
90. Vorder Bruegge WF, Peura DA. Stress-related mucosal damage: review of drug therapy. J Clin Gastroenterol. 1990;12(Suppl 2):S35–40.
91. Sachar H, Vaidya K, Laine L. Intermittent vs continuous proton pump inhibitor therapy for high-risk bleeding ulcers: a systematic review and meta-analysis. JAMA Intern Med. 2014;174:1755–62.
92. Laine L, Jensen DM. Management of patients with ulcer bleeding. Am J Gastroenterol. 2012;107:345–60.
93. Tringali A, et al. Comparing intravenous and oral proton pump inhibitor therapy for bleeding peptic ulcers following endoscopic management: a systematic review and meta-analysis. Br J Clin Pharmacol. 2017;83(8):1619–35.

94. Savides TJ, Jensen DM. Therapeutic endoscopy for non-variceal gastrointestinal bleeding. Gastroenterol Clin N Am. 2000;29(2):465–87. vii
95. Marmo R, Rotondano G, Bianco MA, Piscopo R, Prisco A, Cipolletta L. Outcome of endoscopic treatment for peptic ulcer bleeding: Is a second look necessary? A meta-analysis. Gastrointest Endosc. 2003;57(1):62–7.
96. Tsoi KK, Chan HC, Chiu PW, Pau CY, Lau JY, Sung JJ. Second-look endoscopy with thermal coagulation or injections for peptic ulcer bleeding: a meta-analysis. J Gastroenterol Hepatol. 2010;25(1):8–13.
97. Spiegel BM, Ofman JJ, Woods K, Vakil NB. Minimizing recurrent peptic ulcer hemorrhage after endoscopic hemostasis: the cost- effectiveness of competing strategies. Am J Gastroenterol. 2003;98(1):86–97.
98. Jairath V, Kahan BC, Logan RF, Hearnshaw SA, Dore CJ, Travis SP, Murphy MF, Palmer KR. National audit of the use of surgery and radiological embolization after failed endoscopic haemostasis for non-variceal upper gastrointestinal bleeding. Br J Surg. 2012;99(12):1672–80.
99. Wong TC, Wong KT, Chiu PW, Teoh AY, Yu SC, Au KW, Lau JY. A comparison of angiographic embolization with surgery after failed endoscopic hemostasis to bleeding peptic ulcers. Gastrointest Endosc. 2011;73(5):900–8.
100. Ang D, Teo EK, Tan A, Ibrahim S, Tan PS, Ang TL, Fock KM. A comparison of surgery versus transcatheter angiographic embolization in the treatment of nonvariceal upper gastrointestinal bleeding uncontrolled by endoscopy. Eur J Gastroenterol Hepatol. 2012;24(8):929–38.
101. Ripoll C, Banares R, Beceiro I, Menchen P, Catalina MV, Echenagusia A, Turegano F. Comparison of transcatheter arterial embolization and surgery for treatment of bleeding peptic ulcer after endoscopic treatment failure. J Vasc Interv Radiol. 2004;15(5):447–50.
102. Lai KC, Lam SK, Chu KM, et al. Lansoprazole for the prevention of recurrences of ulcer complications from long-term low-dose aspirin use. N Engl J Med. 2002;346:2033–8.
103. Sung JJ, Lau JY, Ching JY, et al. Continuation of low-dose aspirin therapy in peptic ulcer bleeding: a randomized trial. Ann Intern Med. 2010;152:1–9.
104. Lai KC, Chu KM, Hui WM, et al. Esomeprazole with aspirin versus clopidogrel for prevention of recurrent gastrointestinal ulcer complications. Clin Gastroenterol Hepatol. 2006;4:860–5.
105. Chan FK, Ching JY, Hung LC, et al. Clopidogrel versus aspirin and esomeprazole to prevent recurrent ulcer bleeding. N Engl J Med. 2005;352:238–44.
106. Sanchez-Delgado J, Gene E, Suarez D, et al. Has H. pylori prevalence in bleeding peptic ulcer been underestimated? A meta-regression. Am J Gastroenterol. 2011;106:398–405.
107. D'Amico G, Garcia-Tsao G, Pagliaro L. Natural history and prognostic indicators of survival in cirrhosis: a systematic review of 118 studies. J Hepatol. 2006;44(1):217–31.
108. Merli M, Nicolini G, Angeloni S, Rinaldi V, De Santis A, Merkel C, Attili AF, Riggio O. Incidence and natural history of small esophageal varices in cirrhotic patients. J Hepatol. 2003;38:266–72.
109. Zoli M, Merkel C, Magalotti D, Gueli C, Grimaldi M, Gatta A, Bernardi M. Natural history of cirrhotic patients with small esophageal varices: a prospective study. Am J Gastroenterol. 2000;95:503–8.
110. Vorobioff J, Groszmann RJ, Picabea E, Gamen M, Villavicencio R, Bordato J, Morel I, Audano M, Tanno H, Lerner E, Passamonti M. Prognostic value of hepatic venous pressure gradient measurements in alcoholic cirrhosis: a 10-year prospective study. Gastroenterology. 1996;111:701–9.
111. D'Amico G, Pagliaro L, Bosch J. Pharmacological treatment of portal hypertension: an evidence-based approach. Semin Liver Dis. 1999;19:475–505.
112. North Italian Endoscopic Club for the Study and Treatment of Esophageal Varices. Prediction of the first variceal hemorrhage in patients with cirrhosis of the liver and esophageal varices. A prospective multicenter study. N Engl J Med. 1988;319(15):983–9.
113. Sarin SK, Lahoti D, Saxena SP, Murthy NS, Makwana UK. Prevalence, classification and natural history of gastric varices: a long-term follow-up study in 568 portal hypertension patients. Hepatology. 1992;16:1343–9.
114. Calès P, Pascal JP. Natural history of esophageal varices in cirrhosis (from origin to rupture). Gastroenterol Clin Biol. 1988;12:245–54.
115. Bosch J, Gonzales-Abraldes J, Garcia-Pagan JC. Clinical manifestations and management of bleeding episodes in cirrhotics. In: Textbook of hepatology from basic science to clinical practice, vol. 1; 2007. p. 640–57.
116. Carbonell N, Pauwels A, Serfaty L, Serfaty L, Fourdan O, Lévy VG, Poupon R. Improved survival after variceal bleeding in patients with cirrhosis over the past two decades. Hepatology. 2004;40:652–9.
117. Garcia-Tsao G, Bosch J. Management of varices and variceal hemorrhage in cirrhosis. N Engl J Med. 2010;362(9):823–32.
118. El-Serag HB, Everhart JE. Improved survival after variceal hemorrhage over an 11-year period in the Department of Veterans Affairs. Am J Gastroenterol. 2000;95:3566–73.
119. de Franchis R. Revising consensus in portal hypertension: report of the Baveno V consensus workshop on methodology of diagnosis and therapy in portal hypertension. J Hepatol. 2010;53:762–8.
120. Bernard B, Grangé JD, Khac EN, Amiot X, Opolon P, Poynard T. Antibiotic prophylaxis for the prevention of bacterial infections in cirrhotic patients with gastrointestinal bleeding: a meta-analysis. Hepatology. 1999;29:1655–166.
121. Fernández J, Ruiz del Arbol L, Gómez C, Durandez R, Serradilla R, Guarner C, Planas R, Arroyo V, Navasa M. Nor-floxacin vs ceftriaxone in the prophylaxis of infections in patients with advanced cirrhosis and hemorrhage. Gastroenterology. 2006;131:1049–56.
122. Garcia-Tsao G, Sanyal AJ, Grace ND, Carey WD. Practice Guidelines Committee of American Association for Study of Liver Diseases; Practice Parameters Committee of American College of Gastroenterology. Prevention and management of gastroesophageal varices and variceal hemorrhage in cirrhosis. Am J Gastroenterol. 2007;102(12):922–38.
123. Bañares R, Albillos A, Rincón D, Alonso S, González M, Ruiz-del-Arbol L, Salcedo M, Molinero LM. Endoscopic treatment versus endoscopic plus pharmacologic treatment for acute variceal bleeding: a meta-analysis. Hepatology. 2002;35:609–15.
124. de Franchis R. Updating consensus in portal hypertension: report of the Baveno IV consensus workshop on methodology of diagnosis and therapy of portal hypertension. J Hepatol. 2005;43: 167–76.
125. de Franchis R, Pascal JP, Ancona E, Burroughs AK, Henderson M, Fleig W, Groszmann R, Bosch J, Sauerbruch T, Soederlund C. Definitions, methodology and therapeutic strategies in portal hypertension. A Consensus Development Workshop, Baveno, Lake Maggiore, Italy, April 5 and 6, 1990. J Hepatol. 1992;15(1–2):256–61.
126. D'Amico G, De Franchis R. Upper digestive bleeding in cirrhosis. Post-therapeutic outcome and prognostic indicators. Hepatology. 2003;38:599–612.
127. Chavez-Tapia NC, Barrientos-Gutierrez T, Tellez-Avila F, et al. Meta-analysis: antibiotic prophylaxis for cirrhotic patients with upper gastrointestinal bleeding—an updated Cochrane review. Aliment Pharmacol Ther. 2011;34:509–18.
128. Chen PH, Chen WC, Hou MC, et al. Delayed endoscopy increases re-bleeding and mortality in patients with hematemesis and active esophageal variceal bleeding: a cohort study. J Hepatol. 2012;57:1207–13.

129. Cheung J, Soo I, Bastiampillai R, et al. Urgent vs. non-urgent endoscopy in stable acute variceal bleeding. Am J Gastroenterol. 2009;104:1125–9.
130. Helmy A, Hayes PC. Review article: current endoscopic therapeutic options in the management of variceal bleeding. Aliment Pharmacol Ther. 2001;15:575–94.
131. Villanueva C, Colomo A, Aracil C, Guarner C. Current endoscopic therapy of variceal bleeding. Best Pract Res Clin Gastroenterol. 2008;22:261–78.
132. Park WG, Yeh RW, Triadafilopoulos G. Injection therapies for variceal bleeding disorders of the GI tract. Gastrointest Endosc. 2008;67:313–23.
133. de Franchis R, Primignani M. Endoscopic treatments for portal hypertension. Semin Liver Dis. 1999;19:439–55.
134. Westaby D. Emergency and elective endoscopic therapy for variceal haemorrhage. Baillieres Clin Gastroenterol. 1992;6:465–80.
135. Pushpanathan C, Idikio H. Pathological findings in the esophagus after endoscopic sclerotherapy for variceal bleeding. Am J Gastroenterol. 1986;81(1):9–13.
136. Sarin SK, Nanda R, Sachdev G. Intravariceal versus paravariceal sclerotherapy: a prospective, controlled, randomised trial. Gut. 1987;28(6):657–62.
137. Bhargava DK, Singh B, Dogra R, Dasarathy S, Sharma MP. Prospective randomized comparison of sodium tetradecyl sulfate and polidocanol as variceal sclerosing agents. Am J Gastroenterol. 1992;87(2):182–6.
138. Akriviadis E, Korula J, Gupta S, Ko Y, Yamada S. Frequent endoscopic variceal sclerotherapy increases risk of complications. Prospective randomized controlled study of two treatment schedules. Dig Dis Sci. 1989;34(7):1068–74.
139. Sanowski RA, Waring JP. Endoscopic techniques and complications in variceal sclerotherapy. J Clin Gastroenterol. 1987;9:504–13.
140. Schuman BM, Beckman JW, Tedesco FJ, Griffin JW Jr, Assad RT. Complications of endoscopic injection sclerotherapy: a review. Am J Gastroenterol. 1987;82:823–30.
141. Cohen LB, Korsten MA, Scherl EJ, Velez ME, Fisse RD, Arons EJ. Bacteremia after endoscopic injection sclerosis. Gastrointest Endosc. 1983;29:198–200.
142. Sarles HE, Sanowski RA, Talbert G. Course and complications of endoscopic variceal sclerotherapy: a prospective study of 50 patients. Am J Gastroenterol. 1985;80:595–9.
143. Haynes WC, Sanowski RA, Foutch PG, Bellapravalu S. Esophageal strictures following endoscopic variceal sclerotherapy: clinical course and response to dilation therapy. Gastrointest Endosc. 1986;32:202–5.
144. Baillie J, Yudelman P. Complications of endoscopic sclerotherapy of esophageal varices. Endoscopy. 1992;24(4):284–91.
145. Laine L, Cook D. Endoscopic ligation compared with sclerotherapy for treatment of esophageal variceal bleeding. A meta-analysis. Ann Intern Med. 1995;123(4):280–7.
146. Lo GH. The role of endoscopy in secondary prophylaxis of esophageal varices. Clin Liver Dis. 2010;14:307–23.
147. D'Amico G, Pagliaro L, Pietrosi G, Tarantino I. Emergency sclerotherapy versus vasoactive drugs for bleeding oesophageal varices in cirrhotic patients. Cochrane Database Syst Rev. 2010;3:CD002233.
148. Stiegmann GV, Goff JS, Michaletz-Onody PA, Korula J, Lieberman D, Saeed ZA, Reveille RM, Sun JH, Lowenstein SR. Endoscopic sclerotherapy as compared with endoscopic ligation for bleeding esophageal varices. N Engl J Med. 1992;326:1527–32.
149. Cárdenas A. Management of acute variceal bleeding: emphasis on endoscopic therapy. Clin Liver Dis. 2010;14:251–62.
150. Young MF, Sanowski RA, Rasche R. Comparison and characterization of ulcerations induced by endoscopic ligation of esophageal varices versus endoscopic sclerotherapy. Gastrointest Endosc. 1993;39:119–22.
151. Bosch J, García-Pagán JC. Prevention of variceal rebleeding. Lancet. 2003;361:952–4.
152. Hou MC, Lin HC, Kuo BI, Chen CH, Lee FY, Lee SD. Comparison of endoscopic variceal injection sclerotherapy and ligation for the treatment of esophageal variceal hemorrhage: a prospective randomized trial. Hepatology. 1995;21:1517–22.
153. Sarin SK, Govil A, Jain AK, Guptan RC, Issar SK, Jain M, Murthy NS. Prospective randomized trial of endoscopic sclerotherapy versus variceal band ligation for esophageal varices: influence on gastropathy, gastric varices and variceal recurrence. J Hepatol. 1997;26:826–32.
154. Hou MC, Lin HC, Lee FY, Chang FY, Lee SD. Recurrence of esophageal varices following endoscopic treatment and its impact on rebleeding: comparison of sclerotherapy and ligation. J Hepatol. 2000;32:202–8.
155. Garcia-Pagan JC, Bosch J. Endoscopic band ligation in the treatment of portal hypertension. Nat Clin Pract Gastroenterol Hepatol. 2005;2:526–35.
156. Bolognesi M, Balducci G, Garcia-Tsao G, Gatta A, Gines P, Merli M, Rodes J, Stiegmann GV. Complications in the medical treatment of portal hypertension. Proceedings of the third Baveno international consensus workshop on definitions, methodology and therapeutic strategie. In: de Franchis R, editor. Portal hypertension III. Oxford: Blackwell Science; 2001. p. 180–201.
157. Lo GH, Lai KH, Shen MT, Chang CF. A comparison of the incidence of transient bacteremia and infectious sequelae after sclerotherapy and rubber band ligation of bleeding esophageal varices. Gastrointest Endosc. 1994;40:675–9.
158. Ibrahim M, El Mikkawy A, Mostafa I, et al. Endoscopic treatment of acute variceal hemorrhage by using hemostatic powder TC-325: a prospective pilot study. Gastrointest Endosc. 2013;78:769–73.
159. Gonzalez R, Zamora J, Gomez-Camarero J, et al. Meta-analysis: combination endoscopic and drug therapy to prevent variceal rebleeding in cirrhosis. Ann Intern Med. 2008;149:109–22.
160. Gimson AE, Westaby D, Williams R. Endoscopic sclerotherapy in the management of gastric variceal haemorrhage. J Hepatol. 1991;13:274–8.
161. Sarin SK, Mishra SR. Endoscopic therapy for gastric varices. Clin Liver Dis. 2010;14(2):263–79.
162. Ramesh J, Limdi JK, Sharma V, Makin AJ. The use of thrombin injections in the management of bleeding gastric varices: a single-center experience. Gastrointest Endosc. 2008;68(5):877–82.
163. Przemioslo RT, McNair A, Williams R. Thrombin is effective in arresting bleeding from gastric variceal hemorrhage. Dig Dis Sci. 1999;44(4):778–81.
164. Datta D, Vlavianos P, Alisa A, Westaby D. Use of fibrin glue (beriplast) in the management of bleeding gastric varices. Endoscopy. 2003;35(8):675–8.
165. Zuccaro GJ. Management of the adult patients with acute lower gastrointestinal bleeding. Am J Gastroenterol. 1998;93(8):1202–8.
166. Das A, Ben-Menachem T, Cooper GS, et al. Prediction of outcome in acute lower-gastrointestinal haemorrhage based on an artificial neural network: internal and external validation of a predictive model. Lancet. 2003;362:1261–6.
167. Kollef MH, O'Brien JD, Zuckerman GR, et al. BLEED: a classification tool to predict outcomes in patients with acute upper and lower gastrointestinal hemorrhage. Crit Care Med. 1997;25:1125–32.
168. Strate LL, Orav EJ, Syngal S. Early predictors of severity in acute lower intestinal tract bleeding. Arch Intern Med. 2003;163:838–43.
169. Strate LL, Saltzman JR, Ookubo R, et al. Validation of a clinical prediction rule for severe acute lower intestinal bleeding. Am J Gastroenterol. 2005;100:1821–7.

170. Strate LL, Gralnek IM. ACG Clinical Guideline: Management of patients with acute lower gastrointestinal bleeding. Am J Gastroenterol. 2016;111:459–74.
171. Velayos FS, Williamson A, Sousa KH, et al. Early predictors of severe lower gastrointestinal bleeding and adverse outcomes: a prospective study. Clin Gastroenterol Hepatol. 2004;2: 485–90.
172. Newman J, Fitzgerald JE, Gupta S, et al. Outcome predictors in acute surgical admissions for lower gastrointestinal bleeding. Color Dis. 2012;14:1020–6.
173. Green BT, Rockey DC, Portwood G, et al. Urgent colonoscopy for evaluation and management of acute lower gastrointestinal hemorrhage: a randomized controlled trial. Am J Gastroenterol. 2005;100:2395–402.
174. Jensen DM, Machicado GA. Diagnosis and treatment of severe hematochezia. The role of urgent colonoscopy after purge. Gastroenterology. 1988;95:1569–74.
175. Jensen DM, Machicado GA, Jutabha R, et al. Urgent colonoscopy for the diagnosis and treatment of severe diverticular hemorrhage. N Engl J Med. 2000;342:78–82.
176. American Society for Gastrointestinal Endoscopy. The role of endoscopy in the patient with lower gastrointestinal bleeding. Gastrointest Endosc. 1998;48:685–8.
177. Laine L, Shah A. Randomized trial of urgent vs elective colonoscopy in patients hospitalized with lower GI bleeding. Am J Gastroenterol. 2010;105(12):2636–41.
178. Kouanda AM, Somsouk M, Sewell JL, Day LW. Urgent colonoscopy in patients with lower gastrointestinal bleeding: a systematic review and meta-analysis. Gastrointest Endosc. 2017; https://doi.org/10.1016/j.gie.2017.01.035.
179. American Society for Gastrointestinal Endoscopy. The role of endoscopy in the patient with lower GI bleeding. Gastrointest Endosc. 2014;79(6):875–85.
180. Prakash C, Chokshi H, Walden DT, Aliperti G. Endoscopic hemostasis of in acute diverticular bleeding. Endoscopy. 1999; 31(6):460–3.
181. Foutch PG, Zimmermann K. Diverticular bleeding protu- 59 berance (sentinel clot); clinical implication, histopathological correlation, and result of endoscopic interventions. Am J Gastroenterol. 1996;91(12):2589–93.
182. Bloomfeld RS, Rockey DC, Shetzline MA. Endoscopy therapy of acute diverticular haemorrhage. Am J Gastroenterol. 2001;96(8):2367–72.
183. Ramirez FC Johnson DA, Zierer ST, Walker GJ, Sanowski RA. Successful endoscopic hemostasis of bleeding colonic 61 diverticula with epinephrine injection. Gastrointest Endosc. 1996;43(2):167–70.
184. Simpson PW, Nguyen NH, Lim JK, Soetikno RM. Use of endoclip in the treatment of massive colonic diverticula bleeding. Gastrointest Endosc. 2004;59(3):433–7.
185. Helmrich GA, Stalworth JR, Brown JJ. Angiodysplasia: characterization, diagnosis and advances in treatment. South Med J. 1990;83(12):1450–3.
186. Farrell JJ, Friedman LS. Gastrointestinal bleeding in the elderly. Gastroenterol Clin N Am. 2001;30(2):377–407.
187. Brandt LJ, Spinell MK. Ability of naloxone to enhance the colonoscopy appearance of normal colon vasculature and colon vascular ectasia. Gastrointest Endosc. 1999;49(1):79–83.
188. Parra-Blanco A, Kaminaga N, Kojima T, et al. Colonoscopic polypectomy with cutting current: is it safe? Gastrointest Endosc. 2000;51:676–81.
189. Bustamante-Balen M, Plume G. Role of hemostatic powders in the endoscopic management of gastrointestinal bleeding. World J Gastrointest Pathophysiol. 2014;5:284–92.
190. Karaman A, Torun E, Gursoy S, et al. Efficacy of Ankaferd Blood Stopper in postpolypectomy bleeding. J Altern Complement Med. 2010;16:1027–8.
191. Holster IL, Brullet E, Kuipers EJ, et al. Hemospray treatment is effective for lower gastrointestinal bleeding. Endoscopy. 2014;46:75–8.
192. Huang R, Pan Y, Hui N, et al. Polysaccharide hemostatic system for hemostasis management in colorectal endoscopic mucosal resection. Dig Endosc. 2014;26:63–8.
193. Ibis M, Kurt M, Onal IK, et al. Successful management of bleeding due to solitary rectal ulcer via topical application of Ankaferd blood stopper. J Altern Complement Med. 2008;14:1073–4.
194. Kurt M, Onal I, Akdogan M, et al. Ankaferd Blood Stopper for controlling gastrointestinal bleeding due to distinct benign lesions refractory to conventional antihemorrhagic measures. Can J Gastroenterol. 2010;24:380–4.
195. Jayaraman V, Hammerle C, Lo SK, et al. Clinical application and outcomes of over the scope clip device: initial US experience in humans. Diagn Ther Endosc. 2013;2013:381873.
196. Anthony T, Penta P, Todd RD, et al. Rebleeding and survival after acute lower gastrointestinal bleeding. Am J Surg. 2004;188:485–90.
197. Jaeckle T, Stuber G, Hoffmann MH, et al. Acute gastrointestinal bleeding: value of MDCT. Abdom Imaging. 2008;33:285–93.
198. Zink SI, Ohki SK, Stein B, et al. Noninvasive evaluation of active lower gastrointestinal bleeding: comparison between contrast-enhanced MDCT and 99mTc-labeled RBC scintigraphy. AJR Am J Roentgenol. 2008;191:1107–14.
199. Khanna A, Ognibene SJ, Koniaris LG. Embolization as first-line therapy for diverticulosis-related massive lower gastrointestinal bleeding: evidence from a meta-analysis. J Gastrointest Surg. 2005;9:343–52.
200. Strate LL, Naumann CR. The role of colonoscopy and radiological procedures in the management of acute lower intestinal bleeding. Clin Gastroenterol Hepatol. 2010;8:333–43; quiz e44
201. Strate LL, Syngal S. Predictors of utilization of early colonoscopy vs. radiography for severe lower intestinal bleeding. Gastrointest Endosc. 2005;61:46–52.
202. Vernava AM 3rd, Moore BA, Longo WE, et al. Lower gastrointestinal bleeding. Dis Colon Rectum. 1997;40:846–58.
203. Ansari MZ, Collopy BT, Hart WG, et al. In-hospital mortality and associated complications after bowel surgery in Victorian public hospitals. Aust New Zeal J Surg. 2000;70:6–10.

Updates in Gastrointestinal Emergencies: Inflammatory Conditions and Obstructions

29

Pietro Gambitta, Emilia Bareggi, Francesca Iannuzzi, Domenico Lo Conte, Alessandra D'Alessandro, Alessandro Ballerini, Stefano Pallotta, Antonio Armellino, and Paolo Aseni

Key Points

- The classic triad of sudden onset of abdominal pain, tachycardia, and abdominal rigidity is the hallmark of perforated peptic ulcer (PPU).
- Early diagnosis, prompt resuscitation, and urgent surgical intervention are essential to improve outcomes in PPU.
- Management of PPU is primarily surgical, and different suture techniques for closure of the perforation and cleansing of the abdomen are described. Laparoscopic surgery should be also considered if available.
- Bowel obstruction can occur anywhere in the small or large intestine and could be intraluminal, intramural, or due to extrinsic compression; the main symptoms are abdominal pain in 92% of patients, nausea or vomiting in 82%, and constipation in 81–90%
- Adhesions are the most common cause of small bowel obstruction representing the 70% of the etiology.
- Intussusception or invagination of a proximal segment of bowel into an adjacent distal segment affects mainly children between 6 months and 1 year old. Just 5% of intussusception occur in adults. In 90% of these cases, intussusception is secondary to other pathologies, very often polyps or adenocarcinomas.
- Small bowel occlusion secondary to gallstone ileus represents a surgical emergency. Laparotomy is in general preferred, but laparoscopy and lithotripsy can be also utilized. Three surgical options are described: enterolithotomy alone; enterolithotomy, cholecystectomy, and fistula repair (one stage procedure); and enterolithotomy with cholecystectomy and fistula repair in a second stage
- Non-operative endoscopic reduction of sigmoid volvulus generally carries a lower risk than open surgery although recurrence rate is higher (71%)
- Acute colonic pseudo-obstruction (ACPO) is usually associated with other severe medical conditions, such as abdominal traumas, serious infections, or acute cardiac diseases. ACPO can also be associated with recent surgery, spinal cord injury, hormone dysregulation, electrolyte imbalances, neurological/respiratory/renal disorders, and drugs.
- Patients with complicated acute diverticulitis with large abscesses (>4–5 cm) can be treated by percutaneous drainage combined with antibiotic treatment. Whenever percutaneous drainage of the abscess is not feasible or not available, the Hartmann resection is the surgical procedure advised for managing diffuse peritonitis in critically ill patients and patients with important comorbidities. In stable patients without comorbidities, primary resection with anastomosis with or without a diverting stoma may be performed.

P. Gambitta · E. Bareggi · F. Iannuzzi · A. Ballerini · S. Pallotta
Endoscopy Division, Luigi Sacco Hospital, University of Milan, Milan, Italy

D. L. Conte
Unit of Hepatobiliary and Colorectal Surgical Oncology, Candiolo Cancer Institute, FPO-IRCCS, Torino, Italy

A. D'Alessandro
Department of Clinical Medicine and Surgery, University of Naples Federico II, Naples, Italy

A. Armellino
Endoscopy Division, Ospedale San Leopoldo Mandic di Merate, ASST Lecco, Lecco, Italy
e-mail: a.armellino@ospedale.lecco.it

P. Aseni (✉)
Department of Emergency, ASST Grande Ospedale Metropolitano Niguarda, Milan, Italy

P. Aseni et al. (eds.), *Operative Techniques and Recent Advances in Acute Care and Emergency Surgery*,
https://doi.org/10.1007/978-3-319-95114-0_29

29.1 Complicated Peptic Ulcer: Perforation and Bleeding

29.1.1 Perforated Peptic Ulcer

Peptic ulcer disease (PUD) results from an imbalance between stomach acid-pepsin and mucosal defense barriers and affects four million people worldwide annually [1] with an incidence estimated at around 1.5–3% [2]. Perforated peptic ulcer (PPU) is a serious complication of PUD; it has a lifetime prevalence of about 5% [3], and it leads to a high risk of morbidity and mortality [4], ranging from 1.3 to 20% [5, 6].

NSAIDs, *Helicobacter pylori* (*H. pylori*), physiological stress, smoking, alcohol consumption, corticosteroids, previous history of PUD, gastrinomas, and Zollinger-Ellison syndrome are risks factors for PUD [1, 7, 8].

29.1.1.1 Clinical Features

Symptoms of PUD include abdominal pain, upper abdominal discomfort, and feeling of fullness. Sudden onset of abdominal pain or acute deterioration of the ongoing abdominal pain without resolution is typical of PPU. The classic triad of sudden onset of abdominal pain, tachycardia, and abdominal rigidity is the hallmark of PPU.

29.1.1.2 Diagnosis

An urgent erect anteroposterior chest X-ray is the basic clinical investigation in patients with acute upper abdominal pain; about 75% of PPU have pneumoperitoneum with free air under the diaphragm [9].

CT scan is recommended as it has a diagnostic accuracy as high as 98% [10]. CT scan is performed in the supine position, and intra-abdominal free air is usually seen anteriorly just below the anterior abdominal wall (Fig. 29.1). CT scan must be done even when the X-ray is positive, especially when the clinical presentation is not specific or malignancy is suspected. Oral contrast with CT scan is a useful tool, and if free leak is seen, diagnosis is certain.

Laboratory tests are performed in PPU, not only to establish the diagnosis but to rule out a differential diagnosis and to better understand the possible involvement of different organs [11].

There are about 11 different scoring systems to predict outcome in PPU. The Boey score (parameters evaluated, presentation ≥ or <24 h; presence of preoperative shock; level of comorbidity) and ASA score (parameters evaluated, degree of comorbidity and present systemic disease) are the most commonly validated systems [8, 12].

29.1.1.3 Management

All patients with PPU require prompt resuscitation, intravenous antibiotics, analgesia, proton pump inhibitory medications (PPI), nasogastric aspiration, urinary catheter, and surgical source control.

Several studies have proven triple therapy eradication of *H. pylori* after simple closure of PPU reduced the incidence of recurrent ulcer [13–15]; it is indicated to start with intravenous PPI as soon as the diagnosis is made and start triple oral therapy for *H. pylori* immediately after surgery.

29.1.1.4 Non-operative Management

Some studies have evaluated the feasibility of a conservative management showing that about 40–80% of PPU will seal

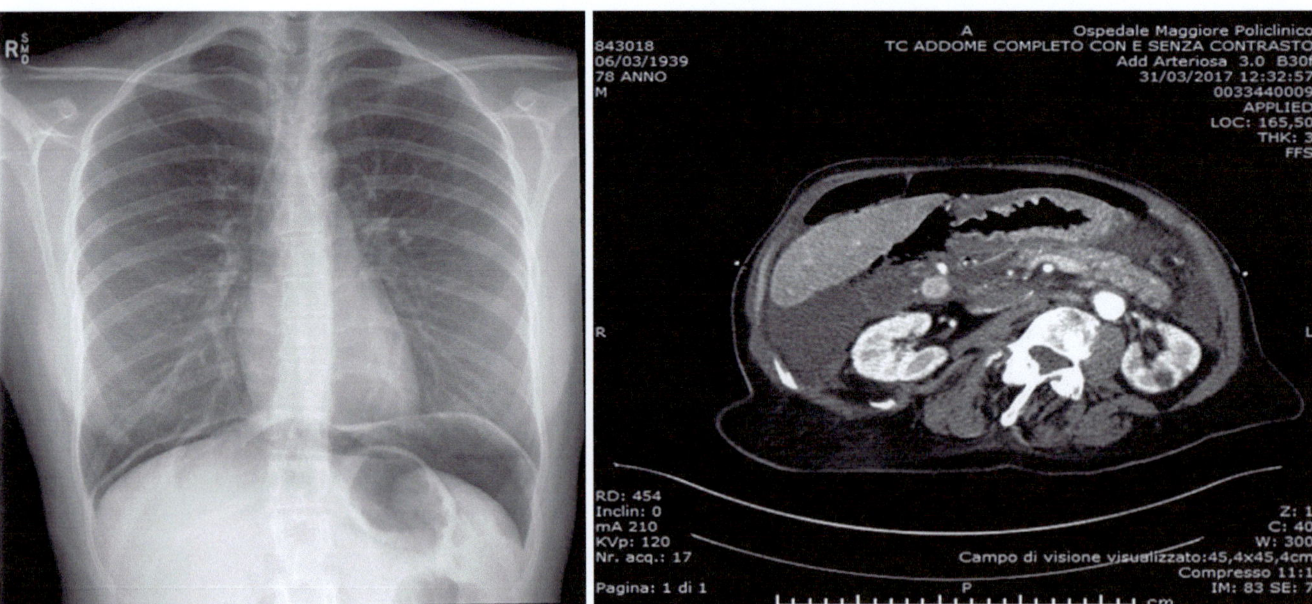

Fig. 29.1 Erect chest X-ray and CT scan with intra-abdominal free air in a patient with PPU

spontaneously and the overall morbidity and mortality are comparable to those operated [2, 16–18]. A non-operative management consists of nasogastric suction, intravenous drip, antibiotics, repeated clinical assessment, and gastrografin study to confirm the absence of leakage. A repeated clinical examination and around-the-clock readiness to operate is fundamental. However, the studies available are few and based on small records. Hence a non-operative management should be conducted only by experienced teams, under trial conditions.

29.1.1.5 Operative Management

Surgery is still the principal way of management. The principal aims of the modern surgery are the closing of the hole and the cleansing of the abdomen. There are several closing techniques: interrupted sutures covered with a pedicled omentum (Cellan-Jones repair), plugging the perforation with a free omental plug (Graham patch), using glue or a mixed technique with a laparoscopic-endoscopic rendezvous.

Laparoscopic exploration should always be done to check the feasibility of the mini-invasive approach, also in case of previous surgery, with the exception of major abdominal distension or unstable patients. It is feasible for holes with a diameter up to 10 mm. It was first performed by Mouret in 1990 for a perforated duodenal ulcer [19]. The mini-invasive approach is believed to reduce the postoperative morbidity and mortality [20]. However, the current evidence remains poor for choosing laparoscopic repair over open surgery. In fact, a recent review of three randomized controlled trials compared laparoscopy with laparotomy [21] failed to demonstrate differences in postoperative morbidity, mortality, and reoperation. The overall conversion rate for laparoscopic surgery is 12.4% mainly due to the size of perforation; a size more than 9 mm is a significant risk factor for conversion [22]. In laparoscopic group the operating time was longer, and recurrent leakage was higher, but the related postoperative pain and length of hospital stay are significantly less, with equivalent costs compared with laparotomy [23].

Patients with a Boey score 3, older than 70 years, and symptoms lasting longer than 24 h should undergo an open surgery [23], while patients with a Boey score of 0–1, ulcer size of less than 10 mm, located on the anterior pyloroduodenal wall, hemodynamically stable, with ASA score less than 3 could benefit from a laparoscopic approach also in the hands of trainees [24, 25].

A 30° scope facilitates the exploration. The first step is the evaluation of the laparoscopic feasibility and the peritoneal liquid sample for bacterial tests. Then a peritoneal toilette with pus aspiration and washing of any abdominal cavity with a low-flow irrigation is useful to reduce the bacterial count. Irrigation is still debated since, according to some authors, it could facilitate a postoperative intra-abdominal collection [26–28].

In case of gastric PPU, a biopsy should be done, especially when a malignancy is suspected; in such patients an oncological resection should be delayed to a second stage. If a suture technique is chosen, an absorbable 2/0 string is more indicated to close the hole with two or three X-made atraumatic stitches. In pateints with frail ulcer edges, or ulcer size greater than 10 mm, it is better to convert to laparotomy. After the simple closure of the defect, an omental pedicle plug seems safer also in the presence of large-sized perforations.

29.1.1.6 Vagotomy and Gastrectomy

Nowadays antiacid procedures like vagotomy and antrectomy are limited to particular situations such as patients with a recurrence of complicated PUD that have already taken PPI and *H. pylori* eradication therapy and patients with a very low compliance or complex duodenal perforated ulcers. Vagotomy alone decreases peak acid output by 50%, whereas vagotomy plus antrectomy decreases peak acid output by 85%. A truncal vagotomy is associated with a high rate of postoperative diarrhea and dumping, while a selective vagotomy, thanks to the preservation of the posterior celiac branches and anterior hepatic branches, has less postoperative morbidity with the same ulcer recurrence rate. However, both procedures damage the pylorus motor function requiring a Heineke-Mikulicz pyloroplasty, in comparison with a highly selective vagotomy preserving the Latarjet's nerves.

When antrectomy is indicated, the gastric ulcer location dictates the extent of resection and the resulting type of reconstruction varying among Billroth I, Billroth II and Roux-en-Y. The mortality related to an urgent gastrectomy is up to 24% [29, 30].

29.1.2 Ulcer Bleeding

Peptic ulcer bleeding is the most likely cause of gastrointestinal bleeding, which is the most common cause of hospitalization in the USA due to gastrointestinal disease. The death rate related has decreased over the past 20 years, ranging from 2.1 to 2.5% in US nationwide database studies [31, 32] to 10% in large, prospective European observational studies [33, 34].

29.1.2.1 Clinical Features and Risk Assessment

Symptoms are often hematemesis or melena associated with abdominal pain and acute weakness. The initial risk assessment, according to vital signs and patient factors, is mandatory. A useful tool to distinguish high-risk and low-risk patients is the Glasgow-Blatchford score. Tachycardia, hypotension, age older than 60 years, and major comorbidities are associated with an increased risk of further bleeding and death. The diagnostic tool is the endoscopy.

29.1.2.2 Management

The initial therapy should be the hemotransfusion when the hemoglobin level is less than 7 g/dL or less than 8 g/dL in case of either symptomatic or stable patients with cardiovascular comorbidities. There is no widespread consensus on the use of high dose of PPI before the endoscopy, strongly recommended only by few guidelines [35–39]. The erythromycin (250 mg intravenously, 30 min before endoscopy) increasing gastric motility could improve the visualization of the gastric mucosa at endoscopy [40].

29.1.2.3 Endoscopic Assessment and Treatment

It is widely accepted that the endoscopy must be done within 24 h [35, 37]. Patients with low risk (normal blood pressure and heart rate and no major comorbidities) should undergo endoscopy during the first 6 h, and if a low-risk endoscopic feature is found, they can be discharged.

Endoscopic features have a key role to predict the risk and to decide the therapeutic strategies (Fig. 29.2). High-risk features such as active bleeding, nonbleeding visible vessel, and adherent clot are positively associated with a higher risk of rebleeding from 25 to 35% [41]. Flat pigmented spots and clean-base ulcers are associated with low rate of rebleeding (5.6% and 0.5%, respectively) [42].

Endoscopic therapy with injection (of epinephrine or alcohol), thermal devices (such as bipolar electrocoagulation probes), or clips should be preferred in patients who have ulcers with active bleeding or a nonbleeding visible vessel. Endoscopic therapy might be considered for ulcers with adherent clots, for which randomized trials show heterogeneous results [41]. If bleeding recurs, endoscopic therapy should be repeated; a randomized trial involving patients with rebleeding after endoscopic therapy showed that surgery was avoided in 73% of cases, and adverse events were significantly less common with endoscopic therapy than with surgery [43]. Transcatheter arterial embolization or surgery is performed if repeat endoscopic therapy fails.

29.1.2.4 Surgical Treatment

Surgical management is limited to those cases of uncontrollable bleeding, and it is mandatory in an old patient with hemodynamic instability (1–2% of ulcer bleeding). This condition takes place more often in the posterior duodenal ulcers near the emergency of the gastroduodenal artery. The main aim is the bleeding control, but there is a consensus on the simultaneous surgical treatment of the peptic disease [2]. The approach is generally in laparotomy; the Kocher's maneuver is paramount to better control the region. A longitudinal pyloro-duodenotomy of 4–5 cm allows the right exposition of the posterior duodenal ulcer, and the hemostasis could be done with two stitches of non-absorbable 3/0 passed through the full thickness of the

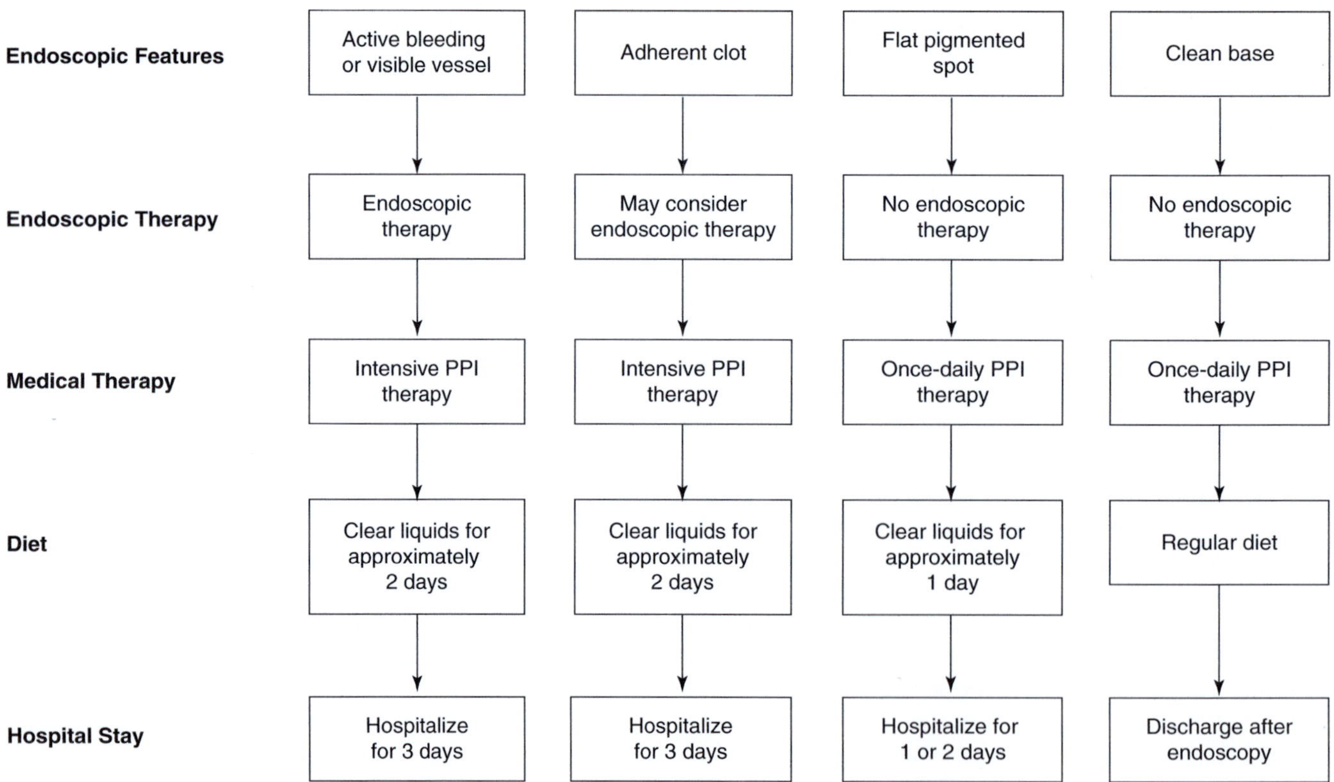

Fig. 29.2 Flow chart of initial treatment of patients with ulcer bleeding, according to the endoscopic features of the ulcer

ulcer and two other stitches placed in the healthy field outside the ulcer to control the gastroduodenal artery, taking care to avoid iatrogenic injuries of the bile duct and papilla. If this strategy is not effective, another possibility is to isolate the gastroduodenal artery on the upper edge of the duodenum directly on its origin from the common hepatic artery and tie it with two stitches of nonabsorbable 3/0. Then if the bleeding is still not under control, the pancreaticoduodenal branch on the inferior edge of the duodenum must also be tied.

Then a transversal pyloroplasty is made; if it cannot be done, a longitudinal pyloroplasty with vagotomy can be performed. A gastroenteroanastomosis can be required due to an increased risk of pyloric stenosis. If the duodenum wall is very frail, impeding a secure closing, a duodenal or antral exclusion could be made closing the duodenum above the ulcer with a linear stapler, and completing the procedure with vagotomy, gastroenteroanastomosis, and controlled duodenal fistula using a Foley or a Pezzer probe.

29.2 Bowel Obstruction

Bowel obstruction is the interruption of the physiological flow in the cephalocaudal sense of the intestinal contents. It may be caused by a mechanical obstruction (mechanical ileus) or by the alteration of intestinal motility (adynamic ileus). The cause of acute mechanical obstruction can be grouped as follows:

- Intraluminal (gallstones, bezoar, foreign bodies, fecal stones, parasites)
- Intramural (congenital atresia, IBD, neoplasia, intussusception endometriosis)
- Extrinsic compression (peritoneal carcinomatosis, peritoneal adhesions, hernias, volvulus)

29.2.1 Clinical Presentation

The symptoms most commonly associated with bowel obstruction are abdominal pain in 92% of patients, nausea or vomiting in 82%, and constipation in 81–90% [44, 45].

Physical examination of the abdomen can show bowel distension, hyperactive bowel sound in the early phase of the obstruction, and hypoactive bowel sound or its absence in the late phase. Fever and peritonism may be signs of a perforative complication or strangulation. The presence of an incarcerated abdominal or a groin hernia should always be investigated and ruled out. A digital rectal examination should be performed to identify fecal impaction or rectal mass or the presence of blood and mucus.

Laboratory exams can show leukocytosis, high level of C-reactive protein, and electrolytes disorders. Metabolic acidosis and high level of lactate should suggest ischemic damage and strangulation.

A plain abdominal X-ray can confirm the suspect of obstruction: bowel distension and air-fluid levels are typical radiological signs of bowel obstruction. The presence of free air in the X-ray can also show a perforation, and can lead to the site of obstruction, but very rarely can demonstrate the cause of obstruction. Abdominal US can offer particular advantage for the diagnosis of proximal duodenal or jejunal obstruction since a plain abdominal X-ray is often normal because frequent vomiting causes lack of air in the obstructed tract.

A CT scan must be performed to individuate the cause of obstruction and can lead to the correct diagnosis and treatment.

29.2.2 Adhesive Small Bowel Obstruction

Adhesions are the most common cause of small bowel obstruction representing the 70% of the etiology [46].

The management of adhesive obstruction is controversial because surgery can remove the cause but can provoke new adhesions, whereas conservative treatment doesn't remove the cause.

If there are signs of sepsis or strangulation, peritonism, severe leukocytosis, high fever, and high lactate, emergency surgery must be considered.

In the other cases, conservative management can be performed. It involves nasogastric tube, intravenous fluid administration, electrolytes re-equilibration, and clinical observation.

Conservative treatment shouldn't be prolonged more than 72 h. After 72 h without resolution, surgery is recommended. In the presence of complications such as signs of sepsis, strangulation, or peritonism, abdominal exploration and surgical treatment are recommended [47].

In stable patients without complications who can be observed without surgery, water-soluble contrast enema can be administrated orally with diagnostic and therapeutic intent. In fact, sometimes, the laxative property of the contrast can solve the obstruction and reduce the hospitalization and the need for surgery [48, 49]. A control X-ray of the abdomen should be planned after 24 h: the progression of the contrast in the colon is a predictive sign of resolution.

Open surgery is preferred when there is a clinical suspicion of strangulation, perforation, and a very dense adhesive disease and when there is a very severe bowel distension.

In selected patients, laparoscopy can be performed, especially when a single adhesive lace is suspected. Laparoscopy seems to have some advantages when compared to open

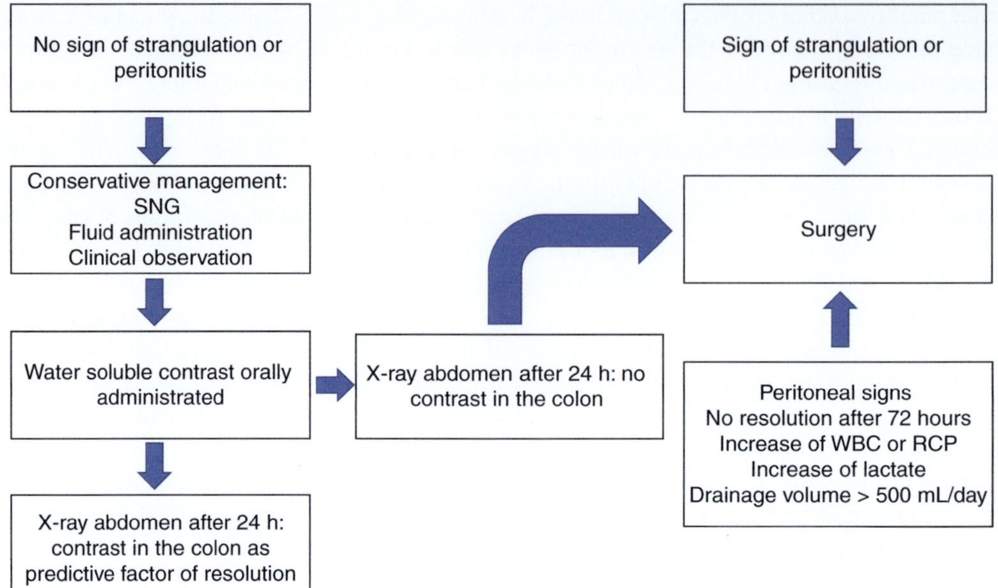

Fig. 29.3 Algorithm for the management of adhesive small bowel obstruction

-surgery such as less postoperative pain, faster return of intestinal function, shorter hospitalization, decreased post-operative adhesion formation [50].

If there is strangulation, perforation, or ischemic damage, ileal resection must be performed.

The extension of adhesiolysis is debated: some surgeons prefer to perform a complete adhesiolysis; others prefer to limit the lysis of those adhesions responsible for the obstruction (Fig. 29.3).

29.2.3 Intussusception

Intussusception is the invagination of a proximal segment of the bowel into an adjacent distal segment.

The majority of patients are children between 6 months and 1 year old. Just 5% of intussusception occurs in adults. In 90% of these cases, intussusception is secondary to other pathologies, very often polyps or adenocarcinomas [51].

The clinical presentation of adult intussusception varies considerably. In children, the classic presentation comprises a triad of symptoms: cramping abdominal pain, bloody diarrhea, and a palpable tender mass. Bloody diarrhea and palpable mass are rare. In adults, the presenting symptoms are less specific and consistent with partial obstruction. The principal symptoms are cramping abdominal pain and vomiting. However preoperative clinical diagnosis, in adults, can be evident in only 50% of cases [52].

The plain X-ray of the abdomen can be the first exam performed, but it can show just an obstruction without leading to diagnosis. Ultrasonography is useful for the diagnosis, especially in children. The classical imaging features include the "target" sign on the transverse view and the "pseudo-kidney" sign or "hayfork" sign in the longitudinal view [53]. However, ultrasonography needs a very expert operator, and obesity or bowel distension represents an obstacle for the diagnosis.

CT scan is currently considered as the most sensitive radiologic method to confirm intussusception, with a reported diagnostic accuracy ranging from 58 to 100% [54]. As well as ultrasonography, CT can show a "target" sign, a very useful indication to localize the intussusception and the possible associated secondary disease.

Some 70–80% of all intussusceptions in the pediatric population may be successfully managed non-operatively by reduction with air- or liquid-contrast enemas under fluoroscopic or US guidance. In the other cases or when radiological or clinical signs of strangulation are evident, emergency surgery must be performed. If a segmental bowel gangrene is suspected, resection with primary anastomoses must be performed.

Due to a significant risk of associated pathologies, especially malignant neoplasms, which can be found in 65% of elderly patients [55], non-operative management is non-indicated in adults and bowel resection with primary anastomosis should be the procedure of choice.

29.2.4 Gallstone Ileus

Gallstone ileus is a mechanical intestinal obstruction due to gallstone impaction within the gastrointestinal tract. The gallstone moves from the gallbladder into the small bowel obstructing the lumen, often in the ileocecal valve. Past biliary colic can be described by 50% of patients with gallstone ileus [56]. X-ray of the abdomen can demonstrate a small bowel obstruction but cannot lead to the etiology. A CT scan may demonstrate a gallstone in the bowel lumen with retro-dilatation of the bowel loops (92.6% of cases), pneumobilia (88.9%), ectopic gallstone (81.5%), air-fluid levels (37%), and the biliodigestive fistula (14.8%).

The CT scan has a sensitivity of 93%, but the rate of a correct preoperative diagnosis is reported in less than 70% of cases [57].

Gallstone ileus represents a surgical emergency. Laparotomy is in general preferred, but laparoscopy and lithotripsy have also been reported [58, 59]. The kind of intervention is still debated. There are three options: enterolithotomy alone, enterolithotomy associated with cholecystectomy and fistula repair (one stage procedure), and enterolithotomy in the first stage and cholecystectomy and fistula repair in a second stage. Bowel resection is sometimes needed in case of focal small bowel gangrene or perforation. The enterotomy in combination with the extraction of the stone solves the obstruction but is associated with a recurrence rate of 17% [60]. The one-stage combined procedure of enterotomy, cholecystectomy, and fistula repair avoids the risk of recurrence but is associated with a high incidence of morbidity and mortality [61, 62].

To resolve the acute obstruction many authors suggest that the simple enterolithotomy is the best option with the lowest mortality and morbidity rate [63]. One-stage procedure is recommended in patients with acute cholecystitis or gangrene of the gallbladder and low-risk patients [64]. The two-stage procedure should be considered in patients with recurrent gallstone ileus.

Endoscopic removal of the stone in the duodenum, ileum, or jejunum by endoscopy with or without YAG laser lithotripsy has been reported [65–67]. Endoscopy in elderly patients with poor general condition cannot be considered a standard procedure since it has several limitations as the distance of the gallstone from the mouth or anus (Figs. 29.4, 29.5, and 29.6).

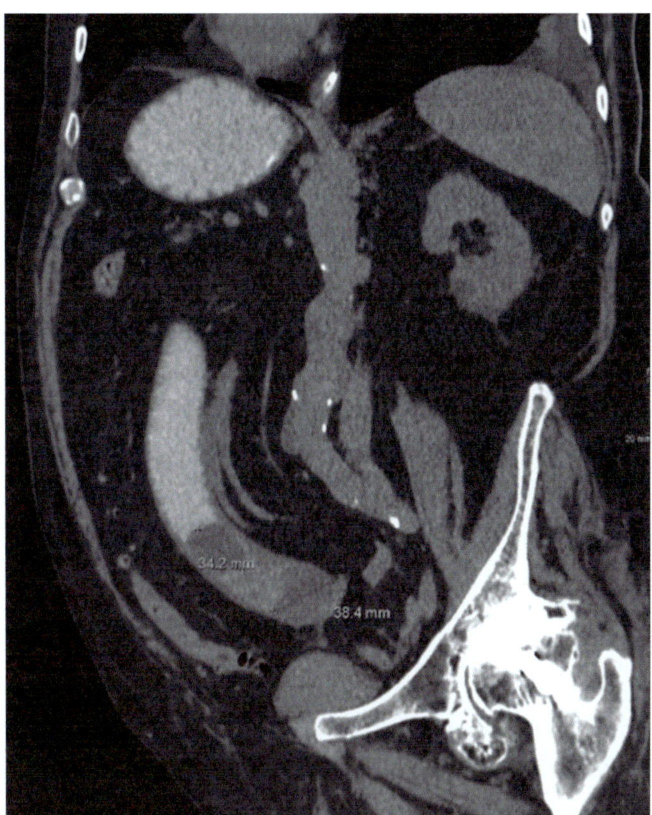

Fig. 29.4 CT scan of a gallstone ileus

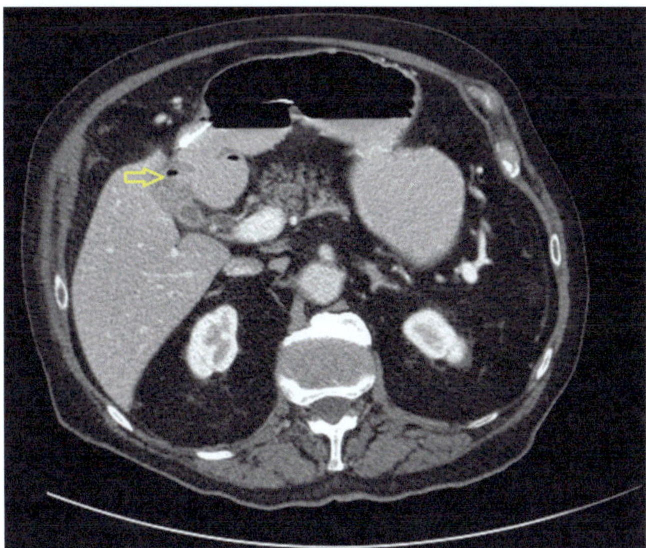

Fig. 29.5 Gallbladder-duodenal fistula with air in the gallbladder

29.3 Colonic and Gastric Volvulus

Gastric and colonic volvulus are rare clinical entity defined as an abnormal rotation of the stomach or sigmoid colon of more than 180°, which creates a closed-loop obstruction that can result in incarceration and strangulation. The rotation involves the mesentery reducing the vascular supply to the viscera. Then, when it is not recognized and treated promptly, the volvulus in its acute presentation may provoke an ischemic damage with consequent perforation and gangrene.

Obstructive symptoms such as abdominal pain and distension, complete constipation, nausea, and vomiting are the usual clinical presentation. Fever, peritonism, elevated white cells blood count, C-reactive protein, lactate, or symptoms of sepsis may suggest ischemic or perforative complications. A plain abdominal X-ray can show bowel distention, ileal or colonic, depending on the anatomical site of the volvulus. Sometimes an “omega loop sign” or a “coffee bean sign” are present. CT scan of the abdomen can demonstrate the rotation of the tract of the bowel and his mesentery. The presence of *pneumatosis intestinalis* in the bowel wall may suggest

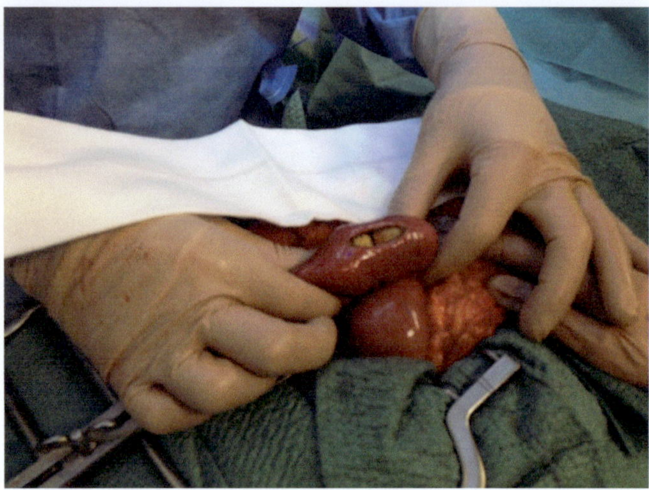

Fig. 29.6 Gallstone ileus: enterotomy and extraction of stones

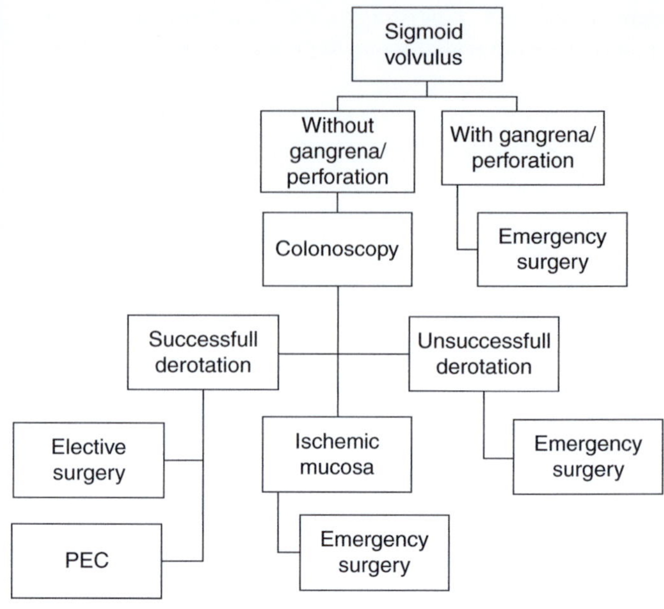

Fig. 29.7 Algorithm for the management of colonic volvulus

ischemic injury. Sigmoid colon is the most frequent site of colonic volvulus (60.9% of colonic volvulus). Ileocecal volvulus is less frequent (34.5%). Transverse colon and splenic flexure volvulus are rare conditions (3.6% and 1%, respectively) [68].

29.3.1 Colonic Volvulus

Colonic volvulus represents the third cause of colonic obstruction, after tumors and diverticula [69]. The principal risk factor is a long sigmoid colon with an elongated mesentery, pregnancy, and previous abdominal surgery. Some studies suggest that colonic volvulus may also be associated with Hirschsprung disease [70]. In the absence of ischemia or perforation, a conservative treatment should be considered especially in elderly patients [71]. The presence of perforation or ischemic colitis represents a surgical emergency, and a sigmoid resection, with or without primary anastomosis, should be performed. Emergency surgery in these patients is associated with a high morbidity and mortality rate [72].

Surgery should be delayed in the absence of peritonitis or ischemic colitis, and colonoscopy with decompression and colonic derotation should be the first choice. The role of endoscopy is both diagnostic and therapeutic. A stenosis with spiral twist "sphincter-like" of the mucosa is an endoscopic sign of colonic volvulus. The endoscopic view of an ischemic mucosa represents an indication for emergency surgery. In the absence of colonic ischemia, a derotation should be performed with a success rate ranging from 79 and 81% [73].

Although non-operative reduction of sigmoid volvulus generally carries a lower risk than open surgery, recurrence rates are higher. The recurrence rate in patients treated with non-operative management is 71% with a mortality of 36% [74].

These data suggest that even patients successfully treated without surgery should be considered for elective surgery. Sigmoid resection with Hartmann procedure or one-stage resection with primary anastomosis depending on intraoperative findings shows the lowest rate of recurrence [75]. Sigmoidectomy with primary anastomosis is the best option for definitive treatment [76]. In an emergency clinical setting, in the presence of colonic ischemia, perforation or fecal peritonitis sigmoidectomy with primary anastomoses is usually not recommended in favor of the Hartmann procedure which is associated with the lowest morbidity and mortality.

An alternative technique to reduce the risk of recurrence after endoscopic derotation is the percutaneous endoscopic colostomy (PEC). This is a mini-invasive technique, which can be performed under intravenous sedation. Under endoscopic view, using PEG kit, sigmoid colon is fixed to the abdominal wall [77]. There are few data on this technique. PEC has less morbidity and mortality than surgery, but there is still no sufficient data that prove his effectiveness on the recurrence rate. According to literature, PEC should be reserved for elderly patients or patients who are unfit for surgery [78] (Figs. 29.7 and 29.8).

29.3.2 Gastric Volvulus

Gastric volvulus (GV) is an abnormal torsion of the stomach of more than 180°, which creates a closed-loop obstruction resulting in incarceration and strangulation. GV is classified based on the axis of torsion, organo-axial type, mesentero-axial type, and a combined type. It could be primary or secondary to diaphragm congenital defects or a hiatal hernia.

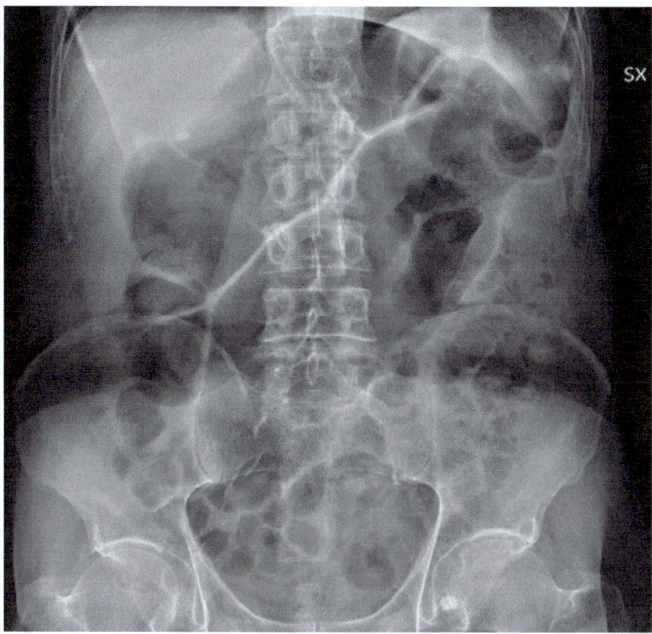

Fig. 29.8 Colonic volvulus, coffee bean sign

Clinical presentation of acute volvulus includes vomiting and abdominal pain. It represents a surgical emergency, for the high risk of ischemic injury of the gastric wall and consequent perforation. Chronic volvulus could be completely asymptomatic or poorly symptomatic, and serious complications are very rare so a conservative management can be considered [79, 80].

In acute volvulus, a plain abdominal X-ray can show just a gastric distension. CT scan is necessary to demonstrate the torsion and the type of volvulus.

The presence of subdiaphragmatic free air represents an indication of emergency surgery.

Early endoscopy is recommended to evaluate an eventual ischemia of the wall. When there are no signs of ischemic or perforative injury, endoscopic reduction of gastric volvulus is effective in the majority of patients [81].

The maneuver is performed pushing the endoscope in the second portion of the duodenum, through the twisted part. Then the endoscope should be pulled back, twisting on the right. This maneuver should be performed with combined endoscopic and radioscopic view [82].

However, surgery should be considered in any case for the high risk of recurrence.

In case of ischemia of gastric mucosa, perforation, or unsuccessful attempt of endoscopic derotation, emergency surgery is required.

The aims of surgery are:

- Derotate the stomach.
- Resect ischemic area of the stomach.
- Prevent the recurrence.

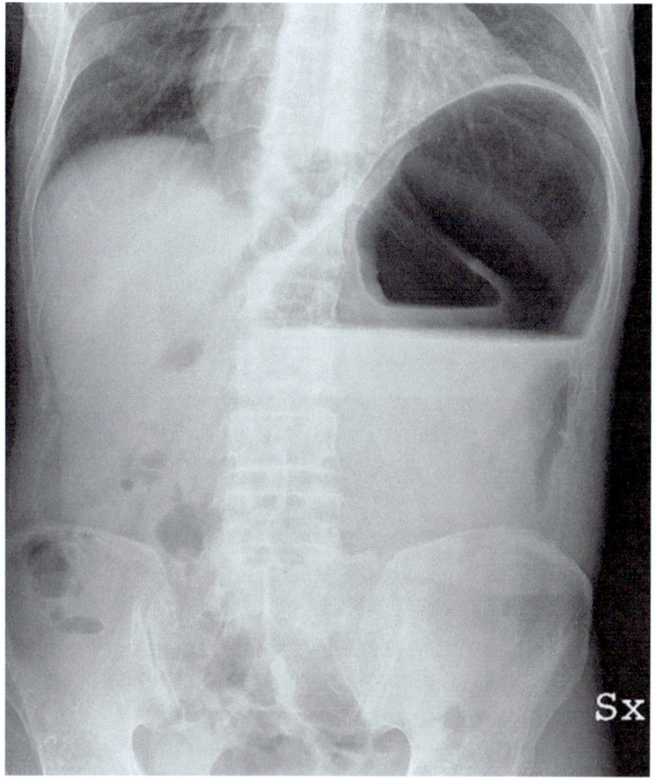

Fig. 29.9 Gastric volvulus: plain abdominal X-Ray

As described by Tanner [83], there are several surgical options:

- Diaphragmatic hernia repair
- Simple gastropexy
- Gastropexy with division of the gastrocolic omentum (Tanner's operation)
- Partial gastrectomy
- Fundoantral gastrogastrostomy
- Repair of the diaphragmatic eventration (Figs. 29.9 and 29.10)

29.4 Colonic Pseudo-obstruction (CPO)

Colonic pseudo-obstruction is a condition characterized by a clinical picture of an obstructive syndrome, in the absence of any demonstrable mechanical obstruction [84]. According to presentation, this syndrome can be divided in acute (ACPO) and chronic (CCPO) form; the former, also known as Ogilvie's syndrome, is defined by acute and rapid colonic dilatation, while the latter is characterized by recurrent episodes of bowel obstruction, without severe colonic distention, and associated with recurrent abdominal pain/bloating in the absence of anatomical abnormality which may explain

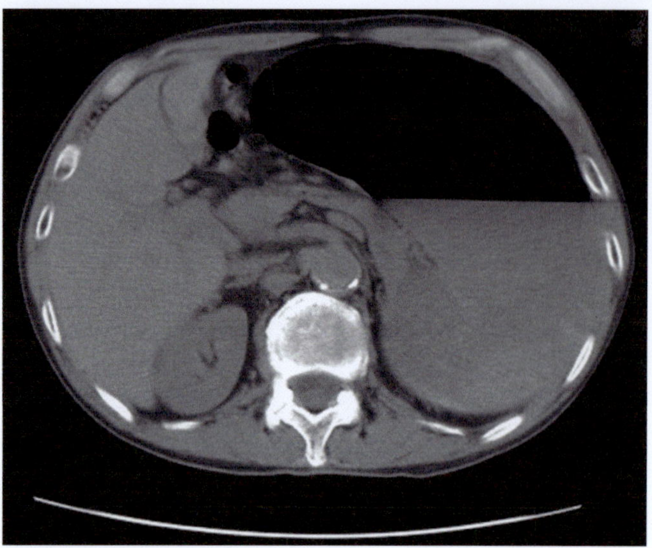

Fig. 29.10 Gastric volvulus. CT scan

the symptoms. Differently from the chronic presentation, the ACPO may represent a life-threatening condition, due to the high risk of perforation and ischemia [86, 87].

The pathophysiological mechanisms underlying acute clinical presentation are still poorly identified. Several studies suggest that an imbalance of autonomic nervous system may determine a lower parasympathetic and/or a higher sympathetic tone, with a consequent reduction of intestinal motility. In several patients, a clear impairment of myenteric plexus has also been demonstrated, especially in subjects with neurological or autoimmune comorbidities. ACPO is usually associated with other severe medical conditions, such as abdominal traumas, serious infections, acute cardiac diseases and neoplasia (small cell lung cancer. multiple myeloma, leukaemia, retroperitoneal tumour invasion of lumbar sympathetic nervous system. In addition, ACPO can also be associated with recent surgery, spinal cord injury, hormonal dysregulation (hypothyroidism and diabetes), electrolyte imbalances (hyponatremia, hypo/hypercalcemia), neurological/respiratory/renal disorders, and drugs (anti-depressants, opiates, anticholinergics, anti-parkinsonian agents). Rarely, autoimmune syndromes, such as systemic lupus erythematosus (SLE) and systemic sclerosis (SS), or hematologic diseases, like multiple myeloma, may induce an acute colonic adynamic ileus. Only in 5–10% of patients with ACPO, there is no evidence of other underlying diseases, defining the field of idiopathic pseudo-obstructions, usually related to a specific form of intestinal neuropathies [87–89].

29.4.1 Diagnosis

The diagnostic algorithm is the same for other obstructive syndromes, and the diagnosis is confirmed when mechanical bowel obstruction is excluded. Computed tomography (CT) is the gold standard diagnostic test for these patients. The demonstration of diffuse dilatation with the absence of a transition zone with dilated fluid-, air-, or air-fluid-filled loops above collapsed loops of bowel distally can suggest ACPO. CT can also detect air into the peritoneal cavity in cases of associated perforation.

During patients' evaluation, a careful estimation of colonic distention should be made; in particular, since the caecum has thinner walls and requires less pressure to increase in size, its length must be exactly defined [90, 91]. Treatment of underlying condition is mandatory in ACPO. Hence all cardiac/respiratory/renal/neurologic and electrolyte disorders should be carefully evaluated and, if possible, treated. A "nihil per os" (NPO) should be maintained with nasogastric tube decompression until the colonic function returns [92].

29.4.2 Treatment

Conservative treatments represent the first therapeutic choice in the absence of perforation or ischemic signs. Medical approach is based on the increase of parasympathetic tone, using cholinesterase inhibitors, e.g., neostigmine, and prokinetic agents, e.g., erythromycin and metoclopramide. Hutchinson et al. have reported a positive role of the sympathetic blocker guanethidine, before the administration of neostigmine [93]. An initial response is usually observed after 3–5 min from the IV administration of these drugs. Since APCO is associated with severe other medical conditions, cholinesterase inhibitors should be administered under cardiac monitoring, and the use of these drugs is contraindicated in patients with bradycardia, severe hypotension, or active bronchospasm [94].

The endoscopic approach has been recently suggested as the first choice treatment. Colonoscopy decompression has a success rate of 75–85%, thus reducing the adverse side effects related to cholinesterase inhibitors. However, decompressive colonoscopy may be insidious in these patients, due to the impossibility to perform bowel preparation and the necessity of minimal air insufflation. On the other hand, colonoscopy also has a diagnostic role, allowing the evaluation of mucosal ischemic signs (e.g., ulcers, submucosal hemorrhage, yellow exudates). Moreover, several studies have demonstrated that achieving caecal intubation is not necessary. Indeed, an adequate decompression can also be obtained from the transverse colon. Recurrence rate after endoscopic decompression is high, ranging from 20 to 60%, and usually repeated colonoscopy is required. For this reason, some authors suggest the positioning of long indwelling tubes, which reduce the recurrence rate but frequently become obstructed [95, 96].

To reduce the risk of recurrence after medical or endoscopic treatment, some authors evaluated the use of polyethylene glycol (PEG) electrolyte-balanced solution after the resolution of acute distension, showing a significant decrease of relapse; however further evidence is needed [97].

In the absence of complications, the conservative approach should be continued for 3–6 days, in case of medical failure or worsening of colon dilatation, a surgical approach should be considered [87]. Colonic perforation, especially at caecum level, is associated with a high risk of mortality (up to 40%). In case of severe dilatation without ischemia, an open percutaneous or laparoscopic cecostomy can be considered [98, 99].

In the presence of perforation, peritonitis, sepsis, or mucosal ischemic signs, urgent laparotomy is indicated. In these patients the necrotic or ischemic area should be resected, and the choice between primary anastomosis or a diversion procedure depends on the presence of perforation and extent of fecal contamination. Particular attention should be paid to fluid infusion during surgical intervention since ACPO may cause a critical colonic liquid sequestration with a high risk of hypovolemic complications [100, 101]

29.5 Acute Colonic Diverticulitis

Acute left-sided colonic diverticulosis is common in Western countries; however, its prevalence is increasing throughout the world, probably because of changes in lifestyle [102]. Although left-sided colonic diverticulosis is more common among elderly patients, a dramatic rise in its incidence has been seen in the younger age groups during recent years [103]. Data from Western countries suggest that about one-fifth of patients with acute diverticulitis are under the age of 50 years [104–106]. Recent data suggest that lifetime risk of developing acute left-sided colonic diverticulitis (ALCD) is only about 4% of all patients with diverticulosis [107]. Evaluation of patients with ALCD is a common problem in the emergency setting with a different severity clinical condition, ranging from localized diverticular inflammation to perforation and fecal peritonitis. There is a lack of well-conducted randomized clinical trials in ALCD, and a large amount of evidence in the literature is of low quality and sometimes conflicting. Since daily decisions in the diagnosis and treatment of acute diverticulitis depend on clinicians' personal preferences rather than evidence-based medicine, the World Society of Emergency Surgery (WSES) developed a classification and a set of recommendations for the management of acute diverticulitis, graded by the levels of evidence available [108–110]. Part of this confusing evidence is related to the fact that the surgical classification (Hinchey) didn't take into consideration computed tomography (CT) evidence- and CT-guided treatments [111]. The widespread availability of CT led to several modifications of the Hinchey classification as, for example, the Neff [112], Sher [113], Ambrosetti [114], Kaiser [115], Mora Lopez [116], and Sallinen [117] classifications, which led to confusing comparisons among studies (Table 29.1). In 2015 a working group of the WSES on acute diverticulitis published a proposal for a new CT-based classification for ALCD [108]. It

Table 29.1 Different classification reported for acute colonic diverticulitis

Classifications of acute diverticulitis by Hinchey et al. into four grades, based on the surgical findings of abscesses and peritonitis
Stage 1 Pericolic abscess
Stage 2 Pelvic, intra-abdominal, or retroperitoneal abscess
Stage 3 Generalized purulent peritonitis
Stage 4 Generalized fecal peritonitis
Neff et al.: based on CT findings
Stage 0 Uncomplicated diverticulitis : diverticula, thickening of the wall, increased density of the pericolic fat
Stage 1 Locally complicated with local abscess
Stage 2 Complicated with pelvic abscess
Stage 3 Complicated with distant abscess
Stage 4 Complicated with other distant complications
Sher et al.: modification of Hinchey classification
Stage 1 Pericolic abscess
Stage 2a Distant abscesses amendable for percutaneous drainage
Stage 2b Complex (pelvic, intra-abdominal, or retroperitoneal) abscesses associated with a possible fistula
Stage 3 Generalized purulent peritonitis
Stage 4 Generalized fecal peritonitis
Ambrosetti et al.: determined by CT scan
Moderate : wall thickening of ≥5 mm, pericolic fat stranding
Severe: wall thickening abscess formation, extraluminal air, extraluminal contrast leak
Kaiser et al. : modified Hinchey classification according to specific CT findings
Stage 0 Mild clinical diverticulitis
Stage 1a Confined pericolic inflammation
Stage 1b Confined pericolic abscess
Stage 2 Pelvic or distant intra-abdominal abscess
Stage 3 Generalized purulent peritonitis
Stage 4 Fecal peritonitis at presentation
Mora-Lopez et al.: modified Neff, based on CT findings
Stage 0 Uncomplicated diverticulitis: diverticula, thickening of the wall, increased density of the pericolic fat
Stage 1a Localized pneumoperitoneum in the form of air bubbles
Stage 1b Local abscess (<4 cm)
Stage 2 Complicated with pelvic abscess (>4 cm)
Stage 3 Complicated with distant abscess, outside pelvis
Stage 4 Complicated with other distant complications, abundant pneumoperitoneum
and/or intra-abdominal free liquid
Sallinen at al.: clinical, radiologic, and physiologic parameters
Stage 1 Uncomplicated diverticulitis
Stage 2 Complicated diverticulitis with small abscess (<6 cm)
Stage 3 Complicated diverticulitis with large abscess (≥6 cm) or distant intraperitoneal or retroperitoneal air
Stage 4 Generalized peritonitis without organ dysfunction
Stage 5 Generalized peritonitis with organ dysfunction
WSES acute diverticulitis working group 2015 based on CT scan findings
Uncomplicated
Stage 0 Diverticula, thickening of the colonic wall, or increased density of the pericolic fat
Complicated
Stage 1a Pericolic air bubbles or little pericolic fluid without abscess (within 5 cm from inflamed bowel segment)
Stage 1b Abscess ≤4 cm
Stage 2a Abscess >4 cm
Stage 2b Distant air (>5 cm from inflamed bowel segment)

(continued)

Table 29.1 (continued)

Classifications of acute diverticulitis by Hinchey et al. into four grades, based on the surgical findings of abscesses and peritonitis
Stage 3 Diffuse fluid without distant free air (no hole in colon)
Stage 4 Diffuse fluid with distant free air (persistent hole in colon)

divides acute diverticulitis into uncomplicated and complicated. In the event of uncomplicated acute diverticulitis (stage 0), the infection does not extend to the peritoneum, and a CT scan shows diverticula, thickening of the colonic wall, or increased density of the pericolic fat. In complicated acute diverticulitis, the infectious process proceeds beyond the colon. The WSES further divides complicated diverticulitis into 6 stages (1a, 1b, 2a, 2b, 3, 4) depending on the presence of pericolic air bubbles or little pericolic fluid (stage 1a) plus abscess ≤4 cm (stage 1b), abscess >4 cm (2a), distant air (>5 cm from inflamed bowel segment, stage 2b), diffuse fluid without distant free air (no hole in the colon, stage 3), or diffuse fluid with distant free air (persistent hole in the colon, stage 4). The WSES working party paper on ALCD was later developed into a set of recommendations for the management of acute diverticulitis, graded in accordance with the levels of evidence available [109, 110, 118].

29.5.1 Diagnosis

An accurate assessment of the patients by a careful clinical evaluation, laboratory inflammation markers, and radiological findings is recommended to identify the best treatment for each patient with ALCD (Fig. 29.1) because the clinical diagnosis of ALCD alone is not sufficiently accurate for patients with suspected diverticulitis. Pain in the lower left abdomen on physical examination and values of C-reactive protein (CRP) >50 mg/L suggests a diagnosis of ALCD, and the clinical suspicion should be solved by a CT scan of the abdomen and pelvis. CT has high sensitivity and specificity and can assess the severity of diverticulitis which is the main information for planning a specific treatment. Abdominal ultrasound (US) may be a useful alternative in the initial evaluation of potentially pregnant or young patients with suspected ALCD. The US has wide availability and easy accessibility, and it may have satisfactory sensitivity and specificity when performed by an expert operator. A step-up approach with CT performed after an inconclusive or negative US may be a safe approach for patients suspected of ALCD.

29.5.2 Therapy of the Immunocompromised Patient

An immunocompromised patient is a patient who does not have the ability to respond normally to infections because of an impaired or weakened immune system. For this reason, immunosuppression is associated with an increase in the complication rate in patients with ALCD. Therefore, elective sigmoid resection after an episode of ALCD should be recommended in immunocompromised patients in the absence of major contraindications.

29.5.3 Treatment of Uncomplicated Acute Diverticulitis

Antimicrobial therapy can be avoided in immunocompetent patients with uncomplicated diverticulitis without systemic manifestations of infection. Patients with CT findings of pericolic air or small fluid collection should be managed by antimicrobial therapy. If patients need antimicrobial therapy, oral administration may be acceptable. Outpatient management is suggested for patients with uncomplicated acute diverticulitis, with no comorbidities. All these patients should be clinically monitored as outpatients and re-evaluated within 7 days to assess for resolution of the inflammatory processes. Earlier revaluation is necessary if the clinical condition deteriorates.

29.5.4 Treatment of Complicated Acute Diverticulitis

Patients with small diverticular abscesses (<4–5 cm) may be treated with antibiotics alone. Patients with large abscesses (>4–5 cm) can best be treated by percutaneous drainage combined with antibiotic treatment (Recommendation 1 C). Whenever percutaneous drainage of the abscess is not feasible or unavailable, based on the clinical conditions, patients with large abscesses can be initially treated by antibiotic therapy alone. However, careful clinical monitoring in an out- or inpatient setting is mandatory. In patients with diverticular abscesses treated conservatively, early colonic evaluation (4–6 weeks) should be planned. Endoscopists and patients usually dislike this recommendation because of the higher risk of iatrogenic perforation. In patients with CT-proven uncomplicated diverticulitis treated conservatively and without other risk factors, early follow-up colonoscopy is not required. Patients aged 50 years or older should participate in colorectal cancer screening programs. Patients with CT findings of distant air without diffuse fluid may be treated by conservative treatment only in selected cases. However, there is a risk of treatment failure, and emergency surgery may be required. Careful monitoring in an inpatient setting is mandatory. A CT scan should be repeated early on the basis of the clinical and laboratory evaluation. If the conservative treatment fails in patients with distant air without diffuse fluid, surgical resection and anastomosis with or without stoma or Hartmann resection is suggested according to the patient clinical conditions and comorbidities. Laparoscopic peritoneal lavage and drainage should not be considered the treatment of choice in patients with generalized peritonitis. Hartmann resection is the surgical procedure advised for managing diffuse peritonitis in critically ill patients and patients with important comorbidities. However, in stable patients without comorbidities, primary resection with anastomosis with or without a diverting stoma may be performed. Emergency laparoscopic sigmoidectomy for the treatment of perforated diverticulitis with generalized peritonitis is feasible in selected patients provided this is performed by experienced surgeons. Damage control surgery strategy may be suggested for clinically unstable patients with diverticular peritonitis (severe sepsis/septic shock).

29.5.5 Elective Surgery

Patient-related factors and not the number of previous episodes of diverticulitis should be considered in planning elective sigmoid resection in patients with ALCD treated conservatively. After a conservatively treated episode of ALCD, an elective sigmoid resection should be planned in high-risk patients, such as immunocompromised patients. The antimicrobial regimen will depend on the underlying clinical condition of the patient, the pathogens presumed to be involved, and the risk factors indicative of major resistance patterns. Discontinuation of antimicrobial treatment should be based on clinical and laboratory criteria, and a short period of postoperative antimicrobial therapy in complicated ALCD is suggested if the source control has been adequately obtained.

29.5.6 Future Areas of Development

The management of patients with ALCD is evolving although a clear understanding of the mechanism underlying recurrence is lacking. Observational studies show that lifestyle factors such as BMI and physical activity can influence the risk of development of acute diverticulitis. Whether these modifications can reduce this risk requires evaluation by controlled trials and planning appropriate adequately powered trials is challenging. An area of ongoing interest is the potential prevention of recurrent episodes of acute diverticulitis by mesalazine associated or not to some probiotics.

29.6 Inflammatory Bowel Diseases (IBD)

Crohn's disease (CD) and ulcerative colitis (UC) are two chronic conditions characterized by inflammation, immunologically mediated, of the gastrointestinal tract.

In CD, the inflammation extends through the entire thickness of the bowel wall from the mucosa to the serosa and usually can interest all the gastrointestinal tracts; it can evolve as mild or moderate inflammatory condition or as severe penetrating (fistulization) or stricturing disease. UC involves specifically colon and rectum and is characterized by localization of inflammation on superficial layers (mucosa and submucosa) of the colon, affecting a variable extent of the large bowel, with a way of spreading from distal to proximal segments.

Both diseases are characterized by relapsing and remitting course and could be associated with intestinal and extraintestinal complications.

These conditions are primarily treated medically, but in patients who become refractory to medical therapy or develop severe complications, surgery may be required.

29.6.1 UC

Patients who develop one or more life-threatening complications require immediate surgery. These complications include colonic perforation, life-threatening gastrointestinal bleeding, and toxic megacolon.

Patients with a severe presentation of UC have frequent loose bloody stools (≥6 per day) with severe abdominal pain and evidence of systemic toxicity, as demonstrated by the presence of fever, tachycardia, anemia, elevated C-reactive protein (CRP), and rapid weight loss.

Fulminant colitis refers to a subgroup of patients with severe ulcerative colitis who have more than ten stools per day, continuous bleeding, abdominal pain, distension, and acute, severe systemic symptoms.

Such patients are at high risk of progressing to toxic megacolon and bowel perforation. Usually, in those patients with clinical signs of systemic toxicity, therapy may include intravenous steroids (prednisolone and methylprednisolone) and intravenous antibiotics (e.g., ciprofloxacin and metronidazole). Bowel rest is recommended in patients with presence of fulminant disease. Nutritional support should be considered in patients who are malnourished. Enteral nutrition is preferred in such patients because it is associated with fewer complications than parenteral nutrition and because it does not deprive the colon of short-chain fatty acids needed for the metabolism and repair of colonic epithelial cells.

In most cases, acute flares of severe colitis respond to medical therapy, and up to 80% of patients with severe colitis will avoid surgical treatment [119]. Patients who have no meaningful clinical response to intravenous glucocorticoids within 7–10 days are considered steroid refractory and should either be proposed for treatment with endovenous immunosuppressants or immunomodulators, such as cyclosporine or an antitumor necrosis factor (anti-TNF) agents. Approximately 25–35% of ulcerative colitis patients will ultimately require surgery for either a complication of the disease or inadequate control of symptoms [120].

Colonic perforation is a rare complication, but patients who develop signs of actual or impending perforation should receive emergent surgery and require immediate colectomy. The associated mortality rate of perforation in UC patients is between 27 and 57% [121].

The development of hemodynamic instability or multi-organ failure is also predictive of a poor outcome. Massive colorectal bleeding occurs in a small percent of patients with UC during their disease course, with the need for immediate surgery. Early signs of multi-organ dysfunction, including disproportionate tachycardia, tachypnea, oliguria, jaundice, hypoxemia, and mental confusion, should prompt an aggressive therapeutic approach including early colectomy [122].

Toxic megacolon, defined by a transverse colon diameter exceeding 6 cm, in UC has been reported in 7–17% of patients requiring hospitalization and is thought to have a lifetime incidence of 0.5–2.5%. Most surgeons consider toxic megacolon to be an indication for emergent colectomy [123].

Surgical management of UC, in the emergent setting, is aimed at removing the inflamed bowel while minimizing morbidity. Total colectomy with a temporary terminal ileostomy is the procedure of choice and can be considered a safe procedure with a low mortality in the absence of a perforation (0–4%) despite a high postoperative complication rate ranging from 23 to 33% [124].

Some surgeons consider that proctectomy in the emergent setting should be avoided [125]. In fact, these patients are often nutritionally depleted, anemic, and on high-dose steroids, which increases the risk of anastomotic complications.

Currently, in elective condition, the most frequent procedure performed, for ulcerative colitis, is the restorative proctocolectomy with ileal pouch-anal anastomosis (IPAA). Its primary benefits are the removal of disease up to the anal transition zone, maintenance of a normal pathway for defecation, and avoidance of a permanent stoma. Despite some morbidities, like pouchitis and increasing number of stools, IPAA is an exceptionally durable and well-tolerated procedure which results in a markedly improved quality of life. Two large, retrospective cohort studies from the Cleveland Clinic and Mayo Clinic have shown that it is a relatively safe procedure, with a low perioperative mortality rate of 0.2–1.0% [126].

29.6.2 CD

Unlike colitis, is characterized by transmural inflammation of the gastrointestinal tract; approximately 80% of patients with CD have small bowel involvement, usually in the distal ileum, with 30% of patients having ileitis exclusively, 50% ileocolitis, and 20% a disease limited to the colon. In contrast to rectal involvement in patients with UC, one-half of CD patients with colitis have sparing of the rectum.

Although advances in the medical management of CD have decreased the need for surgery, it is estimated that between 70 and 90% of Crohn's patients will need a surgical intervention during their life [127]. Within 15 years of diagnosis, 70% of patients may require one or multiple surgical procedures.

The surgical management of CD has changed considerably during the last decades as a result of developments in medical therapy.

The care of CD is primarily a medical therapy. Drugs are evolving rapidly, and symptomatic clinical response may be achieved by second- or third-line medical therapy. So surgery nowadays may be considered as a treatment of last resort. This carries a significant risk because those patients who need surgery will have a more complicated disease and are likely to be at higher risk of septic complications. An essential part of surgical management involves the selection of patients for surgery. Nutritionally compromised patients are likely to benefit from a period of preoperative nutritional support and often require parenteral nutrition support. Some patients with clinical signs of sepsis are likely to benefit from treatment of the septic state, together with nutritional support. Multidisciplinary discussions of therapeutic strategies of individual cases, to optimize medical treatment and surgical timing, are strongly recommended especially for the management of patients with complicated CD, to obtain optimal patient outcome over a lifelong perspective. The specific surgical managements available are multiple, and selection of the most appropriate modality depends on several patient and disease factors.

Sometimes in patients with complicated CD, surgery at an early stage is an effective alternative to medical therapy; for example, patients with abscesses because of internal fistulas (enteric-bladder-vaginal) and/or stenotic bowel segments need surgery at a relatively early stage of the disease rather than after prolonged immunosuppressive treatment which may increase the risk of sepsis and lead to compromised healing capacity [128].

Surgery plays an integral role in treating the complications of CD. However, operative resection is not curative, and, because of the high rate of disease recurrence after segmental bowel resection, the guiding principle of surgical management of CD is the preservation of intestinal length and function. The indications for surgery in patients with small bowel Crohn's disease are failure of medical management and complications of the disease.

Failure of medical management remains the most common indication for surgery in patients with small bowel Crohn's disease. Failure is defined by symptoms that cannot be controlled or progress with maximum medical therapy or in the presence of side effects and the inability of the patient to maintain compliance with a medical regimen.

The most common complication of CD, occurring in 30–50% of patients, is small bowel obstruction [129]. Acute obstruction is more likely to be the result of active inflammation and will often resolve with medical management. In patients with a partial or complete obstruction, refractory to nonsurgical management, surgical intervention is required. Chronic obstruction, which is usually the result of a fixed fibrostenotic intestinal strictures following repeated bouts of inflammation and fibrosis, usually require surgical management. Surgical options include resection of the strictured bowel and stricturoplasty.

Preservation of intestinal length is an important issue, and stricturoplasty represents an alternative to resection and can reduce the risk of short bowel syndrome. Indications for stricturoplasty include short fibrous strictures, diffuse involvement of the small bowel involving multiple strictures, a stricture in someone who has short bowel syndrome or a history of multiple prior small bowel resections, patients with a rapid recurrence of CD manifested as obstruction, or patients with duodenal Crohn's disease. For long strictures (>10 cm) or multiple strictures in proximity, surgical resection with primary anastomosis is required. Stricturoplasties should be avoided in patients with stricture close to a site of resection, in the presence of a perforation, fistula, and phlegmon at the site of stricture. Carcinoma and active bleeding with mucosal disease are also contraindications to stricturoplasty.

Localized ileocecal CD with obstructive symptoms, but without significant evidence of active inflammation, should be treated primarily by surgery. If, however, the patient has had previous ileocecal resection and anastomotic stenosis has occurred, endoscopic dilatation could be tried before undergoing to another intestinal resection. Other complications of CD that may require emergent operative intervention include free perforation, abscesses, fistulae, toxic megacolon, and massive bleeding.

More than 10% of patients with Crohn's disease have an intraabdominal or pelvic abscess during their lifetime. Many patients at risk for perforation or abscess are on corticosteroid therapy, which is known to suppress peritoneal signs and fever and mask the presenting signs of infection. CT scan helps to confirm the diagnosis. Abscesses must be drained, either surgically or percutaneously, and treated with broad-spectrum antibiotics. Although surgical drainage is more often successful, attempting percutaneous drainage may spare an operation to some patients. If an abscess contains enteric contents, it is less likely to resolve without surgical resection.

Fistulas with associated abscess or stricture are other common complications of small bowel CD that require surgery. Enteroenteric fistulas are the most common type of fistula and may be relatively asymptomatic unless a large segment of intestine is bypassed or complications of obstruction arise. Enteroenteric, enterocutaneous, enterovesical, and rectovaginal fistulae are often treated initially according to the principles of fistula healing and medical therapy. If medical therapy is unsuccessful, resection of the involved bowel is required in symptomatic patients.

The surgical management of enteroenteric fistulas generally involves resection of the primary site that has active disease and simple debridement and primary closure of the secondary site, which is usually normal. Enteral fistulas to the vagina and urinary bladder often require primary site resection with repair of the secondary site. Ileosigmoid fistulas may represent an exception to this rule. A minimal sigmoid resection can be performed with minimal morbidity [130].

Less common indications for surgery in small bowel CD include perforation, bleeding, and cancer.

Free perforation is associated with a high mortality, if not treated, and surgical management should involve resection rather than repair. Massive hemorrhage due to Crohn's disease is a rare indication for surgery. Adenocarcinoma of the small intestine is quite rare but increased 12- to 60-fold when compared to the general population. Prognosis is generally poor due to the often advanced stage of disease at the time of diagnosis.

As in small bowel CD, indications for surgery in colonic CD can be grouped into complications of the disease and failure of medical therapy. Indications specific to colonic disease include toxic colitis and development of dysplasia or colorectal cancer. Obstruction from colonic strictures may be present in as many as 17% of patients with Crohn's colitis [131].

The treatment of obstruction and fistula of the colon may differ from that in the small bowel. Benign strictures may be adequately treated by endoscopic balloon dilatation. Stricturoplasty in the colon is not recommended, particularly for the increased risk of cancer in a colonic stricture. Endoscopic dilatation of stenosis in Crohn's disease is the preferred technique for the management of accessible short strictures. Endoscopic dilatation is effective and safe, especially for recurrence after ileocolonic resections, delaying surgery by a mean of 3 years. If surgery is necessary for localized colonic disease (less than a third of patients with colon involvement), then a resection limited to the affected part is preferable. Two segmental resections can be considered for patients with an established indication for surgery when macroscopic disease affects both ends of the colon.

Toxic colitis in CD has a similar presentation to that in UC. Operative indications include perforation, lack of improvement with medical management, fulminant colitis, massive bleeding, and hemodynamic instability. As with ulcerative colitis, the most common procedure for toxic colitis in CD patients is subtotal colectomy and terminal ileostomy. Toxic megacolon and massive bleeding are much less common complications but may require urgent bowel resection when present. Total abdominal colectomy with a Hartmann pouch has been advocated for fulminant toxic megacolon; this allows future restoration of bowel continuity with a sphincter-preserving ileorectal anastomosis. However, a permanent ileostomy may ultimately be required to treat recurrent rectal disease.

Older age at diagnosis of CD, duration of disease (greater than 8 years), and extent of disease (pancolitis) are risk factors for the development of dysplasia or cancer [132].

As with ulcerative colitis, surgery is indicated for a proven malignancy, high-grade dysplasia, or dysplasia associated with nonadenoma-like lesions or mass in colonic CD. Diagnosis and management of low-grade dysplasia are still controversial.

When assessing fistulas involving the colon, it is important to determine the primary site of the fistula. Endoscopic evaluation of the colonic mucosa should be performed. Entero-colonic fistulas are often a result of primary small bowel disease, with the colon only secondarily involved. In these circumstances, it is generally preferable to debride the colonic side of the fistula and close the defect rather than perform a colonic resection.

Perianal disease, including fissures, fistulas, and abscesses, are common problems in the Crohn's population and can have both typical and atypical presentations. Fissures, fistulae, and abscess may be multiple and recurrent, and repeat operations may lead to sphincter damage and incontinence. Damage of even a small amount of sphincter muscle can lead to severe morbidity.

A true abscess requires drainage. Treatment of fistulas depends on the anatomy of the fistula, the amount of sphincter complex involved, as well as the status of the patient's fecal and gas continence. Treatment options include setons, fistula plugs, and mucosal advancement flaps. When a fistula tract can be identified, a seton can be used to prevent premature skin closure and recurrent abscesses. These setons should be left in place for an extended period (up to 6–12 months) to allow complete epithelialization of the tract as visualized by MRI or EUS. In cases where severe perianal disease has destroyed the sphincter, proctectomy with permanent ileostomy may be the only surgical option.

Assuming that CD is still the primary diagnosis, these patients may be assessed for diversion: there is evidence that fecal diversion helps the resolution of perianal disease, at least temporarily [133]. Although as many as 80% of patients with perianal Crohn's manifestations will respond to diversion, relapse may occur despite a stoma, and restoration of intestinal continuity occurs in a minority of patients.

References

1. Zelickson MS, Bronder CM, Johnson BL, Camunas JA, Smith DE, Rawlinson D, Von S, Stone HH, Taylor SM. Helicobacter pylori are not the predominant etiology for peptic ulcers requiring an operation. Am Surg. 2011;77:1054–60.
2. Zittel TT, Jehle EC, Becker HD. Surgical management of peptic ulcer disease today—indication, technique, and outcome. Langenbecks Arch Surg. 2000;385:84–96.
3. Vaira D, Menegatti M, Miglioli M. What is the role of Helicobacter pylori in complicated ulcer disease? Gastroenterology. 1997;113:S78–84.
4. Bas G, Eryilmaz R, Okan I, Sahin M. Risk factors of morbidity and mortality in patients with perforated peptic ulcer. Acta Chir Belg. 2008;108:424–7.
5. Boey J, Choi SK, Poon A, Alagaratnam TT. Risk stratification in perforated duodenal ulcers. A prospective validation of predictive factors. Ann Surg. 1987;205:22–6.
6. Rajesh V, Chandra SS, Smile SR. Risk factors predicting operative mortality in perforated peptic ulcer disease. Trop Gastroenterol. 2003;24:148–50.
7. Chey WD, Wong BC. American College of Gastroenterology guideline on the management of Helicobacter pylori infection. Am J Gastroenterol. 2007;102:1808–25.
8. Vergara M, Catalán M, Gisbert JP, Calvet X. Meta-analysis: role of Helicobacter pylori eradication in the prevention of peptic ulcer in NSAID users. Aliment Pharmacol Ther. 2005;21:1411–8.
9. Grassi R, Romano S, Pinto A, Romano L. Gastro-duodenal perforations: conventional plain film, US and CT findings in 166 consecutive patients. Eur J Radiol. 2004;50:30–6.
10. Kim HC, Yang DM, Kim SW, Park SJ. Gastrointestinal tract perforation: evaluation of MDCT according to perforation site and elapsed time. Eur Radiol. 2014;24:1386–93.
11. Di Saverio S, Bassi M, Smerieri N, Masetti M, Ferrara F, Fabbri C, Ansaloni L, Ghersi S, Serenari M, Coccolini F, Naidoo N, Sartelli M, Tugnoli G, Catena F, Cennamo V, Jovine E. Diagnosis and treatment of perforated or bleeding peptic ulcers: 2013 WSES position paper. World J Emerg Surg. 2014;9:45.
12. Thorsen K, Søreide JA, Søreide K. Scoring systems for outcome prediction in patients with perforated peptic ulcer. Scand J Trauma Resusc Emerg Med. 2013;21:25.
13. Ng EK, Lam YH, Sung JJ, Yung MY, To KF, Chan AC, Lee DW, Law BK, Lau JY, Ling TK, Lau WY, Chung SC. Eradication of Helicobacter pylori prevents recurrence of ulcer after simple closure of duodenal ulcer perforation: randomized controlled trial. Ann Surg. 2000;231:153–8.
14. Kate V, Ananthakrishnan N, Badrinath S. Effect of Helicobacter pylori eradication on the ulcer recurrence rate after simple closure of perforated duodenal ulcer: retrospective and prospective randomized controlled studies. Br J Surg. 2001;88:1054–8.
15. Tran TT, Quandalle P. Long term results of treatment by simple surgical closure of perforated gastroduodenal ulcer followed by eradication of Helicobacter pylori. Ann Chir. 2006;131:502–3.
16. Crofts TJ, Park KG, Steele RJ, Chung SS, Li AK. A randomized trial of nonoperative treatment for perforated peptic ulcer. N Engl J Med. 1989;320:970–3.
17. Bucher P, Oulhaci W, Morel P, Ris F, Huber O. Results of conservative treatment for perforated gastroduodenal ulcers in patients not eligible for surgical repair. Swiss Med Wkly. 2007;137:337–40.
18. Berne TV, Donovan AJ. Nonoperative treatment of perforated duodenal ulcer. Arch Surg. 1989;124:830–2.
19. Mouret P, François Y, Vignal J, Barth X, Lombard-Platet R. Laparoscopic treatment of perforated peptic ulcer. Br J Surg. 1990;77:1006.
20. Song KY, Kim TH, Kim SN, Park CH. Laparoscopic repair of perforated duodenal ulcers: the simple "one-stitch" suture with omental patch technique. Surg Endosc. 2008;22:1632–5.
21. Sanabria A, Villegas MI, Morales Uribe CH. Laparoscopic repair for perforated peptic ulcer disease. Cochrane Database Syst Rev. 2013;(2):CD004778.
22. Bertleff MJ, Lange JF. Laparoscopic correction of perforated peptic ulcer: first choice? A review of literature. Surg Endosc. 2010;24:1231–9.
23. Wright GP, Davis AT, Koehler TJ, Scheeres DE. Cost-efficiency and outcomes in the treatment of perforated peptic ulcer disease: laparoscopic versus open approach. Surgery. 2014;156:1003–7.

24. Thorsen K, Glomsaker TB, von Meer A, Søreide K, Søreide JA. Trends in diagnosis and surgical management of patients with perforated peptic ulcer. J Gastrointest Surg. 2011;15:1329–35.
25. Shelat VG, Ahmed S, Chia CL, Cheah YL. Strict selection criteria during surgical training ensures good outcomes in laparoscopic omental patch repair (LOPR) for perforated peptic ulcer (PPU). Int Surg. 2015;100:370–5.
26. Lau H. Laparoscopic repair of perforated peptic ulcer: a meta-analysis. Surg Endosc. 2004;18:1013–21.
27. Whiteside OJ, Tytherleigh MG, Thrush S, Farouk R, Galland RB. Intra-operative peritoneal lavage—who does it and why? Ann R Coll Surg Engl. 2005;87:255–8.
28. Schein M, Gecelter G, Freinkel W, Gerding H, Becker PJ. Peritoneal lavage in abdominal sepsis. A controlled clinical study. Arch Surg. 1990;125:1132–5.
29. Lanng C, Palnaes Hansen C, Christensen A, Thagaard CS, Lassen M, Klaerke A, Tønnesen H, Ostgaard SE. Perforated gastric ulcer. Br J Surg. 1988;75:758–9.
30. Seow JG, Lim YR, Shelat VG. Low serum albumin may predict the need for gastric resection in patients with perforated peptic ulcer. Eur J Trauma Emerg Surg. 2017;43(3):293–8.
31. Abougergi MS, Travis AC, Saltzman JR. The in-hospital mortality rate for upper GI hemorrhage has decreased over 2 decades in the United States: a nationwide analysis. Gastrointest Endosc. 2015;81(4):882–888.e1.
32. Laine L, Yang H, Chang SC, Datto C. Trends for incidence of hospitalization and death due to GI complications in the United States from 2001 to 2009. Am J Gastroenterol. 2012;107:1190–5.
33. Hearnshaw SA, Logan RFA, Lowe D, Travis SPL, Murphy MF, Palmer KR. Acute upper gastrointestinal bleeding in the UK: patient characteristics, diagnoses and outcomes in the 2007 UK audit. Gut. 2011;60:1327–35.
34. Nahon S, Hagège H, Latrive JP, et al. Epidemiological and prognostic factors involved in upper gastrointestinal bleeding: results of a French prospective multicenter study. Endoscopy. 2012;44:998–1008.
35. Gralnek IM, Dumonceau JM, Kuipers EJ, et al. Diagnosis and management of nonvariceal upper gastrointestinal hemorrhage: European Society of Gastrointestinal Endoscopy (ESGE) Guideline. Endoscopy. 2015;47(10):a1–46.
36. Hwang JH, Fisher DA, Ben-Menachem T, et al. The role of endoscopy in the management of acute non-variceal upper GI bleeding. Gastrointest Endosc. 2012;75:1132–8.
37. Laine L, Jensen DM. Management of patients with ulcer bleeding. Am J Gastroenterol. 2012;107:345–60.
38. Barkun AN, Bardou M, Kuipers EJ, et al. International consensus recommendations on the management of patients with nonvariceal upper gastrointestinal bleeding. Ann Intern Med. 2010;152:101–13.
39. National Institute for Health and Clinical Excellence. Acute upper gastrointestinal bleeding: management. London: National Clinical Guideline Centre at the Royal College of Physicians; 2012.
40. Bai Y, Guo JF, Li ZS. Meta-analysis: erythromycin before endoscopy for acute upper gastrointestinal bleeding. Aliment Pharmacol Ther. 2011;34:166–71.
41. Laine L, McQuaid KR. Endoscopic therapy for bleeding ulcers: an evidence-based approach based on meta-analyses of randomized controlled trials. Clin Gastroenterol Hepatol. 2009;7:33–47.
42. Laine L, Peterson WL. Bleeding peptic ulcer. N Engl J Med. 1994;331:717–27.
43. Lau JYW, Sung JJY, Lam Y, et al. Endoscopic retreatment compared with surgery in patients with recurrent bleeding after initial endoscopic control of bleeding ulcers. N Engl J Med. 1999;340:751–6.
44. Cheadle WG, Garr EE, Richardson JD. The importance of early diagnosis of small bowel obstruction. Am Surg. 1988;54(9):565–9.
45. Markogiannakis H, Messaris E, Dardamanis D, Pararas N, Tzertzemelis D, Giannopoulos P, Larentzakis A, Lagoudianakis E, Manouras A, Bramis I. Acute mechanical bowel obstruction: clinical presentation, etiology management and outcome. World J Gastroenterol. 2007;13(3):432.
46. Mullan CP, Siewert B, Eisenberg RL. Small bowel obstruction. AJR Am J Roentgenol. 2012;198(2):W105–17.
47. Di S, et al. Bologna guidelines for diagnosis and management of adhesive small bowel obstruction (ASBO): 2013 update of the evidence-based guidelines from the world society of emergency surgery ASBO working group. World J Emerg Surg. 2013;8:42.
48. Choi HK, Law WL. Therapeutic value of gastrografin in adhesive small bowel obstruction after unsuccessful conservative treatment: a prospective randomized trial. Ann Surg. 2002;236:1–6.
49. Abbas S, Bissett IP, Parry BR. Oral water soluble contrast for the management of adhesive small bowel obstruction. Cochrane Database Syst Rev. 2007;(3).
50. Li MZ, Lian L, Xiao LB, Wu WH, He YL, Song XM. Laparoscopic versus open adhesiolysis in patients with adhesive small bowel obstruction: a systematic review and meta-analysis. Am J Surg. 2012;204(5):779–86.
51. Marinis A, Yiallourou A, Samanides L, Dafnios N, Anastasopoulos G, Vassiliou I, Theodosopoulos T. Intussusception of the bowel in adults: a review. World J Gastroenterol. 2009;15(4):407–11.
52. Reijnen HA, Joosten HJ, de Boer HH. Diagnosis and treatment of adult intussusception. Am J Surg. 1989;158:25–8.
53. Boyle MJ, Arkell LJ, Williams JT. Ultrasonic diagnosis of adult intussusception. Am J Gastroenterol. 1993;88:617–8.
54. Takeuchi K, Tsuzuki Y, Ando T, Sekihara M, Hara T, Kori T, Kuwano H. The diagnosis and treatment of adult intussusception. J Clin Gastroenterol. 2003;36:18–21.
55. Haas EM, Etter EL, Ellis S, Taylor TV. Adult intussusception. Am J Surg. 2003;186(1):75–6.
56. Clavien PA, Richon J, Burgan S, Rohner A. Gallstone ileus. Can J Surg. 1990;77:737–42.
57. Turner AR, Bhimji SS. Ileus, gallstone. [Updated 2017 Oct 6]. In: StatPearls [Internet]. Treasure Island, FL: StatPearls Publishing; 2018. Available from: https://www.ncbi.nlm.nih.gov/books/NBK430834/
58. Sackmann M, Holl J, Haerlin M, Souerbruch T, Hoermann R, Heinkelein J, et al. Gallstone ileus successfully treated by shockwave lithotripsy. Dig Dis Sci. 1991;36:1794–5.
59. Soto D, Evan SJ, Kavic MS. Laparoscopic management of gallstone ileus. J Soc Laparosc Surg. 2001;5:279–85.
60. Ravikumar R, Williams JG. The operative management of gallstone ileus. Ann R Coll Surg Engl. 2010;92:279–81.
61. Rodriguez-Sanjuan JC, Casado F, Fernandez MJ, Morales DJ, Naranjo A. Cholecystectomy and fistula closure versus enterolithotomy alone in gallstone ileus. Br J Surg. 1997;84:834–7.
62. Halabi WJ, Kang CY, Ketana N, Lafaro KJ, Nguyen VQ, Stamos MJ, Imagawa DK, Demirijan AN. Surgery for gallstone ileus: a nationwide comparison of trends and outcomes. Ann Surg. 2014;259(2):329–35.
63. Ploneda-Valencia CF, Gallo-Morales M, Navarro-Muniz E, Bautista-Lopez CA, de la Cereda-Trujillo LF, Rea-Azpeitia LA, Lopez-Lizarraga CR. Gallstone ileus: an overview of the literature. Rev Gastroenterol Mex. 2017;82(3):248–54.
64. Nuno-Guzman CM, Marin-Contreras ME, Fiqueroa-Snachez M, Corona JL. Gallstone ileus, clinical presentation, diagnostic and treatment approach. World Gastrointestinal Surg. 2016;8(1):65–76.
65. Tauris P. Gallstone ileus revealed by endoscopy. Endoscopy. 1977;9(2):104–6.
66. Bedogni G, Contini S, Meinero M, Pedrazzoli C, Piccinini GC. Pyloroduodenal obstruction due to a biliary stone (Bouveret's Syndrome) managed by endoscopic extraction. Gastrointest Endosc. 1985;31(1):36–8.
67. Alsolaiman MM, Reitz C, Nawaras AT, Rodgers JB, Maliakkal BJ. BMC Gastroenterol. 2002;2(1):15–8.
68. Ballantyne GH. Review of sigmoid volvulus: historyand results of treatment. Dis Colon Rectum. 1982;25(5):494–50.

69. Grossmann EM, Longo WE, Stratton MD, Virgo KS, Johnson FE. Sigmoid volvulus in Department of Veterans Affairs Medical Centers. Dis Colon Rectum. 2000;43(3):414–8.
70. Ranjan A, Jain V, Sharma S, Gupta DK. Sigmoid volvulus: an uncommon complication of Hirschsprung's disease. BMJ Case Rep. 2016;2016.
71. Safioleas M, Chatziconstantinou C, Felekouras E, Stamatakos M, Papaconstantinou I, Smirnis A, Safioleas P, Kostakis A. Clinical considerations and therapeutic strategy for sigmoid volvulus in the elderly: a study of 33 cases. World J Gastroenterol. 2007;13(6):921–4.
72. Tan KK, Chong CS, Sim R. Management of acute sigmoid volvulus: an institution's experience over 9 years. World J Surg. 2010;34(8):1943–8. https://doi.org/10.1007/s00268-010-0563-8.
73. Ifversen AK, Kjaer DW. More patients should undergo surgery after sigmoid volvulus. World J Gastroenterol. 2014;20(48): 18384–9. https://doi.org/10.3748/wjg.v20.i48.18384.
74. Larkin JO, Thekiso TB, Waldron R, Barry K, Eustace PW. Recurrent sigmoid volvulus—early resection may obviate later emergency surgery and reduce morbidity and mortality. Ann R Coll Surg Engl. 2009;91:205–9.
75. Bagarani M, Conde AS, Longo R, Italiano A, Terenzi A, Venuto G. Sigmoid volvulus in West Africa: a prospective study on surgical treatments. Dis Colon Rectum. 1993;36:186–90.
76. Suleyman O, Kessaf AA, Ayhan KM. Sigmoid volvulus: long-term surgical outcomes and review of the literature. S Afr J Surg. 2012;50(1):9–15.
77. Al-Alawi IK. Percutaneous endoscopic colostomy: a new technique for the treatment of recurrent sigmoid volvulus. Saudi J Gastroenterol. 2010;16(2):120–1.
78. Choi D, Carter R. Endoscopic sigmoidopexy: a safer way to treat sigmoid volvulus? J R Coll Surg Edinb. 1998;43(1):64.
79. Frank L, Moran A, Beaton C. Use of percutaneous endoscopic colostomy (PEC) to treat sigmoid volvulus: a systematic review. Endosc Int Open. 2016 Jul;4(7):E737–41.
80. Hsu YC, Perng CL, Chen CK, Tsai JJ, Lin HJ. Conservative management of chronic gastric volvulus: 44 cases over 5 years. World J Gastroenterol. 2010;16(33):4200–5.
81. Zuiki T, Hosoya Y, Lefor AK, Tanaka H, Komatsubara T, Miyahara Y, Sanada Y, Ohki J, Sekiguchi C, Sata N. The management of gastric volvulus in elderly patients. Int J Surg Case Rep. 2016;29:88–93. https://doi.org/10.1016/j.ijscr.2016.10.058. Epub 2016 Oct 27.
82. Tsang TK, Walker R, Yu DJ. Endoscopic reduction of gastric volvulus: the alpha-loop maneuver. Gastrointest Endosc. 1995;42:244–8.
83. Tanner NC. Chronic and recurrent volvulus of the stomach with late results of "colonic displacement". Am J Surg. 1968;115(4):505–15.
84. Ballantyne GH. Review of sigmoid volvulus: history and results of treatment. Dis Colon Rectum. 1982;25(5):494–50.
85. Coulie B, Camilleri M. Intestinal pseudo-obstruction. Annu Rev Med. 1999;50:37–55.
86. Alwan MH, van Rij AM. Acute colonic pseudo-obstruction. Aust N Z J Surg. 1998;68(2):129–32.
87. Bernardi MP, Warrier S, Lynch AC, Heriot AG. Acute and chronic pseudo-obstruction: a current update. ANZ J Surg. 2015;85(10):709–14.
88. Durai R. Colonic pseudo-obstruction. Singapore Med J. 2009;50: 237–44.
89. De Giorgio R, Sarnelli G, Corinaldesi R, Stanghellini V. Advances in our understanding of the pathology of chronic intestinal pseudo-obstruction. Gut. 2004;53:1549–52.
90. De Giorgio R, Cogliandro RF, Barbara G, Corinaldesi R, Stanghellini V. Chronic intestinal pseudo-obstruction: clinical features, diagnosis, and therapy. Gastroenterol Clin North Am. 2011;40(4):787–807.
91. Choi JS, Lim JS, Kim H, Choi JY, Kim MJ, Kim NK, et al. Colonic pseudoobstruction: CT findings. AJR Am J Roentgenol. 2008;190(6):1521–6.
92. Laine L. Management of acute colonic pseudo-obstruction. N Engl J Med. 1999;341(3):192–3.
93. Hutchinson R, Griffiths C. Acute colonic pseudo-obstruction: a pharmacological approach. Ann R Coll Surg Engl. 1992;74(5):364–7.
94. Paran H, Silverberg D, Mayo A, Shwartz I, Neufeld D, Freund U. Treatment of acute colonic pseudo-obstruction with neostigmine. J Am Coll Surg. 2000;190(3):315–8.
95. Geller A, Petersen BT, Gostout CJ. Endoscopic decompression for acute colonic pseudo-obstruction. Gastrointest Endosc. 1996;44:144–50.
96. Harrison ME, Anderson MA, Appalaneni V, et al. The role of endoscopy in the management of patients with known and suspected colonic obstruction and pseudo-obstruction. Gastrointest Endosc. 2010;71:669–79.
97. Sgouros SN, Vlachogiannakos J, Vassiliadis K, Bergele C, Stefanidis G, Nastos H, et al. Effect of polyethylene glycol electrolyte balanced solution on patients with acute colonic pseudo obstruction after resolution of colonic dilation: a prospective, randomised, placebo controlled trial. Gut. 2006;55(5):638–42.
98. Benacci JC, Wolff BG. Cecostomy: therapeutic indications and results. Dis Colon Rectum. 1995;38:530–4.
99. Ramage JI, Baron TH. Percutaneous endoscopic cecostomy: a case series. Gastrointest Endosc. 2003;57:752–5.
100. Ross SW, Oommen B, Wormer BA, Walters AL, Augenstein VA, Heniford BT, Sing RF, Christmas AB. Acute colonic pseudo-obstruction: defining the epidemiology, treatment, and adverse outcomes of Ogilvie's syndrome. Am Surg. 2016;82(2):102–11.
101. Dorudi S, Berry AR, Kettlewell MG. Acute colonic pseudo-obstruction. Br J Surg. 1992;79(2):99–103.
102. Weizman AV, Nguyen GC. Diverticular disease: epidemiology and management. Can J Gastroenterol. 2011;25:385–9.
103. Schoetz DJ. Diverticular disease of the colon: a century-old problem. Dis Colon Rectum. 1999;42:703–9.
104. Collins D, Winter DC. Modern concepts in diverticular disease. J Clin Gastroenterol. 2015;49:358–69.
105. Warner E, Crighton EJ, Moineddin R, Mamdani M, Upshur R. Fourteen-year study of hospital admissions for diverticular disease in Ontario. Can J Gastroenterol. 2007;21:97–9.
106. Jamal Talabani A, Lydersen S, Endreseth BH, Edna TH. Major increase in admission- and incidence rates of acute colonic diverticulitis. Int J Colorectal Dis. 2014;29:937–45.
107. Shahedi K, Fuller G, Bolus R, Cohen E, Vu M, Shah R, et al. Long-term risk of acute diverticulitis among patients with incidental diverticulosis found during colonoscopy. Clin Gastroenterol Hepatol. 2013;11:1609–13.
108. Sartelli M, Moore FA, Ansaloni L, Di Saverio S, Coccolini F, Griffiths EA, et al. A proposal for a CT driven classification of left colon acute diverticulitis. World J Emerg Surg. 2015;10:3.
109. Guyatt G, Gutterman D, Baumann MH, Addrizzo-Harris D, Hylek EM, Phillips B, et al. Grading strength of recommendations and quality of evidence in clinical guidelines: report from an American College of Chest Physicians task force. Chest. 2006;129:174–81.
110. Brozek JL, Akl EA, Jaeschke R, Lang DM, Bossuyt P, Glasziou P, et al. Grading quality of evidence and strength of recommendations in clinical practice guidelines: Part 2 of 3. The GRADE approach to grading quality of evidence about diagnostic tests and strategies. Allergy. 2009;64:1109–16.
111. Hinchey EJ, Schaal PH, Richards MB. Treatment of perforated diverticular disease of the colon. Adv Surg. 1978;12:85–109.
112. Neff CC, vansonnenberg E. CT of diverticulitis. Diagnosis and treatment. Radiol Clin North Am. 1989;27:743–52.
113. Sher ME, Agachan F, Bortul M, Nogueras JJ, Weiss EG, Wexner SD. Laparoscopic surgery for diverticulitis. Surg Endosc. 1997;11:264–7.

114. Ambrosetti P, Becker C, Terrier F. Colonic diverticulitis: impact of imaging on surgical management—a prospective study of 542 patients. Eur Radiol. 2002;12:1145–9.
115. Kaiser AM, Jiang JK, Lake JP, Ault G, Artinyan A, Gonzalez-Ruiz C, et al. The management of complicated diverticulitis and the role of computed tomography. Am J Gastroenterol. 2005;100:910–7.
116. Mora Lopez L, Serra Pla S, Serra-Aracil X, Ballesteros E, Navarro S. Application of a modified Neff classification to patients with uncomplicated diverticulitis. Colorectal Dis. 2013;15:1442–7.
117. Sallinen VJ, Leppäniemi AK, Mentula PJ. Staging of acute diverticulitis based on clinical, radiologic, and physiologic parameters. J Trauma Acute Care Surg. 2015;78:543–51.
118. Sartelli M, et al. WSES Guidelines for the management of acute left sided colonic diverticulitis in the emergency setting. World J Emerg Surg. 2016;11:37.
119. Katz JA. Medical and surgical management of severe colitis. Semin Gastrointest Dis. 2000;11:18–32.
120. Berg DF, Bahadursingh AM, Kaminski DL, Longo WE. Acute surgical emergencies in inflammatory bowel disease. Am J Surg. 2002;184:45–51.
121. Greenstein AJ, Barth JA, Sachar DB, Aufses AH Jr. Free colonic perforation without dilatation in ulcerative colitis. Am J Surg. 1986;152:272–5.
122. Caprilli R, Latella G, Vernia P, Frieri G. Multiple organ dysfunction in ulcerative colitis. Am J Gastroenterol. 2000;95:1258–62.
123. Latella G, Vernia P, Viscido A, Frieri G, Cadau G, Cocco A, Cossu A, Tomei E, Caprilli R. GI distension in severe ulcerative colitis. Am J Gastroenterol. 2002;97:1169–75.
124. Alves A, Panis Y, Bouhnik Y, Maylin V, Lavergne-Slove A, Valleur P. Subtotal colectomy for severe acute colitis: a 20-year experience of a tertiary care center with an aggressive and early surgical policy. J Am Coll Surg. 2003;197:379–85.
125. Khubchandani IT, Kontostolis SB. Outcome of ileorectal anastomosis in an inflammatory bowel disease surgery experience of three decades. Arch Surg. 1994;129:866–9.
126. Fazio VW, Ziv Y, Church JM, Oakley JR, Lavery IC, Milsom JW, Schroeder TK. Ileal pouch-anal anastomoses complications and function in 1005 patients. Ann Surg. 1995;222:120–7.
127. Gardiner KR, Dasari BV. Operative management of small bowel Crohn's disease. Surg Clin North Am. 2007;87:587–610.
128. Dignass A, Van Assche G, Lindsay JO, Lémann M, Söderholm J, Colombel JF, Danese S, D'Hoore A, Gassull M, Gomollón F, Hommes DW, Michetti P, O'Morain C, Öresland T, Windsor A, Stange EF, Travis SP. The second European evidence-based consensus on the diagnosis and management of Crohn's disease: current management. J Crohns Colitis. 2010;4(1):28–62.
129. Hurst RD, Molinari M, Chung TP, Rubin M, Michelassi F. Prospective study of the features, indications, and surgical treatment in 513 consecutive patients affected by Crohn's disease. Surgery. 1997;122:661–7; discussion 667–668.
130. Fazio VW, Wilk P, Turnbull RB Jr, Jagelman DG. The dilemma of Crohn's disease: ileosigmoidal fistula complicating Crohn's disease. Dis Colon Rectum. 1977;20:381–6.
131. Yamazaki Y, Ribeiro MB, Sachar DB, Aufses AH Jr, Greenstein AJ. Malignant colorectal strictures in Crohn's disease. Am J Gastroenterol. 1991;86:882–5.
132. Maykel JA, Hagerman G, Mellgren AF, Li SY, Alavi K, Baxter NN, Madoff RD. Crohn's colitis: the incidence of dysplasia and adenocarcinoma in surgical patients. Dis Colon Rectum. 2006;49:950–7.
133. Hong MK, Craig Lynch A, Bell S, Woods RJ, Keck JO, Johnston MJ, Heriot AG. Faecal diversion in the management of perianal Crohn's disease. Colorectal Dis. 2011;13(2):171–6.

Updates in the Management of Acute Pancreatitis

30

Giampaolo Perri, Giovanni Marchegiani, and Claudio Bassi

Key Points

- Definition of acute pancreatitis (AP) is based on the fulfillment of "two out of three" of the following criteria: clinical (upper abdominal pain), laboratory (serum amylase or lipase >3 upper limit of normal), and/or imaging.
- There are three grades of severity of acute pancreatitis, namely, the mild, the moderately severe, and the severe.
- Systemic inflammatory response syndrome (SIRS) is advised to predict severe acute pancreatitis at admission, while systemic organ dysfunction is a main determinant of clinical outcome.
- Local complications of acute pancreatitis include acute peripancreatic fluid collections, pancreatic pseudocysts, acute necrotic collections, and walled-off necrosis. Each collection may be either sterile or infected.
- Initial management of acute pancreatitis consists of supportive care with fluid resuscitation, pain control, and nutritional support.
- Invasive intervention should be delayed whenever possible until at least 4 weeks after initial presentation to allow the collection to become "walled-off."
- Primarily, image-guided percutaneous catheter drainage or endoscopic transluminal drainage, followed, if necessary, by endoscopic or surgical necrosectomy represent the optimal interventional strategy for patients with suspected or confirmed infected necrosis.
- Late, well-organized, and predominantly fluid collections are usually managed by endoscopic or laparoscopic transgastric drainage.
- Early ERCP is no longer recommended in AP, regardless of disease severity, in the absence of coexisting biliary sepsis.

30.1 General Description

Acute pancreatitis (AP) is an acute inflammatory process of the pancreas. Although its pathogenesis is still not completely understood, several conditions are known to induce AP, with gallstones and chronic alcohol abuse accounting for two-thirds or more cases in the United States [1], where AP is the leading gastrointestinal cause of hospitalization [2].

For most of the cases, AP is a self-limiting illness. In uncomplicated attacks, management involves appropriate supportive care until resolution, followed by treatment of the precipitating cause, reducing the chance of a future attack. For a minority of patients, AP is a life-threatening condition that results in prolonged hospital admission and significant mortality, requiring early recognition of the high-risk group and multidisciplinary management of complications in centers of high expertise.

Mortality ranges from 3% in patients with interstitial edematous pancreatitis to 17% in patients who develop pancreatic necrosis [3, 4]. Mortality within the first 2 weeks (early death) is usually due to systemic inflammatory response syndrome (SIRS) and organ failure, while after this time frame, it is usually due to local pancreatic complications related to pancreatic necrosis and sepsis [5, 6].

G. Perri · G. Marchegiani (✉) · C. Bassi
Department of Surgery, Pancreas Institute, Verona University Hospital, Verona, Italy
e-mail: giovanni.marchegiani@ospedaleuniverona.it; Claudio.bassi@univr.it

P. Aseni et al. (eds.), *Operative Techniques and Recent Advances in Acute Care and Emergency Surgery*,
https://doi.org/10.1007/978-3-319-95114-0_30

Early triage, improvements in intensive care management, nutritional support, and timely and appropriate intervention for local complications with less invasive approaches at high-volume centers have led to the drop of the overall mortality during the last decades.

30.2 Clinical Presentation, Diagnosis, and Severity Assessment

Patients with AP present with persistent, severe, epigastric abdominal pain. The pain is often radiating to the back, associated with nausea and vomiting, and may persist for several hours.

In patients with hereditary, metabolic, or alcoholic AP, the onset of pain may be less abrupt, and the pain itself may be poorly localized than in patients with gallstone pancreatitis.

The degree of systemic disturbance is variable, as well as the physical findings of severe cases, such as abdominal tenderness, obstructive jaundice (due to choledocholithiasis or edema of the pancreatic head), and ecchymotic discoloration due to retroperitoneal bleeding.

Per the 2012 revision of the Atlanta classification, the definition of acute pancreatitis (AP) is based on the fulfillment of "two out of three" of the following criteria (regardless of etiology): clinical (upper abdominal pain), laboratory (serum amylase or lipase >3 upper limit of normal), and/or imaging (computed tomography (CT), magnetic resonance (MR), ultrasonography (US)) criteria [7].

Cross-sectional imaging may be useful but not strictly necessary to diagnose acute pancreatitis. Exceptions include a prolonged period between onset of symptoms and presentation (lipase and amylase may have normalized), unconscious patients, or suspicion of duodenal perforation.

In general, AP can be subdivided into two types (Table 30.1):

Table 30.1 Radiologic/pathologic classification of AP

Interstitial edematous pancreatitis	Necrotizing pancreatitis
Acute inflammation of the pancreatic parenchyma and peripancreatic tissues, without recognizable tissue necrosis	Inflammation associated with pancreatic or peripancreatic necrosis

This represents a radiologic and pathologic classification, to be distinguished from a clinical assessment of severity. Defining the severity of AP is crucial to stratify patients into subgroups, based on the presence of transient or persistent organ failure and local or systemic complications, allowing for appropriate early triage to intensive care units (ICUs) and selection of patients for specific interventions.

The revised Atlanta classification [7] defines three grades of severity of pancreatitis (Table 30.2):

Table 30.2 Grades of severity of AP according to the revised Atlanta classification [7]

Mild AP	Moderately severe AP	Severe AP
Absence of organ failure or local complications	Presence of transient organ failure (resolving within 48 h) or local complications developing in the absence of organ failure	Presence of persistent organ failure (>48 h) with or without local complications

Local complications of acute pancreatitis include peripancreatic fluid collections, pancreatic pseudocysts, acute necrotic collections, and walled-off necrosis [7]. Organ failure (OF) is defined as a score of two or more for any one of three organ systems (respiratory, cardiovascular, or renal) using the modified Marshall scoring system [8].

Many predictive models (e.g., APACHEII, Ranson, and modified Glasgow score) have been developed to predict the clinical outcome of AP during the early hours after hospital admission, based on clinical, laboratory, and radiologic risk factors [9].

Per the IAP/APA guidelines [10], systemic inflammatory response syndrome (SIRS) is advised to predict severe AP at admission and persistent SIRS at 48 h; identifying patients at risk of developing systemic organ dysfunction represents a main determinant of clinical outcome [11].

SIRS is defined by the presence of two or more of the following four criteria (Table 30.3):

Table 30.3 Definition of SIRS [12]; two or more of the criteria should be present

SIRS
• Temperature <36 °C or >38 °C
• Heart rate >90/min
• Respiratory rate >20/min
• White blood cells (<4 × 10^9/L, >12 × 10^9/L) or 10% bands

Other scores can be used only 24–48 h after the disease onset and have not been shown to be consistently superior to the assessment of SIRS or the APACHE II score.

30.3 Management of Acute Pancreatitis

30.3.1 Management of the Early Phase

The initial evaluation of AP should comprehend a clinical examination to assess for early fluid losses, organ failure (cardiovascular, respiratory, or renal compromise), and severity, with the measurement of the SIRS score and APACHE II score. Patients with severe AP should be admitted to an intensive care unit (ICU) for optimal support.

Amylase and lipase value is useful for the diagnosis, but serial measurements in patients with acknowledged AP are not useful to predict severity, prognosis, or following management.

Since the extent of pancreatic and peripancreatic necrosis may only become apparent 72 h after the onset of AP, cross-sectional imaging (e.g., abdominal computed tomography (CT) scan) is not recommended at initial presentation if the diagnosis is already established.

Initial management of AP consists of supportive care with fluid resuscitation, pain control, and nutritional support.

30.3.1.1 Fluid Resuscitation

In the initial stages (within the first 12–24 h) of acute pancreatitis, fluid replacement has been associated with a reduction in morbidity and mortality [13–15] with decreased rates of persistent SIRS and organ failure.

Current guidelines [10] recommend Ringer's lactate for initial fluid resuscitation in acute pancreatitis; a multicenter RCT demonstrated that resuscitation with Ringer's lactate decreased the incidence of SIRS when compared to resuscitation with normal saline in 40 patients with acute pancreatitis [16]. A fluid infusion rate of 5–10 mL/kg/h is recommended, until resuscitation goals are reached. A total infusion of 2500–4000 mL in the first 24 h will likely suit, as an overly aggressive fluid therapy was demonstrated to increase morbidity and mortality [17, 18]. Resuscitation goals should be guided by restoration of physiologic homeostasis using markers such as pressure and flow parameters, urine output, lactate, mixed venous oxygen saturation, and base deficit.

30.3.1.2 Pain Control

Pain is a predominant symptom in AP and should be treated with analgesics according to its duration and severity. A review by the Cochrane has examined five randomized trials comparing different analgesics in AP, founding no evidence of increased complications related to opioid use [19], scaling down the historical concern about their potential (for morphine in particular) to induce sphincter of Oddi spasm and exacerbate the severity of AP. Opioids were instead associated with a reduction in the need for supplementary analgesia, and therefore remains the treatment of choice for the vast majority of patients.

Protracted, severe pain may require administration of opioids through a specific patient-controlled analgesia (PCA) pump.

30.3.1.3 Nutritional Support

Oral feeding in predicted mild pancreatitis can be restarted once abdominal pain is decreasing and inflammatory markers are significantly improving. Those patients can often be managed with intravenous hydration alone since recovery occurs rapidly (usually within 1 week).

Enteral tube feeding, either via naso-jejunal or nasogastric route [20, 21], should be the primary therapy in patients with predicted severe acute pancreatitis requiring nutritional support; two meta-analyses demonstrated enteral nutrition's superiority in decreasing systemic infections, multi-organ failure, need for surgical intervention, and mortality when compared with parenteral nutrition [22, 23]. The reasons for such superiority might be explained by a reduction of bacterial translocation and consequent infection of pancreatic necrosis, as enteral feeding contributes to gut barrier function and the higher rate of complications associated with the parenteral route, including line sepsis. Moreover, enteral feeding is also less expensive than parenteral nutrition. Parenteral nutrition can be administered in acute pancreatitis as a second-line therapy if naso-jejunal tube feeding is not tolerated and nutritional support is further required.

30.3.2 Management of Systemic Complications

30.3.2.1 Antibiotics

A secondary infection of pancreatic necrosis appears in about the 40% of patients with necrotizing AP, leading to a second peak in mortality between 2 and 4 weeks after the disease onset. However, international guidelines do not recommend intravenous antibiotic prophylaxis for the prevention of infectious complications in acute pancreatitis [10]. A Cochrane review and a meta-analysis of 14 RCTs showed no benefits from antibiotic prophilaxis [24, 25]. Probiotic prophylaxis and selective gut decontamination are not currently recommended for the prevention of infectious complications.

Intravenous antibiotics should be given in case of suspected infection of necrotizing pancreatitis or extrapancreatic infections; when an infection is suspected, antibiotics should be started while the source of the infection is being determined.

30.3.2.2 Organ Failure

The most common systemic complication in AP is single or multiple organ failure (OF). Regardless of its etiology, OF often requires transfer to the ICU and could be represented by respiratory, cardiovascular, renal, and intestinal severe dysfunction. Noninvasive respiratory support or mechanical ventilation, volume resuscitation, and vasoactive agents with invasive monitoring and dialysis could be required.

Gastrointestinal failure manifests as nausea, vomiting, and abdominal distension and occurs because of reduced perfusion, with a failure to tolerate enteral nutrition and the breakdown of the gut barrier function, with bacterial translocation leading eventually to infected pancreatic necrosis.

30.3.2.3 Abdominal Compartment Syndrome

Abdominal compartment syndrome (ACS) is defined as a sustained intraabdominal pressure greater than 20 mmHg (with or without abdominal arterial perfusion pressure <60 mmHg) that is associated with new-onset OF [26].

According to the available international guidelines, measurement of intra-abdominal pressure via the bladder should be considered in patients with severe acute pancreatitis associated with mechanical ventilation, especially in case of clinical deterioration, as intra-abdominal hypertension (IAH) contributes to the development of OF.

The first approach for the treatment should be medical, targeting the main contributors to IAH like hollow viscera volume (with nasogastric drainage, prokinetics, rectal tubes, and endoscopic decompression, if necessary), intravascular and extravascular volume status, and abdominal wall compliance (analgesia, sedation, and neuromuscular blockade if necessary).

Due to the risk of infecting a previously sterile pancreatic necrosis and the significant fluid losses that may occur in the open abdomen, invasive decompression should only be used after a multidisciplinary discussion in patients with a sustained intra-abdominal pressure >25 mmHg with a new onset of organ failure refractory to medical therapy. Invasive treatment options include percutaneous catheter drainage of ascites, midline laparostomy, bilateral subcostal laparostomy, or subcutaneous midline fasciotomy.

30.3.3 Management of Local Complications

The revised Atlanta classification [7] divides AP into three discrete grades of severity (mild, moderately severe, and severe) based on the absence or presence of systemic and/or local complications.

Furthermore, local complications are categorized based on the time from presentation (< or >4 weeks) and on the presence of necrosis (Table 30.4). Each collection may be in addiction, sterile, or infected.

Acute, non-necrotic fluid collections develop during the first days of AP, usually without a defined wall, and remain asymptomatic. They resolve spontaneously without the need for drainage, as only less than 10% of acute fluid collections persist beyond 4 weeks as pancreatic pseudocysts [27]. Failure of resolution could be related to the presence of necrosis or main pancreatic duct (MPD) interruption.

Intervention for an acute necrotic collection in the first weeks has a high risk of mortality and morbidity [28]. Invasive intervention (i.e., percutaneous catheter drainage, endoscopic transluminal drainage/necrosectomy, minimally invasive or open necrosectomy) should be delayed whenever possible until at least 4 weeks after initial presentation to allow the collection to become "walled-off," following a philosophy expressed by the "3D" concept: delay, drain, and debride.

Common indications for intervention in necrotizing AP, according to the IAP guidelines [10], are indicated in Table 30.5:

Pancreatic infection is a leading cause of morbidity and mortality in acute necrotizing pancreatitis, affecting one-third of patients with pancreatic necrosis [29], often later in the clinical course (10 days) [30, 31].

The presence of gas in peripancreatic collections at CT is considered as evidence of infected necrosis, irrespective of the source of the gas [32]. Fine needle aspiration of collections to detect bacteria is not routinely indicated, because of the high risk of false-negative results [33] and lack of evidence assessing the possible benefits in shortening the period to diagnosis of infection and tailoring the antibiotic treatment.

Traditionally, primary open necrosectomy has been the treatment of choice in infected necrotizing AP. Nowadays, there is consensus in the current literature toward a principle of early organ and nutritional support, followed ideally by

Table 30.4 Local complications in AP according to 2012 revised Atlanta classification [7]

Time	Necrosis −	Necrosis +
<4 weeks	*Acute peripancreatic fluid collection* (Peripancreatic fluid associated with interstitial edematous pancreatitis with no associated peripancreatic necrosis)	*Acute necrotic collection* (A collection containing variable amounts of both fluid and necrosis; the necrosis can involve the pancreatic parenchyma and/ or the extrapancreatic tissues)
>4 weeks	*Pancreatic pseudocyst* (An encapsulated collection of fluid with a well-defined inflammatory wall usually outside the pancreas with minimal or no necrosis)	*Walled-off necrosis* (A mature, encapsulated collection of pancreatic or extrapancreatic necrosis that has developed a well-defined inflammatory wall)
Infection	Each collection type may be sterile or infected	

Table 30.5 Indications for intervention in necrotizing AP according to the IAP/APA guidelines [10]

Common indications	Uncommon indications
• Clinically suspected/ documented infected necrosis with clinical deterioration (preferably when walled-off/>4 weeks) • In the absence of documented infected necrosis, ongoing organ failure for several weeks after the onset of AP (preferably when walled-off/>4 weeks)	• Abdominal compartment syndrome • Ongoing acute bleeding • Bowel ischemia • Ongoing gastric outlet, intestinal, or biliary obstruction due to mass effect from large walled-off necrosis (>4–8 weeks) • Persistent symptoms (pain, "unwellness") in patient with walled-off necrosis without signs of infection (>8 weeks) • Disconnected duct syndrome (>8 weeks)

delayed minimally invasive intervention within a step-up approach, whenever possible.

A fluid collection with minimal or no necrotic component that became persistent ("true" pancreatic pseudocysts) is very uncommon. The great majority of persistent pancreatic collections, especially when requiring intervention, has at least a small amount of necrosis with varying degrees of fluid content.

Indication for sterile, necrotizing AP is gastric, intestinal, or biliary obstruction due to mass effect or persistent symptoms (e.g., pain, "persistent unwellness") in patients without signs of infection, arbitrarily >4–8 weeks after onset of acute pancreatitis.

Furthermore, a disconnected duct syndrome (i.e., full transection of the pancreatic duct in the presence of pancreatic necrosis) seems to be very common in patients during the follow-up after necrotizing pancreatitis, most of them requiring an intervention later than 8 weeks after the acute attack [34].

Conventional management of late pancreatic collections was by open pancreatic cystogastrostomy, but with the development in interventional radiology, therapeutic endoscopy, and minimal access surgery, new minimally invasive techniques have been employed as alternatives to the traditional approach. Late, well-organized, and predominantly fluid collections are usually managed by endoscopic or laparoscopic transgastric drainage. There is a consistent degree of overlap between the early and late patient populations, most studies in the literature including heterogeneous groups.

30.3.3.1 Percutaneous, Endoscopic, and Surgical Step-Up Approach

Primarily, image-guided percutaneous (retroperitoneal) catheter drainage (Fig. 30.1) or endoscopic transluminal drainage (Fig. 30.2), followed, if necessary, by endoscopic or surgical necrosectomy, represents the optimal interventional strategy for patients with suspected or confirmed infected necrosis.

The PANTER (PAncreatitis, Necrosectomy versus sTEp-up appRoach) trial from the Dutch Pancreatitis Study Group, a multicenter RCT accounting 88 patients with (suspected) infected necrotizing pancreatitis, demonstrated how this approach decreased death or major complications, as well as costs, when compared to primary open necrosectomy [35].

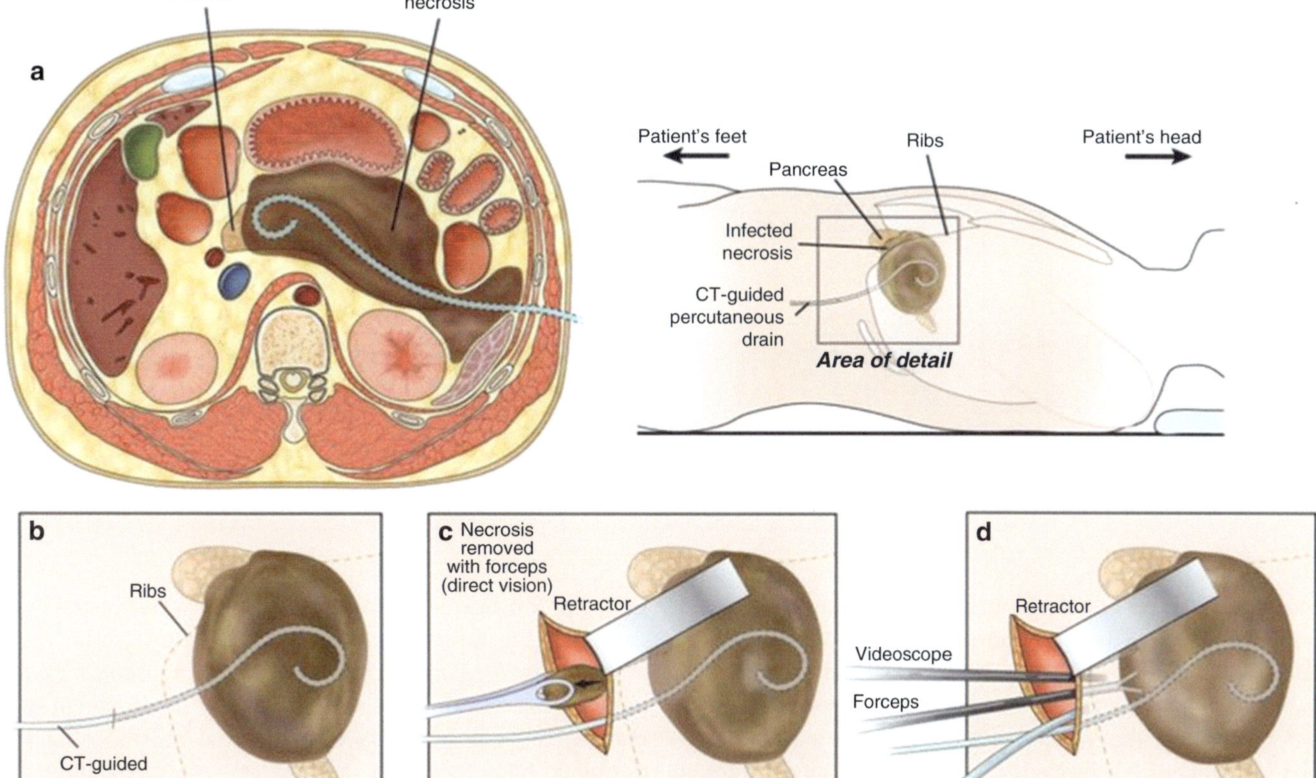

Fig. 30.1 Surgical step-up approach. (**a**) Peripancreatic collection drained by a percutaneous catheter inserted through the left retroperitoneal space. (**b**) Detail of CT-guided percutaneous drain. (**c**) First necrosis removal under direct vision, following the percutaneous drain. (**d**) Video-assisted retroperitoneal debridement (VARD). *Courtesy of S van Brunschot* et al., *Dutch Pancreatitis Study Group* [37]

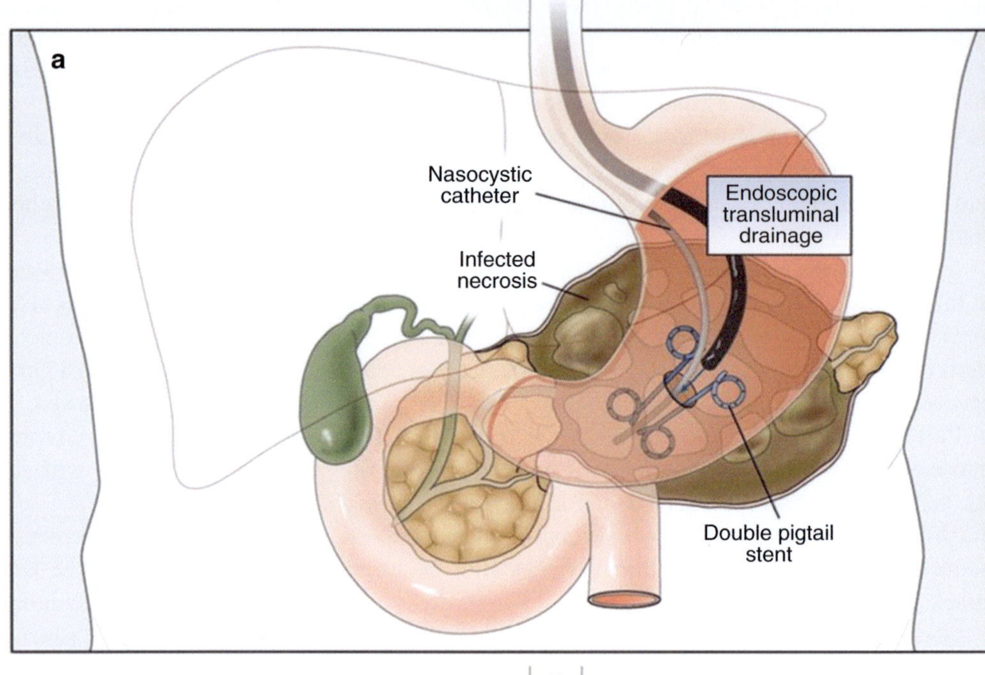

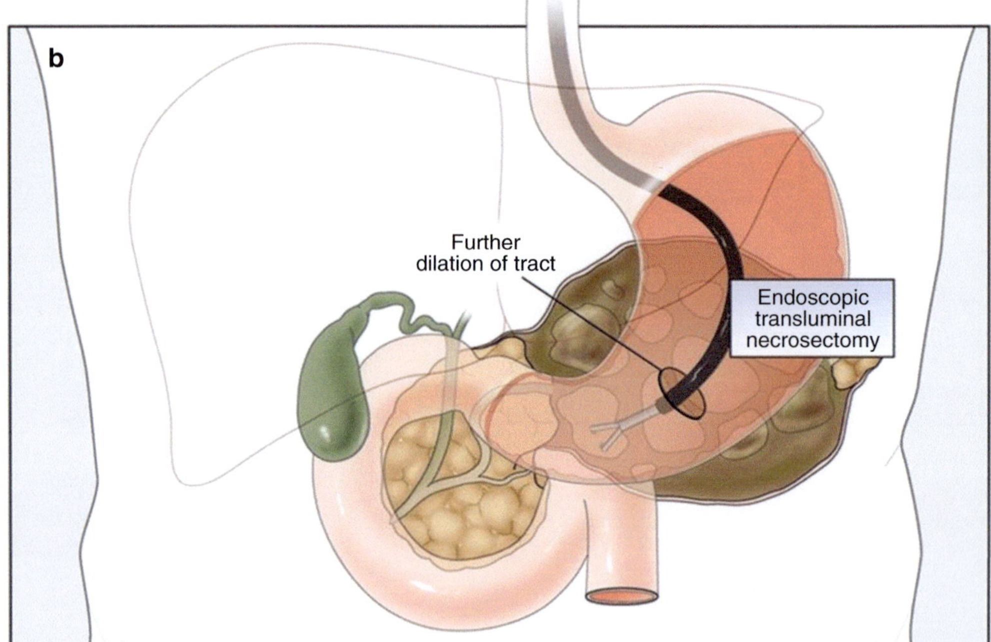

Fig. 30.2 Endoscopic step-up approach. (**a**) Endoscopic transluminal drainage (ETD) followed by (**b**) endoscopic transluminal necrosectomy (ETN) *Courtesy of S van Brunschot* et al., *Dutch Pancreatitis Study Group* [37]

Indeed, 35% of patients in the trial were successfully managed with percutaneous drainage alone and did not require subsequent debridement. Left retroperitoneal catheter drainage can facilitate minimally invasive retroperitoneal necrosectomy. After placement, the catheters undergo vigorous manual irrigation with isotonic saline every several days, creating a "closed circuit" of lavages, combined with contrast CT scans to follow the necrotic debridement and, if necessary, the placement of progressively larger-bore catheters (up to 24–28 French).

Even if percutaneous catheter drainage seems to be technically feasible in >95% of patients with infected necrosis [35], a promising alternative gaining worldwide popularity is natural orifice transluminal endoscopic surgery (NOTES) for drainage and/or necrosectomy purpose. Endoscopic cystogastrostomy was initially reported for the management of a mature pancreatic abscess with minimal necrosis, but the technique has evolved in the past 10 years, extending the indication also for debridement of necrosis.

First, the collection is punctured through the gastric wall, followed by balloon dilatation of the tract. Two double-pigtail stents and a nasocystic catheter for continuous postoperative irrigation are usually placed (endoscopic transluminal drainage). Later, the cystostomy tract is dilated, the collection is entered with an endoscope, and necrosectomy is performed (endoscopic transluminal necrosectomy).

Several trials are testing NOTES efficacy compared to minimally invasive intervention (the early pilot PENGUIN [36] trial and the ongoing TENSION [37] trial from the Dutch Study Group) showing at least an equivalence between the two procedures.

The choice of initial percutaneous or endoscopic drainage is largely based on the position of the collection, with some authors suggesting to approach lateral collections and those extending behind the colon from the left or right flank and to prefer endoscopic drainage for those medial collections where a percutaneous route is compromised by overlying the bowel, spleen, or liver.

As discussed before, transgastric EUS-guided drainage is also the treatment of choice for late, persistent pancreatic collections, especially when mainly fluid. If catheter or endoscopic drainage fails, the optimal method of necrosectomy is still debated [38]. Minimally invasive necrosectomy seems to be associated with a decreased risk of complications and death as compared to open necrosectomy [39]. Several minimally invasive approaches have been described for surgical necrosectomy, including percutaneous minimally invasive retroperitoneal (MIRP) [40] necrosectomy, video-assisted retroperitoneal debridement (VARD) [41], and laparoscopic cystogastrostomy [42].

30.3.3.2 Video-Assisted Retroperitoneal Debridement (VARD)

VARD [41] is a drain-guided, minimally invasive retroperitoneal procedure requiring a 5 cm flank incision (Fig. 30.1). Using the retroperitoneal drain for guidance, the collection is entered, and loosely adherent necrosis is removed under video assistance (using a 0° laparoscope). The cavity is cleared of the infected/purulent material using a standard suction device. At the end of the procedure, two large-bore surgical drains are inserted, and a continuous postoperative lavage system is installed.

30.3.3.3 Laparoscopic Cystogastrostomy

In large, organized, solid, predominant post-acute collections, EUS-guided transgastric approach is at risk of inadequate drainage, with the necessity of repeated interventions. The improvements of laparoscopic operative technique and equipment have refocused interest on the potential of a single laparoscopic intervention. The current technique has evolved from the intragastric approach to a true laparoscopic transgastric approach [42], which requires an anterior gastrotomy for access and cystogastrostomy creation through the posterior gastric wall.

30.3.3.4 Laparoscopic Open Necrosectomy

Open necrosectomy is currently practiced and remains popular even with the increasing experience in minimally invasive approaches, especially in case of failure of those first-line treatments, extended infected necrosis (>50% of the pancreas), or severe acute complications (intestinal perforation, ACS, intracavitary bleeding).

The abdomen is entered though a midline or a bilateral subcostal incision preferred for minimizing contamination of the lower abdomen and allowing lateral access. The pancreas is exposed by dividing the gastrocolic ligament or gastrohepatic omentum by accessing into the lesser sac, allowing for manual necrosectomy.

In terms of necrosectomy, all described procedures are generally similar, being the main differences in terms of how they prevent recurrence of an infected collection within the debridement cavity.

In classical open necrosectomy approach with open packing, as described in 1987 by Bradley [43], the abdomen remains open following the debridement, and the cavity is packed with a laparostomy, with drains in place, allowing for resolution with healing by secondary intention. This open packing technique has been reported to have higher incidence of incisional hernias, bleeding, fistulae, and mortality rates [44].

For these reasons, the concept has been re-elaborated to mimic the step-up approach, with a first intervention aimed to a more conservative debridement, followed by planned reinterventions with sequential pack changes, in response to the bleeding and fistulation that can arise following aggressive necrosectomy. The pancreatic bed is drained or packed, and the abdomen is closed by suturing mesh or a zipper to the fascial edges of the wound [45].

Open necrosectomy could also be followed by closed packing, where a thorough debridement and infected tissue removal is followed by a primary closure of the abdomen, with the goal to achieve sepsis control and minimize the need for reoperation or subsequent drainage [46, 47]. Silicone drains (Jackson-Pratt) may be placed and removed sequentially. After debridement, reconstruction of a closed peripancreatic compartment is also possible, by suturing the gastrocolic and duodenocolic ligaments over large-bore drains, allowing side to side continuous lavage [48].

30.3.4 Management of Underlying Conditions Predisposing to Acute Pancreatitis

30.3.4.1 ERCP and Cholecystectomy

Controversy still exists regarding the role and timing of endoscopic retrograde cholangiopancreatography (ERCP) in gallstone pancreatitis. A recent meta-analysis of 7 RCTs including 757 patients found no evidence of benefits of early routine ERCP in the attempt of avoiding mortality or local/systemic complications, regardless of the predicted severity of biliary AP [49]. Therefore, early ERCP is no longer recommended in acute pancreatitis, regardless of disease severity, in the absence of coexisting biliary sepsis/cholangitis.

For patients with evidence of biliary obstruction and AP, without signs of cholangitis, evidence is still lacking. Early ERCP remains recommended in the presence of jaundice and SIRS, while patients with jaundice without SIRS can be managed with observation for 24–48 h. ERCP is therefore reserved for those cases in which bilirubin levels arise after the acute attack or persist as elevated, as in most of the cases, a spontaneous passage of stones causes only a temporary jaundice. This last group of patients could benefit of MRCP or EUS to assess the presence or absence of persistent ductal stones.

Cholecystectomy should be delayed in patients with peripancreatic collections until the collections either resolve or if they persist beyond 6 weeks, a timeline after which cholecystectomy can be safely performed [50].

On the other hand, cholecystectomy during index admission for mild biliary pancreatitis appears safe and is recommended over interval cholecystectomy, as demonstrated by a recent RCT [51], reducing the rate of recurrent gallstone-related complications, with a very low risk of cholecystectomy-related complications.

Case Scenario

A 54-year-old male patient admitted to the ICU for severe biliary AP with no clinical signs of sepsis was treated with initial fluid resuscitation and enteral nutrition.

After initial stabilization, the patient was then transferred to the gastroenterology unit and underwent ERCP with sphincterotomy. A CT scan performed 3 weeks after the presentation showed extended (>50% of the pancreatic gland) walled-off sterile necrosis (Fig. 30.3). The patient was at that time asymptomatic, and oral food intake was administered.

1. What would be the preferred treatment?
   A. Follow-up with CT scan at 7–10 days
   B. Percutaneous drainage
   C. Endoscopic cystogastrostomy
   D. Open necrosectomy

Four days later, the patient presented clinical and laboratory signs of sepsis. An urgent CT scan was repeated (Fig. 30.4).

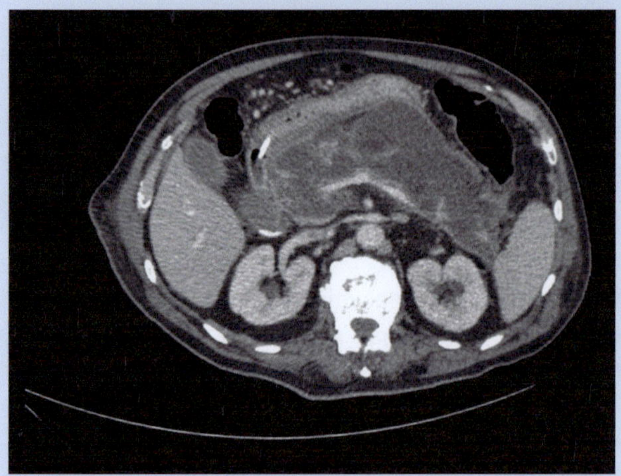

Fig. 30.3 Third week CT scan

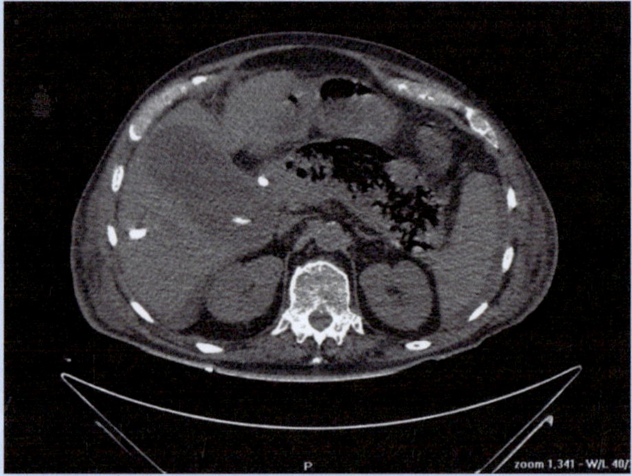

Fig. 30.4 CT scan performed while the patient presented with sepsis showed gas in peripancreatic collections

2. What would be the preferred treatment?
   A. Conservative treatment with parenteral antibiotics
   B. Percutaneous drainage
   C. Laparoscopic cystogastrostomy
   D. Open necrosectomy

The infected necrotic collection was drained via a percutaneous drainage (20F) (Fig. 30.5).

Cultural examination of the necrotic output permitted a targeted antibiotic treatment.

The patients developed persistent sepsis associated with hemodynamic instability despite the previously described treatment.

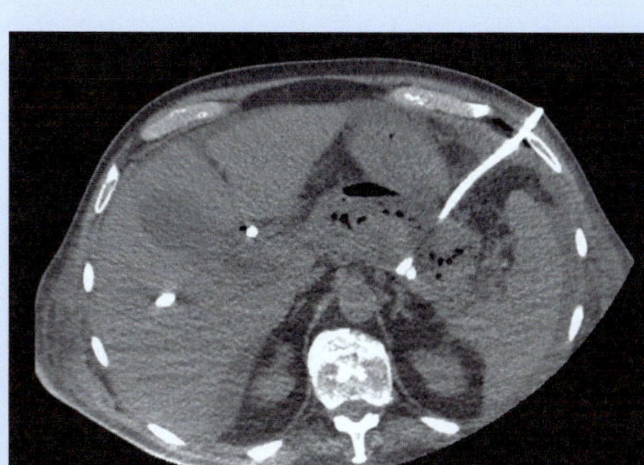

Fig. 30.5 Percutaneous 20F drainage with a left-side access

3. What would be the next step of intervention (extended pancreatic infected necrosis, sepsis)?
   A. Change of antibiotic therapy
   B. Percutaneous drainage with larger-bore drain
   C. Endoscopic transluminal drainage and necrosectomy
   D. Open necrosectomy

Please see Chap. 58 for the correct answer.

References

1. Yadav D, Lowenfels AB. Trends in the epidemiology of the first attack of acute pancreatitis: a systematic review. Pancreas. 2006;33:323–30.
2. Peery AF, Dellon ES, Lund J, et al. Burden of gastrointestinal disease in the United States: 2012 update. Gastroenterology. 2012;143:1179.
3. Singh VK, Bollen TL, Wu BU, et al. An assessment of the severity of interstitial pancreatitis. Clin Gastroenterol Hepatol. 2011;9:1098.
4. van Santvoort HC, Bakker OJ, Bollen TL, et al. A conservative and minimally invasive approach to necrotizing pancreatitis improves outcome. Gastroenterology. 2011;141:1254.
5. Gloor B, Müller CA, Worni M, et al. Late mortality in patients with severe acute pancreatitis. Br J Surg. 2001;88:975.
6. Mutinga M, Rosenbluth A, Tenner SM, et al. Does mortality occur early or late in acute pancreatitis? Int J Pancreatol. 2000;28:91.
7. Banks PA, et al. Classification of acute pancreatitis—2012: revision of the Atlanta classification and definitions by international consensus. Gut. 2013;62:102–11.
8. Marshall JC, et al. Multiple organ dysfunction score: a reliable descriptor of a complex clinical outcome. Crit Care Med. 1995;23:1638.
9. Gomatos IP, et al. Prognostic markers in acute pancreatitis. Expert Rev Mol Diagn. 2014;14:333–46.
10. Working Group IAP/APA Acute Pancreatitis Guidelines. IAP/APA evidence-based guidelines for the management of acute pancreatitis. Pancreatology. 2013;13:e1.
11. Buter A, et al. Dynamic nature of early organ dysfunction determines outcome in acute pancreatitis. Br J Surg. 2002;89:298–302.
12. American College of Chest Physicians/Society of Critical Care Medicine consensus conference: definitions for sepsis and organ failure and guidelines for the use of innovative therapies in sepsis. Crit Care Med. 1992;20:864–74.
13. Talukdar R, et al. Early management of severe acute pancreatitis. Curr Gastroenterol Rep. 2011;13:123.
14. Trikudanathan G, et al. Current controversies in fluid resuscitation in acute pancreatitis: a systematic review. Pancreas. 2012;41:827.
15. Gardner TB, et al. Faster rate of initial fluid resuscitation in severe acute pancreatitis diminishes in hospital mortality. Pancreatology. 2009;9:770.
16. Wu BU, et al. Lactated Ringer's solution reduces systemic inflammation compared with saline in patients with acute pancreatitis. Clin Gastroenterol Hepatol. 2011;9:710–7.
17. Mao EQ, et al. Fluid therapy for severe acute pancreatitis in acute response stage. Chin Med J. 2009;122:169–73.
18. Mao EQ, et al. Rapid hemodilution is associated with increased sepsis and mortality among patients with severe acute pancreatitis. Chin Med J. 2010;123:1639–44.
19. Basurto Ona X, et al. Opioids for acute pancreatitis pain. Cochrane Database Syst Rev. 2013;(7):CD009179.
20. Eatock FC, et al. A randomized study of early nasogastric versus nasojejunal feeding in severe acute pancreatitis. Am J Gastroenterol. 2005;100:432–9.
21. Kumar A, et al. Early enteral nutrition in severe acute pancreatitis: a prospective randomized controlled trial comparing nasojejunal and nasogastric routes. J Clin Gastroenterol. 2006;40:431–4.
22. Al-Omran M, et al. Enteral versus parenteral nutrition for acute pancreatitis. Cochrane Database Syst Rev. 2010;(1):CD002837.
23. Petrov MS, et al. Enteral nutrition and the risk of mortality and infectious complications in patients with severe acute pancreatitis: a meta-analysis of randomized trials. Arch Surg. 2008;143:1111–7.
24. Villatoro E, et al. Antibiotic therapy for prophylaxis against infection of pancreatic necrosis in acute pancreatitis. Cochrane Database Syst Rev. 2010;(5):CD002941.
25. Wittau M, et al. Systematic review and meta-analysis of antibiotic prophylaxis in severe acute pancreatitis. Scand J Gastroenterol. 2011;46:261–70.
26. Kirkpatrick AW, et al. Intra-abdominal hypertension and the abdominal compartment syndrome: updated consensus definitions and clinical practice guidelines from the World Society of the Abdominal Compartment Syndrome. Intensive Care Med. 2013;39:1190–206.
27. Lenhart DK, Balthazar EJ. MDCT of acute mild (nonnecrotizing) pancreatitis: abdominal complications and fate of fluid collections. AJR Am J Roentgenol. 2008;190:643.
28. Mier J, et al. Early versus late necrosectomy in severe necrotizing pancreatitis. Am J Surg. 1997;173:71–5.
29. Banks PA, Freeman ML, Practice Parameters Committee of the American College of Gastroenterology. Practice guidelines in acute pancreatitis. Am J Gastroenterol. 2006;101:2379.
30. Beger HG, Bittner R, Block S, Büchler M. Bacterial contamination of pancreatic necrosis. A prospective clinical study. Gastroenterology. 1986;91:433.
31. Bradley EL 3rd, Allen K. A prospective longitudinal study of observation versus surgical intervention in the management of necrotizing pancreatitis. Am J Surg. 1991;161:19.

32. Buchler M, et al. Acute pancreatitis: when and how to operate. Dig Dis. 1992;10:354–62.
33. Rodriguez JR, Razo AO, Targarona J, Thayer SP, Rattner DW, Warshaw AL, et al. Debridement and closed packing for sterile or infected necrotizing pancreatitis: insights into indications and outcomes in 167 patients. Ann Surg. 2008;247:294–9.
34. Beck WC, Bhutani MS, Raju GS, Nealon WH. Surgical management of late sequelae in survivors of an episode of acute necrotizing pancreatitis. J Am Coll Surg. 2012;214:682–8.
35. van Santvoort HC, et al. A step-up approach or open necrosectomy for necrotizing pancreatitis. N Engl J Med. 2010;362:1491–502.
36. Bakker OJ, et al. Endoscopic transgastric vs surgical necrosectomy for infected necrotizing pancreatitis: a randomized trial. JAMA. 2012;307:1053–61.
37. van Brunschot S, et al. Transluminal endoscopic step-up approach versus minimally invasive surgical step-up approach in patients with infected necrotising pancreatitis (TENSION trial): design and rationale of a randomised controlled multicenter trial [ISRCTN09186711]. BMC Gastroenterol. 2013;13:161.
38. Sorrentino L, Chiara O, Mutignani M, et al. Combined totally mini-invasive approach in necrotizing pancreatitis: a case report and systematic literature review. World J Emerg Surg. 2017;12:16.
39. Raraty MG, Halloran CM, Dodd S, Ghaneh P, Connor S, Evans J, et al. Minimal access retroperitoneal pancreatic necrosectomy: improvement in morbidity and mortality with a less invasive approach. Ann Surg. 2010;251:787–93.
40. Carter CR, et al. Percutaneous necrosectomy and sinus tract endoscopy in the management of infected pancreatic necrosis: an initial experience. Ann Surg. 2000;232:175–80.
41. Horvath KD, et al. A technique for laparoscopic-assisted percutaneous drainage of infected pancreatic necrosis and pancreatic abscess. Surg Endosc. 2001;15:1221–5.
42. Gibson SC, et al. 'Step-port' laparoscopic cystogastrostomy for the management of organized solid predominant post-acute fluid collections after severe acute pancreatitis. HPB (Oxford). 2014;16:170–6.
43. Bradley EL 3rd. Management of infected pancreatic necrosis by open drainage. Ann Surg. 1987;206:542–50.
44. Heinrich S, et al. Evidence-based treatment of acute pancreatitis: a look at established paradigms. Ann Surg. 2006;243:154–68.
45. Radenkovic DV, et al. Planned staged reoperative necrosectomy using an abdominal zipper in the treatment of necrotizing pancreatitis. Surg Today. 2005;35:833–40.
46. Pezzilli R, et al. A prospective multicentre survey on the treatment of acute pancreatitis in Italy. Dig Liver Dis. 2007;39:838–46.
47. Fernandez-del Castillo C, et al. Debridement and closed packing for the treatment of necrotizing pancreatitis. Ann Surg. 1998;228:676–84.
48. Wig JD, et al. Closed lesser sac lavage in the management of pancreatic necrosis. J Gastroenterol Hepatol. 2004;19:1010–5.
49. Tse F, Yuan Y. Early routine endoscopic retrograde cholangiopancreatography strategy versus early conservative management strategy in acute gallstone pancreatitis. Cochrane Database Syst Rev. 2012;5:CD009779.
50. Nealon WH, Bawduniak J, Walser EM. Appropriate timing of cholecystectomy in patients who present with moderate to severe gallstone-associated acute pancreatitis with peripancreatic fluid collections. Ann Surg. 2004;239:741–9.
51. da Costa DW, Bouwense SA, Schepers NJ. Same-admission versus interval cholecystectomy for mild gallstone pancreatitis (PONCHO): a multicentre randomised controlled trial. Lancet. 2015;386(10000):1261–8.

31 Updates in the Management of Cholecystitis, Cholangitis, and Obstructive Jaundice

Mattia Garancini, Alessandro Redaelli, Marco Dinelli, Davide Leni, Davide Fior, and Vittorio Giardini

Key Points

- Management of cholecystitis, cholangitis, and obstructive jaundice should invite the clinician to take into account the different but synergistic points of view of the surgeons, endoscopists, and interventional radiologists.
- Most patients with acute cholecystitis should be offered laparoscopic cholecystectomy as soon as possible on their first admission; if cholecystectomy is indicated but cannot be performed within 7 days from onset of symptoms, it should be delayed 45–60 days after symptom onset.
- Patients' risk stratification and severity grading following the international guidelines of acute cholecystitis are an important parameter; a clearer stratification of risk parameters for severity of cholecystitis and a stratification in terms of patients' comorbidities, malnutrition, and reduced functional reserve can help in choosing the best clinical/surgical management of complex cases and improve the patients' outcome.
- ERCP is recognized as the first-line treatment of cholangitis to provide bile drainage after well-managed sepsis and systemic complications; as alternative approaches (in particular in case of failed ERCP), EUS-guided drainage is an emerging procedure with fewer severe adverse events compared to percutaneous biliary drainage.

M. Garancini (✉) · V. Giardini
Unit of Advanced Laparoscopic Surgery, Department of General Surgery II, San Gerardo Hospital, Monza (MB), Italy

A. Redaelli · M. Dinelli
Department of Interventional Endoscopy, San Gerardo Hospital, Monza (MB), Italy
e-mail: a.redaelli@asst-monza.it; m.dinelli@asst-monza.it

D. Leni · D. Fior
Department of Radiology, San Gerardo Hospital, Monza (MB), Italy
e-mail: d.leni@asst-monza.it; d.fior@asst-monza.it

31.1 Introduction

The treatment of hepatic and biliary emergency represents a clinical challenge for the acute care surgeons, endoscopists, and interventional radiologists. The complexity of the biliary anatomy and the potentially high risk of bleeding and iatrogenic damage during invasive procedures make the management of hepatic and biliary emergency a risky undertaking.

Acute calculous cholecystitis is initially a chemical inflammation; nevertheless, it is quite regularly complicated by bacterial invasion from the gut. Polymicrobial infections are frequently observed. Bactibilia occurs in at least 60% of the early stage of acute cholecystitis (particularly in the elderly) and may result in severe septic complications. Similarly, the acute inflammation and infection of the biliary tree mostly result from a combination of biliary obstruction and bacterial growth in bile. Progressive biliary obstruction causes an increase in intraductal pressure, which eventually leads to cholangio-venous and cholangio-lymphatic reflux. Translocation of bacteria from the biliary tree into the bloodstream may result in a septic shock, a potentially fatal complication. Consequently, outlining a clinical algorithm for the diagnostic and therapeutic pathway for every single patient is of paramount importance.

In this chapter, we discuss the recent updates in the management of cholecystitis, cholangitis, and obstructive jaundice taking into account the different but synergistic

P. Aseni et al. (eds.), *Operative Techniques and Recent Advances in Acute Care and Emergency Surgery*,
https://doi.org/10.1007/978-3-319-95114-0_31

points of views from the surgeons, endoscopists, and interventional radiologists.

31.2 Cholecystitis

Acute calculus cholecystitis (ACC) is a very common disease; in developed countries, 10–15% of the adult population is affected by gallstones, and ACC occur in 20% of patients with symptomatic disease, with wide variation in severity [1–5]. The publication in 2007 of the Tokyo Guidelines for the management of acute cholangitis and cholecystitis in the *Journal of Hepato-Biliary-Pancreatic Surgery* represented the first comprehensive report stating diagnostic criteria, severity assessment, and treatment criteria for acute cholecystitis [6]; this article represents a cornerstone for following international guidelines. Since 2007 several other algorithms were proposed for the treatment of ACC; one of the most comprehensive and reliable is the 2016 WSES guidelines in acute calculous cholecystitis [7] (Fig. 31.1). Treatment of ACC traditionally includes antibiotics, cholecystectomy, and cholecystostomy. Several areas of uncertainty persist on this topic, in particular concerning the diagnostic criteria, the best antimicrobial therapy to be managed, the evaluation of associated common bile duct stones, the identification of "high-risk" patients, the surgical timing, and the type of treatment including the surgical procedure. The type of surgical approach is not more considered a matter of discussion since laparoscopic cholecystectomy must be considered a preferable option versus open cholecystectomy. This statement is supported by a high quality of evidence. Nevertheless, it's recommended that surgeons should never hesitate to convert to open surgery to prevent injuries when they experience technical difficulties during the procedure.

With the aim to report an extensive update, all of these arguments will be here discussed point by point.

31.2.1 Diagnostic Criteria

There are no critical updates in recent literature. There is no single clinical or laboratory finding with sufficient diagnostic accuracy to establish or exclude ACC. The diagnosis of ACC can be based on a combination of clinical history, a complete clinical examination, laboratory tests, and imaging studies. In the presence of clinical suspicion, the finding of an inflamed gallbladder (wall thickening >3 mm, wall edema, distension of the gallbladder, peri-cholecystic fat density, peri-cholecystic fluid collection) containing stones is the cornerstone for an appropriate diagnosis, and abdominal ultrasound (AUS) represents the most important tool to reach full evidence. A large meta-analysis published in 2012 indicated heterogeneity in the diagnostic performance of AUS, showing for this procedure a sensitivity of 81% (95% CI, 75–87%) and a specificity of 83% (95% CI, 74–89%) [8]. Diagnostic accuracy of magnetic resonance imaging (MRI) is similar to one of AUS; hepatobiliary iminodiacetic acid scan (HIDA scan) has the highest sensitivity and specificity

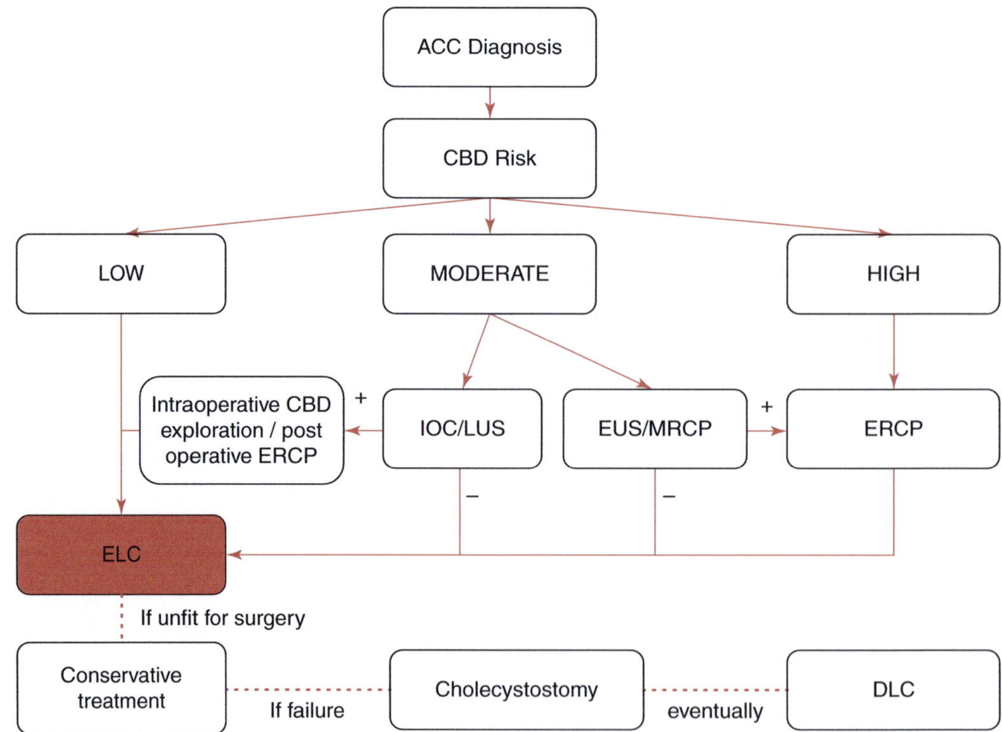

Fig. 31.1 Comprehensive algorithm for the treatment of acute calculous cholecystitis. ACC from the 2016 WSES guidelines on acute calculous cholecystitis [7]. *ACC* acute calculous cholecystitis; *CBD* common bile duct; *DLC* delayed laparoscopic cholecystectomy; *ELC* early laparoscopic cholecystectomy; *ERCP* endoscopic retrograde cholangiopancreatography; *EUS* endoscopic ultrasound; *IOC* intraoperative cholangiography; *LUS* laparoscopic ultrasound; *MRCP* magnetic resonance cholangiopancreatography

for acute cholecystitis, although its scarce availability, the long time required to perform the test, and exposure to ionizing radiation limit its use.

31.2.2 Surgical Timing

The optimal timing of elective laparoscopic cholecystectomy (ELC) in patients with ACC is still controversial. Some authors recommend to perform surgery within 24 h of hospital admission, others as soon as possible, and some others within 72 h–7 days from the symptom onset [9–14]. Early surgery is associated with a lower risk of major bile duct injury, a similar conversion rate, and a shorter total hospital length of stay and prevents a 20% risk of recurrent gallstone symptoms within 3 months from the initial diagnosis of cholecystitis [9, 15–17]. Nevertheless, the analyzed trials lack a homogeneous definition of early surgical treatment. "Early" has been variably defined as anywhere from 24 h to 7 days after either the onset of symptoms or the time of diagnosis at hospital admission [9–17]. We can, however, conclude, as Banz et al. do, that there is no advantage to delaying surgical intervention during the initial admission. Banz et al. in their retrospective database of more than 4000 patients have shown that laparoscopic cholecystectomy, if done beyond 6 days from onset of symptoms of acute cholecystitis, results in a significantly higher morbidity in the form of conversion to open surgery, overall postoperative complications, and duration of hospital stay [18]. Most patients with ACC should be offered laparoscopic cholecystectomy as soon as this is feasible on their first admission. De Mestral et al. [15] in their population-based analysis of more than 20,000 patients of ACC have shown that ELC (within 7 days of symptom onset) showed half the incidence of bile duct injury and shorter hospital stay compared with delayed cholecystectomy (more than 7 days of symptom onset). The development of fibrosis in Calot's triangle following resolution of initial bout of inflammation after ACC has been considered the main causal factor for a technically difficult surgery and is associated with higher bile duct injury (Fig. 31.2). Indeed, even in the absence of clear demonstration in this sense, laparoscopic cholecystectomy should be delayed in case of more than 6–7 days of symptom onset; delayed cholecystectomy should be performed 45–60 days after symptom onset. Besides, there is a further problem concerning the adherence to these recommendations. Several studies reported an ELC rate of 15–40% of the whole ACC population, suggesting that the current guidelines and recommendations for ELC in ACC may have some difficulties to be accepted in the clinical practice mainly due to the unpredictable availability of operatory rooms and surgeons.

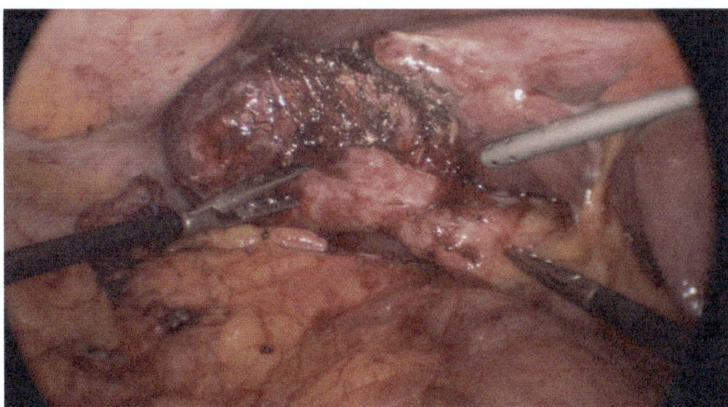

Fig. 31.2 Elective laparoscopic cholecystectomy after several episodes of relapsing ACC previously treated with antibiotics in another hospital. The surgical procedure has been managed with anterograde technique for the presence of marked Calot's triangle inflammation and fibrosis

31.2.3 Antimicrobial Therapy

Regarding the best antimicrobial therapy in case of ACC, the first item to be discussed is the opportunity for surgical treatment (cholecystectomy) rather than drainage (cholecystostomy) to remove the septic focus. This aspect should be discussed for each patient with the surgeon, in order to conclude the presence of surgical indication basing on surgical timing and the type of patients (high-risk patients or not). Antibiotics should be suggested as supportive care; they constitute the primary therapy in patients undergoing delayed surgery or observation. When employed for treating the first episode of ACC, they showed a high rate of relapse. When possible, surgery is more effective than antibiotics alone in the treatment of ACC [7]. On the other hand, the type of bacteria affecting the patients is similarly of great importance. Empiric antibiotic regimens demonstrated to be adequate in only two-thirds of patients. There might be a trend for poorer outcome in patients treated with inadequate antibiotic agents, emphasizing the importance of tailoring antibiotic treatment. Bile culture and the results of local antimicrobial susceptibility testing (local antibiogram) are useful in this perspective and can precisely individuate specific bacteria involved in cholecystitis in 60% of the patients and 7–31% of blood cultures. Bile and blood samples should be sent to culture in all cases of acute cholecystitis excepting those with grade I severity. Escherichia coli strains represent the most commonly isolated bacteria (almost 30% of bile cultures and 43% of blood cultures. The concordance between empiric treatment coverage and culture isolate susceptibility was 67.6%. In most discordant cases, the isolates were *Enterobacter* spp. (40.9%) and *Enterococcus* spp. (31.8%). Among patients treated with antibiotics, the in-hospital mortality rate is reported to be 2% in patients with concordant treatment compared with 14% for patients with discordant treatment (p = 0.09) [19, 20]. When cholecystectomy is

Table 31.1 The antibiotics usually used to treat biliary tract infections and their biliary penetration ability (indicated as the ratio of bile to serum concentrations) [21]

Good penetration efficiency (≥1)		Low penetration efficiency (<1)	
Antibiotics	Bile/serum	Antibiotics	Bile/serum
Piperacillin–tazobactam	60	Cefotaxime	0.75
Tigecycline	38	Meropenem	0.75
Amoxicillin–clavulanate	30	Ceftazidime	0.5
Ciprofloxacin	30	Vancomicin	0.5
Ampicillin–sulbactam	9	Amikacin	0.3
Ceftriaxone	5	Gentamicin	0.3
Levofloxacin	5	Cefepime	0.1
Penicillin G	5	Imipenem	0.01
Cefazolin	3		
Clyndamicin	3		
Doripenem	1.17		
Ceforoxime	1		
Metronidazole	1		

performed, antimicrobial therapy can be stopped within 24 h since the source of infection is controlled; moderate-severe ACC should be treated with antimicrobial therapy even after cholecystectomy is performed, and therapy should be continued until the patient is afebrile, with a normalized white count and without abdominal findings [20].

Moreover, the decision of which antibiotic should be chosen must take into account the penetration ability in the biliary system of each antibiotic (penetration efficiency is reported in Table 31.1 [21]). The duration of therapy should be strictly evaluated periodically to avoid the unnecessarily use of broader-spectrum agents to prevent the emergence of antimicrobial resistance. A recent article reported among 136 gram-negative bacterial isolated (mostly *E. coli*, *Klebsiella* spp., *Enterobacter* spp.) an antimicrobial resistance of 49.3, 20.6, 8, 4.4, 4.4, 13.2, and 33.8% (range: 0–100%) for, respectively, cefazolin, cefuroxime, ceftriaxone, ceftazidime, gentamicin, levofloxacin, and ampicillin–sulbactam.

31.2.4 Associated Common Bile Duct Stone

The presence of common bile duct stones (CBDS) is reported to occur in 10–20% in case series of cholelithiasis, with lower incidence during ACC ranging from 5 to 15% of the patients [22–24]. Alteration of biochemical parameters is frequently associated to cholecystitis; for this reason, it can be difficult to identify patients with synchronous common bile duct stones. Normal liver biochemical tests have a negative predictive value of 97%. Meanwhile, the positive predictive value of any abnormal biochemical liver test is only 15% [25]. Specificity of serum bilirubin level for common bile duct stones (CBDS) is 60% with a cutoff level of 1.7 mg/dL and 75% with a cutoff level of 4 mg/dL [26]. Some authors

Table 31.2 Predictive factors and risk classes for choledocholithiasis [27]

Risk class	Predictive factors
Moderate	• Abnormal liver biochemical test other than bilirubin • Age older than 55 years • Clinical gallstone pancreatitis
Strong	• Common bile duct diameter >6 mm (with gallbladder in situ) • Bilirubin level 1.8–4 mg/dL
Very strong	• Evidence of common bile duct stone at AUS • Clinical ascending cholangitis • Bilirubin >4 mg/dL

propose a classification of predictive risk factors for choledochal lithiasis. Following this classification (reported in Table 31.2), patients can be stratified in three classes of risk: "high," in the presence of any very strong factor; "low," in the absence of risk factor; and "intermediate," for all other patients [27]. Indeed, since the rate of patients with ACC and synchronous CBDS is relevant, several authors include the possibility of choledocholithiasis within their algorithms for the treatment of ACC. At this respect, we report the comprehensive algorithm reported by Ansaloni et al. in 2016 (Fig. 31.1) describing the pre-, intra-, and postoperative possibilities to individuate and treat choledocholithiasis [7].

31.2.5 Patients' Risk Stratification and Severity Grading of ACC

Patients' risk stratification should result from an integration between the severity of cholecystitis with the anamnesis in terms of comorbidities, malnutrition, and reduced functional reserve. In patients with severe comorbidities or reduced functional reserve, in particular, in the presence of severe cholecystitis, treatments alternative to early cholecystectomy could be of benefit and should be taken into account. In this sense, we have previously presented the option of antimicrobial therapy, and we will later discuss the option of cholecystostomy. Anyway, it is desirable to identify the parameters to stratify the risk of surgery in this setting of patients. Patients' age >80, Mannheim peritonitis index ≥29, and comorbidities are significantly associated with a high postoperative morbidity, while increased age and low white blood count are significantly related to mortality in gangrenous cholecystitis [28]. Diabetes mellitus does not contraindicate urgent surgery but is associated with an increased risk of postoperative morbidity (in particular cardiovascular events, renal failure, and infective complication) and mortality (4.4% vs. 1.4%). Moreover, in patients with diabetes, ELC is associated with lower rate of surgical site infections and reduced hospital stay compared to open counterpart and should be consequently pursued [28, 29]. In pregnant women in the presence of mild ACC, ELC should be the first-line approach. In terms of patients' stratification and consequent therapeutic approach, TG13 suggest ELC as the first-line treatment in grade I ACC; meanwhile in grade II ACC, elective cholecystectomy is suggested as the first-line treatment just if advanced laparoscopic techniques are available and after the improvement of the acute inflammatory process. If a patient does not respond to initial medical treatment, urgent or early gallbladder drainage is required. In patients with surgical risk, observation (follow-up without cholecystectomy) after improvement with initial medical treatment could be indicated. In grade III (severe) ACC accompanied by organ dysfunction, urgent or early gallbladder drainage should be performed [30].

The 2016 WSES guidelines appear to suggest a more extended indication for surgical treatment of ACC. Surgery in general and laparoscopic approach in particular should initially be always attempted except in case of absolute anesthesiology contraindications or septic shock (the only cases with the real indication to antibiotic therapy alone or cholecystostomy). In the presence of advanced inflammation, gangrenous gallbladder, or any setting of the "difficult gallbladder" in whom the anatomy is difficult to recognize and main bile duct injuries are more likely, laparoscopic or open subtotal cholecystectomy is a valid option [7]. The therapeutic algorithm for patients with ACC should include a systematic determination of the degree of cholecystitis and surgical risk assessment. In this sense, actual guidelines for ACC treatment need to be reviewed, and they should include clear risk stratification parameters for severity of cholecystitis and a stratification of patients' comorbidities, malnutrition, and reduced functional reserve. Table 31.3 shows the severity grading of acute cholecystitis proposed by Tokyo Guidelines of 2013 [30].

Table 31.3 TG13 severity grading for acute cholecystitis [30]

Severity class	Criteria
Grade III (severe) acute cholecystitis	• Cardiovascular dysfunction requiring dopamine or norepinephrineinfusion
	• Neurological impairment (consciousness)
	• Respiratory distress (PaO_2/FiO_2 ratio/300)
	• Oliguria or serum creatinine >2 mg/dL
	• PT–INR >1.5
	• Platelet count <100,000/mm^3
Grade II (moderate) acute cholecystitis	• Elevated white blood cell count (>18,000/mm^3)
	• Palpable tender mass in the right upper abdominal quadrant
	• Duration of complaints >72 h
	• Marked local inflammation (gangrenous cholecystitis, peri-cholecystic abscess, hepatic abscess, biliary peritonitis, emphysematous cholecystitis)
Grade I (mild) acute cholecystitis	Does not meet the criteria of "grade III" or "grade II" acute cholecystitis. Grade I can also be defined as acute cholecystitis in a healthy patient with no organ dysfunction and mild inflammatory changes in the gallbladder, making cholecystectomy a safe and low-risk operative procedure

31.2.6 Alternatives Options for High-Risk Patients: Radiologic-Assisted Cholecystostomy

Although cholecystectomy is generally safe, the mortality rate in patients with significant comorbidities and high-risk for surgery ranges between 14 and 30% [31, 32]. Therefore, as an interim management, high-risk patients may be treated with decompression of gallbladder combined with broad-spectrum antibiotics. Surgical cholecystostomy, introduced by Bobbs [33], was the only available method for gallbladder compression for more than a century. In recent years, percutaneous cholecystostomy (PC), a technique that consists of percutaneous catheter placement in the gallbladder lumen under imaging guidance, has become an alternative to surgical cholecystostomy. PC for acute cholecystitis was first reported in 1980 when it was performed in a patient with empyema of the gallbladder [34]. Since then, PC has been performed as an alternative treatment to cholecystectomy and surgical cholecystostomy in high-risk patients with acute cholecystitis [35–38]. Percutaneous cholecystostomy is mainly indicated in calculous or acalculous cholecystitis, but it could be useful also in cholangitis and biliary obstruction as a treatment procedure or for opacification of the biliary tree. It may also provide a potential route for stone extraction. PC may play an important role as an easy method in the diagnostic visualization of the biliary tree, if the cystic duct is patent [39]. PC is usually accomplished successfully and can be performed under intravenous sedation and local anesthesia either at the radiology department or bedside after antibiotic coverage. Coagulopathy, if present, should be corrected with transfusions of fresh frozen plasma or platelets or both. Under aseptic conditions and US guidance, using local anesthesia, the procedure is carried out by using either modified Seldinger technique or trocar technique. 18 to 22G Chiba needles can be used to puncture the gallbladder while the patient is laying on his/her hospital bed or the fluoroscopy table if the interventional radiologist wants to control the placement of the tube with fluoroscopy. US guidance is enough for almost all procedures, but CT guidance may also be used. Access to the gallbladder is confirmed by aspiration of bile. For confirmation also, not more than 5 mL of iodinated contrast material may be injected avoiding possible exacerbation of sepsis. After placing the suitable guide wire through the needle into the gallbladder (this may be confirmed either with US or fluoroscopy), 6–10 French pigtail catheters are placed. PC is considered technically successful when the pigtail catheter loop is visualized either sonographically or fluoroscopically in the gallbladder lumen.

Bile sample should be obtained for cultures. The catheter is sutured to the skin, placed on gravity drainage, and then flushed daily with 5–10 mL of sterile saline to avoid occlusion. If the cholecystostomy is performed at the bedside, a single stick trocar can also be used to place a catheter into the gallbladder under ultrasonographic guidance. There is a large range of drainage systems which are suitable for PC, and locking loop catheters can be used to reduce the risk of dislodgment as the catheter dislodgment tends to occur in a higher rate here than in other organs. Technical success rate is very high ranging from 95 to 100% [36, 40, 41]. The reasons for the technical failure may be porcelain gallbladder or thickened gallbladder wall which can make the gallbladder puncture impossible [42]. Other reasons are small gallbladder lumen either filled with stones or not which does not accommodate pigtail catheter [41], bowel loop in between, lack of operator's experience, and suboptimal patient cooperation [43].

Two approaches have been utilized in accessing the gallbladder. One is transhepatic puncture and in particular, if possible, the "bare area" of the liver portion attached to the liver by connective tissue and not covered by peritoneum. However, the bare area cannot be reliably imaged or punctured. The other one is the transperitoneal puncture, entering the free peritoneal surface of the gallbladder wall.

The transhepatic approach is preferable in the absence of severe liver disease and coagulopathy [36, 40, 43] because of the catheter stability and decreased bile leakage. The transperitoneal approach may be chosen to prevent injury to the hepatic parenchyma and minimize potential bleeding and infectious complications in the presence of severe liver disease and coagulopathy.

Using anchoring device with transperitoneal approach allows greater stability and minimizes bile leakage by securing the gallbladder to the abdominal wall [44]. On the other hand, performing transperitoneal access may be difficult if massive ascites or colon interposition is present [45–48].

No difference had been found in the complication rates between the patients drained either with transhepatic or transperitoneal procedure [39, 43]. Tract formation is critical after PC to avoid bile leakage and peritonitis. It was reported that for mature tract development, 2 weeks is required when the transhepatic approach is used, whereas 3 weeks in transperitoneal approach. Tract maturation after the transhepatic approach was found to be significantly faster [43].

Several days after the procedure, transcatheter cholangiography may be performed to assess the patency of cystic duct, the presence of gallstones, and catheter position. If stones are observed in the common bile duct, they can be removed by endoscopic papillotomy [49].

Tract formation is crucial, and no data are available about the optimal timing of tube removal. Recently some authors published a systematic review of 50 published studies about the timing of tube removal, but no critical outcomes (success, morbidity, mortality, recurrence rate) were associated with drain removal (varying from 2 to 193 days). In the same study, the authors reported their experience on 35 patients followed up for 16 months after percutaneous drainage (clinical success 97.1%, morbidity 34.3% including 8 tube dislodgment, 30 days mortality of 11.4%, and recurrence rate 12.1%) without demonstrating any correlation of outcomes with timing of tube removal [50]. Since the recurrence rate of ACC has been reported to be approximately 25–33% [51, 52], prophylactic treatment for recurrence such as percutaneous gallstone extraction should be considered in inoperable patients with the calculous disease before catheter removal. In patients in whom long-term catheter drainage is maintained, change of catheter every 3 months is necessary. Response rates to PC in the literature are between the range of 56–100% [42, 46, 53–56]. This variation is due to different patient populations and lower rates in the critically ill intensive care patients in whom the diagnosis of ACC is difficult [46]. Response rates to PC are statistically higher in patients with clinical signs and symptoms referable to the gallbladder and right upper quadrant. When the gallbladder is the only focus of infection, the response is remarkable. A poor response is most likely due to severe concomitant systemic disease.

Notwithstanding, widely adopted practice, the percutaneous drainage lacks solid evidence in the specific clinical setting of "high-risk" patients. Gurusamy et al. [5] analyzed the only two RCTs published comparing percutaneous drainage versus early or late cholecystectomy and percutaneous drainage versus conservative treatment in high-risk patients. No differences were measured in the surgically treated population between early and delayed treatments regarding mortality or morbidity nor in the study comparing conservative treatment versus percutaneous drainage; then no demonstrable superiority of one strategy could be defined. Complications associated with PC usually occur immediately or within days and include bleeding, vagal reactions, sepsis, bile peritonitis, pneumothorax, perforation of the intestinal loop, secondary infection or colonization of the gallbladder, and catheter dislodgment [36–38]. Late complications have been reported as catheter dislodgment and recurrent cholecystitis [38].

Overall major and minor complication rates were reported to range from 3 to 8% and 4 to 13%, respectively [37, 39]. Catheter dislodgment reported as the most common complication [56] may be due to inadequate fixation of the catheter, patient movement, and failure to protect the catheter during the transportation. Biliary peritonitis due to bile leakage occurs with a rate of 2.5% and may be prevented with catheter removal after the mature tract formation.

Thirty-day mortality rate varies from 0 to 25% [37, 54, 57], and fatal outcomes are often associated with sepsis and significant comorbidities. Figures 31.3 and 31.4 show PC images.

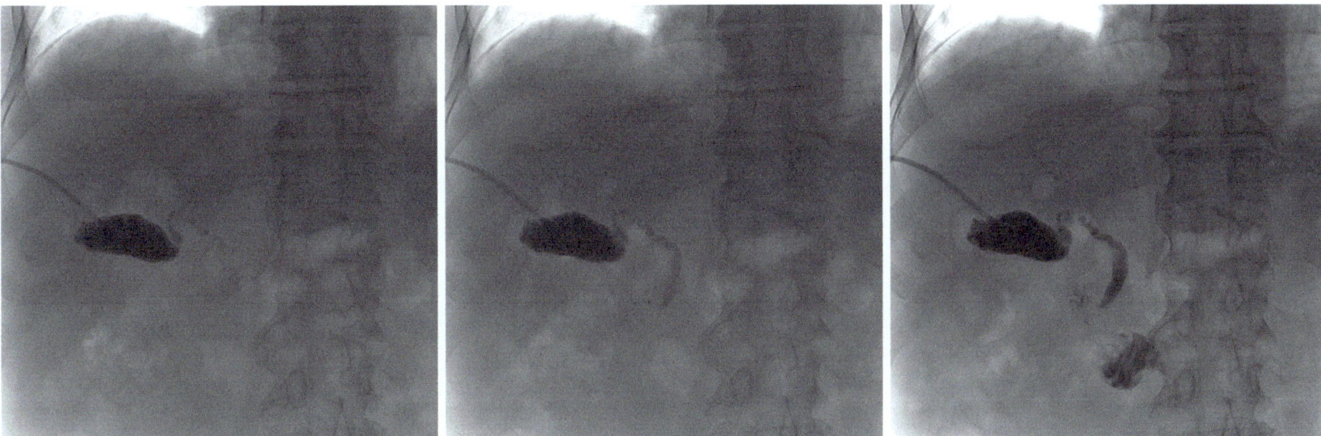

Fig. 31.3 Percutaneous cholangiography transcholecystostomic catheter. Percutaneous cholangiography through a percutaneous transcholecystostomic catheter demonstrates a few stones inside the lumen of the gallbladder not occluding the cystic duct. Choledocus is not significantly dilated and the passage of contrast medium in duodenus is regular. Patient can remove the catheter if there is no clinical contraindication

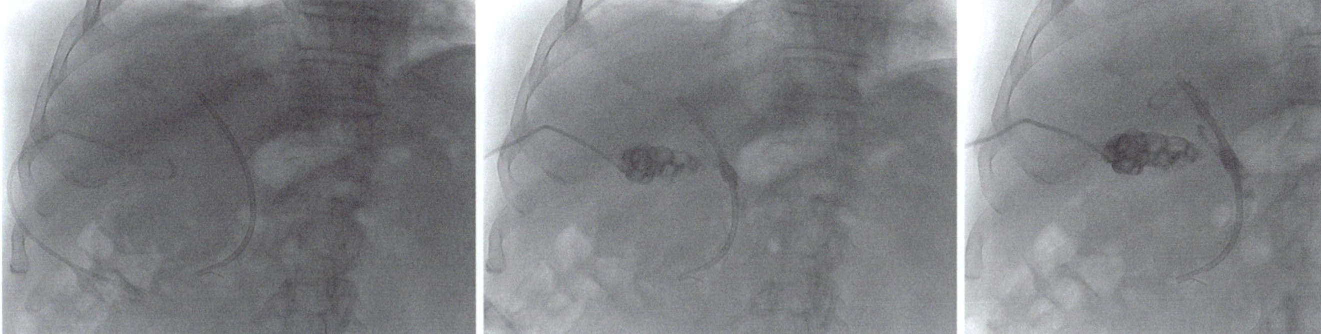

Fig. 31.4 Percutaneous cholangiography transcholecistostomic catheter demonstrates a few stones inside the lumen of the gallbladder not completely occluding the cystic duct. Choledocus is slightly dilated and isolated stones are visible also near plastic biliary stent. No opacification of the duodenus was recorded during the examination

31.2.7 Alternative Options for High-Risk Patients: Endoscopic Gallbladder Drainage

After the introduction of self-expanding stents, endoscopic drainage for acute cholecystitis is an alternative therapeutic option [58, 59]. The older approach was through the papilla during an endoscopic retrograde cholangiopancreatography (ERCP), with or without sphincterotomy, inserting a naso-gallbladder (NGBD) 5–7 Fr drainage, which permits to control the aspirated bile and eventually to rinse the gallbladder or a 6–10 Fr double pigtail stent. Both procedures are usually performed with a temporary intent to bridge the patient to definitive surgery [60]. Retrospective data shows a pooled technical success of 80.9% (range 74.7–86.2%) and a clinical response of 75.3% (range 68.6–81.2%) of such procedures. Reported adverse effects range from 0 to 14% including post-ERCP pancreatitis, perforation of cystic duct or gallbladder, worsening of sepsis, death, and drain dislodgment. Few data have been collected on recurrence rate; only an Italian study reported 20% rate of recurrences (median follow-up: 17 months) [61]. Regarding stent placement, technical success is reported in 91.1–98.7% and clinical success in 81.2–93.2% of patients; those rates are higher than the ones reported with NGBD, probably because the stent was often inserted after drainage removal in more stable patients. The emergent strategy is to use echoendoscopy and a gastric or duodenal window to drain the gallbladder with the same technical approach used in the presence of pseudocyst or pancreatic fluid collections. Briefly, under the guidance of a linear-array echoendoscope, the gallbladder body is punctured (avoiding vessels) passing through the antrum or the neck through the duodenal bulb. Then, a guide wire is inserted, a fistula is created, and after dilatation, an endoscopic nasobiliary drainage (ENBD) or an expandable metallic stent can be inserted under radiological guidance. Recently, dedicated stents with bilateral flanges designed to provide anchorage between non-adherent lumen structures have been developed: this has improved the procedure which does not need radiological control. Endoscopic ultrasound (EUS)-guided drainage can be performed in the presence of ascites and with altered coagulation. Bile leakage is prevented by recently introduced stents; moreover, stent migration in the gastrointestinal lumen should not be considered a dangerous event because the fistula formation with stomach or bowel is quickly stable after drainage [62].

In 2012 Jang et al. [63] published the results of the first RCT comparing PC and EUS-guided gallbladder drainage (GBD) in 59 patients with ACC non-responder to medical treatment and unsuitable for urgent surgery. EUS drainage was done with a 5 Fr nasobiliary catheter. Jang et al. reported for EUS-GBD versus PC similar clinical success rate (100% vs. 96%) and no significant difference in adverse events occurrence (7% vs. 3%), including the need to perform a subsequent cholecystectomy (9% vs. 12%). Discomfort or pain after drainage was indeed significantly reduced in EUS-treated patients. In 2014 Choi et al. [64] published the results of a retrospective study on EUS drained ACC with metallic expandable stent (1 cm diameter, external flares of 22 mm) and partially covered in 63 patients focusing on long-term management. Initial clinical success was 98.4%, and the three procedural adverse events (perforation or peritonitis) were treated conservatively. Fifty-six out of 63 patients were eligible for long-term follow-up (median 275 days, range 40–1185 days). The rate of re-intervention was 3.6%; distal migration of the stents (two patients) was asymptomatic; fracture of the stent or case of food impaction was treated with a restenting. Half of the patients died during the follow-up due to cardiovascular events or malignancy: the remaining 28 patients had a cumulative stent patency rate of 86% at 3 years (median of 458 days, range 151–1185 days). No procedure-related deaths were reported, and 96.4% of the patients had no recurrence of cholecystitis. Irani et al. [65] selected retrospectively 15 patients unfit for surgery and treated with lumen apposing stent in 14 cases through a duodenal access: technical success was 93% and clinical success was 100%, with a median follow-up of 160 days. Recently Walter et al. [66] reported long-term results of a cooperative prospective study on 30 patients using lumen-apposing stents designed to be deployed without the need of devices exchange during endoscopy and radiological assistance. Intentionally, stents were left in situ for 3 months. Technical success was 90% (27 patients) and clinical success 96% (26 patients). In two cases (7%), ACC recurred due to stent obstruction. The stent was removed in 50% of patients after a mean of 91 days, while in the other 50%, the removal was not possible (five patients died before, two stent overgrowth, eight other causes), but no adverse effects have been recorded (mean time 364 days). Mortality at 30 days was 7%, and cumulative stent-related adverse event rate was 30% (the patients selected for the study were all unfit for surgery). Theo et al. [67] conducted a retrospective 1:1 matched cohort analysis of 118 cases unfit for cholecystectomy, treated by PC or EUS drainage reporting similar technical and clinical success rate, no differences in recurrence rates, and a similar 30-day mortality, but a significantly higher rate of severe adverse events in the percutaneous approach population (74.6% vs. 23.7%), mainly related to tube displacement, and a subsequent need of hospital readmissions. Penas-Herrero et al. reported in a recent review on 155 published patients with ACC treated by EUS drainage (plastic stents, nasobiliary catheters, metallic self-expanding stents, and lumen-apposing stents) an overall technical and clinical success of, respectively, 97.45% and 99.34%, with adverse events occurring in less than 8% of patients. No significant differences were measured among different types of stent performance (for plastic stent 100% technical success/100% clinical success, for nasobiliary drains 97.4/100%, and for metal stents 98.51/98.5%), nor in terms of adverse events rate [58]. Interestingly cumulative long-term results in 33 patients with a minimum follow-up of 3 months showed no recurrence of cholecystitis (28 cases with stent left in situ). Patil et al. [59] reviewed the published results of lumen-apposing stents in 78 patients, and the technical combined success was 97% with a clinical combined success rate of 99.6%, while no significant complications have been reported. Thus, EUS-guided gallbladder drainage can be considered a well-established alternative strategy for the "bridge to cholecystectomy" treatment of ACC; moreover, after the introduction of recent lumen-apposing new stents, it appears in a long-term perspective a promising first-line treatment for unfit or high-risk surgical patients. Figure 31.5 shows pictures of an EUS-guided gallbladder drainage.

31.3 Cholangitis

31.3.1 Etiology and Physiopathology

Acute cholangitis is a systemic infectious disease characterized by acute inflammation and infection in the bile ducts resulting from a combination of biliary obstruction and bacterial growth in bile.

The classic presentation is fever, pain, and jaundice, but no more than 50–70% of patients have all the mentioned signs (Charcot's triad); hypotension and mental confusion often represent the only onset symptoms in elderly patients. Diagnostic and grading criteria have been proposed by Japanese authors [68]. Cholangitis should be suspected by clinical presentation (Charcot's triad has a high sensitivity)

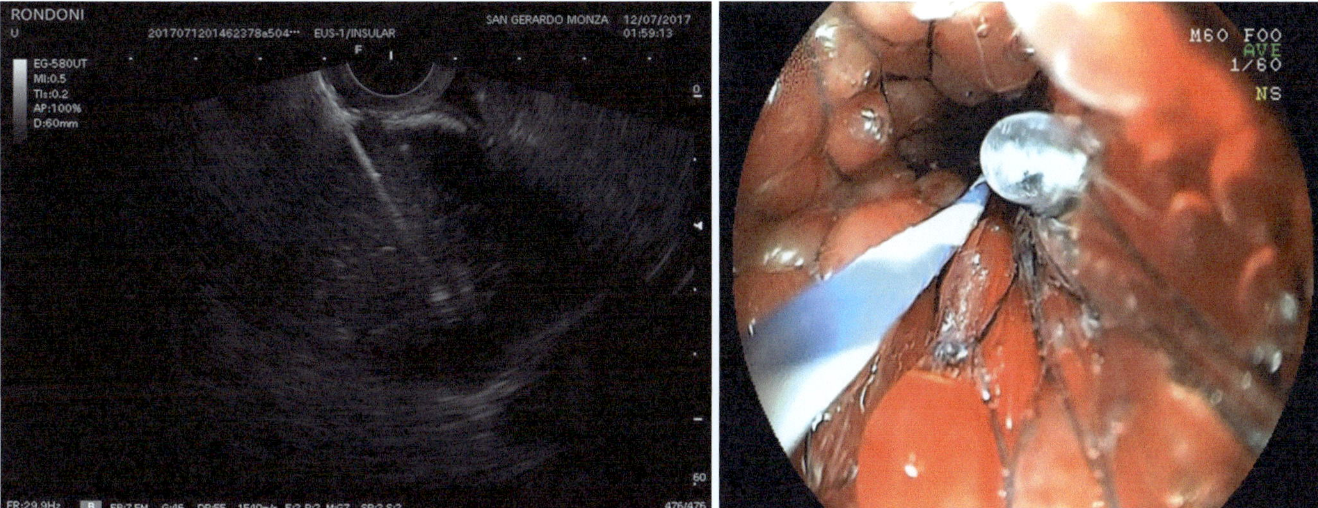

Fig. 31.5 EUS-guided passage of the needle and intra-gallbladder release of the distal part of the stent; subsequent endoscopic appearance of the stent at the distal antrum

and routine blood test (presence of signs of inflammation and cholestasis). The diagnosis becomes definite if imaging reveals stones, strictures, tumors, present or previous stents inducing bile duct dilatation, or previous papillotomy. In this sense, the diagnosis of cholangitis must be confirmed with ultrasonography, CT scan with contrast (suggested as the most effective imaging method for the diagnosis of etiology and complication of acute cholangitis), and/or MRI. Translocation of bacteria into the bloodstream may result in septicemia, an often fatal complication of acute cholangitis. The treatment of sepsis related to cholangitis includes resuscitation approach to be performed within 6 h from the onset and involving blood cultures and subsequent broad-spectrum antibiotic administration. In the event of hypotension and/or serum lactate >4 mmol/L, an initial minimum of 20 mL/kg of crystalloid is required. Vasopressors for patients with hypotension showing no response to initial fluid resuscitation can also be necessary. Biliary obstruction can result from various etiologies, such as choledocholithiasis (28–70%), benign stenoses (5–28%), malignant stenoses (10–57%), biliary stent obstruction (up to 20%), strictured bilio-enteric anastomoses, and parasitic colonization of the bile duct. It is not always clear how bacteria enter an obstructed biliary system, unless interventions such as surgery, endoscopic retrograde cholangiopancreatography (ERCP), or percutaneous transhepatic cholangiography (PTC) have been performed, resulting in the loss of the physiologic barrier between the bile duct and intestine [69]. Severity grading of cholangitis following TG13 guidelines is reported in Table 31.4 [68]. Comprehensive algorithm for the treatment of cholangitis from the TG13 guidelines is reported in Fig. 31.6 [74].

Table 31.4 Severity assessment of cholangitis according to Tokyo Guidelines TG13 [68]

Severity grade of cholangitis	Patients with at least one of the following
Severe cholangitis—grade III	• Cardiovascular dysfunction requiring dopamine infusion
	• Neurological impairment (consciousness)
	• Respiratory distress
	• Oliguria or serum creatinine >2 mg/dL
	• PT–INR >1.5
	• Platelet count <100,000/mm^3
Moderate cholangitis—grade II	• Abnormal white cells count >12,000/<4000 per mm^3
	• Fever =/>39 °C
	• Age =/>75 years
	• Total bilirubin =/>5 mg/dL
	• Hypoalbuminemia
Mild cholangitis—grade I	Patients not meeting the criteria of "grade III (severe)" or "grade II (moderate)" acute cholangitis at initial diagnosis

31.3.2 Treatment Options

Treatment ERCP is recognized as the first-line treatment to be performed within 24 h in the presence of severe cholangitis to provide bile drainage after well-managed sepsis and systemic complications. Urgent (within 24 h) biliary intervention in the management of mild to moderate acute cholangitis caused by common bile ducts stones is related to benefits in terms of shorter stay in hospital and shorter time consumed for control of infection and would also be recommended [70]. When ERCP is not a viable option, such as in case of patients with Roux-en-Y reconstruction or those with

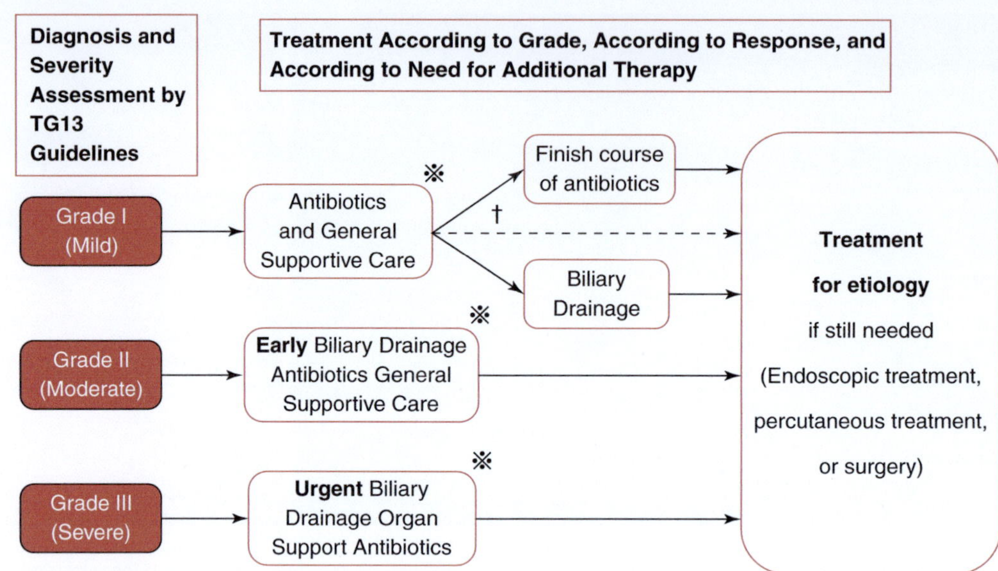

Fig. 31.6 Comprehensive algorithm for the treatment of cholangitis from the TG13 guidelines for diagnosis and severity grading of acute cholangitis [74]

esophageal or upper gastrointestinal obstruction, or finally if ERCP fails, alternative approaches as percutaneous biliary drainage or EUS-guided procedures are necessary for diagnosis and treatment. In the literature, ERCP-related reported mortality ranges from 2 to 65%, but in recent years, general mortality dropped to less than 15% remaining not negligible as 20–30% in severe forms. A recent study [71] focused on procedural interventions in 981 acute cholangitis episodes in 810 patients, confirmed the prognostic value of Tokyo Guidelines but separating patients in high and low risk according to a cutoff level of 0.7% death individual risk, and indicated different drainage strategies as elective (>24 h), early (within 24 h), and urgent (within hours or at admission). No prospective data on this model are however available. Interestingly, organ failure remains the strongest predictor of mortality (OR 47.1), and among the factors contributing to failure, mental confusion has the highest impact (OR 37.6, eight times higher compared to patients without mental confusion). Assessing the interventions, insufficient drainage, and percutaneous approach has a relatively high impact (OR, respectively, of 4.5 and 2.4). Optimal timing for ERCP has been recently evaluated in a prospective study published by How et al. [72] on 199 patients admitted for acute cholangitis, 58% with more than one comorbidity, and 23% having malignant disease already submitted to previous drainage (stent placement). In this study hospital stay was confirmed to be longer in the group submitted to ERCP after 48 h (median 9.1 days) than in the group of early (<48 h) ERCP (median 6.5 days), increasing by 1.44 days for every day ERCP was delayed. Mortality has been influenced (OR 3.6) by delaying ERCP after 72 h and by malignancy (OR 11.3) according to other published studies [73].

Recent studies focused on critical analysis and controversial aspects of TG13 guidelines underline the need to include in the flowchart other endoscopic tools such as balloon enteroscopy-assisted ERCP and EUS-BD [74–76]. Growing evidence of successful unconventional endo-therapy (enteroscopy-assisted ERCP and EUS-guided biliary drainage) is the topic of the review by Tsuchiya et al. [76]. Single and double balloon-assisted enteroscopies are used in altered postsurgery anatomy with clinical success ranging from 61 to 98%. Enteroscopy-assisted ERCP has been compared in a recent retrospective multicentric study [77] with EUS-guided biliary drainage in patients with altered surgical anatomy. Ninety-eight patients were submitted to enteroscopy-assisted ERCP (49) or EUS-BD (49), and EUS-guided approach has been demonstrated technically (98 vs. 65.3%—OR 12.48) and clinically (88 vs. 59.1%—OR 2.4) superior with a procedural time significantly reduced. EUS-guided biliary drainage has been extensively reviewed [78, 79] as for the EUS drainage of the gallbladder. EUS approach can be used as rendezvous technique of inserting a guide deep into the small bowel to be grasped by an endoscope or can be used to do a direct transluminal access to the left liver (hepato-gastrostomy, hepato-jejunostomy, or hepato-duodenostomy), creating a stable fistula and inserting ad hoc stents leaving at least 3 cm of the stent into the gastrointestinal lumen. Stents can also be pushed across the biliary stricture in an antegrade fashion through the papilla or the anastomosis. In 2016 Kahn et al. published a systematic review and meta-analysis to evaluate the cumulative efficacy and safety of EUS-BD and to compare the two approaches of extrahepatic or intrahepatic approach and transluminal methods of EUS-BD [80]. Pooled rates for technical success (90%) and adverse event occurrence (17%) have been calculated. Distal biliary strictures and trans-papillary drainage were associated with higher success rate: intrahepatic approach was associated with higher risk of adverse effects. Other authors analyzed 9 studies (483 patients) to compare percutaneous biliary drainage to EUS-guided endoscopic drainage. Technical success was comparable, but EUS-treated patients had fewer adverse events and re-intervention, with a better clinical outcome, inducing to conclude that EUS-guided drainage could be considered the first-line rescue therapy in cases of failure of traditional ERCP to achieve biliary drainage [81].

Baniya et al. reviewed 6 studies comparing percutaneous transhepatic biliary drainage and EUS approach after failed ERCP (312 patients were included). Even in this meta-analysis, technical and clinical success rates were not significantly different, while EUS approach had a better profile for severe adverse events. Authors concluded that EUS drainage is rapidly changing the strategy after failed ERCP because it is less invasive and more physiologic; furthermore, it provides better absorption of nutrients, prevents external drainage, and requires fewer re-interventions. Moreover, it can be done in the same ERCP session if retrograde access fails [82].

Focusing on technical aspects [78], no differences have been reported in success or complication rates among different anatomical approaches, so the choice of drainage route remains unclear when both are possible, while rendezvous technique seems less successful.

Gallbladder drainage can also be used as an alternative strategy to decompress biliary tree. Overall, higher rates of adverse events have been recorded with intrahepatic route and when plastic stents have been inserted, in particular in terms of bile leakage.

Finally, EUS-BD has always been considered a rescue therapy, but the lower procedural time and the high clinical success performance suggest that EUS-guided therapy will become elective strategy in altered anatomy by surgery or neoplasia (after stenting).

Case Scenario

You are asked to see a 70-year-old febrile and lethargic patient complaining pain in upper right quadrant of the abdomen, Murphy's sign positive. With the exception of two previous hospitalizations for left inguinal hernia repair and pneumonitis, respectively, the patient has no known medical problems. The patient was recently initiated on vasopressors to achieve hemodynamic stability. Positive laboratory tests showed an alkaline phosphatase level of 600 IU/L, total bilirubin level of 6 mg/dL (conjugated 4.5), white blood cell count of 20,000, oliguria with a creatinine value of 2.2 mg/dL, and a platelet count of 90,000/mmμL. A transabdominal ultrasound and a subsequent computed tomography showed an intra- and extrahepatic dilatation of the biliary tree, with a common bile duct of up to 16 mm, sustained by a gallstone in its distal portion, and a calculus cholecystitis with a wall thickness up to 7 mm. The patient has been receiving full-spectrum antibiotics for 36 h.

1. How could be graded the cholangitis of the discussed patients following the TG13?
   A. Severe cholangitis—grade III.
   B. Moderate cholangitis—grade II.
   C. Mild cholangitis—grade I.
   D. There are no parameters for the diagnosis of cholangitis.
2. Which of the following recommendations should you follow?
   A. Change of antimicrobial agents.
   B. Emergency cholecystectomy.
   C. Endoscopic retrograde cholangiopancreatography.
   D. Endoscopic retrograde cholangiopancreatography plus cholecystostomy.
   E. Endoscopic retrograde cholangiopancreatography plus possible cholecystostomy followed by early or delayed cholecystectomy.
3. In case of failed ERCP, which are potential alternatives?
   A. Percutaneous biliary drainage.
   B. EUS-guided endoscopic drainage.
   C. Balloon enteroscopy-assisted ERCP.
   D. All of the abovementioned procedure could be indicated.
4. After the treatment of cholangitis, which is the best surgical timing for cholecystectomy?
   A. Laparoscopic cholecystectomy as soon as possible.
   B. Delayed open cholecystectomy 45–60 days after symptom onset.
   C. Laparoscopic cholecystectomy within 7 days from onset of symptoms is the best option; otherwise delayed 45–60 days after symptom onset.
   D. Cholecystectomy is not indicated.

Please see Chap. 58 for the correct answer.

References

1. Gracie WA, Ransohoff DF. The natural history of silent gallstones: the innocent gallstone is not a myth. N Engl J Med. 1982;307:798–800.
2. Shaffer EA. Epidemiology and risk factors for gallstone disease: has the paradigm changed in the 21st century? Curr Gastroenterol Rep. 2005;7:132–40.
3. Kratzer W, Mason RA, Kächele V. Prevalence of gallstones in sonographic surveys worldwide. J Clin Ultrasound. 1999;27:1–7.
4. Pedersen G, Hoem D, Andrén-Sandberg A. Influence of laparoscopic cholecystectomy on the prevalence of operations for gallstones in Norway. Eur J Surg. 2002;168:464–9.
5. Everhart JE, Khare M, Hill M, Maurer KR. Prevalence and ethnic differences in gallbladder disease in the United States. Gastroenterology. 1999;117(3):632.
6. Hirota M, Takada T, Kawarada Y, Nimura Y, Miura F, Hirata K, et al. Diagnostic criteria and severity assessment of acute cholecystitis: Tokyo guidelines. J Hepatobiliary Pancreat Surg. 2007;14(1):78–82.
7. Ansaloni L, Pisano M, Coccolini F, Peitzmann AB, Fingerhut A, Catena F, et al. WSES guidelines on acute calculous cholecystitis. World J Emerg Surg. 2016;11:25.
8. Kiewiet JJ, Leeuwenburgh MM, Bipat S, Bossuyt PM, Stoker J, Boermeester MA. A systematic review and meta-analysis of diagnostic performance of imaging in acute cholecystitis. Radiology. 2012;264:70.
9. Gutt CN, Encke J, Köninger J, Harnoss JC, Weigand K, Kipfmüller K, et al. Acute cholecystitis: early versus delayed cholecystectomy, a multicenter randomized trial (ACDC study, NCT00447304). Ann Surg. 2013;258(3):385–93.
10. Agresta F, Ansaloni L, Baiocchi GL, Bergamini C, Campanile FC, Carlucci M, et al. Laparoscopic approach to acute abdomen from the Consensus Development Conference of the Società Italiana di Chirurgia Endoscopica e nuove tecnologie (SICE), Associazione Chirurghi Ospedalieri Italiani (ACOI), Società Italiana di Chirurgia (SIC), Società Italiana di Chirurgia d'Urgenza e del Trauma (SICUT), Società Italiana di Chirurgia nell'Ospedalità Privata (SICOP), and the European Association for Endoscopic Surgery (EAES). Surg Endosc. 2012;26(8):2134–64.
11. Lee AY, Carter JJ, Hochberg MS, Stone AM, Cohen SL, Pachter HL. The timing of surgery for cholecystitis: a review of 202 consecutive patients at a large municipal hospital. Am J Surg. 2008;195(4):467–70.
12. Casillas RA, Yegiyants S, Collins JC. Early laparoscopic cholecystectomy is the preferred management of acute cholecystitis. Arch Surg. 2008;143(6):533–7.
13. Cameron IC, Chadwick C, Phillips J, Johnson AG. Management of acute cholecystitis in UK hospitals: time for a change. Postgrad Med J. 2004;80(943):292–4.
14. Senapati PS, Bhattarcharya D, Harinath G, Ammori BJ. A survey of the timing and approach to the surgical management of cholelithiasis in patients with acute biliary pancreatitis and acute cholecystitis in the UK. Ann R Coll Surg Engl. 2003;85(5):306–12.
15. de Mestral C, Rotstein OD, Laupacis A, et al. Comparative operative outcomes of early and delayed cholecystectomy for acute cholecystitis: a population-based propensity score analysis. Ann Surg. 2014;259:10–5.
16. de Mestral C, Rotstein OD, Laupacis A, et al. A population-based analysis of the clinical course of 10,304 patients with acute cholecystitis, discharged without cholecystectomy. J Trauma Acute Care Surg. 2013;74:26–30. discussion 30–31.
17. Gurusamy K, Samraj K, Gluud C, et al. Meta-analysis of randomized controlled trials on the safety and effectiveness of early versus delayed laparoscopic cholecystectomy for acute cholecystitis. Br J Surg. 2010;97:141–50.
18. Banz V, Gsponer T, Candinas D, Guller U. Population-based analysis of 4113 patients with acute cholecystitis: defining the optimal time-point for laparoscopic cholecystectomy. Ann Surg. 2011;254:964–70.
19. Nitzan O, Brodsky Y, Edelstein H, Hershko D, Saliba W, Keness Y, Peretz A, Chazan B. Microbiologic data in acute cholecystitis: ten years' experience from bile cultures obtained during percutaneous cholecystostomy. Surg Infect (Larchmt). 2017;18(3):345–9.
20. Gomi H, Solomkin JS, Takada T, Strasberg SM, Pitt HA, Yoshida M, et al. TG13 antimicrobial therapy for acute cholangitis and cholecystitis. J Hepatobiliary Pancreat Sci. 2013;20(1):60–70.
21. Chang K-K, Chang C-L, Tai F-T, Wang C-H, Lin R-C. Empiric antibiotic choices for community-acquired biliary tract infections. Adv Digest Med. 2014;1(2):54–9.
22. Peng WK, Sheikh Z, Paterson-Brown S, Nixon SJ. Role of liver function tests in predicting common bile duct stones in patients with acute calculous cholecystitis. Br J Surg. 2005;92:1241–7.
23. Khalfallah M, Dougaz W, Bedoui R, Bouasker I, Chaker Y, Nouira R, et al. Validation of the Lacaine-Huguier predictive score for choledocholithiasis: prospective study of 380 patients. J Visc Surg. 2012;149(1):e66–72.
24. Csendes A, Burdiles P, Diaz JC, Maluenda F, Korn O, Vallejo E, Csendes P. Prevalence of common bile duct stones according to the increasing number of risk factors present. A prospective study employing routinely intraoperative cholangiography in 477 cases. Hepatogastroenterology. 1998;45(23):1415–21.
25. Yang MH, Chen TH, Wang SE, Tsai YF, Su CH, Wu CW, et al. Biochemical predictors for absence of common bile duct stones in patients undergoing laparoscopic cholecystectomy. Surg Endosc. 2008;22:1620–4.
26. Barkun AN, Barkun JS, Fried GM, Ghitulescu G, Steinmetz O, Pham C, et al. Useful predictors of bile duct stones in patients undergoing laparoscopic cholecystectomy. Ann Surg. 1994;220:32–9.
27. ASGE Standards of Practice Committee, Maple JT, Ben-Menachem T, Anderson MA, Appalaneni V, Banerjee S, et al. The role of endoscopy in the evaluation of suspected choledocholithiasis. Gastrointest Endosc. 2010;71(1):1–9.
28. Heng Y, Leng J, Tan J, Chen K, Dong J. Proper surgical techniques approved for early laparoscopic cholecystectomy for non-critically ill elderly patients with acute cholecystitis. Hepatogastroenterology. 2013;60:688–91.
29. Karamanos E, Sivrikoz E, Beale E, Chan L, Inaba K, Demetriades D. Effect of diabetes on outcomes in patients undergoing emergent cholecystectomy for acute cholecystitis. World J Surg. 2013;37:2257–64.
30. Yokoe M, Takada T, Strasberg SM, Solomkin JS, Mayumi T, Gomi H, et al. Tokyo guidelines revision committee. TG13 diagnostic criteria and severity grading of acute cholecystitis (with videos). J Hepatobiliary Pancreat Sci. 2013;20(1):35–46.
31. Houghton PWG, Jenkinson LR, Donaldson LA. Cholecystectomy in the elderly: a prospective study. Br J Surg. 1985;72:220–2.
32. Frazee RC, Nagorney DM, Mucha P Jr. Acute calculous cholecystitis. Mayo Clin Proc. 1989;64:163–7.
33. Sparkman RS. Bobbs centennial: the first cholecystostomy. Surgery. 1967;61:965–71.
34. Radder RW. Ultrasonically guided percutaneous catheter drainage for gallbladder empyema. Diagn Imaging. 1980;49:330–3.
35. McGahan JP, Lindfors KK. Percutaneous cholecystostomy: an alternative to surgical cholecystostomy for acute cholecystitis. Radiology. 1989;173:481–5.
36. VanSonnenberg E, D'Agostino HB, Goodacre BW, Sanchez RB, Casola G. Percutaneous gallbladder puncture and cholecystostomy: results, complications and caveats for safety. Radiology. 1992;183:163–70.
37. Gervais DA, Mueller PR. Percutaneous cholecystostomy. Semin Intervent Radiol. 1996;13:35–43.

38. Van Overhagen H, Meyers H, Tilanus HW, Jeekel J, Lameris JS. Percutaneous cholecystostomy for patients with acute cholecystitis and an increased surgical risk. Cardiovasc Intervent Radiol. 1996;19:72–6.
39. Vogelzang RL, Nemcek AA. Percutaneous cholecystostomy: diagnostic and therapeutic efficacy. Radiology. 1988;168:29–34.
40. Garber SJ, Mathleson JR, Cooperberg PL, Mac Farlane JK. Percutaneous cholecystostomy: safety of the transperitoneal route. J Vasc Interv Radiol. 1994;5:295–8.
41. Chopra S, Dodd DG, Mumbover AL, Chintapalli KN, Schwesinger WH, Sirinek KR, et al. Treatment of acute cholecystitis in noncritically ill patients at high surgical risk: comparison of clinical outcomes after gallbladder aspiration and percutaneous cholecystostomy. Am J Roentgenol. 2001;176:1025–31.
42. England RE, McDermott VG, Smith TP, Suhocki PV, Payne CS, Newman GE. Percutaneous cholecystostomy: who responds? Am J Roentgenol. 1997;168:1247–51.
43. Hatjidakis AA, Karampekios S, Prassopoulos P, Xynos E, Raissaki M, Vasilakis SI, et al. Maturation of the tract after percutaneous cholecystostomy with regard to the access route. Cardiovasc Intervent Radiol. 1998;21:36–40.
44. Cope C. Percutaneous subhepatic cholecystostomy with removal anchor. Am J Roentgenol. 1988;151:1129–32.
45. Picus D, Burns MA, Hicks ME, Darcy MD, Vesely TM. Percutaneous management of persistently immature cholecystostomy tracts. J Vasc Interv Radiol. 1993;4:97–102.
46. Warren LP, Kadir S, Dunnick NR. Percutaneous cholecystostomy: anatomic considerations. Radiology. 1988;168:615–6.
47. Corbett CRR, Fyte NCM, Nicholis RJ, Jackson BT. Bile peritonitis after removal of T-tubes from the common bile duct. Br J Surg. 1986;73:641–3.
48. Vauthey N, Lerut J, Martini M, Becker C, Gersch P, Blumgart LH. Indications and limitations of percutaneous cholecystostomy for acute cholecystitis. Surg Gynecol Obstet. 1993;176:49–54.
49. Safrany L, Cotton PB. Endoscopic management of choledocholithiasis. Surg Clin North Am. 1982;62:825–36.
50. Macchini D, Degrate L, Oldani M, Leni D, Padalino P, Romano F, Gianotti L. Timing of percutaneous cholecystostomy tube removal: systematic review. Minerva Chir. 2016;71(6):415–26.
51. Van Steenbergen W, Ponette E, Marchal G, Pelemans W, Aerts R, Fevery J. Percutaneous cholecystostomy for acute complicated cholecystitis in elderly patients. Am J Gastroenterol. 1990;85:1363–7.
52. Sugiyama M, Tokuhara M, Atomi Y. Is percutaneous cholecystostomy the optimal treatment for acute cholecystitis in the very elderly? World J Surg. 1998;22:459–63.
53. Browning PD, Mc Gahan JP, Gersovich EO. Percutaneous cholecystostomy for suspected acute cholecystitis in the hospitalized patient. J Vasc Interv Radiol. 1993;4:531–8.
54. Chang L, Moonka R, Stelzner M. Percutaneous cholecystostomy for acute cholecystitis in veteran patients. Am J Surg. 2000;180:198–202.
55. Raissaki M, Hatzidakis AA, Prassopoulos P, Bakandaki A, Vrachassotakis N, Vasilakis SJ, et al. Late complication following percutaneous cholecystostomy: retained abdominal wall gallstone. Eur Radiol. 2000;10:1284–6.
56. Patel M, Miedema BW, James MA, Marshall JB. Percutaneous cholecystostomy is an effective treatment for high-risk patients with acute cholecystitis. Am Surg. 2000;66:33–7.
57. Avrahami R, Badani E, Watemberg S, et al. The role of percutaneous transhepatic cholecystostomy in the management of acute cholecystitis in high-risk patients. Int Surg. 1995;80:111–4.
58. Penas-Herrero I, de la Serna-Higuera C, Perez-Miranda M. Endoscopic ultrasound-guided gallbladder drainage for the management of acute cholecystitis. J Hepatobiliary Pancreat Sci. 2015;22:35–43.
59. Patil R, Ona MA, Papafragkakis C, Arnand S, Duddempudi S. Endoscopic ultrasound-guided placement of the lumen apposing self expandable metallic stent for gallbladder drainage : a promising technique. Ann Gastroenterol. 2016;29:162–7.
60. Itoi T, Coelho-Prabhu N, Baron TH. Endoscopic gallbladder drainage for management of acute cholecystitis. Gastrointest Endosc. 2010;71:1038–45.
61. Mutignani M, Iacopini F, Perri V, et al. Endoscopic gallbladder drainage for acute cholecystitis: technical and clinical results. Endoscopy. 2009;41:539–46.
62. Gurusuamy KS, Rossi M, Davidson BR. Percutaneous cholecystectomy for high-risk surgical patients with acute calculous cholecystitis. Cochrane Database Syst Rev. 2013;12(8).
63. Jang JW, Lee SS, Song TJ, et al. Endoscopic ultrasound-guided transmural and percutaneous trans hepatic gallbladder drainage are comparable for acute cholecystitis. Gastroenterology. 2012;142:805–11.
64. Choi JH, Lee SS, Choi JH, Park DH, Seo DW, Lee SK, Kim MH. Long-term outcomes after endoscopic ultrasonography-guided gallbladder drainage for acute cholecystitis. Endoscopy. 2014;46(8):656–61.
65. Irani S, Baron TH, Grimm IS, Kashab MA. EUS-guided gallbladder drainage with a lumen apposing metal stent. Gastrointest Endosc. 2015;82(6):1110–5.
66. Walter D, Teoh AY, Itoi T, et al. EUS-guided gallbladder drainage with a lumen-apposing metal stent : a prospective long-term evaluation. Gut. 2016;65:6–8.
67. Teho AY, Serna C, Penas I, et al. Endoscopic ultrasound-guided gallbladder drainage reduces adverse events compared to percutaneous cholecystostomy in patients who are unfit for cholecystectomy. Endoscopy. 2017;49:130–8.
68. Kiriyama S, Takada T, Strasberg SM, et al. TG13 guidelines for diagnosis and severity grading of acute cholangitis. J Hepatobiliary Pancreat Sci. 2012;20:24.
69. Kimura Y, Takada T, Kawarada Y, et al. Definitions, pathophysiology, and epidemiology of acute cholangitis and cholecystitis: Tokyo guidelines. J Hepatobiliary Pancreat Surg. 2007;14:15.
70. Jang SE, Park SW, Lee BS, Shin CM, Lee SH, Kim JW, Jeong SH, Kim N, Lee DH, Park JK, Hwang JH. Management for CBD stone-related mild to moderate acute cholangitis: urgent versus elective ERCP. Dig Dis Sci. 2013;58(7):2082–7.
71. Schneider J, Hapfelmeier A, Thores S, et al. Mortality risk for acute cholangitis (MAC) : a risk prediction model for in-hospital mortality in patients with acute cholangitis. BMC Gastroenterol. 2016;16:15.
72. Hou L, Laine L, Motamedi N, et al. Optimal timing of ERCP in acute cholangitis. J Clin Gastroenterol. 2017;51(6):534–8.
73. Kashab M, Tariq A, Tatiq U, et al. Delayed and unsuccessful ERCP are associated with worse outcomes in patients with acute cholangitis. Clin Gastroenterol Hepatol. 2012;10:1157–61.
74. Miura F, Takada T, Strasberg SM, Solomkin JS, Pitt HA, Gouma DJ, Garden OJ, Büchler MW, et al. TG13 flowchart for the management of acute cholangitis and cholecystitis. J Hepatobiliary Pancreat Sci. 2013;20(1):47–54.
75. Sun Z, Zhu Y, Zhu B, Xu G, Zhang N. Controversy and progress for treatment of acute cholangitis after Tokyo guidelines (TG13). Biosci Trends. 2016;10:22–6.
76. Tsuchiya T, Sofuni A, Tsuji S, et al. Endoscopic management of acute cholangitis according to TG13. Dig Endosc. 2017;29(s2):94–9.
77. Khashab MA, El Zein MH, Sharzehi K, et al. EUS-guided biliary drainage or enteroscopy-assisted ERCP in patients with surgical anatomy and biliary obstruction: an international study. Endoscopy. 2016;4:1322–7.
78. Minaga K, Kitano M. Recent advances in endoscopic ultrasound-guided biliary drainage. Dig Endosc. 2018;30(1):38–47.

79. Moole H, Bechtold ML, Forcione D, Puli SR. A meta-analysis and systematic review : success of EUS guided biliary stunting in patients with inoperable malignant biliary strictures and a failed ERCP. Medicine. 2017;96:3.
80. Kahn MA, Akbar A, Naron TH, et al. Endoscopic ultrasound-guided biliary drainage: a systematic review and meta-analysis. Dig Dis Sci. 2016;61:684–703.
81. Sharaiha RZ, Kahn MA, Kamal F, et al. Efficacy and safety of EUS-guided biliary drainage in comparison with percutaneous biliary drainage when ERC fails: a systematic review and meta-analysis. Gastrointest Endosc. 2017;85(5):904–14.
82. Baniya R, Upadhaya S, Madala S, et al. Endoscopic ultrasound-guided biliary drainage versus percutaneous transhepatic biliary drainage after failed endoscopic retrograde cholangiopancreatography: a meta-analysis. Clin Exp Gastroenterol. 2017;10:67–74.
83. Altman A, Zangan SM. Benign biliary strictures. Semin Intervent Radiol. 2016;33(4):297–306.
84. Lin H, Li S, Liu X. The safety and efficacy of nasobiliary drainage versus biliary stenting in malignant biliary obstruction: a systematic review and meta-analysis. Medicine (Baltimore). 2016;95:e5253.
85. Iacono C, Ruzzenente A, Campagnaro T, Bortolasi L, Valdegamberi A, Guglielmi A. Role of preoperative biliary drainage in jaundiced patients who are candidates for pancreatoduodenectomy or hepatic resection: highlights and drawbacks. Ann Surg. 2013;257(2):191–204.
86. Davids PH, Groen AK, Rauws EA, et al. Randomised trial of self-expanding metal stents versus polyethylene stents for distal malignant biliary obstruction. Lancet. 1992;340:1488–92.
87. Almadi MA, Barkun A, Martel M. Plastic vs. self-expandable metal stents for palliation in malignant biliary obstruction: a series of meta-analyses. Am J Gastroenterol. 2017;112:260–73.
88. Chen MY, Lin JW, Zhu HP, et al. Covered stents versus uncovered stents for unresectable malignant biliary strictures: a meta-analysis. Biomed Res Int. 2016;2016:6408067.
89. Ekkelenkamp VE, de Man RA, Ter Borg F, et al. Prospective evaluation of ERCP performance: results of a nationwide quality registry. Endoscopy. 2015;47:503–7.
90. Sportes A, Camus M, Greget M, Leblanc S, Coriat R, Hochberger J, Chaussade S, Grabar S, Prat F. Endoscopic ultrasound-guided hepaticogastrostomy versus percutaneous transhepatic drainage for malignant biliary obstruction after failed endoscopic retrograde cholangiopancreatography: a retrospective expertise-based study from two centers. Therap Adv Gastroenterol. 2017;10(6):483–93.
91. Nguyen-Tang T, Binmoeller KF, Sanchez-Yague A, et al. Endoscopic ultrasound (EUS)-guided transhepatic anterograde self-expandable metal stent (SEMS) placement across malignant biliary obstruction. Endoscopy. 2010;42:232–6.
92. Kawakubo K, Isayama H, Kato H, et al. Multicenter retrospective study of endoscopic ultrasound-guided biliary drainage for malignant biliary obstruction in Japan. J Hepatobiliary Pancreat Sci. 2014;21:328–34.

32 Updates in Non-traumatic Urological Emergencies

Angelo Naselli, Stefano Paparella, and Pierpaolo Graziotti

Key Points

- Renal colic and concomitant sepsis are a life-threatening condition; it must be recognized early to start treatment as soon as possible; immediate drainage either by ureteral stenting or percutaneous puncture in case of suspected or known infection is mandatory and is only a part of the treatment.
- Drainage of the bladder either by suprapubic puncture or indwell urethral catheterization is mandatory in case of acute urinary retention; bedside cystoscopy may help in difficult urethral catheterization if suprapubic puncture is contraindicated.
- Testicular torsion should be recognized among causes of acute scrotum mainly by clinical history and physical examination; ancillary diagnostic tests should never delay intervention also in equivocal cases.
- Differentiate between high- and low-flow priapism by means of clinical history, physical examination and penile blood gas examination; immediate treatment for low-flow priapism is mandatory.
- Fournier's gangrene delayed surgical treatment may cause death of the patient even if broad-spectrum antibiotics are started immediately; it is mandatory to recognize early signs of necrosis of the perineum, keeping in mind that skin necrosis may occur lately.
- Poor response to antibiotic treatment in a diabetic patient with a pyelonephritis should immediately arouse suspicion of emphysematous infection of the kidney and prompt a computed tomography scan for the diagnosis.
- Poor response to antibiotic treatment of prostatitis should arouse the suspicion of emphysematous prostatitis; transrectal ultrasound and/or computed tomography scan of the pelvis is necessary to obtain a diagnosis.
- Normalizing glycaemia level in subjects with uncontrolled diabetes is a mandatory step of the treatment of any infectious urological conditions.

A. Naselli · S. Paparella · P. Graziotti (✉)
Urology Department, San Giuseppe Hospital, Multimedica Group, Milan, Italy
e-mail: angelo.naselli@auro.it; stefano.paparella@multimedica.it

32.1 Renal Colic

32.1.1 Diagnosis

Renal colic is a frequent cause of access to emergency department. The basic patient's assessment consists of patient medical history, visit, urine dipstick test, collecting a serum blood sample for blood cell count and to measure the level of creatinine, uric acid, (ionized) calcium, sodium, C-reactive protein (and procalcitonin if available), glucose and lactate [1].

Common renal colic symptoms are acute flank/hypochondrium pain, acute groin pain (likely linked to renal pelvis, ureteropelvic junction, lumbar ureter stones) and/or iliac pain and/or urinary urgency and frequency (likely linked to pelvic ureter stones). Macroscopic haematuria may be concomitant. Microscopic haematuria or leucocytes are common findings of the urine dipsticks.

Patients with a suspected renal colic and without sign or symptoms of systemic inflammatory response syndrome (SIRS) must be screened for stone in urinary tract.

Bedside ultrasound imaging is a fast, safe and cheap first-line assessment tool [2].

P. Aseni et al. (eds.), *Operative Techniques and Recent Advances in Acute Care and Emergency Surgery*,
https://doi.org/10.1007/978-3-319-95114-0_32

It may identify hydronephrosis, stone in the pelvis, in the ureteropelvic junction and the distal tract of the ureter. About 80% of the cases do not require further imaging with substantial reductions in radiation exposure and imaging costs [3].

However, ultrasound has a lower accuracy in respect to computed tomography. Particularly, hydronephrosis on ultrasound had relatively low positive and negative predictive values, around 0.7–0.8, respectively, for the presence or absence of a ureteral stone [4].

The performance of kidney-ureter-bladder radiography (KUB) is relatively poor; sensitivity and specificity range from 40 to 80%. Moreover, the detection capability of alternative diagnosis of acute flank pain is unsatisfactory, particularly in the female, being well under 10% [5–7].

Therefore, CT may be necessary to obtain a correct diagnosis. Ultra-low or low-dose computed tomography showed a sensitivity of 90/100% and a specificity of 86/100% regarding urolithiasis in a recent systematic review, while radiation exposure was significantly reduced with respect to standard CT. Average radiation dose ranged from 1 to 1.5 millisieverts. Nevertheless, it may not be as effective in detecting stones <3 mm in size or in patients with a body mass index of >30 kg/m^2 [8].

However, if the pre-test probability of stone disease, a combination of clinical, laboratory suspicion, ultrasound and (when available) KUB findings, at the index visit is not significantly higher than the pre-test probability of alternative diagnoses, standard CT should be preferred. As a matter of fact, low-dose CT accuracy in the detection of alternative diagnoses is unknown [9].

Stones can be classified according to plain X-ray appearance [kidney-ureter-bladder (KUB) radiography] as well as by density (Hounsfield units) measured by CT which is likewise efficient in this regard. Non-contrast-enhanced CT can be used to classify stones according to density, inner structure and composition. Thus, if an active treatment of the stone is planned, CT is mandatory. It gives a precise measure of stone size, location, distance from the skin and particularly of its density. Moreover, a contrast CT may be necessary to assess the urinary tract morphology before planning complex procedures [10, 11].

In case of pregnant woman or children, the use of CT should be avoided. Ultrasound fails to detect urinary stone in up to 40% of paediatric cases. Low-dose CT particularly is an option only if magnetic resonance (MR) is not available and in extremely urgent cases. As a matter of fact, they may be replaced efficiently by MR urography, which may require sedation or anaesthesia in children. MR shows the level of obstruction and identifies stones as filling defects (as well as urography) [12, 13].

Patients with renal colic complicated by a suspected or ascertained infection must be *immediately* screened for SIRS. SIRS should be disclosed by means of standard international criteria assessment. The presence of at least two of the subsequent criteria is suggestive of SIRS: temperature (>38 or < 36), pulse (>90), respiratory rate (>20), white blood cell count >12 or <4 × 10^9/L, blood glucose (>120 mg% not if diabetics), new confusion/drowsiness, plasma C-reactive protein >2 SD above the normal value and plasma procalcitonin >2 SD above the normal value.

SIRS associated with a suspected or confirmed infection is an uncomplicated sepsis. If one or more organ dysfunction is found, a severe sepsis is diagnosed. The most serious form of sepsis is the septic shock (*lactate* >4 mmol/L at any time point or severe, uncontrolled hypotension) [14].

Mortality related to uncomplicated sepsis, severe sepsis and septic shock is, respectively, 10%, 35% and 50% [15].

32.1.2 Treatment Priority in an Emergency Setting

(a) Patients without SIRS/sepsis and stone size <7 mm:
  - Pain relief.
  - According to patient preference, after and adequate information, medical expulsive therapy or active treatment (SWL, ureterorenoscopy).

(b) Patients without SIRS/sepsis and stone size >6 mm:
  - Pain relief.
  - Active treatment (SWL, ureterorenoscopy, PCNL); expulsive medical therapy has a low change of having a good outcome and should not be proposed unless the patient refuses any active treatment.

(c) Patients with SIRS/sepsis:
  - Pain relief and imaging must not delay urosepsis treatment which includes kidney drainage.

(d) Obstructive anuria, oligoanuria (patients with one kidney or bilateral obstruction):
  - Pain relief and imaging must not delay anuria treatment.
  - Immediate kidney drainage and sepsis treatment when concomitant.

32.1.3 Treatment Modality

32.1.3.1 Pain Relief

Non-steroidal anti-inflammatory drugs (NSAIDs) are superior to placebo in reducing pain by 50% in a large meta-analysis. Opioids are equally efficient to reach an adequate pain control. However, they have significantly more side effects, particularly pethidine. Moreover, antispasmodics and hyoscine, also in combination with NSAID, do not improve NSAID efficiency. Among NSAIDs, indomethacin was the less effective. Therefore, NSAID should be the first choice of pain treatment. Antispasmodics and hyoscine should not be used. Opioids should be deserved as a second choice [15, 16].

A recent Cochrane meta-analysis demonstrates that patients with larger stones benefit from alpha-blocker oral therapy. They increase the likelihood of spontaneous passage of ureteral stones (relative risk 1.57, confidence interval 1.17–2.27), irrespective of the stone level, and improve pain control (number of pain episodes −0.74, confidence interval −1.28 to −0.21) [17].

Kidney drainage (or immediate stone treatment) should be discussed with the patient (see the following paragraph), in case of uncontrolled pain, despite pharmacological therapy.

32.1.3.2 Urosepsis Treatment

Urological sepsis needs a multidisciplinary approach.

The following recommendations of the “surviving sepsis campaign” guidelines involve particularly the urologists:

- Obtain routine microbiologic cultures (at least two sets of blood cultures, aerobic and anaerobic) before starting antimicrobial.
- Start antimicrobials as soon as possible after recognition and within 1 h for both sepsis and septic shock.
- Empiric broad-spectrum therapy with one or more antimicrobials for patients presenting with sepsis or septic shock to cover all likely pathogens (including bacterial and potentially fungal or viral coverage) is strongly recommended.
- Shorter courses of antimicrobial are appropriate in some patients, particularly those with rapid clinical resolution following effective source control of intra-abdominal or urinary sepsis and those with anatomically uncomplicated.
- Start pharmacologic prophylaxis (unfractionated heparin [UFH] or low-molecular-weight heparin [LMWH]) against venous thromboembolism (VTE) in the absence of contraindications.
- Any required source control intervention be implemented as soon as medically and logistically practical after the diagnosis is made (immediate kidney drainage).

Kidney drainage may be obtained by ureteral stenting or percutaneous nephrostomy (PCN) placement of the kidney.

Outcomes and complications are similar. The slightly increased risk of bacteraemia following ureteral stenting is balanced by the slightly increased risk of major complications following PCN, which reaches 5% of cases [18]. Indeed, PCN should be preferred in extremely urgent cases because it can be performed immediately in the emergency room by ultrasound guidance and with local anaesthesia.

A treatment algorithm should include a first-line assessment clinical history, physical examination, laboratory data [9] and ultrasound assessment. In controversial situation, a CRP level >28 mg/L suggests an occult or early sepsis and should indicate immediate kidney drainage [19].

32.1.3.3 Obstructive Anuria/Oligoanuria with or Without Urosepsis

See the previous paragraph regarding kidney drainage and urosepsis management (Figs. 32.1 and 32.2).

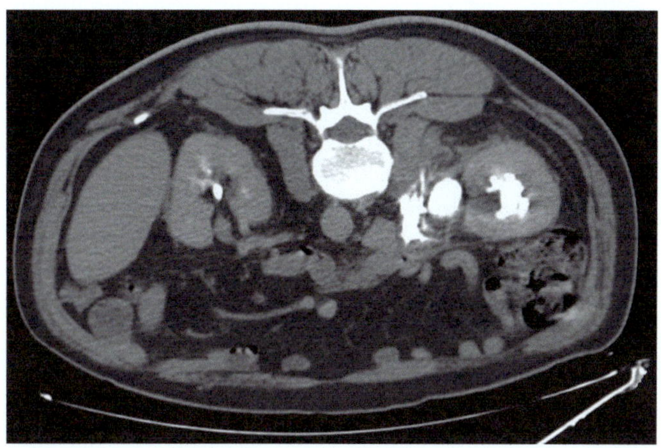

Fig. 32.1 A case of mild symptomatic renal colic followed by subtle urosepsis occurrence the day after the first access to the emergency room. CT scan shows urine extravasation. Drainage by ureteral stenting was performed

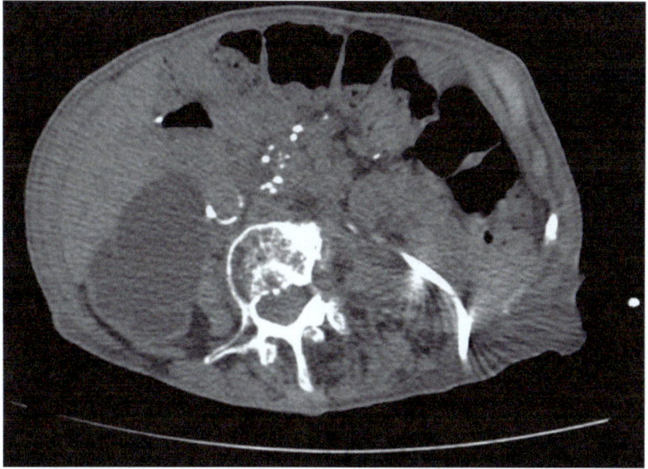

Fig. 32.2 A case of obstructive oligoanuria and sepsis. The right kidney was not working because of an inveterate ureteral obstructing stone. The patient presented left renal colic, oligoanuria and signs and symptoms of severe sepsis. Immediate drainage was performed by percutaneous drainage. The procedure was difficult because of severe scoliosis and colic interposition

32.2 Acute Urinary Retention

32.2.1 Diagnosis

Acute urinary retention (AUR) is a frequent urological emergency and an important public health issue which affects mainly men. AUR is associated with increased mortality, especially in men aged 45–54 with respect to general population. It has been estimated that up to "1 to 10" men in their 70s will experience AUR. The risk increases further to "3 to 10" in the population with moderate to severe urinary symptoms [20, 21]. Clinical symptoms are lower abdominal pain, swelling, and inability to pass urine. Physical examination discloses a hypogastric palpable mass, dull at percussion. It must include digital rectal examination to assess size and consistency of the prostate and presence or absence of constipation. As stated before, lower urinary tract symptoms may precede or not AUR. If diagnosis is equivocal, bedside ultrasound may help in discriminating AUR.

32.2.2 Treatment

Bladder must be immediately drained either by urethral or suprapubic catheterisation. No statistically significant difference between the two techniques has been detected in the past. Overall, suprapubic drainage has less incidence of urinary infection, urethral stricture, and allows trial without catheter removal, whereas urethral drainage has lower risk of serious complications like bowel perforation and sepsis [22, 23].

In case of active bleeding from the urethra, severe urethral stricture, false passages/channels, bladder neck contracture, locally advanced pelvic cancer, anasarca (glans not visible into a swollen prepuce), presence of penile prosthesis or malfunctioning implants for incontinence in the male and early loss of catheter after radical prostatectomy or cystectomy, urethral catheterisation may be impossible if not contraindicated. Indeed, suprapubic drainage should be avoided in patients with concomitant anticoagulant therapy or with known coagulopathy, a small contracted bladder and surgical scarring of the lower abdominal wall [24].

It must be emphasized that 30-day mortality related to suprapubic catheterization is around 1% likewise in some major urological surgical procedures like cystectomy or prostatectomy [25].

Indeed, serious complications by urethral catheterization are rarely reported, even if possible, including urethral/penis damage, Fournier's gangrene, haemorrhage, sepsis and death [26–29].

If suprapubic drainage is not feasible and urethral catheterization impossible, even with the aid of perineal compression or by lifting the prostatic urethra with digital rectal exploration, a trial with blind guide wire insertion should be performed. If it fails the procedure should be repeated with the help of a flexible cystoscopy under direct vision. Filiform and related procedures should not be employed. If flexible cystoscopy is not available or fails, the patient should be treated in the operating room. Pain relief in the meanwhile could be obtained by emptying the bladder by means of a simple suprapubic puncture with a needle [24].

If the procedure is performed in a sterile manner, routine antibiotic prophylaxis is not needed [30].

32.3 Acute Scrotal Pain

32.3.1 Diagnosis

Testicular torsion occurs mainly in prepuberal or young adults [31], even if it may also occur in older subjects. As a matter of fact, up to a quarter of cases have more than 31 years [32]. Sporadic cases in older people, aged more than 50 and 60 years, have been reported [33, 34]. Testicular torsion is caused by twisting of the spermatic cord within the tunica vaginalis. It involves the whole spermatic cord only in infants. Firstly, venous blood flow stops. Eventually, venous and arterial pressure equalizes, and arterial flux comes to an end causing ischaemia and then necrosis. Ischaemia usually occurs about 4 h after torsion and is sure within 24 h. Detorsion is necessary to revert the process. It is successful in more than 90% cases if performed within 6 h, 50% within 12 h and less than 10% after 1 day [35].

Diagnosis is based on clinical history and physical examination. While assessing a patient, it should be kept in mind that up to 40% of cases of acute scrotum in a boy is a torsion [36].

Alternative diagnosis of acute scrotum is trauma, epididymitis/orchitis, incarcerated hernia, varicocele, idiopathic scrotal oedema, and torsion of the appendix testis, the most frequent being epididymitis and appendix torsion.

The proportion of testicular torsion in acute scrotum is around 70%, whereas it is about 10% for epididymitis and appendix torsion in young boys [35, 37]. However, it should be underlined that a peak of incidence of testicular torsion, epididymitis and hydatid torsion has been, respectively, measured within 1 year, around 5 years and 10 years of life when they represent the most frequent cause of acute scrotum. Since then, testicular torsion remains the most important aetiology for young adults.

Testicular torsion causes an acute pain in the scrotum, sometimes irradiating in inguinal region and even in iliac fossa. It usually does not recognize any precipitating cause. Epididymitis and appendix torsion may develop the same symptom. Tenderness of the epididymis and pyuria and a hard and tender nodule of the upper pole of the testis, leaving posteriorly the epididymis, may help in discriminating testicular torsion. Moreover, the appendix torsion can be followed by the onset of the "blue dot sign", a blue discoloration of the skin corresponding to the palpable nodule. In both cases the testis size remains comparable to the healthy one where it increases in torsion. Testicular torsion frequently causes a shortening of the spermatic cord. Therefore, the affected testis may appear higher. This sign is highly specific. Finally, the cremasteric reflex may only be elicited in non-torsion cases of acute scrotum with a sensitivity near 100% [38].

Doppler ultrasound has a significant accuracy in discriminating testicular torsion from alternative diagnosis. Its sensitivity and specificity are around 90% [39].

Scintigraphy using technetium 99 m pertechnetate has a 100% probability to detect torsion. Indeed, it may be not always available and cause a significant delay in the diagnosis and should be deserved to assess undescended testis [40].

However, if clinical history and physical examination are suggestive of torsion, the patient must be immediately treated, and ancillary imaging procedures should be avoided [41].

32.3.2 Treatment

Detorsion may be performed manually, rotating the testis from left to right for the right testis and from the right to left for the left testis. More than one 360° grade rotation may be necessary. Anaesthesia with lidocaine injected in the spermatic cord may help as well as bland sedation. Pain must be relieved immediately, and return of the arterial and venous flux should be documented [42].

If it fails or the outcome is uncertain, surgical exploration should be performed immediately. If the physician is not experienced with manual detorsion, it should not be attempted, and surgical exploration should be done. If the testis is not viable, it should be removed [43].

32.4 Priapism

32.4.1 Definition, Pathogenesis and Classification

Priapism is a persistent and painful erection lasting more than 4 h that is not related to sexual arousal or relieved by sexual intercourse [44]. There are two types of priapism: low-flow and high-flow.

Low-flow priapism, or ischaemic priapism (95% of all priapism episodes), results from decreased venous and lymphatic drainage of the corpus cavernosum. High-flow priapism is less likely to be ischaemic and is most often caused by a traumatic arterial laceration. The main complication of prolonged priapism is erectile dysfunction, especially in recurrent ischaemic priapism, due to inflammation and fibrosis of the corpus cavernosum [44, 45]. Most cases of low-flow priapism in adults are secondary to medication or drug use. Abuse of alcohol and cocaine can be related to the onset of priapism. Some drugs are also involved in the development of priapism: psychiatric medications (chlorpromazine, trazodone, thioridazine and other selective serotonin reuptake inhibitors—SSRIs) and blood pressure medications such as hydralazine, prazosin and calcium channel blockers [46, 47]. Ischaemic priapism occurs relatively often (up to 35%) after intracavernous injections of papaverine-based combinations, while it is rare (< 1%) after prostaglandin E1 monotherapy. Priapism is rare in men who have taken PDE5Is (sildenafil, vardenafil and tadalafil) with only sporadic cases reported [48]. Blood dyscrasias and hypercoagulable states (such as sickle cell disease, thalassemia, polycythaemia, vasculitis) can cause low-flow priapism. Sometimes neurologic conditions may be the trigger (spinal stenosis, spinal cord lesions or trauma, multiple sclerosis). Indeed, priapism resulting from metastatic or regional infiltration is rare [44, 48]. Infections (toxin-mediated) (i.e. scorpion sting, spider bite, rabies, malaria) are another rare cause of low-flow priapism. The most common cause of high-flow priapism is arteriovenous fistula formation secondary to perineal trauma [44, 48]. Priapism may occur at all ages. The incidence rate of priapism in the general population is low (0.5–0.9 cases per 100,000 person-years) [49]. In patients with sickle cell disease, the prevalence of priapism is up to 3.6% in patients <18 years of age [50] increasing up to 42% in patients ≥18 years of age [51].

32.4.2 Diagnosis

Patients present with an erect, tender penis and soft glans, unrelated to sexual arousal [52]. High-flow state is usually less painful and carries a smaller risk of ischaemia [47]. The diagnostic challenge lies in differentiating high- from low-flow states through patient history, as the treatment differs greatly. Generally, high-flow priapism patients will have a recent history of perineal trauma. These patients usually seek treatment later in the course as they do not typically experience intense pain, as opposed to low-flow patients [44]. Penile blood gas examination, aspirated from the corpus cavernosum, may help in discriminating between high- and low-flow states. Low-flow priapism is a hypoxic state, so blood appears dark and dusky; instead non-ischaemic priapism aspirate is well oxygenated and bright red. An ischaemic penile blood gas typically reveals a partial pressure of oxygen (PO2) < 30 mmHg, a partial pressure of carbon dioxide (PCO_2) > 60 mmHg and a pH < 7.25, whereas a non-ischaemic state will closely mimic normal arterial blood. Colour duplex ultrasonography may help. There will be an absence of blood flow in the cavernous arteries in ischaemic priapism. Additionally, a fistula or pseudoaneurysm may be discovered by ultrasound in the high-flow state [46]. The role of MRI in the diagnostic evaluation of priapism is controversial and limited to postemergency assessment. It may be helpful to assess the viability of the corpora cavernosa and the presence of penile fibrosis [53]. Complete blood count (CBC), coagulation studies and a sickle cell screen should be assessed [44]. Haemoglobin electrophoresis and reticulocyte count can reveal sickle cell abnormalities or thalassemia and are indicated for all priapism patients unless the cause of priapism is definitively known. Finally, a urine toxicology screen for illicit drugs is useful when suspected [46].

32.4.3 Treatment

Emergency medical intervention is required to minimize potential irreversible consequences, such as corporal fibrosis and permanent erectile dysfunction (ED) [54]. The duration of priapism represents the most significant predictor of the development of ED. Interventions beyond 48–72 h since onset may help to relieve erection and pain but have little benefit in preventing ED. The first step in the management of priapism, regardless of the cause, is always hydration and analgesia. If the patient has an acute sickle cell crisis, fluids and analgesia with supplemental oxygen may lead to detumescence [44].

Historically, several first-line treatments have been described for low-flow (ischaemic) priapism; however, there is lack of evidence of benefit for such measures. Treatment is often heterogeneous and varies depending on the patient's response. A schematic summary of treatment is composed of (1) initial conservative measures, (2) cavernosal irrigation, (3) intracavernosal therapy and (4) surgical therapy. The treatment is sequential, and the physician should move on to the next stage if the prior treatment fails.

1. Initial conservative measures include local anaesthesia of the penis, the insertion of wide-bore butterfly (16–18G) and the aspiration of cavernosal blood until bright red arterial blood is obtained.
2. Cavernosal irrigation should be performed with 0.9% w/v saline solution. Irrigation can be alternated with aspiration.
3. Intracavernosal therapy includes injection of intracavernosal adrenoceptor agonist. Current first-line therapy is phenylephrine with aliquots of 200 micrograms being injected every 5–10 min until detumescence is achieved (maximum dose of phenylephrine is 1 mg within 1 h). The dose of phenylephrine should be reduced in children. It can result in significant hypertension and should be used with caution in men with cardiovascular disease, and monitoring of pulse, blood pressure and electrocardiogram (ECG) is advisable in all patients during administration and for 60 min afterwards. Its use is contraindicated in men with a history of cerebrovascular disease and significant hypertension [55]. Pharmacological agents include sympathomimetic drugs or alpha-adrenergic agonists. Options for intracavernosal sympathomimetic agents include phenylephrine, etilephrine, ephedrine, epinephrine, norepinephrine and metaraminol, with a resolution rate of up to 80% [48, 56, 57]. The use of intracavernosal adrenalin injection alone has also been sporadically reported [58] as well as oral or subcutaneous terbutaline sulphate and intracavernosal injection of methylene blue [59, 60].
4. If there is immediate recurrence after aspiration, the next step is a surgical shunt between the corpora spongiosa and cavernosum. Penile prosthesis implantation should be considered if priapism has last for more than 36 h [45, 48, 62].

For high-flow priapism, the treatment strategy is much different. This type of priapism is non-ischaemic as arterial blood flow is intact. Thus, it is not usually an emergency and invasive treatment may be delayed. The goal is to preserve penile function. Treatment with selective arterial embolization using an autologous clot is highly effective with normal sexual function restoration in 86% of cases [61].

32.5 Fournier's Gangrene

32.5.1 Definition and Pathogenesis

Fournier's gangrene is a necrotizing fasciitis of the perineal, perianal or genital areas. It is usually caused by a polymicrobial infection. Fournier's gangrene is a relatively uncommon disease, but it can affect all ages and both genders. It is life-threatening with a mortality rate of 13–22% despite timely and aggressive therapy [63, 64]. The necrotizing fasciitis frequently stems from an infection of the anorectum (30–50%), uro-genitalia (20–40%) or genital skin (20%) [65]. Trauma to these regions is a possible source of infection (instrumentation, perineal trauma, recent catheterization). Fournier's gangrene has been shown to be strongly associated with diabetes, chronic alcoholism, human immunodeficiency virus (HIV), chronic steroid abuse, cytotoxic drugs and lymphoproliferative diseases [66]. A malnutrition situation associated with lower socio-economic status (and a poor perineal hygiene) has also been shown to be related to the development of Fournier [66]. The underlying principle of all these conditions is compromised host immunity creating a favourable environment to establish infection. Additionally, the infection is most aggressive when both aerobic and anaerobic bacteria are involved [47]. The process begins locally with infection in the skin and spreads down the fascial planes where inflammation, ischaemia and necrosis occur. The infectious organisms trigger an inflammatory response resulting in an obliterative endarteritis of the surrounding vasculature. Subsequent thrombosis of the nutrient vessels and a resultant reduction in blood flow to this region leads to tissue ischaemia. The reduced oxygen tension of the tissues promotes further anaerobic bacteria proliferation and fascial necrosis and digestion. The low oxygen content and necrosis potentiate the effects of the anaerobic bacteria and cause rapid dissemination of the infection [47]. Clinical investigations have highlighted the polymicrobial nature of this infection. *Streptococcus*, *Staphylococcus*, *Klebsiella* and *Escherichia* are commonly identified by wound cultures; involvement of *Clostridium* sp. is now less common [67].

32.5.2 Diagnosis

Patients typically present with genital induration, pain, erythema, swelling and crepitus. Systemic features such as fever, rigor and tachycardia are often present. In up to 40% of cases, the onset of the disease is more insidious resulting in delayed diagnosis and management [68]. Examination may reveal purulent discharge, crepitus and patches of necrotic tissue with surrounding oedema. Cutaneous manifestations tend to appear later in the disease process as these patches progress to florid gangrene [68]. Advanced Fournier's gangrene can extend through the fascial planes ascending as high as the torso and descending to the thigh. The location of the portal of entry and anatomy of the fascial planes determine the extent of the infection [69]. It's important an accurate history, revealing diabetes, chronic alcohol abuse, HIV, steroid abuse, lymphoproliferative disease, malignancy or recent catheterisation, instrumentation and perineal trauma. These factors should increase the suspicion of Fournier's. Although the diagnosis of Fournier's gangrene is only certain after surgical exploration, laboratory studies (Table 32.1) and radiological evaluation are important tools in risk assessment and in cases of diagnostic uncertainty. Plain radiographs, ultrasonography, computed tomography (CT) and magnetic resonance imaging (MRI) may demonstrate air in the soft tissue planes as well as help determine the extent of the disease. The use of imaging modalities must not delay surgical intervention [70].

Table 32.1 Common investigation findings and prognostic factors in Fournier's gangrene

Complete blood count	• Leucocytosis; WBC count >15.4 × 10^9 L
	• Haemoglobin <11 g/dL
	• Haematocrit <20/>60%
Biochemistry panel	• Serum Na <135 mmol/L
	• Glucose level > 10 mmol/L
	• Serum creatinine >141 μmol/L
	• Serum K < 2.5/>7 mmol/L
	• Bicarbonate <15/>52 mmol/L
	• Reduced serum Mg
Raised serum lactate	
Raised inflammatory markers	• CRP >150 mg/L
DIC panel	• Sepsis induced coagulopathy
Urea >18 mg/dL	
Arterial blood gas	• Acidosis (possibly due to hypo/hyperglycaemia or septic disturbance)

32.5.3 Treatment

Treatment of Fournier's gangrene relies on an aggressive medical and surgical approach. Medical treatment includes rapid fluid resuscitation and broad-spectrum antibiotics to cover Gram-positive, Gram-negative, *Clostridium* and anaerobes. A parenteral broad-spectrum antibiotic regime is required, on presentation in the management of Fournier's gangrene. Subsequent culture and sensitivity results may modify the choice of antibiotics. Currently there are no recommendations for optimal antibiotic therapy in Fournier's gangrene, and patient management depends on local hospital guidelines. Particularly, patients affected by uncontrolled diabetes (who represents a large portion) should be treated in order to obtain reasonable glycaemia level to help the recovery from infection [47]. Surgical debridement is mandatory and must be performed as soon as possible. It should be followed by aggressive wound care with frequent dressing changes and re-debridement if required. Suprapubic catheterization may be necessary depending on the extent of the damage. Consensus from case series suggests that surgical debridement should be early (<24 h) and complete, as delayed and/or inadequate surgery results in higher mortality rate [70]. The early and radical removal of necrotic and devitalized tissue is the crucial step in halting progression of the infection. Even a few hours of delay increases the risk of death [71]. In a retrospective analysis of 72 patients with Fournier's gangrene, Kabay et al. highlighted that a time delay in surgical debridement was associated with significant mortality [72]. It's important to consider that the extension of the infection cannot be judged by the degree of cutaneous necrosis and surgical exploration is imperative. A careful and close observation of the wound and repeated debridement are necessary measures to control the infection.

A mean of 3.5 debridement operations per patient has been suggested to be necessary for adequate infection control [73]. The rapid and aggressive pathological process underlying Fournier's gangrene and the eventual surgical debridement can result in large scrotal, perineal and abdominal defects. The choice of surgical reconstruction is based on the characteristics of the damage. The use of scrotal skin flaps [74], split-thickness skin grafts [75], fasciocutaneous perforator flaps [76] and myocutaneous flaps [77] has all been described in the literature. Adjunctive treatments such as pooled immunoglobulin and hyperbaric oxygen have traditionally been used for Fournier's, although randomized controlled trials of effectiveness are lacking. Hyperbaric oxygen therapy is thought to hasten tissue healing by optimizing the immune system's activity through fibroblast proliferation, maximizing neutrophil function, reducing oedema and increasing intracellular transport of antibiotics [78]. However, adjunctive treatments such as pooled immunoglobulin and hyperbaric oxygen remain uncertain and should not be used routinely [79–81] (Fig. 32.3).

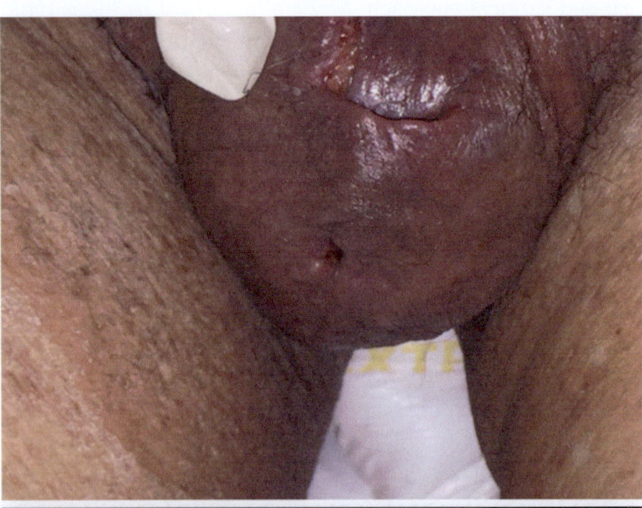

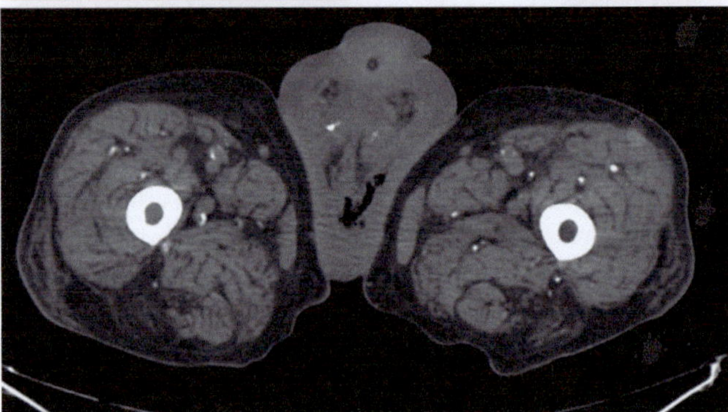

Fig. 32.3 Subtle presentation of Fournier's gangrene. The first diagnosis in the emergency was epididymitis in uncontrolled diabetes with mild fever. Thereafter, physicians observed a fast extending erythema and swelling of the scrotal skin, reaching the pubic area. A CT scan showed air in the scrotum. Immediate surgical exploration was performed

32.6 Emphysematous Pyelonephritis

32.6.1 Definition and Pathogenesis

Emphysematous pyelonephritis (EPN) is a rare type of acute necrotising infection of the kidney with high mortality rate (up to 50%). It is an acute and severe infection of the renal parenchyma and perirenal tissue, which results in gas within the renal parenchyma, collecting system or perinephric tissue [82–86].

It was first described in 1898 by Kelly and Mac Callum [87], but the term "emphysematous pyelonephritis" was first used in 1962 by Schultz and Klorfein [88]. The results of recent meta-analysis showed that EPN has a 3:1 female to male ratio and occurs predominantly in patients with diabetes mellitus (DM), with an incidence of 85% [89]. The increased occurrence in women is presumably because of their increased susceptibility to urinary tract infections [83]. DM gives a combination of high tissue glucose concentrations, impaired tissue perfusion and the presence of gas-producing organisms, the ideal environment for developing EPN [90]. The high tissue glucose level acts as a substrate for the microorganisms to produce hydrogen and carbon dioxide by fermentation [90].

32.6.2 Diagnosis

The most common symptoms are fever/chills and rigors, pyuria, dysuria and flank pain, with a high incidence of leucocytosis. These symptoms and signs are nonspecific and cannot differentiate EPN from the usual pyelonephritis. Crepitus in the lumbar region, though exceedingly rare, can suggest the presence of EPN. In the absence of specific signs, poor response to antibiotic treatment in a diabetic patient with a pyelonephritis should immediately arouse suspicion of this life-threatening infection and prompt an early computed tomography (CT) of the abdomen for the diagnosis and plan treatment. CT was the diagnostic test of choice, with a 100% detection rate. Therefore, once EPN is suspected, CT must not be delayed to confirm the diagnosis. Various radiological classifications have been suggested based on CT. Wan et al. [85] described two distinct radiological classifications of EPN, while Huang and Tseng [91] classified EPN into four categories. The most common causative organism for EPN is *E. coli*, isolated in 47–90% of the patients; the other commonly involved organisms include *P. mirabilis*, *K. pneumoniae*, *Enterococcus* species and *P. aeruginosa* [84, 91, 92]. Some predictors of poor outcome in EPN are thrombocytopenia, azotaemia and haematuria [93]. Initial presentations of thrombocytopenia, altered consciousness, severe proteinuria, shock (systolic BP <90 mmHg) and extension of infection to the perinephric space are significantly associated with mortality [91]. A recent meta-analysis has reported that over 54% of patients who had shock as a presenting symptom, finally died from EPN [89].

32.6.3 Therapy

All the patients should be managed medically, with antibiotics, diabetic control and fluids at presentation. If the patient is showing signs of shock or end-organ failure that is not responding to medical management, then a consultation with an intensive care specialist for early supportive care and admission to a high-dependency unit is useful, as the evidence suggests these patients have the highest mortality rates.

Once the diagnosis of EPN is established, the clinician should consider the best strategy treatment. The treatment of EPN is controversial. There are many different treatment options: emergency nephrectomy (EN), percutaneous drainage (PCD) and medical management alone (MM). Drainage procedures include an early drainage of obstructed systems (in case of urolithiasis) or pararenal infected fluid and gas. Traditionally, early nephrectomy has been considered the treatment of choice in EPN with few reports suggesting increased mortality with medical therapy as compared to surgery [94]. However, surgery is often poorly tolerated in EPN due to poor hemodynamic status; the mortality rate in a series by Ahlering et al. advocating emergency nephrectomy was 42% [95]. Kapoor et al. have also reported that early nephrectomy is associated with higher mortality rates than an initial conservative approach [96]. In 1996, Chen et al. reported that antibiotic therapy combined with CT-guided percutaneous drainage was an acceptable alternative to nephrectomy [97]. In that study, most patients received medical and percutaneous therapy, and only two patients required nephrectomy. A few reports have been published with mortality rates stratified by risk variables, delineating which patients need more aggressive management than others [89, 96, 98]. However, these were based on relatively few patients, and they also had varying results for the same risk variable. Anyway, they remain the only available guide to aid clinicians in managing EPN. The treatment of EPN has evolved over the years from invasive surgery to more conservative approaches due to the availability of better imaging modalities, potent antibiotics and image-guided drainage. Over the last two decades, improvements in management techniques have drastically reduced the mortality rate of EPN to 21% [86–99]. A recent meta-analysis has shown that compared to emergency nephrectomy, percutaneous drainage and medical management alone are associated with a significantly lower mortality rate [89]. If PCD or MM is not improving the patient's condition, then open drainage (OD) must be considered before considering a nephrectomy [89].

32.7 Emphysematous Prostatitis

32.7.1 Definition and Pathogenesis

Emphysematous prostatitis (EP) is a rare condition that is characterized by gas and abscess accumulation in the prostate. The first case of EP was reported in 1983 by Mariani et al. [100]. Prostatic abscess is an infrequent condition that can be diagnosed at an early stage with advanced diagnostic modalities such as ultrasound, computed tomography (CT) or magnetic resonance imaging (MRI). The majority of patients present in the fifth or sixth decade of life and have predisposing factors, which may include diabetes mellitus, hepatic cirrhosis, immunosuppressed status, bladder outlet obstruction, prior genitourinary tract instrumentation or bladder catheterization [101, 102]. The mortality rate was up to 30% in the pre-antibiotic era. The current reported mortality rate varies from 3 to 18% [101, 102]. However recent studies suggest a higher mortality rate, about 25% [103].

32.7.2 Diagnosis

Emphysematous infections are typically defined and diagnosed by radiological imaging. The incidence of reported cases has increased due to a greater use of abdominal–pelvic imaging and a deeper awareness of such infections. However, the number of these emphysematous urinary tract infections (UTIs) might still be under-reported and underdiagnosed because imaging modalities are not routinely used. There are no pathognomonic symptoms or signs. The major presentation is lower urinary tract infection with symptoms of dysuria, frequency and urgency [101]. Fever, acute urine retention and perineal pain may subsequently appear. Rectal examination typically reveals a soft and fluctuant prostate with increased prostate size. Because the presenting symptoms of emphysematous prostatitis are nonspecific, patients are often treated for simple urinary tract infection. Proper diagnosis, however, should be based on clinical history, rectal examination and imaging modalities [104]. Since the diagnosis is often difficult to confirm by history and physical examination alone, radiological imaging can be important in the diagnosis and management. Transrectal ultrasound is the most widely used technique in the diagnosis of prostatic abscess and in the guidance of aspiration and drainage [105]. CT and MRI are superior for demonstrating extra-prostatic penetration, the extent of the pelvic inflammatory process and other possible infectious sources, regardless of the cost-effectiveness [106]. The bacterial flora and aetiology of prostatic abscess have changed from Gram-positive infections (associated with complications of ineffectively treated gonorrhoea) to Gram-negative infections associated with urinary obstruction [100]. Sending material for culture (pus, urine, blood, and/or a fragment of the prostate) is important in order to identify the etiologic agent, especially for immunosuppressed patients because they usually present with uncommon germs [107]. Urine culture may be negative unless the abscess opens into the urethra or bladder. The reported etiologic microorganisms in gas-forming infections of the genitourinary tract include *Escherichia coli*, *Klebsiella* species, *Proteus mirabilis*, *Citrobacter* species, *Pseudomonas aeruginosa*, *Bacteroides fragilis* and yeast. Gas in body tissues is usually associated with the presence of anaerobic infection. However, Gram-negative facultative anaerobes can also produce gas by fermenting glucose in necrotic tissues [100, 108–111].

32.7.3 Therapy

Most of the available data on prostatic abscess are from case reports, and the diagnostic and therapeutic routine has not been standardized. Review of individual cases allows some general observations regarding treatment of abscesses, which generally consists of parenteral antimicrobial therapy and abscess drainage [112]. Antibiotic treatments with a third-generation cephalosporin or quinolone alone, or in combination with metronidazole or gentamicin, have been reported. Prolonged administration of antibiotics for 4–6 weeks is essential to completely eradicate the pathogens [113]. Surgical drainage is the most important step in the treatment of prostatic abscess; nevertheless the best method of drainage remains somewhat controversial [105]. Abscess drainage may be performed by transurethral resection of the prostate (TURP), open perineal incision or TRUS-guided trans-perineal needle aspiration [113]. The transurethral approach should be proposed in selected patients who are hemodynamically stable and able to tolerate the anaesthesia. At the acute infectious stage, this should be done very carefully because hydrostatic pressure during the transurethral procedure may push pathogens from the urothelium into the systemic blood stream and lead to sepsis or septic shock. Only when primary aspiration is done and the patient is stable should TURP be arranged to remove the residual abscess. Transrectal aspiration of a prostatic abscess could be performed under TRUS guidance and local anaesthesia. However, this procedure may be hard to perform precisely for EP patients because ultrasound waves are reflected by gas, and there is interference of acoustic shadow from prostate calcification and air collections, as occurred in our case one. Open perineal incision has been reported, although the patient eventually died [108]. CT-guided transcutaneous (trans-perineal or trans-gluteal) abscess drainage for EP is suggested, because the abscess can be drained more precisely and more thoroughly than US-guided drainage or aspiration. Some studies found that the use of transrectal ultrasound in diagnosis and minimally invasive therapeutic management allowed complete success to be achieved with shortened hospital stay [105–107]. In patients with acute urine retention secondary to acute prostatitis or prostatic abscess, urine flow should be diverted with a suprapubic cystostomy tube because urethral instrumentation may aggravate sepsis. However, in some cases when cystostomy is contraindicated, a urethral catheter could be carefully used instead. At present, there is no consensus on the duration of cystostomy insertion. Once a cystostomy is performed, the reported duration of placement is variable from 6 weeks to 3 months [103].

References

1. Fwu CW, Eggers PW, Kimmel PL, Kusek JW, Kirkali Z. Emergency department visits, use of imaging, and drugs for urolithiasis have increased in the United States. Kidney Int. 2013;83:479–86.
2. Park YH, Jung RB, Lee YG, Hong CK, Ahn JH, Shin TY, Kim YS, Ha YR. Does the use of bedside ultrasonography reduce emergency department length of stay for patients with renal colic? A pilot study. Clin Exp Emerg Med. 2016;3(4):197–203.
3. Sternberg KM, Littenberg B. Trends in imaging use for the evaluation and followup of kidney stone disease: a single center experience. J Urol. 2017;198(2):383–8. https://doi.org/10.1016/j.juro.2017.01.072.
4. Sternberg KM, Pais VM Jr, Larson T, Han J, Hernandez N, Eisner B. Is hydronephrosis on ultrasound predictive of Ureterolithiasis in patients with renal colic? J Urol. 2016;196(4):1149–52. https://doi.org/10.1016/j.juro.2016.04.076.
5. Heidenreich A, Desgrandschamps F, Terrier F. Modern approach of diagnosis and management of acute flank pain: review of all imaging modalities. Eur Urol. 2002;41(4):351–62.
6. Kennish SJ, Bhatnagar P, Wah TM, Bush S, Irving HC. Is the KUB radiograph redundant for investigating acute ureteric colic in the non-contrast enhanced computed tomography era? Clin Radiol. 2008;63(10):1131–5.
7. Sarofim M, Teo A, Wilson R. Management of alternative pathology detected using CT KUB in suspected ureteric colic. Int J Surg. 2016;32:179–82. https://doi.org/10.1016/j.ijsu.2016.06.047. Epub 2016 Jun 30.
8. Rob S, Bryant T, Wilson I, Somani BK. Ultra-low-dose, low-dose, and standard-dose CT of the kidney, ureters, and bladder: is there a difference? Results from a systematic review of the literature. Clin Radiol. 2017;72(1):11–5.
9. Xiang H, Chan M, Brown V, Huo YR, Chan L, Ridley L. Systematic review and meta-analysis of the diagnostic accuracy of low-dose computed tomography of the kidneys, ureters and bladder for urolithiasis. J Med Imaging Radiat Oncol. 2017;61:582.
10. el-Assmy A, Abou-el-Ghar ME, el-Nahas AR, Refaie HF, Sheir KZ. Multidetector computed tomography: role in determination of urinary stones composition and disintegration with extracorporeal shock wave lithotripsy—an in vitro study. Urology. 2011;77(2):286–90.
11. Lotan E, Weissman O, Guranda L, Kleinmann N, Schor R, Winkler H, Portnoy O. Can unenhanced CT findings predict interventional versus conservative treatment in acute renal colic? Am J Roentgenol. 2016;207(5):1016–21.

12. Palmer JS, Donaher ER, O'Riordan MA, Dell KM. Diagnosis of pediatric urolithiasis: role of ultrasound and computerized tomography. J Urol. 2005;174(4 Pt 1):1413–6.
13. Muthusami P, Bhuvaneswari V, Elangovan S, Dorairajan LN, Ramesh A. The role of static magnetic resonance urography in the evaluation of obstructive uropathy. Urology. 2013;81(3):623–74.
14. Levy MM, Fink MP, Marshall JC, Abraham E, Angus D, Cook D, Cohen J, Opal SM, Vincent JL, Ramsay G. International sepsis definitions conference. 2001 SCCM/ESICM/ACCP/ATS/SIS international sepsis definitions conference. Intensive Care Med. 2003;29(4):530–8.
15. Holdgate A, Pollock T. Systematic review of the relative efficacy of non-steroidal anti-inflammatory drugs and opioids in the treatment of acute renal colic. BMJ. 2004;328(7453):1401.
16. Afshar K, Jafari S, Marks AJ, Eftekhari A, MacNeily AE. Nonsteroidal anti-inflammatory drugs (NSAIDs) and non-opioids for acute renal colic. Cochrane Database Syst Rev. 2015;(6):CD006027.
17. Hollingsworth JM, Canales BK, Rogers MA, Sukumar S, Yan P, Kuntz GM, Dahm P. Alpha blockers for treatment of ureteric stones: systematic review and meta-analysis. BMJ. 2016;355:i6112.
18. Ramsey S, Robertson A, Ablett MJ, Meddings RN, Hollins GW, Little B. Evidence-based drainage of infected hydronephrosis secondary to ureteric calculi. J Endourol. 2010;24(2):185–9. https://doi.org/10.1089/end.2009.0361.
19. Angulo JC, Gaspar MJ, Rodríguez N, García-Tello A, Torres G, Núñez C. The value of C-reactive protein determination in patients with renal colic to decide urgent urinary diversion. Urology. 2010;76(2):301–6.
20. Jacobsen SJ, Jacobson DJ, Girman CJ, Roberts RO, Rhodes T, Guess HA, Lieber MM. Natural history of prostatism: risk factors for acute urinary retention. J Urol. 1997;158(2):481–7.
21. Emberton M, Fitzpatrick JM. The Reten-World survey of the management of acute urinary retention: preliminary results. BJU Int. 2008;101(Suppl 3):27–32.
22. Ichsan J, Hunt DR. Suprapubic catheters: a comparison of suprapubic versus urethral catheters in the treatment of acute urinary retention. Aust N Z J Surg. 1987;57(1):33–6.
23. Horgan AF, Prasad B, Waldron DJ, O'Sullivan DC. Acute urinary retention. Comparison of suprapubic and urethral catheterisation. Br J Urol. 1992;70(2):149–51.
24. Villanueva C, Hemstreet GP 3rd. Difficult male urethral catheterization: a review of different approaches. Int Braz J Urol. 2008;34(4):401–11.
25. Ahluwalia RS, Johal N, Kouriefs C, Kooiman G, Montgomery BS, Plail RO. The surgical risk of suprapubic catheter insertion and long-term sequelae. Ann R Coll Surg Engl. 2006;88(2):210–3.
26. Radhakrishnan S, Marsh R, Sheikh N, Johnson P, Greene D. Urethral catheter induced pseudoaneurysm of the bulbar artery. Int J Urol. 2005;12(10):922–4.
27. Kondo H, Yamada T, Kanematsu M, Kako N, Goshima S, Yamamoto N. Embolization for massive urethral hemorrhage. Abdom Imaging. 2007;32(2):262–3.
28. Mamarelis G, Moris D, Vernadakis S. Fournier's gangrene after urethral rupture: an uncommon complication of a common procedure. Am Surg. 2014;80(5):E150–1.
29. Davis NF, Quinlan MR, Bhatt NR, Browne C, MacCraith E, Manecksha R, Walsh MT, Thornhill JA, Mulvin D. Incidence, cost, complications and clinical outcomes of iatrogenic urethral catheterization injuries: a prospective multi-institutional study. J Urol. 2016;196(5):1473–7.
30. Canes D. Male urethral catheterization. N Engl J Med. 2006;355(11):1178–9.
31. Barada JH, Weingarten JL, Cromie WJ. Testicular salvage and age-related delay in the presentation of testicular torsion. J Urol. 1989;142(3):746–8.
32. Anderson JB, Williamson RC. Testicular torsion in Bristol: a 25-year review. Br J Surg. 1988;75(10):988–92.
33. Tang YH, Yeung VH, Chu PS, Man CW. A 55-year-old man with right testicular pain: too old for torsion. Urol Case Rep. 2017;11:74–5.
34. Seo YM, Myung NH, Hong JH. Missed spermatic cord torsion in an old man. Korean J Urol. 2013;54(10):718–20.
35. Davenport M. ABC of general surgery in children. Acute problems of the scrotum. BMJ. 1996;312(7028):435–7.
36. Watkin NA, Reiger NA, Moisey CU. Is the conservative management of the acute scrotum justified on clinical grounds? Br J Urol. 1996;78(4):623–7.
37. McAndrew HF, Pemberton R, Kikiros CS, Gollow I. The incidence and investigation of acute scrotal problems in children. Pediatr Surg Int. 2002;18(5–6):435–7.
38. Kadish HA, Bolte RG. A retrospective review of pediatric patients with epididymitis, testicular torsion, and torsion of testicular appendages. Pediatrics. 1998;102(1 Pt 1):73–6.
39. Kravchick S, Cytron S, Leibovici O, Linov L, London D, Altshuler A, Yulish E. Color Doppler sonography: its real role in the evaluation of children with highly suspected testicular torsion. Eur Radiol. 2001;11(6):1000–5.
40. Kodali SK, Abdullah ZS, Sharma P, Khan MU, Naeem M. Missed torsion in undescended testes detected by scintigraphy: testicular scintigraphy a decisive complementary tool. Clin Nucl Med. 2013;38(1):58–9.
41. Ringdahl E, Teague L. Testicular torsion. Am Fam Physician. 2006;74(10):1739–43.
42. Cornel EB, Karthaus HF. Manual derotation of the twisted spermatic cord. BJU Int. 1999;83(6):672–4.
43. Sidler D, Brown RA, Millar AJ, Rode H, Cywes S. A 25-year review of the acute scrotum in children. S Afr Med J. 1997;87(12):1696–8.
44. Rosenstein D, McAninch J. Urologic emergencies. 1. Med Clin North Am. 2004;88:495–518.
45. Montague DK, et al. American Urological Association guideline on the management of priapism. J Urol. 2003;170(4 Pt 1):1318–24.
46. Burnett AL, Bivalacqua TJ. Priapism current principles and practice. 2. Urol Clin North Am. 2007;34:631–42.
47. Wagner MJ. 3. PEER VII: Physician's evaluation and educational review in emergency medicine. ACEP; 2006 (revised 2007).
48. Broderick GA, et al. Priapism: pathogenesis, epidemiology, and management. J Sex Med. 2010;7(1 Pt 2):476–500.
49. Eland IA, et al. Incidence of priapism in the general population. Urology. 2001;57(5):970–2.
50. Furtado PS, et al. The prevalence of priapism in children and adolescents with sickle cell disease in Brazil. Int J Hematol. 2012;95(6):648–51.
51. Olujohungbe AB, et al. A prospective diary study of stuttering priapism in adolescents and young men with sickle cell anemia: report of an international randomized control trial—the priapism in sickle cell study. J Androl. 2011;32(4):375–82.
52. Samm BJ, Dmochowski RR. Urologic emergencies. 5. Postgrad Med. 1996;100:187–200.
53. Ralph DJ, et al. The use of high-resolution magnetic resonance imaging in the management of patients presenting with priapism. BJU Int. 2010;106(11):1714–8.
54. El-Bahnasawy MS, et al. Low-flow priapism: risk factors for erectile dysfunction. BJU Int. 2002;89(3):285–90.
55. Muneer A, et al. Investigating the effects of high-dose phenylephrine in the management of prolonged ischaemic priapism. J Sex Med. 2008;5(9):2152–9.
56. Burnett AL, et al. J Sex Med. 2013;10(1):180–94.
57. Roberts JR, et al. Intracavernous epinephrine: a minimally invasive treatment for priapism in the emergency department. J Emerg Med. 2009;36(3):285–9.

58. Keskin D, et al. Intracavernosal adrenalin injection in priapism. Int J Impot Res. 2000;12(6):312–4.
59. Hubler J, et al. Methylene blue as a means of treatment for priapism caused by intracavernous injection to combat erectile dysfunction. Int Urol Nephrol. 2003;35(4):519–21.
60. Gupta A, et al. Successful use of terbutaline in persistent priapism in a 12-year-old boy with chronic myeloid leukemia. Pediatr Hematol Oncol. 2009;26(1):70–3.
61. Numan F, Cantasdemir M, Ozbayrak M, et al. Posttraumatic nonischemic priapism treated with autologous blood clot embolization. J Sex Med. 2008;5:173–9.
62. Burnett AL. Surgical management of ischemic priapism. J Sex Med. 2012;9(1):114–20.
63. Samm BJ, Dmochowski RR. Urologic emergencies. Postgrad Med. 1996;100:187–200.
64. Cohen MS. Current experience and management of Fournier's gangrene. Lecture presented at: 78th Annual Meeting of the Am Urol Assoc; 1983.
65. Eke N. Fournier's gangrene: a review of 1726 cases. Br J Surg. 2000;87:718–28.
66. Pastore AL, Palleschi G, Ripoli A, et al. A multistep approach to manage Fournier's gangrene in a patient with unknown type II diabetes: surgery, hyperbaric oxygen, and vacuum assisted closure therapy: a case report. J Med Case Rep. 2013;7:1.
67. Ulug M, Gedik E, Girgin S, et al. The evaluation of microbiology and Fournier's gangrene severity index in 27 patients. Int J Infect Dis. 2009;13:e424–30.
68. Grabe M, Bjerklund-Johansen TE, Botto H, et al. Fournier's gangrene. In: Guidelines on urological infections. Arnhem: European Association of Urology (EAU); 2011; p. 76–8.
69. Ndubuisi E, Raphael JE. Fournier's gangrene. http://cdn.intechopen.com/pdfs-wm/18914.pdf. Accessed Dec 2014.
70. Proud D, et al. Are we getting necrotizing soft tissue infections right? A 10-year review. ANZ J Surg. 2014;84:468.
71. Thwaini A, Khan A, Malik A, et al. Fournier's gangrene and its emergency management. Postgrad Med J. 2006;82:516–9.
72. Kabay S, Yucel M, Yaylak F, et al. The clinical features of Fournier's gangrene and the predictivity of the Fournier's gangrene severity index on the outcomes. Int Urol Nephrol. 2008;40:997–1004.
73. Chowla SN, Gallop C, Mydio JH. An analysis of repeated surgical debridement. Eur Urol. 2003;43:572–5.
74. Ferreira PC, et al. Fournier's gangrene: a review of 43 reconstructive cases. Plast Reconstr Surg. 2007;119:175–84.
75. Maguina P, Palmieri TL, Greenhalgh DG. Split thickness skin grafting for recreation of the scrotum following Fournier's gangrene. Burns. 2003;29:857–62.
76. Lee SH, Rah DK, Lee WJ. Penoscrotal reconstruction with gracilis muscle flap and internal pudendal artery perforator flap transposition. Urology. 2012;79:1390–4.
77. Tremp M, Meyer Zu Schwabedissen M, Schaefer DJ, et al. The combined pedicled anterolateral thigh and vastus lateralis flap as filler for complex perineal defects. Ann Plast Surg. 2015;75(1):66–73.
78. Janane A, Hajji F, Ismail TO, et al. Hyperbaric oxygen therapy adjunctive to surgical debridement in management of Fournier's gangrene: usefulness of a severity index score in predicting disease gravity and patient survival. Actas Urol Esp. 2011;35:332–8.
79. Chennamsetty A, et al. Contemporary diagnosis and management of Fournier's gangrene. Ther Adv Urol. 2015;7:203.
80. Jallali N, et al. Hyperbaric oxygen as adjuvant therapy in the management of necrotizing fasciitis. Am J Surg. 2005;189:462.
81. Mallikarjuna MN, et al. Fournier's gangrene: current practices. ISRN Surg. 2012;2012:942437.
82. Narlawar RS, Raut AA, Nagar A, Hira P, Hanchate V, Asrani A. Imaging features and guided drainage in emphysematous pyelonephritis: a study of 11 cases. Clin Radiol. 2004;59:192–7.
83. Shokeir AA, El-Azab M, Mohsen T, El-Diasty T. Emphysematous pyelonephritis: a 15-year experience with 20 cases. Urology. 1997;49:343–6.
84. Tang HJ, Li CM, Yen MY, Chen YS, Wann SR, Lin HH, et al. Clinical characteristics of emphysematous pyelonephritis. J Microbiol Immunol Infect. 2001;34:125–30.
85. Wan YL, Lee TY, Bullard MJ, Tsai CC. Acute gas-producing bacterial renal infection. Correlation between imaging findings and clinical outcome. Radiology. 1996;198:433–8.
86. Somani BK, Nabi G, Thorpe P, Hussey J, Cook J, N'Dow J. Is percutaneous drainage the new gold standard in the management of emphysematous pyelonephritis? Evidence from a systematic review. J Urol. 2008;179:1844–9.
87. Kelly HA, MacCallum WG. Pneumaturia. JAMA. 1898;31:375–81.
88. Schultz EH Jr, Klorfein EH. Emphysematous pyelonephritis. J Urol. 1962;87:762–6.
89. Aboumarzouk et al. Emphysematous pyelonephritis: time for a management plan with an evidence-based approach. Arab J Urol. 2014;12:106–15.
90. Kuzgunbay B, Turunc T, Tokmak N, Dirim A, Aygun C, Ozkardes H. Tailored treatment approach for emphysematous pyelonephritis. Urol Int. 2011;86:444–7.
91. Huang J-J, Tseng C-C. Emphysematous pyelonephritis: clinicoradiological classification, management, prognosis, and pathogenesis. Arch Intern Med. 2000;160:797–805.
92. Lu YC, Chiang BJ, Pong YH, Huang KH, Hsueh PR, Huang CY, et al. Predictors of failure of conservative treatment among patients with emphysematous pyelonephritis. BMC Infect Dis. 2014;14:418.
93. Wan YL, Lo SK, Bullard MJ, Chang PL, Lee TY. Predictors of outcome in emphysematous pyelonephritis. J Urol. 1998;159:369–73.
94. Cook DJ, Achong MR, Dobranowski J. Emphysematous pyelonephritis. Complicated urinary tract infection in diabetes. Diabetes Care. 1989;12:229–32.
95. Ahlering TE, Boyd SD, Hamilton CL, Bragin SD, Chandrasoma PT, Lieskovsky G, et al. Emphysematous pyelonephritis: a 5-year experience with 13 patients. J Urol. 1985;134:1086–8.
96. Kapoor R, Muruganandham K, Gulia AK, Singla M, Agrawal S, Mandhani A, et al. Predictive factors for mortality and need for nephrectomy in patients with emphysematous pyelonephritis. BJU Int. 2010;105:986–9.
97. Chen MT, Huang CN, Chou YH, Huang CH, Chiang CP, Liu GC. Percutaneous drainage in the treatment of emphysematous pyelonephritis: 10-year experience. J Urol. 1997;157:1569–73.
98. Tienza A, Hevia M, Merino I, Velis JM, Algarra R, Pascual JI, et al. Case of emphysematous pyelonephritis in kidney allograft: conservative treatment. Can Urol Assoc J. 2014;8:E256–9.
99. Ubee SS, McGlynn L, Fordham M. Emphysematous pyelonephritis. BJU Int. 2011;107:1474–8.
100. Mariani AJ, Jacobs LD, Clapp PR, Hariharan A, Stams UK, Hodges CV. Emphysematous prostatic abscess: diagnosis and treatment. J Urol. 1983;129:385–6.
101. Granados EA, Riley G, Salvador J, et al. Prostatic abscess: diagnosis and treatment. J Urol. 1992;148:80–2.
102. Liu KH, Lee HC, Chuang YC, et al. Prostatic abscess in southern Taiwan: another invasive infection caused predominantly by Klebsiella pneumoniae. J Microbiol Immunol Infect. 2003;36:31–6.
103. Wen S-C, Juan Y-S, Wang C-J, et al. Emphysematous prostatic abscess: case series study and review. Int J Infect Dis. 2012;16:e344–9.
104. Arger PH. Computed tomography of the lower urinary tract. Urol Clin North Am. 1985;12:677–86.
105. Lim JW, Ko YT, Lee DH, et al. Treatment of prostatic abscess: value of transrectal ultrasonographically guided needle aspiration. J Ultrasound Med. 2000;19:609–17.

106. Chou YH, Tiu CM, Liu JY, et al. Prostatic abscess: transrectal color Doppler ultrasonic diagnosis and minimally invasive therapeutic management. Ultrasound Med Biol. 2004;30:719–24.
107. Oliveira P, Andrade JA, Porto HC, et al. Diagnosis and treatment of prostatic abscess. Int Braz J Urol. 2003;29:30–4.
108. Lin DC, Lin YM, Tong YC, et al. Emphysematous prostatic abscess after transurethral microwave thermotherapy. J Urol. 2001;166:625.
109. Lu DC, Lei MH, Chang SC, et al. Emphysematous prostatic abscess due to Klebsiella pneumoniae. Diagn Microbiol Infect Dis. 1998;31:559–61.
110. Bartkowski DP, Lanesky JR. Emphysematous prostatitis and cystitis secondary to Candida albicans. J Urol. 1988;139:1063–5.
111. Bae GB, Kim SW, Shin BC, et al. Emphysematous prostatic abscess due to Klebsiella pneumoniae: report of a case and review of the literature. J Korean Med Sci. 2003;18:758–60.
112. Patel NP, Lavengood RW, Fernandes M, et al. Gas-forming infections in genitourinary tract. Urology. 1992;39:341–5.
113. Collado A, Palou J, Garcia-Penit J, Salvador J, De La Torre P, Vicente J. Ultrasound-guided needle aspiration in prostatic abscess. Urology. 1999;53:548–52.

Updates in the Management of Ob-Gyn Emergencies

33

Antonio Ragusa, Alessandro Svelato, Mariarosaria Di Tommaso, Sara D'Avino, Denise Rinaldo, and Isabella Maini

Key Points

- Every physician can manage obstetric and gynecological emergency/urgency effectively following the suggestions collected in this chapter.
- Diagnosis is more important than therapy. All efforts must be employed to find the causes of illness and so perform an etiological therapy.
- Never postpone an instrumental diagnosis because the woman is pregnant.
- Never postpone surgery because the woman is pregnant, especially if the condition is life-threatening.
- The vast majority of obstetric and gynecological emergency/urgency needs a multidisciplinary approach, so teamwork is the priority.
- Sometimes it is necessary to perform an empirical treatment waiting for the definitive results of exams that will guide a targeted therapy.
- To act promptly is the key to solve emergency/urgency.
- Simulation and continuous training are mandatory to improve skills in the management of emergency/urgency.

33.1 Management of Gynecological Emergencies

33.1.1 Ovarian Cysts

The major causes of ovarian cyst complications, frequently representing an emergency, are:

- Ovarian torsion
- Ruptured ovarian cyst (also corpus luteum rupture)

33.1.1.1 Ovarian Torsion

Ovarian torsion refers to the complete or partial rotation of the ovary on its ligamentous supports, resulting in the impedance of its blood supply. The fallopian tube often twists along with the ovary; when this occurs, it is referred to as adnexal torsion [1]. Isolated torsion of the fallopian tube is less common but may also occur [2].

Epidemiology and Risk Factors

Torsion is one of the most common surgical emergencies, preceded by ectopic pregnancy, corpus luteum rupture with hemorrhage, pelvic inflammatory disease, and appendicitis [3]. Its exact incidence is unknown.

A. Ragusa (✉) · A. Svelato · S. D'Avino
Department of Obstetrics and Gynecology, Massa Carrara General Hospital, Massa, Italy

M. Di Tommaso
Department of Health Science, University of Florence, Florence, Italy
e-mail: mariarosaria.ditommaso@unifi.it

D. Rinaldo
Department of Obstetrics and Gynecology, "Bolognini" General Hospital, Bergamo, Italy

I. Maini
Department of Obstetrics and Gynecology, Fondazione MBBM, Ospedale S. Gerardo, Monza, Italy

P. Aseni et al. (eds.), *Operative Techniques and Recent Advances in Acute Care and Emergency Surgery*,
https://doi.org/10.1007/978-3-319-95114-0_33

The primary risk factor is an ovarian mass, particularly a mass that is 5 cm in diameter or larger [4–6]. Torsion is more likely to occur with benign cysts rather than malignant lesions, possibly because malignant masses are more likely to be fixed [6–8]. Since many of these masses are associated with functional cysts, the risk of torsion is higher in women of reproductive age, during pregnancy, and in women undergoing ovulation induction.

Clinical Presentation

Clinical presentation is characterized by the acute onset of moderate to severe pelvic pain, often with nausea and vomiting, in a woman with an adnexal mass. Torsion may also occur in the absence of an adnexal mass [8–10].

Diagnosis

An abdominal and pelvic examination should be performed. Most patients exhibit pelvic and/or abdominal tenderness [5, 6, 8].

A serum human chorionic gonadotropin, hematocrit, white blood cell count, and electrolyte panel should be taken. Ultrasound is the imaging study of choice.

The presence of these findings varies across patients:

- Rounded and enlarged ovary with heterogeneous stroma (due to edema and vascular and lymph engorgement), often abnormally located anterior to the uterus [11, 12] (Fig. 33.1).
- Multiple small peripheral follicles are thought to be due to displacement caused by edema.
- The "whirlpool sign" on Doppler grayscale, which represents the twisted vascular pedicle (round hyperechoic structure with concentric hypoechoic stripes or a tubular structure with internal heterogeneous echoes) [13, 14].
- Decreased or absent Doppler flow within the ovary [15–17].

Management

The mainstay of treatment of ovarian torsion is a swift operative evaluation to preserve ovarian function, avoiding necrosis that occurs in some hours of vessel occlusion [18]. For most premenopausal patients with ovarian torsion, detorsion and ovarian conservation are recommended. Cystectomy is often performed if a benign mass is present. Oophorectomy should be reserved for dead tissue and is reasonable for postmenopausal women [19] or when ovarian conservation is not technically possible.

Management of torsion in pregnancy is similar to that in nonpregnant patients but may be technically more difficult given the size of the gravid uterus [20].

33.1.1.2 Ruptured Ovarian Cyst

Rupture of an ovarian cyst is a common occurrence in women of reproductive age. Physiologic cysts, such as a follicular or corpus luteal, or pathologic cysts may rupture. Ovarian cyst rupture results in a release of cyst fluid or blood that may irritate the peritoneal cavity [21].

Epidemiology and Risk Factors

The incidence of ruptured ovarian cysts is uncertain. Some data suggest that 4% of women will be admitted to the hospital for an ovarian cyst by the age of 65 [21].

Clinical Presentation

Rupture of an ovarian cyst is associated with a sudden onset of unilateral lower abdominal pain. The classic presentation is the sudden onset of severe focal lower quadrant pain, often following sexual intercourse [22].

Diagnosis

Sonographic findings contribute to the diagnosis. A finding of a combination of an ovarian cyst and blood or a significant amount of serous fluid in the pelvis makes the diagnosis highly likely. An ovarian cyst may or may not be visualized,

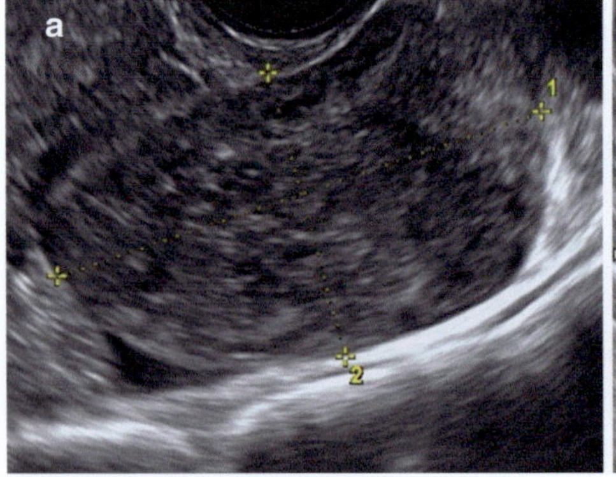

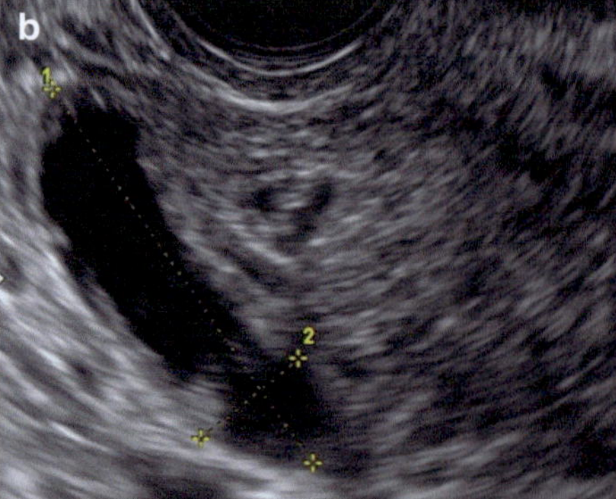

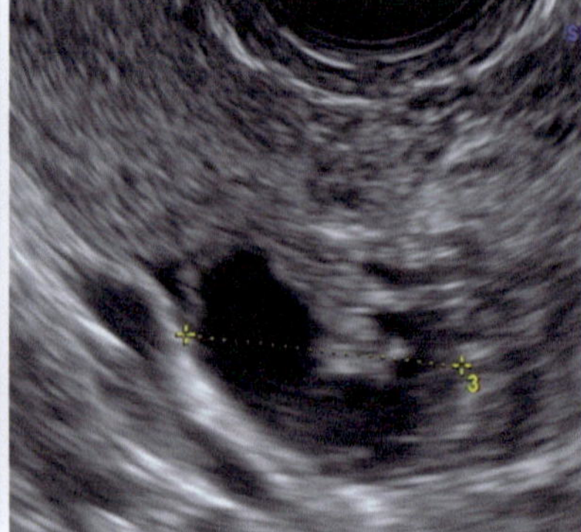

Fig. 33.1 A case of adnexal torsion. The ovary is enlarged, the stroma is heterogeneous (**a**).The swollen salpinx can be seen medial to the ovary (**b**). Courtesy of Daniela Giuliani, MD

since it may collapse after cyst rupture. Checking human chorionic gonadotropin is useful in order to exclude ectopic pregnancy. Ruptured ovarian cysts do occur in pregnant women, but ectopic pregnancy is more likely to be life-threatening than cyst rupture and should be excluded first.

Management

For women with an uncomplicated rupture of an ovarian cyst, the observation rather than surgical intervention is recommended. These patients can usually be managed as outpatients as long as they are hemodynamically stable without a significant drop in hematocrit. They should return if increased pain or light-headedness occurs. Oral analgesia is given as needed. Non-hemorrhagic cyst fluid is usually reabsorbed within 24 h and symptoms typically resolve within a few days. Follicular and corpus luteum cysts account for most of these cases.

Laparoscopic surgery, rather than laparotomy, is performed to control a hemorrhage if the patient's clinical condition is unstable [23].

In pregnant women, the rupture of an ovarian cyst is most likely to occur in the first or early second trimester. Conservative management is preferable in pregnancy, as for nonpregnant patients. If surgery is necessary due to pain or hemorrhage, laparoscopy is a reasonable approach [24].

33.1.2 Uterine Fibroids

Uterine myomas are benign growths which originate from smooth muscle tissue and connective tissue on the walls of the uterus [25]. Their growth is affected by estrogens, growth hormones, and progesterone [26].

They are the most common benign gynecological pathology, with an incidence of between 20 and 77% in premenopausal women, but the real incidence is not known as more than 50% of these tumors are asymptomatic [27, 28].

Their symptoms can include abnormal bleeding, heavy menstrual bleeding, pain, a feeling of compression, and urinary symptoms [29, 30].

A bimanual gynecological examination is often used in the first instance to verify if the patient has uterine fibroids [29].

Uterine fibroids are often suspected in a premenopausal woman when an enlarged uterus or mass is palpated during a pelvic examination or when she reports heavy menstrual bleeding [31]. Ultrasonography is the standard confirmatory test because it can easily and inexpensively differentiate a fibroid from a pregnant uterus or an adnexal mass [31].

The need for further imaging depends on the clinical findings in the patient. In women with heavy menstrual bleeding, ultrasonographic examination after the infusion of saline into the endometrial cavity can identify the extent of intracavitary fibroids [32].

Magnetic resonance imaging (MRI) with gadolinium contrast can provide information on devascularized (degenerated) fibroids and the relationship of fibroids to the endometrial and serosal surfaces. This relationship influences the choice among uterine-sparing treatment options [31].

Possible complications of uterine fibroids include colliquative necrosis and torsion [32, 33]. Colliquative necrosis occurs more frequently during pregnancy due to the rapid growth of the fibroid, which makes the blood supply that reaches the fibroid insufficient [32, 33]. The said condition can result in intense localized abdominal pain, mild leukocytosis, and less frequently hyperpyrexia, nausea, and sickness. The diagnosis becomes suspected on the basis of clinical and ultrasound findings [26, 32]. The latter can show the colliquative necrosis of the fibroid, which has irregular non-vascularized hypoechoic areas with regard to myomas, along with peripheral vascularization with high impedance (pseudo-capsule) and pain caused by the pressure of the ultrasound probe [10]. Adnexal torsion, appendix abscess, and adnexal abscess are to be considered in differential diagnosis.

Another possible complication is the torsion of pedunculated subserous myoma with consequent necrosis. This causes acute abdominal pain.

The nature of symptoms leads to the choice of therapy. There is no evidence to support routine treatment of symptomatic fibroids [34].

The treatment of these conditions is initially conservative and involves the administration of paracetamol or FANS, hydration, and possible antibiotic therapy.

If this therapy does not solve the problem, surgical removal of myoma via laparoscopic or laparotomy can be performed.

33.1.3 Acute Pelvic Inflammatory Disease

Pelvic inflammatory disease (PID) is caused by an infection ascending from the vagina and endocervix, causing endometritis, salpingitis, parametritis, oophoritis, ovarian tube abscesses, and/or pelvic peritonitis [35]. The responsible causal agents are microorganisms that are transmitted sexually, such as *Neisseria gonorrhoeae*, *Chlamydia trachomatis*, *Mycoplasma genitalium*, and other microorganisms that are present in the vaginal flora (i.e., anaerobic, G. vaginalis, *Haemophilus influenzae*, *E. coli*, other enteric gram-negative bacteria, *Streptococcus agalactiae*) [36]. Moreover, cytomegalovirus (CMV), *M. hominis*, *U. urealyticum*, and *M. genitalium* could also be associated with some cases of PID, also not transmitted sexually [37–39].

Connected risk factors are [40]:

- Young age
- Multiple partners
- Instrumental interventions on the uterus and pelvis/disruption of the cervical barrier
- Pregnancy termination—abortion
- The insertion of an intrauterine device in the previous 6 weeks
- Hysterosalpingography
- In vitro fertilization

There is no real symptom or pathognomonic sign of PID [41].

It can often start in asymptomatic form. A diagnostic suspect can be considered in the presence of any of the following clinical signs and/or symptoms:

- Lower abdominal pain, usually bilateral
- Deep dyspareunia
- Abnormal bleeding: postcoital, intermenstrual, and menorrhagia
- Vaginal discharge

Clinical Signs

- Abdominal pain with possible leg involvement
- Cervical motion tenderness
- Uterine tenderness
- Adnexal tenderness
- Oral temperature >101 °F (>38.3 °C)

Complications

- Tubo-ovarian abscess and pelvic peritonitis
- Fitz-Hugh-Curtis syndrome with by pain in the right upper quadrant together with perihepatitis [42]. A delay in diagnosis or treatment can increase the risk of long-term sequelae such as ectopic pregnancy, sterility, and chronic pelvic pain [41]

Differential Diagnosis

- Extrauterine pregnancy (a pregnancy test is recommended for all women with suspected PID) [43].
- Acute appendicitis.
- Endometriosis: the relationship between the symptoms and the menstrual cycle can be useful [43].
- Rupture or twist of ovarian cysts.
- Urinary tract infection—often linked to dysuria.

33.1.3.1 Diagnosis

There is no sensitive and specific anamnestic note, instrumental exam, or lab test for the diagnosis of acute PID [44].

Additional criteria used to improve the specificity of clinical criteria and support a diagnosis of PID are:

- Vaginal cervical swab for gonorrhea and chlamydia. A positive result supports the diagnosis of PID. Lack of infection does not exclude PID [45].
- An increase in white blood cells (WBC) [40] and PCR support the diagnosis but are not specific and can often be normal in slight to moderate PID.
- A transvaginal scan can highlight fluid collection or tubular ovarian complexes.

When there is a diagnostic doubt, laparoscopy may be useful to exclude other pathologies. It enables to take samples from the salpinges and Douglas and can provide information regarding the severity of the condition. It is, however, invasive, and pelvic organs may seem normal in mild disease [46].

An endometrial biopsy should be performed, with Nelaton related to aspiration syringe and sterile technique, in women who undergo laparoscopy that does not provide visual evidence of salpingitis, because endometritis may be the only sign of PID [44].

Other image techniques can be used if the clinical diagnosis is uncertain, in the case of serious illness or those unresponsive to therapy [41].

33.1.3.2 Management

Treatment must provide empirical and broad-spectrum coverage of probable pathogenic agents [44] such as *Neisseria gonorrhoeae* (i.e., cephalosporin), *Chlamydia trachomatis* (i.e., tetracycline, macrolides), and anaerobic bacteria (i.e., metronidazole) [40].

Cases of light to moderate PID, with suspected clinically or microbiologically confirmed, in patients without signs of sepsis, hemodynamically stable with pain controlled by common analgesics, without ovarian tube abscesses, can be managed as outpatients with oral therapy [47]. The optimal duration of the treatment is not known, but most of the clinical studies indicate a response after 10–14 days of therapy. The patients must be reassessed within 72 h. A lack of clinical improvement can indicate the need for further investigation or hospital treatment.

Hospitalization is indicated in the case of PID during pregnancy, lack of response to oral treatment intolerance to the oral treatment, clinically severe disease (hemodynamically unstable, pain, nausea, and vomiting, fever, acute abdomen), ovarian tube abscess, and impossibility of excluding emergency surgery. In these cases, parenteral therapy is indicated [44].

Partners of women with PID should undergo screening tests for gonorrhea and chlamydia. Abstention from unprotected sexual intercourse is recommended until both the partner and patient have completed the treatment.

33.1.4 Pelvic Endometriosis

Endometriosis can be defined as the presence of endometrial glands and stroma in ectopic locations, primarily the pelvic peritoneum, ovaries, fallopian tubes, vagina, cervix, uterosacral ligaments, and rectovaginal septum [48] but also in extrapelvic sites, i.e., laparotomy scars, pleura, lungs, diaphragm, kidneys, spleen, gallbladder, nasal mucosa, spinal canal, stomach, or breast [49]. Ectopic tissues respond to normal cyclic hormonal stimulation as they have the same steroid receptors as normal endometrium. Microscopic internal bleeding, with subsequent inflammatory response, neovascularization, and fibrosis formation is responsible for the clinical consequences of this disease [50].

Epidemiology: this condition affects 6–10% of women of childbearing age, with a prevalence of 38% in infertile women and 71–87% of women with chronic pelvic pain [51]. The incidence remains stable, although improved recognition may have led to an increased diagnosis rate.

Risk factors include family history, early menarche, short menstrual cycles and prolonged flow, heavy bleeding, nulliparity, delayed childbearing, and anatomic alterations [52].

Etiology: the cause of endometriosis is still unclear. Several theories have tried to explain this condition, but none of them have been fully proved [48, 53]. Leading theories include metaplastic conversion of coelomic epithelium and hematogenous or lymphatic dispersion of endometrial cells, but it is more likely to be a combination of these [54].

In 1927, Sampson proposed his theory of retrograde menstruation through the fallopian tubes into the peritoneal cavity, so causing endometriosis. Later, this was found to be a common physiologic phenomenon that could not appropriately explain the onset of endometriosis, although it probably increases the risk of developing this condition.

More recently, research has focused on the role played by the immune system in the pathogenesis of endometriosis [55]; women with this disorder have increased humoral immune responsiveness and macrophage activation, as well as decreased cell-mediated immunity with diminished T-cell and natural killer cell responsiveness.

Meyer suggested another theory regarding metaplasia [56]: endometrium and peritoneum derive from the same coelomic wall epithelium, which can transform into endometrial-type glands in response to unknown stimuli; this could explain endometriosis in unusual sites and in women who have undergone total hysterectomy and are not taking estrogen replacement.

Symptoms: the presentation of endometriosis is highly variable and ranges from debilitating pelvic pain and infertility to no symptoms [57]: pain can include dysmenorrhea, dyspareunia, and dyschezia, depending on the site involved [51, 58]. There is an overlap of symptoms with many conditions, both gynecological and not.

Sterility is another important consequence of endometriosis (20–30% of patients): it can be caused by adherences or by a decreased production of oocytes [59]; periovarian and peritubal adhesions can interfere mechanically with ovum transport, peritoneal endometriosis interferes with tubal motility, corpus luteum function, and folliculogenesis. Aromatase is believed to raise prostaglandin E levels via an increased cyclooxygenase-2 expression. Endometriosis can also cause a decrease in fertility by binding more sperm to the ampullary epithelium and so affecting sperm-endosalpingeal interactions [60].

Diagnosis: pelvic ultrasonography, MRI, and CT scanning are usually useful in the case of advanced disease with endometrial cyst formation or anatomic distortion. Visualization of endometrial implants is the definitive method of diagnosis, mainly by laparoscopy.

Differential diagnosis can be carried out for appendicitis, diverticulitis, urinary tract infections and cystitis (by urinalysis and urine culture), chlamydia infections, gonorrhea and pelvic inflammatory disease (by cervical Gram stain and cultures), ectopic pregnancy, ovarian cyst, and ovarian torsion (by ultrasound).

Staging: the American Society for Reproductive Medicine classification of endometriosis is the most widely used staging system [61] (Figs. 33.2 and 33.3). Point scores are assigned according to the number and size of lesions and their bilaterality, as well as to the associated adhesion formation. This is a method of recording laparoscopic findings. This classification does not correlate with pain and other symptoms. It can also be used to monitor a patient's response to therapy, although it requires laparoscopic or, less frequently, laparotomic surgery both initially and for follow-up.

Treatment: as endometriosis depends on a woman's cyclic production of menstrual hormones, an improvement in this condition can be achieved by suppressing the hormonal

REVISED AMERICAN SOCIETY FOR REPRODUCTIVE MEDICINE CLASSIFICATION OF ENDOMETRIOSIS 1985

Patient's Name ______________________ Date: ______________________

Stage I (Minimal)	1-5	Laparoscopy ________ Laparotomy ________ Photography ________
Stage II (Mild)	6-15	Recommended Treatment ________
Stage III (Moderate)	16-40	________
Stage IV (Severe)	>40	

Total ________ Prognosis ________

	ENDOMETRIOSIS	< 1 cm	< 1 – 3 cm	> 3 cm
Peritoneum	Superficial	1	2	4
	Deep	2	4	6
Ovary	R Superficial	1	2	4
	Deep	4	16	20
	L Superficial	1	2	4
	Deep	4	16	20
	POSTERIOR CULDESAC OBLITERATION	Partial		Complete
		4		40
	ADHESIONS	< 1/3 Enclosure	1/3-2/3 Enclosure	> 2/3 Enclosure
Ovary	R Filmy	1	2	4
	Dense	4	8	16
	L Filmy	1	2	4
	Dense	4	8	16
Tube	R Filmy	1	2	4
	Dense	4	8	16
	L Filmy	1	2	4
	Dense	4*	8*	16

*If the fimbriated end of the fallopian tube is completely enclosed, change the point assignment to 16.

Additional Endometriosis: ________ Associated Pathology: ________

To be used with normal tubes and ovaries — Left, Right

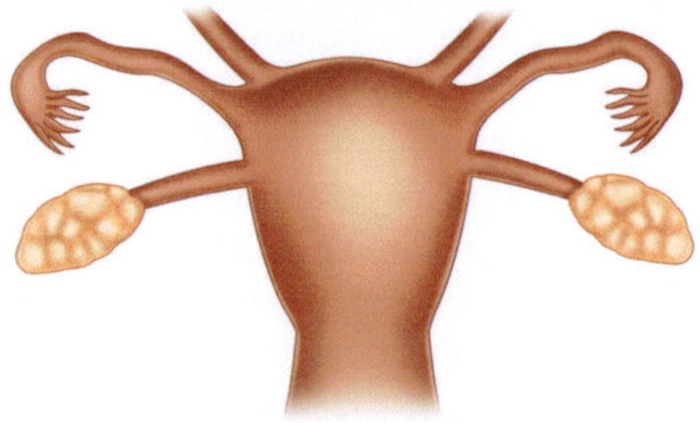

To be used with abnormal tubes and/or ovaries — Left, Right

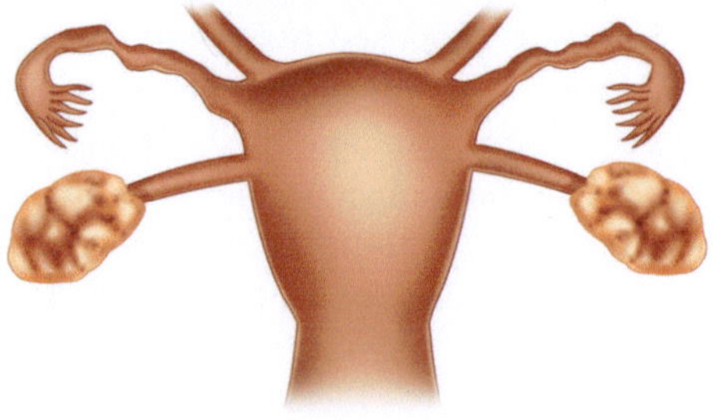

Fig. 33.2 American Society for Reproductive Medicine revised classification of endometriosis, 1985 [61]

rhythm. Gonadotropin-releasing hormone (GnRH) agonists, androgens, progestins, and oral contraceptive pills can be prescribed for this purpose. Nonsteroidal anti-inflammatory agents have not been proven to have any benefit in placebo-controlled trials [62].

Surgical management of endometriotic lesions usually provides pain relief and an improvement of symptoms [63], with a non-predictable improvement of pregnancy rates.

With conservative surgery, the aim is to remove visible endometriotic implants and lyse peritubal and periovarian

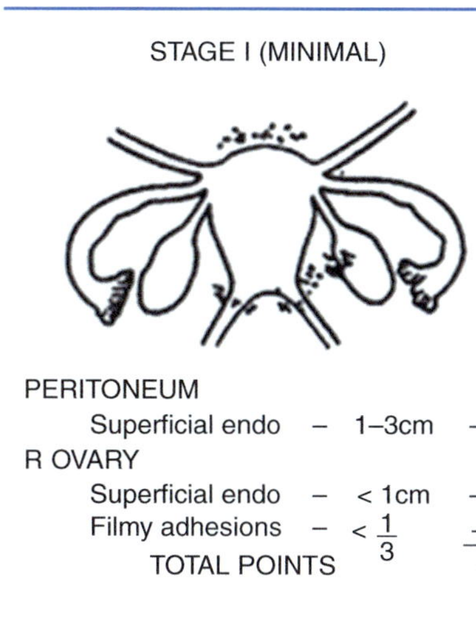

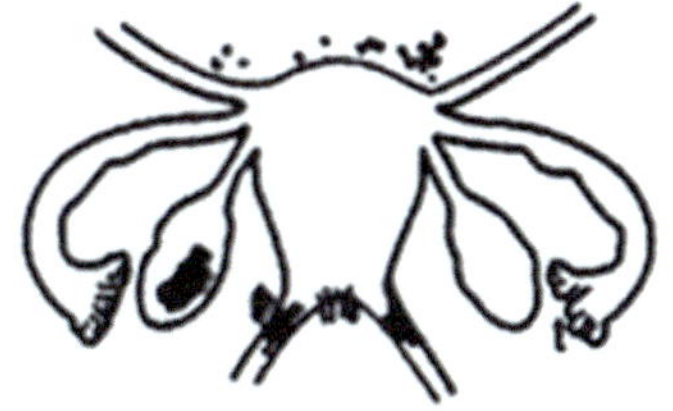

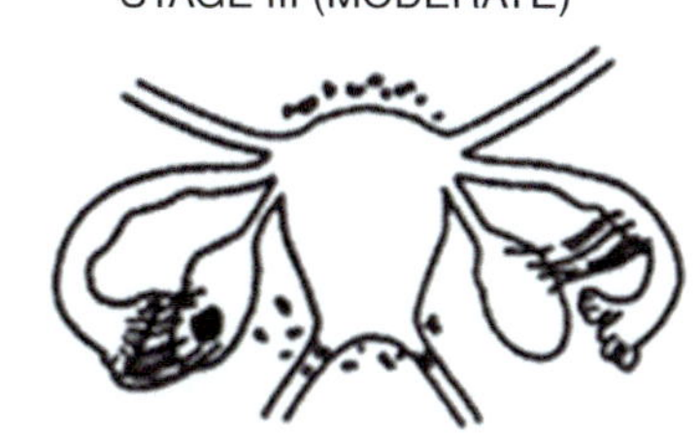
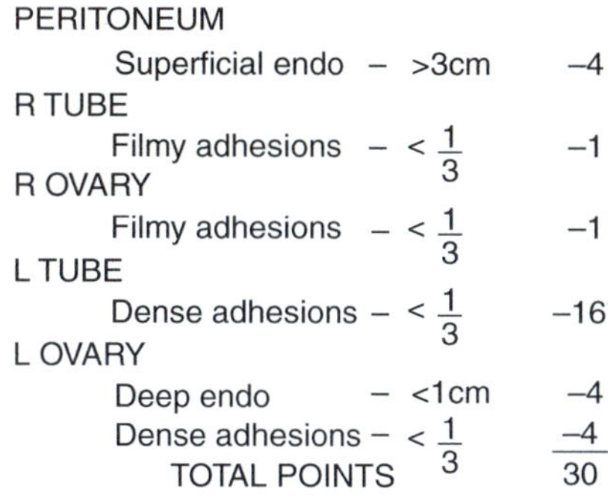

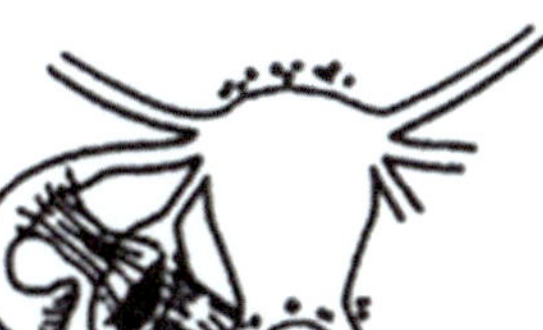
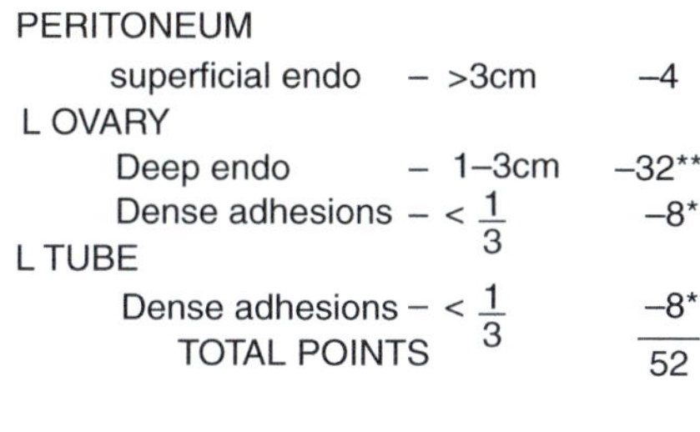

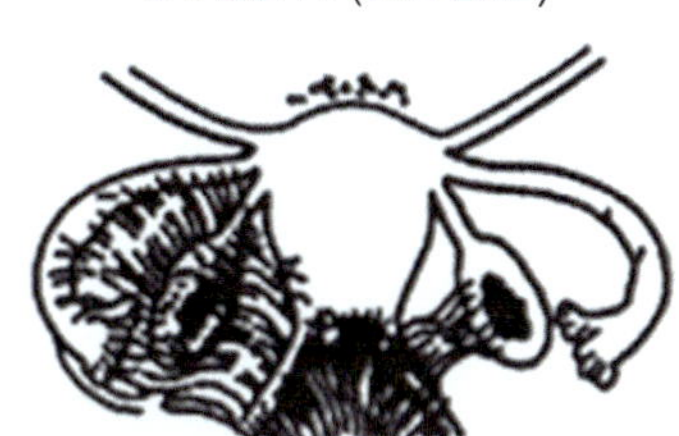

Fig. 33.3 American Society for Reproductive Medicine revised classification of endometriosis, 1985 [61]

adhesions with a laparoscopic approach. Ablation can be performed with laser or electrodiathermy. These techniques were shown to be effective for relieving pelvic pain in 87% of patients [64].

The indication for semiconservative surgery is mainly for women who have no desire for future childbearing, are too young for surgical menopause, and are in strong need of pain relief. Such surgery consists of hysterectomy and cytoreduction of pelvic endometriosis.

Radical surgery includes total hysterectomy with bilateral oophorectomy and cytoreduction of visible endometriosis. Adhesiolysis is performed to recover mobility and normal intrapelvic relationships.

33.1.5 Severe Vaginal Bleeding

Severe vaginal bleeding is a condition that may be related to many etiologies, both functional and structural. It can take place during menstrual flow, as an increased blood loss, or between two menstrual flows. These situations are, respectively, called menorrhagia and metrorrhagia.

Munro in 2011 proposed a classification system for abnormal uterine bleeding (AUB) in non-gravid women of reproductive age that was officially approved by FIGO [65]. This system is called "PALM-COEIN," as an acronym of the nine categories of causes of vaginal bleeding (Fig. 33.4):

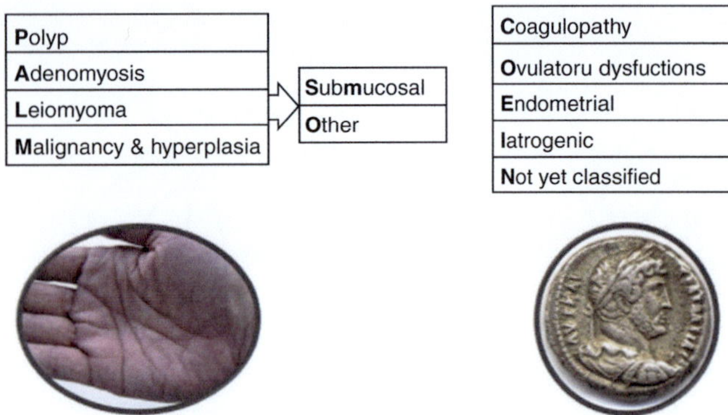

Fig. 33.4 A simple way to remember the causes of AUB; the first four (PALM) are structural anomalies; the others are not related to structural anomalies [65]

Polyp
Adenomyosis
Leiomyoma
Malignancy and hyperplasia
Coagulopathy
Ovulatory dysfunction
Endometrial
Iatrogenic
Not yet classified

Polyps: both endometrial and endocervical. These formations have a variable vascular, glandular, fibromuscular, and connective tissue; they are usually asymptomatic but can also bleed [66]. Polyps are usually benign, but a small minority may have atypical or malignant features [67]. A therapeutic approach consists of removal, mostly by hysteroscopy.

Adenomyosis: the relationship between AUB and adenomyosis is still unclear; adenomyosis can be assessed with MRI and ultrasonography, but as the latter is more available in common practice, it is proposed that ultrasound criteria comprise the minimum requirements for inclusion in the PALM-COEIN system.

Leiomyoma: this is a benign fibromuscular formation of myometrium, also known as fibroid or myoma. There is a high prevalence of this benign tumor worldwide, and it is often asymptomatic. Fibroids can be classified according to their number, size, and location, but the PALM-COEIN system just includes the categorization of intramural and subserosal lesions. They are usually removed, with relief of symptoms, if present [68].

Malignancy and hyperplasia: atypical hyperplasia and malignancy are quite uncommon but are a significant cause of vaginal bleeding that requires further investigation and classification according to the WHO and FIGO system [69].

Coagulopathy: this term includes the spectrum of systemic disorders of hemostasis that may cause vaginal bleeding, i.e., von Willebrand disease (VWD). It is particularly important to consider this cause, as it has been proven that coagulation disorders can often be forgotten in differential diagnosis of vaginal bleeding [70, 71]. These conditions require a hematologic approach and specific treatment. Coagulopathy can also be caused by medications; this case would enter the "Iatrogenic" category, but, since women taking these drugs usually have a hemostasis disorder, it is still included in the "Coagulopathy" category [65].

Ovulatory dysfunction: this is a common cause of AUB, generally manifesting as a combination of unpredictable timing of bleeding and variable amount of flow. Disorders of ovulation may be present as a variety of menstrual issues, from amenorrhea, through light and infrequent spotting, to episodes of extremely heavy menstrual bleeding (HMB), requiring medical or even surgical intervention. Some ovulatory disorders have a clear endocrinological etiology, i.e., hypothyroidism, polycystic ovary syndrome, mental stress, hyperprolactinemia, anorexia, obesity, weight loss, or extreme exercise. In some cases, the disorder can be iatrogenic, due to gonadal steroids or phenothiazines and tricyclic antidepressants [65].

Endometrial: if abnormal bleeding takes place in the context of regular menstrual bleeding, characteristic of ovulatory cycles, and if no other causes are identified, the cause is probably a primary disorder of the endometrium. There could be a deficit in the endometrial production of vasoconstrictors, such as endothelin 1 and prostaglandin F2α, or an accelerated lysis of the endometrial clot for augmented levels of plasminogen activator, with an increased concentration of molecules promoting vasodilation, i.e., prostaglandin E2 (PGE2) and prostacyclin (PGI2) [72–74]. Unfortunately, it is not possible to measure these abnormalities at present. Other secondarily disorders can cause endometrial bleeding, such as inflammation or infection of endometrial tissue, problems in the uterine phlogistic response and disorders in local vasculogenesis. The role played by inflammation in uterine bleeding is still not clear: a retrospective evaluation of women with chronic endometritis could not assess a correlation between inflammation and AUB [75, 76], but there is data that supports a relationship between AUB and *Chlamydia trachomatis* infection [77]. An involvement of endometrium as a cause of abnormal uterine bleeding should probably be a diagnosis of exclusion.

Iatrogenic: there are several possible iatrogenic causes of vaginal bleeding, by intrauterine devices, both medicated or not, and a multitude of drugs. Gonadal steroid therapy is very commonly an agent of AUB, which in this case is called "breakthrough bleeding (BTB)." Systemically administered steroids, such as progestins, estrogens, and androgens, have a therapeutic effect on the hypothalamic-pituitary-ovarian axis and directly affect the endometrium itself. These drugs are used as hormonal contraceptives, and bleeding is usually due to their periodic withdrawal. BTB is more frequent in smokers, because of an enhanced hepatic metabolism that decreases the levels of circulating steroids [78]. Systemic agents involved in dopamine metabolism can cause uterine bleeding, secondary to ovulation problems. Tricyclic antidepressants, such as amitriptyline and nortriptyline, and phenothiazines reduce serotonin uptake and thus interfere with the dopamine metabolism [79]. Finally, severe vaginal bleeding is a common side effect of anticoagulant drugs, such as warfarin, heparin, and low molecular weight heparin (LMWH), but as previously stated, these cases are included in the "Coagulopathy" category.

Not yet classified: this category comprises many disorders of the endometrium that may contribute to AUB but which have not been properly studied yet, so their role is still unknown.

33.1.6 Vulvar Abscesses

Vulvar abscesses are a common gynecological problem caused by infection of the cute or of the subcutaneous tissue of the vulva. The most common vulvar abscesses, which occur in about 2% of women, are Bartholin gland cysts [80]. Recent prevalence estimates and risk factors are difficult to define. Data from literature point to bacterial infections in 57% of cases, with *E. coli* as the most frequent single agent, followed by streptococci [81].

The patient has severe pain and swelling. On physical examination, the abscess looks like a warm and soft mass, fluctuating in the lower vestibular area.

Rare serious complications can include infections such as systemic infection, sepsis, and secondary bleeding.

Possibly treatment includes antibiotic therapy selected on an empirical basis involving drainage, use of CO_2 laser to carry out ablation of the cyst, fenestration or excision of the gland, fistulization to create an opening for a new duct, marsupialization, or excision of the Bartholin gland.

Despite the numerous types of treatment available, recurrences are frequent [82], and the healing process is prolonged and involves the interruption of daily activities, sexual intercourse, as well as discomfort for the female patient.

33.1.6.1 Fine-Needle Aspiration

Recurrences after 6 months range from 0 to 38%. Compared to alcohol sclerotherapy, this method has been associated with about as twice as high frequency of recurrence [83].

33.1.6.2 Alcohol Sclerotherapy

Irrigation with alcohol al 70% for 5 min, after evacuation of the cavity of the cyst. Recurrence at 7 months ranges from 8 to 10% [84]. Average healing time: 1 week.

Complications: transient hyperthyroidism, hematoma, and tissue necrosis [84].

33.1.6.3 Drainage

Incision and drainage are quite a fast and simple procedure that provides immediate relief to the patient, with a failure rate of 13% [85]. Definite drainage can be carried out by positioning a Word catheter for 4–6 weeks, or marsupialization to recreate the orifice of the duct, enabling continuous drainage.

33.1.6.4 Fistulization

The technique for creating a new, epithelialized outflow tract for an obstructed Bartholin duct was by placing either a 14-French Foley catheter, a Jacobi ring, or a Word catheter near the Bartholin gland duct. The Word catheter is inflated with 3 mL of saline solution and is left in place for 4–6 weeks. The Jacobi ring is a rubber catheter, fashioned into a ring from an 8-French T tube threaded over a 2-0 silk suture that enters and leaves the cyst or abscess through two separate incisions [86].

Recurrence after 6 months ranges from 4 to 17%.

The most common adverse event is the premature loss of the Word catheter.

Healing takes place on average after about 3 weeks.

33.1.6.5 Marsupialization

Incision of the vestibular skin and the cyst wall, emptying the cyst, preserving the new orifice. Suture of the wall of the cyst to the edges of the incision of the skin.

Healing takes place on average in less than 2 weeks.

Complications: rare hemorrhage (11%).

Compared to patients treated using incision and drainage, those undergoing marsupialization heal more slowly, without any significant difference in recurrence [87].

33.1.6.6 Carbon Dioxide Laser

With the aim of creating an opening of the orifice of the duct in the skin of the vulvar area, outpatient treatment of vulvar abscesses using a CO_2 laser was described [88–90].

The cysts and/or abscess is emptied and then vaporized [88].

Recurrence ranges from 2 to 20%.

Complications: heavy bleeding (2–8%) after the ablation of the gland using a laser [90].

33.1.6.7 Excision of the Gland

The average duration of the procedure is 20–60 min.

Recurrences at 2 years range from 0 to 3%.

Average healing time 11 days.

Complications: bleeding (2–8%), fever (24%), and dyspareunia (8–16%) [88].

The choice of treatment for Bartholin's gland cysts remains difficult [81].The ideal treatment is fast and safe, performed in outpatient regime, using local anesthesia, with a low rate of recurrence and fast healing.

All therapies described are carried out as outpatient procedure, using local anesthesia or block of the pudendal nerve, with an average duration of about 20 min. Average healing time is 2 weeks or less. Adverse events are generally rare and are not life-threatening. Regardless of the treatment, recurrences occur in less than 20% of patients, with few exceptions (the highest percentage is for those after aspiration only).

The best treatment has still not been identified, and in existing literature, the best intervention among those described previously has not been defined. The operator can, therefore, choose the suitable treatment on the basis of the patient's characteristics (symptoms, age, size of abscess, etc.), the resources of the hospital where he/she is working, and his/her experience [81].

33.1.7 Sexual Violence

33.1.7.1 Definition

Violence against women is a major public health and human rights concern. Sexual violence is defined as, "any sexual act, attempt to obtain a sexual act, unwanted sexual comments or advances, or acts to traffic women's sexuality, using coercion, threats of harm or physical force, by any person regardless of relationship to the victim, in any setting, including but not limited to home and work" [91].

33.1.7.2 Prevalence

Studies show that most victims are female, and that the violence is generally committed by a man, and that many victims know their tormentor [91]. Global statistics show that between 13 and 61% of women 15–49 years old report that an intimate partner has physically abused them at least once in their lifetime [92]. There is significant under-reporting of sexual violence. The reasons for nonreporting are complex and multifaceted but typically include fear of retribution or ridicule and a lack of confidence in investigators, police, and health workers. Sexual violence has a significant negative impact on the health of populations. The main consequences are listed in Table 33.1 [91].

33.1.7.3 Clinical Assessment

The victim must have a safe and protected environment, and all those involved must have received suitable training with regard to communicating with victims of sexual violence.

Table 33.1 Consequences of sexual violence [91]

Unwanted pregnancy
Illegal abortion
Sexually transmitted infections (STI), including HIV/AIDS
Sexual dysfunction
Infertility
Pelvic inflammatory disease
Urinary infections
Dangerous sexual practices
Depression, substance abuse, post-traumatic stress disorder (PTSD), and suicide

Clinical assessment must be carried out by expert personnel, and, when possible, the victim must have the possibility to choose the sex of the examiner.

Complete assessment in the case of sexual violence includes [93]:

- Consent to clinical examination
- Remote and recent medical history, including the description of the events, gynecological obstetric history
- Physical examination
- Detailed examination of the genito-anal apparatus
- Recording and classification of the identified lesions
- Collection and preservation of biological samples
- Forensic report

In women, genital trauma is more easily seen behind the posterior vulvar commeasure, labia minora, hymen, and/or fossa navicularis (fossa of vestibule of vagina).

The most frequent types of genital trauma include [91]: Lacerations (Fig. 33.5)

- Bruising
- Abrasions
- Redness and swelling (Fig. 33.6)

The most frequent non-genital traumas include:

- Hematomas and bruises
- Lacerations

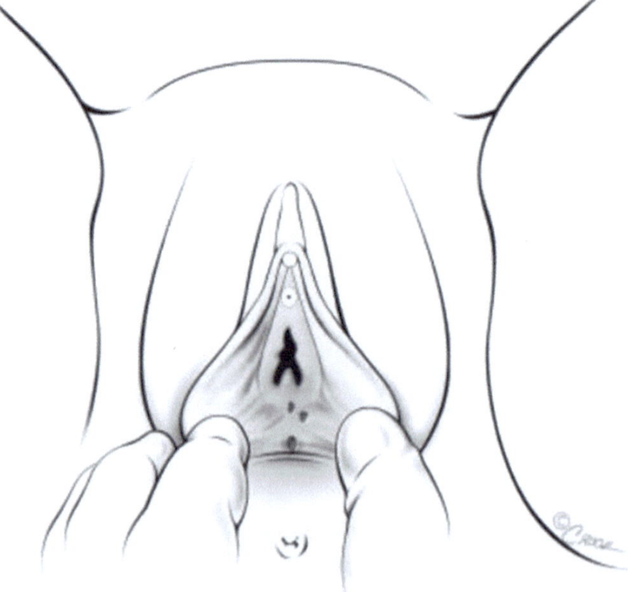

Fig. 33.5 Multiple lacerations near the vulvar posterior commissure (With permission of World Health Organization, Guidelines for medico-legal care of victims of sexual violence, 2003)

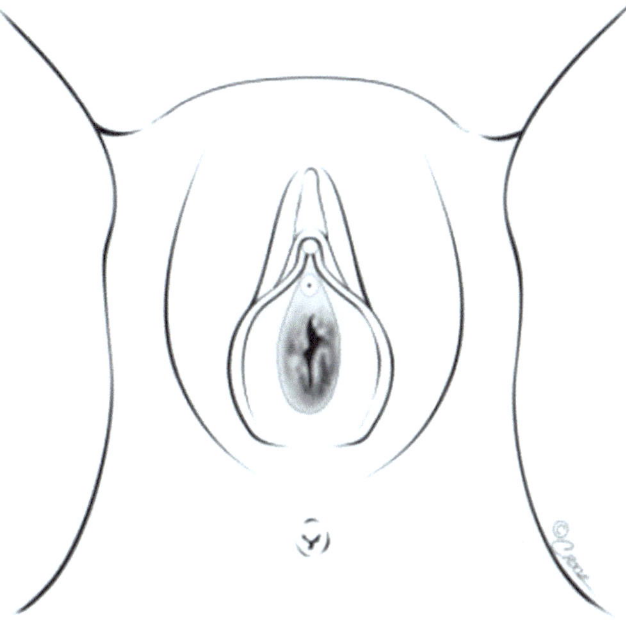

Fig. 33.6 Swelling of the hymen (With permission of World Health Organization, Guidelines for medico-legal care of victims of sexual violence, 2003)

– Signs of tying the wrists, ankles, and neck
– Signs of bites, fingers, and belts
– Anal or rectal trauma

On the basis of the facts and the information provided by the patient and by investigators, the doctor can decide which type of samples to take. Ideally, the samples must be taken within 24 h from the attack. In fact, after 72 h the possibility of obtaining reliable samples is reduced (Table 33.2) [93].

The presence of semen is confirmed by sampling using a swab, followed by microscopic examination (Table 33.3). The swab must be inserted delicately beyond the hymen, taking care not to touch the external parts (Fig. 33.7). In the case of suspected ejaculation inside the mouth, since the sperm

Table 33.2 Persistence of biological evidences

Type of assault	Persistence of biological evidences
Kissing, licking, biting	48 h or longer
Oral penetration	48 h
Vaginal penetration	7 days
Digital penetratiom	12 h
Anal penetration	72 h

Table 33.3 Shows the samples that are more frequently taken in the case of sexual violence [91]

Site	Material	Equipment	Sampling instructions	Notes
Anus (rectum)	Semen	Cotton swabs and microscope slides	Use swab and slides to collect and plate material; lubricate instruments with water, not lubricant	1
	Lubricant	Cotton swab	Dry swab after collection	
Blood	Drugs	Appropriate tube	Collect 10 mL of venous blood	2
	DNA (victim)	Appropriate tube	Collect 10 mL of blood	
Clothing	Adherent foreign materials (e.g. semen, blood, hair, fibres)	Paper bags	Clothing should be placed in a paper bag(s). Collect paper sheet or drop cloth. Wet items should be bagged separately	3
Genitalia	Semen	Cotton swabs and microscope slide	Use separate swabs and slides to collect and plate material collected from the external genitalia, vaginal vault and cervix; lubricate speculum with water not lubricant or collect a blind vaginal swab (see Fig. 33.11)	1
Hair	Comparison to hair found at scene	Sterile container	Cut approximately 20 hairs and place hair in sterile container	4
Mouth	Semen	Cotton swabs, sterile container (for oral washings) or dental flossing	Swab multiple sites in mouth with one or more swabs (see Fig. 33.12). To obtain a sample of oral washings, rinse mouth with 10 mL water and collect in sterile container	1
	DNA (victim)	Cotton swab		5
Nails	Skin, blood, fibres, etc. (from assailant)	Sterile toothpick or similar or nail scissors/clippers	Use the toothpick to collect material from under the nails or the nail(s) can be cut and the clippings collected in a sterile container	6
Sanitary pads/ tampons	Foreign material (e.g. semen, blood, hair)	Sterile container	Collect if used during or after vaginal or oral penetration	7
Skin	Semen	Cotton swab	Swab sites where semen may be present	1
	Saliva (e.g. at sites of kissing, biting or licking), blood	Cotton swab	Dry swab after collection	
	Foreign material (e.g. vegetation, matted hair or foreign hairs)	Swab or tweezers	Place material in sterile container (e.g. envelope, bottle)	
Urine	Drugs	Sterile container	Collect 100 mL of urine	2

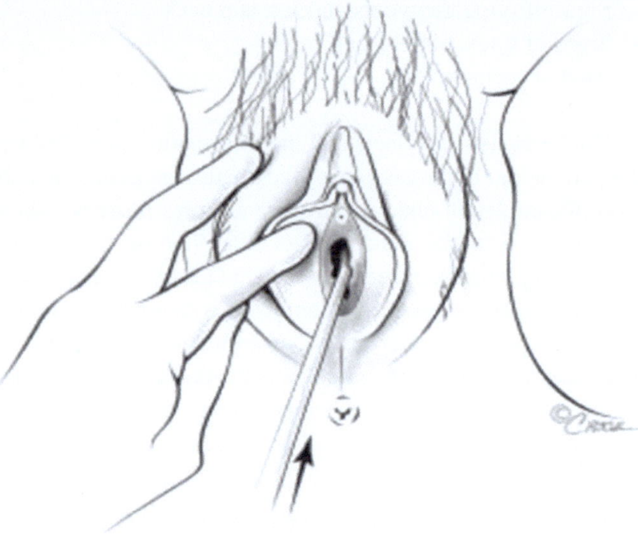

Fig. 33.7 Vaginal swab (With permission of World Health Organization, Guidelines for medico-legal care of victims of sexual violence, 2003)

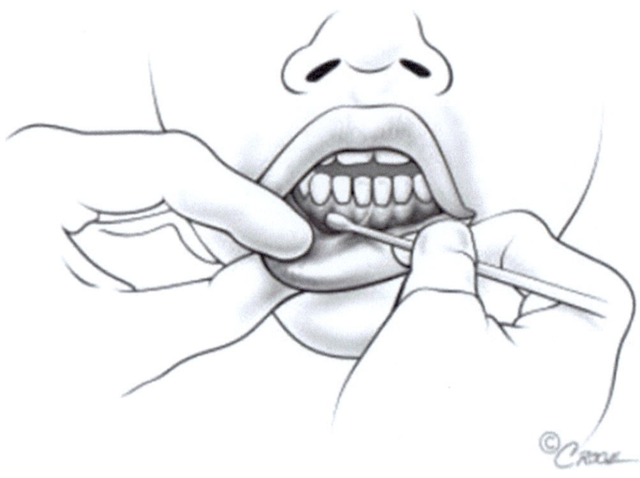

Fig. 33.8 Mouth swab (With permission of World Health Organization, Guidelines for medico-legal care of victims of sexual violence, 2003)

and semen tend to collect in the spaces between the teeth and the edges of the gums, it is important to take samples using a swab placed in the space between the teeth (Fig. 33.8).

Those who wish to report the assault to the police immediately should be encouraged to do so. The wishes of those who disclose recent sexual assault but do not wish to report the offense to the police should be respected. They should be offered an examination with collection of DNA and other evidence, without police involvement. This gives patients the opportunity to consider their options and report the assault at a later date [93].

33.1.7.4 Treatment and Follow-Up

Aims of the treatment are:

- Prevention of sexually transmitted diseases
- Prevention of HIV/AIDS infection
- Emergency contraception
- Psychological and social support [91]

33.2 Management of Ob-Gyn Emergencies

33.2.1 Antepartum Hemorrhage

33.2.1.1 Introduction

Antepartum hemorrhages are defined as a blood loss from the genitals during the second part of the pregnancy and complicate 2–5% of pregnancies. They can be divided into placental abruption hemorrhages (40%), placenta previa (20%), local causes (10%), vasa previa (0.5%), and uncertain origin (30%) [94].

33.2.1.2 Placenta Previa

Placenta abruption is found in 1% of pregnancies, more frequently during young maternal ages [95, 96].

The most predictive risk factor is abruption in a previous pregnancy. Other risk factors for placental abruption include: pre-eclampsia, fetal growth restriction, non-vertex presentations, polyhydramnios, advanced maternal age, multiparity, low body mass index (BMI), pregnancy following assisted reproductive techniques, intrauterine infection, premature rupture of membranes, abdominal trauma (both accidental and resulting from domestic violence), smoking and drug misuse (cocaine and amphetamines) during pregnancy. First trimester bleeding increases the risk of abruption later in the pregnancy [97].

The clinical picture is characterized on the basis of the entity of the bleeding at three levels [95, 96]:

- Level 1 characterized by slight vaginal bleeding, mild uterine contraction and the absence of cardiotocographic changes;
- Level 2 characterized by slight to moderate vaginal bleeding, more intense uterine contractions and the presence of cardiotocographic changes;
- Level 3 characterized by heavy vaginal bleeding, uterine contractions with the characteristics of from tachysistole and tetanic, intense abdominal pain and clear pathological CTG, conditions that can lead to the death of the fetus.

Diagnosis is clinical. Bleeding, which is not present in 20-30% of cases, is generally dark red. The pain is acute, continuous or intermittent, and localization is related to the position of the placenta. If the placenta is posterior, an acute lower lumbar pain may be the only symptom. Uterine contractile activity is hyperkineticc, or even hypertonic and tetanic in more serious cases. Nausea e sickness could also be among the symptoms [98].

A scan used in the diagnosis of *placental abruption* is not a very sensitive technique, even if specific [99]. Cardiotocography is not always useful in initial phases, but it becomes increasingly more pathological when the abruption involves at least half of the placental bed. The most frequent changes are severe variable decelerations, late decelerations, bradycardia and the reduction in variability [100].

Placental abruption involves a high level of perinatal mortality and morbidity and can cause rare, but serious maternal and fetal complications [95, 96]. Maternal complications include: mortality (1%), hypovolemic shock (5%), acute renal failure (0.5–1.5%), disseminated intravascular coagulation (CID) (10%), postpartum hemorrhages (25%) and recurrence (8–25%).

Placenta previa is a condition in which the placenta is positioned in the lower uterine segment and can reach or cover, partially or completely, the internal uterine orifice. There is an incidence of 0.3% in single pregnancies [94]. On the basis of the topography, four possible eventualities can be highlighted:

1. Low-lying placenta, ending in the lower uterine segment
2. Marginal placenta previa, which reaches or is less than 2 cm from the edge of internal uterine orifice
3. Partial placenta previa, which partially covers the internal uterine orifice
4. Central placenta previa, which completely covers the internal uterine orifice

The risk factors for placenta previa are previous placenta previa, previous cesarean section, previous uterine surgery, pregnancies using medically assisted procreation techniques, twin pregnancies, smoking, cocaine, multiparity, and advanced maternal age [94].

Patients with placenta previa usually come for a checkup because of bleeding without pain at about the beginning of the third trimester [101, 102]. On examination, the uterus appears decontracted, not painful and normal. In the beginning, the bleeding is bright red and is very light; the onset of symptoms is often slow and insidious and occurs weeks before labor; in one-third of the cases, patients do not have any blood loss until the start of labor. The differential diagnosis with placental abruption can be particularly insidious.

The diagnosis of placenta previa is usually carried out via transvaginal scan, which is more precise than a transabdominal scan.

The complications connected to placenta previa can be both maternal and fetal. The maternal complications are maternal mortality (0.03%), antepartum hemorrhage, intrapartum hemorrhage, hysterectomy, postpartum hemorrhage, sepsis, and thrombophlebitis. Fetal complications are perinatal mortality (4–8%), prematurity, and delayed intrauterine growth.

33.2.1.3 Antepartum Hemorrhage: Management

All patients with blood loss after 20 weeks must be transported to the delivery room. The two primary objectives are the hemodynamic evaluation of the mother and the assessment of the well-being of the fetus. Two large venous accesses must be put in place for hematocrit and blood typing sampling. The clinical situation can differ according to whether or not there is a state of shock. Once the patient has been stabilized and fetal conditions assessed, the cause of the bleeding must be investigated. The clinical situation depends on the extent of the blood loss, on the period of the pregnancy during which it takes place, and on the degree of maternal-fetal compromise.

33.2.2 Postpartum Hemorrhage

33.2.2.1 Introduction

The World Health Organization defines primary postpartum hemorrhage (PPH) as blood loss greater than or equal to 500 mL within 24 h of a vaginal delivery. PPH is regarded as severe if the blood loss exceeds 1000 mL; in a cesarean section, blood loss equal to or greater than 1000 mL can be defined as anomalous [103]. Secondary PPH is defined as abnormal bleeding from the genital tract from 24 h after delivery until 12 weeks postpartum [104, 105].

PPH is one of the most frequent causes of mortality and morbidity in the obstetric population globally [103].

The causes of PPH can be manifold. In clinical practice, they are summarized as the “4 Ts” [106]:

- Tone (uterine atony)
- Tissue (retained placenta and abnormal placental implantation)
- Trauma (uterine rupture, cervical laceration, uterine inversion, or birth canal lacerations)
- Thrombin (blood coagulation disorders)

The fundamentals of PPH treatment are:

1. Maintenance of uterine contractility, obtained by physical or pharmacologic means
2. Maintenance or support of circulation with proper hydration
3. Prevention or treatment of the established hemorrhagic coagulopathy

Intervention should be made in the "golden hour" to increase the chances of survival of the patient [104, 107].

33.2.2.2 Medical Management of PPH

The first action to be taken in the case of PPH is to request the cooperation of other medical and paramedic staff. While waiting for support, an assessment of the extent of the bleeding through retroplacental bag, gauze, and drapes is advised [108, 109].

Simultaneous with the assessment of blood loss is the need to begin the monitoring of vital signs: blood pressure, respiratory rate, heart rate, electrocardiography (ECG), pulse oximetry, temperature, and diuresis through a urinary catheter. Checking should be carried out initially every 10 min, according to the clinical evolution, and then every 30 min [108]. At this stage, a request for blood components should be sent to the transfusion center.

Two large venous access points (16 G or, better, 14 G) should also be established; the use of infusion pumps is preferable. A urinary catheter also needs to be inserted to empty the bladder.

The pharmacologic therapy at this stage includes oxytocin and tranexamic acid (TXA). There is significant variation in practice in this regard. However, oxytocin together with TXA is to be the first choice (20 IU in 500 mL saline in 2 h) [105]. If no effect is observed after 20 min, a second-line uterotonic may have to be given.

Evidence supporting the early use of TXA in massive hemorrhage, at variable dosage of between 1 and 4 g [108–113], has been increasing rapidly.

At the same time, samples regarding blood group have to be taken, and repeated blood counts and basic coagulation tests should be carried out: prothrombin time, partial thromboplastin time, fibrinogen, and antithrombin.

Close monitoring is needed to avoid or correct hypothermia and to measure and avoid acidosis (lactates >2 mmol/L) and desaturation. We suggest that an arterial blood gas analysis be carried out to obtain a baseline hemoglobin level.

The source of bleeding should be established by applying the rule of the 4 Ts [106], and the relevant corrective actions should be determined:

- Tone (bimanual uterine compression, intracavitary uterine tamponade through a hydrostatic balloon catheter, and use of uterotonics). In the absence of a hydrostatic balloon, a latex glove or a condom can be used with good results, as suggested by the FIGO 2012 Guidelines [114]. It should be emphasized that the use of gauze tamponade is now discouraged.
- Tissue (exploration and evacuation of the uterus).
- Trauma (vaginal lacerations and cervix and/or uterine rupture repair).
- Thrombin (in relation to blood coagulation disorders due to thrombin dysfunction; any coagulation defects should be evaluated and corrected with ROTEM/TEG monitoring, if available).

The restoration of the circulating volume by giving the least volume of crystalloids (Ringer-lactate/acetate as the first line) or colloids [115] until the hypoperfusion is corrected, based on an evaluation of the clinical and laboratory variables (sensory state, diuresis, lactates, and deficit base), and speeding up the request of blood products should be carried out only when resolution of the effective hemorrhage is not achieved.

During massive hemorrhage, fibrinogen is one of the first coagulation factors to decrease beyond critical levels. Several recent studies have suggested that fibrinogen is an important predictor of severe PPH [116, 117]. Some guidelines have indicated that fibrinogen concentrate should be the replacement therapy of choice [118].

Transfusion in the presence of the effective PPH is carried out based on clinical indications and not on information obtained from blood chemistry tests.

Cases that do not respond to the therapies described above require a conservative surgical interventionist approach. In case of non-response to the measures outlined thus far, the application of partial or total hysterectomy will be necessary.

33.2.2.3 Surgical Management of PPH

Once the peritoneum has been opened, the integrity of the womb must be checked, carefully examining the uterine walls and aiming at obtaining a contraction of the womb utilizing a prolonged massage [119]. If this massage has no result, a compressive type of intervention must be carried out (B-Lynch or Hayman technique) which solves the problem in more than 85% of cases [120–126].

In the rare cases that B-Lynch or Hayman techniques are not effective, it is necessary to proceed without further delay with a hysterectomy.

B-Lynch

The B-Lynch technique is simple to carry out and has excellent results if the indication is correct. In order to carry out the intervention after a vaginal birth, in the absence of hysterotomy, as in the case of a cesarean section, the prevesical peritoneum must be opened, opening the uterine bladder fold of peritoneum and detaching the bladder downward at least 2 cm. The lower uterine segment must be cut diagonally for 4 cm. The uterus must be exteriorized from the laparotomic breach, proceeding using a monofilament thread of at least 120 cm in length with a rounded needle of more than 48 mm. The anterior part of the uterus is punctured completely on the right side from the dissection of the bladder at least 15 mm from the *hysterotomy*. The needle must come out from the anterior part at least 15 mm above the *hysterotomy*, creating the first "handle" puncturing the posterior segment of the uterus completely by at least 4 cm from the right uterosacral ligament to the left uterosacral ligament, thus creating the second "handle" puncturing the anterior segment of the uterus 15 mm above the *hysterotomy and bringing out* the needle 15 mm below the *hysterotomy* (Fig. 33.9).

Hayman

This case also involves the creation of handles, from 2 to 4, which, unlike the B-Lynch, are not connected to each other. First of all, we proceed, as for B-Lynch, with the detachment of the bladder. Two stitches are then placed on the lower uterine segment, next to each other, taking care to leave a space for secretion (Fig. 33.10).

Ligature of the Hypogastric Artery

Ligature of the hypogastric artery, or when indicated, the uterine artery, is not so useful in solving corporal bleeding, due to the intense branches of the ovarian artery that take blood to the uterus. On the other hand, it is considerably useful in lower uterine segment bleeding, from the cervix and the vagina, and for broad ligament hematoma. It is also very useful in cases of uterine rupture to conclude a hysterectomy, otherwise impossible due to the overflow of blood in the operating area.

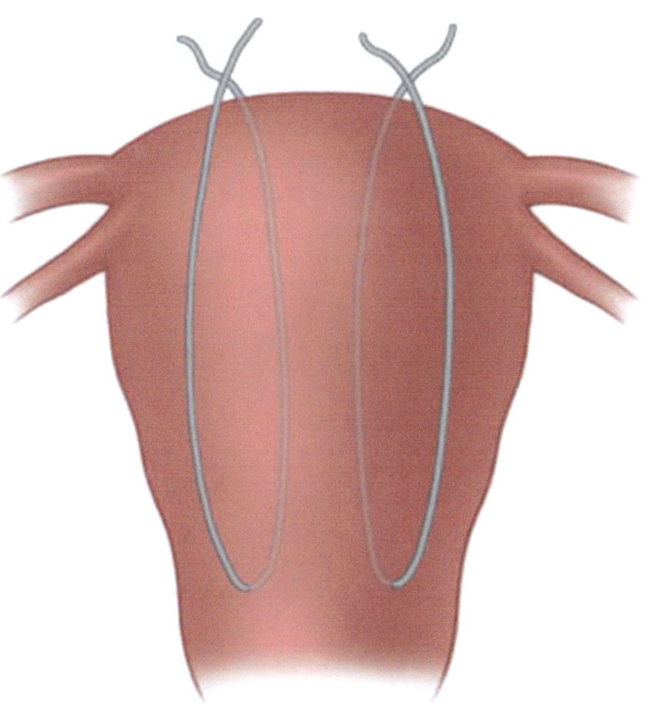

Fig. 33.10 Hayman. Two to four stitches are made in the uterus piercing the lower segment by 15 mm caudal to the real or imagined breach, going through the uterus from front to back and then tying the threads on the bottom of the uterus, confirming that the assistant ensures the volumetric reduction of the uterine size [124, 125] (*With permission of Piccin Editore. From Ragusa A, Crescini C. URGENZE ED EMERGENZE IN SALA PARTO.Padova 2015: Casa Editrice PICCIN Nuova Libreria*)

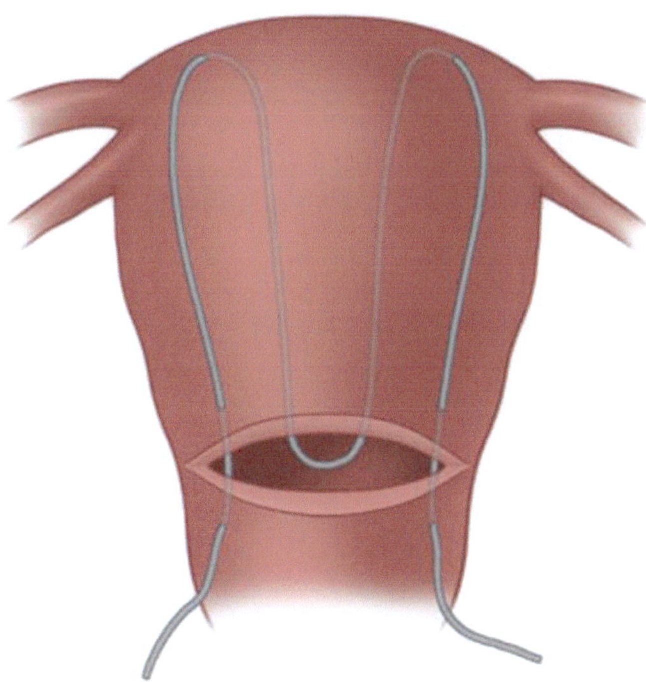

Fig. 33.9 B-Lynch. The two ends of the thread must then be tied slowly using a flat surgical knot, taking care to pull the thread with enough force to compress properly the uterus without tearing it [120–123]. The assistant must help reduce the size of the uterus by compression. After having verified that hemorrhage has stopped, the *hysterotomy* can be sutured. (*With permission of Piccin Editore. From Ragusa A, Crescini C. URGENZE ED EMERGENZE IN SALA PARTO, Padova 2015. Casa Editrice PICCIN Nuova Libreria*)

The first action to be taken is an incision of the broad ligament in the part between the round ligament and the suspensory ligament of the ovary, taking care to remain at the side, above the iliopsoas muscle, so as not to meet veins or the lateral uterine anastomosis of the pelvic vessels. If the uterus is to be sacrificed, it is useful to cut and tie the round ligament. Careful dissection must be performed, leaving the ureter medial, which runs at the back of the broad ligament, and lateral pelvic vessels, until identifying the hypogastric artery that should be kept to the side. At this point, the same hypogastric artery must be followed to the origin of the uterine artery. Proceed from lateral to medial with a curved dissector (right angle), to isolate the artery that is closed with a thread passed by means of a right angle, or using a clip, opening the right angle slightly to be sure to close the artery completely [126].

The numerous anastomoses between uterine artery, lower bladder, and long vaginal bowels are dramatically reduced, obtaining a net decrease in the vascularization of the lower segment, of the cervix and the upper third of the vagina. The risks connected to the closure of the hypogastric artery are gluteal necrosis (if the artery is clamped before the first eminence of the rear trunk), ureter injury, and more bleeding in isolation maneuvers.

Hysterectomy

Subtotal hysterectomy has lower surgical morbidity and is the operation of choice, unless there is trauma to the cervix or lower segment.

If the cervix and paracolpos are not involved as the source of hemorrhage, subtotal hysterectomy should be adequate to achieve hemostasis, which is the objective of the intervention. Additionally, the procedure is safer, faster, easier to carry out, and less likely to cause damage to the bladder or ureters compared with total hysterectomy [103, 127]. However, if the lower segment and paracolpos are involved in the hemorrhage, such as in cases of placenta previa, total hysterectomy will be necessary for hemostasis [103, 127].

33.2.3 Inversion of the Uterus

Uterine inversion is a rare complication of childbirth and happens when the fundus of the uterus descends abnormally through the genital tract, thus turning itself inside out [128–132].

Four grades of uterine inversion are described (Fig. 33.11):

- Grade 1: fundus inverts down to the cervical canal.
- Grade 2: fundus inverts into the vagina.
- Grade 3: fundus is visible at the introitus.
- Grade 4: complete inversion of both the uterus and vagina. Reported incidence ranges from 1/2000 to 1/6400 [128–132]. Maternal mortality can be high as 15% if the condition is not promptly diagnosed and corrected. Factors that have been associated with this condition are summarized in (Table 33.4).

33.2.3.1 Diagnosis

Uterine inversion can be difficult to diagnose, particularly if the fundus is not outside the introitus.

Early recognition is important to enable prompt treatment and to reduce morbidity and mortality [128–132].

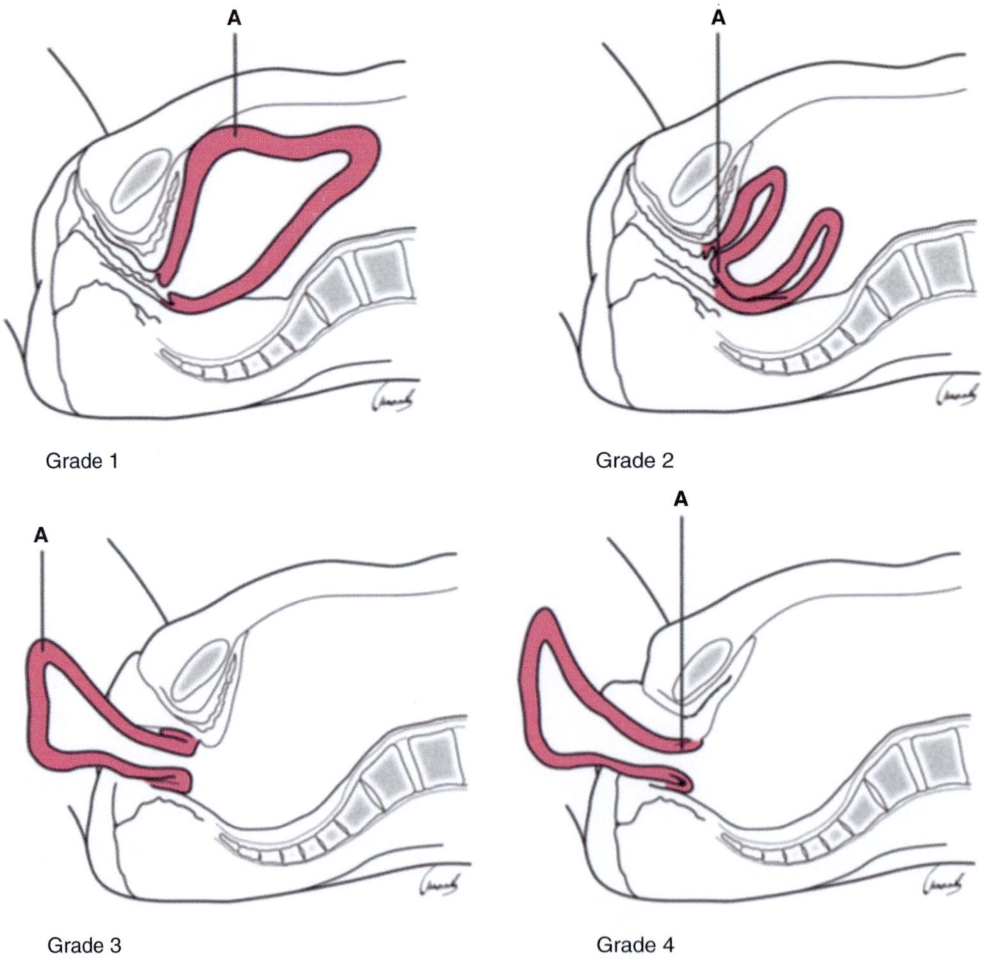

Fig. 33.11 Grades of uterine inversion. (*With permission of Piccin Editore. From Ragusa A, Crescini C. URGENZE ED EMERGENZE IN SALA PARTO, Padova 2015. Casa Editrice PICCIN Nuova Libreria*)

Table 33.4 Risk factors for uterine inversion

Risk factors
Excessive traction on umbilical cord
Short umbilical cord
Inappropriate fundal pressure
Abnormally adherent placenta
Previous uterine inversion
Precipitate labor
Uterine abnormalities
Vaginal birth after cesarean (VBAC)
Fibroids
Connective tissue disorders (e.g., Marfan syndrome, Ehlers-Danlos syndrome)

Symptoms and signs include:

- Development of sudden maternal shock not proportionate to blood loss
- Atonic postpartum hemorrhage (present in over 90% of cases)
- Severe lower abdominal pain in the third stage of labor
- Hypovolemic shock with tachycardia and hypotension
- A mass in the vagina or outside the introitus at vaginal examination
- Uterine fundus not palpable on abdominal examination (a dimple may be appreciated in the fundal area)

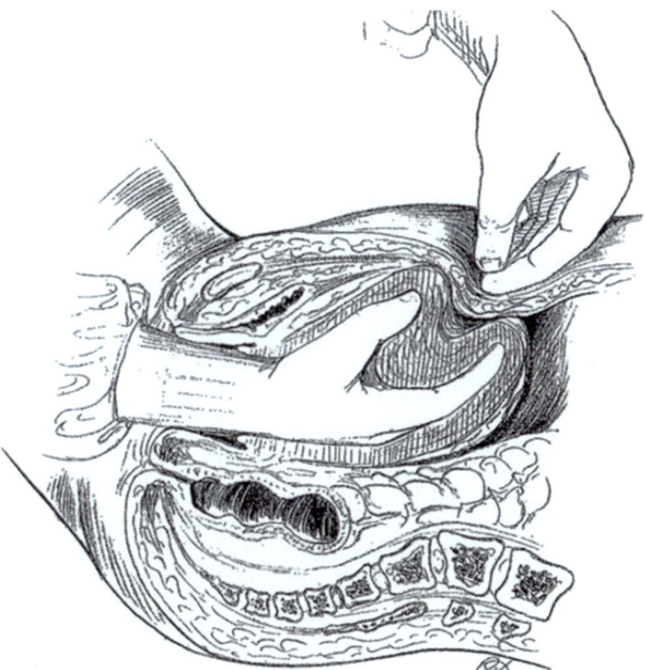

Fig. 33.12 Manual replacement (Johnson maneuver) (*With permission of Piccin Editore. From Ragusa A, Crescini C. URGENZE ED EMERGENZE IN SALA PARTO, Padova 2015. Casa Editrice PICCIN Nuova Libreria*)

33.2.3.2 Management

The treatment of maternal shock should be addressed immediately with standard resuscitation. At the same time, it's crucial to put the uterus into its anatomical position, in order to resolve neurogenic shock. After 30 min a cervical constriction ring may develop, thus making uterine repositioning impossible, so the earlier the restoration, the more likely the success [128–133].

If the placenta is still attached, no attempts to remove should be done, since they may result in major bleeding. Placenta should be removed in theater after the uterus has been replaced [133].

Interventions are:

- Call for senior help.
- Insert two large-bore intravenous cannulae.
- Give high flow oxygen (10 L/min).
- Collect blood and send for crossmatch (4–6 units), full blood count and clotting (consider transfusion).
- Start immediately fluid replacement (at least 1000 mL crystalloids).
- Continuously monitor blood pressure, pulse, respiratory rate, urine output, and O_2 saturation.
- Position urinary catheter.
- Organize appropriate analgesia.
- Try manual replacement first (the Johnson maneuver), preferably under general anesthesia, and if possible, use tocolytic agents (Fig. 33.12).
- Hydrostatic pressure can be used to correct uterine inversion (O'Sullivan technique). Infuse warm saline into the posterior fornix of the vagina via a rubber tube held 2 m above the level of the vagina, in order to distend the vagina and push the fundus upward. To increase the hydrostatic pressure and prevent saline to overflow, it is possible to seal the vaginal orifice with a hand or a Silastic ventouse cup. Uterine rupture should be ruled out first.
- If replacement is successful, administer uterotonics such as oxytocics, and the attendant should keep his hand in the uterine cavity for a few minutes, until a firm contraction occurs to prevent re-inversion.
- After successful replacement, a tamponade balloon catheter can be put inside the uterine cavity to maintain uterine position [134].
- If manual replacement fails, transfer the patient to the operating theater in order to try surgical reduction of the inverted uterus. Different techniques are described [135]. Laparotomy may be required at this point. Upward gentle traction with atraumatic Allis forceps, placed within the dimple of the inverted uterus may be used to achieve replacement to the anatomical position (Huntington's method) (Fig. 33.13). To facilitate this procedure, especially if a cervical ring makes repositioning difficult, is possible to cut vertically the cervical ring posteriorly (where it is less likely to involve the bladder or uterine

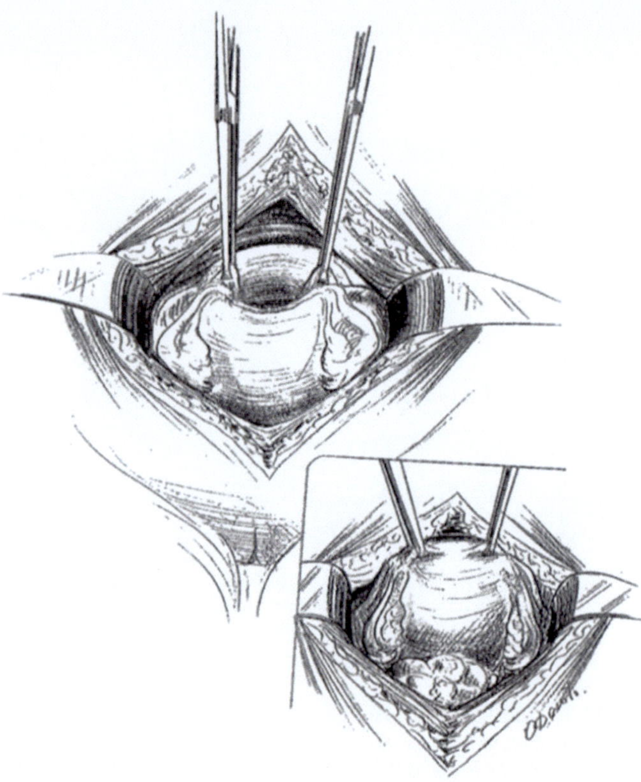

Fig. 33.13 Surgical correction of uterine inversion with Huntington's method (*With permission of Piccin Editore. From Ragusa A, Crescini C. URGENZE ED EMERGENZE IN SALA PARTO, Padova 2015. Casa Editrice PICCIN Nuova Libreria*)

vessels) to aid replacement of the uterus (Haultain's technique). Hysterotomy site is then repaired.

- Antibiotics should be given.
- The patients should be monitored closely since re-inversion of the uterus is frequent.

33.2.4 Prolapsed Umbilical Cord

Cord prolapse is defined as the descent of a loop of umbilical cord below the presenting part, in the presence of ruptured membranes [136–142].

It is an obstetrical emergency and occurs approximately in 0.1–0.6% of all births, while in breech presentations, its incidence can be as high as 1% [136–142].

In cord prolapse, perinatal mortality is due to asphyxia and is caused by mechanical compression of the cord between the presented part and bony pelvis or by spasm of the cord vessels when exposed to cold or manipulations [144, 143].

The interval between diagnosis and birth is significantly related to stillbirth and perinatal death [145].

Perinatal mortality rate has improved and is currently estimated to be 10% or less [144, 143]. The explanations for these better outcomes are the increased availability of cesarean delivery and advances in neonatal resuscitation.

Umbilical cord prolapse primarily occurs in two settings:

1. When the presenting part does not adequately fill the pelvis because of maternal or fetal characteristics
2. When obstetric interventions are performed that dislodge the presenting part are performed

Fetal and maternal factors that have been associated with this condition are summarized in Table 33.5.

It is important to avoid amniotomy unless the fetal head is well-engaged or, if necessary, "needling" the bag for a slower, more controlled release of fluid.

33.2.4.1 Diagnosis

Early diagnosis is important. A cord prolapsed may be obvious when there is a loop of cord protruding through the vulva. However, a prolapsed cord is not always apparent and may only be found on vaginal examination. It can be suspected when there is an abnormal fetal heart rate pattern in the presence of ruptured membranes, particularly if CTG changes start soon after the rupture [136–142]. In 41–67% of cases, it is associated with severe, sudden decelerations, often with prolonged bradycardia, or recurrent moderate to severe variable decelerations.

33.2.4.2 Management

The approach if the baby is alive and of viable gestation is elevation of the presenting part to relieve compression of the cord and expedite delivery, usually by cesarean section [145].

Prompt delivery has been shown to improve outcomes.

Table 33.5 Risk factors for cord prolapse

Risk factors
Breech presentation
Multiparity
Unstable lie
Oblique or transverse lie
Polyhydramnios
Prematurity
Multiple pregnancy
Long cord
Low birth weight (<2500 g)
Amniotomy (especially with a high presenting part)
Sudden rupture of membranes (especially in polyhydramnios)
Internal podalic version
Second twin

- Call for senior help, including an anesthetist, the theater team, and the neonatal team.
- Site a wide-bore intravenous cannula and take blood for group and save and full blood count.
- Administer intravenous fluids.
- Check vitality of the fetus by ultrasound to visualize fetal movements even with the absence of cord pulsation and inaudible fetal heart tones.
- Relieve cord compression by elevating the presenting part. This can be achieved by:

  Digital elevation of the presenting part of the fetus above the pelvic inlet: two fingers or the entire hand should be kept in the vagina until the baby is born.

  Maternal positioning: such as knee-chest facedown position or the exaggerate Sims' position (left lateral with a pillow under the left hip) (Fig. 33.14).

If the cord has prolapsed out from the vagina, an attempt to gently replace it back with minimal handling is possible. There is no sufficient evidence to recommend the practice of covering the cord with gauzes soaked in warm saline. Excessive manipulations of the cord should be avoided.

- Continuous electronic fetal monitoring should be performed, if possible.

  If the cervix is not fully dilated, a cesarean section should be performed [145].

  If the cervix is fully dilated and the obstetrician believes that a vaginal delivery can be performed more rapidly than a cesarean section, it is appropriate to proceed with vaginal delivery. If prerequisites for operative birth are met, ventouse or forceps can be considered.

Regional anesthesia is possible if fetal conditions permit, and the safest method of anesthesia for both the mother and fetus should be considered.

Team training exercises have been shown to shorten the interval between diagnosis and delivery and may lead to improved neonatal outcomes [146–148].

33.2.5 Acute Abdominal Pain During Pregnancy

33.2.5.1 Introduction

Acute abdominal pain during pregnancy has an impact that ranges from 1:500 to 1:635, and 0.2–1% of these patients require surgery [149].

Table 33.6 shows the possible pathologies in relation to the seat of the pain.

33.2.5.2 Acute Appendicitis

The insidence of acute appendicitis during pregnancy is 1 case every 1500–2000 pregnancies and is the cause of 25% of surgery for non-obstetric indications [149, 150].

Diagnosis

The most common symptom is the pain in the lower right quadrant (McBurney point). Associated symptoms include anorexia, nausea, and sickness. A perforated appendix should be suspected if the pain changes from localized to wide-

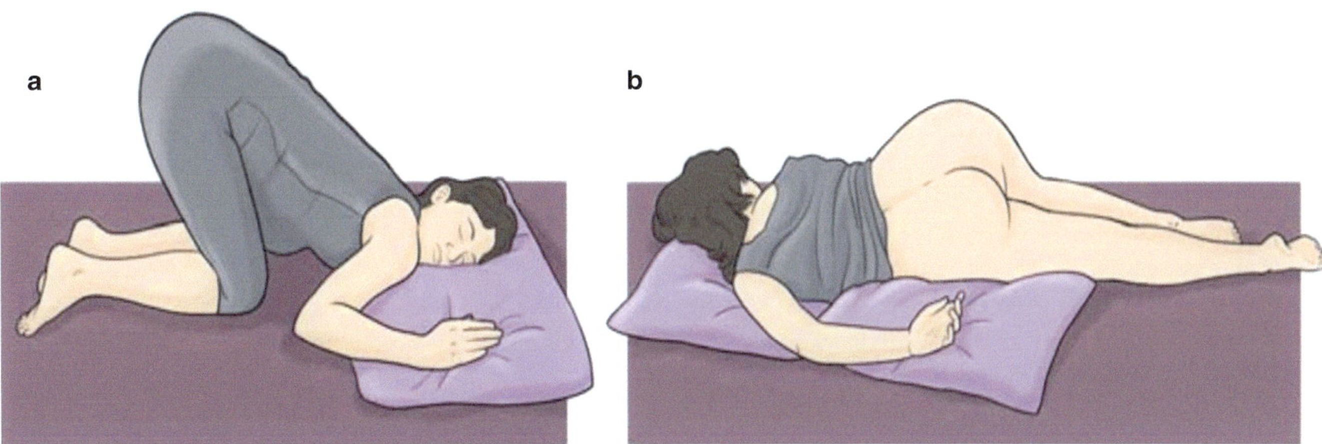

Fig. 33.14 Maternal positioning to relieve cord compression: (**a**) knee-chest facedown position; (**b**) exaggerate Sims' position (left lateral with a pillow under the left hip (*With permission of Piccin Editore. From Ragusa A, Crescini C. URGENZE ED EMERGENZE IN SALA PARTO, Padova 2015. Casa Editrice PICCIN Nuova Libreria*)

Table 33.6 Location of abdominal pain and possible underlying pathologies

Location of the pain	Organs to be considered	Possible causes
Widespread	Any intra-abdominal organ	Irritation of the initial stage of the visceral peritoneum
Left hypochondria	Spleen, pancreas, left splenic flexures of the colon	Heat attack, bleeding or rupture of the spleen, colitis
Epigastrium	Stomach, pancreas, aorta, heart	Gastritis, pancreatitis, dissection or rupture of the aorta, acute myocardial infarction
Right hypochondria	Liver, kidney, right or hepatic of the colon, gallbladder	Hepatitis, cholecystitis, rupture or hepatic hemorrhage, acute fatty *liver* of *pregnancy* (AFLP), HELLP syndrome, preeclampsia imminent
Right side	Right kidney, ascending colon	Pyelonephritis, kidney or ureteric stones, inflammatory bowel disease
Mesogastrium	Transverse colon, appendix (visceral pain in the initial stage), uterus	Appendicitis, gastroenteritis, mesenteric lymphadenitis, acute pancreatitis, postpartum placenta, dehiscence or rupture of the previous uterine scar
Left side	Left kidney, descending colon	Pyelonephritis, kidney or ureteric stones, inflammatory bowel disease
Left iliac ditch	Sigmoid colon, left fallopian tube and ovary	Inflammatory bowel disease, diverticulitis of the sigmoid colon, ectopic pregnancy, tubo-ovarian abscess, ruptured ovarian cyst, adnexal torsion
Hypogastrium	Bladder, uterus	Cystitis, postpartum placenta, dehiscence or breakage of previous uterine scar
Right iliac ditch	Appendicitis, sigmoid colon, right fallopian tube and ovary	Appendicitis, diverticulitis of the sigmoid colon, ectopic pregnancy, tubo-ovarian abscess, ruptured ovarian cyst, adnexal torsion

spread. A retrocecal appendix can cause symptoms at the back or side of the patient [150, 151].

On physical examination a Rovsing sign may be noted [150, 151]. Stiffness and abdominal defense, irritation of the psoas, and rectal and pelvic pain may not be present. Leukocytosis is of little use. However, the predominant neutrophilia (>80%) and an increase in the C-reactive protein may be of help. A scan can identify an inflamed appendix or a periappendiceal abscess. The scan should be performed with the patient in left lateral *decubitus* position. An abnormal appendix has a tubular structure, *non-compressible*, showing *no peristalsis*, with a diameter of more than 6 mm, which originates from the base of the cecum [150].

If the scan is not decisive and diagnostic doubts persist, it indicates a magnetic resonance (MR) should be carried out [150]. A computed tomography (CT) must be used if there are still diagnostic doubts [149, 150].

Management

Surgical intervention should be carried out immediately [152, 153]. Active labor is the only indication to postpone surgery, which will have to be carried out postpartum [152, 153]. There are no indications to perform a cesarean section, except in the case of perforated appendix. Surgery may be carried out via laparoscopy or laparotomy [152, 153]. In the case of laparotomy performed during the first trimester, the incision of the skin must be carried out at the McBurney point [141, 153]. The incision may also be longitudinal, paramedian or median [152, 153]. The incision can also be carried out where pain is felt most [152, 153]. Care must be taken to avoid excessive uterine traction, thus avoiding irritation to the uterine bowels, with consequent onset of contractions. If the appendix is ruptured or there is evidence of peritonitis, a copious intra-abdominal irrigation should be carried out. The positioning of drainage can be taken into consideration to drain the possible abscess. The patient must be administered perioperative antibiotic therapy with second-generation cephalosporins, broad-spectrum penicillins, and carbapenems, together with clindamycin or metronidazole [149–153].

33.2.5.3 Acute Cholecystitis

Gallbladder pathologies have an incidence that ranges from 1:1600 to 1:10,000 pregnancies and are thus the second most common cause of non-obstetric surgical problems [150, 151]. Ninety percent of the cases are caused by an obstruction of the cystic duct by biliary stones or sand [150, 151].

Diagnosis

The symptoms of acute cholecystitis include nausea, sickness, anorexia, intolerance to fatty foods, dyspepsia, and mesogastric pain in the upper right quadrant, expanding to the top of the scapula. The Murphy sign is rare [150, 151]. In more serious cases, the patient may have slight jaundice and signs of sepsis [150, 151]. Lab tests can show an increase in direct bilirubin, transaminase, and bilirubin levels [150, 151].

A scan enables to identify the presence of biliary stones in 95–98% of cases. Moreover, it is also able to highlight signs of acute cholecystitis among which edema of the gallbladder with an increase in wall thickness of more than increase 3 mm, accumulation of peri-cholecystic fluid, biliary stone, and Murphy sign showing in the scan [149, 154]. Magnetic resonance cholangiopancreatography (MRCP) can also be used to confirm the suspicion of biliary stones. Endoscopic retrograde cholangiopancreatography (ERCP) can be used for diagnostic purposes or to perform a sphincterotomy to solve possible pancreatitis, with minimum exposure to ionizing radiation [149, 154].

Management

Symptomatic cholelithiasis is often managed initially using conservative treatment by means of hydration to correct electrolyte, analgesic, anti-inflammatory, and bowel disorders. If there is no improvement after 12–24 h, or there are systemic symptoms, antibiotic treatment must be started with third-generation cephalosporins in combination with metronidazole. If the conservative treatment does not result in any improvement, cholecystectomy surgery is indicated via laparoscopic approach. This method can be used in all phases of pregnancy and has been proven to be safe and well tolerated [154].

33.2.5.4 Intestinal Obstruction

Intestinal obstruction complicates 1 out of 3000 pregnancies and is the third most common cause of for non-obstetric surgical problems. Failure to diagnose an intestinal obstruction is connected to 6% maternal mortality and 25–40% of fetal death [150, 153].

Diagnosis

The most frequent symptoms include acute cramping abdominal pain, constipation, nausea, and sickness. The pregnant abdomen can mask the abdominal distension typical of intestinal obstruction [150, 153].

An X-ray of the abdomen can be of help in the diagnosis and should be carried out in supine and upright position. If the X-ray does not give any confirmation, CT or an MR could be performed which allows to identify and treat volvulus [149, 150, 153].

Management

Conservative management includes initial intestinal decompression by means of nasogastric tube, bowel rest, fluid and electrolyte balance, and enemas. If the conservative management is not successful, or if the patient develops fever, tachycardia, or signs of peritonitis, surgical examination is mandatory. Surgery involves an incision median laparotomy, lysis of intestinal adhesions, bowel decompression, and, in the case of necrotic bowel, bowel resection followed by anastomosis. If the obstruction resolves spontaneously after performing the colonoscopy, surgery is recommended in any case after delivery due to the high risk (>50%) of recurrences [149, 150, 153].

33.2.6 Abdominal Trauma During Pregnancy

33.2.6.1 Introduction

Abdominal trauma during pregnancy is one of the main causes of maternal death [1]. Most of these traumas are caused by domestic violence [155]. Penetrating injuries and those caused by falling make up the main causes of trauma during pregnancy [156]. The management of traumas during pregnancy requires a multidisciplinary approach which involves a trauma surgeon, a specialist in emergency medicine, an obstetrician, and a neonatologist [157].

The management protocol for traumas with regard to a pregnant woman is the same as that for women who are not pregnant. First and foremost, the airways must be managed, bearing in mind that possible intubation could be difficult in pregnant women due to the increase in weight and swelling, characteristic of pregnancy [158]. If the airways are not safe, a nasogastric tube should be put in place [159, 160]. The patient must be positioned on her left side to increase the flow of blood to the heart [161, 162].

Priority must be given to the mother's health over that of the fetus. The patient must be transported to an area with a delivery room if her injuries do not endanger the health of the mother and if the fetus is ≥23 weeks. If the trauma is severe, or if the fetus is less than 23 weeks, the patient must be managed exclusively by the emergency division [157].

33.2.6.2 Signs and Symptoms

It is important to bear in mind that a pregnant woman has a 15% increase in heart rate. Signs of hypovolemic shock may be delayed due to the increase in blood volume [157]. The first sign of hypovolemia is that of tachycardia. In these cases the fetus should be monitored as soon as possible. Signs of peritoneal irritation are rare [163]. Uterine pain is a signal of alarm regarding possible placenta detachment. A vaginal examination must be carried out to confirm fetal presentation, cervical dilation, the length of the cervix, and the level of the presenting part. It is important to remember that in the case of vaginal bleeding in pregnancy of more than 23 weeks, a scan should be carried out before any type of vaginal examination with fingers or speculum, to exclude the possibility of a placenta previa.

33.2.6.3 Management

X-rays of the cervical spine, chest, and pelvis should be requested in the case of trauma [162]. The level of radiation used is very low [164]. Exposure to levels of radiation above 5–10 rad can cause deformities before 18 weeks [164, 165].

Nevertheless, investigations should never be delayed. Computerized tomography (CT) of the abdomen during the third 3-month period causes an absorption of radiation of 3.5 rad, which is below the limit that could cause fetal damage [166]. The use of gadolinium as a contrast medium is not toxic to the fetus and can be used when indicated [167].

Lab tests such as complete blood count and coagulation, with particular attention to fibrinogen, should be requested. In pregnant women, the levels of fibrinogen are higher (circa 4 g/L). Levels are below 2 g/L could be a sign of DIC.

A FAST scan is useful in the case of abdominal trauma to highlight the presence of fluid in the abdomen, and its presence is an indication to carry out an abdominal CT.

In pregnancies of more than 23 weeks, the well-being of the fetus should be assessed by means of monitoring the fetal heartbeat [157].

In the case in which a separation of the placenta is suspected, fetal monitoring for at least 24 consecutive hours is advisable [157].

Possible complications of traumas during pregnancy are feto-maternal hemorrhage, rupture of the uterus, and preterm delivery [157].

33.2.7 Ectopic Pregnancy and Abdominal Pregnancy

33.2.7.1 Definition

Ectopic pregnancies are defined as the implantation of blastocyst embryos outside the uterus [168].

33.2.7.2 Epidemiology

The frequency of ectopic pregnancies has increased as a consequence of the increase in risk factors, and thanks to improved diagnostics, reaching 2% of all pregnancies in the USA and 1.4% in Italy [168].

In subpopulations at risk, the incidence is 3% in pregnancies with medically assisted procreation and 10% in patients with previous ectopic pregnancies.

Ten percent of patients who go to the A&E department during the first trimester because of bleeding and/or pelvic pain will be diagnosed with ectopic pregnancy.

Ectopic pregnancy is still the cause of 4–10% of all maternal deaths (hemoperitoneum).

Table 33.7 shows the risk factors for ectopic pregnancy.

33.2.7.3 Clinical

Classical clinical presentation (45% of cases):

- Abdominal pain (97%)
- Vaginal blood loss (79%)
- Palpable adnexal mass and/or backward mass that fills the Douglas (30%), in women with amenorrhea/positive pregnancy test

Table 33.7 Risk factors for ectopic pregnancy

Degree of risk	Risk factors	Odds ratio
High	Previous ectopic pregnancy	9.3–4.7
	Previous tubal surgery	6.0–11.5
	Tubal ligation	3.0–13.9
	Tubal pathology	3.5–25
	In utero DES exposure	2.4–13
	Current IUD use	1.1–45
Moderate	Infertility	1.1–28
	Previous cervicitis (gonorrhea, chlamydia)	2.8–3.7
	History of pelvic inflammatory disease	2.1–3.0
	Multiple sexual partners	1.4–4.8
	Smoking	2.3–3.9
Low	Previous pelvic/abdominal surgery	0.93–3.8
	Vaginal douching	1.1–3.1
	Early age of intercourse (<18 years)	*1.1–2.5*

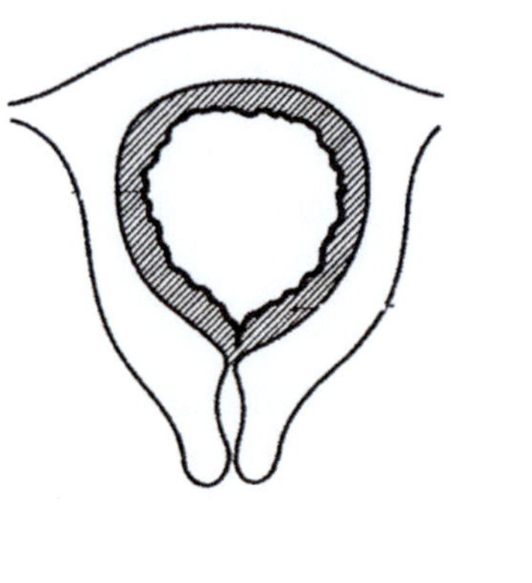
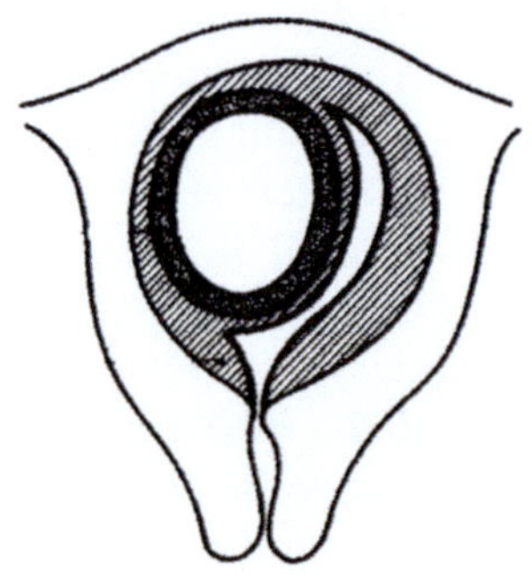
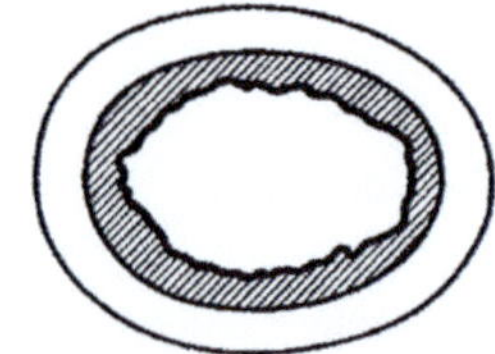
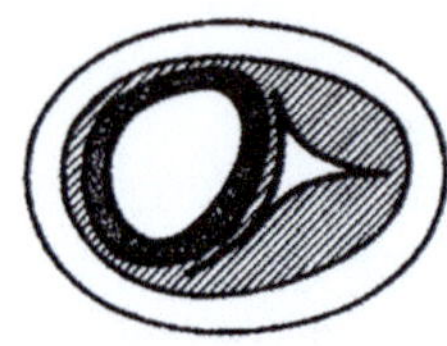

Fig. 33.15 Hyperechoic ring in ectopic pregnancy

33.2.7.4 Diagnosis

Transvaginal Scan

Ten percent of direct evidence of extrauterine implants (gestational vitreous sac with or without embryo); more frequently indirect ultrasound signs, empty uterus (lack of implant endothelium); free liquid in Douglas; and adnexal hyperechoic ring (Fig. 33.15: "bagel sign") [168].

At endometrial level, not tonic, irregular, without the double ring, and absence of embryonic echoes [168].

Significance of Chorionic Gonadotropin Beta Values (β-hCG)

When the scan is not definite, the differential diagnosis is between early endothelial pregnancy, premature abortion at an unknown seat, ectopic pregnancy, and vesicular mole: primary determinant is the serum dosage of β-hCG [169, 170].

- Early intrauterine pregnancy in regular evolution: in 48/72 h the level doubles, in ectopic pregnancy this increase is less, and in vesicular mole the levels are usually much higher.
- Discriminatory area: 2000 UI/L is generally the level above of which, if the pregnancy in the uterus and single, the gestational bag with transvaginal probe is shown (6500 should be seen in transabdominal, while the levels have not been defined for twin pregnancies yet).

33.2.7.5 Management

- Waiting conduct (18–33% GEU spontaneous resolution) does not affect following fertility [168, 171].
- Criteria: asymptomatic patient, first dosage of βHCG < 1000 UI/L, with following dosage at 48–72 h with a decrease of >15%, paraovarian mass <4 cm, endopelvic discharge <100 mL, stability or slow resolution to subsequent ultrasound checks, and patient's compliance [168, 171].
- Medical therapy (about 50% success)
- Criteria: symptomatic patient, first dosage of hCG ≥ 1000 UI/L and <3000 UI/L (3000–5000: risk of failure 5×) even if the subsequent dosage is stable or reduced, first dosage of hCG < 1000 UI/L but subsequent dosage at 48–72 h stable/ decreasing <15%/ increase, paraovarian mass <4 cm, BCF absent, endopelvic discharge <100 mL + stability, or slow resolution to subsequent ultrasound checks [168, 171].

A single dose of methotrexate (MTX) of 50 mg/m^2 via intramuscular injection, followed by weekly monitoring of the hCG and clinical conditions: good response if the decrease is ≥15% between days 4 and 7. If medical therapy fails (14%): possible new medical therapy, programmed or emergency surgery. Table 33.8 shows some precautions to bear in mind during MTX therapy [168, 171].

Table 33.9 shows the effects of the treatment and side effects when using MTX.

- Surgery
- Criteria: severely symptomatic patient, stable or increase in hCG before or after medical therapy, paraovarian mass ≥4 cm, endopelvic discharge ≥100 mL, BCF visualization, and unreliable/noncompliant patient [168, 171].

Conservative (salpingotomy) or demolitive (salpingectomy) surgery: there is no evidence in literature compared to different impacts on reproductive performance; conditions for salpingectomy: severe impairment of tubal anatomy, seat of the ectopic pregnancy (after evaluation of the anatomy of the contralateral tuba), adnexal mass >5 cm, recurrence of homolateral ectopic pregnancy, and uncontrolled hemostasis [168, 171].

If documented trophoblastic peritoneal implants and decrease <50% in hCG during the first day compared to presurgery, administration of MTX 50 mgm^2 IM single dose [168, 171].

Perform anti-D immunoprophylaxis in the case of Rh-negative blood group.

Weekly monitoring of βHCG and clinical conditions are suggested; serial ultrasound examinations are not useful but only at hormonal reset and at 4 months from the resetting. Avoid possible pregnancies for 6 months from the hormonal reset [168, 171].

Table 33.8 Precautions to be taken in the case of MTX therapy

Caveats for physicians and patients regarding the use of methotrexate (MTX)
Avoid intercourse until hCG is undetectable
Avoid pelvic exams and ultrasound during surveillance of MTX therapy
Avoid sun exposure to limit risk of MTX dermatitis
Avoid foods and vitamins containing folic acid
Avoid gas-forming foods because they produce pain
Avoid new conception until hCG is undetectable

ASRM Practice Committee. Treatment of ectopic pregnancy. Fertil Steril 2008

Table 33.9 Treatment and side effects connected to MTX

Effects of the treatment
Increase in abdominal circumference
Increase in hCG at the beginning of the treatment
Vaginal bleeding or spotting
Abdominal pain
Side effects
Epigastric discomfort (heartburn), nausea and sickness
Stomatitis
Dizziness
Severe neutropenia (rare)
Reversible alopecia (rare)
Pulmonary infections (rare)

ASRM Practice Committee. Treatment of ectopic pregnancy. Fertil Steril 2008

33.2.8 Abortion with Hemorrhagic Shock

The definition of abortion is an interruption of a pregnancy prior to the 24 weeks' of gestation [171].

Complications of an abortion are hemorrhagic shock due to severe bleeding and sepsis. Even without complications, an incomplete abortion can become dangerous if treatment is delayed. An accurate initial assessment of the patient is therefore necessary.

The possibility of an abortion must be taken into consideration for fertile women with at least two of the three following symptoms:

- Vaginal bleeding
- Cramps and/or lower abdominal pains
- History of amenorrhea

A transvaginal scan, along with BHCG dosage, should be provided.

Tachycardia and hypotension may be signs of severe hemorrhage or septic shock.

Hemorrhage after an abortion is rare and occurs in less than 1% of cases. The different definitions of postabortion hemorrhage include "blood loss of more than 250 mL," "blood loss of more than 500 mL," "blood loss requiring hospitalization," or "blood loss requiring transfusion" [172, 173].

The risk factors regarding postabortion hemorrhage are:

1. Previous cesarean sections (two or more cesarean sections)
2. Obesity
3. Problems regarding coagulation or hemorrhagic diathesis
4. Abnormalities of the placenta (placental accretion)
5. History of previous postpartum hemorrhage
6. Advanced maternal age
7. Fibroids and/or other uterine abnormalities

Hemorrhage can be caused by atony (52%), intravascular coagulopathy (5%), abnormal placenta (17%), or complications during surgery such as perforation (7%), cervical laceration (12%), and placental tissue retention [174].

Hemorrhage can be one of the most serious and immediate complications of an abortion. Timely intervention and early recognition of the source/cause of the bleeding can reduce the onset of hemorrhagic shock and, therefore, morbidity and mortality.

If bleeding occurs, an assessment of the blood loss must be carried out, with frequent recording of vital parameters (blood pressure and respiratory rate) along with a venous access.

33.2.8.1 Treatment of the Hemorrhage

The first steps to be taken in the case of bleeding include:

1. A physical examination to identify the source/cause of the bleeding (vagina, uterus, cervix)
2. Bimanual examination to evaluate uterine tone
3. Scan to assess the accumulation of blood or retention of tissue

Primary Treatment

In the case of cervical lacerations, carry out surgical repair using absorbable sutures. If the bleeding continues after the sutures, a possible laceration of the uterine artery or uterine perforation should be taken into consideration.

If there is no evidence of cervical lacerations or uterine perforation, uterine massage must be performed. At the same time, uterotonics must be given. The most frequently used drugs for postabortion hemorrhage are methylergometrine maleate [175, 176] and misoprostol; oxytocin and prostaglandins (carboprost) are used less frequently. Methylergometrine maleate, in doses of 0.2 mg im, has a rapid effect (within 5 min) and, if not contraindicated, is the first choice of medication. Misoprostol is also effective in cases of postabortion hemorrhage. The recommended dosages are 800–1000 μg [174] orally or sublingual with more rapid peak concentration [177] compared to rectal administration [178]. Oxytocin is considered as an effective uterotonic, but it can be less useful than other types of medication since, during the first and second trimester, the uterus has fewer receptors for oxytocin.

Secondary Treatment

If bleeding continues after the administration of uterotonics and bimanual massage, place further intravenous access and alert the anesthetist/resuscitator. Assess for signs of shock (heart rate higher than 100 bpm, blood pressure lower than 90 mmHg, cold and sweaty skin cute, respiratory rate higher than 30 per minute, changes in mental condition). Administer high oxygen concentrations. Administer fluids and request lab tests (blood count, coagulation, cross-tests). If the suspected clinical disseminated intravascular coagulation is high, a transfusion of red blood cells (RBC) and fresh frozen plasma must be carried out. The results of the lab tests and the clinical assessment of the patient will indicate the need for a transfusion of RBC, FFP, cryoprecipitate, and platelets.

Revision of the cavity if a scan shows that there is evidence of tissue retention or blood reaccumulation.

If an atony or bleeding of the lower part of the uterus is suspected, a Foley balloon can be put in place, filled with between 30 cc and 80 cc of saline solution, or a Bakri balloon, filled with 120 cc of saline solution [179, 180].

Following Treatment

In the case of failure of primary and secondary treatment, intensive actions such as the embolization of uterine arteries, laparoscopy, laparotomy, and hysterectomy are necessary.

If the radiology service is not available, the next step should be laparotomy. Laparoscopy can be useful if performed by expert surgeons, to confirm the suspected perforation and to repair the continuity of the uterus [180].

Even if not described by literature regarding abortions, it could be reasonable to try to control hemorrhages during abortions to perform bilateral uterine artery ligation and/or a B-Lynch suture, before carrying out a hysterectomy [180].

In conclusion, consultation with an obstetrician/gynecologist is indicated for all patients with a diagnosis of spontaneous or incomplete abortions. Patients with severe hemorrhage or those who are hemodynamically unstable need immediate consultation and treatment.

Case Scenario

A 24-year-old nulliparous woman referred to our emergency room for sudden pelvic pain.

She reported a similar, but milder, episode in the previous 3 months. She also reported mild nausea, without episodes of vomiting, and should adjust regularly.

Her past medical history was negative.

Her last period was 1 month before, and her last gynecological examination was 1 year before without any pathological findings.

Vital parameters at the arrival in ER were normal.

On physical examination we found:

Tenderness at lower abdominal quadrants; Blumberg sign was negative.

Tenderness of right adnexal region.

1. Which emergency is clinically less likely?
   A. Appendicitis
   B. Ectopic pregnancy
   C. Adnexal torsion
   D. PID
2. Which blood test would you perform first?
   A. Blood count + CRP + βHCG
   B. Blood count + βHCG
   C. Blood count + hepatic and renal function
   D. Blood count + CRP

   Blood tests showed neutrophil leukocytosis, normal hemoglobin, high-level CRP, and negative βHCG.
3. Which imaging would you request?
   A. Transvaginal ultrasound
   B. Abdominal ultrasound
   C. Abdominal X-ray
   D. Abdominal CT

   We performed transvaginal ultrasound with these results (Fig. 33.16):
   - Rounded and enlarged ovary, with heterogeneous stroma with multiple small peripheral follicles
   - Decreased Doppler flow within the ovary
   - Tenderness
   - Free fluid

   We suspected an adnexal torsion in a stable patient without acute abdomen.
4. Which other US finding is typical of adnexal torsion?
   A. "Whirlpool" sign
   B. Ground-glass ovarian cyst
   C. "Beads-on-a-string" sign
   D. "Cogwheel" sign
5. Which is the correct management of this patient?
   A. Laparoscopic detorsion within 24–36 h
   B. Laparoscopic oophorectomy
   C. Laparotomic detorsion and ovarian conservation within 24–36 h
   D. Conservative management

The patient underwent laparoscopic adnexal detorsion after a few hours.

An elongated utero-ovarian ligament was found during the intervention. The tube was cake on the ovarian lining ligament, and this had caused the ischemic phenomena of the ovary. The next day the woman was dismissed in good general conditions and postponed to routine outpatient gynecological examination after 3 weeks.

Please see Chap. 58 for the correct answer.

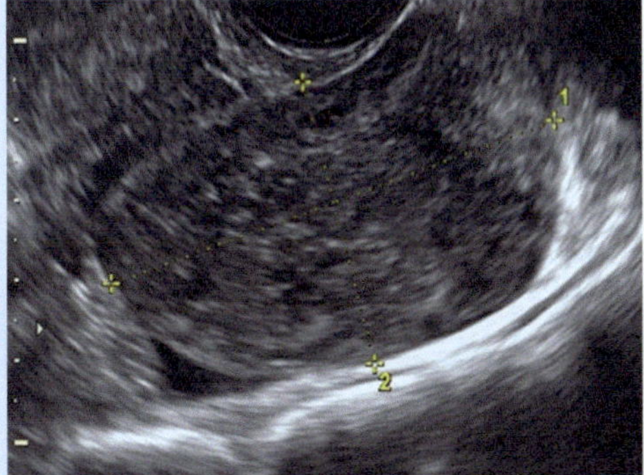
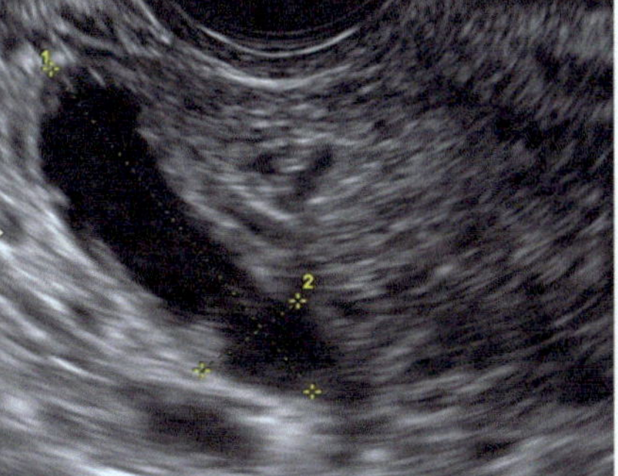
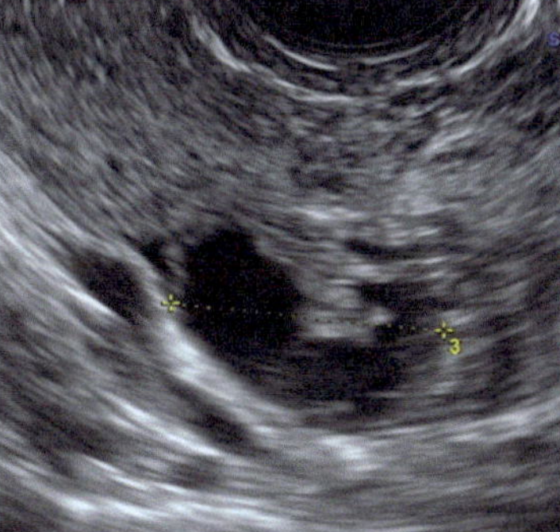

Fig. 33.16 Case scenario: adnexal torsion. The ovary is enlarged; the stroma is heterogeneous. Medial to the ovary is visible the swollen salpinx

Acknowledgments We would like to thank Dr. Marta Betti and Dr. Anna Carli for the collaboration offered in the drafting of this chapter.

References

1. McWilliams GD, Hill MJ, Dietrich CS III. Gynecologic emergencies. Surg Clin North Am. 2008;88:265.
2. Schrager J, Robles G, Platz T. Isolated fallopian tube torsion: a rare entity in a premenarcheal female. Am Surg. 2012;78:118.
3. Bouguizane S, Bibi H, Farhat Y, et al. [Adnexal torsion: a report of 135 cases]. J Gynecol Obstet Biol Reprod (Paris). 2003;32:535.
4. Varras M, Tsikini A, Polyzos D, et al. Uterine adnexal torsion: pathologic and grayscale ultrasonographic findings. Clin Exp Obstet Gynecol. 2004;31:34.
5. Houry D, Abbott JT. Ovarian torsion: a fifteen year review. Ann Emerg Med. 2001;38:156.
6. White M, Stella J. Ovarian torsion: 10 year perspective. Emerg Med Australas. 2005;17:231.
7. Oltmann SC, Fischer A, Barber R, et al. Cannot exclude torsion a - 15year review. J Pediatr Surg. 2009;44:1212.
8. Tsafrir Z, Hasson J, Levin I, et al. Adnexal torsion: cystectomy and ovarian fixation are equally important in preventing recurrence. Eur J Obstet Gynecol Reprod Biol. 2012;162:203.
9. Kokoska ER, Keller MS, Weber TR. Acute ovarian torsion in children. Am J Surg. 2000;180:462.
10. Rousseau V, Massicot R, Darwish AA, et al. Emergency management and conservative surgery of ovarian torsion in children: a report of 40 cases. J Pediatr Adolesc Gynecol. 2008;21:201.
11. Anthony EY, Caserta MP, Singh J, Chen MY. Adnexal masses in female pediatric patients. AJR Am J Roentgenol. 2012;198:W426.
12. Wilkinson C, Sanderson A. Adnexal torsion a multimodality imaging review. Clin Radiol. 2012;67:476.
13. Valsky DV, EshBroder E, Cohen SM, et al. Added value of the grayscale whirlpool sign in the diagnosis of adnexal torsion. Ultrasound Obstet Gynecol. 2010;36:630.
14. Vijayaraghavan SB, Senthil S. Isolated torsion of the fallopian tube: the sonographic whirlpool sign. J Ultrasound Med. 2009;28:657.
15. Albayram F, Hamper UM. Ovarian and adnexal torsion: spectrum of sonographic findings with pathologic correlation. J Ultrasound Med. 2001;20:1083.
16. BenAmi M, Perlitz Y, Haddad S. The effectiveness of spectral and color Doppler in predicting ovarian torsion. A prospective study. Eur J Obstet Gynecol Reprod Biol. 2002;104:64.
17. Lee EJ, Kwon HC, Joo HJ, et al. Diagnosis of ovarian torsion with color Doppler sonography: depiction of twisted vascular pedicle. J Ultrasound Med. 1998;17:83.
18. Taskin O, Birincioglu M, Aydin A, et al. The effects of twisted ischaemic adnexa managed by detorsion on ovarian viability and histology: an ischaemic are perfusion rodent model. Hum Reprod. 1998;13:2823.
19. Jones HW, Jones GS. Novak textbook of gynecology. 10th ed. Baltimore: Wolters Kluwer Lippincott Williams & Wilkins; 1981. p. 471.
20. Mathevet P, Nessah K, Dargent D, Mellier G. Laparoscopic management of adnexal masses in pregnancy: a case series. Eur J Obstet Gynecol Reprod Biol. 2003;108:217.
21. Bottomley C, Bourne T. Diagnosis and management of ovarian cyst accidents. Best Pract Res Clin Obstet Gynaecol. 2009;23:711.
22. Kim JH, Lee SM, Lee JH, et al. Successful conservative management of ruptured ovarian cysts with hemoperitoneum in healthy women. PLoS One. 2014;9:e91171.
23. Teng SW, Tseng JY, Chang CK, et al. Comparison of laparoscopy and laparotomy in managing hemodynamically stable patients with ruptured corpus luteum with hemoperitoneum. J Am Assoc Gynecol Laparosc. 2003;10:474.
24. Reif P, Schöll W, Klaritsch P, Lang U. Rupture of endometriotic ovarian cyst causes acute hemoperitoneum in twin pregnancy. Fertil Steril. 2011;95:2125.e1.
25. Viswanathan M, Hartmann K, McKoy N, Stuart G, Rankins N, Thieda P, Lux LJ, Lohr KN. Management of uterine fibroids: an update of the evidence. Evid Rep Technol Assess (Full Rep). 2007;(154):1–122.
26. Evans P, Brunsell S. Uterine fibroid tumors: diagnosis and treatment. Am Fam Physician. 2007;75(10):1503–8.
27. Vollenhoven B. Introduction: the epidemiology of uterine leiomyomas. Baillieres Clin Obstet Gynaecol. 1998;12(2):169–76.
28. Greenberg MD, Kazamel TI. Medical and socioeconomic impact of uterine fibroids. Obstet Gynecol Clin North Am. 1995;22(4):625–36.
29. Tropeano G, Amoroso S, Scambia G. Non-surgical management of uterine fibroids. Hum Reprod Update. 2008;14(3):259–74.
30. Downes E, Sikirica V, Gilabert-Estelles J, Bolge SC, Dodd SL, Maroulis C, et al. The burden of uterine fibroids in five European countries. Eur J Obstet Gynecol Reprod Biol. 2010;152(1):96–102.
31. Stewart EA. Clinical practice. Uterine fibroids. N Engl J Med. 2015;372(17):1646–55.
32. Munro MG, Critchley HO, Fraser IS. The FIGO classification of causes of abnormal uterine bleeding in the reproductive years. Fertil Steril. 2011;95(7):2204–8.
33. Ouyang DW, Economy KE, Norwitz ER. Obstetric complications of fibroids. Obstet Gynecol Clin North Am. 2006;33(1):153–69.
34. Pérez-López FR, Ornat L, Ceausu I, Depypere H, Erel CT, Lambrinoudaki I, et al. EMAS position statement: management of uterine fibroids. Maturitas. 2014;79(1):106–16.
35. Wiesenfeld HC, Sweet RL, Ness RB, et al. Comparison of acute and subclinical pelvic inflammatory disease. Sex Transm Dis. 2005;32:400–5.
36. Ness RB, Kip KE, Hillier SL, et al. A cluster analysis of bacterial vaginosis-associated microflora and pelvic inflammatory disease. Am J Epidemiol. 2005;162:585–90.
37. Cohen CR, Mugo NR, Astete SG, et al. Detection of *Mycoplasma genitalium* in women with laparoscopically diagnosed acute salpingitis. Sex Transm Infect. 2005;81:463–6.
38. Haggerty CL, Totten PA, Astete SG, et al. *Mycoplasma genitalium* among women with nongonococcal, nonchlamydial pelvic inflammatory disease. Infect Dis Obstet Gynecol. 2006;2006:30184.
39. Jurstrand M, Jensen JS, Magnuson A, et al. A serological study of the role of *Mycoplasma genitalium* in pelvic inflammatory disease and ectopic pregnancy. Sex Transm Infect. 2007;83:319–23.
40. Ross J, Judlin P, Jensen J, International Union Against Sexually Transmitted Infections. 2012 European guideline for the management of pelvic inflammatory disease. Int J STD AIDS. 2014;25(1):1–7. https://doi.org/10.1177/0956462413498714.. Epub 29 Aug 2013
41. Government of Western Australia. Department of Health Benign gynaecology acute pelvic inflammatory disease. Clinical guidelines gynaecology 2015.
42. European Guideline for the Management of Pelvic Inflammatory Disease UK National Guideline for the Management of Pelvic Inflammatory Disease 2011.
43. UK National Guideline for the Management of Pelvic Inflammatory Disease 2011.
44. CDC-Center for Disease Control and Prevention. Sexually transmitted disease treatment guidelines 2015.

45. Workowski KA. Centers for Disease Control and Prevention sexually transmitted diseases treatment guidelines. Clin Infect Dis. 2015;61(Suppl 8):S759–62. https://doi.org/10.1093/cid/civ771.
46. Maleckiene L, et al. Comparison of clinical and laparoscopic diagnoses of pelvic inflammatory disease. Int J Gynaecol Obstet. 2009;104(1):74–17.
47. Ness RB, Trautmann G, Richter HE, et al. Effectiveness of treatment strategies of some women with pelvic inflammatory disease: a randomized trial. Obstet Gynecol. 2005;106(3):573–80.
48. Burney RO, Giudice LC. Pathogenesis and pathophysiology of endometriosis. Fertil Steril. 2012;98(3):511–9.
49. Jubanyik KJ, Comite F. Extrapelvic endometriosis. Obstet Gynecol Clin North Am. 1997;24(2):411–40.
50. Avraham S, Seidman DS. Surgery versus pharmacological treatment for endometriosis. Future Med. 2014;10:161–6.
51. American College of Obstetricians and Gynecologists. Practice Bulletin 114. Management of Endometriosis. Obstet Gynecol. 2010;116(1):223–36.
52. Viganò P, Parazzini F, Somigliana E, Vercellini P. Endometriosis: epidemiology and aetiological factors. Best Pract Res Clin Obstet Gynaecol. 2004;18(2):177–200.
53. Nap AW, Groothuis PG, Demir AY, Evers JLH, Dunselman GAJ. Pathogenesis of endometriosis. Best Pract Res Clin Obstet Gynaecol. 2004;18(2):233–44.
54. Signorile PG, Baldi A. Endometriosis: new concepts in the pathogenesis. Int J Biochem Cell Biol. 2010;42(6):778–80.
55. Mathur S, Peress MR, Williamson HO, et al. Autoimmunity to endometrium and ovary in endometriosis. Clin Exp Immunol. 1982;50(2):259–66.
56. Suginami H. A reappraisal of the coelomic metaplasia theory by reviewing endometriosis occurring in unusual sites and instances. Am J Obstet Gynecol. 1991;165(1):214–8.
57. Schrager S, Falleroni J, Edgoose J. Evaluation and treatment of endometriosis. Am Fam Physician. 2013;87(2):107–13.
58. Kodaman PH. Current strategies for endometriosis management. Obstet Gynecol Clin North Am. 2015;42(1):87–101.
59. Suzuki T, Izumi SI, Matsubayashi H, Awaji H, Yoshikata K, Makino T. Impact of ovarian endometrioma on oocytes and pregnancy outcome in in vitro fertilization. Fertil Steril. 2005;83(4):908–13.
60. Reeve L, Lashen H, Pacey AA. Endometriosis affects spermendosalpingeal interactions. Hum Reprod. 2005;20(2):448–51.
61. American Fertility Society. Revised American Fertility Society classification of endometriosis: 1985. Fertil Steril. 1985;43(3):351–2.
62. Allen C, Hopewell S, Prentice A, Gregory D. Nonsteroidal anti-inflammatory drugs for pain in women with endometriosis (Review). 2010;(2). www.cochranelibrary.com.
63. Jacobson T, Duffy JMN, Barlow D, Konincks PR, Garry R. Laparoscopic surgery for pelvic pain associated with endometriosis. Cochrane Libr. 2010;(11):1–21.
64. Jones KD, Sutton C. Patient satisfaction and changes in pain scores after ablative laparoscopic surgery for stage III-IV endometriosis and endometriotic cysts. Fertil Steril. 2003;79(5):1086–90.
65. Munro MG, Critchley HOD, Broder MS, Fraser IS. FIGO classification system (PALM-COEIN) for causes of abnormal uterine bleeding in nongravid women of reproductive age. Int J Gynecol Obstet. 2011;113(1):3–13.
66. Lieng M, Istre O, Sandvik L, Qvigstad E. Prevalence, 1-Year regression rate, and clinical significance of asymptomatic endometrial polyps: cross-sectional study. J Minim Invasive Gynecol. 2009;16(4):465–71.
67. Anastasiadis PG, Koutlaki NG, Skaphida PG, Galazios GC, Tsikouras PN, Liberis VA. Endometrial polyps: prevalence, detection, and malignant potential in women with abnormal uterine bleeding. Eur J Gynaecol Oncol. 2000;21(2):180–3.
68. Wamsteker K, Emanuel MH, de Kruif JH. Transcervical hysteroscopic resection of submucous fibroids for abnormal uterine bleeding: results regarding the degree of intramural extension. Obstet Gynecol. 1993;82(5):736–40.
69. Tavassoli FA, Devilee P. World Health Organization classification of tumors: pathology and genetics of tumours of the breast and female genital organs. Lyon: IARC Press; 2003.
70. Dilley A, Drews C, Lally C, Austin H, Barnhart E, Evatt B. A survey of gynecologists concerning menorrhagia: perceptions of bleeding disorders as a possible cause. J Womens Health Gend Based Med. 2002;11(1):39–44.
71. Byams VR, Anderson BL, Grant AM, Atrash H, Schulkin J. Evaluation of bleeding disorders in women with menorrhagia: a survey of obstetrician-gynecologists. Am J Obstet Gynecol. 2012;207(4):269.e1–5.
72. Gleeson NC. Cyclic changes in endometrial tissue plasminogen activator and plasminogen activator inhibitor type 1 in women with normal menstruation and essential menorrhagia. Am J Obstet Gynecol. 1994;171(1):178–83.
73. Smith SK, Abel MH, Kelly RW, Baird DT. Prostaglandin synthesis in the endometrium of women with ovular dysfunctional uterine bleeding. Br J Obstet Gynaecol. 1981;88(4):434–42.
74. Smith SK, Abel MH, Kelly RW, Baird DT. A role for prostacyclin (PGi2) in excessive menstrual bleeding. Lancet (London, England). 1981;1(8219):522–4.
75. Heatley MK. The association between clinical and pathological features in histologically identified chronic endometritis. J Obstet Gynaecol. 2004;24(7):801–3.
76. Pitsos M, Skurnick J, Heller D. Association of pathologic diagnoses with clinical findings in chronic endometritis. J Reprod Med. 2009;54(6):373–7.
77. Toth M, Patton DL, Esquenazi B, Shevchuk M, Thaler H, Divon M. Association between chlamydia trachomatis and abnormal uterine bleeding. Am J Reprod Immunol. 2007;57(5):361–6.
78. Rosenberg MJ, Waugh MS, Stevens CM. Smoking and cycle control among oral contraceptive users. Am J Obstet Gynecol. 1996;174(2):628–32.
79. Meijer WEE, Heerdink ER, Nolen WA, Herings RMC, Leufkens HGM, Egberts ACG. Association of risk of abnormal bleeding with degree of serotonin reuptake inhibition by antidepressants. Arch Intern Med. 2004;164(21):2367.
80. Marzano DA, Haefner HK. The Bartholin gland cyst: past, present, and future. J Low Genit Tract Dis. 2004;8:195.
81. Krissi H, Shmuely A, Aviram A, From A, Edward R, Peled Y. Acute Bartholin's abscess: microbial spectrum, patient characteristics, clinical manifestation, and surgical outcomes. Eur J Clin Microbiol Infect Dis. 2016;35(3):443–6.
82. Downs MC, Randall HW Jr. The ambulatory surgical management of Bartholin duct cysts. J Emerg Med. 1989;7:623–6.
83. Cobellis PL, Stradella L, De Lucia E, et al. Alcohol sclerotherapy: a new method for Bartholin gland cyst treatment. Minerva Ginecol. 2006;58:245–8.
84. Kafali H, Yurtseven S, Ozardali I. Aspiration and alcohol sclerotherapy: a novel method for management of Bartholin's cyst or abscess. Eur J Obstet Gynecol Reprod Biol. 2004;112:98–101.
85. Cheetham DR. Bartholin's cyst: marsupialization or aspiration? Am J Obstet Gynecol. 1985;152:569–70.
86. Gennis P, Li SF, Provataris J, et al. Jacobi ring catheter treatment of Bartholin's abscesses. Am J Emerg Med. 2005;23:414–5.
87. Andersen PG, Christensen S, Detlefsen GU, et al. Treatment of Bartholin's abscess. Marsupialization versus incision, curettage and suture under antibiotic cover. A randomized study with 6 months' follow up. Acta Obstet Gynecol Scand. 1992;71:59–62.
88. Penna C, Fambrini M, Fallani MG. CO2 laser treatment for Bartholin's gland cyst. Int J Gynaecol Obstet. 2002;76:79–80.
89. Benedetti Panici P, Manci N, Bellati F, et al. CO2 laser therapy of the Bartholin's gland cyst: surgical data and functional

short- and long-term results. J Minim Invasive Gynecol. 2007;14:348–51.
90. Fambrini M, Penna C, Pieralli A, et al. Carbon-dioxide laser vaporization of the Bartholin gland cyst: a retrospective analysis on 200 cases. J Minim Invasive Gynecol. 2008;15:327–31.
91. World Health Organization. Guidelines for medico-legal care of victims of sexual violence, 2003.
92. Ellsberg M, Jansen HA, Heise L, Watts CH, Garcia-Moreno C, WHO Multi-Country Study on Women's Health and Domestic Violence Against Women Study Team. Intimate partner violence and women's physical and mental health in the WHO multicountry study on women's health and domestic violence: an observational study. Lancet. 2008;371(9619):1165–72. https://doi.org/10.1016/S0140-6736(08)60522-X.
93. UK National Guidelines on the Management of Adult and Adolescent Complainants of Sexual Assault; 2011.
94. Ragusa A, Crescini C. URGENZE ED EMERGENZE IN SALA PARTO. Padova: Casa Editrice PICCIN Nuova Libreria; 2015. p. 197–211.
95. Oyelese Y, Ananth CV. Placental Abruptio. Obstet Gynecol. 2006;108(4):1005–16.
96. Yeo L, Vintzleos A. Placenta Abruptio. Philadelphia: Lippincott, Williams & Wilkins; 2004.
97. Royal College of Obstetricians and Gynaecologists. Antepartum haemorrhage. RCOG 2011. Green-top guidelines N° 63.
98. Tikkanen M. Etiology, clinical manifestations, and prediction of placental abruption. Acta Obstet Gynecol Scand. 2010;89(6):732–40.
99. Glantz C, Purnell L. Clinical utility of sonography in the diagnosis and treatment of placental abruption. J Ultrasound Med. 2002;21(8):837–40.
100. Usui R, Matsubara S, Ohkuchi A, Kuwata T, Watanabe T, Izumi A, et al. Fetal heart pattern reflecting the severity of placental abruption. Arch Gynecol Obstet. 2008;277(3):249–53.
101. Oyelese Y, Smulian JC. Placenta previa, placenta accreta and vasa previa. Obstet Gynecol. 2006;107(4):927–41.
102. Royal College of Obstetricians and Gynaecologists. Placenta praevia, placenta praevia accreta and vasa praevia: diagnosis and management. RCOG 2011. Green-top guidelines N° 27.
103. WHO recommendations for the prevention and treatment of postpartum haemorrhage. 2012. http://apps.who.int/iris/bitstream/10665/75411/1/9789241548502_eng.pdf. Last accessed 06 Jun 2017.
104. Royal College of Obstetricians and Gynaecologists (RCOG). Prevention and management of postpartum haemorrhage. Green-top Guideline N. 52. 2009. https://www.rcog.org.uk/en/guidelines-research-services/guidelines/gtg52/. Last accessed 06 Jun 2017.
105. Mousa HA, Blum J, Abou El Senoun G, Shakur H, Alfirevic Z. Treatment for primary postpartum haemorrhage. Cochrane Database Syst Rev. 2014;(2):CD003249.
106. Mukherjee S, Sabaratnam A. Post-partum haemorrhage. Obstet Gynaecol Reprod Med. 2009;19:121–16.
107. Meir JY, Natale N, Arisi E, et al. Emorragia post-partum: linee guida per la prevenzione, Diagnosi e il trattamento. Linee guida AOGOI. I libri dell'AOGOI. Cento, Ferrara: Editeam; 2009. p. 23–49
108. Abdul-Kadir R, McLintock C, Ducloy AS, et al. Evaluation and management of postpartum hemorrhage: consensus from an international expert panel. Transfusion. 2014;54(7):1756–68.
109. Pavord S, Maybury H. How I treat postpartum hemorrhage. Blood. 2015;125(18):2759–70.
110. Ducloy-Bouthors AS, Jude B, Duhamel A, et al. High-dose tranexamic acid reduces blood loss in postpartum haemorrhage. Crit Care. 2011;15(2):R117.
111. Sentilhes L, Deneux-Tharaux C. Prophylactic tranexamic acid in addition to uterotonics may prevent blood loss for vaginal and caesarean deliveries. Evid Based Med. 2016;21(3):97.
112. Butwick AJ. Postpartum hemorrhage and low fibrinogen levels: the past, present and future. Int J Obstet Anesth. 2013;22(2): 87–91.
113. Edwards P, Shakur H, Barnetson L, et al. Central and statistical data monitoring in the Clinical Randomisation of an Antifibrinolytic in Significant Haemorrhage (CRASH-2) trial. Clin Trials. 2014;11(3):336–43.
114. Lalonde A, International Federation of Gynecology and Obstetrics. Prevention and treatment of postpartum hemorrhage in low-resource settings. Int J Gynaecol Obstet. 2012;117(2):108–18.
115. AIFA. Nota informativa importante concordata con l'EMA e l'AIFA: Restrizione d'uso di HES (medicinali contenenti amido idrossietilico). 2013. http://www.agenziafarmaco.gov.it/it/content/nota-informativa-importante-sulla-restrizione-d%E2%80%99uso-di-hes-medicinali-contenenti-amido-idros. Last accessed 06 Jun 2017.
116. Charbit B, Mandelbrot L, Samain E, et al. The decrease of fibrinogen is an early predictor of the severity of postpartum hemorrhage. J Thromb Haemost. 2007;5(2):266–73.
117. Collins PW, Lilley G, Bruynseels D, et al. Fibrin-based clot formation an early and rapidly available biomarker for progression of postpartum hemorrhage: a prospective cohort study. Blood. 2014;124(11):1727–36.
118. Kozek-Langenecker SA, Afshari A, Albaladejo P, et al. Management of severe perioperative bleeding: guidelines from the European Society of Anaesthesiology. Eur J Anaesthesiol. 2013;30(6):270–382.
119. Hofmeyr GJ, Abdel-Aleem H, Abdel-Aleem MA. Uterine massage for preventing postpartum haemorrhage. Cochrane Database Syst Rev. 2013;(7):CD006431.
120. Allam MS, B-Lynch C. The B-Lynch and other uterine compression suture techniques. Int J Gynecol Obstet. 2005;89(3):236–41.
121. B-Lynch C, Coker A, Lawal AH, Abu J, Cowen MJ. The B-Lynch surgical technique for the control of massive postpartum haemorrhage: an alternative to hysterectomy? Five cases reported. Br J Obstet Gynaecol. 1997;104(3):372–5.
122. Baskett TF. Uterine compression sutures for postpartum hemorrhage: efficacy, morbidity, and subsequent pregnancy. Obstet Gynecol. 2007;110(1):68–71.
123. Price N, B-Lynch C. Technical description of the B-Lynch brace suture for treatment of massive postpartum hemorrhage and review of the published cases. Int J Fertil Womens Med. 2005;50(4):148–63.
124. Hayman RG, Arulkumaran S, Steer PJ. Uterine compression sutures: surgical management of postpartum hemorrhage. Obstet Gynecol. 2002;99(3):502–6.
125. Ghezzi F, Cromi A, Uccella S, Raio L, Bolis P, Surbek D. The Hayman technique: a simple method to treat postpartum haemorrhage. BJOG. 2007;114(3):362–5.
126. Joshi VM, Otiv SR, Majumder R, Nikam YA, Shirivastava M. Internal iliac artery ligation for arresting postpartum haemorrhage. BJOG. 2007;114(3):356–61.
127. Lethaby A, Mukhopadhyay A, Naik R. Total versus subtotal hysterectomy for benign gynaecological conditions. Cochrane Database Syst Rev. 2012;(4):CD004993.
128. Grady K, Howell C, Cox C. Uterine inversion - chapter23. In: The MOET coursemanual: managing obstetric emergencies and trauma. 2nd ed. London: RCOG Press; 2007.
129. Loeffler F. Postpartum haemorrhge and abnormalities of the third stage of labour. In: Chamberlain G, editor. Turnbull's obstetrics. 2nd ed. Edinburgh: Churchill Livingstone; 1995. p. 729–34.
130. O'Sullivan J. Acute inversion of the uterus. Br Med J. 1945;2: 282–3.

131. Ragusa A, Crescini C, et al. Uterine inversion- Chapter 11. In: Manuale di urgenze ed emergenze in sala parto. 2nd ed. Padova: Piccin Press; 2016.
132. Shah-Hosseini R, Evrard JR. Puerperal uterine inversion. Obstet Gynecol. 1989;73(4):567–70.
133. Watson P, Besch N, Bowes WA Jr. Management of acute and subacute puerperal inversion of the uterus. Obstet Gynecol. 1980;55(1):12–6.
134. Soleymani Majd H, Pilsniak A, Reginald PW. Recurrent uterine inversion: a novel treatment approach using SOS Bakri balloon. BJOG. 2009;116(7):999–1001.
135. Huntington JL, Irving FC, Kellog FS. Abdominal reposition in acute inversion of the puerperal uterus. Am J Obstet Gynecol. 1928;15:34–40.
136. Boyle JJ, Katz VL. Umbilical cord prolapse in current obstetric practice. J Reprod Med. 2005;50(5):303–6.
137. Draycott T, Winter C, Crofts J, et al., editors. Module 8. Cord prolapse in: PROMPT: practical obstetric multi professional training course manual. London: RCOG Press; 2008. p. 117–24.
138. Goswami K. Umbilical cord prolapse. In: Grady K, Howell C, Cox C, editors. Managing obstetric emergencies and trauma. The MOET course manual. 2nd ed. London: RCOG Press; 2007. p. 233–7.
139. Koonings PP, Paul RH, Campbell K. Umbilical cord prolapse. A contemporary look. J Reprod Med. 1990;35(7):690–2.
140. Panter KR, Hannah ME. Umbilical cord prolapse: so far so good? Lancet. 1996;347(8994):74. Royal College of Obstetricians and Gynaecologists. Umbilical cord prolapse. Green-top Guideline No.50; April 2008.
141. Siassakos D, Crofts JF, Winter C, Weiner CP, Draycott TJ. The active components of effective training in obstetric emergencies. BJOG. 2009;116(8):1028–32.
142. Usta IM, Mercer BM, Sibai BM. Current obstetrical practice and umbilical cord prolapse. Am J Perinatol. 1999;16(9): 479–84.
143. Murphy DJ, MacKenzie IZ. The mortality and morbidity associated with umbilical cord prolapse. Br J Obstet Gynaecol. 1995;102(10):826–30.
144. Lin MG. Umbilical cord prolapse. Obstet Gynecol Surv. 2006;61(4):269–77.
145. Katz Z, Shoham Z, Lancet M, Blickstein I, Mogilner BM, Zalel Y. Management of labor with umbilical cord prolapse: a 5-year study. Obstet Gynecol. 1988;72(2):278–81.
146. Crofts JF, Ellis D, Draycott TJ, Winter C, Hunt LP, Akande VA. Change in knowledge of midwives and obstetricians following obstetric emergency training: a randomized controlled trial of local hospital, simulation centre and teamwork training. BJOG. 2007;114(12):1534–41.
147. Siassakos D, Fox R, Draycott TJ. Umbilical cord prolapse [Green-top guideline no. 50]. London: RCOG Press; 2008.
148. Siassakos D, Hasafa Z, Sibanda T, Fox R, Donald F, Winter C, et al. Retrospective cohort study of diagnosis-delivery interval with umbilical cord prolapse: the effect of team training. BJOG. 2009;116(8):1089–96.
149. Khandelwal A, Fasih N, Kielar A. Imaging of acute abdomen in pregnancy. Radiol Clin North Am. 2013;51:1005–22.
150. Germain A, Brunaud L. Visceral surgery and pregnancy. J Visc Surg. 2010;147:e129–35.
151. Gilo NB, Amini D, Landy HJ. Appendicitis and cholecystitis in pregnancy. Clin Obstet Gynecol. 2009;52:586–96.
152. ACOG Committee on Obstetric Practice. ACOG Committee Opinion No. 474: Non obstetric surgery during pregnancy. Obstet Gynecol. 2011;117:420–1.
153. Evans SR, Sarani B, Bhanot P, Feldman E. Surgery in pregnancy. Curr Probl Surg. 2012;49:333–88.
154. Knab LM, Boller AM, Mahvi DM. Cholecystitis. Surg Clin North Am. 2014;94:455–70.
155. Kuhlmann RS, Cruikshank DP. Maternal trauma during pregnancy. Clin Obstet Gynecol. 1994;37(2):274–93.
156. Petrone P, Talving P, Browder T, Teixeira PG, Fisher O, Lozornio A, et al. Abdominal injuries in pregnancy: a 155-month study at two level 1 trauma centers. Injury. 2011;42(1):47–9.
157. Vikram K, Parul G, Ranjana K, Umamaheshwar K. Trauma in pregnancy - a review. Adv Res Gastroenterol Hepatol. 2016;2(1):555580.
158. Suresh MS, Wali A. Failed intubation in obstetrics: airway management strategies. Anesthesiol Clin North Am. 1998;16:477–98.
159. Ramsay G, Paglia M, Bourjeily G. When the heart stops: a review of cardiac arrest in pregnancy. J Intensive Care Med. 2013;28(4):204–14.
160. Lockey DJ, Crewdson K, Lossius HM. Pre-hospital anaesthesia: the same but different. Br J Anaesth. 2014;113(2):211–9.
161. Pearlman M, Faro S. Obstetric septic shock: a pathophysiologic basis for management. Clin Obstet Gynecol. 1990;33(3):482–92.
162. American College of Surgeons Committee: on Trauma. Trauma in women. In: Advanced trauma life support for doctors: student course manual. 9th ed. Chicago, Surgeons. 2012;9:259–68.
163. Epstein FB. Acute abdominal pain in pregnancy. Emerg Med Clin North Am. 1994;12(1):151–65.
164. Puri A, Khadem P, Ahmed S, Yadav P, Al-Dulaimy K. Imaging of trauma in a pregnant patient. Semin Ultrasound CT MR. 2012;33(1):37–45.
165. Donnelly EH, Smith JM, Farfán EB, Ozcan I. Prenatal radiation exposure: background material for counseling pregnant patients following exposure to radiation. Disaster Med Public Health Prep. 2011;5(1):62–8.
166. De Santis M, Di Gianantonio E, Straface G, Cavaliere AF, Caruso A, Schiavon F, et al. Ionizing radiations in pregnancy and teratogenesis: a review of literature. Reprod Toxicol. 2005;20(3):323–9.
167. Patel SJ, Reede DL, Katz DS, Subramaniam R, Amorosa JK. Imaging the pregnant patient for nonobstetric conditions: algorithms and radiation dose considerations. Radiographics. 2007;27(6):1705–22.
168. Ray JG, Schull MJ, Urquia ML, You JJ, Guttmann A, Vermeulen MJ, Franco EL, Academic Editor. Major radiodiagnostic imaging in pregnancy and the risk of childhood malignancy: a population-based cohort study in Ontario. PLoS Med. 2010;7(9):e1000337. Published online 7 Sept 2010. https://doi.org/10.1371/journal.pmed.1000337.
169. Sagiv R, Debby A, Feit H, Cohen-Sacher B, Keidar R, Golan A. The optimal cutoff serum level of human chorionic gonadotropin for efficacy of methotrexate treatment in women with extrauterine pregnancy. Int J Gynaecol Obstet. 2012;116(2):101–4.
170. Abe T, Akira S, Negishi Y, Ichikawa M, Nakai A, Takeshita T. Relevance of declines in serum human chorionic gonadotropin levels to the management of persistent ectopic pregnancy. J Obstet Gynaecol Res. 2009;35(5):961–6.
171. Hajenius PJ, Mol F, Mol BW, Bossuyt PM, Ankum WM, van der Veen F. Interventions for tubal ectopic pregnancy. Cochrane Database Syst Rev. 2007.
172. Diagnosis and management of ectopic pregnancy. Green-top guideline no. 21. 2016;123(13):e15–55. https://doi.org/10.1111/1471-0528.14189. First published: 3 Nov 2016.
173. Choudhary N, Saha SC, Gopalan S. Abortion procedures in a tertiary care institution in India. Int J Gynaecol Obstet. 2005;91: 81–6.
174. Steinauer JE, Diedrich JT, Wilson MW, Darney PD, Vargas JE, Drey EA. Uterine artery embolization in postabortion hemorrhage. Obstet Gynecol. 2008;111:881–9.
175. O'Connell K, Jones H, Simon M, Saporta V, Paul M, Lichtenberg E. First-trimester surgical abortion practices: a survey of National Abortion Federation members. Contraception. 2009;79:385–92.

176. O'Connell K, Jones HE, Lichtenberg ES, Paul M. Second-trimester surgical abortion practices: a survey of National Abortion Federation members. Contraception. 2008;78:492–9.
177. Tang O, Schweer H, Seyberth H, Lee S, Ho P. Pharmacokinetics of different routes of administration of misoprostol. Hum Reprod. 2002;17:332–6.
178. Meckstroth K, Whitaker A, Bertisch S, Goldberg A, Darney P. Misoprostol administered by epithelial routes: drug absorption and uterine response. Obstet Gynecol. 2006;108:582–90.
179. Frick AC, Drey EA, Diedrich JT, Steinauer JE. Effect of prior cesarean delivery on risk of second-trimester surgical abortion complications. Obstet Gynecol. 2010;115:760.
180. Olamijulo J, Doufekas K. Intrauterine balloon tamponade for uncontrollable bleeding during first trimester surgical termination of pregnancy. J Obstet Gynaecol. 2007;27:440–1.

34 Acute Aortic Syndrome

Antonino M. Grande, Alessandro Mazzola, Stefano Pirrelli, Adele Valentini, and Eloisa Arbustini

34.1 Introduction

Acute aortic syndrome (AAS) is an expression, formulated by Vilacosta [1, 2] in 1993, which includes various aortic pathologies (Table 34.1) representing surgical or medical emergencies in which the dominant symptom is the "aortic pain." Such pain occurs suddenly and is described as tearing, ripping, and pulsating, sometimes migrating [3].

The syndrome comprises several pathological entities that are closely related and all if not diagnosed and managed in due time are life-threatening: penetrating aortic ulcer (PAU), intramural hematoma (HMI), acute aortic dissection (AAD), pseudoaneurysm formation, retrograde aortic type A dissection postinvasive endovascular procedures (RTAD), and aortic rupture. We should consider that the common denominator of all these conditions is the disruption of the aortic media layer. The main histological features are described in Table 34.2.

Table 34.1 Acute aortic syndrome: emergency situations involving thoracic aorta

- Penetrating aortic ulceration
- Intramural hematoma
- Aortic dissection
- Pseudoaneurysm
- Retrograde aortic type A dissection postinvasive endovascular procedures
- Blunt trauma (acute aortic rupture)

Table 34.2 Definitions

- Penetrating atherosclerotic ulcer is described as an ulcerating atherosclerotic lesion in the intima that penetrates the elastic lamina and can result in the formation of intramural hematoma within the media of the aortic wall
- An intramural hematoma can take place without the trigger tear in the intima and can cause aortic dissection. It is supposed that a hematoma formation can result from rupture of an atherosclerotic plaque and/or spontaneous rupture of vasa vasorum
- Aortic dissection is defined as a separation of the layers within the aortic wall
- Pseudoaneurysm is an aortic wall disruption from where blood leaks through but is contained by the adventitia or surrounding perivascular soft tissue

A. M. Grande (✉)
Department of Cardiac Surgery, IRCCS Fondazione Policlinico San Matteo, Pavia, Italy
e-mail: amgrande@libero.it

A. Mazzola
Cardiac Surgery, IRCCS Multimedica Sesto S. Giovanni, Milano, Italy
e-mail: sandromaz@tin.it

S. Pirrelli
Unit of Vascular Surgery, CardioThoracoVascular Department, Ospedale Carlo Poma, Mantova, Italy
e-mail: stefano.pirrelli@asst-mantova.it

A. Valentini
Radiology IRCCS Fondazione Policlinico San Matteo, Pavia, Italy
e-mail: a.valentini@smatteo.pv.it

E. Arbustini
Center for Inherited Cardiovascular Diseases, IRCCS Fondazione Policlinico San Matteo, Pavia, Italy
e-mail: e.arbustini@smatteo.pv.it

P. Aseni et al. (eds.), *Operative Techniques and Recent Advances in Acute Care and Emergency Surgery*,
https://doi.org/10.1007/978-3-319-95114-0_34

Key Points

- Non-contrast chest CT is very important for the diagnosis of intramural hematoma.
- In patients with chest pain and ST-segment elevation, the diagnosis of aortic dissection should always be kept in mind before administering thrombolytic drugs and considering the possibility of the involvement of the right coronary artery in the dissection.
- To reduce the incidence of malperfusion and brain embolic risk, alternative cannulation sites such as right/left axillary artery and innominate artery have been employed and preferred to the femoral artery. These central cannulation sites share in common the avoidance of retrograde perfusion of the thoracoabdominal aorta when femoral artery cannulation is performed.
- Consider the possibility of malperfusion during each step of the operation, monitor the cerebral and visceral perfusion and promptly adapt the strategies of the cardiopulmonary bypass and surgical technique to avoid ischemic damage to the organs. Malperfusion should be suspected when it is difficult to keep a normal flow and high resistance is found in the arterial line with concomitant low systemic arterial blood pressure measured on the left radial and femoral lines. At the same time INVOS (Near-infrared spectroscopy INVOS; Somanetics, Troy, MI) may show cerebral oxygen desaturation (value <50% from baseline).
- Inspection of the transverse aortic arch is of utmost importance to identify potential intimal entry and reentry tears.
- We recommend an open distal anastomosis without cross-clamping the aorta during cooling and resection of all tears in the ascending aorta and in the arch.
- Clamping the aorta can induce false lumen pressurization leading to propagation of the dissection and malperfusion; clamp itself can cause additional aortic lesions.
- Hemiarch replacement or a total arch replacement? If the entry tear is located in the ascending aorta or the concavity of the aortic arch, a hemiarch replacement offers a safe therapeutic option, especially for the elderly or unstable patient. Entry tears near the origin of the supra-aortic branches suggest a total arch replacement and reimplantation of the arch vessels.

34.2 Penetrating Atherosclerotic Ulcer and Intramural Hematoma

Penetrating atherosclerotic ulcer (PAU) and intramural hematoma (IMH) represent pathologic variations of aortic dissection but are distinct in their presentation, natural history, and prognosis [4].

Pathological mechanism from atherosclerotic lesion implicates the aortic intimal layer ulceration and penetration of the internal elastic lamina of the aortic wall. Aortic layer separation develops IMH and eventually aortic dissection. An IMH can take place without the trigger tear in the intima and can cause aortic dissection (Fig. 34.1). It is supposed that a hematoma formation can result from rupture of an atherosclerotic plaque and/or spontaneous rupture of vasa vasorum [5].

IMH was described by Krukemberg [6] in 1920 as "Dissection without intimal tear"; later in 1985, Yamada [7] suggested the definition of "Aortic dissection without intimal rupture" and unlike the classic dissection there is an intact intima that precludes flow communication [8].

PAU presents a definite hallmark (Figs. 34.2 and 34.3), absence of an intimal flap, and it is often associated with an intramural hematoma (IMH). Furthermore, the same mechanism may produce saccular and fusiform aneurysms and also embolization (Figs. 34.4 and 34.5).

The IMH formation may broaden along the media determining either "double-barreled" or "thrombosed" aortic dissection (see intraoperative images Figs. 34.6 and 34.7). Double-barreled aortic dissection presents a clear communication between the true and false lumens; on the other side, thrombosed aortic dissection shows no opacification of the false lumen at angio-computed tomography (angio-CT) [9].

PAU is most often visualized in older male patients with systemic hypertension (up to 92%), smoking (up to 77%), coronary artery disease (up to 46%), and chronic obstructive pulmonary disease (24–68%). PAU is responsible for about 7.5% (range 2.3–11%) of all cases of acute aortic syndrome, and in ~50% (range 42–61%) of cases, there are concurrent aortic aneurysms [3].

Due to the aging of the population and the increasingly widespread use of computed tomography (CT) and magnetic resonance imaging (MRI), PAU and IMH without an intimal tear are ever more frequently diagnosed especially in older patients who are evaluated for cardiac surgery. Moderate or severe arteriosclerosis of the ascending aorta and aortic arch is present in approximately 15–20% of those older than 50 years and 33% of those 80 years of age or older [10].

The symptoms of PAU are the same as in aortic syndrome, precisely acute intense chest pain, described as tearing, ripping, migrating, or pulsating. Anyway, in certain

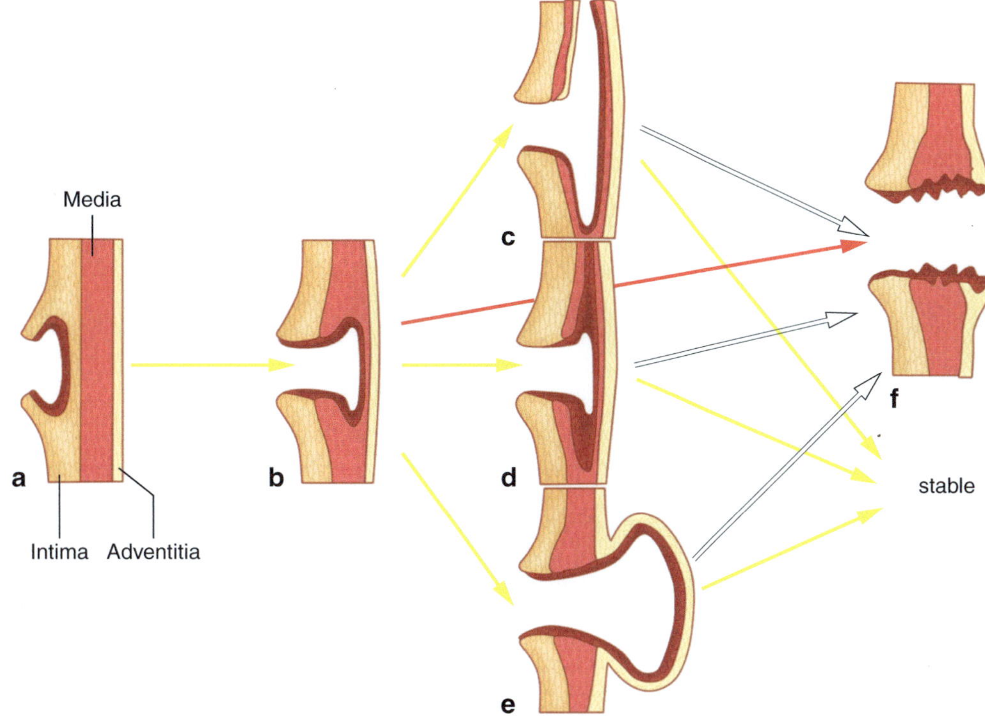

Fig. 34.1 Atheromatous ulcer development and its course. The ulcer occurs in patients with advanced atherosclerosis, and most cases are asymptomatic and confined to the intimal layer (**a**). *Penetrating atherosclerotic ulcer* (PAU) is defined as a deep atheromatous ulcer that penetrates the elastic lamina and the media layers (**b**). PAU can lead to aortic dissection (**c**, **d**), aortic aneurysm (**e**), or rupture (**f**)

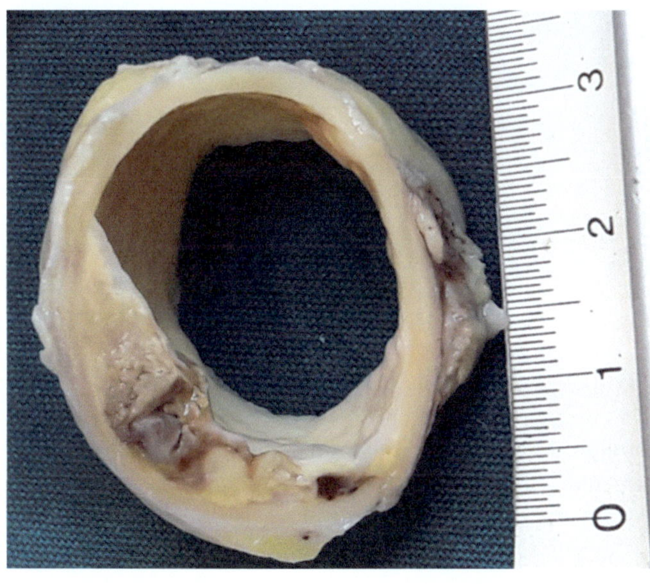

Fig. 34.2 PAU: surgical sample of the ascending aorta in a 71-year-old man who made CT scan to determine cancer staging; PAU was an incidental finding. The large atherosclerotic plaque appeared complicated by a deep ulceration and intraplaque hemorrhage (Reprinted from Grande AM, et al. Penetrating atherosclerotic ulcer of the ascending aorta; Tex Heart Inst J 2018; in press, permission from Tex Heart Inst J)

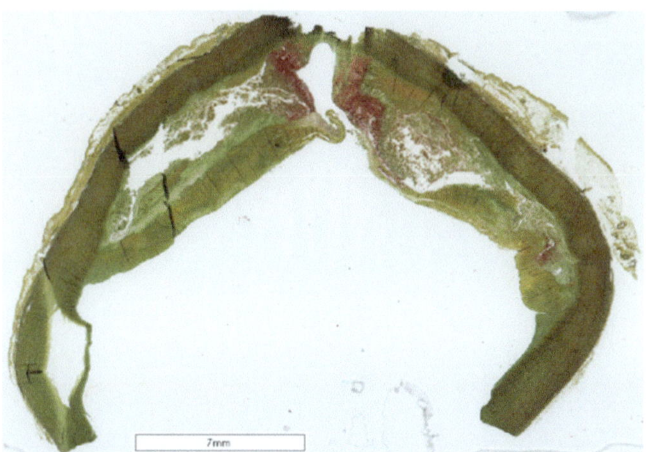

Fig. 34.3 Same case: the figure shows the pathology sample of the aorta. The severe atherosclerotic plaque is complicated by a deep ulceration, which corresponds to the angio-computed tomography imaging (panel X). Movat pentachrome stain (Reprinted from Grande AM, et al. Penetrating atherosclerotic ulcer of the ascending aorta; Tex Heart Inst J 2018; in press, permission from Tex Heart Inst J)

cases, patients can be asymptomatic, and the diagnosis is incidental.

PAU with concomitant IMH localized in the ascending aorta is considered as surgical emergency for the elevated risk of rupture and cardiac tamponade; acute IMH in ascending aorta is treated surgically after diagnosis [11–13]; treatment of PAU and IMH localized in the descending aorta is not always well defined [14].

34.2.1 Diagnosis

In the past angiography was considered the gold standard diagnostic test for aortic lesions, now CT and magnetic resonance imaging (MRI) are considered the most common and precise diagnostic imaging procedures. Non-contrast chest CT is very important for diagnosis because images may show a more hyperdense intramural hematoma than the hypodense lumen area (Fig. 34.8a, b); angio-CT reveals a characteristic smooth circumferential hemathoma appearance. IMH is differentiated from dissection by the lack of an intimal flap.

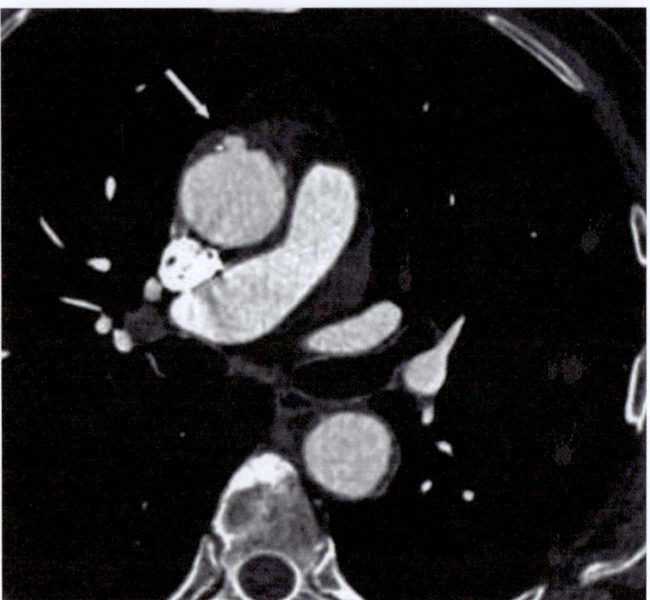

Fig. 34.4 Same case: in CT scan the white arrow indicates PAU that was an incidental finding; the patient had severe atherosclerotic disease involving carotid and coronary arteries (Reprinted from Grande AM, et al. Penetrating atherosclerotic ulcer of the ascending aorta; Tex Heart Inst J 2018; in press, permission from Tex Heart Inst J)

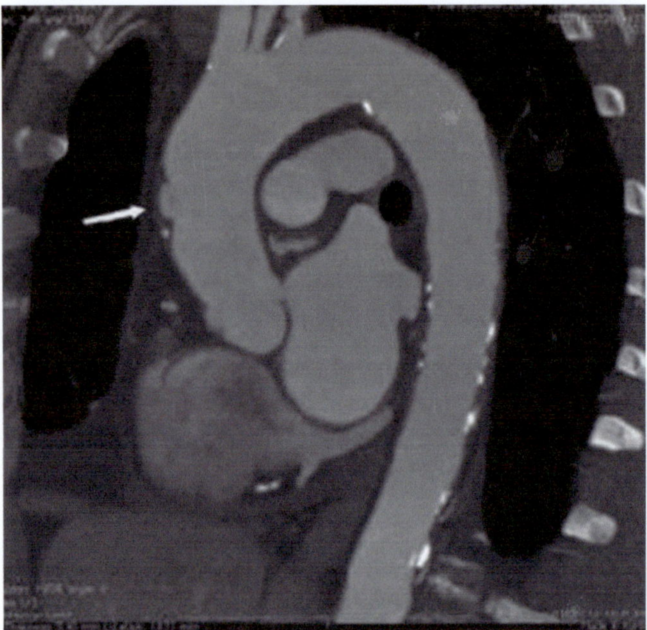

Fig. 34.5 Same case: CT scan, lateral view, the white arrow indicates PAU located in the anterior aspect of ascending aorta. The patient underwent ascending aorta replacement (Reprinted from Grande AM, et al. Penetrating atherosclerotic ulcer of the ascending aorta; Tex Heart J 2018; in press, permission from Tex Heart Inst J)

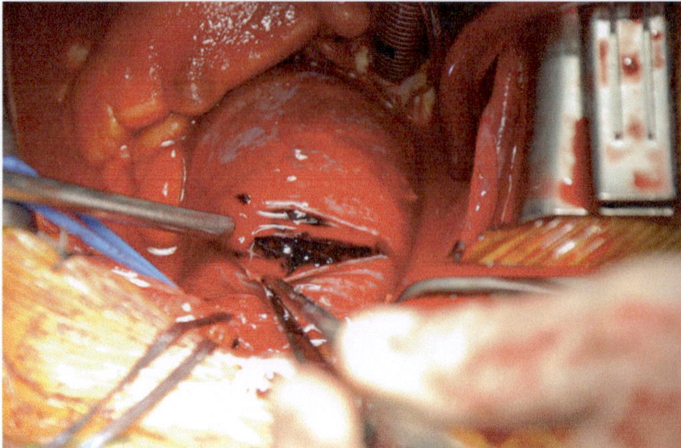

Fig. 34.6 Transverse aortotomy is made in ascending aorta: note the intramural hematoma

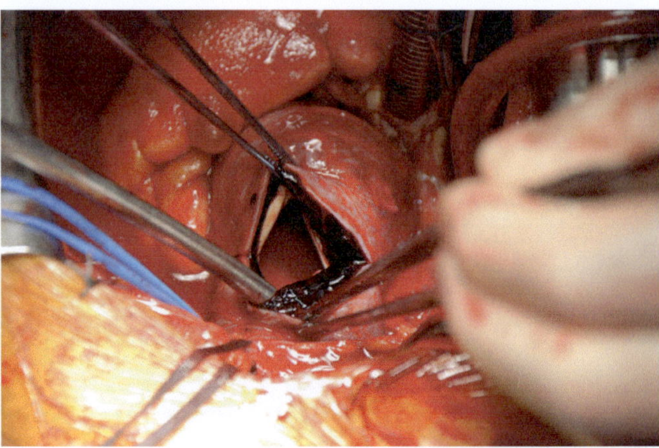

Fig. 34.7 The ascending aortic wall was completely incised, and a "double-barreled" aorta is evident

34.3 Acute Aortic Dissection

Definition. Acute aortic dissection (AAD) is characterized by a sudden development of an intimal tear where the blood flow penetrates into the thickness of the tunica media dissecting the inner from outer layers producing a false lumen. This mechanism eventually produces an aortic wall rupture through the adventitia or by a reentering into the true aortic lumen through another tear. The dissection usually proceeds distally even if a retrograde diffusion is possible.

Various classifications have been proposed, based mainly on the extension of the dissection and/or on the location of the intimal tear, but the DeBakey and Stanford classifications are the two most widely used ways of illustrating the types of aortic dissection.

34.3.1 Classification of Aortic Dissection (Fig. 34.9)

34.3.1.1 DeBakey Classification

- Type I. Intimal tear usually originates in the proximal ascending aorta, and dissection involves ascending aorta, arch, and variable lengths of descending thoracic and abdominal aorta.

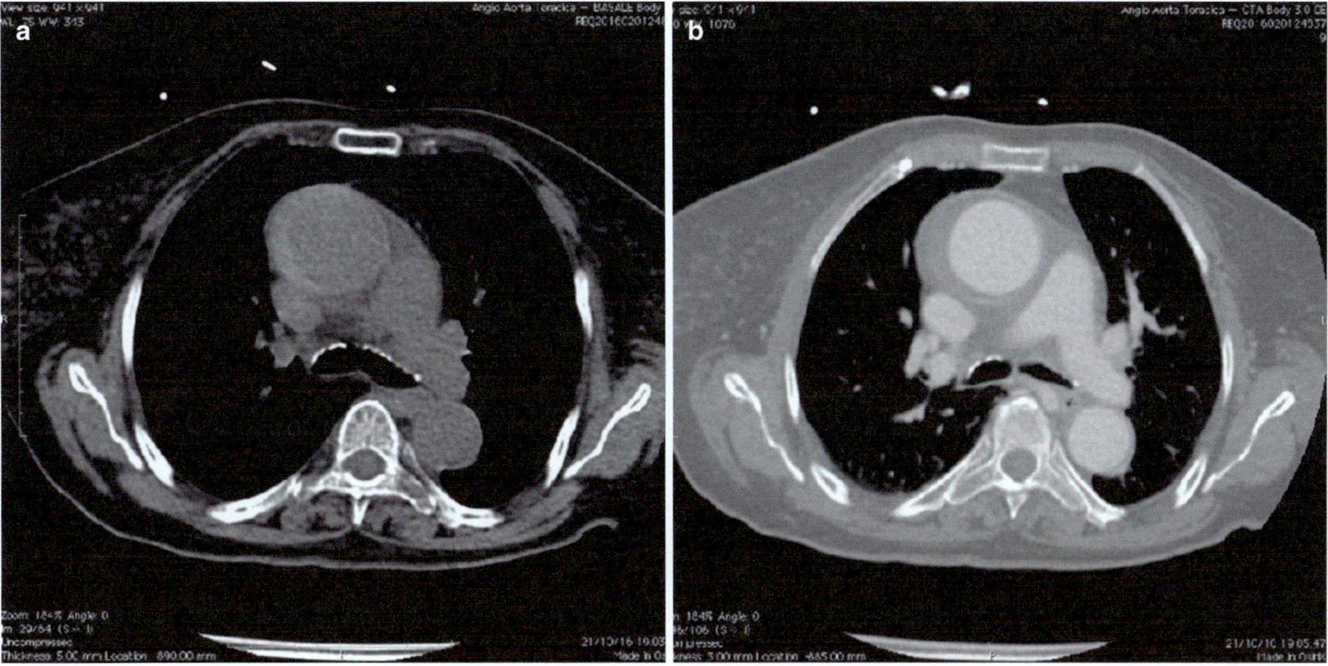

Fig. 34.8 (**a**) Unenhanced CT shows a more hyperdense intramural hematoma than the hypodense lumen area in the ascending aorta. (**b**) Angio-CT

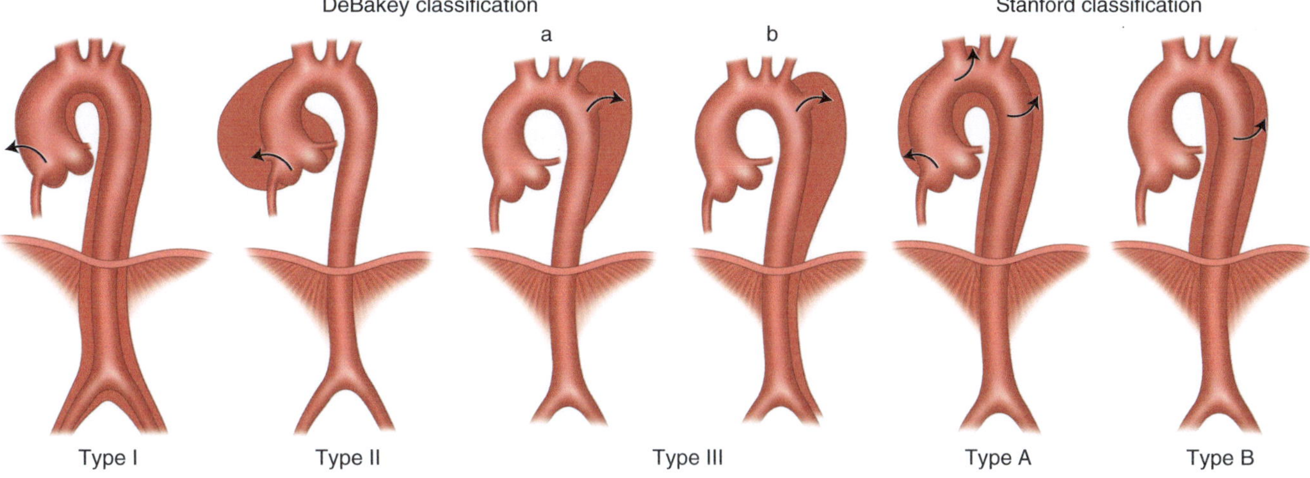

Fig. 34.9 DeBakey and Stanford classification of aortic dissection

- Type II. Dissection is confined to ascending aorta.
- Type III. Dissection may be confined to descending thoracic aorta (type IIIa) or may extend into the abdominal aorta and iliac arteries (type IIIb). Dissection may also extend proximally to involve the arch and the ascending aorta.

34.3.1.2 Stanford Classification

- Type A. All cases in which ascending aorta is involved by dissection, with or without involvement of the arch and descending thoracic aorta.
- Type B. Cases in which only descending thoracic aorta is involved; however, occasionally, dissections originating in the descending thoracic aorta extend proximally (retrograde) to include the aortic arch but not the ascending aorta, and others originating in the aortic arch remain localized or extend distally (antegrade) without involving the ascending aorta.

The Stanford classification considers the extent of dissection, rather than the location of the entry tear [15]; type A indicates involvement of the ascending aorta, with or without involvement of the arch or the descending aorta, regardless of the site of the primary intimal tear, and type B represents all others, or dissections that do not involve the ascending aorta [16].

Furthermore, roughly two-thirds of patients present type A AAD the remainder has type B AAD.

34.3.2 Epidemiology

Incidence of AAD is estimated 6 per hundred thousand per year [17]; it is more frequent in men compared to women [18]. The most common risk factor for AD is systemic hypertension [15]; in the IRAD registry [19], mean age is 63; other well-known risk factors are Marfan, Loeys-Dietz, Turner, Noonan, and Ehlers-Danlos syndromes, cystic medial necrosis, bicuspid aortic valve, aortic coarctation, pregnancy, and previous cardiac surgery [16].

34.3.3 Clinical Presentation

AAD may show several symptoms, and although many of them are typical, it is not rare that the diagnosis is delayed or missed entirely for a confounding medical presentation.

The most common symptom is chest pain that is of sudden onset, severe, tearing, and knifelike. The pain is located in the anterior chest and may migrate to the back and to the abdomen following the dissection path of the AAD. Anterior chest pain is more frequent in type A AAD and type B AAD and presents more often back and abdominal pain. In type B AAD, pain often decreases once adequate blood pressure control is reached. AAD symptoms are summarized in Tables 34.3, 34.4 and 34.5.

Table 34.3 Algorithm for diagnosis and treatment for aortic dissection (AD)

CLINICAL DATE TO ASSESS PROBABILITY SCORE FOR DIAGNOSIS AORTIC DISSECTION (AD)

HISTORY	PAIN	PHYSICAL EXAMINATION
- Marfan, Ehlers-Danlos,	- Chest/back/abdominal	- Differential BP or pulses in arms
- Loves-Dietz syndromes	severe	- Cardiac murmurs / Carotid bruits
- Family history aortic disease	abrupt	- Neurologic deficit
- Aortic valve disease	tearing	- Hypertension
- Aneurysm		- Hypertension / Shock
- Previous cardiac surgery		

the involvement of the above data (from O to 3) it is associated with probability AD

ACUTE CHEST PAIN

↙ ↘

ECG: normal, non ST-segment alterations

ECG: STEM! + coronary angiography → revascularization
If score 2-3 order TTE / AngioTC

Chest X-ray: widened mediastinum → consider history and physical examination

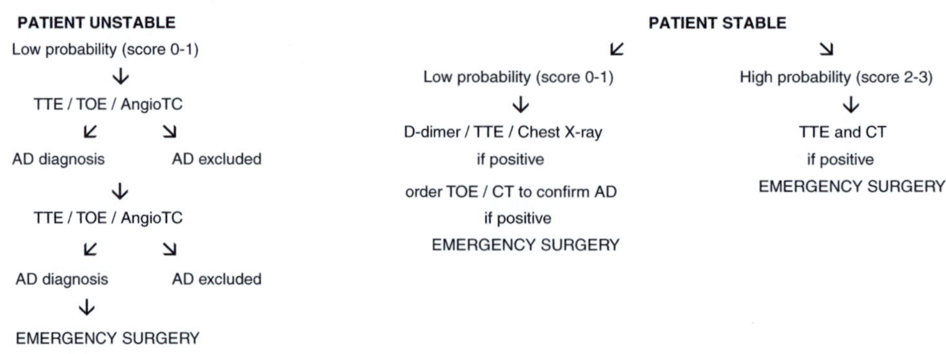

- Initiate immediately BP control therapy
- Negative chronotropic agents
- Pain control drugs (Morphine)

BP blood pressure, *CT* computed tomography, *TTE* transthoracic echocardiography, *TOE* transesophageal echocardiography

Table 34.4 Symptoms and clinical signs type A and type B aortic dissections (modified by 2014 ESC Guidelines)

Symptoms and clinical signs	AAD type A	AAD type B
Chest pain	80%	70%
Back pain	40%	70%
Abrupt onset of pain	85%	85%
Migrating pain	<15%	20%
Aortic regurgitation	40–75%	–
Cardiac tamponade	<20%	–
Myocardial ischemia or infarct	10–15%	10%
Heart failure	<10%	<5%
Pleural effusion	15%	20%
Syncope	15%	<5%
Spinal cord injury	<1%	NR
Mesenteric ischemia	<5%	NR
Acute renal failure	<20%	10%
Lower limb ischemia	<10%	<10%

Table 34.5 Main findings in physical examinations, signs, and laboratory results in aortic dissection diagnosis

Findings and signs	Laboratory results
Systemic blood pressure	Hemoglobin and hematocrit decrease
Cold and clammy skin	Blood urea nitrogen and creatinine
Differential blood pressures or pulses in arms	Troponin I and T
Differential femoral pulses	D-dimer
Neurological signs (somnolence, coma, vision problems, hemispheric neglect, weakness, peripheral paresthesias)	Creatine kinase (reperfusion injury)
Jugular venous distension (cardiac tamponade)	Aspartate transaminase, alanine aminotransferase (liver difference)
Cardiac murmurs (systolic in aortic stenosis and bicuspid valve, aortic diastolic)	Lactate (bowel ischemia)
Carotid bruits or absent carotid pulse	Blood gases
Abdominal findings: tenderness, pain distension, absent bowel sounds	
Oliguria or anuria	

34.3.4 Diagnosis

A careful history and physical examination are the core of diagnostic workup of AAD as it is shown in Table 34.3. Blood pressure (BP) is often >200 mmHg (systolic value); BP <100 mmHg in a patient with cold and clammy skin may suggest a contained aortic rupture and cardiac tamponade. Differential BP and pulses in the arms are signs suggestive of supra-aortic vessel involvement. Carotid bruit or absent carotid pulse may be present in case of neurologic symptoms. A systolic cardiac murmur may be present in case of aortic stenosis (bicuspid valve). A new diastolic murmur along the sternal border can show acute aortic regurgitation. Consider that abdominal pain may be due to splanchnic vessel involvement in AD. Differential femoral pulses and loss of sensation or motor strength in the legs may be related to iliac obstruction by the false lumen.

Electrocardiogram and chest X-ray in acute aortic syndrome are important to rule out other pathologies that present chest pain (e.g., myocardial infarction, pneumothorax, etc.) [20]. In type A dissection, chest X-ray can show a widened mediastinum, but 20–28% of dissections do not present this finding [21, 22]. For this reason, X-ray should not be utilized to diagnose aortic dissection. Cardiac troponin is often high especially in late diagnosis [23].

Transthoracic echocardiography (TTE), M-mode and two-dimensional, presents sensitivity and specificity that range 77–80% and 93–96%, respectively, when the ascending aorta is involved [24–26].

Transesophageal echocardiography (TOE). TOE allows to identify intimal flaps, both entry and re-entry tears along the ascending and descending aorta, thrombus formation in false lumen and, through color Doppler use, antegrade and retrograde flow. The sensitivity and specificity of TOE are 99% and 89% respectively [15], but consider that the results are highly operator-dependent.

The distal portion of the ascending aorta and proximal aortic arch may be inadequately visualized with TOE because of the juxtaposition of the air-filled trachea and right main bronchus, which can lead to false-negative results. Therefore, a short segment of the distal ascending aorta, just before the innominate artery, is concealed from sight (a 'blind spot'). Furthermore, images of the ascending aorta may show artifacts caused by reverberations from the posterior wall of the ascending aorta or the posterior wall of the right pulmonary artery [15]. The diagnostic precision of TOE can be meliorated making a modification which enables the visualization of the distal ascending aorta, aortic arch, and its branches through a fluid-filled balloon placed in the trachea and left main bronchus [27, 28] (Fig. 34.10). The modified technique may enable the dissection type diagnosis and the visualization of the proximal cerebral vessels; in addition, the technique detects true lumen perfusion and cannulation.

Angio-CT provides excellent images and allows to differentiate the different types of acute aortic syndromes: IMH, PAU, and AAD (Figs. 34.4, 34.5, 34.11, 34.12, 34.13, 34.14, and 34.15). Furthermore, multislice helical CT of the heart with retrospective ECG gating gives the opportunity to obtain motion-free images of the aortic root and coronary arteries. Angio-CT should not be limited to the chest but extended to the entire aorta and iliofemoral vessels in order to assess for subclinical malperfusion and to plan the surgical strategy.

Angio-CT has sensitivities of up to 100% and specificities of 98–99% [29–31]. MRI is the preeminent diagnostic test for AAD showing sensitivity and specificity of 98% [32] and allowing entry and reentry site visualization: the true lumen shows signal void, while the false lumen presents higher

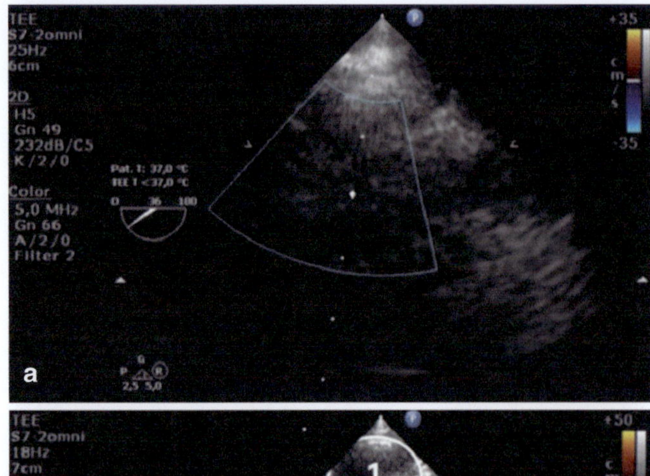

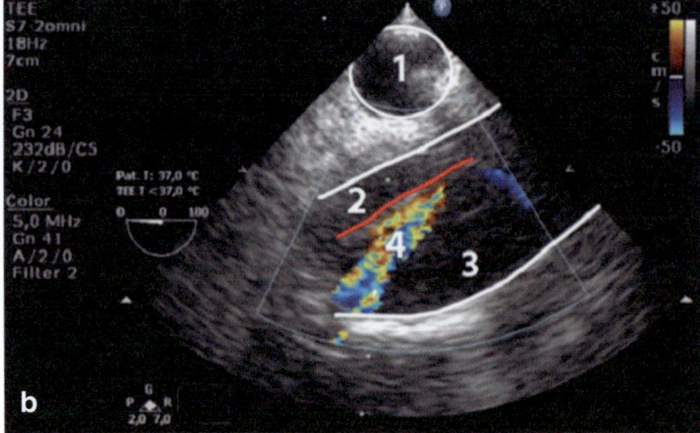

Fig. 34.10 Panel (**a**) modified TEE long- and short-axis (X-plane) view of the distal ascending aorta (DAA), showing an intimal tear. Panel (**b**) same image with color Doppler showing differential flow in the true and false lumen. *1* = trachea with inflated endotracheal balloon; *2* = true lumen; *3* = false lumen; *4* = intimal tear (published with permission by Klomp [28])

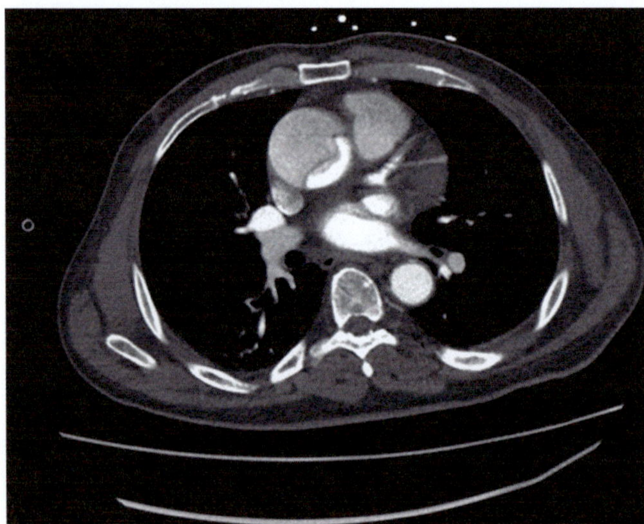

Fig. 34.11 Type A dissection in a 48-year-old male bricklayer: he was evaluated in the emergency department for the abrupt onset of chest pain at work. The dissection starts from the valvar plane, and the false lumen is anterior and lateral compressing on the true lumen

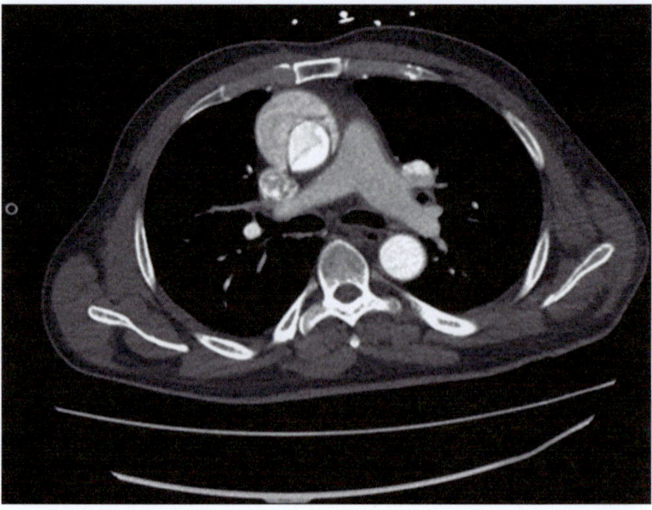

Fig. 34.12 Same case: the false lumen compressing the true lumen, level pulmonary trunk bifurcation

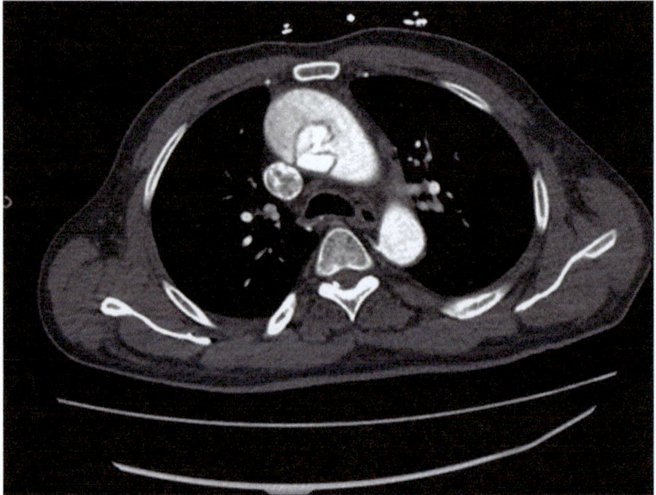

Fig. 34.13 Same case: the true lumen re-expands at the aortic arch level

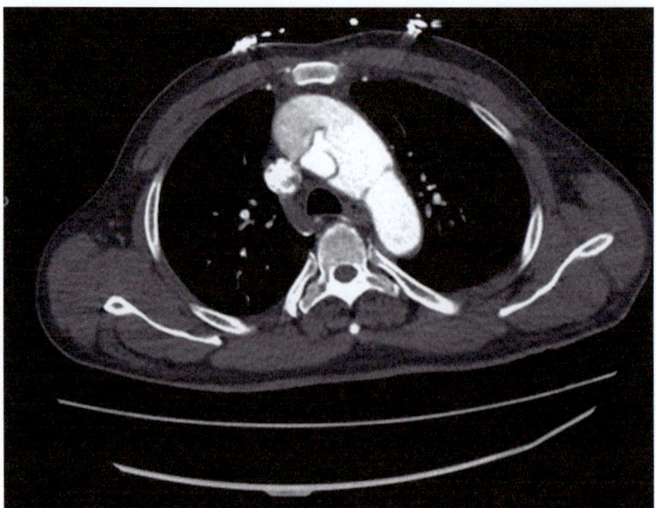

Fig. 34.14 Same case: reentry into the true lumen

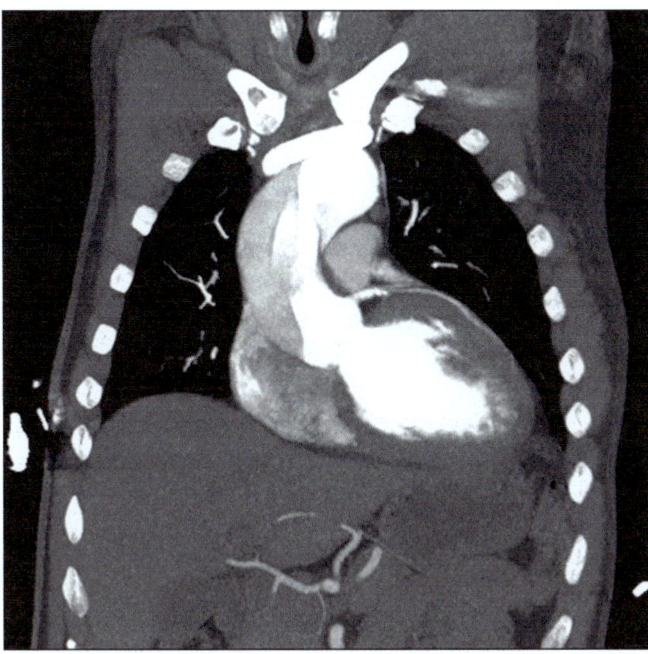

Fig. 34.15 Same case: coronal plane showing blood flow reentry into the true lumen at aortic arch level

signal intensity found in turbulent flow. Note also that in case of complete thrombosis of one lumen, dissection can be obscured and MRI can show more accurately than CT the turbulent flow inside the dissected aorta. The main limitations of MRI are long scan time and the incompatibility with ferromagnetic medical equipment that may hinder its use in many cases, especially in unstable patients.

34.3.5 Treatment

PAU, HMI, type A (or type I and II), and aortic pseudoaneurysm are among the most feared conditions encountered in the emergency department, and the surgical treatment is essentially the same.

The goals of the treatment are:

1. Eliminate the risk of rupture of the "aorta at risk": ***replace*** *the aorta at risk*; the aorta at risk is the ascending for type A dissection and the descending for type B.
2. Eliminate hypertension inside the false lumen: *depressurize the false lumen*; the distal rupture of the intimal flap creates a "reentry" that represents a natural way of depressurization of the false lumen, and generally it is accompanied by a reduction of the pain [15]. The persistence of the pain suggests hypertension of the false lumen, and when this is accompanied by visceral or peripheral ischemia, percutaneous fenestration must be considered.
3. Restore the flow in the aortic branches: antegrade perfusion reduces the risk of malperfusion [15].
4. Promote the thrombosis of the false lumen: thrombosis of the false lumen is a prerequisite for "healing" and remodeling of the aortic wall.

If pericardial tamponade is diagnosed, pericardiocentesis before surgery can be harmful because it may counteract hypotonic hemostasis and eventually cause more pericardial bleeding and intractable tamponade [33].

The surgical technique comprises utilization of cardiopulmonary bypass (CPB), deep hypothermic circulatory arrest, and anterograde cerebral perfusion. The site of arterial cannulation for CPB is still a topic of controversy. Direct central cannulation through the ascending aorta is described [34–36], and it has a theoretical advantage of not changing the natural antegrade blood flow and in doing so avoiding intraoperative malperfusion. Other arterial cannulation sites are the *axillary*, *innominate*, and *femoral* arteries. Axillary artery cannulation for type A dissection is preferred overall the femoral cannulation that establishes a retrograde perfusion presenting a significant risk of atheroembolism, malperfusion, and ischemic leg complications [37]. Venous drainage is achieved through a cannula in the right atrium or in the common femoral vein.

If a patient has evidence of shock due to cardiac tamponade, axillary artery – femoral vein circulatory assistance should be started before the chest is opened. An alternative technique is innominate or brachiocephalic artery cannulation (direct or via a graft) that provides a single-access site both for CPB and antegrade cerebral perfusion (ACP); considering these advantages, several surgeons use the innominate artery cannulation technique [38–43].

Deep hypothermic circulatory arrest and antegrade or retrograde selective cerebral perfusion are employed for cerebral protection.

Central cannulation directly through the ascending aorta. This site allows to establish an antegrade blood flow and accurate position of the tip of the cannula is obtained with epiaortic echo guidance using the Seldinger technique through the non-dissected part of the aortic wall in most cases, usually via the left side of the ascending aorta [36]. Many authors believe this technique may carry the risk of aortic rupture and a higher incidence of stroke and malperfusion [37, 44, 45].

34.3.5.1 Axillary Cannulation

Axillary artery (AA) cannulation is achieved through an 8–10 cm incision below the middle third of the clavicle or in the deltopectoral groove, pectoralis major muscle is split, and the cephalic vein is encountered where it penetrates the fascia to join the axillary vein (Figs. 34.16, 34.17, and 34.18); if necessary, the vein should be divided. Then, the clavipectoral fascia is incised, the pectoralis minor muscle is exposed,

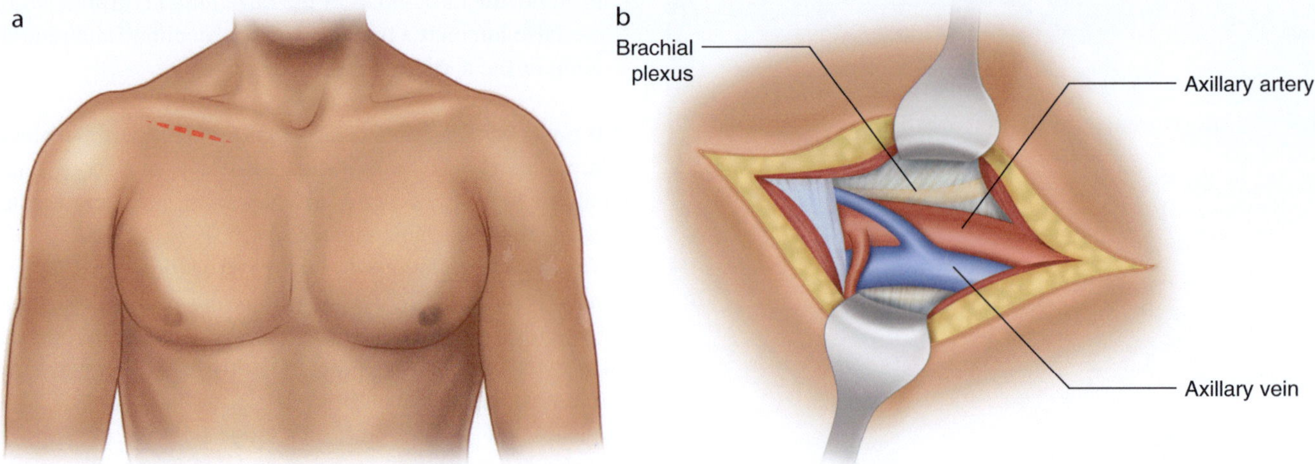

Fig. 34.16 (a) Right axillary artery site incision below the middle third of the clavicle. (b) Brachial plexus, axillary artery, axillary vein

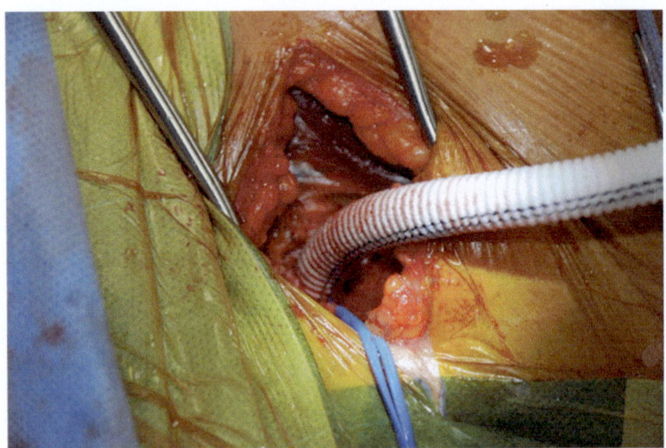

Fig. 34.17 The Dacron graft anastomosed to axillary artery

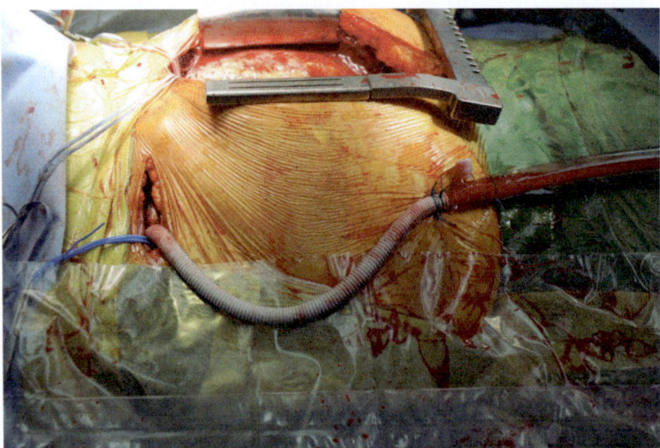

Fig. 34.18 Axillary artery cannulation: a 10 mm Dacron prosthesis is interposed between the axillary artery, and it is connected to the arterial line

arterial branches of the thoracoacromial trunk will be encountered and if necessary divided to gain full access through the fatty tissue overlying the axillary vessels. In the dissection, the axillary vein is usually encountered first. The axillary artery lies superior and deep to the vein and can be easily palpated. The artery is easily exposed and encircled by an umbilical tape; making a gentle traction on the tape will allow the axillary artery to be drawn up into the surgical wound, avoiding contact and damage with the brachial plexus [46].

34.3.5.2 Innominate Artery Cannulation

This cannulation is employed for both arterial return and selective antegrade cerebral perfusion for repair of acute type A aortic dissection. After median sternotomy is made from the sternal notch to the xiphoid process, the thymus is completely dissected off the pericardium and all the thymic vein tributaries draining into the left innominate vein divided, thus exposing the entire length of extrapericardial ascending aorta up to arch vessels. The left innominate vein is identified, taped, and gently moved upward to expose the arch vessels. Then, the innominate artery (IA), the left common carotid artery (LCCA), and the left subclavian artery (LSA) are taped. When direct cannulation is used, a single purse string is placed on the IA at 2 cm away from its origin from the arch.

A graft interposition allows monitoring cerebral perfusion through the same graft by reading the right radial pressure. After systemic heparinization, the IA, or the AA, is partially clamped and an 8 mm polytetrafluoroethylene or Dacron graft is anastomosed in an end-to-side fashion and secured outside the surgical field using silk sutures (Fig. 34.18). The right atrium is cannulated using a single two-stage venous cannula, and cardiopulmonary bypass is started. It is described a direct IA cannulation using a 20 F wire reinforced Medtronic cannula and the tip of the cannula is moved into the proximal arch; the cannula is connected to the arterial line from the circuit [47].

34.3.5.3 Femoral Artery Cannulation

Femoral arterial cannulation was one of the first and once almost exclusively employed, but it is now less and less frequent. One of the main reasons is the higher risk of malperfusion (see below). When the femoral artery is pulseless, the true lumen is compressed by the false one. In this case, suturing an 8 mm graft to the femoral artery can restore the flow in the aortic true lumen and may improve visceral perfusion.

34.3.5.4 Malperfusion

During CPB, malperfusion is suspected when it is difficult to keep a normal flow and high resistance is found in the arterial line with concomitant low systemic arterial blood pressure measured on the left radial and femoral lines. At the same time INVOS (near-infrared spectroscopy INVOS, Somanetics, Troy, MI) may show cerebral oxygen desaturation (value <50% from baseline).

34.3.5.5 Hypothermia in Aortic Arch Surgery

Hypothermia reduces brain metabolic need in order to permit safe periods of circulatory arrest during aortic arch surgery. A consensus from experts in high-volume aortic institutions defined 'profound', 'deep', 'moderate', and 'mild' hypothermia in this way [48] as follows:

Profound hypothermia: ≤14 °C.
Deep hypothermia: 14.1–20 °C.
Moderate hypothermia: 20.1–28 °C.
Mild hypothermia: 28.1–34 °C.

Temperature reduction determines bleeding complications resulting from hypothermia-induced coagulopathy and from increased systemic inflammatory response from prolonged CPB times required for cooling and rewarming [49]. Randomized controlled trials are lacking, most studies are retrospective, and therefore some concern has been reported about the optimal degree of hypothermia during circulatory arrest. Anyway, an increasing number of centers utilize "moderate" or "mild" hypothermia with selective antegrade cerebral perfusion [50–54].

34.3.5.6 Left Ventricle Vent

When CPB is instituted and cooling is started, the left ventricle is vented through a cannula inserted in the right superior pulmonary vein.

34.3.5.7 Technique Without Aortic Clamping

Once AA cannulation is performed, the chest is opened via median sternotomy, pericardium incised and suspended with silk stay sutures. The inspection of the transverse aortic arch (Figs. 34.19 and 34.20) is essential to identify any potential intimal entry and reentry tears. The venous cannula is positioned in the righ atrium. We believe it would be preferable not to cross-clamp the ascending aorta and to perform an open distal anastomosis. David and colleagues suggest that avoidance of aortic cross-clamping during cooling and resection of the primary tear improved early and late outcome [55].

Furthermore, clamping the ascending aorta may cause false lumen pressurization leading to propagation of the

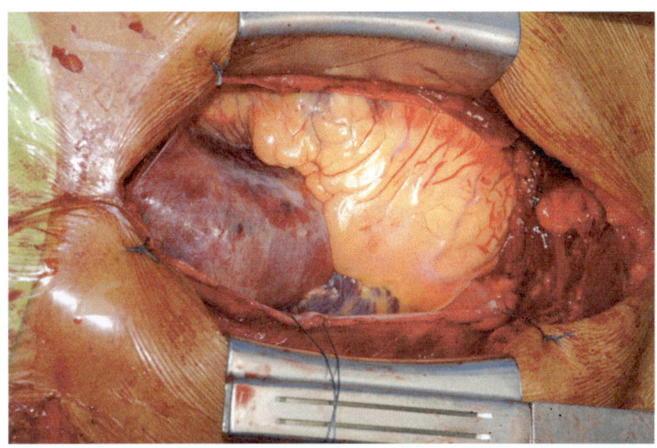

Fig. 34.19 Ascending aorta hematoma in a 79-year-old woman. The patient had a sudden onset of abrupt chest pain that radiated to the back. She was hospitalized, and angio-CT showed type A aortic dissection involving the aortic arch and false lumen thrombosis. Surgical view after sternotomy: the pericardium is opened, and the ascending aorta appears markedly enlarged showing a bluish ecchymosis of its wall

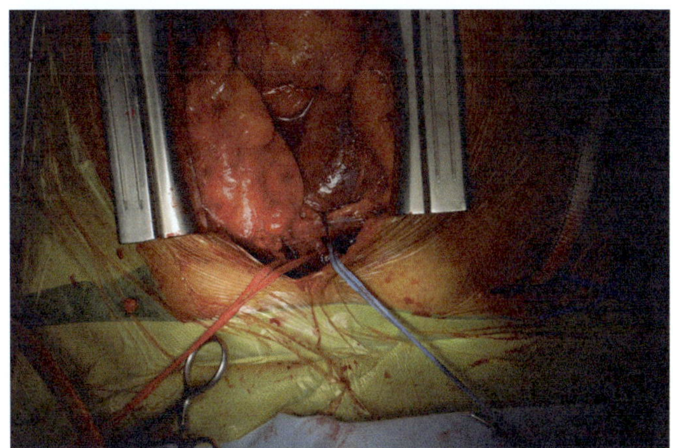

Fig. 34.20 Surgical field preparation: left innominate vein and the innominate artery are encircled by blue and red tape respectively

dissection and malperfusion, but also there is an elevated risk of inducing additional aortic lesions by the clamp itself [56].

The patient is cooled, and circulatory arrest is started when the desired cooling temperature is reached (nasopharyngeal, bladder, or rectal); the patient's head is positioned in Trendelenburg and packed in ice, as well as CO_2 field flooding. With circulatory arrest the aorta is incised , false and true lumens are entered (Figs. 34.21 and 34.22) and cardioplegia is infused in coronary ostia. Selective brain perfusion is started through the right axillary artery, after IA proximal clamping, or via the IA and the left common carotid artery (LCCA) direct cannulation (Fig. 34.23) assuring a flow of 10–15 mL/kg/min and perfusion pressure maintained at 45–60 mmHg. Left subclavian artery (LSA) is blocked with a 6-F Fogarty catheter to prevent the "subclavian steal phenomenon" and excessive back bleeding.

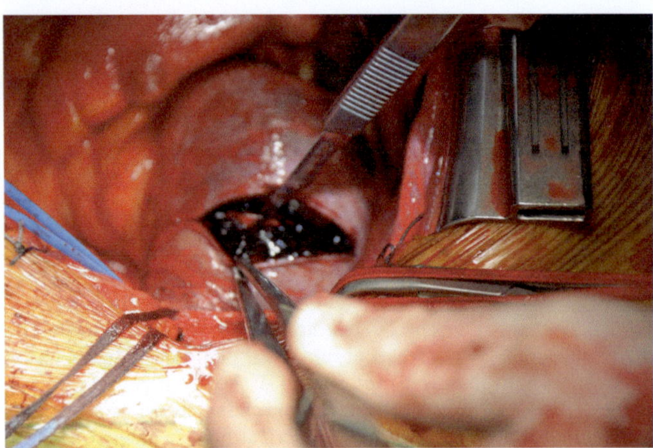

Fig. 34.21 Same case: the ascending aorta is incised

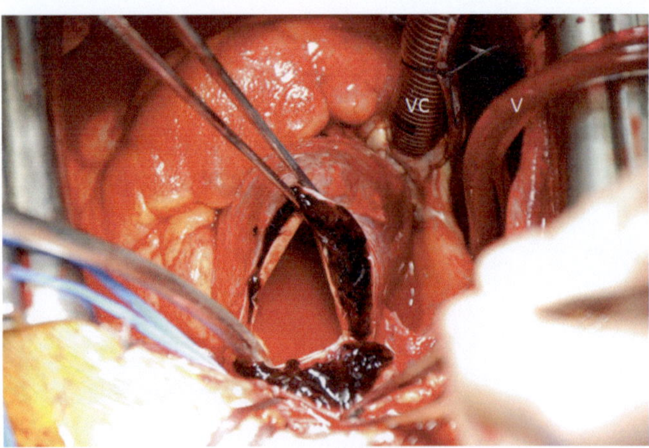

Fig. 34.22 Same case: the ascending aorta was opened (VC, venous cannula in right atrium; V, vent positioned in right superior pulmonary vein)

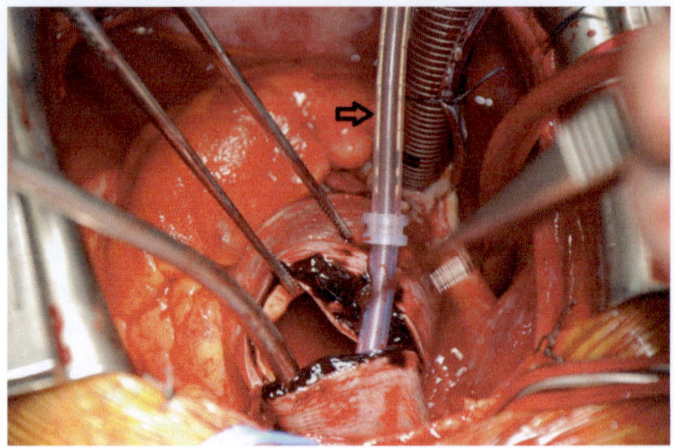

Fig. 34.23 Same case: the black arrow indicates the cannula for cerebral perfusion positioned in the left common carotid artery

34.3.5.8 Technique Using Aortic Clamping

We discourage aortic clamping but sometimes it may necessary in case of massive aortic regurgitation and left ventricular distension. Furthermore, few surgeons use to clamp the aorta and, consequently, we describe also this technique. Before the aorta is clamped, it is important to manually check if the aortic cannula (if central cannulation is performed) is correctly in the arch and not in the ascending aorta in order to prevent an accidental clamping; then pump pressure is reduced, and the aorta is cross-clamped midway between the sinotubular junction and the IA, an area that the surgeon will remove. The aorta is incised, the false and true lumens of the aorta are entered, and cardioplegia is injected antegrade into the coronary ostia and/or retrogradely into coronary sinus in order to arrest the heart.

When the desired cooling temperature is reached, the aortic clamp is released and CPB is arrested and cerebral perfusion and protection started.

34.3.5.9 Surgical Decision–Making Strategies

Ascending aorta is opened and precisely inspected, and any intimal tears found must be resected, and any thrombus should be removed (Figs. 34.24, 34.25, 34.26, and 34.27). Once proximal aortic stump has been reinforced, aortic valve competence must be evaluated pouring saline into the root in order to assess if the valve holds the water (Fig. 34.28); acute aortic valve regurgitation can be determined by:

- Aortic root acute dilation from false lumen expansion.
- Aortic valve leaflet disruption caused by dissection.
- Dissection flap prolapsing through the valve.

The aortic root and the coronary ostia are accurately inspected for evaluation of surgical strategy: supracoronary graft anastomosis with aortic valve resuspension (Figs. 34.29) and Bentall procedure with a composite valve graft or with a valve-sparing root replacement; on the other hand, sinus-retaining and valve-conserving techniques are unsuitable in pre-existing root pathology (Marfan syndrome) or annuloaortic ectasia [57].

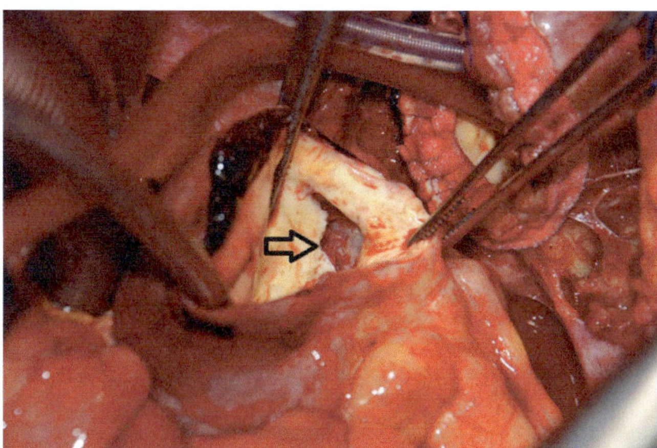

Fig. 34.24 Same case: inspection of the aorta, an intimal tear is seen in the proximal ascending aorta (black arrow)

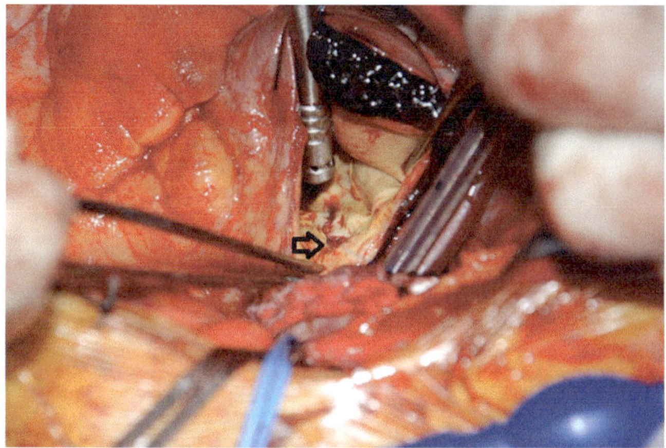

Fig. 34.25 Same case: black arrow shows an intimal tear on the posterior wall of the ascending aorta

34.3.5.10 Distal Aortic Anastomosis

The distal aortic anastomosis is performed first at the healthiest aortic wall, replacing the ascending aorta. If the entry tear is located in the concavity of the aortic arch, a hemiarch replacement should be done, especially in the elderly or unstable patient. If there are entry tears near the origin of the supra-aortic branches or in case of aortic arch enlargement >5 cm, a total arch replacement and reimplantation of the arch vessels should be performed. False lumen is obliterated positioning Teflon (DuPont) felt or pericardial strips internally and externally to buttress the aortic tissue prior to suturing the graft (Fig. 34.30) [58].

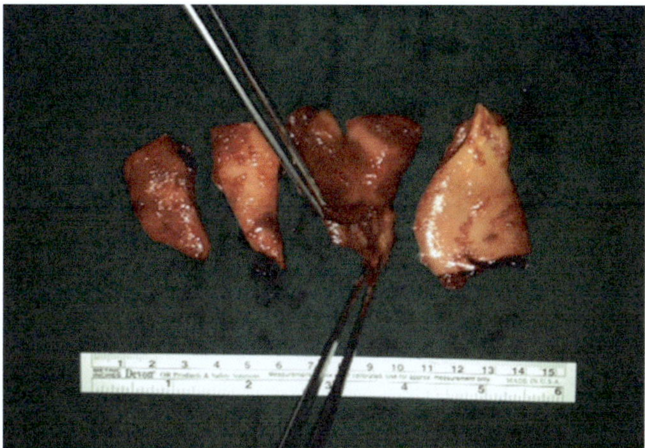

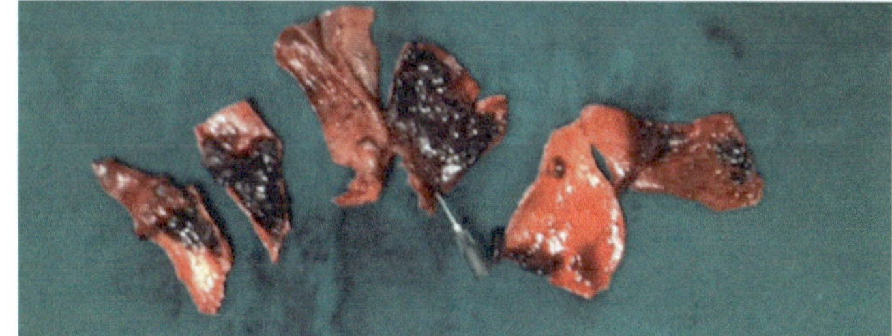

Fig. 34.26 Same case: aortic wall removed. Above, forceps point out the intimal tear; down, the aortic wall is opened; below, the needle indicates the intimal tear and intramural hematoma

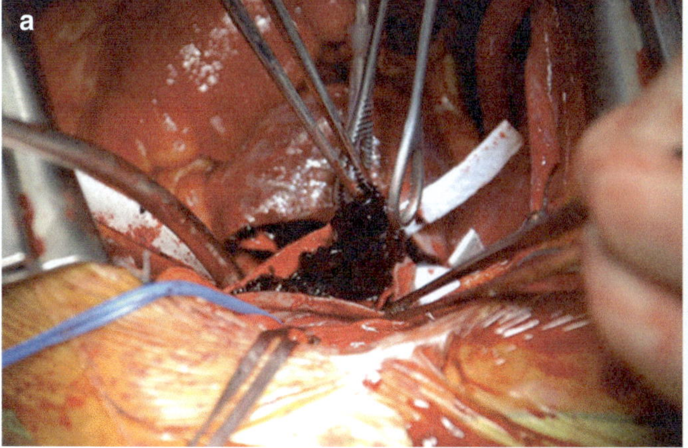

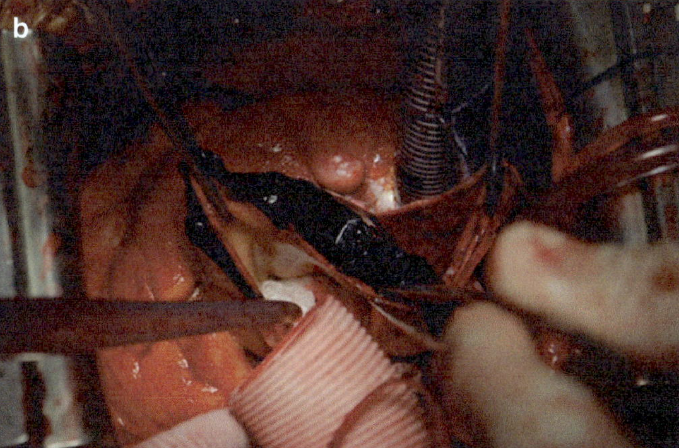

Fig. 34.27 Same case. (**a**) Clots are removed from the distal ortic stump. (**b**) intramural clots removed from proximal aortic stump

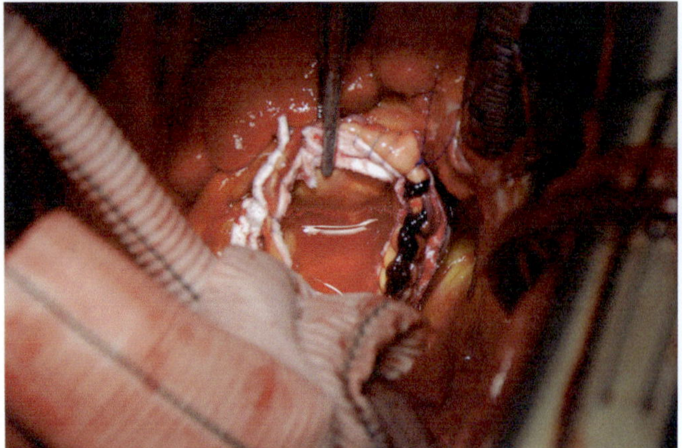

Fig. 34.28 The aortic valve is competent: the valve holds the water

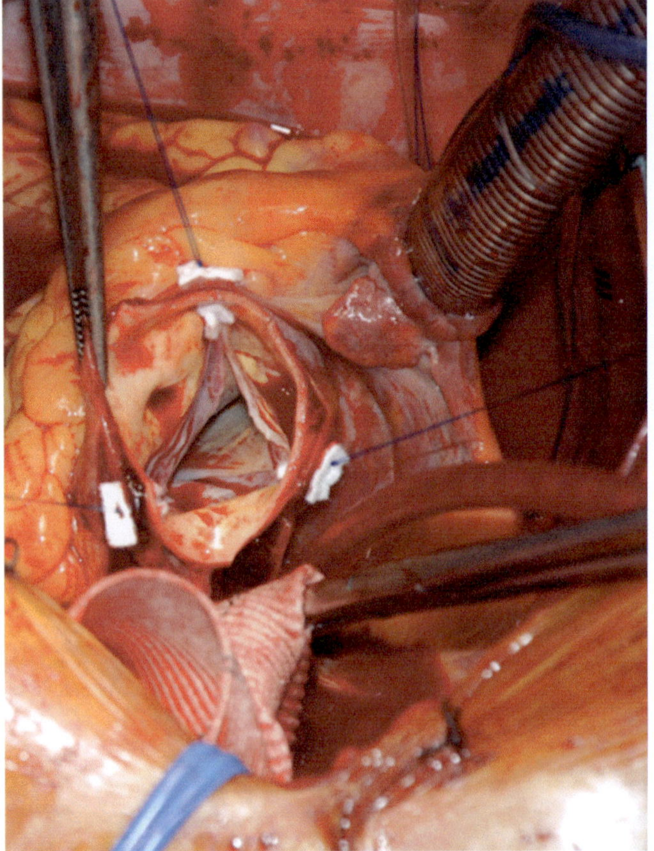

Fig 34.29 The aortic valve is suspended: the three commissures are suspended with Prolene 4–0 reinforced with pledgets; the dissection spares the coronary ostia; the left coronary ostium is evident

The reinforced aortic stump is anastomosed using 3–0 or 4–0 polypropylene suture to a woven polyester graft that has a sidearm (Fig. 34.31). Just before the anastomosis is carried out, the flow in LCCA is stopped and cannula removed, then de-airing is achieved, and the graft is distally clamped. Now the true lumen perfusion and the cerebral circulation are secured by the sidearm branch, connected to the heart-lung machine, favouring false lumen thrombosis. The patient is gradually rewarmed to 36 °C. If necessary, the distal anastomosis is often reinforced with interrupted 4–0 polypropylene pledgeted sutures.

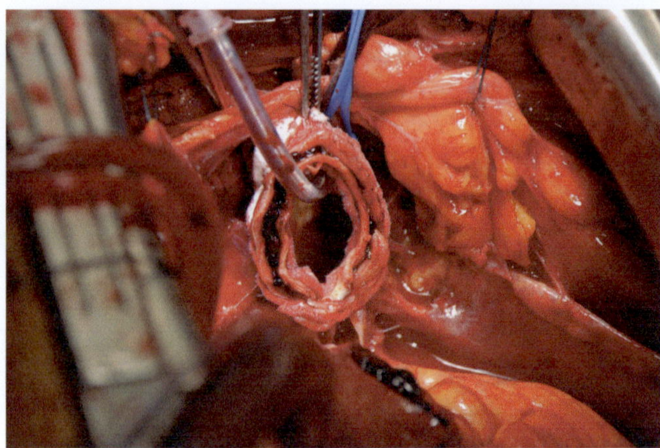

Fig. 34.30 Same case: the distal aorta stump is reinforced with Teflon; in hypothermic circulatory arrest, the cannula is positioned in the left common carotid artery for cerebral perfusion

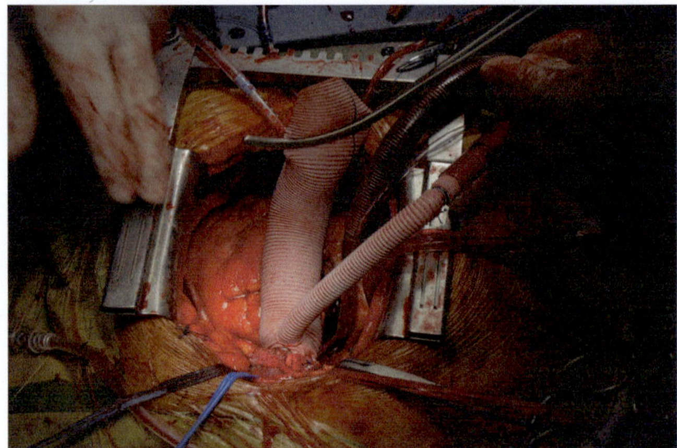

Fig. 34.31 Same case: a bifurcated dacron graft (size 30 mm) was sutured in the distal aortic stump; note the sidearm branch (SB) for antegrade perfusion

If the aortic arch needs to be replaced, the distal end-to-end anastomosis between the woven graft and the descending aorta (beyond the LSA) is accomplished using the "elephant trunk" technique [59, 60].

34.3.5.11 Elephant Trunk (ET) Technique

The aorta is severed just beyond the origin of the LSA, and an island of aortic wall containing the arch vessels is tailored; the left phrenic and left vagus nerves are identified and protected. A polyester graft is prepared as follows (Figs. 34.32 and 34.33):

- A stay suture is positioned at the proximal extremity of the graft.
- The proximal extremity is inverted into the distal 5 cm segment that will remain in the descending aorta (elephant trunk).

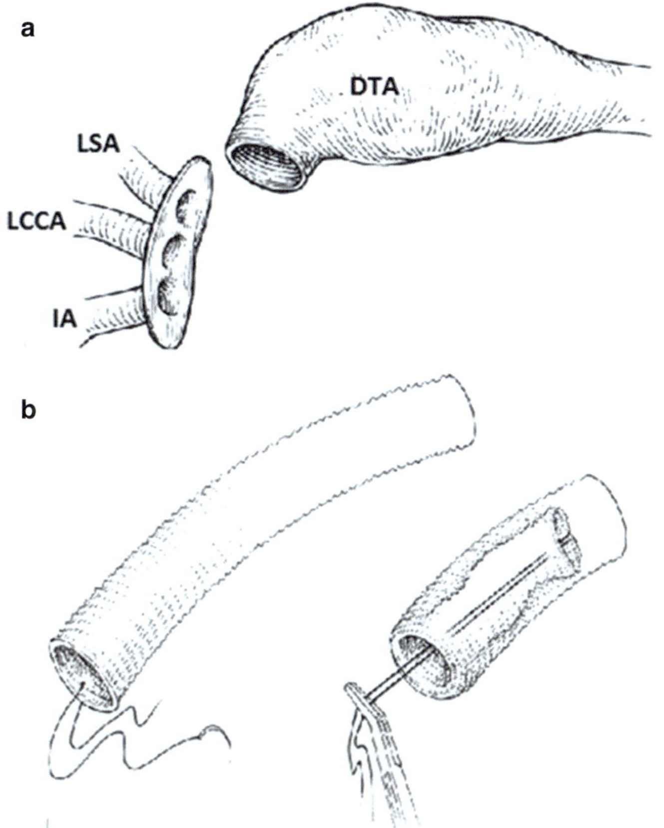

Fig. 34.32 Elephant trunk technique. (**a**) The aorta is severed just distal to the left subclavian artery (LSA), and arch vessels are separated from the aorta tailoring a cuff; (**b**) a stay suture is positioned at the proximal extremity of the graft, and it is invaginated into distal 5 cm segment that will be positioned in descending thoracic aorta (DTA). *LCCA* left common carotid artery, *IA* innominate artery

- The entire graft is inserted into the descending thoracic aorta.
- The graft—descending aorta anastomosis is accomplished.
- At this point the stay suture allows withdrawal of the inverted segment.
- The aortic island containing the supra-aortic vessels is sutured to the graft.
- Proximal anastomosis accomplished.

In this way, the distal portion of the graft is left dangling in the descending aorta allowing an easier second-stage surgery (less tissue dissection and bleeding, clamping the graft distal to LSA) or an endovascular stent graft (Fig. 34.33).

Supra-aortic vessels reimplantation can be achieved suturing "en bloc" an island of aortic wall containing the arch vessels. Alternatively, the three arch vessels are individually sutured to a branched graft; in this case axillary

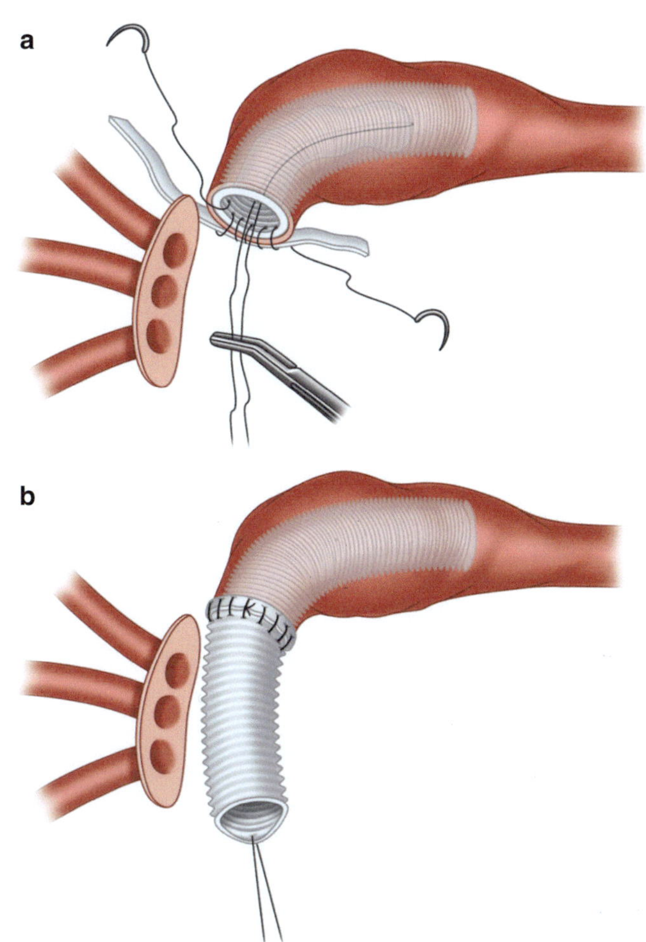

Fig. 34.33 (**a**) The invaginated graft is positioned into DTA; aorta is sutured to doubled-over edge of aortic graft with continuous 3–0 polypropylene suture reinforced with a Teflon strip. (**b**) Applying traction on stay suture, the invaginated tract of graft is pulled out of DTA (*ET* elephant trunk)

artery perfusion is used; the vessels are sequentially sutured (starting from the LSA) to the branches of the particular aortic graft that allows the distal and proximal perfusion by a lateral (fourth) branch during the arterial reimplantation. *Frozen elephant trunk technique* allows to treat in a single time the aneurysm extended from the arch to the descending thoracic aorta with a composite prosthesis constituted by a dacron phrostesis (for the aortic arch) sutured to an endoprosthesis (for the descending thoracic aorta).

34.3.5.12 Proximal Aortic Anastomosis

The graft is anastomosed to a prepared aortic cuff with Teflon strips (Figs. 34.34 and 34.35), or the aortic root is replaced with a composite graft or with a valve-sparing root replacement (see surgical decision-making strategies). The anastomosis is accomplished by a continuous 4–0 polypropylene suture.

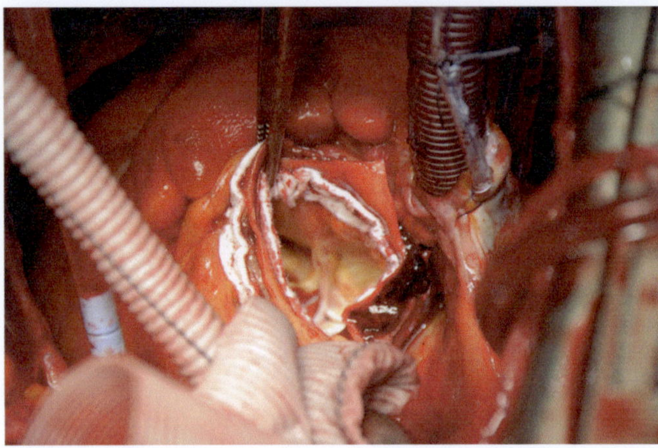

Fig. 34.34 Same case: the proximal aortic stump is reinforced in the inner and outside surface; note the aortic valve

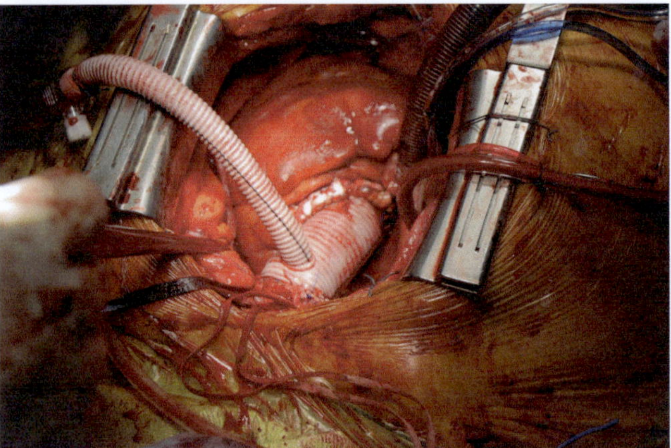

Fig. 34.35 Same case: the proximal anastomosis is completed, note the sidearm branch for anterograde perfusion

The sidearm branch is resected and sutured using polypropylene 4–0; a needle vent is inserted in woven graft for de-airing the prosthesis and the heart.

34.4 Type B Acute Aortic Dissection (AAD)

Surgical treatment in type B AAD historically presents a mortality ranging between 30 and 70%; mortality is now dramatically lowered due to development of endovascular technique, although it remains high in the presence of visceral malperfusion (ranging from 23 to 80%) and in case of aortic rupture.

When the patient is hemodynamically stable, the treatment consists in the first step in the treatment of type B (AAD) consists in stabilising blood pressure using intravenous beta blockers in order to prevent progression of the dissection process and to secure organ perfusion [61].

Surgical or endovascular treatment is necessary in the presence: 1) persistence of pain, 2) hemothorax, 3) visceral or spinal ischemia, 4) retrograde extension into ascending aorta. An aggressive endovascular approach to acute type B dissection has been proposed by some authors [62]. The INSTEAD trial [61] showed no survival advantage of endografting as opposed to medical therapy at 2 years (95.6±2.5% with optimal medical therapy versus 88.9±3.7% with TEVAR (Thoracic Endovascular Aortic Repair) (P = 0.15)). It showed, however, a beneficial impact of stent grafting on aortic remodeling that can be affected positively the long-term outcome.

The aortic fenestration technique is used for decompressing the hypertensive false lumen by producing a hole in the distal part of the dissection flap; in this way there is an outflow from the false lumen and a concomitant reduction of intraluminal pressure, relieving branch vessel obstruction and reducing the risk of progression of the dissection [63]. The technique is utilized in case of visceral malperfusion; in the past treatment was based on surgical intervention on the abdominal aorta creating a resection of the septum between the false and true lumens restoring adequate flow in both sides of the septum. Resection can be associated with the prosthetic replacement of the abdominal aorta with fixation of the distal layers with Teflon felt.

At present, in case of malperfusion, the *endovascular approach* is preferred: the aim of the procedure, performed percutaneously, is to cannulate the false and the true lumen with a guidewire and enlarging it with a balloon angioplasty in order to achieve the same result of surgery. In addition, a stenting of the dissected origin of visceral arteries can guarantee an adequate perfusion.

Endografting is preferred when dissection causes a complete collapse of the true lumen with consequent obstruction of all visceral vessels (see Case 1, Figs. 34.36 and 34.37). In this case, a 10–15 cm in length endograft placement may achieve an adequate flow in the true lumen, closing the proximal entry tear. The procedure is performed under transesophageal echocardiography (TEE) guidance in order to ensure the correct guidewire position inside the lumens. True and false lumens are reached cannulating both femoral arteries under continuous angiographic control: a 7 Fr. X 90 cm introducer sheath, placed in both lumens, may assure a good visualization of the origin of visceral and intercostal arteries, before and after the opening of the endograft. The procedure must be performed with a spinal drainage due to the risk of

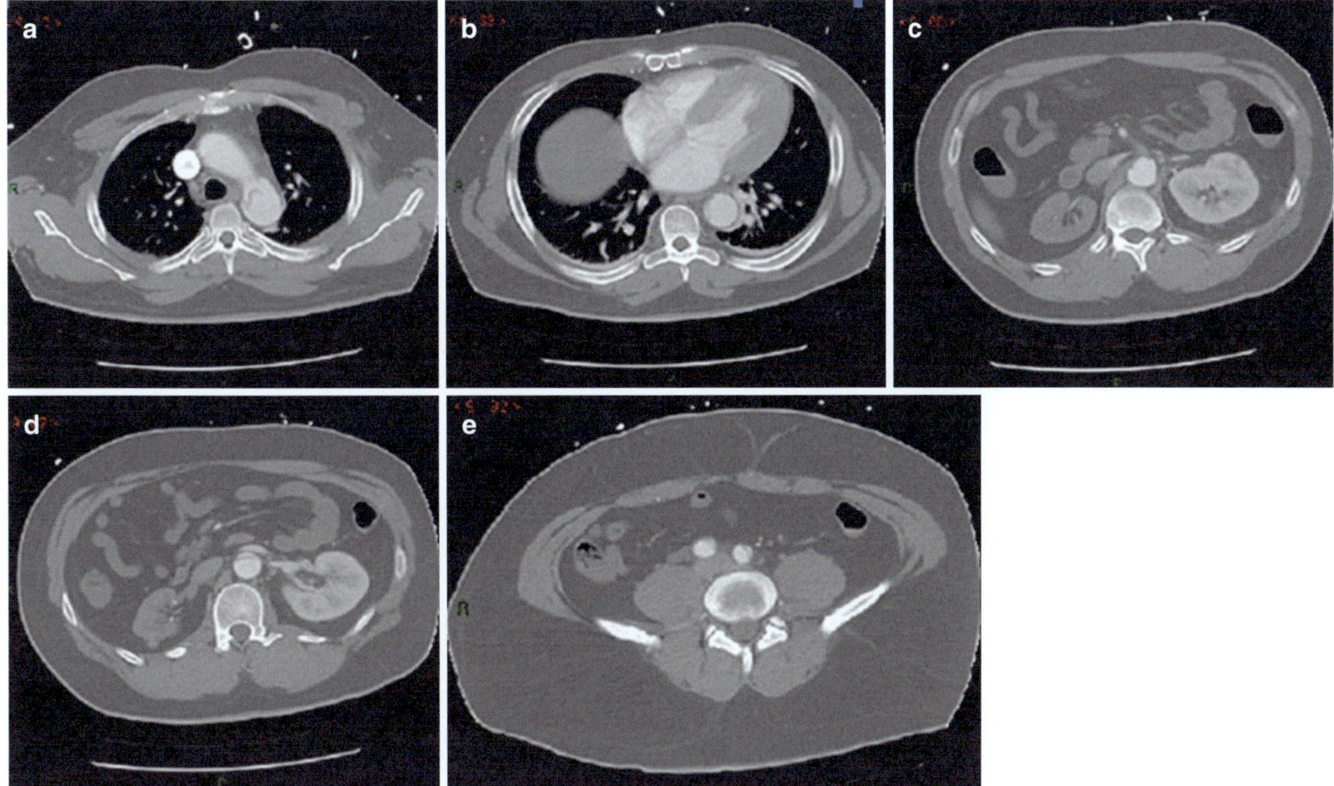

Fig. 34.36 Case 1. (**a**–**e**) CT images show type B aortic dissection in a 34-year-old patient admitted to emergency ward for abdominal pain occurred 15 days before. The true lumen (**c**) completely collapsed with a dynamic occlusion of the superior mesenteric artery. The hypoperfusion (**d**) of the left kidney and the complete absence (**e**) of true lumen in the iliac vessels

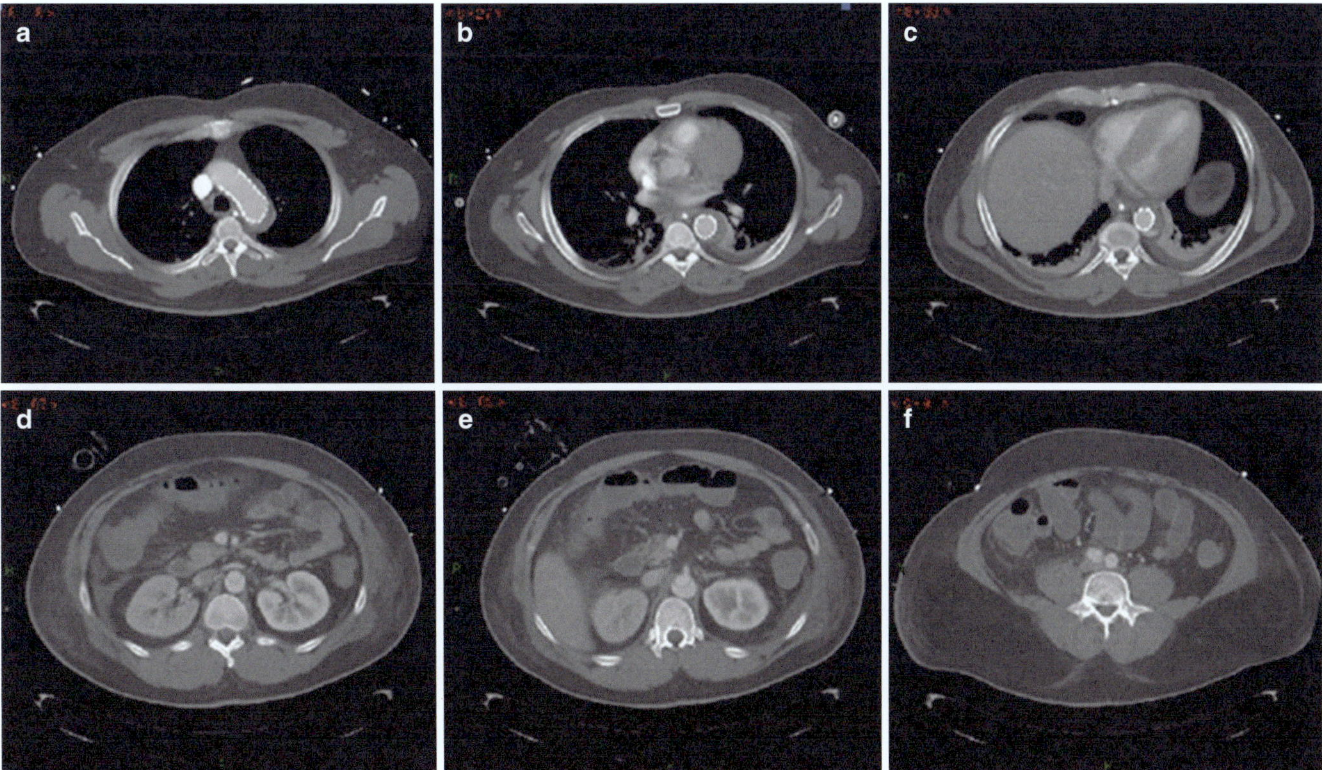

Fig. 34.37 (**a**-**f**) postoperative CT scan after successful deployment in emergency (for an incoming bowel ischemia) of an aortic thoracic endograft with re-expansion of the true lumen and reopening of the superior mesenteric artery and iliac vessels

exclusion of intercostal arteries where the true lumen is expanded. A post-deployment ballooning of the graft is contraindicated because of aortic wall's extreme fragility; moreover, an endograft without proximal and distal bare stents is positioned to minimize the risk of retrograde distal dissection. A medium radial force is preferred to reduce the risk of aortic rupture, especially in genetic disorders (Marfan, Loeys-Dietz patients). Spinal drainage must be prolonged up to 72 h and requires frequent monitoring of lower limb motility and spinal cord pressure.

Chimney technique. The chimney technique was described by Greenberg et al. [64] in 2003. The technique involves deployment of a covered stent parallel to the main aortic stent graft that, protruding proximally likewise a chimney, allows the flow in vital side branches covered by the aortic endovascular graft; the technique can be also successfully used in endografting the false lumen and preserving perfusion of the true lumen. An example is shown in Case 2 (Figs. 34.38, 34.39 and 34.40) where the chimney graft was employed in a 68-year-old man that had a previous aortic arch open surgery. He was admitted for chest pain due to a blister in the false lumen of the descending aorta.

Aortic graft replacement. The open surgical solution is reserved in case of aortic rupture, and operation is done

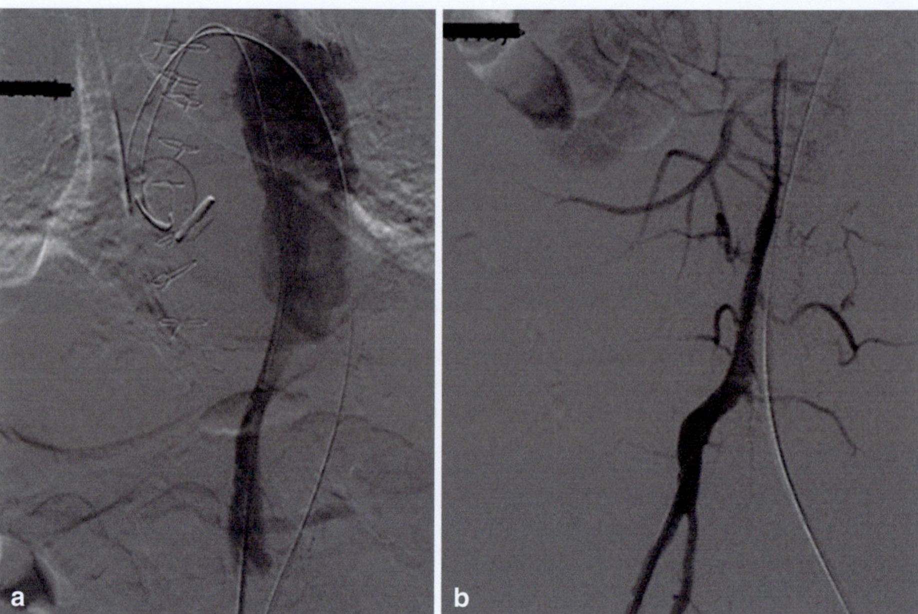

Fig. 34.38 Case 2, (**a**) intraoperative angiogram of a patient that had aortic arch replacement. The patient, a 68-year-old man, was admitted with thoracic pain due to a blister in the false lumen of the descending aorta. Complete view of the false lumen is seen after left femoral artery cannulation. (**b**) Intraoperative angiogram of the true lumen cannulated from the right femoral artery showing the all visceral vessels originate from the true lumen

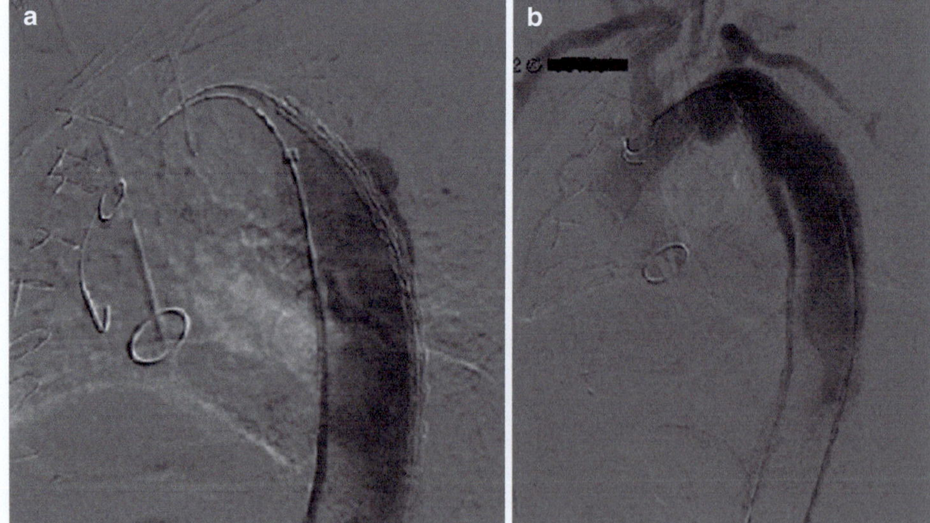

Fig. 34.39 Case 2, (**a**) The endograft in place for stenting of the false lumen. The true lumen has been inserted along the chimney graft to guarantee the perfusion of visceral arteries. (**b**) Postoperative angiograms showing the exclusion of the blister, the perfusion of the true lumen, and false lumen endografting

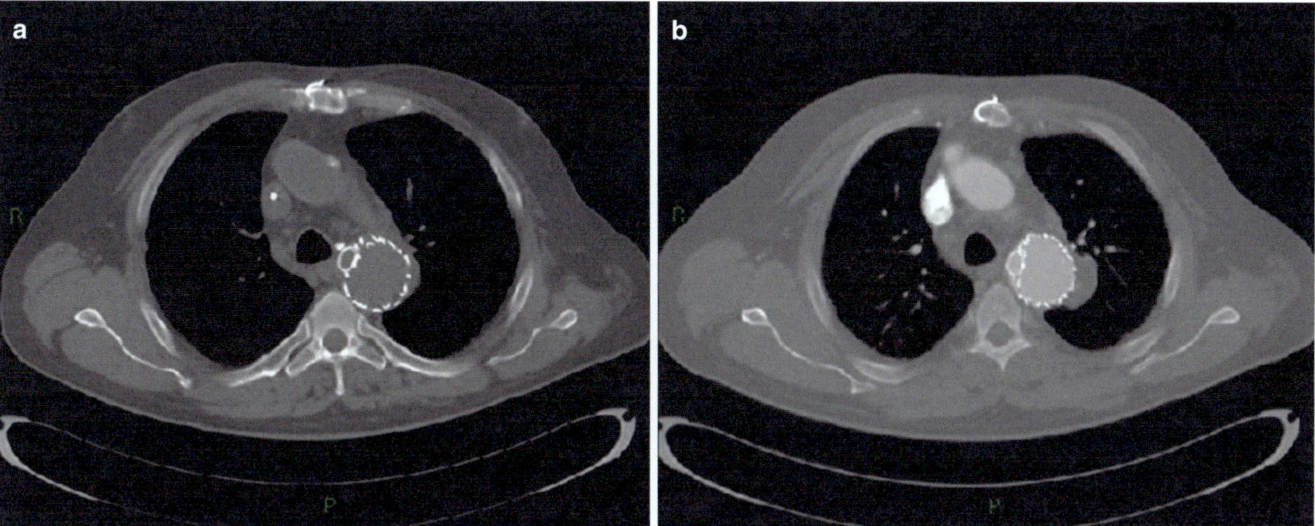

Fig. 34.40 (**a** and **b**) Postoperative CT scan showing the patency (basal and after contrast) of the chimney graft

using extracorporeal circulation. The surgical technique is similar to that described in thoracoabdominal repair: the operation can be carried out by left heart bypass, cardiopulmonary bypass or circulatory arrest and deep hypothermia. A thoracotomy in fifth intercostal space is performed with extension in phreno-laparotomy. All the visceral and spinal cord supply vessels are identified; once the proximal and distal control of the aorta is achieved, the extracorporeal circulation is started and aorta crossclamped.

Upon the completion of the proximal anastomosis suturing a Dacron graft to the aortic stump, the clamp is moved to the level of the diaphragm and, after the complete removal of the internal flap, spinal cord supply vessels are identified and sutured to the graft. The operation is completed with the progressive reattachment of the visceral vessels with Teflon felt ring reinforcement and glue apposition. During this time visceral perfusion can be performed through the derivation of the extracorporeal arterial line.

In case of type B retrograde dissection, the treatment is that for type A dissection.

34.5 Pseudoaneurysm

Thoracic aortic pseudoaneurysm (TAP) or false aneurysm is considered in AAS: there is a common denominator, a breach in the aortic wall where blood leaks through but is contained by the adventitia or surrounding perivascular soft tissue. The risk of rupture is higher than that of a true aneurysm of comparable size due to poor support of the aneurysm wall, and thus TAP is considered immediately for intervention. TAPs often occur in cardiac surgery cases and are associated with anastomosis or cannulation site of the vessel, leading to a poor healing process and defects in the layers of the wall [65, 66] (see Figs. 34.41, 34.42, 34.43, 34.44, 34.45 and 34.46). Furthermore, any traumatic, inflammatory, or infectious event can be associated with the development of a TAP [67]. The use of BioGlue has been involved in the postoperative formation of TAP; the inflammatory reaction to the BioGlue components is considered responsible for the aortic wall damage [68, 69]. Endovascular procedures may determine TAP or AAD in an aortic wall involved in the atherosclerotic process, particularly with the use of endografts with proximal bare stents [70].

34.6 Retrograde Type A Aortic Dissection Postinvasive Endovascular Procedures

"Retrograde type A aortic dissection" (RTAD) is defined as a dissection that originates distally to the ascending aorta with retrograde flap progression into the ascending aorta. It was a known complication during conventional cardiac surgery, but recently, it has been described as one of the most alarming complication after thoracic aortic endovascular repair (TEVAR) and should be included in acute thoracic aortic syndrome.

We present a clinical case showing this frightening complication in a young woman affected by Loeys-Dietz patient with a Kommerell's diverticulum and a bronchial artery aneurysm (Figs. 34.47, 34.48 and 34.49).

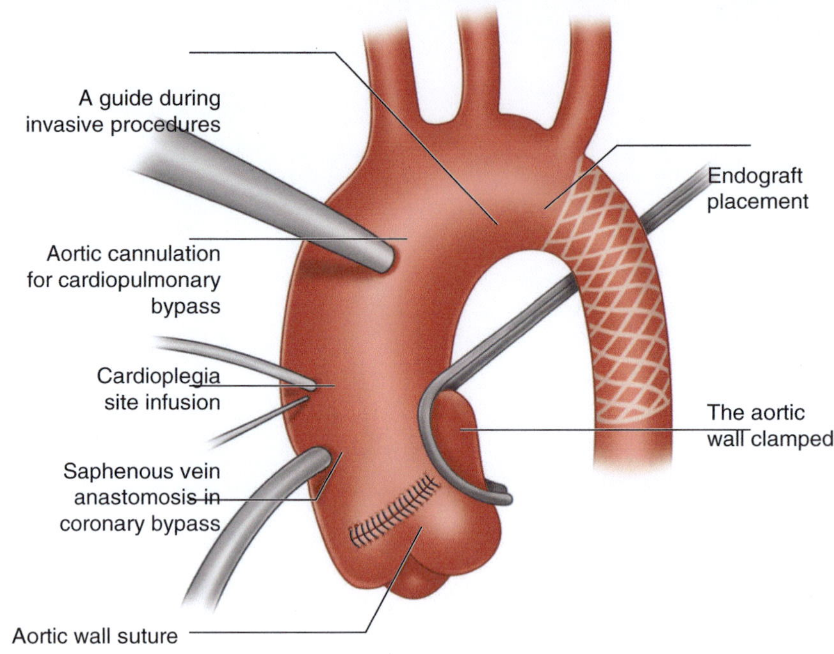

Fig. 34.41 The picture illustrates the main causes that can determine a pseudoaneurysm formation

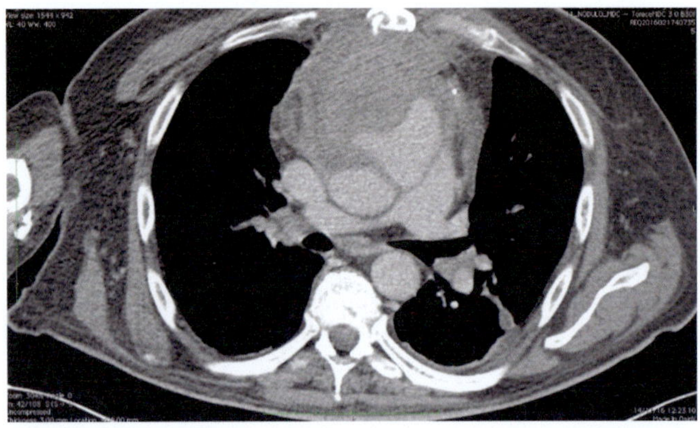

Fig. 34.42 Ascending aorta pseudoaneurysm. A 60-year-old man had an aortic valve replacement (bioprosthesis) and triple coronary bypass; the procedure was complicated by sternal wound infection that required a sternal rewiring. Anyway 6 weeks later, due to sternal instability and dark blood drainage from the wound, the patient underwent angio-CT that showed a huge pseudoaneurysm just underneath the sternal plane, compressing the cardiac structures (right pulmonary artery is absolutely flattened)

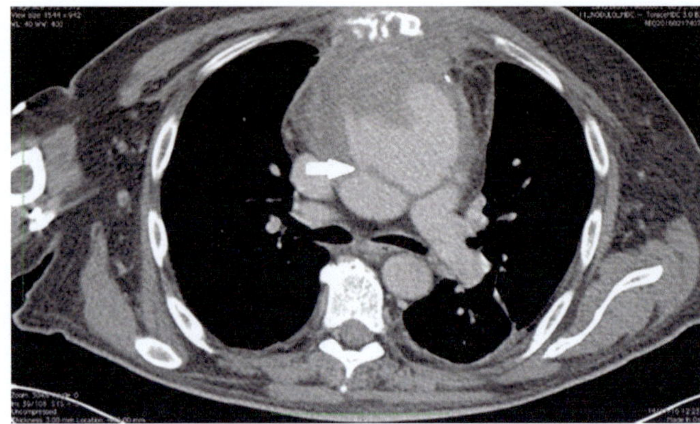

Fig. 34.43 The white arrow shows the blood passage from aorta to the pseudoaneurysm

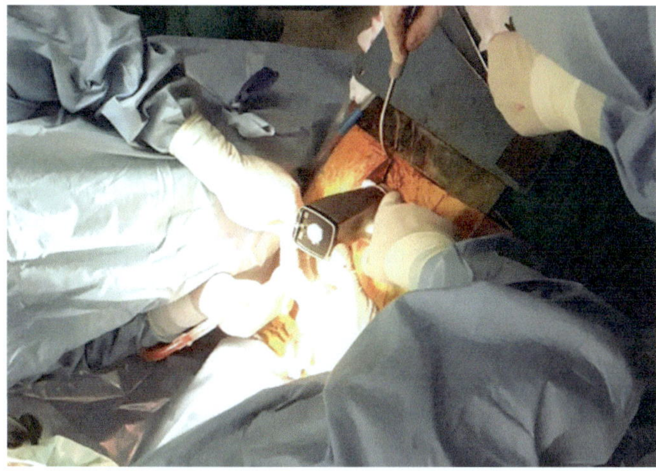

Fig. 34.44 At surgery, extracorporeal circulation is established via the femoral approach with access gained prior to initiation of the sternotomy. The sternum is lifted directly upward as it is divided using an oscillating saw

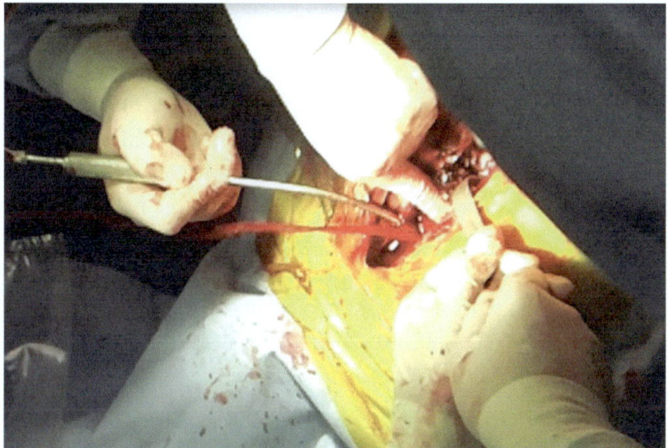

Fig. 34.45 The sternum is lifted gently upward, and while attempting to carefully separate adhesions, the pseudoaneurysm was entered causing massive bleeding. The patient was immediately cooled

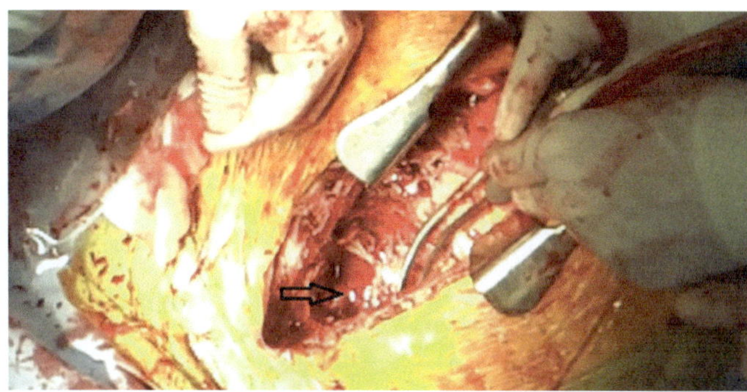

Fig. 34.46 The aorta was found bleeding from the previous cannulation site, responsible for pseudoaneurysm formation. The arrow indicates the pledgets sutured on this point

34.7 Blunt Trauma: Acute Aortic Rupture

Traumatic rupture of the thoracic aorta is a potentially lethal lesion occurring in 10–30% of death due to blunt thoracic trauma, and it is the second cause of death after head injury [71, 72]. The thoracic aorta lesions are often a result of sudden deceleration and occur most frequently in motor vehicle accidents. Approximately 90% of the lesions take place at the aortic isthmus; the remaining 10% is distributed between the ascending aorta, aortic arch, and distal descending aorta. In most cases a sudden deceleration determines a forward shift of the ascending and descending aorta, while the ligamentum arteriosum and the great vessels hold the isthmus and the transverse arch, thus stressing the area of the isthmus and causing a tear of the aortic wall [73]. The tear can involve all the layers of the aortic wall with transection of the aorta or only the intimal layer. Part or all of the circumference of the aortic wall can be involved. If the aortic adventitia remains intact, a pulsating hematoma forms.

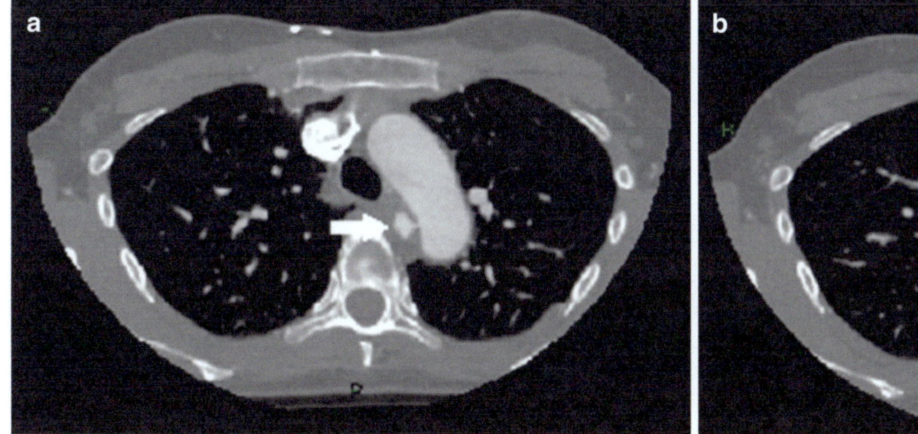

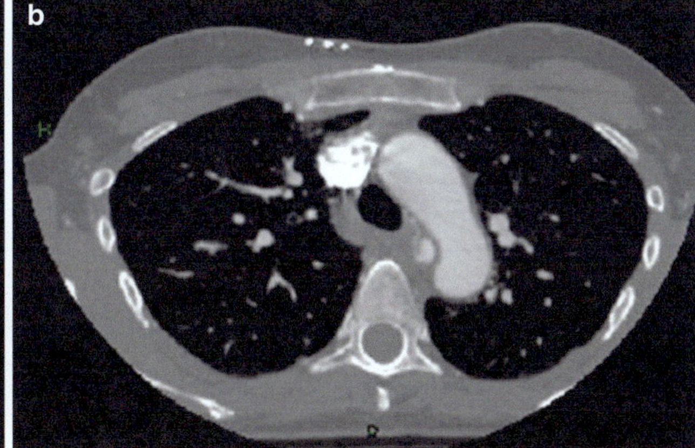

Fig. 34.47 (**a**) Spiral CT showing in Loeys-Dietz patient with a Kommerell's diverticulum, the white arrow indicates the bronchial artery aneurysm

Treatment has evolved from performing emergent open repair with clamp and sew technique to using circulatory support, medical management, and, at the present time, endovascular repair. Moreover, it is important to consider that multi-trauma patients often may not tolerate open surgery for concomitant severe injuries, and endovascular procedure appears the most attractive treatment also in terms of mortality, incidence of spinal cord ischemia, renal insufficiency, and graft infection.

Fig. 34.48 (a) Intraoperative angiogram in the same patient showing the previous stenting of the right lusoria subclavian artery (S) and white arrow shows the iatrogenic retrograde aortic dissection

The trauma can cause a complete rupture of the aortic layers, and if the mediastinal pleura remains intact, an enormous amount of blood pours into the pleural cavity causing hemothorax with immediate signs and symptoms of hemorrhagic shock. Alternatively, if the adventitial layer remains intact, a minor amount of blood is poured outside the aorta, the mediastinal hematoma is smaller, and the patient may be hemodynamically stable.

34.7.1 Diagnosis

The hemothorax, a very common complication after a thoracic trauma, must be continuously evaluated. To drain the pleural space allows lung expansion, anyway insertion of a chest drainage should be avoided when there are clinical and radiological signs indicative of an aortic dissection or transection. In this case, intercostal drainage can lead to rapid patient exsanguination. Thus, in these patients, drainage should be deferred until confirmation of the diagnosis is obtained. The possibility to delay the surgery in multi-trauma patients, treating first the concomitant lesions, reduces the perioperative mortality and morbidity. In the conscious patients, the symptoms can help the diagnosis: the presence of an interscapular or retrosternal pain is very significative. Some clinical signs are: bruit in the second intercostal space, arterial pulse asymmetry and arterial pressure difference between upper and lower limbs and between the two upper limbs.

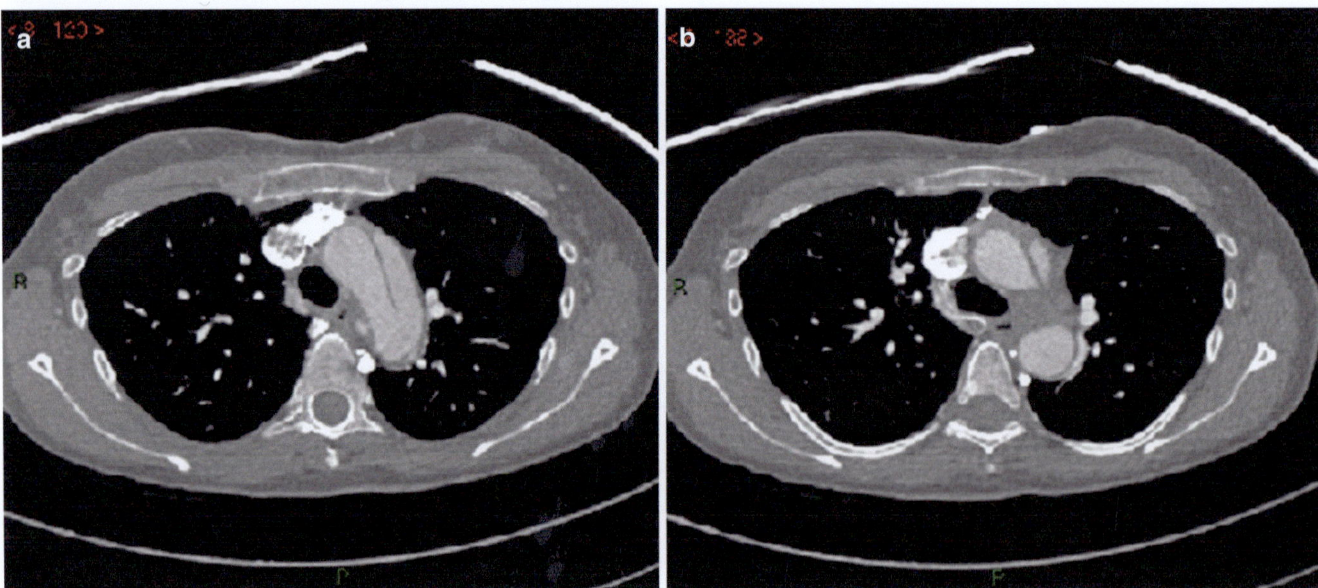

Fig. 34.49 (a and b) Spiral CT showing a retrograde dissection of the aortic arch caused by Terumo guidewire during the attempt of embolization of the aneurysm of the bronchial artery

Chest X-ray may show left hemothorax opacification and rightward shift of the mediastinum, signs that are not diagnostic of aortic rupture because hemothorax may be due to traumatic injuries of heart chambers, intercostal vessels, pulmonary vessels, etc. Helical angio-CT allows to identify the precise place of the aortic laceration and all the findings indicative of aortic rupture: extravasation of contrast, intimal flaps, mural thrombus, para-aortic hematoma, wall thickening, pseudoaneurysm, and pseudocoarctation [74]. Transesophageal echocardiography gives not only aortic images but also important information about cardiac activity, valve function and pericardial effusion.

If adequate treatment is not started, up to 50% of the initial survivors die within the first 72 h [75].

Multiple organ injuries are often found in patients with traumatic aortic rupture, such as closed head injury, multiple rib fractures, pulmonary contusions in 38%, upper limb fractures, pelvic injuries, liver injuries and spleen rupture, spine fractures, and spinal cord injuries.

The best time for repair a blunt thoracic aortic injury is unclear; anyway delayed repair is often pursued and associated with improved outcomes, but there is always the risk of rupture during observation. A risk score to evaluate aortic stability and predict rupture [76] was developed at the Department of Surgery, University of Maryland Medical Center, (Baltimore, USA). The score was based on evaluating the following factors: admission lactate >4 mM, posterior mediastinal hematoma >10 mm, and lesion/normal aortic diameter ratio >1.4 on the admission CT. All the above factors were independently associated with aortic rupture and the model was 100% sensitive and 84% specific for predicting aortic rupture. No aortic lesions ruptured in patients with fewer than two factors. The CT features directly reflect the severity of the aortic lesion, and the progressive risk for aortic rupture is evaluated; pseudoaneurysms (maximum height, mm, 21 ± 10, stable, vs. 41 ± 17, rupture, $p < 0.001$) reflect greater aortic disruption incidence, and when it is measured by the lesion/normal diameter ratio, size was found as an important independent risk factor for aortic rupture.

34.7.2 Treatment

34.7.2.1 Surgery

The surgical exploration is performed through a left fourth space posterolateral thoracotomy (Fig. 34.50). Once the pleural space is opened and the clots removed, it is important to achieve a rapid control of the isthmic area; the surgical strategy is different and depends mainly on the aortic injury and surgeon's preference; the techniques employed are the following:

- Clamp and sew technique.
- Femoro-femoral partial bypass with the interposition of oxygenator.
- Pulmonary-femoral artery bypass, total bypass.

Surgical repair of the traumatic aortic rupture is achieved through a) direct suturing, b) patch plasty and C) tube-graft interposition.

The main point is to prevent paraplegia and therefore to avoid spinal cord injury; most clinical series have failed to demonstrate a clear benefit; partial bypass and total bypass do not definitely prevent this complication, and it seems that a cross-clamp time limit of 30 min can reduce the incidence of paraplegia [77]; when cross-clamp time is ≥1 h, the probability of paraplegia reaches 80% [78].

34.7.2.2 Blood Supply to Spinal Cord

The frequency of severe neurologic complications has declined, but the rate of postoperative paraplegia is still high, in the range of 5–10% [79–81], and is commonly referred as "Russian roulette" for the vascular surgeon [82] and undoubtedly also for the patient. The vertebral arteries are the main supply of blood to the spinal cord that is furnished by:

- One anterior spinal artery.
- Two posterior spinal arteries.
- Anterior and posterior radicular arteries.
- Arterial vasocorona determined by anastomosis between branches of anterior and posterior arteries.

The ischemic complications are related to damages to the anterior spinal artery. In the lower cord, blood is supplied to the anterior spinal artery by the great anterior radiculomedullary artery, the artery of Adamkiewicz, originating from a left intercostal or lumbar artery in 68–73% of cases and at the level of the 9th to 12th intercostal artery in 62–75%, in the remaining case from T5 and T8 [83].

34.7.2.3 Endovascular Treatment

The first aspect in the endovascular treatment is the size of the native aorta because in most cases these patients are very young; then the size of the access vessels: it is important to consider the possibility of an iliac conduit if the size of the femoral artery is less 5 mm. Furthermore, a

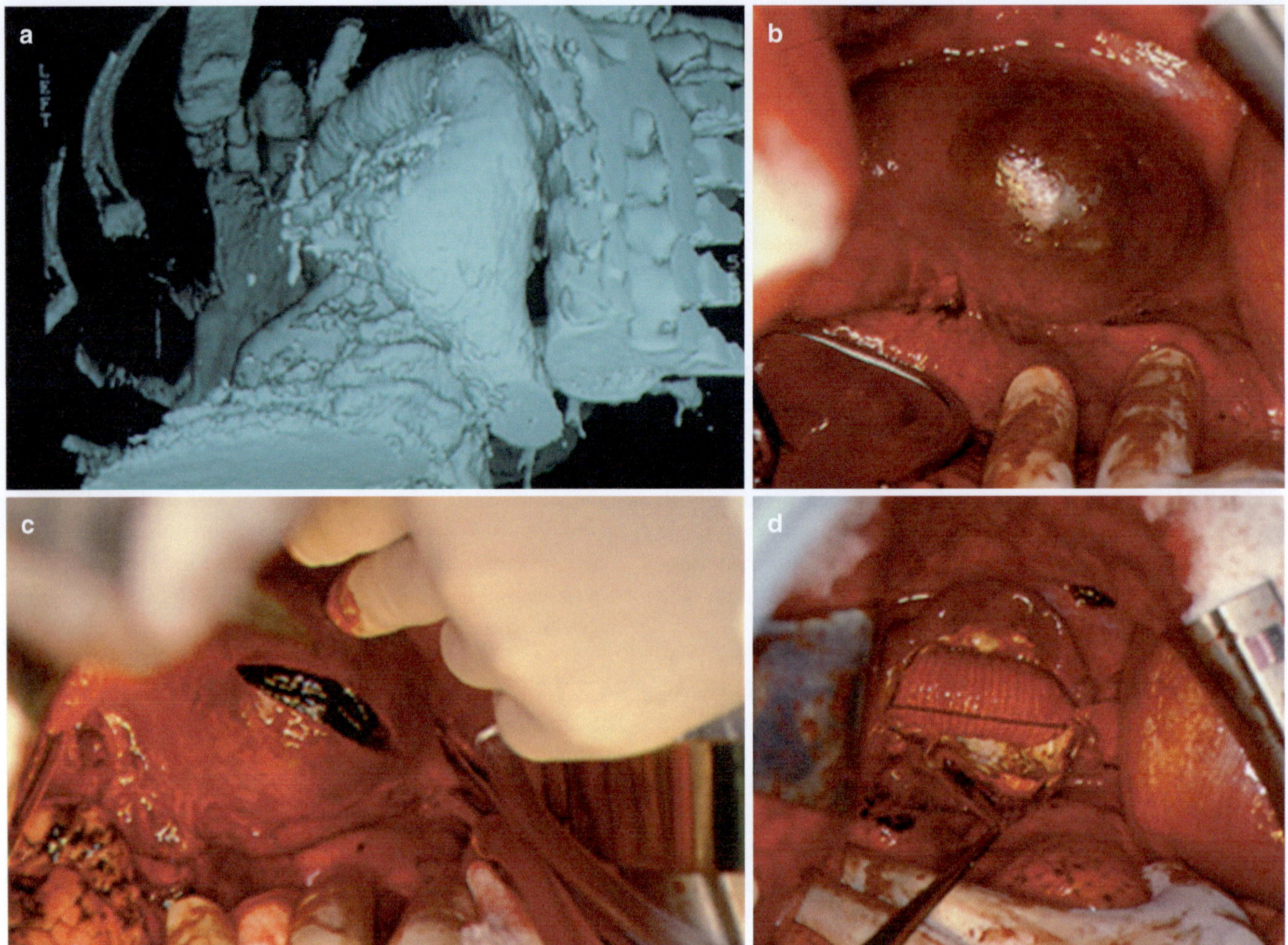

Fig. 34.50 Case 1. (**a**) Helical CT: a dilatation of the isthmic aorta is shown in a post-traumatic rupture. (**b**) At surgery, in the aortic isthmic area the adventitial hematoma. (**c**) The area is incised, and a huge hematoma encircling the aortic disruption is evident. (**d**) Final aspect after reconstruction of the aorta with Dacron graft interposition

size discrepancy along the diseased aorta: in the young patient, there is often a discrepancy in diameter between the aortic arch and the descending aorta. For this reason, a conic graft is often preferred. The endovascular operation is performed trough a femoral incision, and the device is positioned under fluoroscopic control. TE echocardiography is very useful to control the exclusion of the pseudoaneurysm or the dissection site. Anyway, consider that concomitant traumatic lesions of the neck may contraindicate its use. Sometimes it is necessary to proceed to a coverage of the left subclavian artery to ensure enough proximal neck length. For this reason, it is important to monitor the arterial pressure in the left radial artery: the comparison with the right radial pressure can be a good indication of the achieved exclusion of the subclavian artery. The decision whether to perform a carotid-subclavian bypass is based on the clinical evaluation of the left hand vascularization, monitoring the arterial pressure (systolic pressure >50 mmHg). For this reason it is important to monitor the vascularization in the postoperative period and an angiographic catheter can be positioned in the contralateral femoral artery. After the delivery of the graft a post-dilation with a compliant balloon is not routinely necessary [84]. In Figs. 34.51 and 34.52 it is shown an isthmic aortic rupture in a 26-year-old woman treated with endografting.

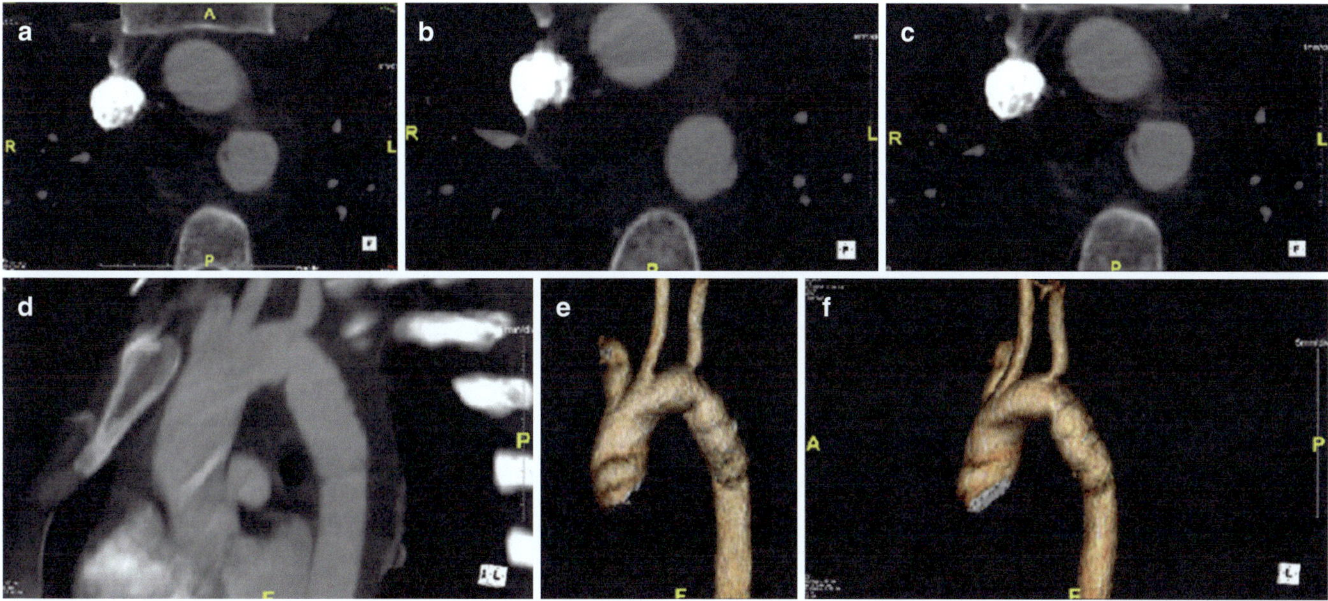

Fig. 34.51 Case 2. (**a**–**f**) Axial and 3D reconstruction showing an aortic dissection at isthmic level

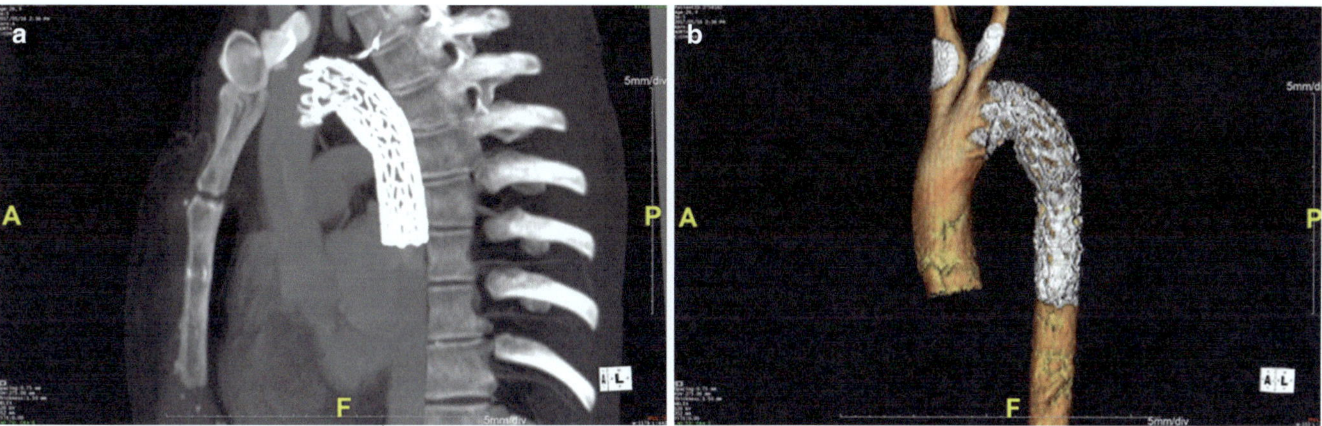

Fig. 34.52 (**a**, **b**) postoperative reconstruction after endografting of the aorta with complete coverage of the left subclavian artery

Case Scenario: Missing the diagnosis

We report two cases where the missed diagnosis determined the patient's death.

Case 1. A 39-year-old man went to the emergency department complaining chest pain that began about 24 h earlier and has not resolved despite painkiller assumption; the pain irradiated to the left arm, the neck, and the back. EKG was normal; chest X-ray showed a slight mediastinal enlargement, and echocardiography diagnosed ectasia in the aortic root and in ascending aorta, mild aortic insufficiency. Cardiac enzymes resulted negatives, an acute coronary syndrome was excluded, and the patient 24 h later was discharged with antacid therapy. He was found dead 4 h later. Autopsy showed cardiac tamponade, cause of death, and type A aortic dissection (Figs. 34.53, 34.54 and 34.55).

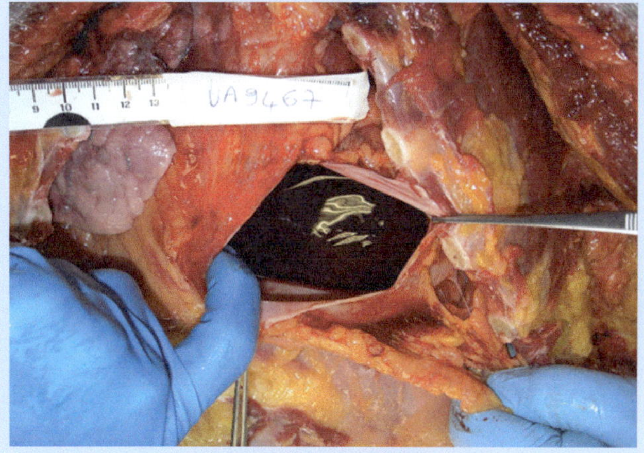

Fig. 34.53 Cardiac tamponade: pericardial cavity is filled with blood and clots

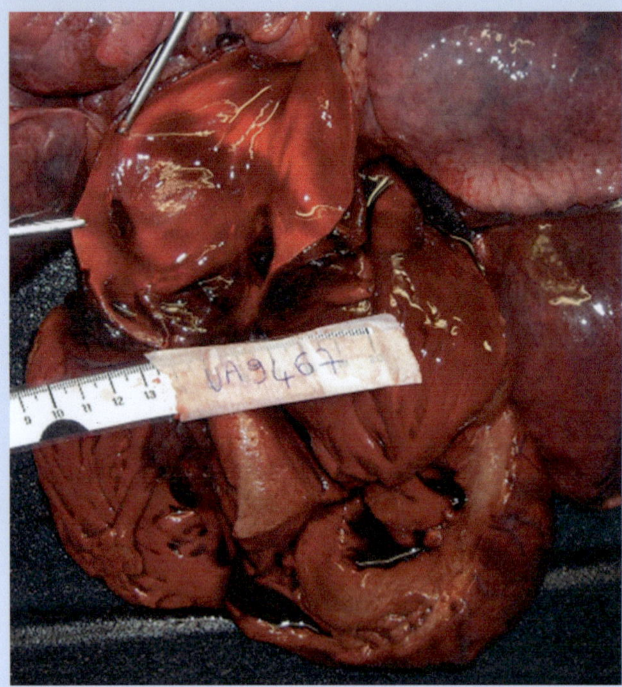

Fig. 34.54 The intimal tear above the noncoronary cusp of the aortic valve

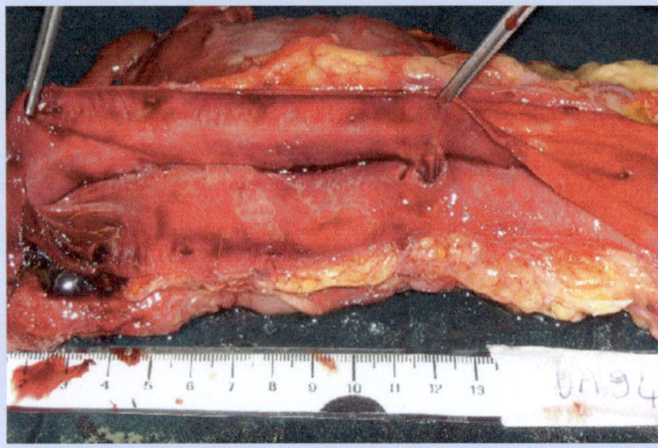

Fig. 34.55 The descending thoracic aorta showing the two lumens: the false pulled by forceps and the true presenting diffuse atherosclerotic plaques

1. Why the diagnosis was missed?
   A. History and physical examination were not considered and angio-CT was not prescribed.
   B. Mediastinal enlargement was not consistent at chest X-ray.
   C. Echocardiography did not show aortic dissection.
   D. Angio-CT was not prescribed.
2. Why transthoracic echocardiography did not help to get the right diagnosis?
   A. Echocardiography showed an aortic ecstasy and not an aortic dissection.
   B. Echocardiography is not indicated in this case.
   C. Cardiac tamponade was not found.
   D. The patient should be always considered examining all findings and signs.

Case 2. A 60-year-old man was admitted to the emergency department with sudden onset of chest pain, hypotension, and diplopia. Laboratory findings were normal, while chest X-ray showed an enlarged mediastinum (Fig. 34.56). Later, the patient reported a significant amelioration of chest pain, and diplopia was his complain that determined the missed diagnosis of type A aortic dissection. The patient was found dead after 5 days.

1. The right diagnosis was missed because:
   A. Patient's history and physical examination were not considered.
   B. Answers a and d.
   C. Transthoracic echocardiography was not prescribed.
   D. Angio-CT was not prescribed.
2. Sign and symptoms of vision problems are rarely found in thoracic aortic dissection.
   A. False.
   B. Vision problems are late.
   C. Vision problems can indicate cerebral perfusion impairment.
   D. Answers a and c.

Please see Chap. 58 for the correct answer.

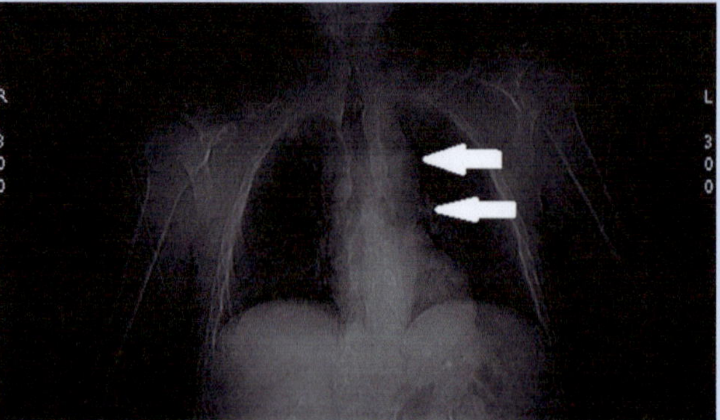

Fig. 34.56 Case 2. Chest X-ray showing a slight mediastinal enlargement (white arrows)

References

1. Vilacosta I, San Roman JA, Aragoncillo P, Ferreirós J, Mendez R, Graupner C, et al. Penetrating atherosclerotic aortic ulcer: documentation by transesophageal echocardiography. J Am Coll Cardiol. 1998;32:83–92.
2. Vilacosta I, San Roman JA. Acute aortic syndrome. Heart. 2001;85:365–8.
3. Lansman SL, Saunders PC, Malekan R, Spielvogel D. Acute aortic syndrome. J Thorac Cardiovasc Surg. 2010;140:S92–7.
4. Coady MA, Rizzo JA, Elefteriades JA. Pathologic variants of thoracic aortic dissections. Penetrating atherosclerotic ulcers and intramural hematomas. Cardiol Clin. 1999;17:637–57.
5. Vilacosta I, Aragoncillo P, Cañadas V, San Román JA, Ferreirós J, Rodríguez E. Acute aortic syndrome: a new look at an old conundrum. Heart. 2009;95(14):1130–9.
6. Krukenberg E. Beitrage zur Frage des Aneurysma dissecans. Beitr Pathol Anat Allg Pathol. 1920;67:329–51.
7. Yamada T, Takamiya M, Naito H, et al. Diagnosis of aortic dissection without intimal rupture by x-ray computed tomography. Nippon Acta Radiol. 1985;45:699–710.
8. Chou AS, Ziganshin BA, Charilaou P, Tranquilli M, Rizzo JA, Elefteriades JA. Long-term behavior of aortic intramural hematomas and penetrating ulcers. J Thorac Vasc Surg. 2016;151:361–73.
9. Roberts WC. Aortic dissection: anatomy, consequences, and causes. Am Heart J. 1981;101:195–214.
10. Wareing TH, Davila-Roman VG, Daily BB, Murphy SF, Schechtman KB, Barzilai B, et al. Strategy for the reduction of stroke incidence in cardiac surgical patients. Ann Thorac Surg. 1993;55:1400–8.
11. Harris KM, Braverman AC, Eagle KA, Woznicki EM, Pyeritz RE, Myrmel T, et al. Acute aortic intramural hematoma: an analysis from the International Registry of Acute Aortic Dissection. Circulation. 2012;126:S91–6.
12. Alomari IB, Hamirani YS, Madera G, Tabe C, Akhtar N, Raizada V. Aortic intramural hematoma and its complications. Circulation. 2014;129:711–6.
13. Ganaha F, Miller DC, Sugimoto K, Do YS, Minamiguchi H, Saito H, Mitchell RS, Dake MD. Prognosis of aortic intramural hematoma with and without penetrating atherosclerotic ulcer: a clinical and radiological analysis. Circulation. 2002;106:342–8.
14. Watanabe S, Hanyu M, Arai Y, Nagasawa A. Initial medical treatment for acute type a intramural hematoma and aortic dissection. Ann Thorac Surg. 2013;96:2142–6.
15. Erbel R, Aboyans V, Boileau C, Bossone E, Bartolomeo RD, Eggebrecht H, Evangelista A, Falk V, Frank H, Gaemperli O, Grabenwöger M, Haverich A, Iung B, Manolis AJ, Meijboom F, Nienaber CA, Roffi M, Rousseau H, Sechtem U, Sirnes PA, Allmen RS, Vrints CJ, ESC Committee for Practice Guidelines. 2014 ESC Guidelines on the diagnosis and treatment of aortic diseases: Document covering acute and chronic aortic diseases of the thoracic and abdominal aorta of the adult. The task force for the diagnosis and treatment of aortic diseases of the European Society of Cardiology (ESC). Eur Heart J. 2014;35:2873–926.
16. Kouchoukos NT, Blackstone EH, Hanley FL, Kirklin JK. Acute Aortic Dissection Chap 25: Kirklin/Barratt-Boyes cardiac surgery morphology, diagnostic criteria, natural history, techniques, results, and indications. Philadelphia: Elsevier Saunders; 2013. p. 942–72.
17. Howard DP, Banerjee A, Fairhead JF, Perkins J, Silver LE, Rothwell PM. Population based study of incidence and outcome of acute aortic dissection and premorbid risk factor control: 10-year results from the Oxford vascular study. Circulation. 2013;127:2031–7.
18. Olsson C, Thelin S, Stahle E, Ekbom A, Granath F. Thoracic aortic aneurysm and dissection: increasing prevalence and improved outcomes reported inanition wide population-based study of more than 14,000 cases from1987 to 2002. Circulation. 2006;114:2611–8.
19. Hagan PG, Nienaber CA, Isselbacher EM, Bruckman D, Karavite DJ, Russman PL, Evangelista A, Fattori R, Suzuki T, Oh JK, Moore AG, Malouf JF, Pape LA, Gaca C, Sechtem U, Lenferink S, Deutsch HJ, Diedrichs H, Marcos y Robles J, Llovet A, Gilon D, Das SK, Armstrong WF, Deeb GM, Eagle KA. The International Registry of Acute Aortic Dissection (IRAD): new insights into an old disease. JAMA. 2000;283:897–903.
20. Mussa FF, Horton JD, Moridzadeh R, Nicholson J, Trimarchi S, Eagle KA. Acute dissection and intramural hematoma. A systematic review. JAMA. 2016;316:754–63.
21. Falconi M, Oberti P, Krauss J, et al. Different clinical features of aortic intramural hematoma versus dissection involving the descending thoracic aorta. Echocardiography. 2005;22:629–35.
22. Harris KM, Strauss CE, Eagle KA, et al. Correlates of delayed recognition and treatment of acute type a aortic dissection. Circulation. 2011;124(18):1911–8.
23. Vagnarelli F, Corsini A, Bugani G, et al. Troponin T elevation in acute aortic syndromes. Eur Heart J Acute Cardiovasc Care. 2016;5:61–71.
24. Mintz GS, Kotler MN, Segal BL, Parry WR. Two dimensional echocardiographic recognition of the descending thoracic aorta. Am J Cardiol. 1979;44:232–8.
25. Khandheria BK, Tajik AJ, Taylor CL, Safford RE, FAJr M, Stanson AW, Sinak LJ, Oh JK, Seward JB. Aortic dissection: review of value and limitations of two dimensional echocardiography in a six-year experience. J Am Soc Echocardiogr. 1989;2:17–24.
26. Iliceto S, Ettorre G, Francioso G, Antonelli G, Biasco G, Rizzon P. Diagnosis of aneurysm of the thoracic aorta. Comparison between two non invasive techniques: two-dimensional echocardiography and computed tomography. Eur Heart J. 1984;5:545–55.
27. van Zaane B, Nierich AP, Buhre WF, Bruinsma GJBB, Moons KGM. Resolving the blind spot of transesophageal echocardiography: a new diagnostic device for visualizing the ascending aorta in cardiac surgery. Br J Anaesth. 2007;98:431–41.
28. Klomp WWJ, Peelen LM, Bruinsma GJBB, van't Hof AWJ, Grandjean JG, Nierich AP. Modified transesophageal echocardiography of the dissected thoracic aorta; a novel diagnostic approach. Cardiovasc Ultrasound. 2016;14:28.
29. Shiga T, Wajima Z, Apfel CC, Inoue T, Ohe Y. Diagnostic accuracy of transesophageal echocardiography, helical computed tomography, and magnetic resonance imaging for suspected thoracic aortic dissection: systematic review and meta-analysis. Arch Intern Med. 2006;166:1350–6.
30. Sommer T, Fehske W, Holzknecht N, Smekal AV, Keller E, Lutterbey G, et al. Aortic dissection: a comparative study of diagnosis with spiral CT, multiplanar transesophageal echocardiography, and MR imaging. Radiology. 1996;199:347–52.
31. Yoshida S, Akiba H, Tamakawa M, Yama N, Hareyama M, Morishita K, et al. Thoracic involvement of type A aortic dissection and intramural hematoma: diagnostic accuracy—comparison of emergency helical CT and surgical findings. Radiology. 2003;228:430–5.
32. Nienaber CA, von Kodolitsch Y, Nicolas V, Siglow V, Piepho A, Brockhoff C, Koschyk DH, Spielmann RP. The diagnosis of thoracic aortic dissection by noninvasive imaging procedures. N Engl J Med. 1993;328:1–329.
33. Isselbacher EM, Cigarroa JE, Eagle KA. Cardiac tamponade complicating proximal aortic dissection: is pericardiocentesis harmful? Circulation. 1994;90:2375–8.
34. Frederick JR, Yang E, Trubelja A, et al. Ascending aortic cannulation in acute type a dissection repair. Ann Thorac Surg. 2013;95:1808–11. https://doi.org/10.1016/j.athoracsur.2012.10.086.
35. Suzuki T, Asai T, Matsubayashi K, et al. Safety and efficacy of central cannulation through ascending aorta for type A aortic dissection. Interact Cardiovasc Thorac Surg. 2010;11:34–7. https://doi.org/10.1510/icvts.2009.231852.

36. Asai T, Suzuki T, Kinoshita T, Sakakura R, Minamidate N, Vigers P. The direct aortic cannulation for acute type A aortic dissection. Ann Cardiothorac Surg. 2016;5:401–3.
37. Tiwari KK, Murzi M, Bevilacqua S, Glauber M. Which cannulation (ascending aortic cannulation or peripheral arterial cannulation) is better for acute type a aortic dissection surgery? Interact Cardiovasc Thorac Surg. 2010;10:797–802. https://doi.org/10.1510/icvts.2009.230409.
38. Huang FJ, Wu Q, Ren CW, Lai YQ, Yang S, Rui QJ, Xu SD. Cannulation of the innominate artery with a side graft in arch surgery. Ann Thorac Surg. 2010;89(3):800–3.
39. Banbury MK, Cosgrove DM 3rd. Arterial cannulation of the innominate artery. Ann Thorac Surg. 2000;69:957.
40. Di Eusanio M, Quarti A, Pierri MD, Di Eusanio G. Cannulation of the brachiocephalic trunk during surgery of the thoracic aorta: a simplified technique for antegrade cerebral perfusion. Eur J Cardiothorac Surg. 2004;26(4):831–3.
41. Ji S, Yang J, Ye X, Wang X. Brain protection by using innominate artery cannulation during aortic arch surgery. Ann Thorac Surg. 2008;86(3):1030–2.
42. Stassano P, Musumeci A, Iannelli G, D'Alise G, Mottola M. A new cannula for innominate artery cannulation. J Thorac Cardiovasc Surg. 2005;130(3):944–5.
43. Preventza O, Bakaeen FG, Stephens EH, Trocciola SM, de la Cruz KI, Coselli JS. Innominate artery cannulation: an alternative to femoral or axillary cannulation for arterial inflow in proximal aortic surgery. J Thorac Cardiovasc Surg. 2013;145(3 Suppl):S191–6.
44. Reece TB, Tribble CG, Smith RL, Singh RR, Stiles BM, Peeler BB, Kern JA, Kron IL. Central cannulation is safe in acute aortic dissection repair. J Thorac Cardiovasc Surg. 2007;133:428–34.
45. Reuthebuch O, Schurr U, Hellermann J, Prétre R, Künzli A, Lachat M, Turina MI. Advantages of subclavian artery perfusion for repair of acute type A dissection. Eur J Cardiothorac Surg. 2004;26:592–8.
46. Neri E, Massetti M, Capannini G, Carone E, et al. Axillary artery cannulation in type A aortic dyssection operations. J Thorac Cardiovasc Surg. 1999;118:324–9.
47. Kaul P. How I do it—sole innominate cannulation for acute type A aortic dissection. J Cardiothorac Surg 2012; 7:125. http://swww.cardiothoracicsurgery.org/content/7/1/125.
48. Yan TD, Bannon PG, Bavaria J, Coselli JS, Elefteriades JA, Griepp RB, Hughes GC, LeMaire SA, Kazui T, Kkpochoukos NT, Misfeld M, Mohr FW, Oo A, Svensson LG, Tian DH. Consensus on hypothermia in aortic arch surgery. Ann Cardiothorac Surg. 2013;2:163–8.
49. Englum BR, Andersen ND, Husain AM, Mathew JP, Hughes GC. Degree of hypothermia in aortic arch surgery—optimal temperature for cerebral and spinal protection: deep hypothermia remains the gold standard in the absence of randomized data. Ann Cardiothorac Surg. 2013;2:184–93.
50. Englum BR, Kamiya H, Hagl C, Kropivinitskaya I, et al. The safety of moderate hypothermic lower body circulatory arrest with selective cerebral perfusion: a propensity score analysis. J Thorac Cardiovasc Surg. 2007;133:501–9.
51. Pacini D, Leone A, Di Marco L, et al. Antegrade selective cerebral perfusion in thoracic aorta surgery: safety of moderate hypothermia. Eur J Cardiothorac Surg. 2007;31:618–22.
52. Suzuki T, Asai T, Nota H, et al. Selective cerebral perfusion with mild hypothermic lower body circulatory arrest is safe for aortic arch surgery. Eur J Cardiothorac Surg. 2013;43(4):e94–8.
53. Zierer A, El-Sayed Ahmad A, Papadopoulos N, et al. Selective antegrade cerebral perfusion and mild (28 degrees C—30 degrees C) systemic hypothermic circulatory arrest for aortic arch replacement: results from 1002 patients. J Thorac Cardiovasc. 2012;144:1042–9.
54. Urbanski PP, Lenos A, Bougioukakis P, et al. Mild-to-moderate hypothermia in aortic arch surgery using circulatory arrest: a change of paradigm? Eur J Thorac Cardiothorac Surg. 2012;41:185–91.
55. David TE, Armstrong S, Ivanov J, et al. Surgery for acute type A aortic dissection. Ann Thorac Surg. 1999;67:1999–2001. discussion 2014-2019.
56. Grabenwoger M, Weiss G. Type A aortic dissection: the extent of surgical intervention. Ann Cardiothorac Surg. 2013;2:212–5.
57. Hussain ST, Svensson LG. Surgical techniques in type A dissection. Ann Cardiothorac Surg. 2016;5:233–5.
58. Coselli JS, LeMaire SA, Walkes J-C. Surgery for acute type A dissection. Oper Tech Thorac Cardiovasc Surg. 1999;4:13–32.
59. Borst HG, Walterbusch G, Schaps D. Extensive aortic replacement using "elephant trunk" prosthesis. Thorac Cardiovasc Surg. 1983;31:37–40.
60. Crawford ES, Coselli JS, Svensson LG, Safi HJ, Hess KR. Diffuse aneurysmal disease (chronic aortic dissection, Marfan, and mega aorta syndromes) and multiple aneurysm. Treatment by subtotal and total aortic replacement emphasizing the elephant trunk operation. Ann Surg. 1990;211:521–37.
61. Nienaber CA, Rousseau H, Eggebrecht H, et al. Randomized comparison of strategies for type B aortic dissection: the INvestigation of STEnt Grafts in Aortic Dissection (INSTEAD) trial. Circulation. 2009;120:2519–28.
62. Swee W, Dake MD. Endovascular management of thoracic dissection. Circulation. 2008;117:1460–73.
63. Hartnell GG, Gates J. Aortic fenestration: a why, when, and how-to guide. Radiographics. 2005;25:175–89.
64. Greenberg RK, Clair D, Srivastava S, Bhandari G, Turc A, Hampton J, et al. Should patients with challenging anatomy be offered endovascular aneurysm repair? J Vasc Surg. 2003;38:990–6.
65. Quevedo HC, Santiago-Trinidad R, Castellanos J, Atianzar K, Anwar A, i Rafeh NA. Systematic review of interventions to repair ascending aortic pseudoaneurysms. Ochsner J. 2014;14:576–85.
66. Razzouk A, Gundry S, Wang N, et al. Pseudoaneurysms of the aorta after cardiac surgery or chest trauma. Am Surg. 1993;59:818–23.
67. Deshpande A, Mossop P, Gurry J, et al. Treatment of traumatic false aneurysm of the thoracic aorta with endoluminal grafts. J Endovasc Surg. 1998;5:120–5.
68. Luk A, David TE, Butany J. Complications of Bioglue postsurgery for aortic dissections and aortic valve replacement. J Clin Pathol. 2012;65:1008–12.
69. Rosu C, Beauieu N, Cartier R, Demers P. Pseudoaneurysm as late complications of hybrid aortic arch repair. Innovations. 2016;11:360–2.
70. Eggebrecht H, Thompson M, Rousseau H, Czerny M, Lonn L, Mehta RH, et al. Retrograde ascending aortic dissection during or after thoracic aortic stent graft placement: insight from the European registry on endovascular aortic repair complications. Circulation. 2009;120(11 Suppl):S276–81.
71. Richens D, Kotidis K, Neale M, Oakley C, Fails A. Rupture of the aorta following road traffic accidents in the United Kingdom 1992-1999. The results of the co-operative crash injury study. Eur J Cardio Thorac Surg. 2003;23:143–8.
72. Bertrand S, Cuny S, Petit P, Trosseille X, Page Y, Guillemot H, et al. Traumatic rupture of thoracic aorta in real-world motor vehicle crashes. Traffic Inj Prev. 2008;9:153–61.
73. Grande AM, Eren EE, Halmann GL, Cooley DA. Rupture of the thoracic aorta: emergency treatment and management of chronic aneurysms. Tex Heart Inst J. 1984;11:244–9.
74. Gavant ML. Helical CT grading of traumatic aortic injuries. Impact on clinical guidelines for medical and surgical management. Radiol Clin North Am. 1999;37:553–74. vi.
75. Demers P, Miller C, Scott Mitchell R, et al. Chronic traumatic aneurysms of the descending thoracic aorta: mid-term results of endovascular repair using first and second-generation stent-grafts. Eur J Cardiothorac Surg. 2004;25:394–400.
76. Harris DG, Rabin J, Kufera JA, Taylor BS, Sarkar R, O'Connor JV, Scalea TM, Crawford RS. A new aortic injury score predicts early rupture more accurately than clinical assessment. J Vasc Surg. 2015;61:332–8.

77. Tatou E, Steinmetz E, Jazayeri S, Benhamiche B, Brenot R, David M. Surgical outcome of traumatic rupture of the thoracic aorta. Ann Thorac Surg. 2000;69:70–3.
78. von Oppell UO, Dunne TT, De Groot MK, Zilla P. Traumatic aortic rupture: twenty-year meta-analysis of mortality and risk of paraplegia. Ann Thorac Surg. 1994;58:585.
79. Coselli JS, LeMaire SA, Miller CC 3rd, et al. Mortality and paraplegia after thoracoabdominal aortic aneurysm repair: a risk factor analysis. Ann Thorac Surg. 2000;69(2):409–14.
80. Estrera AL, Miller CC 3rd, Huynh TT, Porat E, Safi HJ. Neurologic outcome after thoracic and thoracoabdominal aortic aneurysm repair. Ann Thorac Surg. 2001;72(4):1225–31.
81. Cambria RP, Clouse WD, Davison JK, Dunn PF, Corey M, Dorer D. Thoracoabdominal aneurysm repair: results with 337 operations performed over a 15-year interval. Ann Surg. 2002;236(4):471–9.
82. Doppman JL. Paraplegia after surgery for thoracoabdominal aneurysms: Russian roulette for the vascular surgeon [editorial]. Radiology. 1993;189:27–8.
83. Yoshioka K, Niinuma H, Ehara S, Nakajima T, Nakamura M, Kawazoe K. MR angiography and CT angiography of the artery of Adamkiewicz: state of the art. Radiographics. 2006;26:S63–73.
84. Chandrasekhar J, Allada C, O'Connor S, Rahman M, Shadbolt B, Farshid A. Efficacy of non-compliant balloon post-dilation in optimization of contemporary stents: A digital stent enhancement study. IJC Heart & Vessels 2014; 3:43-48.

35 Update in the Management of Non-traumatic Thoracoabdominal Vascular Emergencies

Stefano Pirrelli, Alessandro Mazzola, Giulia Ticozzelli, Isabella Maria Bianchi, Maria di Matteo, and Pietro Quaretti

Key Points

- Under anesthesiological point of view, in emergency always monitor right radial artery (in endovascular repair) and left femoral artery (in open repair) and position a single endotracheal tube in endo-repair or double-lumen in open repair. Always CSF is mandatory, in open repair, while in endo repair only if extensive coverage is expected.
- In emergency, open technique always prepare the patient for extracorporeal cannulation and cooling especially in dissecting aneurysm.
- In emergency, if possible, an endovascular approach is preferable.
- The 24-h availability of various sizes of thoracic graft and cover graft, in your hospital, allows you to treat with an endovascular technique almost all the patients.
- The patient must be treated in centers with experiences in both techniques open and endovascular.

35.1 Epidemiology

Improvement in imaging modalities has led to increased diagnosis and awareness of thoracoabdominal aortic diseases and their potentially lethal outcome. Despite progress in anesthetic and surgical management, open and endovascular repair of the thoracoabdominal aorta has remained a challenging operation with potential catastrophic complications as paraplegia and renal failure. Sound judgment is required to decide whether or not an elective operation is justified. This should be based on an understanding of the natural history of thoracic aortic pathology. Etiology of thoracoabdominal pathology has been divided into two groups, dissecting and nondissecting. Atherosclerotic or degenerative etiology is the main nondissecting etiology for approximately 80% of these aneurysms. Dissecting thoracoabdominal aneurysms have been associated with an increased production of symptoms and an increased risk of death from rupture. The presence of dissection decreased the 5-year survival in patients with TAAA from 71% without dissection to 46% if the aneurysm was associated with dissection. The male-female ratio was established to average 2:1 for nondissecting pathology. This gender ratio increased to an average of 3:1 for dissecting pathology. Gender difference was found to have no impact on the risk of rupture and the expansion rate of aneurysms, while the female sex was found to be associated with an increased risk of postoperative death [1]. Patients often have a high prevalence of comorbidities like hypertension

S. Pirrelli (✉)
Chief Unit of Vascular Surgery, Cardiothoracovascular Department, Asst Mantova, Ospedale Carlo Poma, Mantova, Italy
e-mail: stefano.pirrelli@asst-mantova.it

A. Mazzola
Cardiac Surgery, IRCCS Multimedica Sesto S. Giovanni, Milano, Italy

G. Ticozzelli · I. M. Bianchi
Department of Anesthesia and Intensive Care Unit, Foundation IRCCS Policlinico S. Matteo, Pavia, Italy
e-mail: g.ticozzelli@smatteo.pv.it

M. di Matteo
Department of Anesthesia and Intensive Care Unit, University of Pavia, Pavia, Italy

P. Quaretti
Chief Interventional Radiology Unit, Foundation IRCCS Policlinico S. Matteo, Pavia, Italy
e-mail: p.quaretti@smatteo.pv.it

P. Aseni et al. (eds.), *Operative Techniques and Recent Advances in Acute Care and Emergency Surgery*, https://doi.org/10.1007/978-3-319-95114-0_35

(83%), coronary artery disease (35%), peripheral artery disease, and visceral occlusive disease (25%). Furthermore, chronic renal failure and chronic obstructive pulmonary disease were found to be predictive variables of early postoperative death.

35.2 Classification

Thoracoabdominal aneurysms can be classified according to the Crawford classification into four types with the adjunct of the fifth type by Safi (Fig. 35.1). Type I aneurysm extends from the level of the left subclavian artery to renal arteries. Type II involves the entire thoracic descending aorta at the level of the left subclavian artery, all the visceral branches, and finishes to the iliac arteries. Type III usually begins distal to T6 level extending to the iliac bifurcation. Type IV involves the supra-celiac aorta, at or below the diaphragm, to the iliac bifurcation, Safi's type V starts from middle descending to the renal arteries.

This classification still has an importance since it concerns the extent of the pathology, and it reflects the operative approach. The extent of involvement in the thoracoabdominal aorta is not associated with an increased risk of rupture.

The indication to proceed with operative repair of a TAAA must be based on the available information on the natural history of TAAA and the results of surgical repair. Data on the expansion rate and the risk of rupture of abdominal aortic aneurysms has led to clear recommended indications to proceed with operative repair for a 5 cm and greater or with rapid expansion. The information that a large aneurysm has a higher risk of rupture than a smaller one has been known for decades. The size of the aneurysm plays a role in surgical decision-making only when many other factors must be weighed in the scales of judgment. In a young good-risk patient, it is reasonable to proceed with AAA repair even for an aneurysm smaller than 5 cm although we do know the risk of rupture to be minimal. This rationale does not apply for small thoracoabdominal aneurysm because of the higher operative risk. The main criteria have remained the size. Patients with symptomatic aneurysms greater than 6 cm have a decreased 5-year survival of 61.1% versus 38.2% (size less than 6 cm). The presence of symptoms, of course, increases the risk of rupture. Knowledge of the expansion rate of the aneurysm is essential to properly manage small aneurysms which might be observed with serial CT scan. The estimated change in maximal diameter was found to be 0.43 cm per year. The presence of chronic obstructive pulmonary disease is the only factor associated with an increased expansion rate.

35.3 Diagnosis

Transesophageal echocardiography (TEE) has been the first-choice technique for a long time for the advantage to be performed in emergency and OR. The diagnostic sensibility is very high (98%) similar to NMR and spiral CT; however the specificity is inferior (77%) due to false positive secondary to artifacts in the dilated aorta. Limits are the availability of an expert operator and the reduced visualization of the aortic arch for the presence of the left main bronchus. CT scan represents the diagnostic gold standard for the thoracoabdominal aorta with a sensibility of 94% and a specificity of 87%. The possibility of 3D reconstruction allows evaluating the coronary involvement and the exact morphology of the dissected flap.

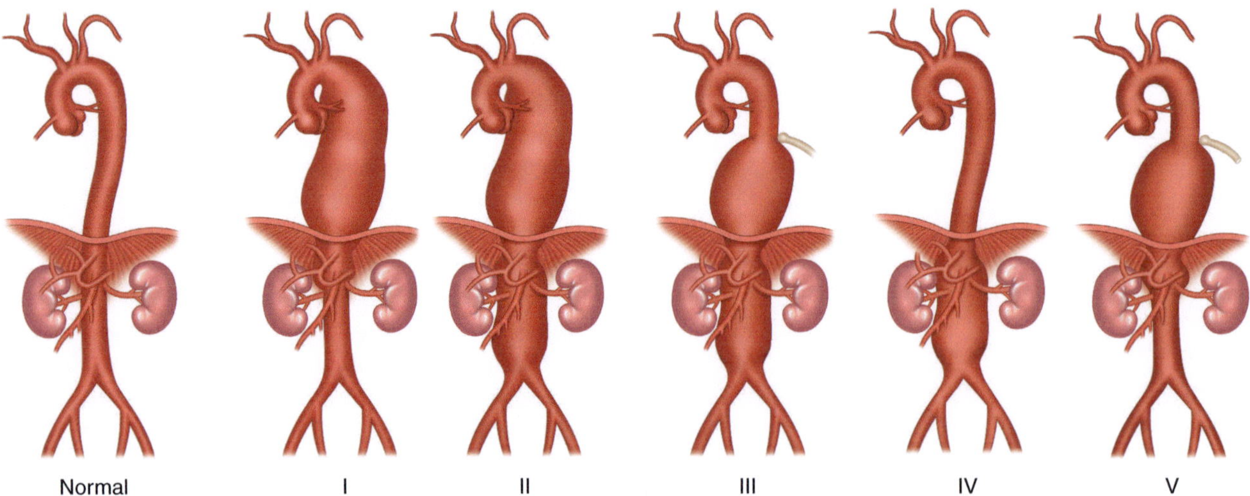

Fig. 35.1 Classification of aneurysms of dissecting and nondissecting origin according to the Crawford in four types with the adjunct of the fifth type by Safi

35.4 Treatment in Emergency

35.4.1 Patient Preoperative Assessment in Emergency

The preoperative assessment is crucial for the anesthesiologist to evaluate the real physiopathological status, evaluating the standard blood tests, stratifying the correlated risk, and, when possible, optimizing the medical therapy to improve the outcome [2].

In an urgent-emergent setting, this could not be possible because of the short period available. So what is the "ideal bundle care" in this situation? The anesthesiologist work must be focalized on feasible and efficient, but not time-consuming, protective organ strategies. *Cardiac* assessment should be used as an important criterion to evaluate the real functional capacity, because a poor one, measured as metabolic equivalents (METs), is associated with an increased incidence of postoperative cardiac events. METs evaluation can be useful to understand if the patient could fit for open repair (with very aggressive surgical approaches such as thoracotomy) or for an endovascular procedure (suitable anatomy), which represents a therapeutic solution for the high-risk patient. Preoperative plasma levels of biomarkers like cardiac troponins T and I, measured even in the postoperative days, are useful due to their sensibility and specificity. Other biomarkers such as pro-BNP and BNP, corrected for factors like renal dysfunction or obesity, should be considered. **Pulmonary** assessment is important too: chest X-ray and arterial blood gas analysis can be performed easily and quickly. The anesthesiologist must know if there is any evidence of tracheal or bronchial compression by the aneurysm. During open repair (OR), one-lung ventilation with a left-side double-lumen endotracheal tube (DLT) is necessary to proceed to left thoracotomy (during AATA type I, II, and III repair). **Renal** assessment is another important issue because of the high risk of renal injury following both the surgical and the endovascular approach. A protocol to prevent contrast-induced nephropathy (including hydration, administration of *N*-acetylcysteine, withdrawal of potential nephrotoxic drugs) must be undertaken as soon as possible. Arterial blood gas analysis can demonstrate a status of metabolic acidosis related to previous renal impairment. The hemostatic status is often altered, due to the vascular pathology and to patients' therapy. Most of the vascular patients take antiplatelet agents. The functional platelet assay could help to identify the therapeutic window to reduce the bleeding risk and to perform one of the most invasive anesthesiological procedures more safely, the cerebrospinal fluid (CFS) drainage [3]. According to the literature, there is a wide range, from 4 to 30%, of patients taking clopidogrel that are not responders to the drug: in this subgroup, with high on-treatment platelet reactivity, we could consider to perform CFS drainage in hemodynamically stable patients. The presence of an anticoagulant therapy with vitamin K antagonists (VKAs) should be checked with laboratory standard tests and, if available, with the point-of-care (POC) viscoelastic tests such as thromboelastography (TEG) or rotational thromboelastogram (ROTEM). The effect of the anticoagulant therapy must be antagonized with the administration of prothrombin concentrate complex (PCC) at the recommended dose of 25 up to 50 UI/kg, related to patient body weight and the INR value, and the administration of vitamin K 10 mg IV. The exact reversal of the drug can be monitored by laboratory standard tests or using POCs. The goal is to achieve an INR value below 1.5 as early as possible. Recent guidelines suggest the use of four-factor PCCs because it is a balanced drug, thanks to the presence of anticoagulant factor proteins C and S. The reversal of direct oral anticoagulants (DOAC) is more complex because the antidote for thrombin inhibitor (dabigatran), idarucizumab, is not widely available and the antidote for direct factor Xa inhibitors (rivaroxaban, apixaban, and edoxaban) is in experimental phase. As first-line therapy, four-factor PCCs can be used. We can monitor the efficacy of the reversal therapy with POC. The PCCs available on market available as three (II, IX, and X) or four factors (II, VII, IX, and X), allow for a rapid re-coagulation of the patient in order to avoid fresh frozen plasma and its transfusional collateral effects, such as hemodilution, allergic reaction, transfusion-related acute lung injury (TRALI), and transfusion acute cardiac overload (TACO) [4]. Once the patient is "recoagulated," we can proceed with the invasive anesthesiological procedures, in stable patients. All these procedures require a short time (up to 1 h) to be performed, and they can be crucial for end-organ protective strategies.

35.4.2 Intraoperative Management

Five-lead electrocardiogram is used to detect early signs of myocardial ischemia through the continuous monitoring of D2-V5 derivations. Right radial (or brachial) and right femoral artery lines are fundamental to measure, respectively, arterial pressure in the upper part of the body and the distal aortic perfusion pressure during partial cardiopulmonary bypass (CPB). Temperature control is important too: bladder and nasopharyngeal probes are required, in order to control a mild permissive hypothermia (core temperature of 32–34 °C) to prevent neurological injuries (paraparesis, paraplegia). The use of intraoperative monitoring with transesophageal echocardiography can help to guide the placement of the venous cannula of the CBP ant to detect any cardiac dysfunction. Because of the possibility of severe bleeding during

OR, a large-bore central catheter must be available (best 12.5 Fr high-flow) and additional central venous line may be disposable (the "double-stick" technique is simple and feasible using echo-guide, providing two large-bore catheters in the same central vein, usually right internal jugular vein). A rapid high-flow infusion device is fundamental to treat blood losses immediately and effectively. A goal-directed hemostatic therapy is essential to optimize the coagulation status and to reduce transfusions. TAAA repair is associated with a major risk of intraoperative bleeding and coagulopathy. This is related to several factors: hypothermia, acidosis, hemodilution, surgical bleeding, heparin administration, and continuous activation of the coagulation with consumption of clotting factors and fibrinogen. Heparin reversal could represent a major challenge for the anesthesiologist, and it could be guided by POCs; TEG and ROTEM can show residual heparin comparing reaction time R-kaolin TEG or clotting time CT-INTEM, respectively, with and without adding heparinase to the cuvette. Other pro-hemorrhagic factors are thrombocytopenia, platelet dysfunction, and hyperfibrinolysis. All these alterations may be monitored and corrected using POC coagulation tests [5]. Thrombocytopenia and platelet dysfunction can be treated with platelet concentrate transfusion; hyperfibrinolysis, monitored by D-dimers, FDP, and viscoelastic tests, can be treated with antifibrinolytic drugs such as tranexamic acid (TXA) at a dose of 12.5 mg/kg. In case of a severe bleeding, fibrinogen is the first factor to decrease critically, and its rapid restoration must be considered. The value of fibrinogen can be measured either by laboratory test (conventional Clauss method) or with POC. The viscoelastic tests measure clot firmness (TEG-MA maximum amplitude, ROTEM-MCF maximum clot firmness), which is determined by fibrinogen and platelets. Fibrinogen levels can be evaluated by using tests (TEG-FF and ROTEM-FIBTEM), which eliminate platelet contribution to clot strength [6]. The trigger value to fibrinogen administration is debated: Ranucci et al. propose a value of 115 mg/dL as a trigger value for fibrinogen supplementation in cardiac surgery [7]. Fibrinogen can be supplemented with different strategies. Fresh frozen plasma (FFP) is widely used to achieve this aim, but it contains fibrinogen at variable concentrations, and, consequently, large volumes are needed (about 30 mL/kg FFP increase fibrinogen concentration by 1 g/L). Hence, fibrinogen concentrate could be an effective and safer alternative, thanks to its high concentration (20 g/L) [8]. However, the concentrate is still not available to treat acquired bleeding in the UK and USA. Thus, we can affirm that the need of transfusion of allogenic blood components may be reduced and optimized targeting "all the prohemostatic strategies" guided by POC viscoelastic test (real-time, bedside, and time-sparing) or standard laboratory test. After the surgical or endovascular planning (aneurysm extension, coverage or reimplantation of left subclavian artery, coverage or reimplantation of the intercostal arteries, status of pelvic circulation, and previous abdominal aortic surgery), we would have to proceed with the insertion of CBF drainage (usually a 16-g needle), just before the final positioning of the patient. It must be inserted at the level of L3–L4, and the cerebrospinal fluid pressure (CBFP) must be monitored in continuous in order to measure the cerebrospinal fluid perfusion pressure.

Table 35.1 Summary of anesthesiological management in urgent-emergent setting of AATA

Anesthetic management in urgent/emergent setting	Endovascular	Open repair
Arterial line	Right radial artery (planned with surgeon)	Right radial and femoral artery
Endotracheal tube	Single endotracheal tube	Left-side double-lumen (verifying the correct position with fiberscope)
Central venous access	Right or left internal jugular vein (echo-guide preferentially)	Right internal jugular vein with "double-stick" technique for seven of two large-bore catheters
Temperature probes	Nasopharyngeal	Nasopharyngeal and bladder
CSF drainage	Yes for extensive aortic coverage, coverage or reimplantation of left subclavian artery	Yes if AATA types I, II, and III
NIRS	Cerebral and spinal	Cerebral and spinal
MEP and SSEP	Not available	Not available
POC	Recommended	Recommended

Ischemic spinal cord injury (SCI) remains the most devastating complication after TAAA repair by any modality. Main risk factors for SCI after TAAA repair are listed in Table 35.1. The risk of SCI may also be described according to the "Crawford classification," [9] even with the recent advances in neuroprotective strategies, and CSF drainage types I and type II remain the categories associated with the highest percentages of SCI (Fig. 35.1). TEVAR offers a less invasive approach, but it is still associated with a significant risk of SCI. Crawford et al. reported a significant increase in the incidence of permanent SCI for ruptured thoracic aneurysm compared to elective repair [10]. In a more recent case series, Gaudino and colleagues reported that the risk of SCI was not significantly higher in the ruptured group [11] (Table 35.2, Fig. 35.2).

Monitoring spinal cord viability is crucial to prevent SCI. The use of motor-evoked potentials (MEPs) and somatosensory-evoked potentials (SSEPs) has been reported to guide therapeutic maneuverers (CSF drainage, MAP augmentation, and CVP lowering) during TAAA repairs. Even though evoked potentials are widely accepted, they are challenging, invasive, and not available for postoperative surveillance. The use of NIRS has been proposed for monitoring

SCI. According to the "collateral network" concept [21], blood supply to the spinal cord is provided by a rich network of intra- and paraspinous arterial collaterals that enables sufficient blood flow when segmental arteries are occluded. NIRS optodes used to detect paraspinous muscle oxygenation may provide an indirect, noninvasive, real-time monitoring of spinal cord blood flow. In particular, monitoring paraspinous vasculature at lumbar level seems to identify spinal malperfusion during TAAA repair. NIRS measurements can be easily performed in the postoperative period for delayed SCI detection [22, 23]. Performing cerebrospinal fluid drainage (CSFD) is suggested as a class I recommendation, level of evidence B in high-risk patients undergoing both open repair and endovascular thoracic aortic repair, by current American Heart Association guidelines [24]. Several studies also support the effects of CSFD in preventing SCI [16, 19, 25–27]. On the other hand, important complications, such as subdural hematoma, have been reported [28, 29]. Complications of CSFD include those related to lumbar puncture, the presence of an indwelling catheter, and those connected to CSF drainage. In the setting of an urgent TAAA repair, CSFD should be used as protective measure only as the emergent situation may allow [30]. In fact, in a situation of hemodynamic instability, CSFD can be impracticable [31] like other organ-protective strategies. Furthermore, in the urgent TAAA repair, the risk associated with CSFD can be even higher because of concomitant coagulopathy or ongoing antiplatelet/anticoagulant therapy. Again, the use of point-of-care coagulation tests and a goal-directed, selective hemostatic approach might guide a safe CSF drain insertion. In literature, there is only a case report of such use of thromboelastometry to guide hemostatic therapy before CSFD placement and extraction in a patient with severe coagulopathy undergoing TEVAR [32]. Insertion of the lumbar CSF drain should ideally be performed in the awake patients, at L2–L4 level. CSF should be drained to maintain a pressure less than 10–15 mmHg. If signs of SCI develop, lowering goal pressure should be considered. In order to minimize the risk of intracranial hypotension and subdural hematoma, no more than 10–15 mL/h should be drained [12, 33]. Initial results with an automated, pressure-controlled system for CSF drainage have been reported. The spinal drain is generally maintained for 48–72 h if no symptoms of SCI develop. In case of delayed SCI, repeated drain placement has to be taken into account.

Table 35.2 Mechanisms of SCI in open repair and during TEVAR (adapted from ETZ [12])

Open repair	Tevar
Prolonged aortic cross-clamping	Covering of the left subclavian artery, intercostal and lumbar segmental arteries, hypogastric and sacral arteries
Decrease in mean arterial pressure	Previous distal aortic surgery
Increased in CSF pressure	Severe peripheral vascular disease
Insufficient distal perfusion	
Arterial steal phenomenon via patent segmental arteries	
Reperfusion injury	
Thrombosis of spinal cord-supplying vessels	

35.4.3 Open Surgical Technique

The surgical approach in emergency does not differ from one of the elective cases. The approach depends on the history of the patient (previous operations) and from the extension of the aneurysm. In case of previous arch surgery with a median sternotomy, it is important to guarantee a proximal control which can be reached through a fourth space left thoracotomy extended with a transversal sternotomy which can give the possibility to proceed to cannulation of

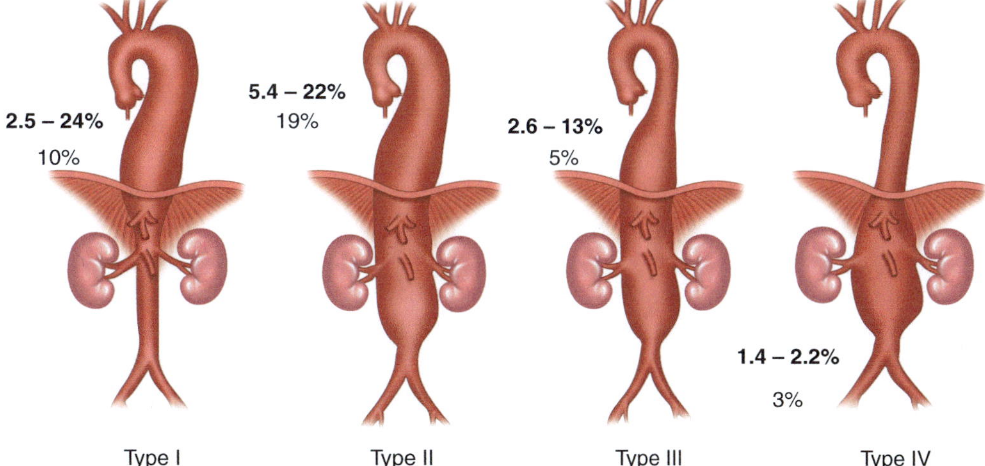

Fig. 35.2 Incidence of SCI according to aneurysm extent reported by experienced centers for TEVAR and open TAAA repair. Yellow figures refer to TEVAR, while black ones represent open repair data [13–20]

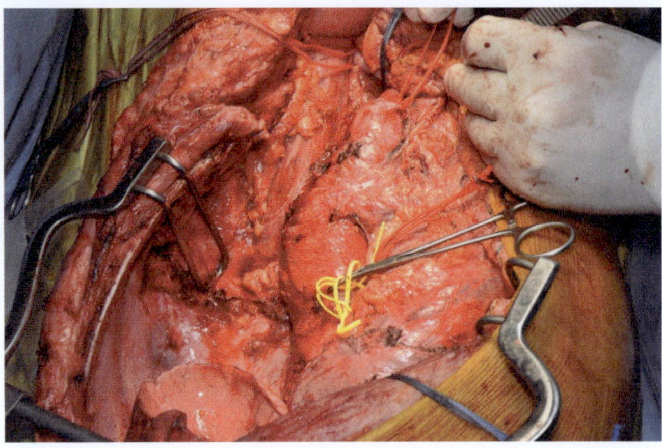

Fig. 35.3 View from the head of the patients: a thoracophrenolaparotomy has been performed and a surgical exposure of the whole thoracoabdominal aorta is reached

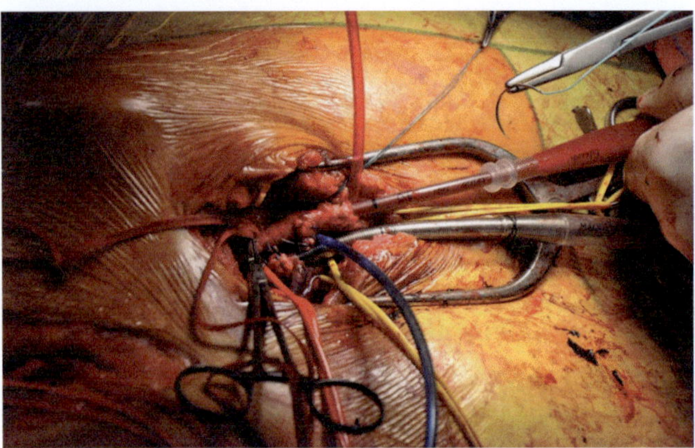

Fig. 35.4 The surgical exposure of femoral vessels can allow the cannulation to start with femoro-femoral extracorporeal circulation

supra-aortic trunks. In this case, the surgical isolation of the left axillary artery can give support for perfusion. The thoracotomy must be extended, depending on the level of the aneurysm in a radial phrenotomy and pararectal laparotomy. A second thoracotomy in the seventh space may be required. Visceral vessels and renal vessels must be accurately isolated at their origin (apart from the right renal artery) with vessel loops to prepare it for cannulation (Fig. 35.3). The aortic bifurcation can be easily reached, and also the origin of the right common iliac artery can be obtained without problems through extra- or transperitoneal space.

The surgical exposure of femoral vessels can allow the cannulation (Fig. 35.4) to start with femoro-femoral extracorporeal circulation.

Once the aorta is clamped proximally, a second clamp can be positioned just 10–15 cm below to guarantee, during the

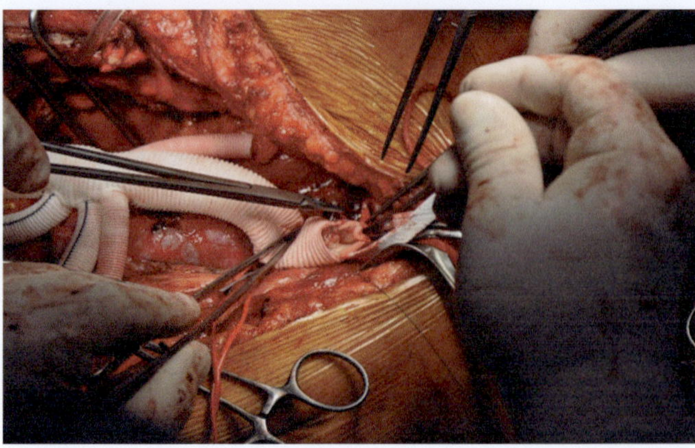

Fig. 35.5 The proximal anastomosis can be done with a 4/0 Prolene and must be reinforced with Teflon pledgets and with a glue

proximal anastomosis, the perfusion of visceral and intercostal arteries. The proximal anastomosis (Fig. 35.5) can be done with a 4/0 Prolene and must be reinforced with Teflon pledgets and with a glue.

The proximal anastomosis can be done with a 4/0 Prolene and must be reinforced with Teflon pledgets and with a glue.

In the thoracoabdominal aorta, a multibranched graft is used and no segment of the native aorta left (Fig. 35.7). This is true especially for genetic disease in which a late dilatation of the aorta can be observed. After the completion of the proximal anastomosis, the clamp is moved down along the aorta above the origin of the celiac axis, and a meticulous reimplantation of the intercostal arteries is achieved (Fig. 35.6).

Once the intercostal anastomosis is completed, a dedicated line of the arterial line is used for blood perfusion of spinal cord (Fig. 35.6).

The anastomosis on the intercostal arteries can be performed variously and reattached on the aortic graft in different shapes: C-shape (Fig. 35.7) or Y-shape (Fig. 35.8). Then the clamp is moved to the aortic bifurcation, the extracorporeal perfusion through the femoral artery is lowered for perfusion of the left hypogastric artery, and a complete separated cannulation of visceral vessels is achieved (Fig. 35.9).

Each visceral vessel is sutured with an end-to-end anastomosis to each branch of the graft and reinforced with a Teflon pledget (Fig. 35.10). After the completion of each anastomosis, the vessel is perfused with antegrade flow from the aortic graft (Fig. 35.11).

Then the diaphragm is reconstructed completely together with the integrity of thoracic and abdominal wall. A double drainage tube is positioned into the pleural space in paravertebral and supradiaphragmatic position and an additional drainage tube into the retroperitoneal space. No need for coverage of the graft.

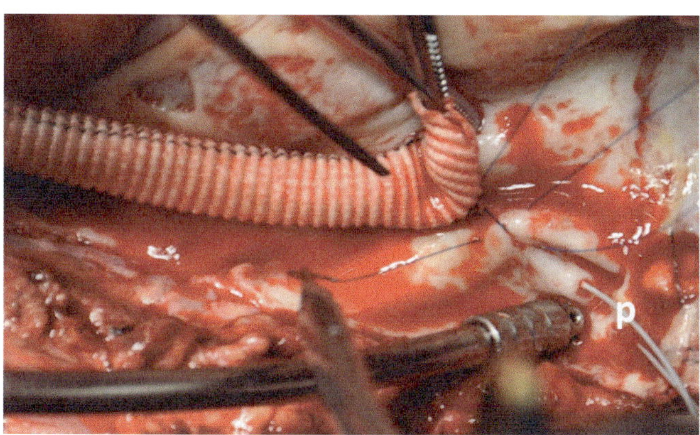

Fig. 35.6 Once the intercostal anastomosis is completed, a dedicated arterial line is used for blood perfusion of spinal cord (p)

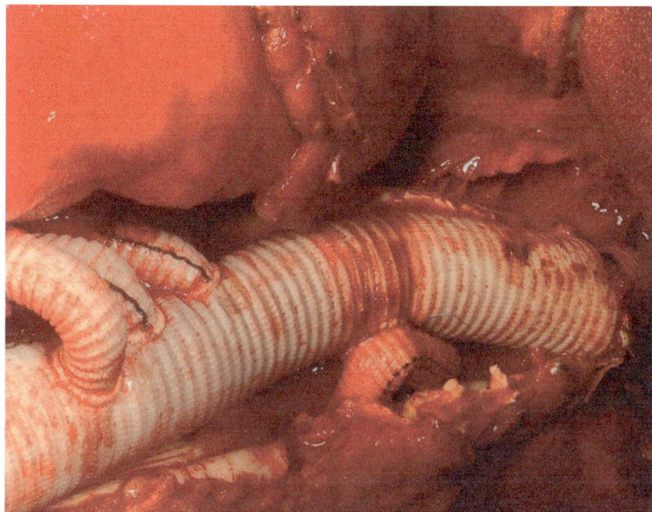

Fig. 35.7 The anastomosis on the intercostal arteries can be performed variously and reattached on the aortic graft in different shapes: C-shape

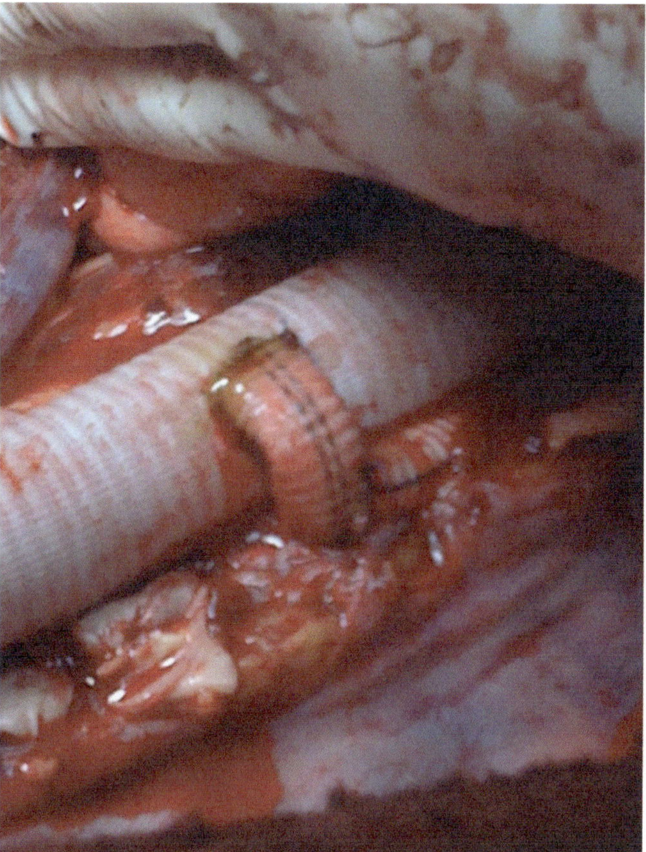

Fig. 35.8 The anastomosis on the intercostal arteries Y-shape

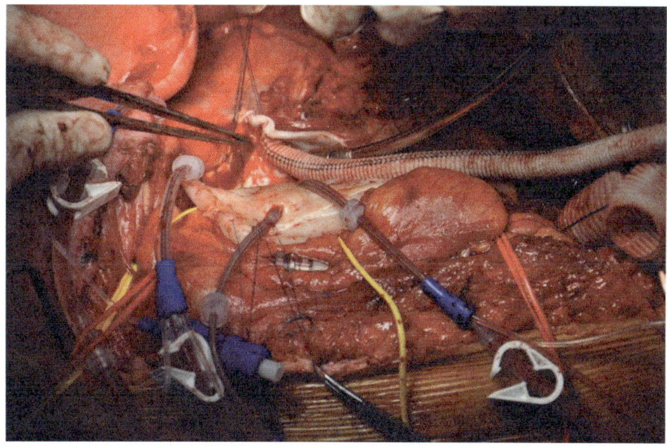

Fig. 35.9 The extracorporeal perfusion through the femoral artery is lowered for perfusion of the left hypogastric artery and a complete separated cannulation of visceral vessels is achieved

35.4.4 Endovascular Techniques in Emergency

In emergency, it is difficult to obtain a fenestrated graft because of the need for customization. So the possibilities of endovascular treatment in emergency are (1) the chimney-sandwich technique for atherosclerotic aneurysm and (2) the exclusion of the false lumen expansion in a patient with previous TEVAR in a dissected aorta.

35.4.4.1 Sandwich Techniques for Atherosclerotic Aneurysms

This technique, first described by Lobato [34], consists in the exclusion of the aneurysm with a double endovascular graft covering all the diseased aorta with revascularization of visceral vessels in the space between the grafts (Fig. 35.12).

With this technique, it is necessary to proceed to a surgical isolation of both the femoral and omeral arteries. In Figs. 35.13 and 35.14 is shown the CT scan of a huge 10 cm of diameter Type III thoracoabdominal aneurysm who arrived in emergency with thoracic pain.

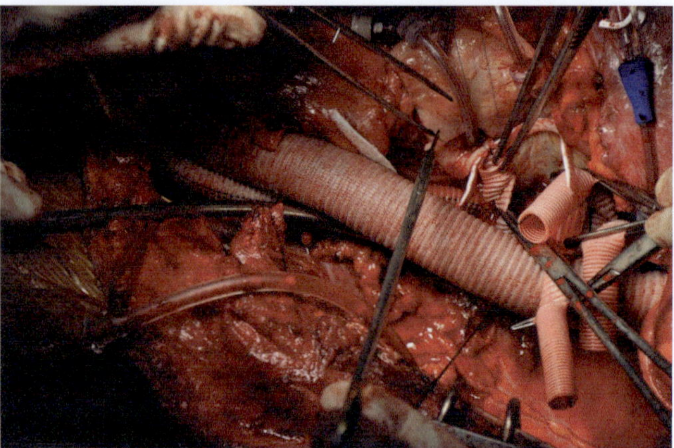

Fig. 35.10 Each visceral vessel is sutured with an end-to-end anastomosis to each branch of the graft and reinforced with a Teflon pledget

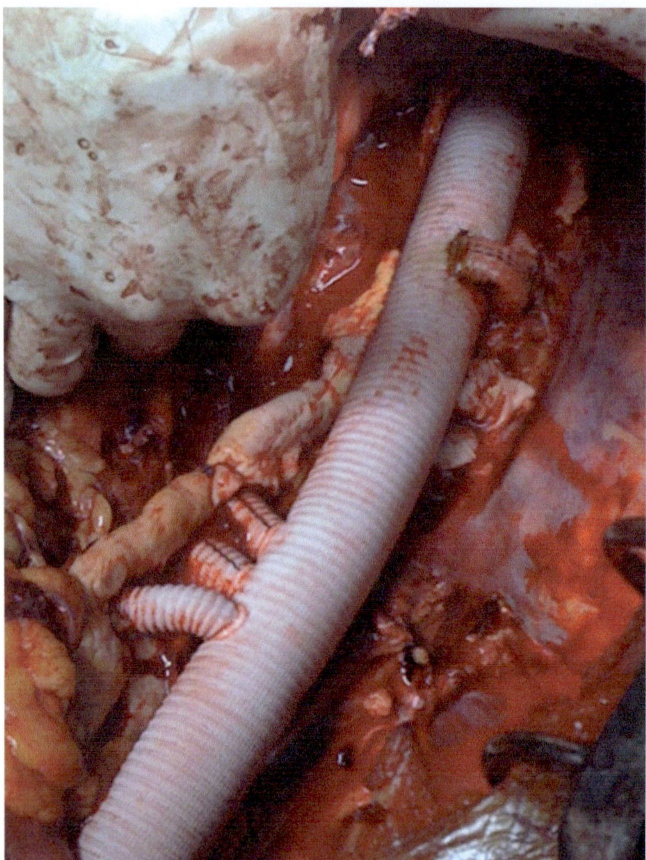

Fig. 35.11 After the completion of each anastomosis, the vessel is perfused with antegrade flow from the aortic graft

In this case, a 12 Fr introducer sheet 30 cm long is bilaterally introduced into the omeral arteries. From each side, it is possible to cannulate the renal arteries and the SMA and celiac trunk (Figs. 35.16, 35.17, and 35.18). Once the visceral vessels are cannulated, the first thoracic graft is advanced through one femoral artery. The graft is released

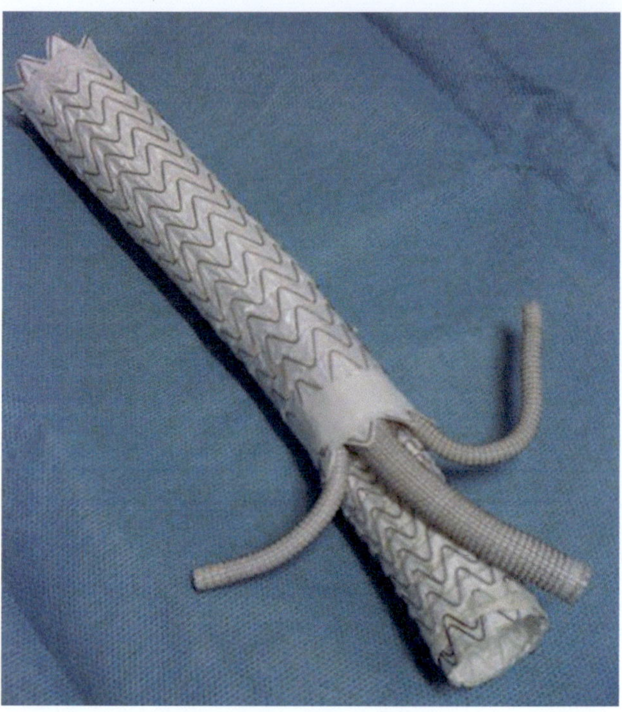

Fig. 35.12 An example of a "sandwich technique" with two thoracic PTFE grafts (Gore™) positioned and cover grafts for visceral vessels

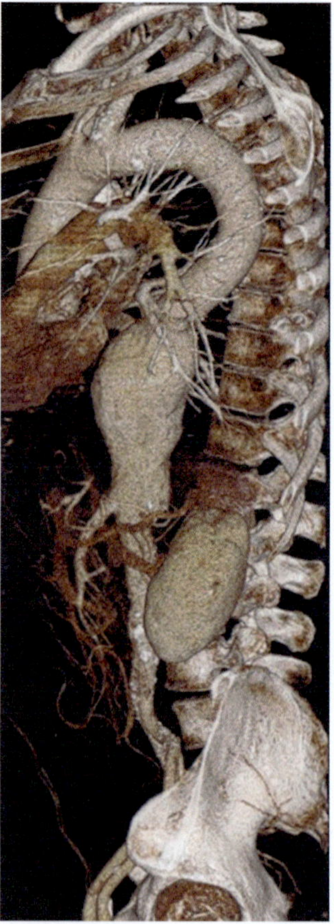

Fig. 35.13 A patient idoneous for the sandwich procedure (pre-op CT scan)

Fig. 35.14 Pre-op CT scan showing occlusion of the celiac axis and a type III TAA

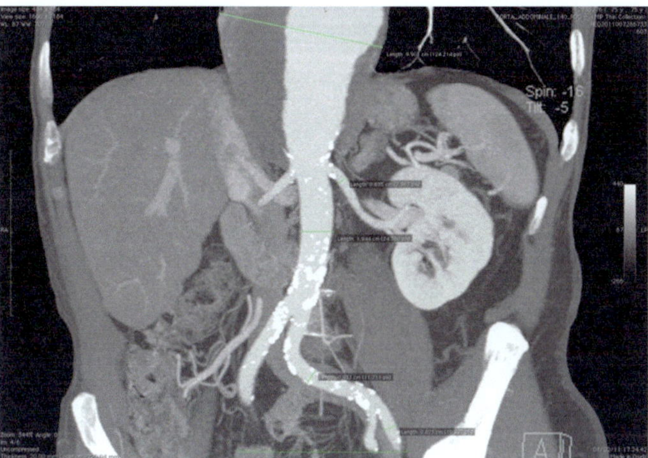

Fig. 35.15 Pre-op CT scan, sagittal view

from the proximal neck down to the origin of the celiac trunk (in the case described, the celiac trunk is occluded as you can see in Fig. 35.12).

After the opening of the first graft and the cannulation of all vessels, the second graft is delivered inside the first one at the level of the origin of the stent grafts for visceral arteries. After the release of the visceral stent graft, a rapid angiographic check is performed to control the patency of the vessels (Figs. 35.17 and 35.18).

Then the introducer is removed and the arteries closed.

In the early postoperative period, it is necessary to perform a CT scan to check the complete thrombosis of the aneurysmal sac because there is still the risk of blood perfusion through the space between the various grafts (gutter). In the CT scan performed after three months, there is the complete exclusion of the aneurysm (Figs. 35.17, 35.18, and 35.19). In the following Figs. 35.19, 35.20, and 35.21, a complete exclusion of the aneurysm is shown with patency of the visceral vessels.

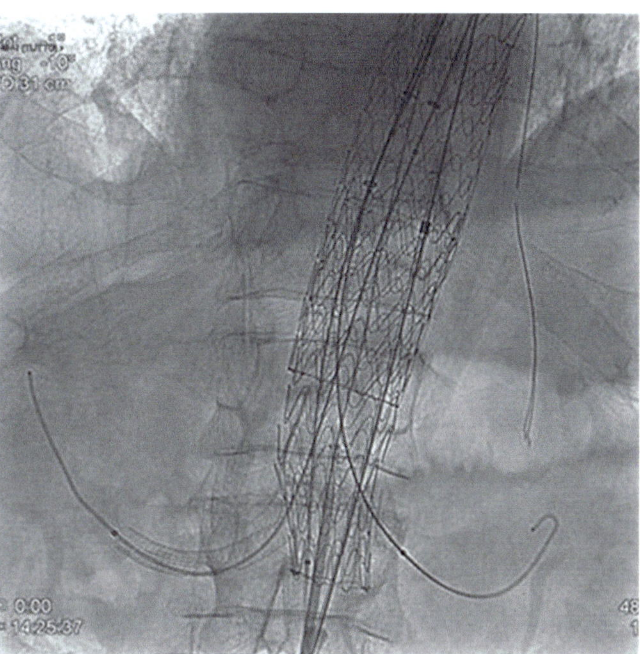

Fig. 35.16 A first thoracic graft has been positioned with the distal end just above the origin of the celiac trunk. The visceral vessel all cannulated from above through the omeral accesses. A second thoracic graft is positioned inside the first one according to Fig. 35.12

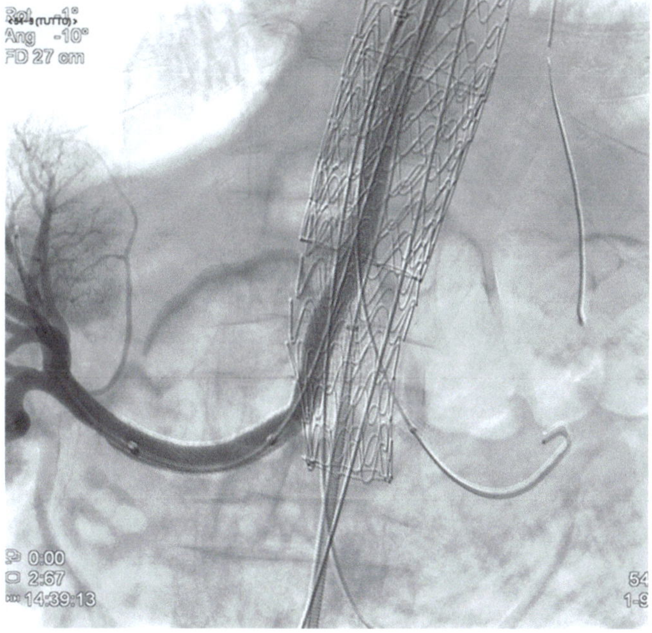

Fig. 35.17 A rapid angiographic check of the right renal artery is made

35.4.4.2 Candy-Plug Technique

This technique is used to exclude the dilated false lumen in a dissected aorta already treated with a frozen elephant trunk technique or a descending aorta endografting (TEVAR) (Figs. 35.22 and 35.23).

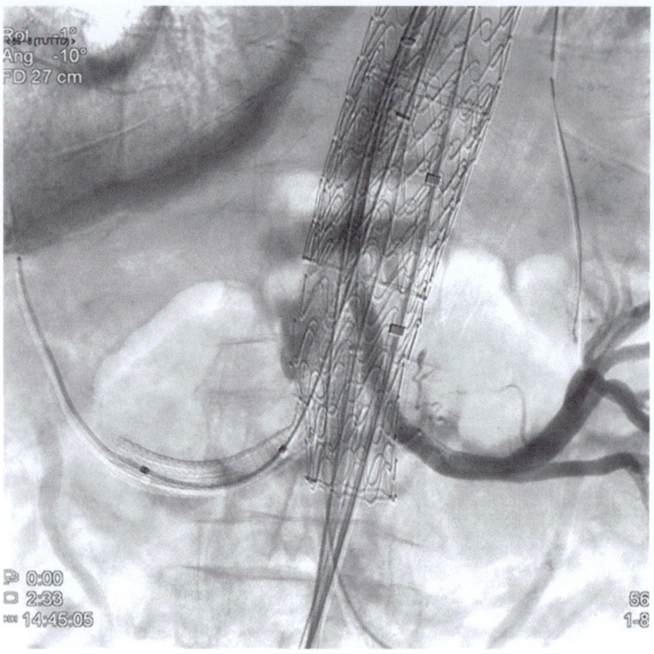

Fig. 35.18 A rapid angiographic check of the left renal artery is made

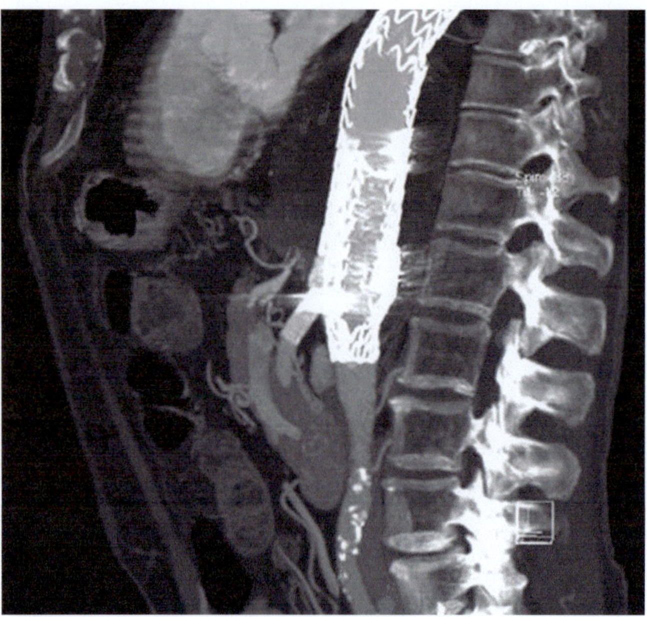

Fig. 35.19 Post-op CT scan showing patency of all the vessels treated

It consists in the positioning of a parallel graft or plug into the false lumen. The graft must be filled up with spiral coils to occlude completely the communication and the reperfusion from the entry tear below the distal end of the previous endovascular graft.

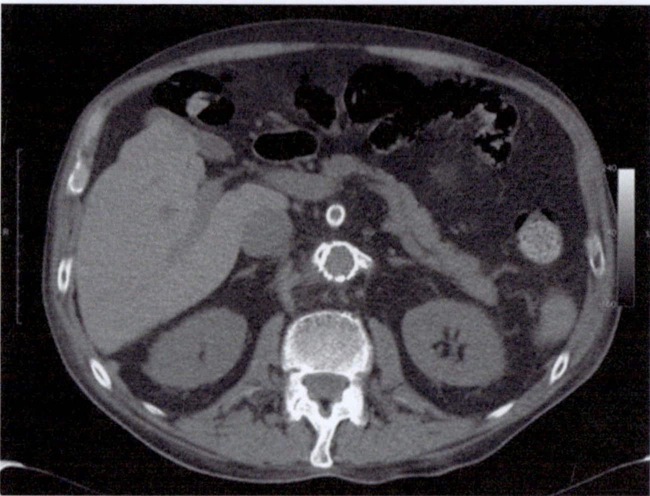

Fig. 35.20 Post-op CT scan showing patency of all the vessels treated

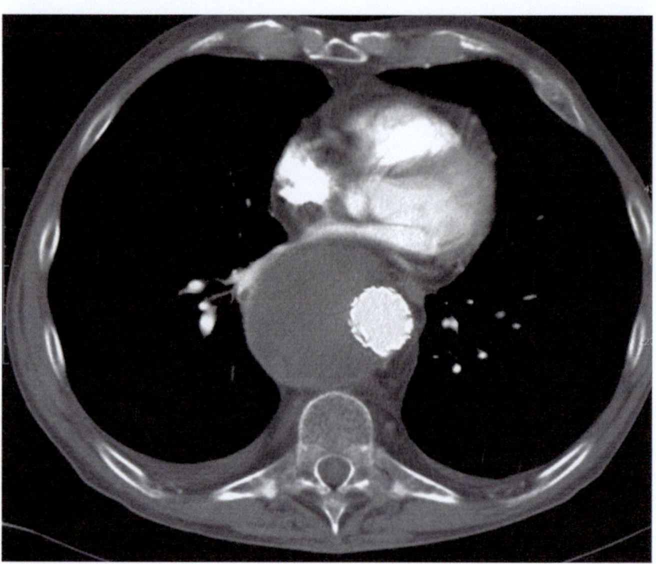

Fig. 35.21 Post-op CT scan showing complete exclusion of the aneurysm

In this case from the femoral artery, it is possible to cannulate the false lumen (Fig. 35.24).

After the cannulation of the false lumen, it is possible to close the false lumen with a plug or spiral coils to close the flow in the false lumen. In the case shown, the false lumen was too large. So we have decided to position a parallel graft and to fill it with spiral coils (Figs. 35.25, 35.26, and 35.27).

In Fig. 35.28 the complete exclusion of the false lumen sac is shown.

Fig. 35.22 Pre-op CT scan showing the endograft positioned into the thoracic aorta for a type A dissecting aneurysm involving the arch (frozen elephant trunk technique)

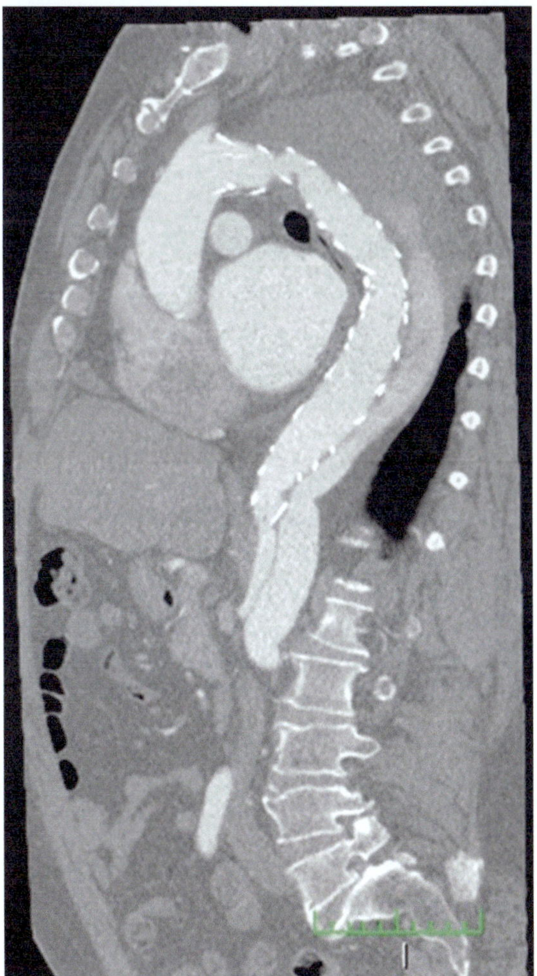

Fig. 35.23 The retroperfusion of the false lumen through a distal reentry tear brought to the enlargement of the false lumen aneurysmatic

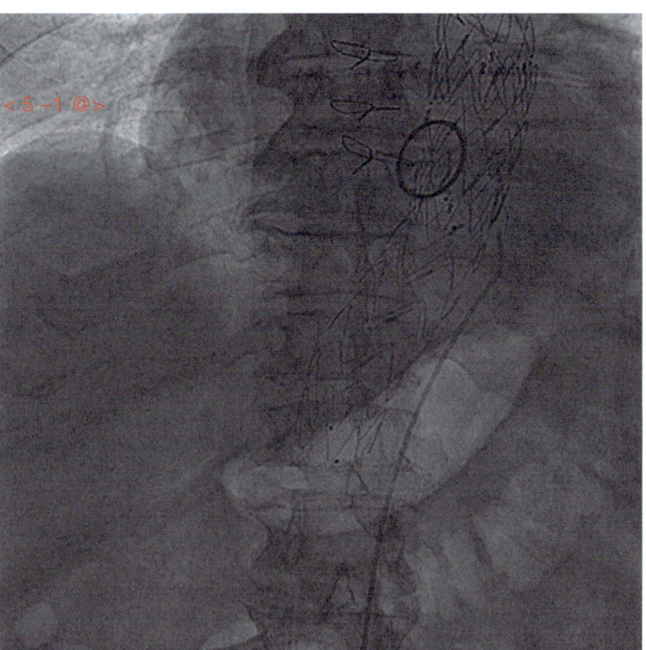

Fig. 35.24 Intraoperative angiographic study showing the cannulation of the false lumen through the femoral artery

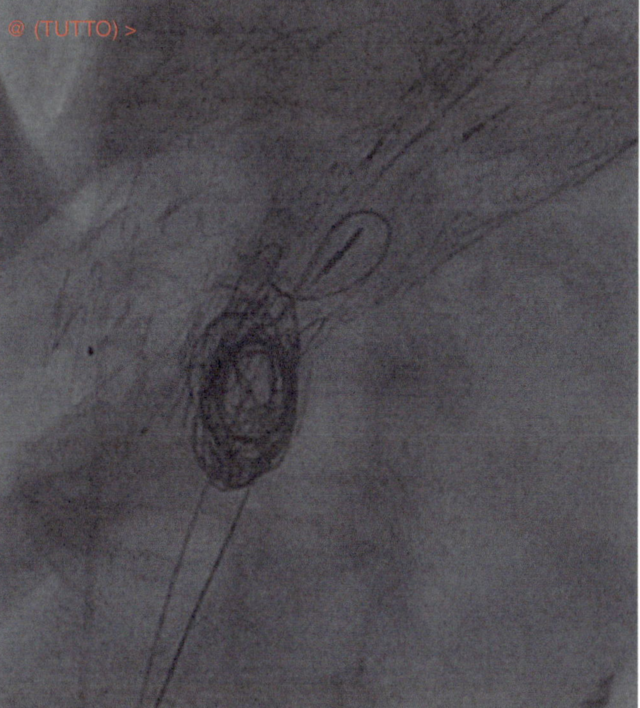

Fig. 35.25 Spiral coils are positioned into the false lumen just above the origin of the reentry tear

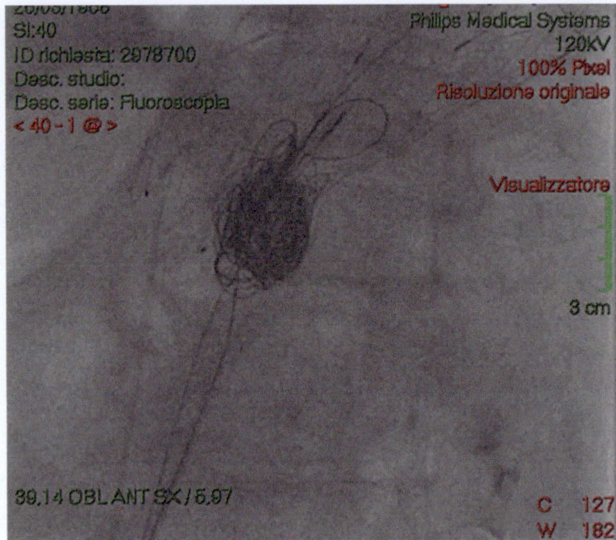

Fig. 35.26 The embolization of the parallel graft at the end of the procedure

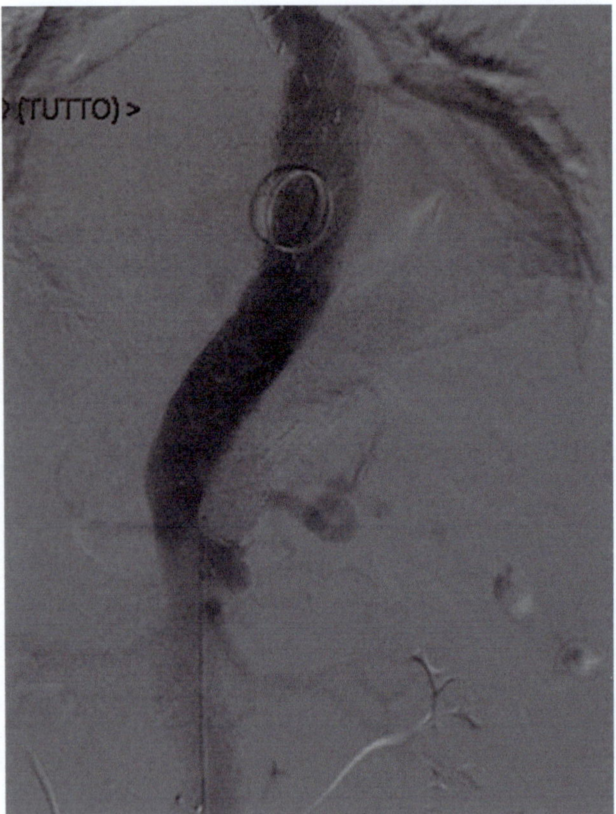

Fig. 35.27 Completion angiography with complete exclusion of the false lumen

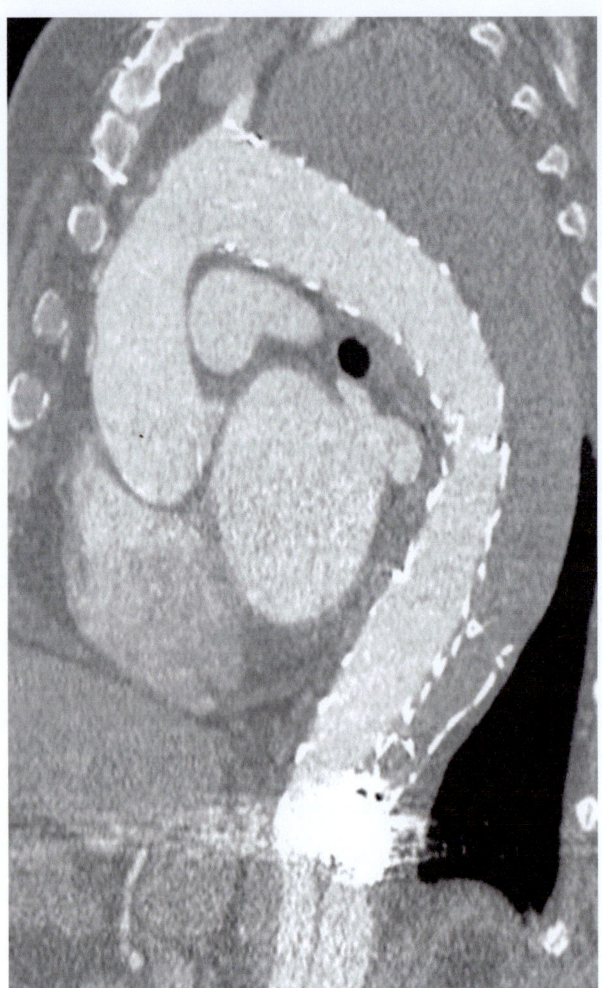

Fig. 35.28 Post-op CT scan showing complete exclusion of the false lumen

Case Scenario

A 47-year-old woman is admitted in emergency ward for thoracic interscapular pain. The patient had a previous diagnosis of type B aortic dissection but with stability of the diameter of the aorta in previous CT scan (Fig. 35.29).

The patient underwent a CT scan.

1. What do you expect?
   A. Aortic rupture.
   B. Aortic re-dissection.
   C. Retrograde dissection.
   D. All the precedent answers are correct.

2. How many aortic lumens can you recognize in the CT scan (Figs. 35.29, 35.30, 35.31, and 35.32)?
   A. 1
   B. 2
   C. 3
   D. More than 3

3. **Which therapy do you** suggest**?**

   A. Medical
   B. Open surgery
   C. Endovascular
   D. Hybrid

Self-Evaluation Questions

1. **Should the anesthesiologist perform the CSF drainage in an urgent-emergent setting of TAAA repair?**
   A. It can be considered only in endovascular repair.
   B. Only for surgical repair.
   C. Always in setting of TAAA repair.
   D. YES, in hemodynamically stable patients. Rescue use of CSF drainage should be reserved for patients with postoperative signs of spinal cord injury and in those taking antiplatelet agents without the possibility to perform a preprocedural platelet functional test.

2. Could POC viscoelastic tests guide a goal-directed hemostatic therapy?

   A. Only the standard laboratory test can be used.
   B. POCs can measure only some features of coagulation setting.
   C. POCs cannot guide the transfusional blood requirements.
   D. POC can monitor real-time during all phases of surgery.

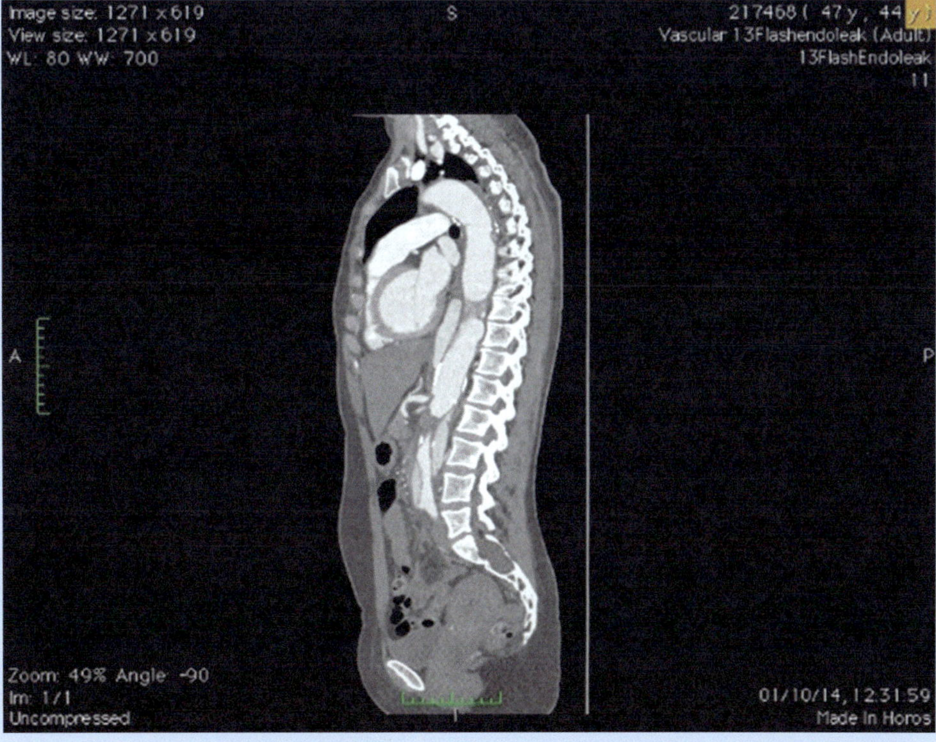

Fig. 35.29 CT pre-op in a patient 47 years old admitted with thoracic pain

3. Could NIRS be useful to monitor indirectly spinal cord perfusion in an urgent-emergent setting of TAAA repair?
   A. It's difficult to perform.
   B. In an urgent-emergent setting, MEP and SSEP are recommended because they can detect early signs of spinal cord hypoperfusion.
   C. Spinal NIRS can be used only in intraoperative setting.
   D. Spinal NIRS is a potential, real-time, noninvasive, and always available technique to monitor the spinal cord perfusion indirectly during and after endovascular or open TAAA repair.

Please see Chap. 58 for the correct answer.

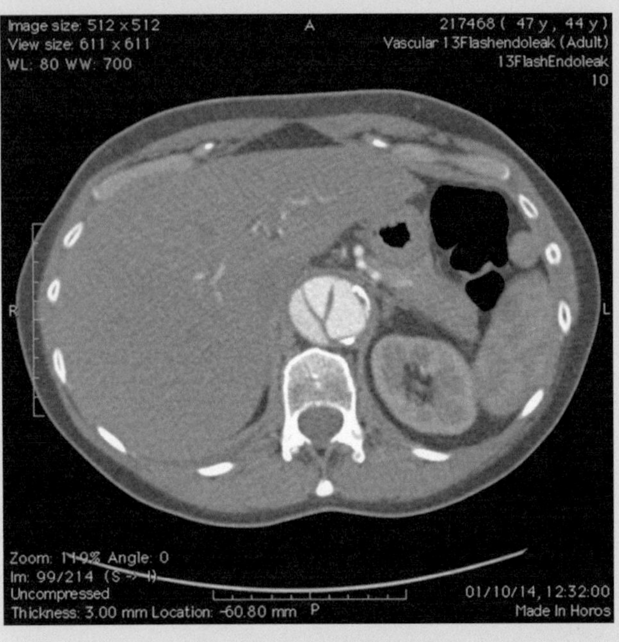

Fig. 35.30 CT pre-op showing a variety of flaps and lumen into the thoracoabdominal aorta

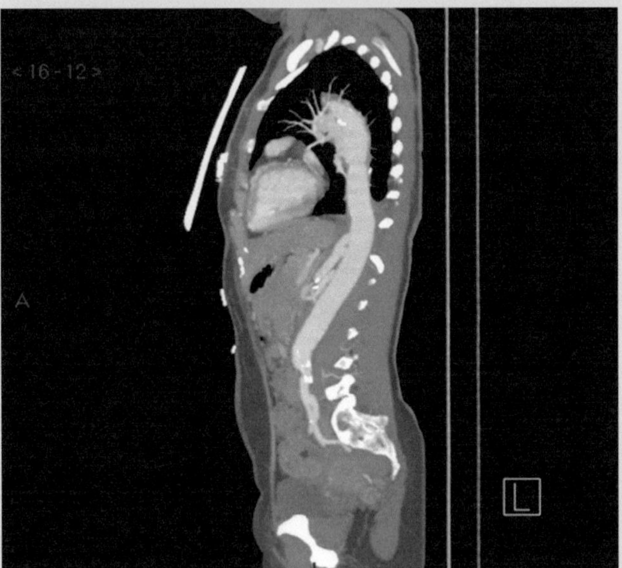

Fig. 35.31 Postoperative CT scan after the replacement of the whole aorta and visceral vessels

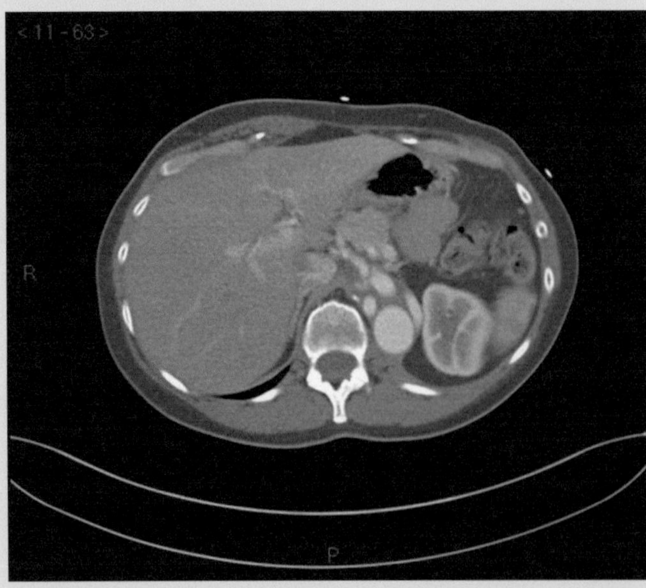

Fig. 35.32 Post-op CT scan with the view of all the visceral vessels completely replaced

References

1. Schepens MAAM, Deafauw JJAM, Hamerlijinck RPHM. Surgical treatment of TAAA by simple cross clamping. Risk factors and late results. J Thorac Cardiovasc Surg. 1994;107:134–42.
2. Anton JM, Herald K. Anesthetic management of open thoracoabdominal aortic aneurysm repair. J Int Anesthesiol Clin. 2016;54(2):76–101.
3. Tantry US, Bonello L, Aradi D, et al. Working group on on-treatment platelet reactivity. J Am Coll Cardiol. 2013;62(24):2261–73.
4. Ranucci M, Sim P. Point-of-care tests for severe hemorrhage. A manual for diagnosis and treatment. 1st ed. Berlin: Springer; 2016.
5. Ortmann E, Rubino A, Altemimi B, Collier T, Besser MW, Klein AA. Validation of viscoelastic coagulation tests during cardiopulmonary bypass. J Thromb Haemost. 2015;13:1207–16.
6. Rahe-Meyer N, Solomon C, Winterhalter M, Piepenbrock S, Tanaka K, Haverich A, Pichlmaier M. Thromboelastometry-guided administration of fibrinogen concentrate for the treatment of excessive intraoperative bleeding in thoracoabdominal aortic aneurysm surgery. J Thorac Cardiovasc Surg. 2009;138(3):694–702. https://doi.org/10.1016/j.jtcvs.2008.11.065. Epub 2009 May 17.
7. Ranucci M, Pistuddi V, Baryshnikova E, Colella D, Bianchi P. Fibrinogen levels after cardiac surgical procedures: association with postoperative bleeding, trigger values, and target values. Ann Thorac Surg. 2016;102(1):78–85.
8. Rahe-Meyer N, Hanke A, Schmidt DS, Hagl C, Pichlmaier M. Fibrinogen concentrate reduces intraoperative bleeding when used as first-line hemostatic therapy during major aortic replacement surgery: results from a randomized, placebo-controlled trial. J Thorac Cardiovasc Surg. 2013;145(Suppl 3):S178–85.
9. Svensson LG, Crawford ES, Hess KR, Coselli JS, Safi HJ. Experience with 1509 patients undergoing thoracoabdominal aortic operations. J Vasc Surg. 1993;17(2):357–70.
10. Crawford ES, Hess KR, Cohen ES, Coselli JS, Safi HJ. Ruptured aneurysm of the descending thoracic and thoracoabdominal aorta. Analysis according to size and treatment. Ann Surg. 1991;213(5):417.
11. Gaudino M, Lau C, Munjal M, Girardi LN. Open repair of ruptured descending thoracic and thoracoabdominal aortic aneurysms. J Thorac Cardiovasc Surg. 2015;150(4):814–23.
12. Etz CD, Weigang E, Hartert M, Lonn L, Mestres CA, Di Bartolomeo R, Bachet JE, Carrel TP, Grabenwöger M, Schepens MA, Czerny M. Contemporary spinal cord protection during thoracic and thoracoabdominal aortic surgery and endovascular aortic repair: a position paper of the vascular domain of the European Association for Cardio-Thoracic Surgery. Eur J Cardiothorac Surg. 2015;47:943–57.
13. Greenberg RK, Lu Q, Roselli EE, Svensson LG, Moon MC, Hernandez AV, et al. Contemporary analysis of descending thoracic and thoracoabdominal aneurysm repair: a comparison of endovascular and open techniques. Circulation. 2008;118:808–17.
14. Conrad MF, Ye JY, Chung TK, Davison JK, Cambria RP. Spinal cord complications after thoracic aortic surgery: long-term survival and functional status varies with deficit severity. J Vasc Surg. 2008;48:47–53.
15. Fehrenbacher JW, Siderys H, Terry C, Kuhn J, Corvera JS. Early and late results of descending thoracic and thoracoabdominal aortic aneurysm open repair with deep hypothermia and circulatory arrest. J Thorac Cardiovasc Surg. 2010;140:S154–60; discussion S85–S90.
16. Coselli JS, LeMaire SA, Koksoy C, Schmittling ZC, Curling PE. Cerebrospinal fluid drainage reduces paraplegia after thoracoabdominal aortic aneurysm repair: result of a randomized clinical trial. J Vasc Surg. 2002;35:631–9.
17. Zoli S, Roder F, Etz CD, Brenner RM, Bodian CA, Lin HM, et al. Predicting the risk of paraplegia after thoracic an thoracoabdominal aneurysm repair. Ann Thorac Surg. 2010;90:1237–44; discussion 45.
18. Sundt TM, Flemming MD, Oderich GS, Torres NE, Li Z, Lenoch J, et al. Spinal cord protection during open repair of thoracic and thoracoabdominal aortic aneurysms using profound hypothermia and circulatory arrest. J Am Coll Surg. 2011;212:678–83; discussion 84–5.
19. Safi HJ, Estrera AL, Miller CC, Huynh TT, Porat EE, Azizzadeh A, et al. Evolution of risk for neurologic deficit after descending and thoracoabdominal aortic repair. Ann Thorac Surg. 2005;80:2173–9; discussion 9.
20. Stone DH, Brewster DC, Kwolek CJ, Lamuraglia GM, Conrad MF, Chung TK, et al. Stent-graft versus open-surgical repair of the thoracic aorta: mid-term results. J Vasc Surg. 2006;44:1188–97.
21. Griepp RB, Griepp EB. Spinal cord perfusion and protection during descending thoracic and thoracoabdominal aortic surgery: the collateral network concept. Ann Thorac Surg. 2007;83(2):S865–9; discussion S890–S892.
22. Etz CD, von Aspern K, Gudehus S, et al. Near-infrared spectroscopy monitoring of the collateral network prior to, during, and after thoracoabdominal aortic repair: a pilot study. Eur J Vasc Endovasc Surg. 2013;46(6):651–6.
23. Luehr M, Mohr FW, Etz CD. Indirect neuromonitoring of the spinal cord by near-infrared spectroscopy of the paraspinous thoracic and lumbar muscles in aortic surgery. Thorac Cardiovasc Surg. 2016;64(04):333–5.
24. Hiratzka LF, Bakris GL, Beckman JA, Bersin RM, Carr VF, Casey DE, et al. 2010 ACCF/AHA/AATS/ACR/ASA/ACA/SCAI/SIR/STS/SVM Guidelines for the diagnosis and management of patients with thoracic aortic disease: a report of the American College of Cardiology Foundation/American Heart Association Task Force on Practice Guidelines, American Association for Thoracic Surgery, American College of Radiology, American Stroke Association, Society of Cardiovascular Anesthesiologists, Society for Cardiovascular Angiography and Interventions, Society of Interventional Radiology, Society of Thoracic Surgeons, and Society for Vascular Medicine. Circulation. 2010;121:e266–369.
25. Svensson LG, Hess KR, D'Agostino RS, Entrup MH, Hreib K, Kimmel WA, et al. Reduction of neurologic injury after high-risk thoracoabdominal aortic operation. Ann Thorac Surg. 1998;66:132–8.
26. Acher CW, Wynn MM, Hoch JR, Kranner PW. Cardiac function is a risk factor for paralysis in thoracoabdominal aortic replacement. J Vasc Surg. 1998;27:821–30.
27. Sugiura J, Oshima H, Abe T, Narita Y, Araki Y, Fujimoto K, Mutsuga M, Usui A. The efficacy and risk of cerebrospinal fluid drainage for thoracoabdominal aortic aneurysm repair: a retrospective observational comparison between drainage and non-drainage. Interact Cardiovasc Thorac Surg. 2017;24(4):609–14.
28. Wynn MM, Mell MW, Tefera G, Hoch JR, Acher CW. Complications of spinal fluid drainage in thoracoabdominal aortic aneurysm repair: a report of 486 patients treated from 1987 to 2008. J Vasc Surg. 2009;49:29–35.
29. Murakami H, Yoshida K, Hino Y, Matsuda H, Tsukube T, Okita Y. Complications of cerebrospinal fluid drainage in thoracoabdominal aortic aneurysm repair. J Vasc Surg. 2004;39:243–5.
30. Loddo P, Degiudici A, Maxia A, Pibiri L, Pisu F, Ruiu G, Zanetti PP. Emergency surgery in thoracoabdominal aneurysms repair. Clinical outcome. G Ital Chir Vasc. 2003;10:255–67.
31. Zanetti PP, Krasoń M, Walas R, Cebotaru T, Popa C, Vintila B, Steiu F. "Open" repair of ruptured thoracoabdominal aortic aneurysm (experience of 51 cases). Pol J Cardiothorac Surg. 2015;12(2):119.

32. Bevilacqua S, Casini A, Galeotti I, Corsoni V, Romagnoli S. Rotational thromboelastometry–guided hemostatic therapy for management of cerebrospinal fluid catheter in patients undergoing endovascular aortic repair. Reg Anesth Pain Med. 2015;40(5):631–4.
33. Fedorow CA, Moon MC, Mutch WA, et al. Lumbar cerebrospinal fluid drainage for thoracoabdominal aortic surgery: rationale and practical considerations for management. Anesth Analg. 2010;111:46–58.
34. Lobato AC, Camacho-Lobato L. Enovascular treatment of complex aortic aneurysms using the sandwich technique. J Endovasc Ther. 2012;19:691–706.

Updates in the Management of Non-traumatic Abdominal Vascular Emergencies (Abdominal Aortoiliac Aneurysms, Intestinal Ischemia, Splanchnic Aneurysms)

36

P. Tracanelli, M. T. Occhiuto, R. Vercelli, A. Rampoldi, and F. Romani

Key Points

- Abdominal aortic aneurysms (AAA) are often asymptomatic and represent an incidental finding on diagnostic imaging.
- Their rupture is an emergency with elevated mortality.
- AAA diameter (≥ 5.5 cm) or symptoms or rapid aneurysm growth (>1 cm/year) require a prompt vascular surgeon evaluation.

36.1 Aortoiliac Aneurysms

Aneurysms involving abdominal aorta and iliac arteries are relatively common and potentially life-threatening.

Aneurysms usually result from degeneration in the media of the arterial wall, leading to a slow and continuous dilatation of the lumen of the vessel.

Most of the abdominal aortic aneurysms (AAA) are asymptomatic and detected as an incidental finding on diagnostic imaging obtained for other reasons. Rupture of an aortic aneurysm represents an emergency that can lead to 100% of mortality if not treated and needs prompt diagnosis and treatment.

P. Tracanelli · M. T. Occhiuto · F. Romani (✉)
Vascular Surgery Division, CardioToracoVascular Department, Niguarda Hospital, Milan, Italy
e-mail: mariateresa.occhiuto@ospedaleniguarda.it; federico.romani@ospedaleniguarda.it

R. Vercelli · A. Rampoldi
Interventional Radiology Unit, Niguarda Hospital, Milan, Italy
e-mail: ruggero.vercelli@ospedaleniguarda.it; antoniogaetano.rampoldi@ospedaleniguarda.it

Historically ruptured abdominal aortic aneurysms (rAAA) were treated with conventional open surgery. Despite significant advances in intensive care unit management and surgical techniques, mortality following repair of ruptured AAA remains high. Following the experience and good results with endovascular treatment in elective setting, operators suggest that also rAAA treatment may be improved using endovascular technique (endovascular aneurysm repair, EVAR). Theoretically, ruptured EVAR (r-EVAR) has several advantages, including the option to perform the entire procedure or parts of the procedure under local anesthesia, avoiding the hypotensive effects of general anesthesia, and the fact that a percutaneous approach minimizes blood loss and avoids laparotomy. But aortic endograft under emergency circumstances presents many challenges, and it's far to be the "gold standard" for ruptured abdominal aneurysms. Among aortoiliac emergencies nowadays, we have to mention the failure of endovascular treatment with the need for open conversion. Surgical techniques of prosthetic explants in case of failure of EVAR are still debated.

36.1.1 Epidemiology, Risk Factors, and Natural History

AAA can be defined as an abdominal aortic diameter of 3.0 cm or more in either anterior-posterior or transverse planes. The prevalence of AAA increases with age; an incidence of 12.5% in men and 5.2% in women between 74 and 84 years of age is reported. A diagnosis of aortic aneurysm is performed in about 700,000 persons in Europe, 220,000 each year. It accounts for approximately 11,000 deaths every year in the United States, with mortality rates from ruptured AAAs reaching up to 90%. Risk factors for AAA are similar to those of other cardiovascular diseases: male sex, smoking, age older than 65 years, coronary artery disease, hypertension,

P. Aseni et al. (eds.), *Operative Techniques and Recent Advances in Acute Care and Emergency Surgery*,
https://doi.org/10.1007/978-3-319-95114-0_36

previous myocardial infarction, peripheral arterial disease, and a family history of AAA. Beyond the inherent risk of rupture, patients with AAA are also at an increased risk of cardiovascular disease and death [1]. The reported growth rate of AAAs is between 30 and 55 mm ranges from 0.2 to 0.3 cm per year, with a wide variation between patients. Larger AAA diameters are associated with higher AAA growth rates. The most important factor related to aneurysm growth rate is smoking. A larger initial aneurysm diameter is a significant and independent risk factor for AAA rupture. Other factors that have been associated with an increased risk of AAA rupture across several studies include female gender, hypertension, AAA expansion rate, and peak AAA wall stress [2].

Rupture of an aortic aneurysm represents an emergency that can lead to 100% of mortality if not treated. The risk of rupture depends on aneurysm diameter (1% between 40 and 49 mm up to 33% for AAA > 7 cm). The incidence of ruptured abdominal aortic aneurysms ranges between 5.6 and 17.5 per 100,000 person-years in Western countries and seems to have declined in the last decade. The overall mortality rate in all patients with a ruptured abdominal aortic aneurysm (rAAA) is around 80%. One-third of all patients with rAAA do not reach the hospital alive, and one-third do not have an intervention. The operative mortality of ruptured aortic aneurysm has not improved significantly in recent years, with mortality rates still ranging from 32 to 80% [3].

36.1.2 Clinical Presentation

The detection of an aortic aneurysm with physical examination is moderately sensitive (sensitivity of 68% and specificity of 75%). The most common finding is palpation of a pulsatile mass around the level of the umbilicus. Abdominal auscultation may reveal the presence of a bruit. Obesity, abdominal distention, and smaller aneurysm size can reduce the accuracy of abdominal palpation. Rarely symptoms due to compression of adjacent structures are described. Lower extremity edema may be related to compression of the inferior vena cava. Rarely aortocaval or aortoenteric fistulae can occur. Lumbar pain related to vertebral lesion may be due to a large dimension aneurysm erosion activity. Compression of bowel may cause gastrointestinal symptoms like dyspepsia, weight loss, or bowel obstruction, as well as ureteral compression that may lead to hydronephrosis. Distal embolization from aortic thrombus or aneurysm complete thrombosis could be the cause of lower limb acute ischemia. Otherwise, most of the aortic aneurysms are asymptomatic, and diagnosis of AAA is often made as an incidental finding on imaging studies, such as abdominal ultrasonography or computed tomography. AAA may be visible on plain radiography if the aneurysm wall is calcified [1].

A ruptured aortoiliac aneurysm is characterized by hypotension, shooting abdominal or back pain, and a pulsatile abdominal mass. This triad may be incomplete or absent, and misdiagnosis can occur in up to 60% of cases [4]. Abdominal pain or other symptoms occurring in a patient known to have or newly diagnosed with AAA can present a clinical dilemma. In surgical series, between 5 and 22% of AAA are symptomatic (Fig. 36.1). In the absence of rupture, pain or other symptoms may indicate rapid expansion causing compression of adjacent structures, or an inflammatory or infected AAA. Symptoms that may be related to AAA include abdominal pain or back pain, signs of acute thromboembolism, and fever. A triad of chronic abdominal pain, weight loss, and elevated erythrocyte sedimentation rate in a patient with an AAA is highly suggestive of an inflammatory aneurysm. Patients with inflammatory aneurysms are often more symptomatic than patients with the more typical AAAs, but the incidence of actual rupture may be lower.

36.1.3 Management and Indication to Treat

The management of AAA depends on the size or diameter of the aneurysm and is a balance between the risk of aneurysm rupture and the operative mortality for aneurysm repair. For very small aneurysms between 3.0 and 3.9 cm, the risk of rupture is very low, and these aneurysms do not require surgical intervention. Two large multicentered randomized controlled trials of early open elective surgery versus surveillance, the UK

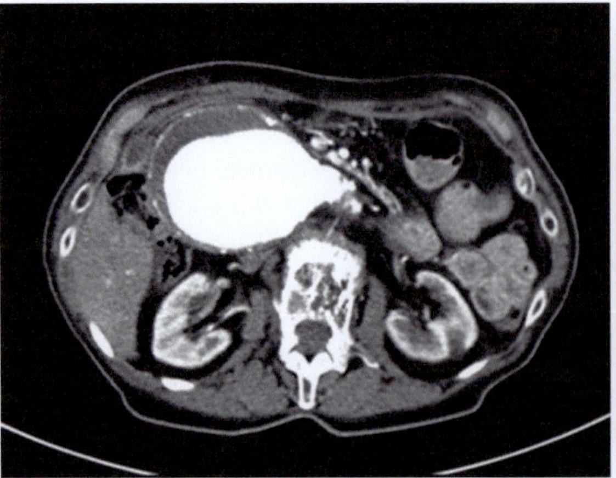

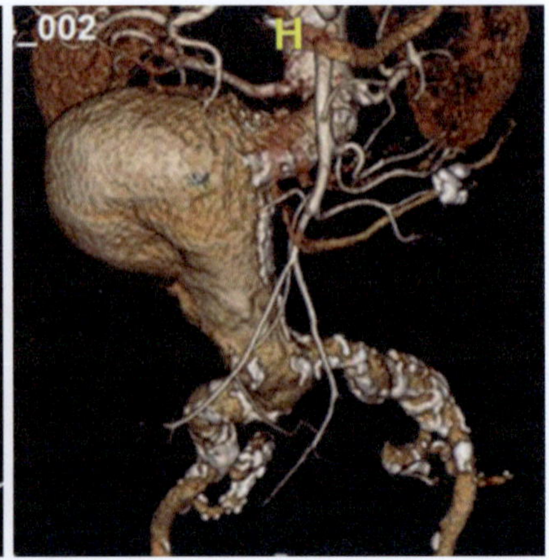

Fig. 36.1 CT scan of a big symptomatic aneurysm

Small Aneurysm Trial (UKSAT) and the American Aneurysm Detection and Management study (ADAM), and a smaller trial of endovascular repair versus surveillance (CAESAR) [5] were performed in order to analyze the management of aneurysms from 4.0 to 5.5 cm in diameter. PIVOTAL trial [6] focused only on the 4.0 and 5.0 cm diameter range and compared early endovascular repair versus surveillance. In the UKSAT no significant difference in all-cause mortality at 5 years between the two groups was registered, and results were similar after 12 years of follow-up. The aneurysm rupture rate was 1% per year in the surveillance group, and the elective mortality rate for open surgery in the immediate repair cohort was 5.6%. Most patients in the surveillance group eventually underwent surgery because of aneurysm enlargement. Cost-effectiveness analyses suggested that surveillance was less costly than early surgery. In the ADAM study, rupture rate in the surveillance group (0.6% per year) and perioperative mortality rate in the surgery group (2.7%) were lower than in the UKSAT [7]. As with other studies, 60% of the surveillance group underwent operative AAA repair because of aneurysm enlargement. The findings of these two trials, summarized in a recent Cochrane review (at 6 years HR 1.11 [95% CI 0.91e1.34]), show the safety and hence benefits of a policy of ultrasonographic surveillance for aneurysms 4.0 e 5.5 cm in diameter [8].

When the diameter of 5.5 cm, measured by ultrasonography, in males is reached or symptoms develop or rapid aneurysm growth is observed (>1 cm/year), immediate referral to a vascular surgeon is recommended. Patients with a higher risk of rupture should be considered for surgery when the maximum aortic diameter reaches 5.0 cm. Females suffer AAA rupture at smaller aortic diameters than males and should be referred to vascular surgeons for assessment at a maximum aortic diameter of 5.0 cm, and aneurysm repair should be considered at a maximum aneurysm diameter of 5.2 cm in females.

Coexisting iliac aneurysms should be treated concurrently with AAA, and aortoiliac aneurysms comprise up to 43% of a specialist vascular surgeon's workload. Isolated iliac aneurysms may be treated by either open or endovascular techniques. Intervention should be considered when the iliac diameter exceeds 3 cm.

In case of symptomatic aneurysms, it's necessary to exclude other sources of symptoms. When no other cause is apparent, an urgent repair is suggested. In the presence of very large AAA (>6.0 cm), treatment is suggested even if the aneurysm is not felt to be the source of symptoms [9–11].

Although AAA repair should be offered to most patients with ruptured AAA, some patients may be at such high risk due to underlying comorbidities that comfort care is appropriate.

36.1.4 Symptomatic and Ruptured AAA

AAA rupture is defined as bleeding outside the adventitia of a dilated aortic wall (Fig. 36.2). Rupture is further classified into free rupture in the peritoneal cavity, often associated to shock and retroperitoneal rupture where the retroperitoneal tissue provides tamponade and reduces temporarily the volume of blood loss. Differentiation between symptomatic and ruptured aneurysms is critical. Symptomatic AAAs are those that have become painful but without breach of the aortic wall and without signs of shock. The inclusion of symptomatic AAAs in data on ruptured AAAs will artificially improve the results of outcomes.

The initial management of the patient with symptomatic (non-ruptured) or ruptured AAA is guided by the hemodynamic status. If a patient with a known aortic aneurysm presents signs of shock and symptoms linked to an aneurysm rupture, further diagnostic does not seem mandatory, and the patient should be immediately transferred to the operating room. Emergency ultrasound scanning can be done to confirm the suspected diagnosis. Most patients with a ruptured abdominal aortic aneurysm who reach the hospital alive are sufficiently stable to undergo computed tomography for further therapy setting. The timing of surgery for patients with symptomatic but unruptured aneurysms remains controversial. For patients determined to have a symptomatic AAA, but for whom repair will be delayed to optimize associated medical conditions, an observation period in intensive care unit setting is indicated.

Patients with AAA who require emergent or urgent aortic surgery for ruptured or symptomatic (non-ruptured) AAA should be treated at a facility where surgical expertise and/or the perioperative resources necessary for major aortic surgery are available (e.g., operating room personnel, an appropriately trained surgeon, perioperative intensive care). For patients who present to a facility where these are not available, transfer to a vascular center with higher levels of hospital resources is appropriate and may result in lower mortality. Outcomes for open surgical repair of ruptured AAA are correlated with surgeon experience with a higher annual caseload of open aneurysm repair per year (non-ruptured and ruptured) correlating with improved outcomes [12–14].

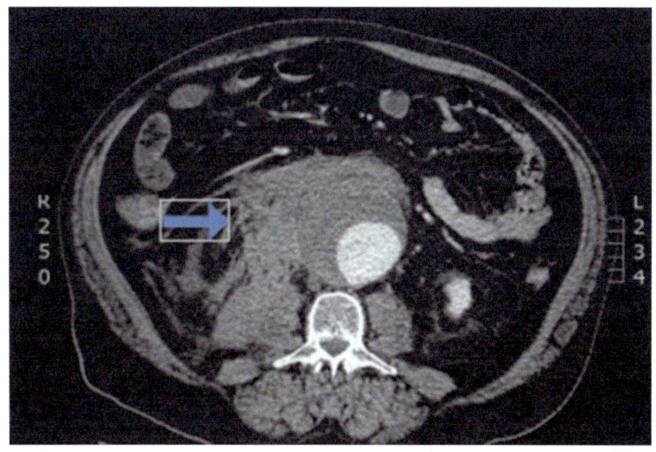

Fig. 36.2 CT scan of retroperitoneal rupture of AAA

36.1.5 Perioperative Management

The treatment of a patient with rAAA requires a multidisciplinary approach to ensure a quick diagnosis, appropriate preoperative and perioperative support, efficient aneurysm repair, and excellent postoperative care. The primary goal in the initial management of patients with rAAA is achieving hemodynamic stability to allow perfusion of the vital organs. Two large-bore peripheral intravenous catheters should be placed in all patients (symptomatic non-ruptured or ruptured AAA) for medication and fluid administration. In hemodynamically unstable patients with ruptured AAA, indirect evidence from the trauma population and one observational study in patients with AAA suggest that allowing a relatively low systolic blood pressure of 80–100 mmHg (permissive hypotension) may prevent further tearing of the aorta and limit blood loss. Dick et al. report that aggressive volume resuscitation of patients with rAAA before proximal aortic control resulted in an increased perioperative risk of death independent of systolic blood pressure [15–17].

Pain control is an important part of management. It is important to keep the patient comfortable, but conscious. In patients who remain severely hypertensive despite adequate pain control, short-acting intravenous beta-blockers can be used to reduce the blood pressure. Laboratory studies including complete blood count, electrolytes, blood urea nitrogen, creatinine, liver function tests, prothrombin time, partial thromboplastin time, and a type and crossmatch should be obtained. Similar to trauma patients with severe ongoing hemorrhage, patients with ruptured AAA often require massive transfusion.

36.1.6 Aneurysm Repair

Two methods of aneurysm repair are currently available: open surgery and endovascular aneurysm repair (EVAR).

Open AAA repair—Open aneurysm repair involves replacement of the diseased aortic segment with a tube or bifurcated prosthetic graft through a midline abdominal or retroperitoneal incision.

EVAR—EVAR involves the placement of modular graft components delivered via the iliac or femoral arteries, which line the aorta and exclude the aneurysm sac from the circulation.

36.1.6.1 Open Surgical Treatment

The most important step in rAAA surgery is the rapid, safe, and effective control of the proximal aorta with a consequent reduction of blood loss. After aortic clamping takes place, the anesthesia team should replace blood loss more aggressively. The aorta may be approached either transperitoneally or through the retroperitoneal space. Self-retaining retractors are used. The bowel is kept warm and, if possible, is not exteriorized. An infrarenal control and clamping if possible are performed. Often a supraceliac control is necessary and allows a quick and safe control of the aorta in a bloodless field. However, it causes a visceral ischemic injury that can contribute to the development of multi-system organ failure. In addition, supraceliac control can increase the cardiac afterload and promote myocardial ischemia. Another method for aortic control is balloon occlusion. Proximal control of the aorta can be carried out by placing a balloon in the proximal aorta without supraceliac exposure. An occlusion balloon can be inserted directly into the aorta or under fluoroscopic guidance through the femoral or brachial artery. Due to the risk of coagulation disorders, dissections should be minimized to reduce injury to blood vessels and other structures. The patient should be kept warm because hypothermia can lead to surgical bleeding and adverse cardiac events. Heparin administration is controversial [18].

Key Points
In rupture abdominal aortic aneurysms

- Hemodynamic status of the patient decides the following steps of treatment.
- Permissive hypotension is necessary to reduce massive bleeding and keep the patient alive.
- In case of hard proximal aortic clamping, use an intra-aortic balloon.
- If abdominal pressure is high, perform a temporary abdominal closure.

For symptomatic, non-ruptured AAAs, perioperative mortality rates are similar to those of elective repair. The mortality associated with ruptured AAA may be as high as 90% when patients who die at home or upon the arrival to the hospital are taken into account. In spite of obvious improvements in prehospital care, cardiovascular anesthesia, and critical care, surgical mortality following open repair of ruptured AAA has changed very little, remaining at approximately 30–50%. Factors that are associated with increased mortality following open repair of ruptured are reported in Table 36.1.

For patients with several prognostic factors for poor outcome, the incidence of serious comorbidities, such as dialysis dependence, colonic ischemia, and myocardial infarction, is high, and the need for surgery related to a complication is

Table 36.1 Factors that are associated with increased mortality following open repair of ruptured AAA

Hypotension with a systolic blood pressure <80 mmHg
Advanced age (>80 years)
Cardiac arrest
Loss of consciousness
Creatinine >1.3 on admission
Ischemic heart disease
Female sex
Hemoglobin <9.0 on admission

also high. The presence of >3 prognostic factors increases the likelihood that the patient will require extended care. For patients older than 80 years old, with renal dysfunction, loss of consciousness, and hemoglobin <9, the chance of survival following open repair of ruptured AAA is almost zero. The presence of multiple risk factors for poor outcome in a patient of advanced age should lead to consideration for comfort care [19–22].

Abdominal compartment syndrome (ACS) is observed in 10–55% of patients after emergent aneurysm repair. An abdominal pressure of more than 20 mmHg in the presence of organ dysfunction is normally used to describe this critical state. Measurement of the intra-abdominal pressure can either be performed by urinary bladder pressure, which is the most frequently used technique, by gastric pressure or by invasive methods like catheterization of the pressure in the vena cava. The debate regarding the timing of and criteria for decompression is ongoing. In past years the concept of temporary abdominal closure with impermeable mesh or Silastic sheeting of a vacuum-assisted closure was prompted. An increased abdominal pressure represents a negative predictive factor for the survival after open repair of a ruptured AAA. Hypotension, high pulmonary compliance, and oliguria can occur in serious cases of ACS. Measurement of the intra-abdominal pressure is recommended, and in case of elevated levels (>20 mmHg) in combination with organ dysfunction, decompressive surgery should immediately be performed. Temporary abdominal closure systems can positively influence the outcome [2].

36.1.6.2 Endovascular Treatment EVAR

Elective endovascular aneurysm repair demonstrates a reduction in perioperative (30-day) morbidity and mortality compared to open repair. There is accumulating evidence that morbidity and mortality following repair of symptomatic or ruptured AAA may also be reduced. The first successful endovascular repair of a rAAA was performed in 1994 by Marin et al. [23] EVAR is less invasive, avoids damage to periaortic and abdominal structures, reduces bleeding from surgical dissection, minimizes hypothermia, and lessens the requirement for deep anesthesia. Because of these potential advantages combined with reports of lower procedural mortality, EVAR has been regarded as superior to OSR for the treatment of rAAA. Observational studies have reported improved short-term survival after EVAR compared with OR, but methodological limitations lead to biased outcomes. Three randomized controlled trials have compared OSR and EVAR in the treatment of patients with rAAA. Hinchliffe et al. observed 32 patients with rAAA, finding a 30-day mortality rate of 53% in the EVAR group and 53% in the OSR group. Moderate or severe operative complications occurred in 77% of the patients in the EVAR group and 80% of the patients in the OSR group. The median total hospital stay in the EVAR group was 10 days, compared to 12 days in the OSR group. Reimerink et al. [24] randomized 116 patients with rAAA to treatment with either OSR or EVAR. The combined rate of death and severe complications at 30 days postsurgery was 42% in the EVAR group versus 47% in the OSR group. The 30-day mortality was 21% among the patients assigned to EVAR compared to 25 of the patients assigned to OSR in this study. In the IMPROVE (Immediate Management of the Patient with Rupture: Open Versus Endovascular repair) trial, 613 patients were prospectively recruited [25]. The 30-day mortality rate was 35.4% (112/316) in the EVAR group and 37.4% (111/297) in the OSR group. The 30-day mortality rate among patients with confirmed ruptures was 36.4% (100/275) in the EVAR group and 40.6% (106/261) in the OSR group. Although these trials had some limitations due to the relatively small number of patients who were recruited, no significant differences were found between EVAR and OSR regarding either the mortality rate or the complication rate. A systematic review and meta-analysis from van Beek et al. including a total of 3769 articles, 3 RCTs, 21 observational studies, and 8 administrative registries estimate the short-term (combined 30-day or in-hospital) survival after EVAR and OR for patients with rRAAA. The results indicate that EVAR is not inferior to OR in patients with a ruptured abdominal aortic aneurysm with regard to short-term survival. This supports the use of EVAR in suitable patients and OR as reasonable alternative [3]. The debate on the trial results is still open. We can say that in the presence of good anatomical features, endovascular expertise and availability of materials EVAR could be an alternative to open repair for rRAAA. For rAAA endovascular treatment, the institution must have a defined program for emergency endovascular surgery with rapid availability of high-quality computed tomography, availability of trained support staff, stock of available endovascular prostheses in a wide range of sizes, and available vascular surgeon appropriately trained in advanced endovascular techniques [26–29].

Technical Notes

A preoperative contrast- enhanced CT scan is almost mandatory. The identification of appropriate proximal and distal sealing zones, as well as evaluation of the iliofemoral access, is critical to success.

Key Points
In rupture abdominal aortic aneurysms

- In case of endovascular treatment, choose a device very familiar to surgeons

In case of unsuitability of iliac access (for low diameters, calcification, or angulations) adjunctive procedures, low-profile delivery systems, or a uni-iliac device have to be considered. If it's possible and available, a bifurcated graft is used to treat the ruptured aneurysm (Fig. 36.3).

This avoids crossover femoral-femoral bypass that usually requires general anesthesia and has a much higher risk of postoperative groin infections. Otherwise, an aorto-uni-iliac implant and femorofemoral bypass can be considered in the situation of hemodynamically unstable patients or when it is difficult to access the contralateral iliac artery due to stenosis, occlusion, or tortuosity (Fig. 36.4).

No studies have thus far have shown any one device to be superior in treating ruptured abdominal aortic aneurysms, and in fact, most devices have been shown to work sufficiently well. The important thing is to use a device that one is very familiar with [30]. Most centers perform r-EVAR under local anesthesia. It is very quick, and it does not affect patient hemodynamics, but patient discomfort and unrest may compromise the procedure and the precise

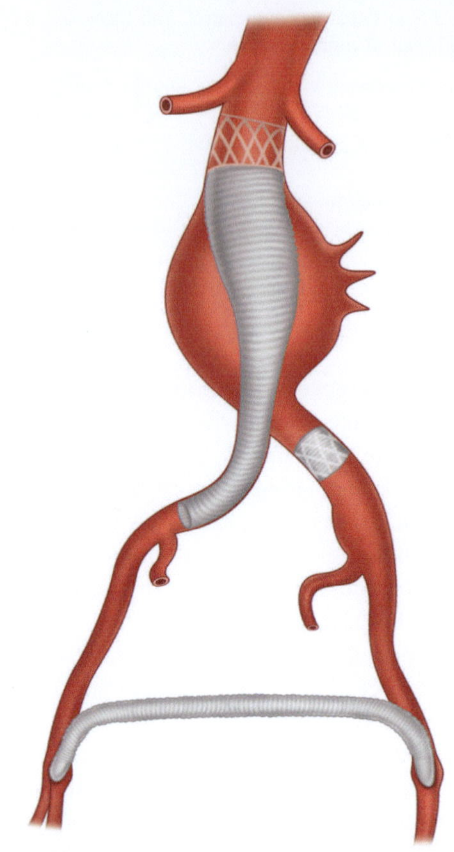

Fig. 36.4 AUI EVAR for rAAA: aorto-uni-iliac endograft with iliac occlusion and femorofemoral bypass

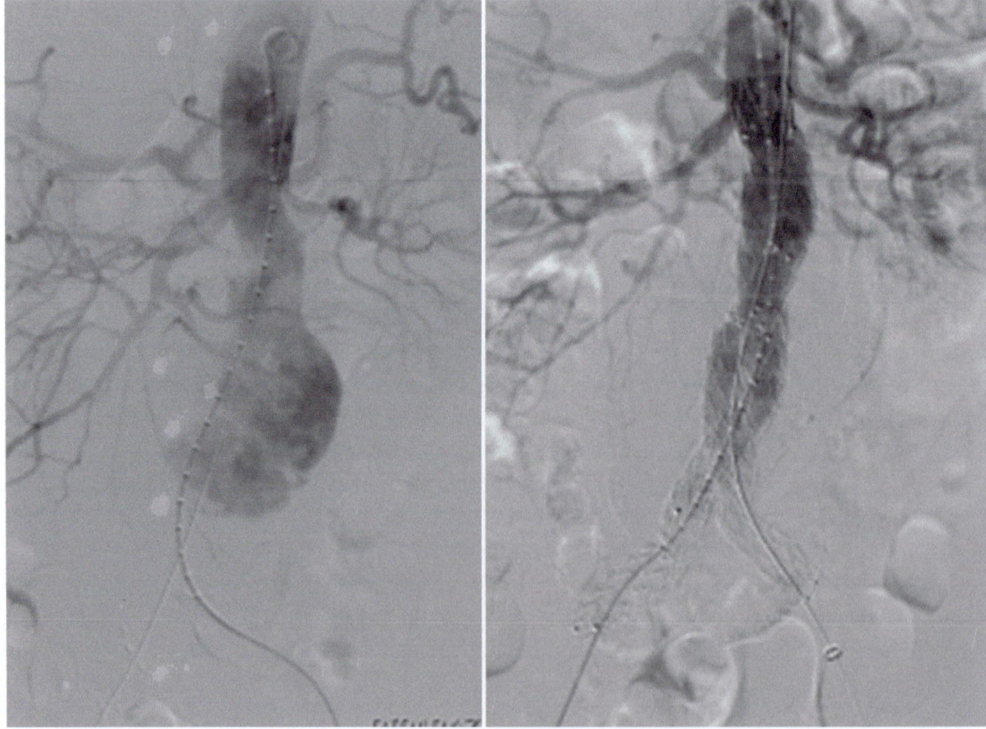

Fig. 36.3 Angiography of bifurcated EVAR for symptomatic AAA

placement of the endograft. The use of percutaneous access is probably best reserved for patients with contained ruptures that are stable.

The use of heparin for anticoagulation during r-EVAR is debatable. Depending on the clinical status of the patient and the expected complexity of the planned repair, anticoagulation must be administered using careful judgment. Close communication with the anesthesiologist and monitoring of the activated clotting time are essential in all cases to individualize heparin use [31–34]. An aortic occlusion balloon is generally used only when severe hemodynamic instability occurs. In case of patient instability, a large balloon for aortic occlusion is positioned (Coda, Cook Medical; Reliant, Medtronic). Balloon inflation should only be carried out when truly necessary (approximately 19–27% of patients) because the use of an occlusion balloon is not without risk and "trash embolization" and aortic rupture from the balloon can occur. The transfemoral approach is the recommended access route for the aortic occlusion catheter. Initially, an axillary approach was suggested because of downward displacement in the aneurysm sac during femoral insertion. Actually, the contralateral femoral access serves as the access route for a sized sheath long enough to support an inflated balloon. Angiography is performed via the sheath, and deployment of the stent graft's main body and ipsilateral leg can be done with the occlusion balloon inflated. Via the ipsilateral side, a new balloon is inflated inside the main body, and the primary suprarenal balloon may now be deflated and withdrawn via the sheath, thereby maintaining circulatory control and also restoring circulation to the visceral branches. Staged declamping upon completion of the procedure is good practice [35].

Severe angulation; short, conical, or wide aortic neck; and thrombosis at the landing zone are all factors that might prevent standard EVAR of an AAA. By using fenestrated or branched stent grafts, sealing can be accomplished at the suprarenal, supramesenteric, or supraceliac levels. But most of these systems are custom-made devices, which limits their use in practice to elective cases. In an acute setting, other techniques are reported.

A chimney or snorkel configuration requires antegrade catheterization from a transbrachial approach to facilitate placement of a covered stent into one or more branch vessels in a parallel course, adjacent to the main intra-aortic stent graft (Fig. 36.5).

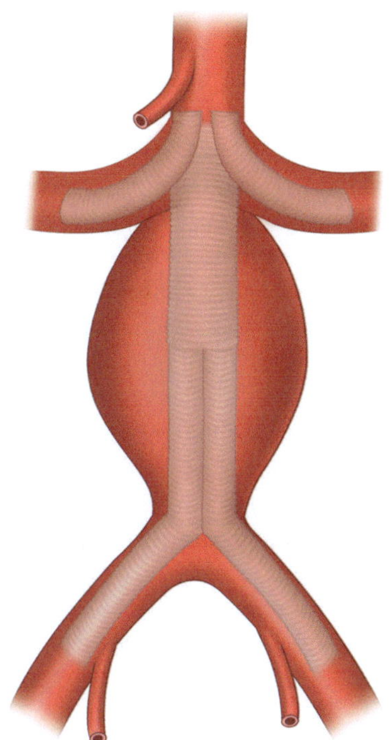

Fig. 36.5 c-EVAR for rAAA: EVAR with chimney technique for renal arteries

The proximal portion of the snorkel stent extends above the proximal edge of the main aortic stent graft, thereby extending the proximal seal zone in a short or no-neck aortic aneurysm. Lachat et al. [36] have described the lift technique as an alternative to the chimney technique. Through a femoral access, followed by an 8-F sheath, the target renal vessel is cannulated, and a chimney graft is advanced 1–2 cm into the renal artery and deployed such that its proximal end faces downward. The distal end is fixed in place with an inflated angioplasty balloon. A stiff guidewire is inserted coaxially through the 8-F sheath, the guidewire is removed from the renal artery, and the 8-F sheath is carefully pushed over the stiff guidewire, lifting the chimney graft upward. With the chimney reoriented cranially, the aortic stent graft is immediately deployed. Use of physician-modified endovascular grafts have been described as a safe and effective alternative for treating patients with juxtarenal aneurysms who have no other alternatives for repair, as well as in ruptured aneurysms. Physician-modified endovascular grafts are performed under sterile conditions and the time required for device manufacture ranges from 30 to 80 min, depending on the number of fenestrations. The system is resheathed, depending on what system has been used [37–39].

Some authors report treatment of rAAA with the Nellix endovascular aneurysm sealing (EVAS) system (Endologix, Irvine, CA, USA). It consists of two identical catheter-based devices with a 10-mm flow lumen being created by two balloon-expandable polytetrafluoroethylene-covered cobalt-chromium stents. The stents are mounted on balloons for deployment and are surrounded by polyurethane endobags. The EVAS device fixes the two stents within the aneurysm sac using the endobags, which are filled with a polyethylene glycol (PEG)-based hydrogel that conforms to the aneurysm flow lumen and solidifies within minutes of delivery, providing fixation and seal at the aortic neck and iliac arteries. Potential advantages of EVAS are related to the possibility to treat a wider range of aortic morphology with a small inventory of devices. Preoperative sizing involving the selection of only a suitable length of the device and the avoidance of contralateral limb cannulation in EVAS may reduce the overall planning and operative procedure duration in certain cases that are very important in the emergency setting. EVAS also provides an option for early hemostasis through endobag inflation with saline while maintaining limb perfusion. A final advantage is the avoidance of type II endoleaks with aneurysm sac sealing.

The potential disadvantages of the EVAS technique for ruptured aneurysm repair include a risk of enlarging a rupture or tearing the aorta with the pressure used to fill the endobags. In addition, there is the potential for failure to seal a ruptured aneurysm due to an inability to generate the required pressure within the ruptured aneurysm sac. The IFU for the Nellix devices specify that they are not suitable for patients with small or large common iliac arteries (<8 or >35 mm, respectively) or those with a large patent flow lumen (>60 mm) within the aneurysm sac.

During EVAR for rAAA, in the presence of inadequate distal landing zone in the common iliac artery, an extension to the external iliac artery is needed.

Preoperative or intraoperative embolization or plug positioning can also be used during EVAR for rAAAs (Fig. 36.6). In select cases, an iliac branch device can be used to preserve internal iliac artery flow.

Abdominal compartment syndrome (ACS) is the major cause of morbidity and mortality after a successful EVAR performed to treat rAAA. Persistent bleeding from the lumbar and inferior mesenteric arteries into the ruptured aneurysm sac in the situation of severe coagulopathy might also contribute to the development of ACS. As reported for open surgery after rAAA recognition and immediate treatment of compartment syndrome is mandatory.

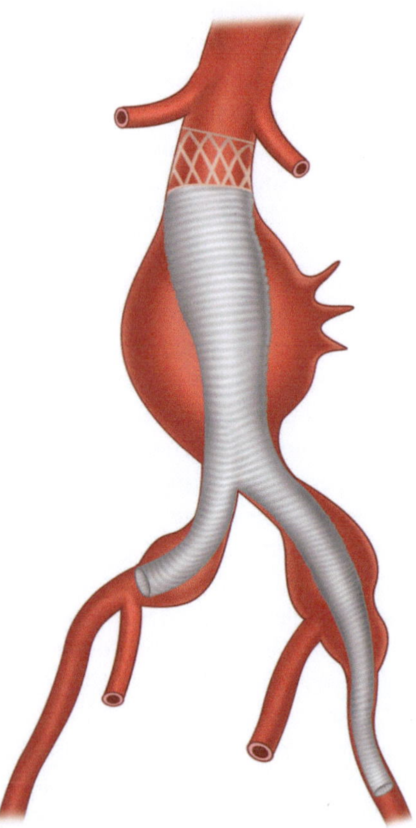

Fig. 36.6 EVAR with a bifurcated graft and embolization of the left internal iliac artery with a plug

36.1.7 Rupture After EVAR

Late failure of endovascular repair secondary to endoleaks, endotension, and sac enlargement, stent graft migration, tear and fracture, or infection continues to be a persistent problem that can result in delayed aneurysm rupture (Fig. 36.7) [40, 41]. Reported rates of abdominal aortic aneurysm (AAA) rupture after EVAR ranging from 0.5 to 1.2% per patient per year [42]. About aortic anatomical features before intervention, larger aneurysm diameter seems to be associated with an increased risk of graft rupture. Not only is the diameter the primary determinant of the risk of primary aneurysm rupture but also a strong predictor of late ruptures, type I endoleak, and aneurysm-related death [43].

Therapeutic approach to post-EVAR rAAA is dependent on the anatomic characteristics and the lesion. While it is ideal to remove all the endograft to eliminate any possible recurrent problems, complete excision is not an easy task. The presence of barbs or hooks, suprarenal fixation stents, or Palmaz stents that are well incorporated into the aorta and inflammatory changes around the aorta and vena cava, left renal vein, and iliac veins may complicate the matter, elevating the complexity of the operation. Complete excision of suprarenal fixation endograft may leave the aortic or arterial wall too thin and denuded, increasing the risk of anastomotic tear. In such cases, partial resection of endograft may significantly reduce the risk of renovisceral ischemia time and adverse outcomes. The endograft remnant can be incorporated in the suture line along with the aortic wall, and it is sewn to the surgical graft. When a total excision of endograft is required, a supraceliac clamping is also required. The reported operative mortality rates for post-EVAR rAAA range widely from 15 to 67%. With the progressive improvement of endovascular technology, its widespread use and long-term follow up, post-EVAR rAAA is

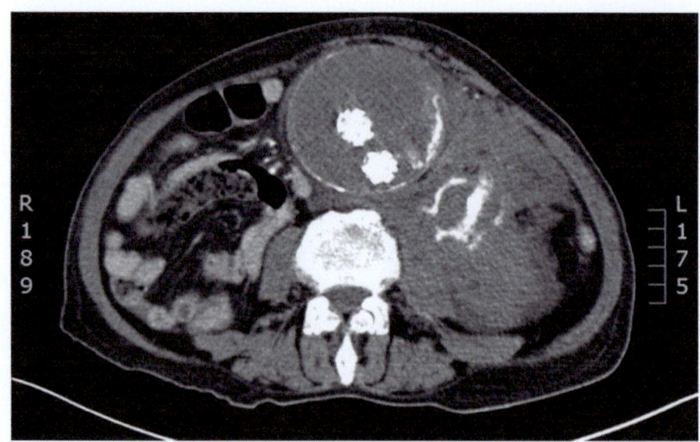

Fig. 36.7 CT scan of rAAA after EVAR

expected to increase in frequency and may lead to more complex endovascular repairs requiring suprarenal fixation or fenestrated endografts. The vascular surgeon should be well equipped to manage this highly lethal condition [43–47].

Key Points

- Ruptured aneurysms require prompt diagnosis and treatment.
- If the patient is sufficiently stable, a CT scan should be performed.
- Aortic clamping is crucial in either possible surgical treatment, open repair, or EVAR.

36.2 Acute Intestinal Ischemia

Acute intestinal ischemia is "a syndrome caused by inadequate blood flow through the mesenteric vessels, resulting in ischemia and eventual gangrene of the bowel wall. Although relatively rare, it is a potentially life-threatening condition" [48]: in fact, actually contemporary reviews show a high mortality, between 60 and 80% [49].

Acute mesenteric ischemia (AMI) can be caused by arterial or venous occlusion; the arterial thrombosis is divided in acute or chronic, in dependence of their onset.

Among acute mesenteric ischemia, we have different etiologies: SMA thromboembolism and mesenteric hypoperfusion syndromes (the most important are nonocclusive mesenteric ischemia and aortic dissection with mesenteric hypoperfusion) [50] (Fig. 36.8).

Nonocclusive mesenteric ischemia (NOMI) is a clinical status, typical of patients with low cardiac output or sepsis, frequently associated with the use of vasoactive/inotropic drugs (often multiple-drug therapies) [50, 51].

36.2.1 Epidemiology and Risk Factors

36.2.1.1 Thrombotic and Embolic AMI

Nowadays population-based studies are not complete because autopsies are rarely performed; actual data refer just to operated patients [50].

AMI frequency was reported to be 17.7% among patients requiring emergency laparotomy and 31% among non-traumatic patients who needed damage-control surgery [52].

Between 1972 and 1982, an epidemiological study conducted with a high autopsy rate (87%) in Sweden (Malmö population) estimated an overall incidence rate of AMI of 12.9% (95% confidence interval, 11.6–14.1) [53].

Figure 36.9 shows the different etiology distribution reported in that study [53].

Today we know that AMI is uncommon, 1–2 per 1000 hospital admissions; it seems to affect especially females (female/male ratio: 3/1), but adjusting for age and gender, we can get similar data.

Patients with AMI are typically between 60 and 70 years old, with some medical comorbidities [49, 54].

Two-thirds of patients with AMI present an acute SMA occlusion, whereas nonocclusive mesenteric ischemia and mesenteric venous thrombosis are less common [52].

History of atrial fibrillation, recent myocardial infarction, congestive heart failure, and peripheral arterial

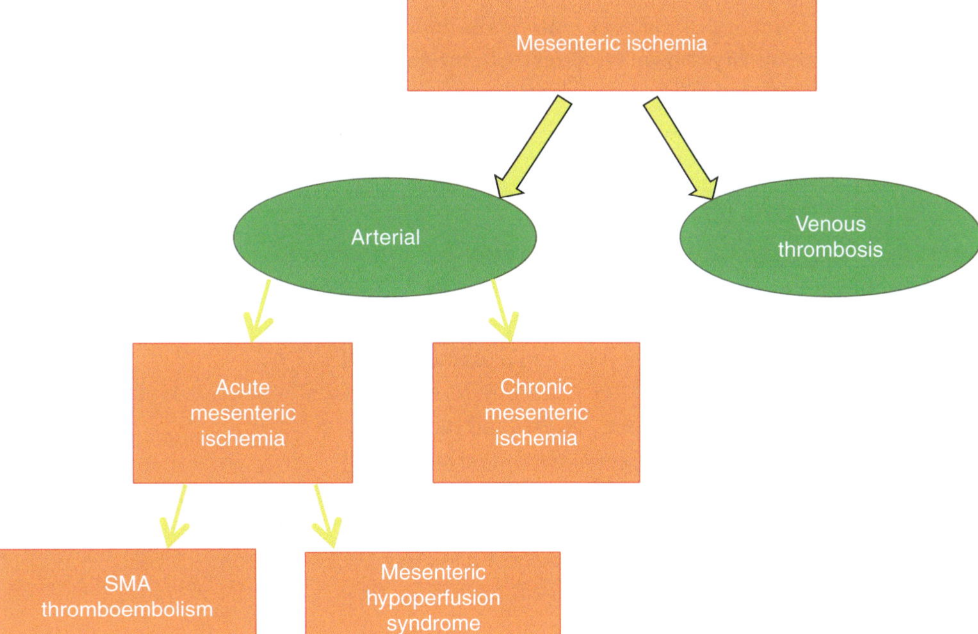

Fig. 36.8 Classification of mesenteric ischemia

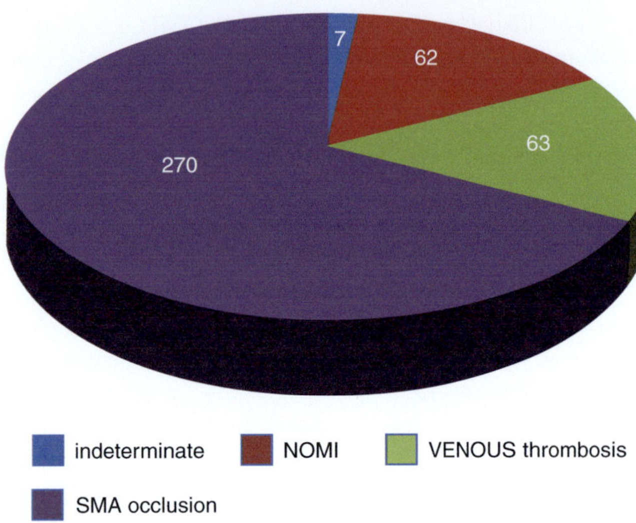

Fig. 36.9 Different etiologies of AMI in Malmö study

emboli are considered clinical risk factors for *embolic* AMI [49, 54].

A history of postprandial abdominal pain, loss of weight, and food intolerance have to make us suspect for an acute thrombotic AMI [49].

Acosta et al. [55] realized a study based on 213 autopsies with cases of SMA occlusion, and they find a ratio embolus/thrombus of 1 [52, 56].

They identified an embolic origin in 80% of patients: the most common findings were atrial fibrillation and synchronous embolism, with embolic dislodgement to renal, splenic, common hepatic, and celiac trunk arteries in 41% of patients.

Thrombotic lesions were frequently associated with old cerebral infarction, aortic wall thrombosis, and disseminated cancer, occlusion, or severe celiac trunk stenosis (in 33% of patients) [55].

Seventy-three percent of patients with SMA thrombotic occlusion had previously shown symptoms of chronic mesenteric ischemia [55].

They also observed that thrombotic occlusions were more proximal than the embolic ones, with larger intestinal infarction [55].

36.2.1.2 Hypoperfusion Syndromes: NOMI

Being clinically not always well defined or easily recognized, NOMI's prevalence isn't clear, even if mixed populations with bowel gangrene show a percentage between 4 and 60%.

Malmö population study defined "NOMI" all those clinical cases where there were no signs of emboli and absence of mesenteric arteries thrombosis, dissection or significant stenosis.

NOMI's incidence was 2/100,000 person-years (in spite of 8.6 for thromboembolic etiologies and 1.8 for MVT); they also reported that NOMI was as fatal as MVT and one-fifth deadly as SMA occlusion.

It's reasonable to think that pharmacological improvements have to lead to a decrease of NOMI, but the rising number of cardiac pump devices has created a new source of NOMI [50, 51].

Another common finding between different experiences is the difficulty to divide NOMI from SMA thromboembolic occlusion without angiography, TC or autoptic exam, because they have common risk factors, such as fatal cardiac failure, recent atrial fibrillation, or surgery.

Most of the patients (often the oldest ones) with NOMI also had SMA (40%) or celiac trunk concomitant stenosis.

About one-fifth presented synchronous infarction in the liver, spleen, or kidney [51, 53].

Mitsuyoshi et al. [57] defined four criteria for early diagnosis of NOMI (Table 36.2): a patient with three of them after cardiovascular surgery or renal replacement therapy is at risk of NOMI; we must require an urgent CT to get an early diagnosis [51].

36.2.1.3 Mesenteric Venous Thrombosis (MVT)

MVT in Malmö study and the most recent ones was 2.7/100,000 person-years, equally affecting males and females, especially from 70 to 79 years, with a mortality rate of 20%.

Risk factors for MVT are divided into three groups: direct injury, local venous congestion or stasis, thrombophilia (Table 36.3) [53, 58].

Table 36.2 Mitsuyoshi et al. criteria for early detection of NOMI

Mitsuyoshi et al. criteria for early diagnosis of NOMI
Symptoms of ileus with slow appearance and an increasing trend
Need of catecholamine administration
An episode of hypotension
Slow increase of transaminase level (LDH included)

Table 36.3 Risk factors for Mesenteric Venous Thrombosis

Direct injury	Local venous congestion/stasis	Thrombophilia
Postsurgical trauma	Portal hypertension/ liver cirrhosis	Activated protein C resistance
Pancreatitis	Heart failure (EF < 20%)	Protein S deficiency
	Obesity (BMI > 40%)	Protein C deficiency
		Lupus anticoagulant
		Cardiolipin antibodies
		Abdominal cancer
		Pancreas cancer
		Liver metastasis
		Metastatic cancer
		Oral contraceptive use/ estrogen substitution
		Extramesenteric previous or synchronous VTE

In these patients, risk factors for early death are intestinal infarction, advanced cancer, pulmonary embolism and hepatorenal failure, elevated age of patient, conditions like malignancy or other comorbidities, and a delay in diagnosis [53, 58].

36.2.2 Diagnosis

The typical AMI clinical trial is characterized, in an elderly patient, by severe abdominal pain without pathological abdominal signs (pain "out of proportion"), bowel emptying, and a source of embolia [50, 52].

These classic symptoms can be absent in 20–25% of cases [52].

Frequently SMA occlusion and MVT are very difficult to be recognized promptly.

There are slight clinical differences among embolic SMA, thrombotic SMA, and MVT, as summarized in Table 36.4.

Independently from AMI etiology, laboratory findings are frequently hemoconcentration, leukocytosis, high anion gap, and lactic acidosis in advanced cases. We can also find elevation of amylase, aspartate aminotransferase, and lactate. All these blood tests are insensitive and nonspecific for AMI [49, 54].

Table 36.4 Clinical different presentation of embolic SMA, thrombotic SMA, and MVT

	Embolic SMA	Thrombotic SMA	MVT
Abdominal pain	Sudden onset	Insidious onset	Insidious onset
Vomiting	+(71%)	+/–	+/–
Diarrhea	+(42%)		y
Bloody stools	+	+/–	
Female genre	++	+	
Age (years old)	>80	>80	<50
Anamnesis of atrial fibrillation	+		
Anamnesis of myocardial infarction	+		
Previous artery embolism	+		
Previous deep vein thrombosis or pulmonary emboli			+
Still-unknown source of emboli	+		
Stroke	+/–	++	
Synchronous embolism	++		
Previous chronic mesenteric ischemia		++	
Pancreatic or hepatic pathologies			+
Coagulation deficit			+

36.2.3 Imaging

About 25% of patients are completely normal at plain x-rays. In advanced cases of AMI, we can see bowel wall edema ("thumb printing") or pneumatosis; x-ray helps to exclude other etiologies of abdominal pain such as bowel obstruction or perforation.

Duplex ultrasonography in the abdominal district can evidence high-grade stenosis of the celiac trunk and SMA, but it's not widespread because it's highly operator-dependent and can't be limited by intestinal gas, typical of nonfasted patients. Then duplex can reach just the proximal part of SMA, but emboli go further, in its distal segments, so this creates the risk of false negative results [49].

Contrast-enhanced computed tomography (CT) represents the examination of choice and has replaced angiography to get the diagnosis [49, 54].

In fact CT allows bowel evaluation and finding AMI etiology (embolic occlusion seems like an oval clot surrounded by contrast in a segment of artery located in the middle and distal part of the main trunk of SMA without significant atheromasic signs, thrombotic lesions present a clot overlying on an atheromasic occlusive lesion at the ostium of SMA) [49, 52].

Otherwise, preoperative CT scan can be used in an endovascular setting to assess the level and orientation of vessels (Fig. 36.10).

Angiography today is important especially for allowing many complementary or stand-alone treatments such as injection of intra-arterial vasodilators, thrombolysis, and angioplasty with or without stenting [49].

Less useful are other diagnostic exams like MRI or laparoscopy; in fact, the first has a CT-inferior resolution, limited to 1 mm (insufficient to see very distal emboli), overestimates the degree of stenosis, and requires significant postprocessing. Moreover, the secondary signs of AMI (indurated fat, bowel wall thickening, etc.) are more difficult to recognize with MRI.

Laparoscopy is quite limited to assess intestinal viability because segmental ischemia can't be seen because of a difficult bowel navigation [49].

36.2.4 Treatment

36.2.4.1 Medical Treatment

Patients with AMI should be treated immediately with an isotonic crystalloid solution, and then, if necessary, invasive monitoring should be started, measuring hourly urine output, continuous central pressure and arterial pressure. A broad-spectrum antibiotic therapy has to be started together with intravenous heparin administration (doubling normal PTT), if not contraindicated [49].

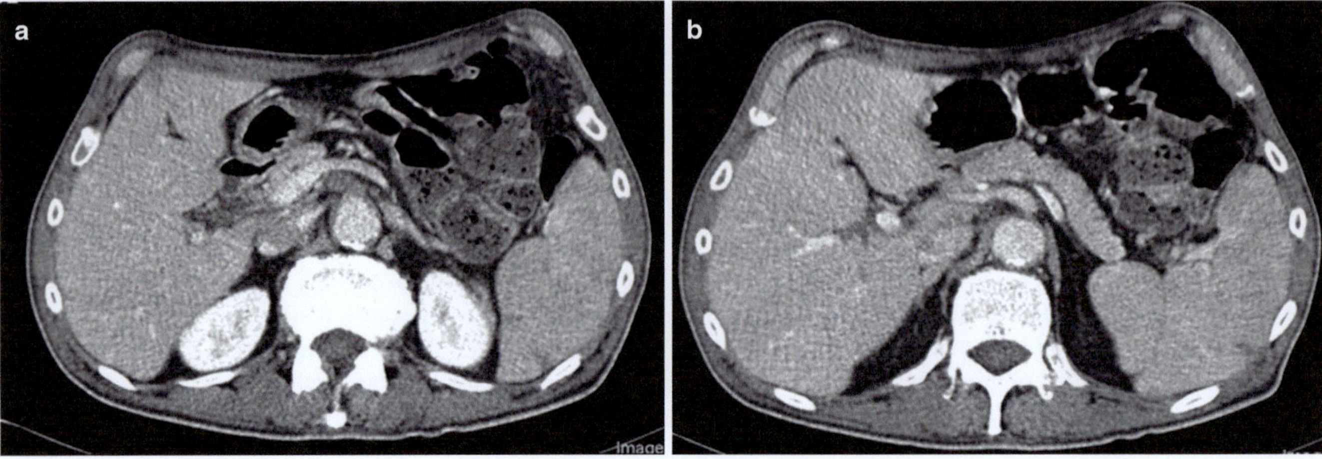

Fig. 36.10 Patient with symptoms of AMI, at CT, occlusion at AMS origin (**a**) and significant stenosis of celiac trunk (**b**)

If these patients develop sepsis and organ dysfunction, they are managed with the awareness that vasopressors can worsen bowel ischemia and visceral vasospasm, so before their administration, we have to verify adequate right heart filling pressures. These patients have a high percentage of fluid sequestration, so it's mandatory to perform serial examination and bladder pressure monitoring to recognize an eventual abdominal compartment syndrome. Dobutamine, lower-dose dopamine, and less epinephrine are considered vasopressors of choice; pure alpha-adrenergic agents shouldn't be used [49].

In MVT anticoagulant therapy is administered to stop the extension of thrombosis, and fibrinolytic drugs try to restore the patency of the affected venous segment [57].

So heparinization starts at the diagnosis, using unfractionated or low molecular weight heparin in therapeutic doses [58].

Literature reports that anticoagulant therapy increases recanalization up to 80% and recommends to consider lifelong treatment in case of prothrombotic risk factors.

It's not well-known how long the patient must be anticoagulated, but in literature, many authors report at least 6 months; after that period, every decision will be tailored to the patient features, considering the MVT etiology.

Risk of bleeding is contained between 1 and 4%; a problem linked to anticoagulation is the risk of intestinal bleeding in case of mucosa necrosis.

A stand-alone medical treatment in MVT is successful in more than 90% of cases [58].

36.2.4.2 Surgical Treatment

Ideally, AMI treatment should require open or endovascular surgery or both.

After clinical and CT evaluation, it's essential to exclude peritonitis and understand the etiology of occlusion (embolic or thrombotic); in case of peritonitis, laparotomy is mandatory.

It's necessary to perform revascularization before sectioning any tract of the bowel, with exception made for cases of intestinal perforation, areas of frank necrosis, or peritoneal soilage, which requires resection of the affected bowel without reanastomosis [49, 52].

Bowel revascularization can be achieved with endovascular, open, or hybrid treatment.

Open Surgery

Open revascularization, through midline laparotomy, can be obtained by surgical embolectomy, endarterectomy, patch angioplasty, or bypass grafting, with final assessement of bowel viability [49].

Key Points

In case of SMA bypass

- Perform a "lazy-C" bypass to avoid aortic clamping and prevent kinking.
- The more the length is, the more the graft has a good lie.
- Perform end-to-end anastomosis to improve graft patency.
- Choose vein graft in case of peritoneal contamination.

With a laparotomic access, it is possible to remove with a Fogarty catheter the thrombotic material even from the mesenteric vein, which runs parallel and right to its artery at the lower border of the pancreas, easily reached after lifting up the transverse colon. Laparotomy also allows to perform a bowel resection if required. In case of venous ischemia, it can be more difficult to distinguish the line between vital and ischemic tissue, as the border can be more diffuse than in the arterial ischemic case. In case of doubt or peritoneal contamination, it's better to exteriorize the bowel ends and perform an anastomosis in a second time.

So a second look surgery could be reasonable, with good results also reported for laparoscopic second looks [49].

Patient has to be prepared and draped including both legs (at least until the knee) in case harvesting great saphenous vein or superficial femoral vein should be required [49].

A vertical midline incision is performed; an anterior or a more lateral surgical approach allows to expose SMA, depending on the etiology of AMI; the first is best for embolic etiologies or patent SMA, and the latter is useful for thrombotic occlusion and/or SMA disease [49].

SMA Embolectomy

SMA embolectomy requires exposition of the anterior wall of the vessel, reached elevating the omentum and transverse colon and mobilizing the small bowel to the right.

The peritoneum is sectioned with a horizontal incision at the base of the transverse mesocolon (without mobilizing the fourth portion of duodenum or Treitz ligament).

During dissection of the superior mesenteric vein (to the right of SMA), autonomic nerve fibers and small lymphatics are exposed, and they are sacrificed to expose SMA. To see the proximal segment of SMA, even the inferior pancreatic border can be carefully mobilized, preserving the splenic vein and its tributaries from the pancreas, too.

So SMA and all the branches included are isolated from the middle to the right colic branches; after systemic heparinization a transversal or longitudinal arterectomy is performed (the latter will require a patch angioplasty).

Ideally it would be better to extract thrombus just venting the proximal tract of SMA, but, if it's necessary, an embolectomy balloon catheter can be also used (the most employed are 3 Fr or 4 Fr); distal segment can be treated with a 2 or 3 Fr catheter of the same kind. Sometimes passing through small distal multiple branches can be difficult; in alternative or adjunct, the surgeon can place a hand on either side of the mesentery and "milk" embolic material out of the arteries.

After complete thrombus removal, we can suture the arteriotomy as previously described [49].

SMA Bypass

In this case, a major tract of the artery is exposed, using a lateral access to SMA, passing above the fourth portion of the duodenum and opening the peritoneum lateral to the duodenum itself, along with the aorta and the left or right common iliac artery.

Graft orientation depends on the features of the inflow vessels (and their degree of atheromasic lesions) and the overall lie of the graft.

One of the most used graft orientations is the "lazy-C": it's a retrograde configuration, with a graft that originates from the right iliac artery and allows to avoid any aortic clamping and prevent kinking (Fig. 36.11).

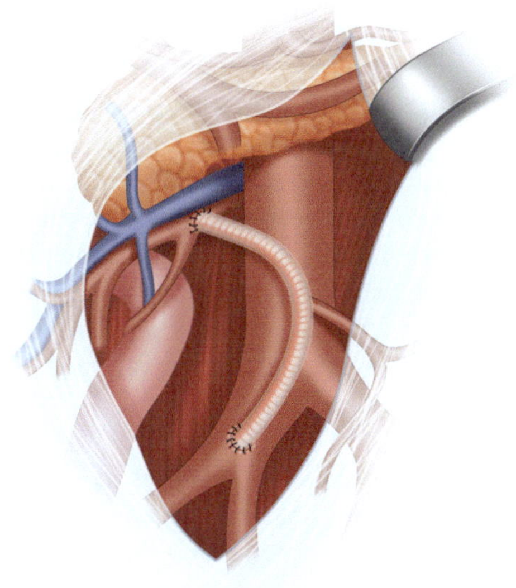

Fig. 36.11 The "lazy-C" bypass from SMA to the right common iliac artery

It's also possible to perform lazy-C grafts originating from the left iliac artery or the distal infrarenal aorta. The more the bypass length is, the more it has a good lie; graft patency results in better performing end-to-end graft to SMA anastomosis.

Anterograde bypass has to be considered if distal inflow sources are not ideal, because of their high degree of atheromasic disease, while the supraceliac aorta is generally relatively free of atheromasic lesion; another advantage is that this graft configuration is not easily prone to kinking.

Disadvantages are that supraceliac aorta is more complex to be isolated, so it requires a great technical effort, spending more time, and if partial clamping isn't possible, with aortic cross clamping, a hemodynamic and physiological stress is produced [49].

Bypass is generally performed with prosthetic grafts of 6–8 mm in Dacron or PTFE; there's no evidence that synthetic bypasses have a better patency than biological ones.

The degree of abdominal contamination leads to choice of graft; in particular, in case of significant peritoneal soilage, the use of vein is preferred; primary options are great saphenous vein or femoral veins. Veins require an additional effort for their harvesting that can be dangerous for critically ill patients; they also show a more elevated risk of kinking and external compression, because of their smaller diameters and the same features of their venous wall.

If there's no alternative to synthetic grafts, Kazmer's technique can be performed, consisting in covering a retrograde prosthetic bypass with an omental flap passed through the transverse mesocolon.

Hybrid Approach: Retrograde Open Mesenteric Stent (ROMS)

It's a hybrid technique proposed by Wyers et al. that consists in opening horizontally or longitudinally the peritoneum at the base of the transverse colon; SMA is isolated, and a local thromboendarterectomy is performed, and then the artery is closed with a patch (in vein or bovine pericardium) angioplasty that helps to easily realize a retrograde cannulation of SMA with a long flexible sheath to the aorta. In the end, SMA is stented to reduce the number of restenoses [49, 59].

This technique allows to reach a good result in SMA revascularization in a faster and easier way, exploring bowel viability at the same time [49].

36.2.4.3 Endovascular Techniques in Acute AMI

Endovascular treatment of AMI has widespread extensive use of multidetector CT angiography and the great progress in endovascular techniques reached in the last two decades [59].

> **Key Points**
> In endovascular treatment of AMI
>
> - Move cautiously catheters to avoid dislodgment of proximal clot.
> - After stenting, measurement of residual pressure gradient across the stent allows to avoid early restenosis.

The most used is a percutaneous femoral access, while a brachial one is used just when SMA takeoff is very sharp or when a proximal stenotic lesion is the origin of occlusion (in this case brachial approach gives us a better angle of access and less risk of dissection).

To get a good imaging, a 5 Fr pigtail catheter is generally preferred, positioned at T12 level. Generally Omnipaque 300 g/mL or Visipaque 270 mg/mL is used, but in patients with impaired renal function, we can choose CO_2 at the beginning, to see the main mesenteric arteries. 1 mg glucagon is injected to stop bowel movements, and then images are acquired by abdominal aortogram in lateral and anteroposterior views, using 20–25 mL of contrast at a rate of 20 mL/s. Once identified the visceral arteries origins, selective catheterism is performed. Caution is needed, avoiding to dislodge eventual proximal clot with catheterization; after controlling with few contrast to have reached the correct position, an angiography will be realized to see the peripheral filling and the venous return (with 15–18 mL of volume at 5–7 mL/s).

SMA and celiac trunk catheters with longer tips can be used to make easier distal access to these vessels. Heparin is administered to achieve an ACT of 250–300 s (generally it's used 100 U/kg) [59].

Aspiration embolectomy: If imaging shows a proximal SMA, embolus an antegrade approach is the first choice: the SMA will be catheterized with a reverse curve catheter and a hydrophilic 0.035-inch guidewire that has to be changed with a stiffer one. Sometimes it is possible to exchange directly the stiffer wire on the reverse curve catheter.

When the wire has been positioned, an introducer with the removable hub (a 7 Fr 45 cm or 8–9 Fr guiding catheter) can be left proximal to the embolus. Inside this, a 4–6 Fr catheter is introduced and aspiration with a manual 20-mL syringe starts, together with sheath withdrawal. In this way, the clot removal can be performed.

Many passages of the aspiration sheath in a to-and-from motion are required to achieve complete clot aspiration; for every passage of the wire out of the femoral sheath, it's necessary to remove its hub to be sure that there's no residual embolic material in the introducer. It's also possible to use a double-lumen aspiration catheter, with one channel for the wire and the other for aspiration; they are useful for difficult access, while their limit is that they remove small amounts of clots compared with large lumen sheets alone [59].

SMA Thrombolysis

Thrombolysis is rarely used alone to treat AMI because it usually needs a long time to clear the obstruction and in case of bowel necrotic disease it could cause severe gastrointestinal bleeding [58].

In literature, there are many combined treatments of thrombolysis with other percutaneous thrombectomy devices [58].

For instance, frequently thrombolysis is performed together with mechanical methods of clot removal, to restore vessel patency rapidly; in fact it is useful to complete the effect of a mechanical removement of thrombotic material in residual or very distal clots.

Thrombolysis increases the risk of gastrointestinal bleeding, and it's contraindicated when laparotomy is necessary; so this treatment is reserved just for those patients with low suspicion of transmural intestinal infarction [59].

In MVT it can be preferably administered as an intrathrombotic treatment using a transhepatic portography to place the catheter in the thrombus; in this way the risk of bleeding and the administered thrombolytic dose can be reduced; in alternative SMA it can be used to administer the drug.

In particular, the aspiration sheath can be left in the proximal SMA (catheter embolectomy has been realized previously) and placed a multi-side hole infusion catheter in the SMA, performing a local thrombolysis with rTPA at 0.5–1 mg/h rate. After 12 h the angiographic result can be controlled, and it can be decided to stop or continue the treatment [59].

Stenting

Stenting of visceral arteries takes place in case of proximal stenosis or occlusion; percutaneous transluminal angioplasty

(PTA) alone, for its low patency rate and its risk of dissection, is not recommended.

At first passing across the lesion is necessary; it can't be easy with a femoral access; in this case, a brachial access can be used with a 4 Fr Headhunter catheter. The following step is introducing a 1.5 mm balloon on a Simmons catheter and dilating the lesion after aspiration and/or thrombolysis.

We have to choose the right balloon for the right lesion because the different features of the devices make them more or less adequate to a different degree of calcified lesions (e.g., Teflon-coated balloons are useful for lesions with difficult access, because of their slipperiness).

It's wise to stent an occlusive lesion with a balloon-expandable stent, stronger than self-expandable nitinol stents, very useful for ostial stenosis and avoiding post-dilatation recoil. For SMA and celiac trunk, stents of 7–9 mm diameters are a good choice, while smallest devices can compromise long-term patency. After stenting, angiography and pressure measurement are performed: a residual pressure gradient across the stent of more than 12 mmHg requires additional PTA and/or stenting to avoid restenosis (Fig. 36.12) [59].

36.2.4.4 Assessment of Bowel Viability

After revascularization it's necessary to assess the extent and severity of intestinal ischemia; before any decision, it's necessary to wait at least 20–30 min of reperfusion [49].

Key Points

- During bowel resection for necrosis, exteriorize the bowel ends and perform an anastomosis in a second time.

Valuating bowel viability is not easy; in fact, intestinal segments prone to irreversible necrosis can appear quite normal, and segments bound to recover after revascularization can seem ischemic [49].

Laparotomy allows to see bowel condition, and it's the first choice method because it's safer and quicker than the same laparoscopy, which is limited in evaluating extensive intestinal paralysis with distended bowel loops.

Assessment of bowel viability is based mainly on clinical judgment and timely reevaluation, with the aim to save the greatest length of intestinal loops as possible [49].

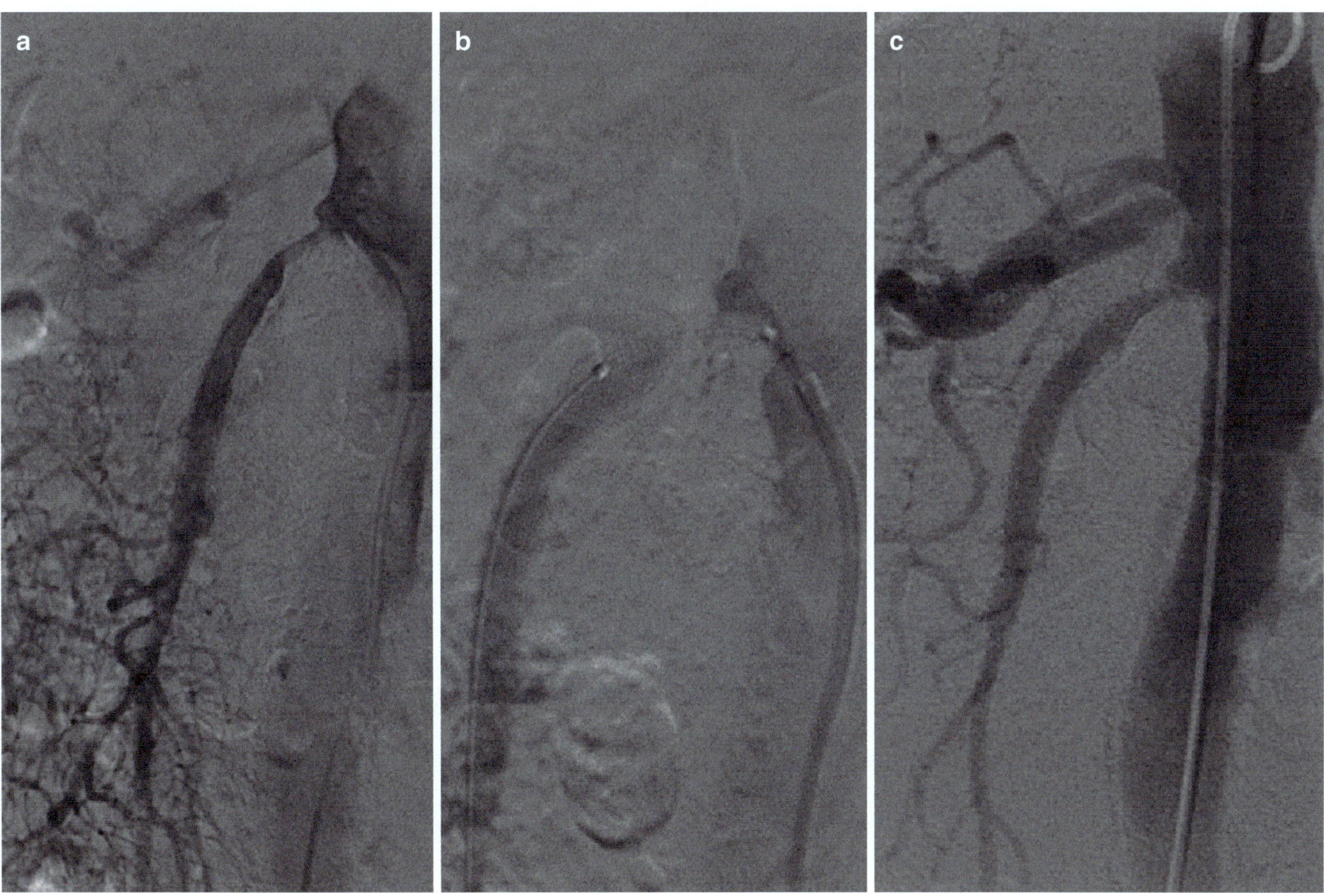

Fig. 36.12 Patient with AMI: at angiography significant AMS stenosis (**a**), stented with a balloon-expandable stent 6 × 18 mm, without reaching the nominal diameter (**b**). Residual pressure gradient across the stent is <12 mmHg; procedure is ended with clinical success (AMI resolution)

The surgeon has to remind that at first-look surgery it is difficult to determine bowel viability with certainty; at the end of the first operation, he has to decide if a second look is required to assess newly bowel viability and extend intestinal resection only if it's strictly necessary. So he typically will leave bowel transected ends stapled shut without reanastomosis [49].

Rarely it's advisable to perform a third look, before final bowel anastomosis is realized [49].

Bowel loops are evaluated looking for color and aspect of the bowel serosa, dilatation of intestinal loop, peristalsis, bleeding from cut surfaces, and visible or palpable pulsations in the mesenteric arcade [49, 50].

A continuous wave 9–10 MHz Doppler can be useful to detect nonviable segments.

Another method uses fluorescein and a perfusion fluorometer or a laser Doppler flowmeter to get an accurate quantification of a segment perfusion.

After revascularization, splanchnic vasospasm can persist for a variable period, worsening bowel ischemia; to reduce this phenomenon, papaverine can be administered into SMA.

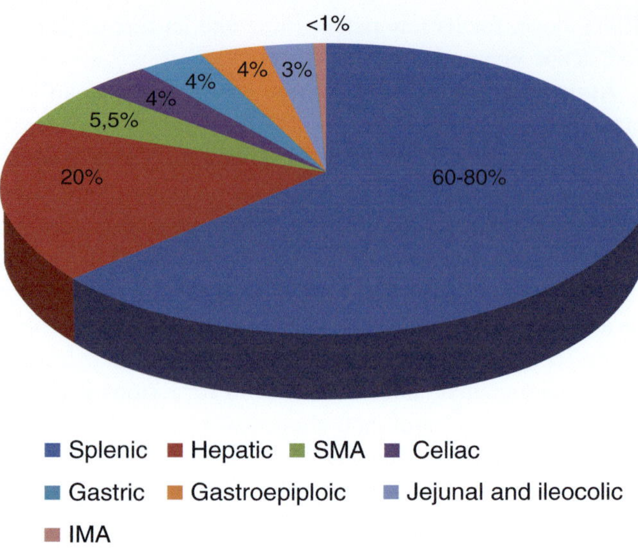

Fig. 36.13 Percentage of involvement of different arteries in visceral arteries

36.3 Splanchnic Aneurysms

Splanchnic aneurysms are intra-abdominal aneurysms of the celiac trunk; gastroduodenal, pancreatic, splenic, superior, or inferior mesenteric artery; and renal arteries and their branches [60].

> **Key Points**
> - In VAAs endovascular treatment is important to occlude their collaterals to avoid carefully the aneurysmatic sac. continues to be perfused

36.3.1 Epidemiology

They are rare, often asymptomatic, incidental findings at TC or MRI, but sometimes they can require an emergency treatment in case of rupture [11, 21]. Rupture is documented in about 25% of them, with an elevated mortality rate of 70% [61].

They can involve visceral arteries with different incidence, as shown in Fig. 36.13 [60].

The rising number of endovascular procedure in the liver and kidney today has increased the number of intrahepatic and renal aneurysms [60].

True visceral aneurysms are divided from pseudoaneurysms: the first are dilatation involving all the three layers of the arterial wall; they can be sacciform or fusiform, mainly caused by atherosclerosis, fibrodysplasia, or connective tissue diseases [61].

The latter are dilatation lacking a complete arterial wall; they represent lesion with an elevated risk of rupture, independently from their size.

Imaging shows us typical signs of atherosclerosis (for exwall calcification) in true visceral aneurysms, while pseudoaneurysms appear like a round contrast-enhanced arterial lesion next to an artery [60, 61].

36.3.2 Etiology

Thirty-two percent of VAAs are due to atherosclerosis, while medial degeneration is responsible for 24% of them, with its reduced number of smooth muscle cells and reduction or fragmentation of fibers. Other etiologies are abdominal and surgical trauma (22%) and infectious or inflammatory diseases (10%). In the pre-antibiotics era, most of VAAs had mycotic and/or inflammatory causes, often in association with endocarditis.

Other causes can be connective tissue diseases, such as Marfan or Ehlers-Danlos syndrome, hereditary hemorrhagic telangiectasia, Osler-Weber-Rendu disease, Kawasaki syndrome, and fibromuscular dysplasia.

Some systemic diseases can also give diffuse vascular anomalies and multiple aneurysms, such as Still disease, systemic LES, Hashimoto thyroiditis, and polyarteritis nodosa.

Finally, pregnancy and portal hypertension are considered risk factors for splenic and hepatic aneurysms [60, 62, 63].

Pseudoaneurysms can result from trauma, inflammation, infection, and vasculitis, or they can be iatrogenic. Moreover, pancreatitis, with the release of pancreatic enzymes, may produce destruction of the arterial wall, resulting in pseudoaneurysms of the splenic, hepatic, gastroduodenal, and pancreaticoduodenal arteries [60].

Visceral aneurysm rupture is a life-threatening condition, with an elevated mortality rate of up to 30% in emergency; rupture can be associated with intra- or retroperitoneal bleeding, gastrointestinal bleeding, or bleeding into adjacent organs. An important number of ruptures occur after other medical procedures [16].

Many authors considered a diameter superior to 2 cm or three times greater than the respective normal artery as mandatory for the treatment of any visceral aneurysm, but different experiences show that the risk of rupture doesn't depend only on aneurysm size but also from its localization, rate of growth, and underlying pathology. Some centers also consider their morphological aspect, believing that wall calcification indicates a long-standing lesion and can be a sign of aneurysmal stability. Instead a signal of impending rupture is rapid size increase [60, 62].

36.3.3 Diagnosis and Imaging

Computed tomography is the first-line imaging modality for patients with abdominal pain in the emergency department. All patients with a suspect of impending rupture of VAA should undergo to CT scan imaging [60].

36.3.4 Treatment

VAAs can be treated with open or endovascular approaches. Management depends mainly on the location of the aneurysm, with an endovascular approach that is the first choice in aneurysms involving the parenchymal branches of the hepatic, splenic, renal, or pancreaticoduodenal arteries [60].

Open and endovascular treatments of VAAs share the common goal of preventing aneurysm expansion and rupture or repairing the ruptured ones. This purpose is best accomplished by excluding the aneurysm from the arterial circulation and pressure. In case of adequate collateral flow, surgical management consists of ligation of the parent artery proximal and distal to the aneurysm. Otherwise, bypasses or grafts should be required [60].

Endovascular treatment can lead to isolation of the aneurysm from the arterial circulation: this goal can be achieved through different techniques.

Aneurysmatic large arteries can be "trapped" between coils placed first distally and then proximally to the aneurysm (Fig. 36.14a). For smaller aneurysms the distal artery or its branches can be occluded with large particles, placing also coils in the larger proximal part of the parent artery. In this way, the aneurysmatic lesion will be excluded from the circulation. We have to pay attention to occlude also other collaterals that could continue to perfuse the aneurysmatic sac (Fig. 36.14b) [60].

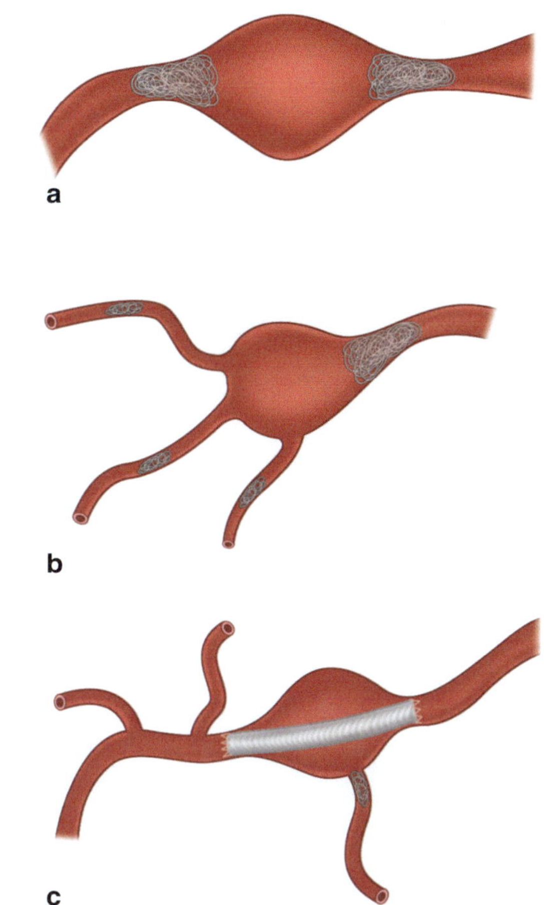

Fig. 36.14 Treatment of aneurysmatic large arteries with coils

Coils are useful also for **saccular aneurysms with a narrow neck**: these devices can be used to fill the sac, constrained by its same neck; in case of **wider neck**, the lesion can be treated using a stent-assisted coil placement.

This technique consists of positioning a stent across the aneurysm neck (Fig. 36.14c) and then filling the sac with coils introduced through the interstices of the stent, which in turn avoid coils migration [60].

Glue or thrombin can be added to fill the sac with the coils into.

Thrombin injection can also be chosen to treat VAA: under CT or ultrasonographic guidance, a 20–22 gauge needle is introduced into the sac, and thrombin is injected until the aneurysmatic or **pseudoaneurysmatic lesion** has no more flow. This method is frequently used for small peripheral traumatic pseudoaneurysms of the liver, spleen, or kidney or for treating pancreaticoduodenal aneurysms [60].

For those VAAs where **preserving arterial perfusion is necessary**, we can use covered stents, useful for arteries of at least 6 mm of diameter; their use is limited by size and stiffness of their delivery systems, which make them not so advisable to be placed in distal tortuous vessels [60].

36.3.5 Follow-Up

Independently of treatment a careful postprocedural surveillance is necessary to exclude any enlargement or reperfusion of the aneurysmatic sac from collateral branches; a good follow-up can be realized with ultrasound and CT scan, performed at 1, 3, 6, 9, and 12 months [60].

36.3.6 Splenic Artery Aneurysms (SAAs)

36.3.6.1 Epidemiology

SAAs represent the 60% of VAAs, their real prevalence is difficult to establish because they are mainly asymptomatic. Autoptic findings suggest a prevalence from 0.1 to 10.4% [62, 64, 65].

Concomitant visceral aneurysms have been detected in 3% of patients, while non-visceral aneurysmatic lesions have been found in 14% of patients (this percentage includes renal artery dilatations) [66].

They are four times more common in women than in men, in particular, in women with multiple pregnancies. In fact, the hormonal changes typical of pregnancy leads to structural weakness of the vessels wall, and portal congestion produces an increase of wall stress. These factors give a combination of medial hyperplasia and fragmentation of the elastic lamina. The same pathophysiology is associated with splenic arteries developed in patients with portal hypertension that counts a prevalence of 10% in lienal aneurysms [60, 62, 64–66].

Other different etiological factors attributed to aneurysm formation include angiodysplasia, pregnancy, atherosclerosis, diabetes, intracranial aneurysm, polyarteritis nodosa, alpha-1-antitrypsin deficiency, and infective factors.

Frequently they are asymptomatic, most of them are identified incidentally, or in case of rupture, this event is associated with a 25% mortality which increases to 75% among pregnant women with fetal mortality of 95%. In pregnant women with splenic aneurysms, two-thirds of them rupture in the third trimester followed by the second trimester; at the time of rupture, most lesions are more than 2.5 cm, but also smaller aneurysms have become symptomatic [67].

36.3.6.2 Clinical Diagnosis

Rupture can be sudden or in two stages, the latter (20–25% of cases) is characterized by an acute abdominal pain, with a brief stable period (from 6 to 96 h) followed by collapse. These clinical features are due to an initial rupture in the lesser sac, contained by omentum and/or blood clots that block foramen of Winslow, and then it is followed by free rupture into greater sac, when the tension within the lesser sac increases.

In 13% of patients, we assist to secondary erosion of the aneurysm into adjacent viscera, causing gastrointestinal bleeding due to rupture into the stomach, colon, or pancreatic duct. Rupture communicating with the splenic vein can lead to an arteriovenous fistula, with portal hypertension, or even mesenteric steal syndrome and ischemia of the small intestine [65–67].

In case of rupture, the patient refers acute abdominal pain in epigastrium or left hypochondrium, sometimes with the Kehr's sign.[1] Nausea, vomiting, and collapse can be associated. In pregnant women ruptured aneurysmatic lienal artery can be misdiagnosed with placental abruption [65, 67].

The natural history of untreated splenic artery aneurysms remains poorly defined; no consensus on a size criterion for aneurysm treatment in asymptomatic patients has been found. For many years splenic aneurysms greater than 2 cm in low-risk patients must be repaired; this dogma was based mainly on several small retrospective reviews of patients with splenic aneurysm rupture, but today has fallen into disuse [64–66].

Another common practice is that patients with childbearing potential or undergoing liver transplantation need aneurysm repair, independently of their size. Stanley et al. have proposed a reasonable approach that consists in treating elected patients with a mortality less than 0.5%, based on the fact that rupture risk is 2% associated with 25% of operative mortality in emergency [66]. Also enlarging aneurysms and aneurysms 2.5–3 cm or more in diameter may require treatment [67].

36.3.6.3 Diagnosis

In suspect of rupture of splenic aneurysm, CT scan or digital subtraction angiography are indicated, in order to define the exact site of the lesion, its collateral branches and the source of bleeding, and to find out other eventual visceral aneurysms [65].

Surgical treatment can involve open, laparoscopic, or endovascular surgery, in dependence of the presentation, location (many of them are placed in the mid-distal part of the artery), and size of the aneurysm.

It is important to preserve the spleen in order to save immunological function [65]. However, there is evidence that ligature or embolization of lienal artery alters the spleen function, even if it is preserved.

[1] Pain in the tip of the left shoulder.

Surgical treatment of SAA includes ligation or resection for aneurysms in the proximal or middle segment of the splenic artery. Short gastric arteries and pancreatic arcade provide flow to the distal splenic artery, so bypass surgery is not necessary [65].

Complete or partial splenectomy can be performed in case of a lesion near the hilum or involving intrasplenic branches; sometimes in emergency partial, pancreatectomy can be necessary too. In this case, mortality rate rises to 20% versus 5% in elective surgery, with highest percentages in emergency.

The approach to the splenic artery can be through an anterior or a lateral route; the second has an increased risk of splenic infarction because it can compromise short gastric and left gastroepiploic vessels.

A safe and feasible treatment is the laparoscopic one, in the hand of a well-experienced surgeon with the help of intraoperative ultrasound. Even in this case, the operator can choose between an anterior and a lateral route, with lateral approach that is the first choice for central and distal aneurysms. Laparoscopic technique is contraindicated in unstable patients.

Endovascular trapping is a good alternative to open surgery for asymptomatic or symptomatic aneurysms without signs of frank rupture (Fig. 36.15) [60, 64, 66].

Complications include coils migration and distal infarction, abscess formation, and, rarely, rupture of the aneurysm. Recanalization can occur in up to 12.5% of patients. Embolization can also fail for technical reasons, in particular in case of extreme tortuous splenic artery [65].

After endovascular treatment we can also observe the so-called "postembolization syndrome," a combination of fevers, abdominal pain, ileus, and pancreatic inflammation, observed in 30–80% of patients, that resolves within 4–5 days after the procedure [64, 66].

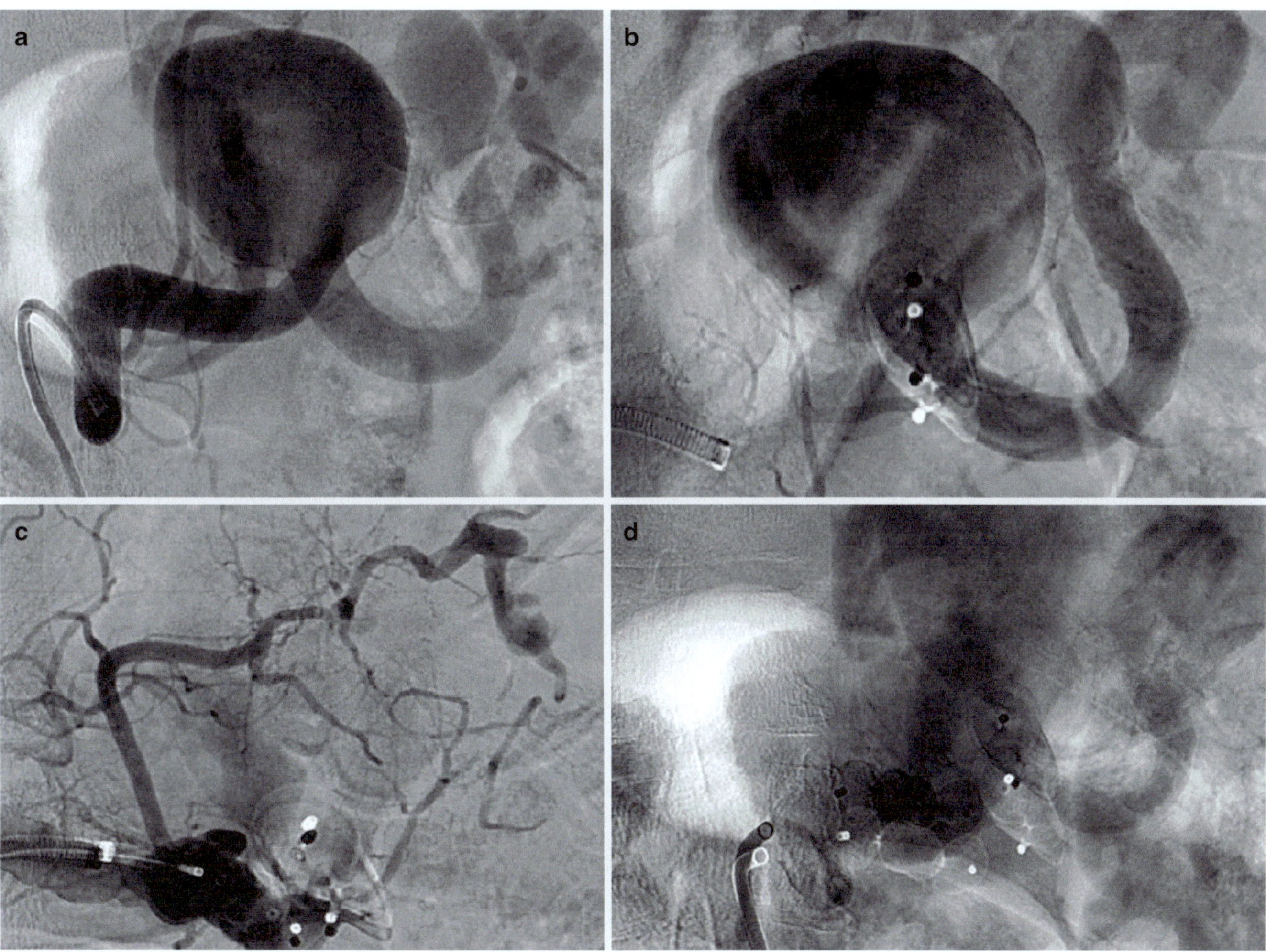

Fig. 36.15 Patient with symptomatic splenic aneurysm seen at CT and confirmed by angiography (**a**); plugs are positioned in the afferent and efferent vessel (**b**); at last we can see complete exclusion of the aneurysm, with revascularization from gastric artery and immediate perfusion of the superior segment of spleen (**c**, **d**)

36.3.7 Hepatic Aneurysms

36.3.7.1 Epidemiology

Hepatic artery aneurysms are the second most common kind of VAAs, with a major prevalence in men (3:2), involved in 66% of cases the extrahepatic tract of the artery, often with a degenerative or dysplastic etiology. Intrahepatic branch aneurysms (3%) instead show a traumatic or iatrogenic history or are associated with infections or vasculitis. Twenty percent of these VAAs can show both intra- and extraparenchymal involvement.

As for the splenic ones, true hepatic artery aneurysms are most commonly due to medial degeneration and secondary atherosclerosis.

They generally affect the patient in their sixth decade of life. Concomitant aneurysms in the visceral or non-visceral arteries are associated, respectively, for 31 and 42% [60, 66].

Key Points

In hepatic artery aneurysms

- Perform a temporary occlusion of the vessel; in case of signs of ischemia, reconstruct the artery, especially in low-risk patients with small-diameter gastroduodenal artery.
- In case of strong surrounding inflammation and proximity to the common bile duct, repair the aneurysm proceeding from the inside.
- In patients with large segments of the liver at risk or baseline liver dysfunction, intrahepatic endovascular embolization is contraindicated.

Rupture has been reported in 20–80% of hepatic aneurysms, with mortality rates from 21 to 35%; that's why an aggressive approach is required to treat these lesions [60].

Pseudoaneurysms represent about 25% of all the hepatic aneurysm cases described in the literature; they are secondary to blunt or to penetrate traumatic injury or iatrogenic.

They become symptomatic medially 5.7 months after injury, with hemobilia, abdominal pain, and jaundice.

36.3.7.2 Diagnosis

Most of hepatic aneurysms are asymptomatic, incidentally diagnosed at CT scan or angiography, but some of them can become symptomatic: in fact, rapid expansion of the aneurysmatic sac produce severe abdominal or back pain in the patient, and large aneurysm can give an extrahepatic compression of the biliary tree.

Aneurysmatic decompression in the biliary tree is quite frequent, while rupture into the peritoneal sac or manifesting with gastrointestinal bleeding is rarer.

One-third of symptomatic patients present the so-called triad of Quincke, characterized by epigastric pain, hemobilia, and obstructive jaundice.

It's not clear which risk factors can be associated to rupture, and its same prevalence is difficult to establish. Hypertension is the commonest comorbidity, while fibromuscular dysplasia or polyarteritis nodosa puts the patient at high risk for hepatic artery aneurysm formation.

These conditions are associated with an increased risk of rupture; we find them in about 50% of ruptured hepatic aneurysms [60, 66].

36.3.7.3 Imaging and Treatment

As for splenic aneurysms, anatomical location of the lesion deeply influences its own surgical treatment.[2] Angiography or CT scan can delineate potential anatomical variants and the exact position of the aneurysmatic sac, evaluating also collateral vessels [66].

When lesion involves the common hepatic artery, the aneurysmatic sac can be ligated or resected theoretically without any reconstruction, because the gastroduodenal and right gastric branches should provide a good perfusion; in literature are reported different experiences that describe central liver necrosis after treating a hepatic proximal lesion.

For this reason, in low-risk patients, arterial reconstruction with autogenous conduit has been suggested, in particular where the gastroduodenal artery is small. Many authors describe the use of intraoperative ultrasound to assess significant changes in hepatic vascularization, before performing a definitive ligation [60, 66].

Surgical treatment of more distal extrahepatic lesion, with the involvement of the proper hepatic or proximal right or left hepatic arteries, requires direct arterial reconstruction with autogenous vein.

Some authors also suggest repairing the aneurysm proceeding from the inside of the sac, in case of strong surrounding inflammation and proximity to the common bile duct [60, 66].

Endovascular management of intrahepatic aneurysms is the treatment of choice: transcatheter coil occlusion or embolization is less invasive than open surgery and allows to avoid hepatic resection.

Ischemic complications are minimal thanks to the collateral blood flow and oxygen delivery coming from the portal vein. We have to remind that patients with large segments of liver at-risk or baseline liver dysfunction are not good candidates for intrahepatic endovascular embolization [60, 66].

Endovascular repair is also for extrahepathic lesions: common hepatic artery aneurysms placed proximal to the origin of the gastroduodenal and right gastric arteries can be embolized by coils with a percutaneous access.

[2]Treatment is the same for aneurysm or pseudoaneurysm; now we'll indicate both lesions with the term "aneurysm."

The proper hepatic artery can be treated with covered stent, but only in absence of excessive tortuosity and if we can find an adequate landing zone.

36.3.8 Gastroduodenal and Pancreaticoduodenal Aneurysms

Aneurysms and pseudoaneurysms often are complications of acute or chronic pancreatitis and pancreatic surgery or have a dysplastic or degenerative etiology. Mainly asymptomatic, some of them can lead to gastrointestinal or intra- or retroperitoneal bleeding. Their treatment today is mainly endovascular, through the sac embolization and a careful search and occlusion of all their collateral vessels.

36.3.9 Celiac Trunk Aneurysms

They represent 4% of all VAAs, often with a degenerative nature, frequently (20%) associated with aortic aneurysms and other visceral aneurysms (40%). They equally affect males and females in the fifth decade of life.

Their real risk of rupture is still unknown; today it is estimated to be about 13%, with a mortality of 100% in emergency, that has led to an aggressive surgical management that can include aneurysmectomy, aneurysmorrhaphy, or ligation, with or without arterial reconstruction or endovascular treatment[3] (Fig. 36.16).

36.3.10 SMA Aneurysms

They represent the 5.5% of all VAAs, generally placed in the proximal 5 cm of the artery.

They affect mainly men in their fifth decade of life and present an increasing trend in prevalence. They can be mycotic or caused by inflammation, trauma, arterial dissection, vasculitis, or dysplasia or degenerative disease. These aneurysms are often symptomatic, showing acute and colic upper abdominal pain, associated to nausea or vomiting; about half of the patients present a palpable pulsating abdominal mass.

The high risk of rupture of this lesion (50%) makes them prone to be surgically treated; techniques are the same as that described for celiac trunk aneurysms [60].

Key Points
AMI and symptomatic VAAs

- Because of their high mortality rate, they represent an emergency condition and should be treated urgently.
- CT scan is the exam of choice for all patients with severe abdominal pain and clinical suspect of AMI, renal artery ischemia, or symptomatic VAAs.
- The treatment of choice is the endovascular one, because it is effective and less invasive than open surgery, with exception made for AMI with bowel necrosis when laparotomic access is mandatory to assess intestinal viability.

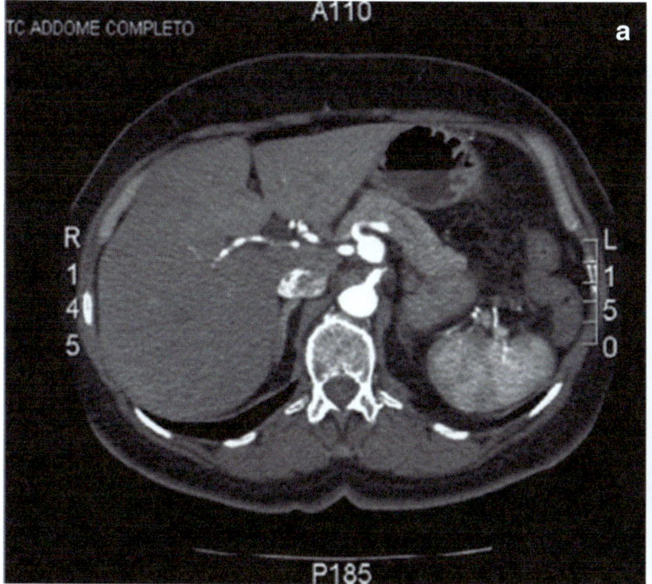

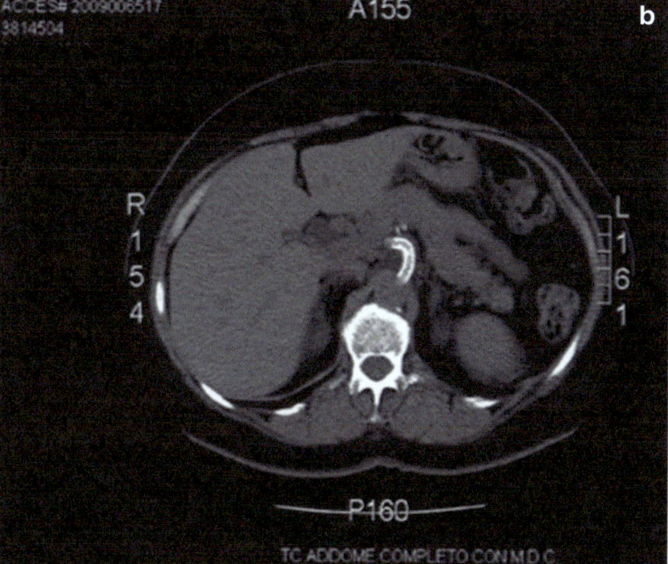

Fig. 36.16 Celiac trunk aneurysm (**a**) treated with a covered stent in the hepatic artery and excluding with coils splenic artery (**b**)

[3]As for other VAAs, their site and morphology condition the kind of treatment (mainly embolization or placement of covered stent).

The lesion frequently is in the proximal tract of SMA or celiac trunk: the lack of a landing zone limits the use of coils or covered stents. Simple ligation in these lesions is possible thanks to the extensive collateral circulation between the two vessels, through the pancreatic arcades. Revascularization with venous or prosthetic graft or direct arterial reconstruction is necessary for patients with a ruptured aneurysm and bowel ischemia or preoperative signs or symptoms of intestinal ischemia [60].

Case Scenario

A. A 60-year-old woman with persistent increasing abdominal pain for 2 months. She refers worsening epimesogastric pain in the last 2 days. Previous medical history: CAD, hypertension, and diabetes.

Vital signs and physical exam result are within normal limits except for abdominal pain.

ECG and screening for myocardial infarction are negative. The abdominal US reveal a turbulent blood flow at the origin of the celiac trunk, but the vessel wall is not well defined.

1. **Which is your diagnostic suspect?**
   A. Myocardial infarction
   B. Celiac trunk stenosis vessels disease
   C. Celiac trunk aneurysm
   D. Both C and D
   E. None of the previous answers

2. **What is the right imaging test for this patient?**
   A. No imaging but analgesic therapy should be started.
   B. Contrasted US abdomen imaging.
   C. MR abdomen imaging.
   D. CT abdomen imaging.
   E. All the previous answers.

3. **Imaging revealed…** (Fig. 36.17)
   A. Abdominal aortic aneurysm
   B. Celiac trunk aneurysm
   C. Celiac trunk stenosis
   D. Both B and C
   E. None of the previous answers

4. **Considering this diagnosis what would you also have to exclude also at CT scan?**
   A. Signs of aneurysmatic rupture
   B. Associated VAAs
   C. Associated abdominal aortic aneurysms
   D. All the previous answers

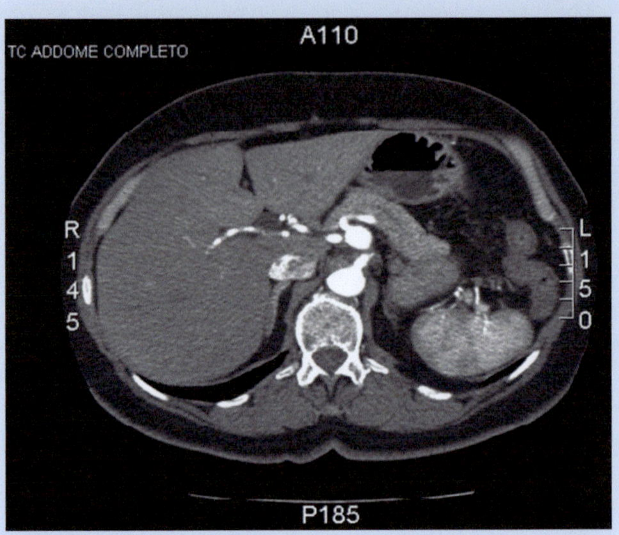

Fig. 36.17 CT scan of the patient

5. **Considering CT findings and clinical assessment, how do you treat the patient?**
   A. Conservative approach, as she has a 1.5 cm celiac trunk symptomatic aneurysm, but she's not of childbearing age, and there are no signs of rupture.
   B. Urgent endovascular treatment (coils embolization) of the aneurysmatic lesion.
   C. Urgent open surgical treatment.
   D. None of the previous answers.

Please see Chap. 58 for the correct answer.

References

1. Hirsch AT, Haskal ZJ, Hertzer NR, et al. ACC/AHA 2005 Practice guidelines for the management of patients with peripheral arterial disease (lower extremity, renal, mesenteric, and abdominal aortic): a collaborative report from the American Association for Vascular Surgery/Society for Vascular Surgery, Society for Cardiovascular Angiography and Interventions, Society for Vascular Medicine and Biology, Society of Interventional Radiology, and the ACC/AHA Task Force on Practice Guidelines. Circulation. 2006;113(11):e463–654.
2. Moll FL, Powell JT, Fraedrich G, Verzini F, Haulon S, Waltham M, van Herwaarden JA, Holt PJE, van Keulen JW, Rantner B, Schlösser FJV, Setacci F, Ricco J-B. Management of abdominal aortic aneurysms clinical practice guidelines of the European Society for Vascular Surgery. Eur J Vasc Endovasc Surg. 2011;41:S1–S58.
3. van Beek SC, Conijn AP, Koelemay MJ, Balm R. Endovascular aneurysm repair versus open repair for patients with a ruptured abdominal aortic aneurysm: a systematic review and meta-analysis of short-term survival. Eur J Vasc Endovasc Surg. 2014;47(6):593–602.
4. Akkersdijk GJ, van Bockel JH. Ruptured abdominal aortic aneurysm: initial misdiagnosis and the effect on treatment. Eur J Surg. 1998;164(1):29–34.
5. Cao P. Comparison of surveillance vs aortic endografting for small aneurysm repair (CAESAR) trial: study design and progress. Eur J Vasc Endovasc Surg. 2005;30:245–51.

6. Ouriel K. The pivotal study: a randomised comparison of endovascular repair versus surveillance in patients with smaller abdominal aortic aneurysms. J Vasc Surg. 2009;49:266–9.
7. Powell JT, Brown LC, Forbes JF, Fowkes FG, Greenhalgh RM, Ruckley CV, et al. Final 12-year follow-up of surgery versus Management of Abdominal Aortic Aneurysms S45 surveillance in the UK small aneurysm trial. Br J Surg. 2007;94:702–8.
8. Ballard DJ, Filardo G, Fowkes G, Powell JT. Surgery for small asymptomatic abdominal aortic aneurysms. Cochrane Database Syst Rev. 2008;(4):CD001835.
9. Sullivan CA, Rohrer MJ, Cutler BS. Clinical management of the symptomatic but unruptured abdominal aortic aneurysm. J Vasc Surg. 1990;11:799.
10. Franks S, Lloyd G, Fishwick G, et al. Endovascular treatment of ruptured and symptomatic abdominal aortic aneurysms. Eur J Vasc Endovasc Surg. 2006;31:345.
11. Antonello M, Lepidi S, Kechagias A, et al. Glasgow aneurysm score predicts the outcome after emergency open repair of symptomatic, unruptured abdominal aortic aneurysms. Eur J Vasc Endovasc Surg. 2007;33:272.
12. Karthikesalingam A, Holt PJ, Vidal-Diez A, et al. Mortality from ruptured abdominal aortic aneurysms: clinical lessons from a comparison of outcomes in England and the USA. Lancet. 2014;383:963.
13. Cho JS, Kim JY, Rhee RY, et al. Contemporary results of open repair of ruptured abdominal aortoiliac aneurysms: effect of surgeon volume on mortality. J Vasc Surg. 2008;48:10.
14. Dua A, Upchurch GR Jr, Lee JT, et al. Predicted shortfall in open aneurysm experience for vascular surgery trainees. J Vasc Surg. 2014;60:945.
15. Dick F, Erdoes G, Opfermann P, Eberle B, Schmidli J, von Allmen RS. Delayed volume resuscitation during initial management of ruptured abdominal aortic aneurysm. J Vasc Surg. 2013;57:943–50.
16. IMPROVE Trial, Powell JT, Thompson SG, et al. The Immediate Management of the Patient with Rupture: Open Versus Endovascular repair (IMPROVE) aneurysm trial, IMPROVE trialists. Acta Chir Belg. 2009;109:678.
17. Reimerink JJ, Hoornweg LL, Vahl AC, et al. Controlled hypotension in patients suspected of a ruptured abdominal aortic aneurysm: feasibility during transport by ambulance services and possible harm. Eur J Vasc Endovasc Surg. 2010;40:54.
18. Veith FJ, Cayne NS, Berland TL, Mayer D, Lachat M. Open surgical and endovascular management of ruptured abdominal aortic aneurysm. In: Moore WS, editor. Vascular and endovascular surgery: a comprehensive review. 8th ed. Philadelphia: Elsevier/Saunders; 2013. p. 685–90.
19. Biancari F, Hobo R, Juvonen T. Glasgow Aneurysm Score predicts survival after endovascular stenting of abdominal aortic aneurysm in patients from the EUROSTAR registry. Br J Surg. 2006;93:191.
20. Sarac TP, Bannazadeh M, Rowan AF, et al. Comparative predictors of mortality for endovascular and open repair of ruptured infrarenal abdominal aortic aneurysms. Ann Vasc Surg. 2011;25:461.
21. Pol RA, Reijnen MM, Zeebregts CJ. Outcome after open repair of ruptured abdominal aortic aneurysm in patients >80 years old: a systematic review and meta-analysis. World J Surg. 2011;35:2575.
22. Scarcello E, Ferrari M, Rossi G, et al. A new preoperative predictor of outcome in ruptured abdominal aortic aneurysms: the time before shock (TBS). Ann Vasc Surg. 2010;24:315.
23. Marin ML, Veith FJ, Cynamon J, et al. Initial experience with transluminally placed endovascular grafts for the treatment of complex vascular lesions. Ann Surg. 1995;222:449–65.
24. Reimerink JJ, Hoornweg LL, Vahl AC, et al. For the AJAX Investigators. Endovascular repair versus open repair of ruptured abdominal aortic aneurysms: a multicenter randomized controlled trial. Ann Surg. 2013;258:248–56.
25. IMPROVE Trial Investigators, Powell JT, Sweeting MJ, et al. Endovascular or open repair strategy for ruptured abdominal aortic aneurysm: 30 day outcomes from IMPROVE randomised trial. BMJ. 2014;348:f7661.
26. Moore R, Nutley M, Cina CS, et al. Improved survival after introduction of an emergency endovascular therapy protocol for ruptured abdominal aortic aneurysms. J Vasc Surg. 2007;45:443–50.
27. Mehta M, Kreienberg PB, Roddy SP, et al. Ruptured abdominal aortic aneurysm: endovascular program development and results. Semin Vasc Surg. 2010;23:206–14.
28. Van Herzeele I, Sevdalis N, Lachat M, et al. Team training in ruptured EVAR. J Cardiovasc Surg. 2014;55:193–206.
29. Ohki T, Veith FJ, Shaw P, et al. Increasing incidence of mid and long-term complications after endovascular graft repair of AAAs: a note of caution based on a 9-year experience. Ann Surg. 2001;234:323–34.
30. Larzon T, Skoog P. One hundred percent of ruptured aortic abdominal aneurysms can be treated endovascularly if adjunct techniques are used such as chimneys, periscopes and embolization. J Cardiovasc Surg. 2014;55:169–78.
31. Badger S, Bedenis R, Blair PH, et al. Endovascular treatment for ruptured abdominal aortic aneurysm. Cochrane Database Syst Rev. 2014;7:CD005261.
32. Holst J, Resch T, Ivancev K, et al. Early and intermediate outcome of emergency endovascular aneurysm repair of ruptured infrarenal aortic aneurysm: a single-centre experience of 90 consecutive patients. Eur J Vasc Endovasc Surg. 2009;37:413–9.
33. Malina M, Veith F, Ivancev K, Sonesson B. Balloon occlusion of the aorta during endovascular repair of ruptured abdominal aortic aneurysm. J Endovasc Ther. 2005;12:556–9.
34. Veith FJ, Lachat M, Mayer D, et al. Collected world and single center experience with endovascular treatment of ruptured abdominal aortic aneurysms. Ann Surg. 2009;250:818–24.
35. Malina M, Holst J. Balloon control for ruptured AAAs: when and when not to use? J Cardiovasc Surg. 2014;55:161–7.
36. Lachat M, Bisdas T, Rancic Z, et al. Chimney endografting for pararenal aortic pathologies using transfemoral access and the lift technique. J Endovasc Ther. 2013;20:492–7.
37. Oderich GS, Ricotta JJ 2nd. Modified fenestrated stent grafts: device design, modifications, implantation, and current applications. Perspect Vasc Surg Endovasc Ther. 2009;21:157–67.
38. Starnes BW. Physician-modified endovascular grafts for the treatment of elective, symptomatic, or ruptured juxtarenal aortic aneurysms. J Vasc Surg. 2012;56:601–7.
39. IMPROVE Trial Investigators. The effect of aortic morphology on peri-operative mortality of ruptured abdominal aortic aneurysm. Eur Heart J. 2015;36(21):1328–34.
40. Hinnen JW, Koning OHJ, van Bockel JH, Hamming JF. Aneurysm sac pressure after EVAR: the role of endoleak. Eur J Vasc Endovasc Surg. 2007;34:432–41.
41. Schermerhorn ML, O'Malley AJ, Jhaveri A, Cotterill P, Pomposelli F, Landon BE. Endovascular vs. open repair of abdominal aortic aneurysm in the Medicare population. N Engl J Med. 2008;358:464–74.
42. Peppelenbosch N, Buth J, Harris PL, van Marrewijk C, Fransen G, EUROSTAR Collaborators. Diameter of abdominal aortic aneurysm and outcome of endovascular aneurysm repair: does size matter? A report from EUROSTAR. J Vasc Surg. 2004;39:288–97
43. Chaar CI, Eid R, Park T, Rhee RY, AbuHamad G, Tzeng E, et al. Delayed open conversions after endovascular abdominal aortic aneurysm repair. J Vasc Surg. 2012;55:1562–9.
44. Mehta M, Paty PS, Roddy SP, Taggert JB, Sternbach Y, Kreienberg PB, et al. Treatment options for delayed AAA rupture following endovascular repair. J Vasc Surg. 2011;53:14–20.
45. Turney EJ, Steenberge SP, Lyden SP, Eagleton MJ, Srivastava SD, Sarac TP, et al. A single center's first 100 late endovascular aneurysm repair expla nts. J Vasc Surg. 2013;57(5):25S.
46. May J, White GH, Stephen MS, Harris JP. Rupture of abdominal aortic aneurysm: concurrent comparison of outcome of those occurring after endovascular repair versus those occurring without

previous treatment in an 11-year single-center experience. J Vasc Surg. 2004;40:860–86.
47. de Bruin JL, Brownrigg JRW, Karthikesalingam A, Patterson BO, Holt PJE, Hinchliffe RJ, Morgan RA, Loftus IM, Thompson MM. Endovascular aneurysm sealing for the treatment of ruptured abdominal aortic aneurysms. J Endovasc Ther. 2015;22(3): 283–7.
48. Dang CV, Su M, et al. Acute mesenteric ischemia. Medscape, drug and diseases-general surgery. 2016.
49. Wyers CW. Acute mesenteric ischemia: diagnostic approach and surgical treatment. Semin Vasc Surg. 2010;23:9–20.
50. Acosta S, Bjorck M. Modern treatment of acute mesenteric ischaemia. Br J Surg. 2014;101(1):e100–8.
51. Bjorck M, Wanhainen A. Nonocclusive mesenteric hypoperfusion syndromes: recognition and treatment. Semin Vasc Surg. 2010;23:54–64.
52. Acosta S. Surgical management of peritonitis secondary to acute superior mesenteric artery occlusion. World J Gastroenterol. 2014;20(29):9936–41.
53. Acosta S. Epidemioloy of mesenteric vascular disease: clinical implications. Semin Vasc Surg. 2010;23:4–8.
54. Ryer EJ, Kalra M, et al. Revascularization for acute mesenteric ischemia. J Vasc Surg. 2012;55:1682–9.
55. Acosta S, Ögren M, et al. Clinical implications for the management of an acute thromboembolic occlusion of the superior mesenteric artery. Autopsy findings in 213 patients. Ann Surg. 2005;241:516–22.
56. Sharafuddin MJ, Nicholson RM, et al. Endovascular recanalization of total occlusions of the mesenteric and celiac arteries. J Vasc Surg. 2012;55:1674.
57. Mitsuyoshi A, Obama K, et al. Early diagnosis and management of mesenteric ischemia with an emphasis on pharmacotheraphy. Aliment Pharmacol Ther. 2005;21:201–15.
58. Bergqvist D, Svensson PJ. Treatment of mesenteric vein thrombosis. Semin Vasc Surg. 2010;23:65–8.
59. Resch T, Acosta S, et al. Endovascular techniques in acute arterial mesenteric ischemia. Semin Vasc Surg. 2010;23:29–35.
60. Nosher JL, Chung F, et al. Visceral and renal artery aneurysms: a pictorial essay on endovascular therapy. Radiographics. 2006;26:1687–704.
61. Lopez VM, Glauser J. A case of renal artery thrombosis with renal infarction. J Emerg Trauma Shock. 2010;3(3):302–8.
62. Pitton MB, Dappa E, et al. Visceral artery aneurysms: incidence, management, and outcome analysis in a tertiary care center over one decade. Eur Radiol. 2015;25:2004–14.
63. Gehlen JML, Heeren PAM, et al. Visceral artery aneurysm. Vasc Endovasc Surg. 2011;45(8):681–7.
64. Hogendoorn W, Lavida A, et al. Open repair, endovascular repair, and conservative management of true splenic artery aneurysms. J Vasc Surg. 2014;60:1667–76.
65. Bizueto-Rosas H, Barajas-Colón JA, et al. Multiple aneurysms splenic; surgical exclusion with conservation of the spleen. Cir Cir. 2016;84(1):58–64.
66. Berceli SA. Hepatic and splenic artery aneurysms. Semin Vasc Surg. 2005;18:196–201.
67. Sadat U, Dar O, et al. Splenic artery aneurysms in pregnancy—a systematic review. Int J Surg. 2008;6:261–5.

37 Mechanical Complications of Acute Myocardial Infarction

Antonino M. Grande and Alessandro Mazzola

Key Points

- Mechanical complications after myocardial infarction are very difficult to diagnose especially in patients who present with severe respiratory distress and shock.
- Quick diagnosis is vital, and it is obtained by echocardiography.
- Patients should undergo emergency surgical treatment.
- The infarcted myocardium is friable, and the endocardium may be covered in part by mural thrombi. Therefore, before aortic cross-clamping, carefully manipulate the heart in order to prevent dislodging necrotic tissues and thrombi.
- The use of the intra-aortic balloon pump and vasodilator drugs decreases both systolic arterial pressure (afterload) and left ventricular end-diastolic pressure (preload), increasing at the same time cardiac output. In this way, chances of survival are significantly improved until surgical treatment.

37.1 Introduction

The main acute mechanical complications (MC) of acute myocardial infarction (AMI) are:

- Ventricular septal rupture (VSR)
- Free wall rupture (FWR)
- Ischemic mitral regurgitation (IMR)

A. M. Grande (✉)
Department of Cardiac Surgery, IRCCS Fondazione Policlinico San Matteo, Pavia, Italy
e-mail: amgrande@libero.it

A. Mazzola
Cardiac Surgery, IRCCS Multimedica Sesto S. Giovanni, Milano, Italy

The occurrence of the MC after AMI is associated with an increased early and late mortality [1]. Anyway, the clinical introduction of primary percutaneous coronary intervention (PCI) has markedly declined the incidence of MC to less than 1%, including VSR (0.17%), FWR (0.52%), and IMR (0.26%). MC are very difficult to diagnose, especially in an emergency situation in patients who present with severe respiratory distress and shock. As matter of fact, echocardiography allows a rapid and precise diagnosis followed by emergency surgery. Intra-aortic balloon pump (IABP) insertion and vasodilator infusion reduce afterload increasing, at the same time, cardiac output.

37.2 Ventricular Septal Rupture (VSR)

Although percutaneous coronary intervention has been making VSR after AMI increasingly rare, mortality remains high. Postmyocardial infarction VSR is most commonly localized in the anterior or apical section of the ventricular septum (VS) as a consequence of anterior AMI. In about 20–40% of patients who had inferior AMI, the VSR is localized in the posterior portion of VS. VSR often occurs with complete occlusion of a coronary artery, in the majority of cases, the left anterior descending coronary artery (LAD), and usually collateral coronary circulation is poor [2]. In the past, before thrombolysis and PCI, VSR occurred in 1–2% of patients who had an AMI, generally within a week the onset of infarction [3, 4]. VSR determines shunting of blood from the left to the right ventricle, and the overall shunt volume depends on the pressure gradient across it and on the size of the defect. VSR eventually produces right ventricular failure and cardiogenic shock; left ventricular failure may be caused by AMI extent.

Physical examination reveals a holosystolic murmur, best heard at the left sternal edge, and a parasternal thrill may be present; it is important a differential diagnosis with mitral insufficiency due to papillary rupture where the murmur is

P. Aseni et al. (eds.), *Operative Techniques and Recent Advances in Acute Care and Emergency Surgery*,
https://doi.org/10.1007/978-3-319-95114-0_37

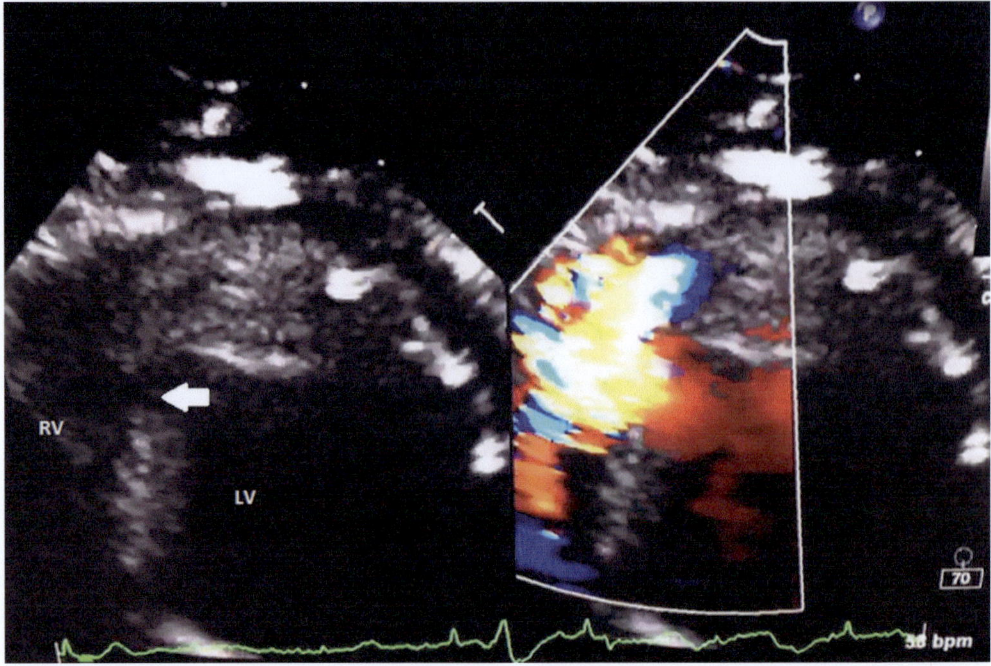

Fig. 37.1 In the left panel, the white arrow shows VSR; in the left panel, color Doppler flow demonstrates a large turbulent left-to-right flow. *VSR* ventricular septal rupture, *RV* right ventricle, *LV* left ventricle

loudest at the apex. Electrocardiogram shows anterior or inferior infarction with ST elevation (STEMI), and chest X-ray may highlight an enlarged heart and pulmonary congestion. Echocardiography with color Doppler flow (Fig. 37.1) is mandatory for diagnosis, showing the VSR site/size and estimating the left-to-right shunt volume.

37.2.1 VSR Surgical Repair

Surgery is done on an emergency basis after diagnosis. IABP insertion and vasodilator drug infusion can stabilize the patient determining an afterload reduction and cardiac output increase.

After median sternotomy, cardiopulmonary bypass is established via venous bicaval cannulation and arterial cannulation of the distal portion of the ascending aorta. The aorta is cross-clamped; cardioplegic solution is infused in ascending aorta but also through the coronary sinus route due to the acute coronary occlusion. Concomitant myocardial revascularization should be done whenever significant coronary artery disease is present and the vessel periphery is suitable. Then, the left ventriculotomy is carried out through the infarcted area in the anterior or apical aspect of the ventricle. The infarcted area is easily recognized by placing a suction probe after the institution of cardiopulmonary bypass: the recent infarcted area and/or a thinned scar of an old myocardial infarct pucker defining the limits within the incision is made. When VSR is located anteriorly, ventriculotomy is done about 1 cm lateral to the left anterior descending (LAD) coronary artery (Fig. 37.2). The septal defect is located below the incision (Fig. 37.3). At this point two surgical repairs are most commonly used.

(a) *Daggett technique*. This technique was introduced in 1977 by Willard M. Daggett [5]. The defect is repaired by suturing a patch of autologous or bovine pericardium. The ventricular septum is not resected, and the patch is tailored for the shape of the defect, covering the adjacent intact septum. The patch is sutured on the LV side of the septum using pledgeted mattress sutures, generally 3.0 polypropylene suture, with pledgets positioned on the right ventricular aspect of the defect. The patch can also be sutured with a continuous 3.0 or 4.0 polypropylene suture. Infarctectomy or aneurysmectomy is performed, and the ventriculotomy is closed using buttressed sutures; if the excised area is too large, a polyester or pericardial patch is sutured.
(b) *David technique*. This is the infarct exclusion technique introduced in 1987 by Tirone E. David [6]: a patch of autologous or bovine pericardium or Dacron is employed to separate the left ventricle from the VSR. Essentially, a new left ventricle is made realizing a new septum beside VSR that is inglobated in the right ventricle. The patch is sutured starting from the inferior border of VSR, and the suture is continued cephalad; stitches are passed through normal myocardium, and also the mitral annulus may be used to secure the patch to healthy tissue (Fig. 37.4) [7]. The ventriculotomy is eventually closed using buttressed sutures (Fig. 37.5).

In case of posterior VSR, it is important to know right ventricular function because the right ventricle is often involved; furthermore, mitral valve function should be assessed and, consequently, evaluated prior to a valve repair/substitution procedure. Posterior VSR is more difficult to expose and repair: the heart is lifted out of pericardial cavity,

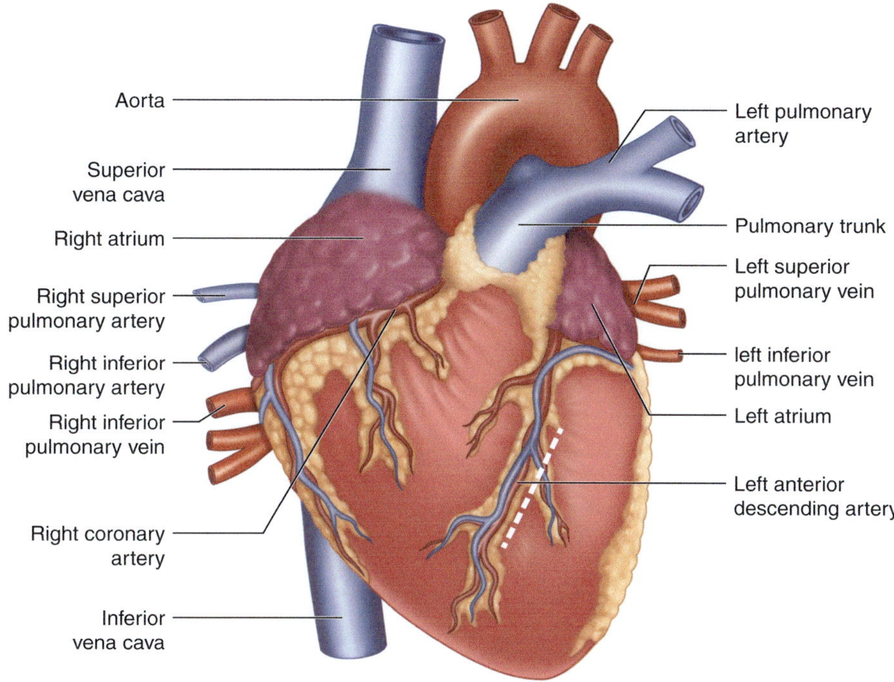

Fig. 37.2 Dashed line marks the incision area, about 1 cm beside the left anterior coronary artery

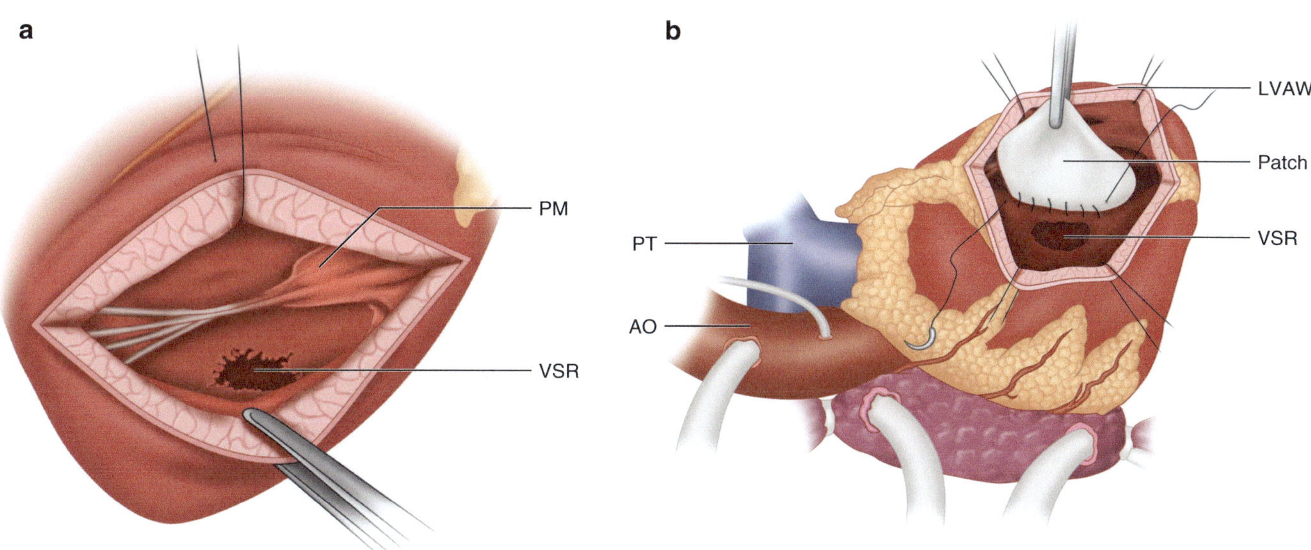

Fig. 37.3 Surgeon view. (**a**) The left ventricle is opened 1 cm lateral to left anterior descending coronary artery ventricular septal rupture (*VSR*) is located underneath the incision. (**b**) the patch is sutured starting for the posterior border of VSR using a 3-0 continuous polypropylene (papillary muscle (*PM*), left ventricle anterolateral wall (*LVAW*))

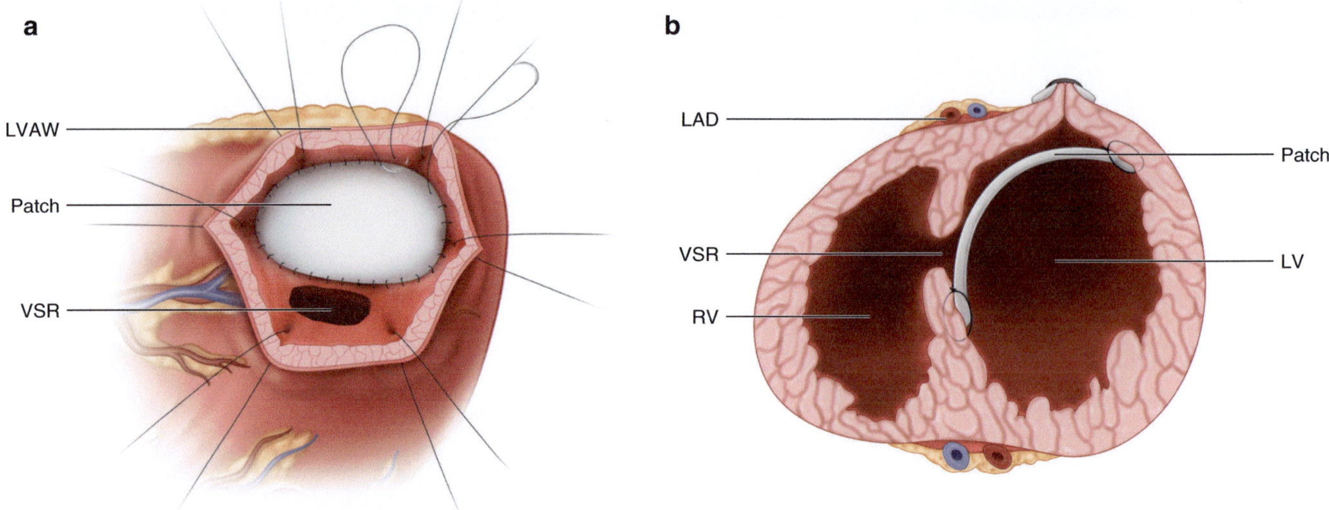

Fig. 37.4 (**a**) Suture line is continued into the LVAW. (**b**) Transverse section of the heart: David's technique allows to exclude LV from the infarcted myocardium (right ventricle (*RV*), left ventricle (*LV*))

Fig. 37.5 The left ventriculotomy is closed using buttressed sutures

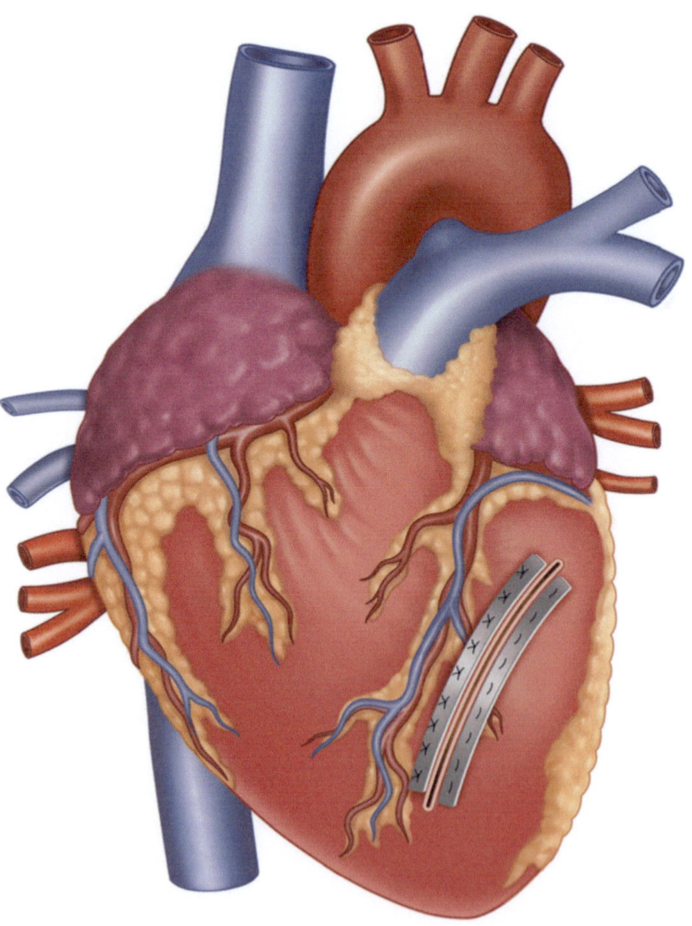

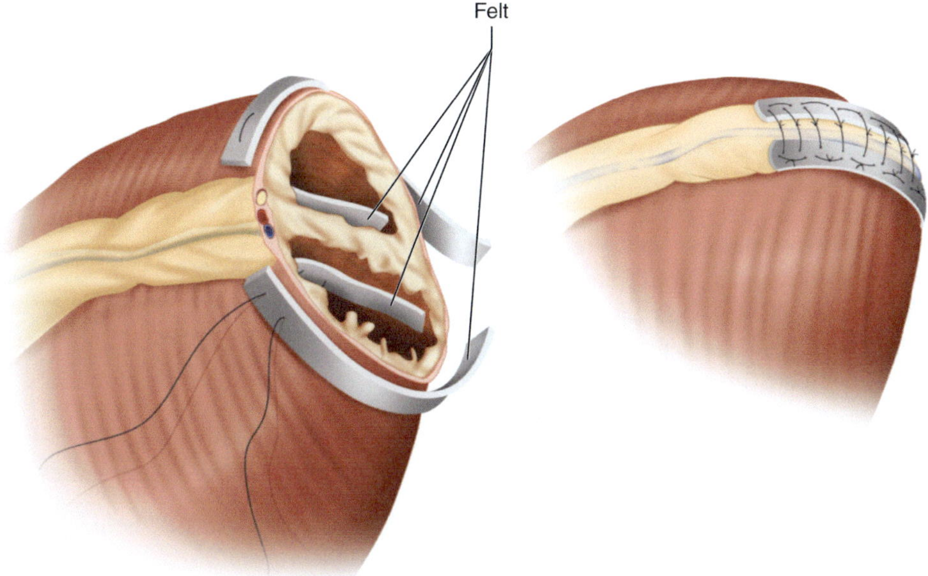

Fig. 37.6 VSR in the apical portion of the septum: the procedure is directly done by amputating the apex of the heart, together with the involved portion of the ventricular septum. The closure is performed by applying strips of polytetrafluoroethylene felt on each side of the septum and on edges of both ventricles

and the left ventricle is incised; VSD is approached through an incision in infarcted left ventricle parallel to the posterior descending coronary artery. The patch is positioned in the same fashion on the left ventricular side.

When the VSR is situated in the apical portion of the septum with an apical AMI, the procedure is directly done amputating the apex of the ventricle, together with the involved portion of the ventricular septum (Fig. 37.6).

It is remarkable to read what Dr. David said in 2012 at the 48th Annual Meeting of the Society of Thoracic Surgeons, Fort Lauderdale, FL, Jan 28–Feb 1, 2012: "… I was able to change the classical technique of infarctectomy and patches with a stiff Dacron graft (DuPont, Wilmington, DE) developed by Bill Daggett in Boston to a more conservative approach whereby we simply opened the infarct and excluded the infarcted muscle and ruptured septum by using a soft patch such as pericardium secured to the healthy endocardium around the infarct. We named the technique "infarct exclusion," and we were able to dramatically reduce, at least my personal mortality, particularly in patients with posterior septal rupture, who had the highest mortality 20–30 years ago …" [8].

37.3 Free Wall Rupture (FWR)

Left ventricular FWR is one of the most lethal complications following myocardial infarction. It occurs 4–10 times more often than rupture of the interventricular septum or of a papillary muscle, two conditions for which surgical treatment is widely applied. However, surgical treatment of cardiac rupture remains a surgical challenge for the high mortality even before the diagnosis is made.

FWR generally occurs between 1 and 7 days after AMI, a *blow out type rupture* determines the sudden patient's death for cardiac tamponade; FWR is more often a gradual process, starting with small areas of endocardial necrosis, allowing formation of hematomas that progressively dissect through the necrotic myocardium into the pericardium, resulting in tamponade and cardiogenic shock. FWR occurs in most cases on the lateral or anteroapical left ventricle. In the FRW the myocardial necrotic tissue appears weakened and friable, not ensuring stable anchoring sites for sutures; therefore, it is often necessary to sacrifice viable areas of myocardium with the result of significant reduction of LV dimensions. Various surgical techniques have been utilized, including pericardial patch placement with epicardial sutures or applying biological glue, infarctectomy with patch placement and ventricular wall reconstruction, pledgeted sutures without infarctectomy, and pericardial, Dacron, Gore-Tex, or Teflon patches adhered with biologic glue or sutures [9]. New techniques allow to preserve the left ventricular cavity size and viable myocardial tissue around the FWR. Sutureless techniques include gelatin-resorcinol-formaldehyde (GRF glue: Cardial, Saint-Etienne, France) applied to a bovine pericardial patch (Impra, Tempe, AZ, USA) [10] and collagen fleece with fibrinogen-based impregnation [11] (Tachocomb; Nycomed Pharma, Linz, Austria).

37.3.1 Clinical Case

A 78-year-old man was transferred from a smaller hospital with cardiac tamponade and aortic dissection diagnosis. Central venous pressure was 20 mmHg, he had anuria, and his face and his upper chest were extensively cyanotic. The chest was entered through a median sternotomy (Fig. 37.7). The neck vessels were isolated before pericardial incision (Figs. 37.8 and 37.9). Peripheral extracorporeal circulation was started after femoral vessels' cannulation. The pericardium was opened, no aortic dissection was found, and blood and clots were removed. A fissuration was found on the lateral aspect of the left ventricle (Fig. 37.10). Repair was accomplished on the beating heart in order to minimize ischemia and to allow assessment of wall function: a wide Teflon patch was applied using gelatin-resorcinol-formaldehyde biological glue (Figs. 37.11 and 37.12).

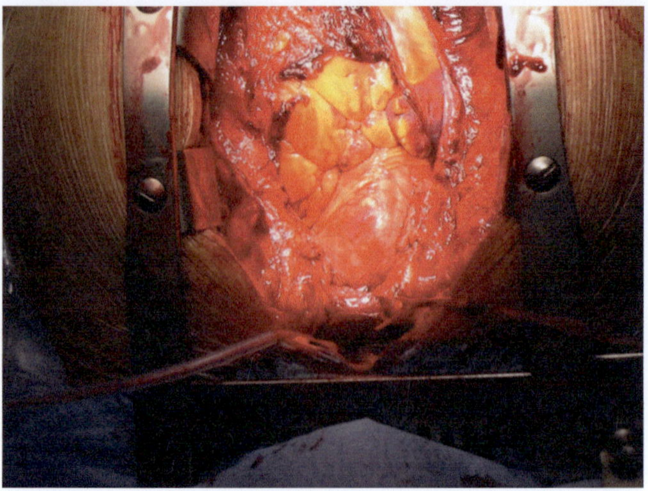

Fig. 37.9 The heart, anterior aspect, after blood and clots removal

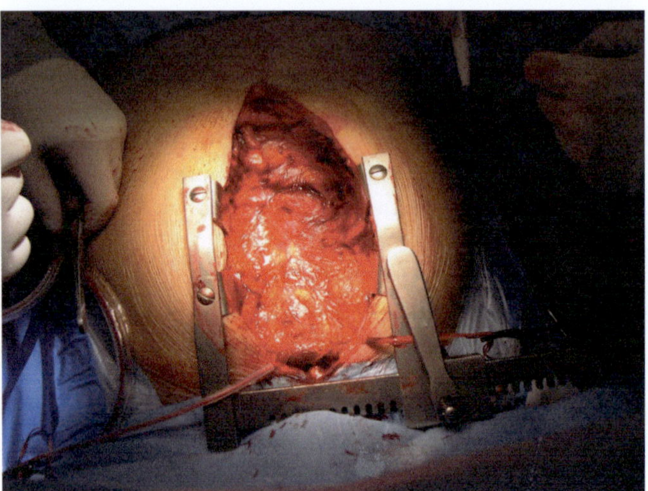

Fig. 37.7 After median sternotomy left innominate vein and brachiocephalic artery are encircled

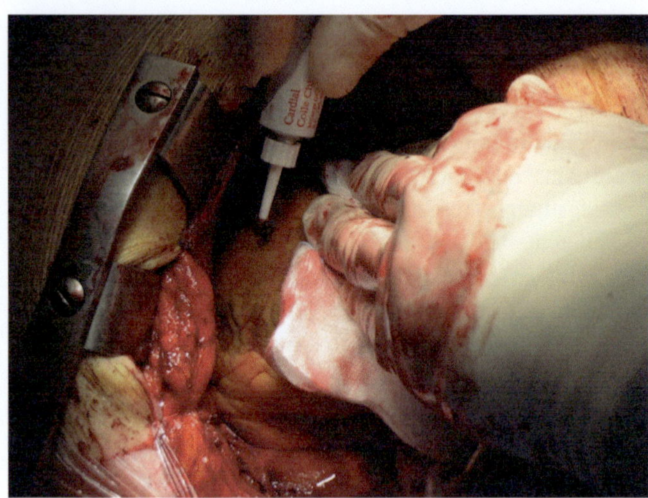

Fig. 37.10 A fissuration was found on the lateral aspect of the left ventricle

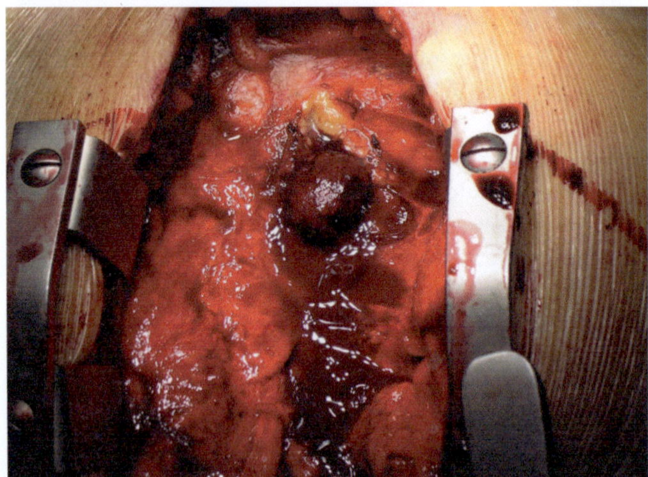

Fig. 37.8 The pericardium is incised and large amounts of blood and clots are removed

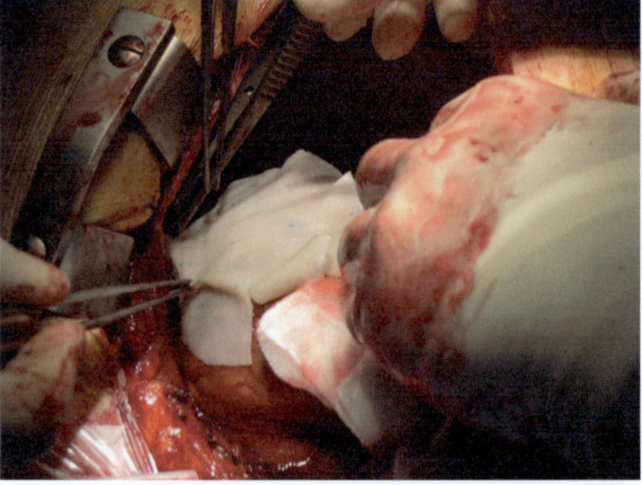

Fig. 37.11 Repair was accomplished on the beating heart in order to minimize ischemia and to allow assessment of wall function: a wide Teflon patch was applied using gelatin-resorcinol-formaldehyde biological glue

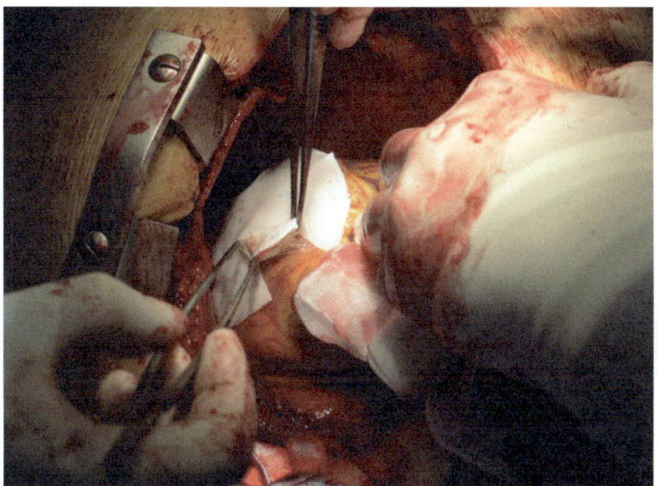

Fig. 37.12 Teflon patch applied to the left ventricle

37.4 Ischemic Mitral Regurgitation (IMR)

In the acute phase of acute myocardial infarction (AMI), IMR is caused either by papillary muscle dysfunction/rupture or rupture of chordae. Papillary muscle rupture may occur from a few hours to 14 days after acute myocardial infarction, and its incidence is about 1% [12] and increases exponentially in fatal AMI %.

37.4.1 Etiology

Majority of patients presents inferoposterior AMI; the posteromedial papillary muscle is involved more frequently than anterolateral papillary muscle, this is in about 75% of cases. This depends on the different blood supply: the posteromedial muscle is perfused by the posterior descending artery, while the anterolateral muscle is perfused by both the left anterior descending and left circumflex coronary arteries. For this reason, posteromedial papillary muscle rupture occurs more frequently with relatively small infarcts [13].

37.4.2 Symptoms

Acute mitral regurgitation is usually characterized by sudden pulmonary edema, hypotension, and cardiogenic shock.

Diagnosis. The diagnosis is often difficult to make; echocardiography, transthoracic and transesophageal (Figs. 37.13 and 37.14), is essential also in differentiating between papillary muscle rupture and left ventricular dysfunction. Chest X-ray shows pulmonary congestion, an enlarged heart, and often bilateral pleural effusion. Right heart catheterization, positioning a Swan-Ganz catheter, will show a prominent "v wave," and it is important to exclude a left-to-right shunt (differential diagnosis with VSR).

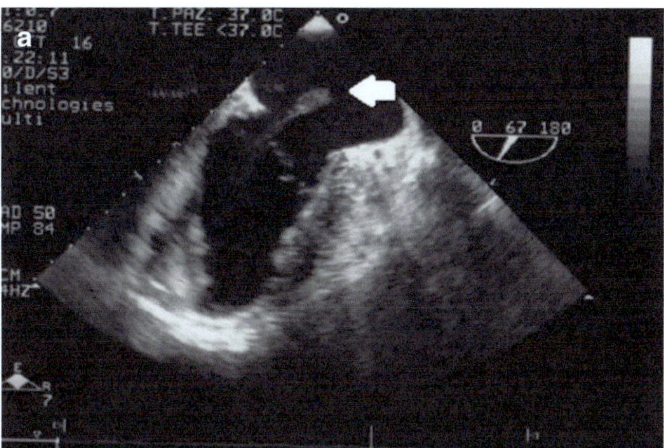

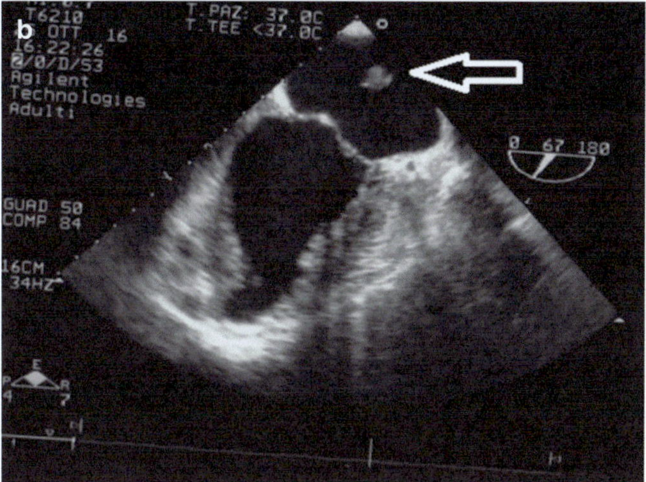

Fig. 37.13 In panel A and B, transesophageal echocardiogram showing a free-floating appendage, attached to the mitral valve, in the left atrium (white arrows). The prolapsing appendage is the ruptured portion of the papillary muscle

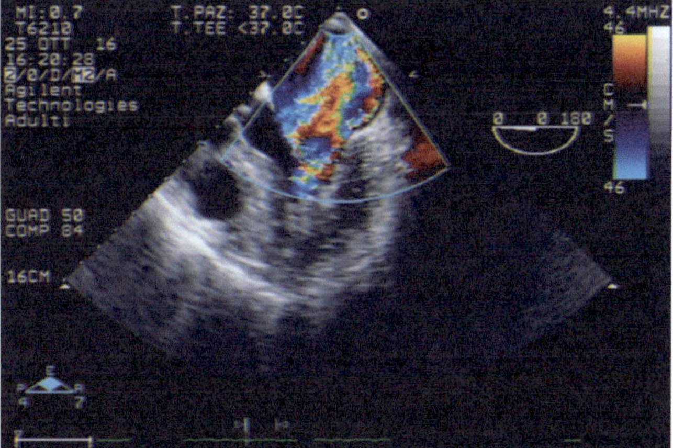

Fig. 37.14 Doppler color flow shows severe mitral regurgitation

37.4.3 Surgery

It is mandatory to try to stabilize the patient positioning intra-aortic balloon pump. Surgery is performed on an emergency basis immediately after diagnosis. In Figs. 37.13, 37.14, 37.15, 37.16, 37.17, and 37.18 we report the clinical case of a 66-year-old man who developed IMR 4 days after posterior AMI. He had sudden pulmonary edema and congestive heart failure; echocardiography showed massive mitral regurgitation (Fig. 37.14), and intra-aortic balloon pump was immediately positioned. Coronary angiography revealed circumflex coronary artery occlusion and LAD proximal critical disease. At surgery a saphenous sequential coronary bypass to obtuse marginal and LAD coronaries was first performed; then the mitral valve was exposed, the ruptured posteromedial papillary muscle was excised (Figs. 37.17 and 37.18), and the mitral valve was replaced with a mechanical prosthesis.

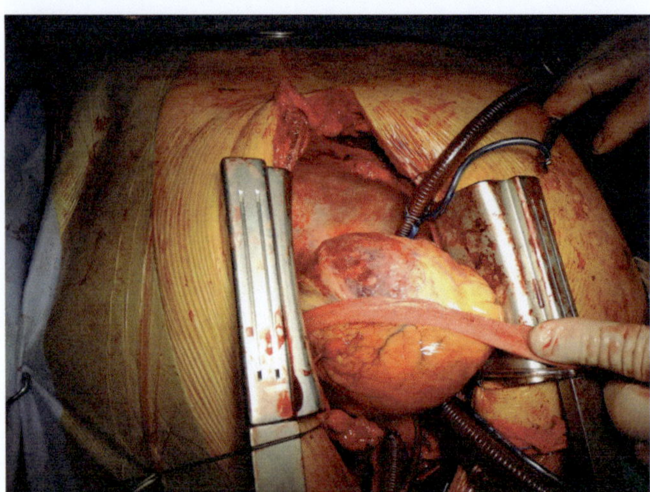

Fig. 37.15 Inferoposterior myocardial infarction

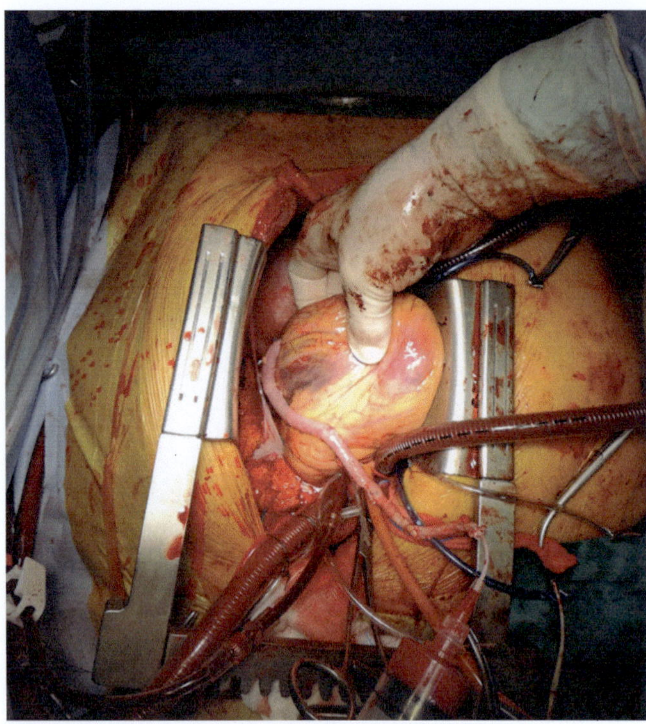

Fig. 37.16 Saphenous vein graft to obtuse marginal and left anterior descending arteries in the sequential fashion

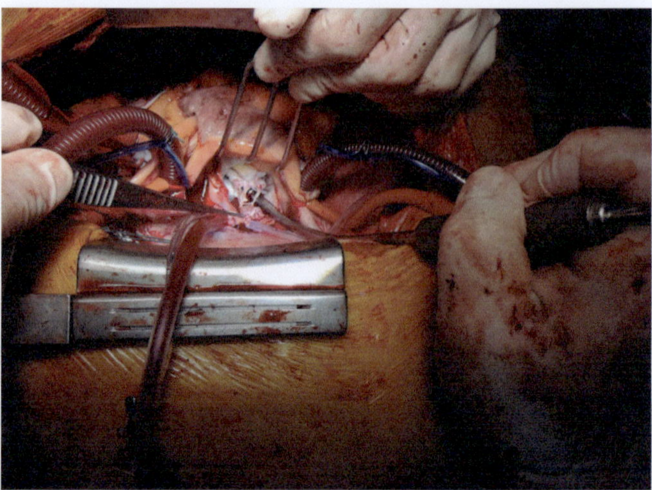

Fig. 37.17 The posteromedial papillary muscle is completely resected

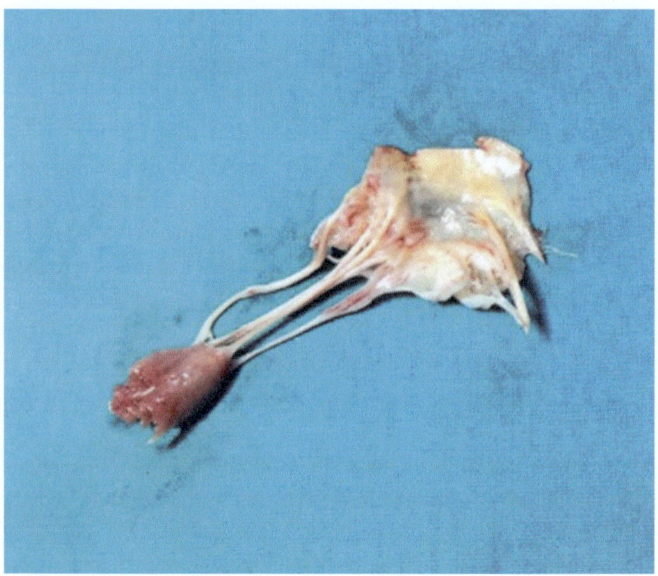

Fig. 37.18 The ruptured apical portion of the posteromedial papillary muscle after surgical excision

Mitral valve repair is often performed in IMR; anyway it is interesting to observe the results of “the mitral valve repair versus replacement for severe ischemic mitral regurgitation trial” [14] where 251 patients with severe ischemic MR were randomized to mitral valve repair or chordal-sparing mitral valve replacement. The primary end point was the left ventricular end-systolic volume index (LVESVI) at 12 months and secondary endpoints were major adverse cardiac and cerebrovascular events, mortality, degree of residual MR, functional status, and quality of life. It is remarkable to note that recurrence of moderate or severe MR at 1 year was 32.6% in the repair group and only 2.3% in the replacement group ($P < 0.001$). In patients that had valve repair, the LVESVI was 64.1 ± 23.9 mL/m^2 in those with recurrent MR versus 47.3 ± 23.0 mL/m^2 in those without recurrent MR ($P < 0.001$). These results suggest that valve repair can dramatically improve LVESVI, but a multidisciplinary team should analyze all the preoperative findings that can indicate and predict a long-lasting repair. Otherwise it is advisable to perform a mitral valve replacement procedure.

37.5 When the Diagnosis Is Missed

You will find hereafter some clinical cases where the missed diagnosis determined the patient's death.

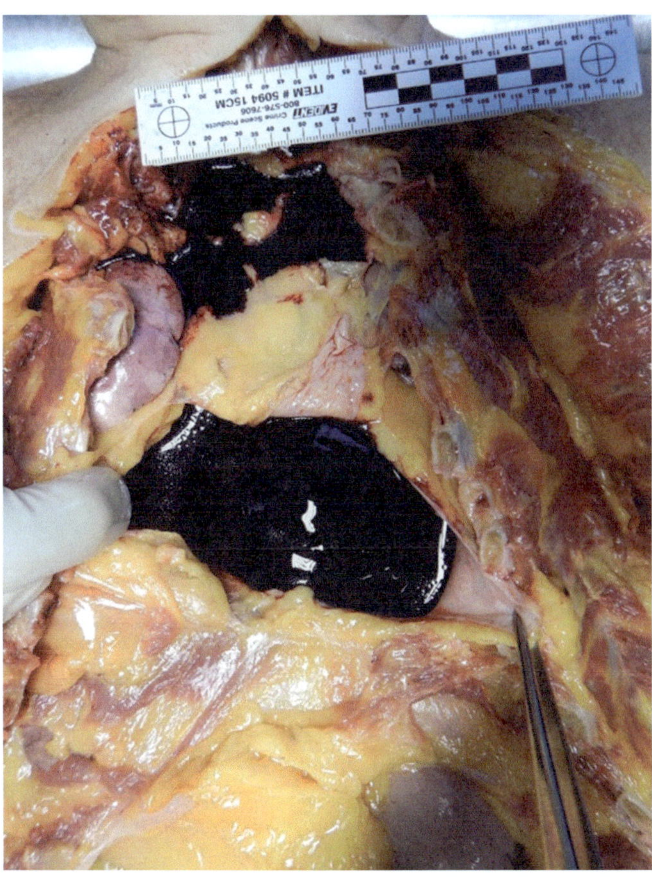

Fig. 37.19 Clinical case 1. Upon removal of the sternal plastron, the lungs were expanded, without adhesions in the pleural cables; the pericardium was intact and contained about 200 mL of blood, partially coagulated

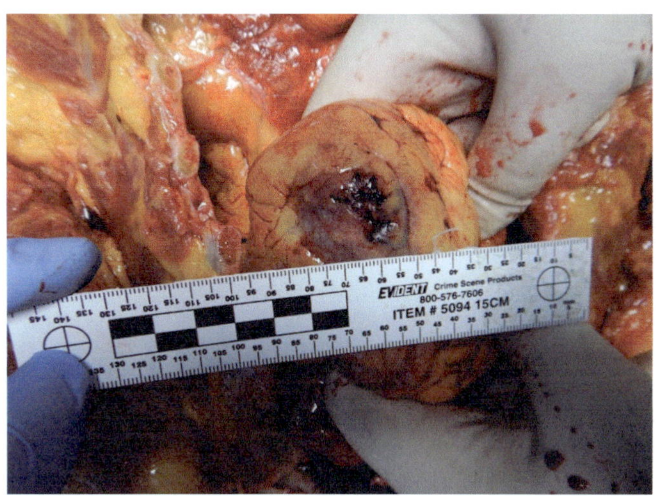

Fig. 37.20 A continuous solution, 3 × 4 cm, of the full thickness of the free wall was found in the left ventricle apex

Case 1 (Figs. 37.19, 37.20, and 37.21) shows the case of an 83-year-old woman, with a history of systemic arterial hypertension, that while on vacation has been complaining of nausea, vomiting, slight epigastric pain, and paresthesias in her left arm over the past several days. Her physician found orthostatic hypotension and rib pain when pressing the left side of her ribcage; her doctor doubted her symptoms, AMI diagnosis missed, and the woman was found dead the same day. Upon removal of the sternal plastron, the lungs were expanded, without adhesions in the pleural cables; the pericardium was intact and contained about 200 mL of blood, partially coagulated. A continuous solution, 3 × 4 cm, of the full thickness of the free wall was found in the left ventricle apex (Fig. 37.21).

Case 2 (Figs. 37.22, 37.23, and 37.24). An asymptomatic 67-year-old man, heavy smoker and with diabetes 2, was found dead at home. At autopsy cardiac tamponade was found; the pericardium contained 420 mL of blood; there were extensive adhesions between the pericardium and inferoposterior portion of the left ventricle, the heart weighed 495 g. The left ventricular posterior wall showed an old infarcted area causing a scar tissue, containing all the myocardial layers, and a pseudoaneurysm with a diameter of 4.5 × 5 cm, its wall thickness being <1 mm. Histopathologic examination showed that the structure contained only pericardial and fibrous elements in its wall; myocardial tissue couldn't be observed. In the apical portion of the pseudoaneurysm, there was an oval perforation, 1.5 × 1 cm. Left anterior descending artery had a 50% stenosis, while right coronary artery and left circumflex artery were hardened by severe atherosclerosis and calcification.

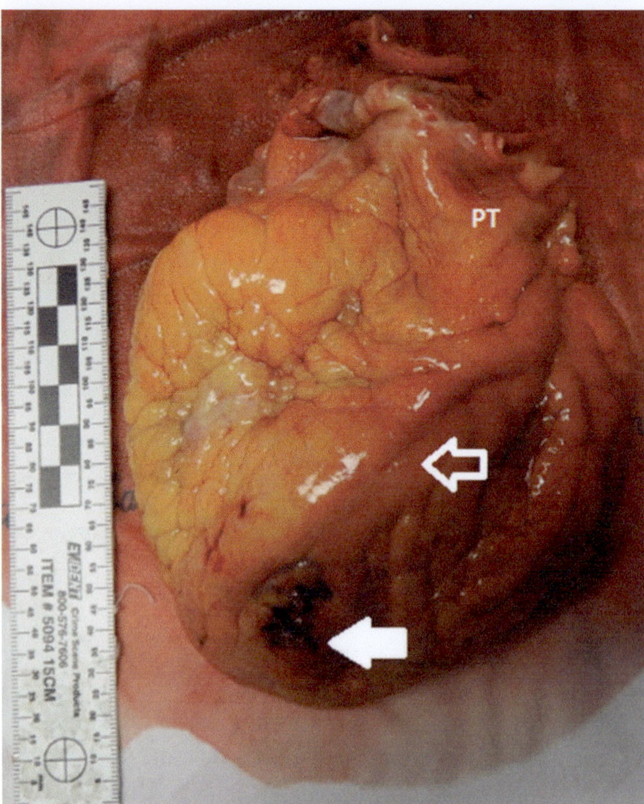

Fig. 37.21 Same case in Fig. 37.20. *PT* pulmonary trunk, hollow arrow left anterior descending artery, solid arrow free wall rupture

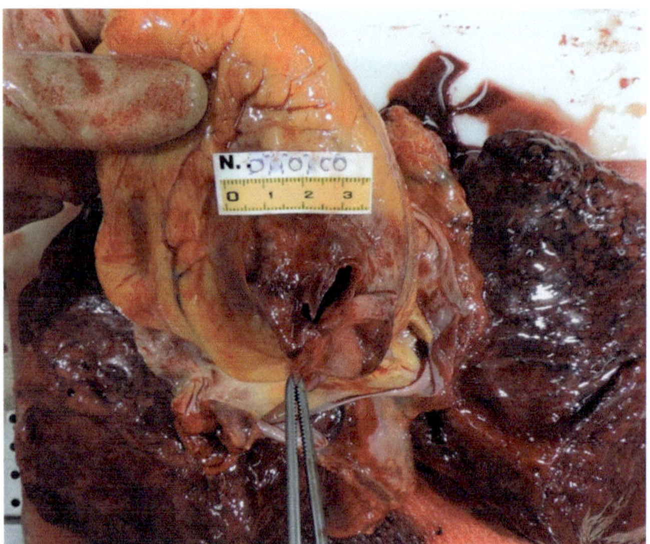

Fig. 37.22 Clinical case 2. At autopsy a pseudoaneurysm in the infero-posterior aspect of the left ventricle, diameter 4.5 × 5 cm, thickness at the same point <1 mm. In the apical portion of the pseudoaneurysm, there is an oval perforation, 1 × 1.5 cm

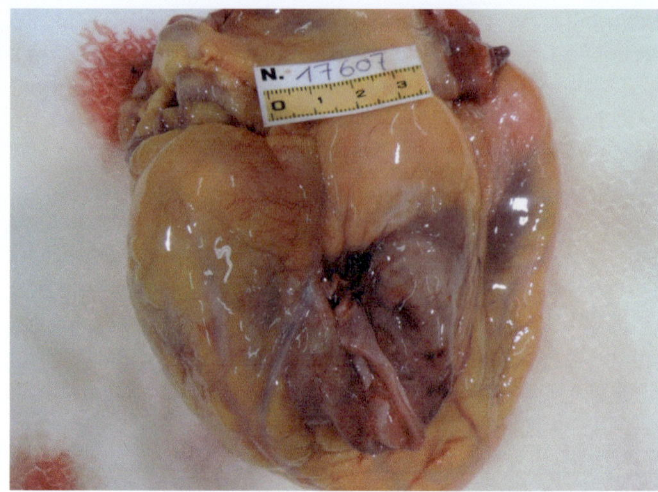

Fig. 37.23 Clinical case 2. Posterior aspect of the heart

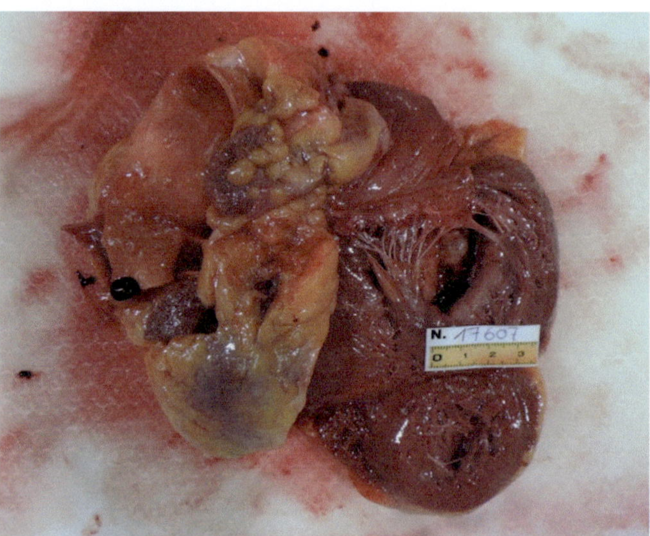

Fig. 37.24 Internal aspect of left ventricle: underneath the medial-posterior papillary muscle, a clot covering the ruptured pseudoaneurysm can be observed

References

1. French JK, Hellcamp AS, Armstrong PW, Cohen E, Kleiman NS, O'Connor CM, Holmes DR, Hochman JS, Granger CB, Mahaffey KW. Mechanical complications after percutaneous coronary intervention in ST-elevation myocardial infarction (from APEX-AMI). Am J Cardiol. 2010;105:59–63.
2. Skehan JD, Carey C, Norrell MS, de Belder M, Balcon R, Mills PG. Patterns of coronary artery disease in post-infarction ventricular septal rupture. Br Heart J. 1989;62:268–72.

3. Pohjola-Sintonen S, Muller JE, Stone PH, et al. Ventricular septal and free wall rupture complicating acute myocardial infarction: experience in the Multicenter Investigation of Limitation of Infarct Size. Am Heart J. 1989;117(4):809–18.
4. Radford MJ, Johnson RA, Daggett WM Jr, et al. Ventricular septal rupture: a review of clinical and physiologic features and an analysis of survival. Circulation. 1981;64(3):545–53.
5. Daggett WM, Guyton RA, Mundth ED, Buckley MJ, McEnany MT, Gold HK, Leinbach RC, Austen WG. Surgery for post-myocardial infarct ventricular septal defect. Ann Surg. 1977;186:233–40.
6. David TE, Feindel CM, Ropchan GV. Reconstruction of the left ventricle with autologous pericardium. J Thorac Cardiovasc Surg. 1987;94:710–4.
7. Arnaoutakis GJ, Conte JV. Repair of postinfarct ventricular septal defect: anterior apical ventricular septal defect. Oper Tech Thorac Cardiovasc Surg. 2014;19(1):96–114. www.optechtcs.com/article/S1522-2942(14)00052-X/pdf.
8. Arnaoutakis GJ, Zhao Y, George TJ, Sciortino CM, McCarthy PM, Conte JV. Surgical repair of ventricular septal defect after myocardial infarction: outcomes from the society of thoracic surgeons national database. Ann Thorac Surg. 2012;94:436–44; discussion 443–4.
9. Lee HM, Lee YT, Kim WS, Jeong DS, Park PW, Sung K. Surgical treatment of post-infarction left ventricular free wall rupture: three cases review. Korean J Thorac Cardiovasc Surg. 2013;46:357–61.
10. Vohra HA, Chaudhry S, Satur CM, Heber M, Butler R, Ridley PD. Sutureless off-pump repair of post-infarction left ventricular free wall rupture. J Cardiothorac Surg. 2006;1:11.
11. Nishizaki K, Seki T, Fujii A, Nishida Y, Funabiki M, Morikawa Y. Sutureless patch repair for small blowout rupture of the left ventricle after myocardial infarction. Jpn J Thorac Cardiovasc Surg. 2004;52:268–71.
12. Clements SD, Story WE, Hurst JW, Craver JM, Jones EL. Ruptured papillary muscle. A complication of myocardial infarction: clinical presentation, diagnosis, and treatment. Clin Cardiol. 1985;8:93–103.
13. Antman EM, Morrow DA. Chapter 55: ST-segment elevation myocardial infarction: management. In: Bonow RO, editor. Braunwald's heart disease—a textbook of cardiovascular medicine. 9th ed. Philadelphia: Saunders; 2011. p. 1150.
14. Acker MA, Parides MK, Perrault LP, et al. Mitral-valve repair versus replacement for severe ischemic mitral regurgitation. N Engl J Med. 2014;370:23–32.

Updates in the Management of Cardiogenic Shock in Acute Coronary Syndrome

38

Maurizio Ferrario, Tiziana Spezzano, Marco Ferlini, Antonio Sciortino, Fabrizio Gazzoli, and Antonino M. Grande

Key Points

- Do not hesitate to position ECMO before cardiovascular and respiratory parameters are irreversibly worsened.
- If PCI is unsuccessful and the patient is hemodynamically unstable, do not delay coronary bypass surgery.
- When ECMO is needed, choose the best cannulation site for the patient.

38.1 Introduction

Cardiogenic shock is a complex clinical status characterized by a progressive multi-organ dysfunction determined by the failure of the heart to deliver an adequate amount of blood to the tissues.

Cardiogenic shock is described hemodynamically as a persistent, i.e., for at least 30 min, hypotension (systolic blood pressure <90 mmHg or mean arterial pressure 30 mmHg) with severe reduction in cardiac index (<1.8 L/min/m^2 without support or <2.0–2.2 L/min/m^2 with inotropic support) and adequate or elevated filling pressures (left ventricular end-diastolic pressure >18 mmHg or right ventricular end-diastolic pressure >10–15 mmHg) [1].

M. Ferrario · T. Spezzano · M. Ferlini
Cardiology, IRCCS Fondazione Policlinico San Matteo, Pavia, Italy
e-mail: m.ferrario@smatteo.pv.it

A. Sciortino · F. Gazzoli · A. M. Grande (✉)
Department of Cardiac Surgery, IRCCS Fondazione Policlinico San Matteo, Pavia, Italy
e-mail: amgrande@libero.it

Clinically it is associated with clinical signs of hypoperfusion as decreased urinary output, altered mental status, and peripheral vasoconstriction with cold extremities.

The diagnosis of cardiogenic shock is made when myocardial dysfunction is viewed in the absence of other causes such as hemorrhage, sepsis, pulmonary embolism, tamponade, aortic dissection, and preexisting valvular disease.

38.2 Incidence

Cardiogenic shock is the most common cause of death in patients with acute myocardial infarction. It complicates approximately 5–10% of cases with acute myocardial infarction [2, 3]. Cardiogenic shock seems to occur more frequently among patients with ST-segment elevation myocardial infarction (STEMI). It was observed that shock developed in 7.5% of patients with STEMI and 2.5% of patients with non-ST-segment elevation myocardial infarction (NSTEMI). The reason for this difference is likely due to the rapid cell necrosis that occurs in the course of STEMI compared to the slower cell loss in NSTEMI [3–5].

38.3 Pathophysiology

Ischemia due to decreased coronary perfusion leads to muscle hypoxia and necrosis which compromises myocardial contractility. This leads to decreased cardiac output and a subsequent drop in the arterial blood pressure. Simultaneously, the body's sympathetic system responds to the reduced blood pressure by increasing peripheral vasoconstriction and heart rate leading to decreased perfusion at the tissue level and increasing cardiac oxygen demand. So it is a vicious circle of causal factors that all reinforce one another [3].

P. Aseni et al. (eds.), *Operative Techniques and Recent Advances in Acute Care and Emergency Surgery*,
https://doi.org/10.1007/978-3-319-95114-0_38

38.4 Etiology

Left ventricular dysfunction (LD) is the most common cause of cardiogenic shock, occurring in 74.5% of patients, followed by acute mitral regurgitation (8.3%), ventricular septal rupture (4.6%), isolated right ventricular shock (3.4%), tamponade or cardiac rupture (1.7%), and other causes (8%) [3].

38.5 Clinical Presentation

At clinical presentation, if left ventricular dysfunction (LVD) is the etiology of cardiogenic shock, most patients show signs of congestion such as jugular venous distention (JVD), orthopnoea, and rales in the lung field. For these patients, volume loading will not result in a beneficial hemodynamic effect, and diuretics and inotropic support should be initiated. By contrast, if right ventricular failure is the underlying cause, then JVD and Kussmaul's sign are present, and pulmonary rales are not found; for patients with silent lung syndrome, administration of fluids can be considered to obtain optimal cardiac filling pressures and increase cardiac output. The clinical presentation is summarized in the four classes of Forrester. This classification of the different hemodynamic profile is not only diagnostic but also therapeutic [6] (Fig. 38.1).

38.6 Predisposing Factors for Cardiogenic Shock

The SHOCK trial registry shows that the predisposing factors are [3]:

- Left anterior descending artery was found to be the most frequently involved artery unrelated to the time of shock onset.
- Severe coronary artery disease, such as triple-vessel disease, precedes shock development.
- Heart rate, systolic blood pressure, and Killip class at presentation.
- Age, diabetes, previous infarction, and reduced ejection fraction.
- Infarct size and anterior infarction.

38.7 Medical Stabilization or Early Revascularization?

After the publication of the results of the SHOCK trial [7], we have witnessed the reduction in the incidence of cardiogenic shock due to early revascularization.

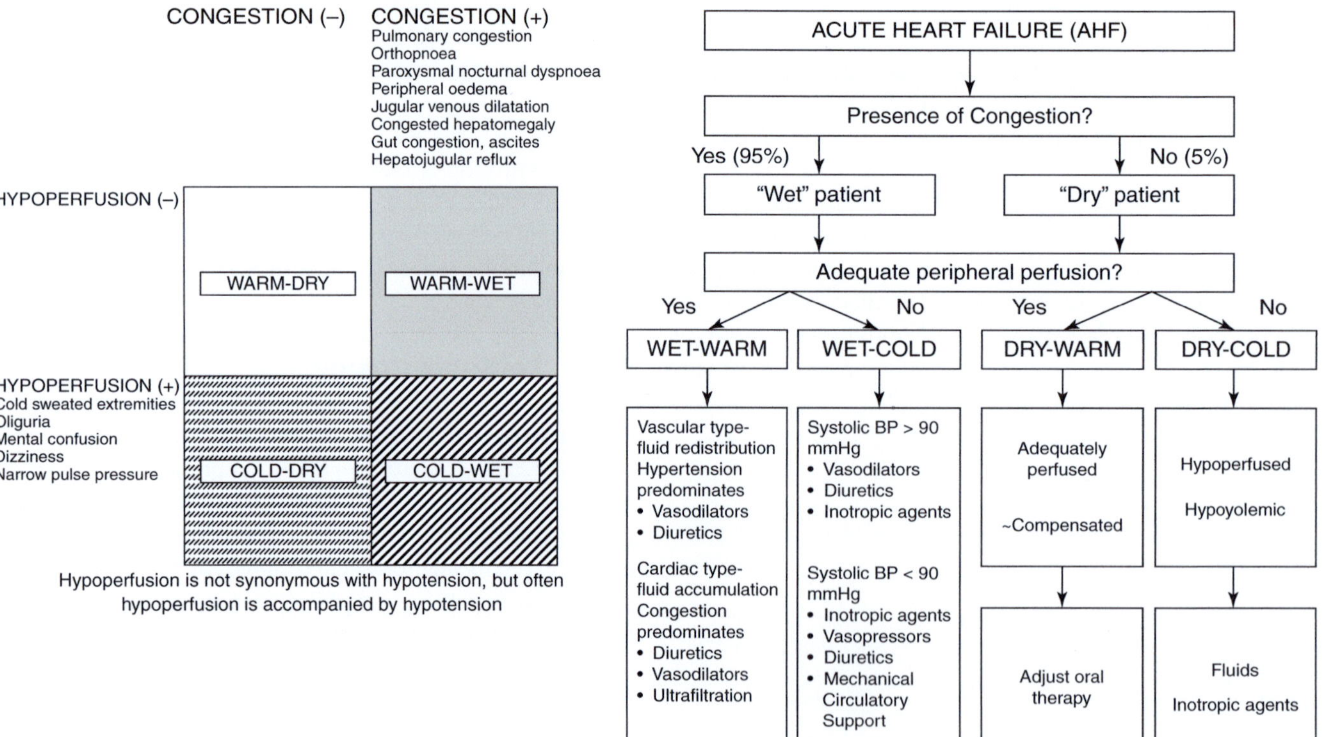

Fig. 38.1 Management of patients with acute heart failure based on clinical profile during an early phase. (Modified from *2016 ESC Guidelines for the diagnosis and treatment of acute and chronic heart failure*)

In the 'Should we emergently revascularize Occluded Coronaries for Cardiogenic Shock' (SHOCK) [7] trial, patients with cardiogenic shock were randomly assigned to initial medical stabilization or early revascularization. Although the primary endpoint, all-cause mortality at 30 days, did not differ between the initial medical stabilization and early revascularization group, there was a significant decrease in mortality after 1 and 6 years in patients assigned to early revascularization. So, coronary revascularization should be performed as soon as possible after AMI and shock onset [8]. Among patients assigned to initial medical stabilization in the SHOCK trial, thrombolytic therapy was associated with an improved 12-month survival. However, thrombolysis alone results in relatively low rates of reperfusion in patients in whom shock is already established. Consequently, triage and immediate transfer to a PCI-capable facility with on-site cardiac surgical backup is recommended for patients with AMI-related cardiogenic shock [9].

38.8 Particular Patient Group

Multi-vessel disease: More than 70% of STEMI patients in cardiogenic shock have significant multi-vessel coronary artery disease. The optimal revascularization strategy for patients with multi-vessel disease and cardiogenic shock is, however, not clear. In contrast to recommendations in hemodynamically stable patients, current European guidelines recommend multi-vessel percutaneous coronary intervention (PCI) for patients in cardiogenic shock and in the presence of multiple, truly critical (~90% diameter) stenoses or highly unstable lesions (angiographic signs of possible thrombus or lesion disruption) if there is persistent ischemia after PCI of the supposed culprit lesion [10]. Complete revascularization is an independent predictor of survival to discharge in STEMI patients with multi-vessel coronary disease and cardiogenic shock [11–13].

38.9 Shock After Myocardial Reperfusion

Early reperfusion by primary PCI or thrombolysis can limit myocardial infarct size by restoration of blood flow. However, primary PCI must occur as soon as possible, i.e., in little more than 120 min after onset of symptoms to provide substantial benefit. Late reperfusion causes increased peri-infarction hemorrhage, edema, and contraction-band necrosis [2]. The "no-reflow" phenomenon is more likely to occur if reperfusion is delayed and negates the benefit of epicardial vessel patency. Flow to the margins of the infarct is determined by perfusion pressure during diastole (mean diastolic aortic pressure minus LV diastolic pressure), coronary vascular resistance, and the presence of collateral circulation. As cardiac output falls and LV end-diastolic pressure rises, perfusion of the peri-infarct zone is further compromised. In the SHOCK trial, 86% of patients received an intra-aortic balloon pump (IABP) in an attempt to stabilize their condition and improve the safety of revascularization. Currently, doubts exist as to whether the IABP can influence outcome following acute myocardial infarction with or without cardiogenic shock.

38.10 Mechanical Complications Causing Cardiogenic Shock

Myocardial disruption, i.e., ventricular septal rupture, free wall rupture, or papillary muscle rupture with mitral regurgitation, precipitates in cardiogenic shock and presents suddenly after transmural infarction.

38.10.1 Interventricular Septal Rupture

In the era before reperfusion therapy, interventricular septal rupture occurred in 1–3% [14]. The actual annual incidence is 0.25–0.31% [15]. The incidence of septal rupture was similar for anterior and inferior myocardial infarction. Patients with hypertension, diabetes mellitus, chronic angina, or previous myocardial infarction were less likely to experience this complication, because prior ischemia leads to myocardial preconditioning, decreasing the likelihood of transmural myocardial necrosis and septal rupture. When acute hemodynamic derangement progresses to cardiogenic shock, the thrill and murmur fade as turbulent transseptal flow decreases in response to poor LV function. Doppler echocardiography differentiates between septal or free wall rupture and mitral regurgitation. The ACC/AHA guidelines recommend immediate operative intervention regardless of clinical status. Pending transfer to the operating room, medical management comprises hemodynamic support with an IABP, inotropes, and afterload reduction. Diuretics are used for pulmonary congestion, and oxygenation is maintained using oxygen by mask, positive airway pressure, or mechanical ventilation. Maintenance of arterial blood pressure with vasopressors must be balanced against the need to moderate shunt fraction by reducing systemic vascular resistance. These patients are at very high risk, and the surgical team must have appropriate experience [16].

38.10.2 Free-Wall Rupture

Cardiac rupture was the leading cause of death in the age of thrombolysis in patients aged >75 (54%).Urgent pericardiocentesis followed by surgical repair provides the best chance of survival in patients with free wall rupture [16].

38.10.3 Papillary Muscle Rupture

The posteromedial papillary muscle is the papillary that most frequently undergoes breakage due to its single vascularization (from right or circumflex coronary artery). The anterolateral muscle instead of being vascularized by two vessels (left anterior descending and circumflex coronary) is less vulnerable. For this reason, mitral regurgitation is most common with inferior infarction followed by partial or total papillary rupture. Papillary muscle dysfunction can be managed medically by reducing LV afterload with an IABP or vasodilators. When mitral regurgitation is severe, early surgery is preferable using techniques to reimplant the flail papillary muscle. Prosthetic valve replacement is a less satisfactory, but frequently, a compelling alternative [16, 17].

Case Scenarios

Case scenario n. 1. Extracorporeal membrane oxygenation (ECMO) as a long-term bridge to heart transplantation for ST-elevation myocardial infarction complicated by refractory cardiogenic shock

A 43-year-old man with acute anterior STEMI was referred to primary PCI: two overlapped stents, one on distal left main (LMCA) and the other on ostial left anterior descending (LAD) coronary artery, were successfully implanted. Five days later, an episode of chest pain with associated anterolateral ST-elevation occurred (Fig. 38.2), quickly jeopardizing clinical conditions to a state of cardiogenic shock (CS). Inotropic support was started, and IABP was positioned in order to sustain the failing circulation. Emergency coronary angiography showed LMCA stent thrombosis. Multiple manual thrombus-aspiration and kissing-balloon angioplasty were performed on LMCA, LAD, and circumflex, restoring patency of all the three main epicardial vessels, but with persistent slow flow (TIMI 2) (Figs. 38.3, 38.4 and 38.5). Despite all the timely treatments, patient's conditions remained critical: mean arterial pressure was 50 mmHg, urine output <0.5 mL/h/kg, blood lactates 10 mmol/L with ongoing IABP, and high-dose inotropic and vasoactive support (inotropic score = 150). Left ventricular (LV) ejection fraction (EF) was estimated 5–10%.

Upon multidisciplinary collegial discussion (cardiologists, intensivists, cardiac surgeons), within 4 h from the shock state onset, femorofemoral VA-ECMO was instituted, in a mildly sedated and spontaneously breathing patient. Full extracorporeal support (2.5–3.0 L/min/m^2) restored tissue perfusion and organ functions within 24 h, allowing for rapid inotropic drugs tapering and withdrawal. Initial congestive pulmonary edema was effectively treated with a 24-h cycle of low-dose inotropic support, forced diuresis, and helmet continuous positive airway pressure. LV overload and pulmonary congestion were thereafter closely monitored with daily echocardiographic (Fig. 38.6) and lung ultrasound evaluations. Direct left heart venting was never indicated. A likely heparin-induced thrombocytopenia imposed the use of lepirudin for systemic anticoagulation. Prevention of leg ischemia was obtained bypassing the femoral artery cannulation site with a small anterograde catheter.

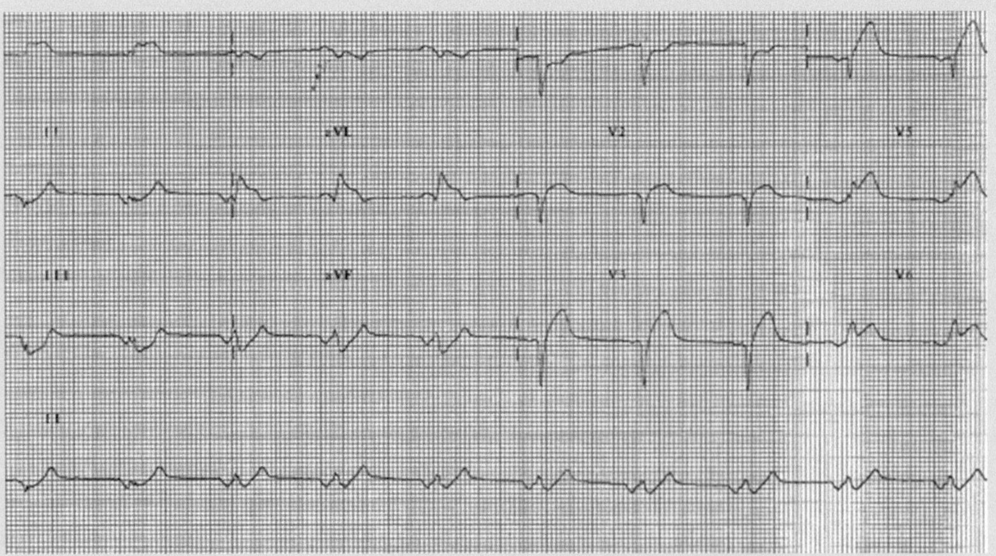

Fig. 38.2 ECG showing ST-segment elevation in the anterolateral leads

We were able to maintain the patient awake and spontaneously breathing, with the advantage of easier and careful neurological monitoring, and avoiding the risk of ventilator-acquired pneumonia. Despite ongoing antibiotic prophylaxis, on day 15, a persistent bacteremia prompted an oxygenator and extracorporeal circuit change, with subsequent regression of the septic state.

Despite overall clinical improvement, there was no significant recovery of heart function, and the attempts to ECMO weaning failed. The patient was hence placed on heart transplant waiting list with status I priority and kept on ECMO until organ availability. After 27 days, heart transplantation was performed using Shumway's technique, and patient was finally weaned from VA-ECMO after total 662 h of cardiopulmonary support. He was discharged from hospital after complete functional recovery. At 30 months, he is still asymptomatic, with a good quality of life.

Case scenario n.2. Cardiac arrest, advanced cardiovascular life support, unsuccessful PCI, and coronary bypass

On June 23, 2015, at 08:07 pm, a 69-year-old man had a loss of consciousness during a tennis match. Bystanders immediately started basic life support (BLS) maneuvers. Using an automated external defibrillator (AED), revealing ventricular fibrillation (VF), they dispensed one ineffective shock.

Ten minutes after the event, the ambulance arrived and started advanced cardiovascular life support (ACLS).

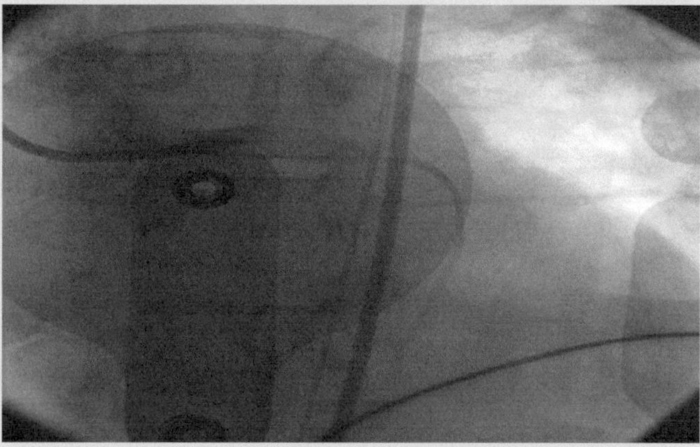

Fig. 38.3 Coronary angiography showing LM total occlusion caused by stent thrombosis

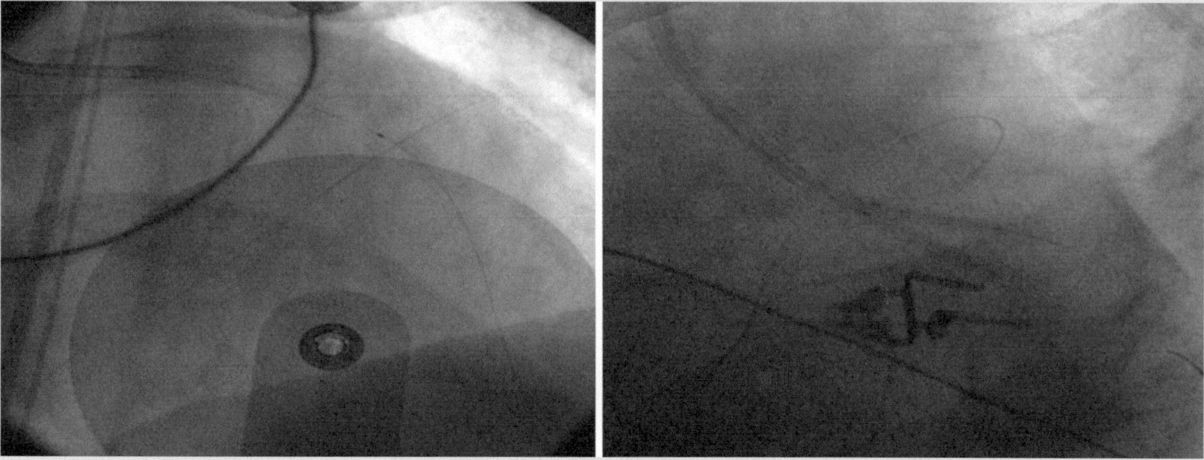

Fig. 38.4 Manual thrombus-aspiration with catheter Export 7F (Medtronic®) and multiple single and kissing-balloon angioplasty performed on LM, LAD, LCX, and ramus

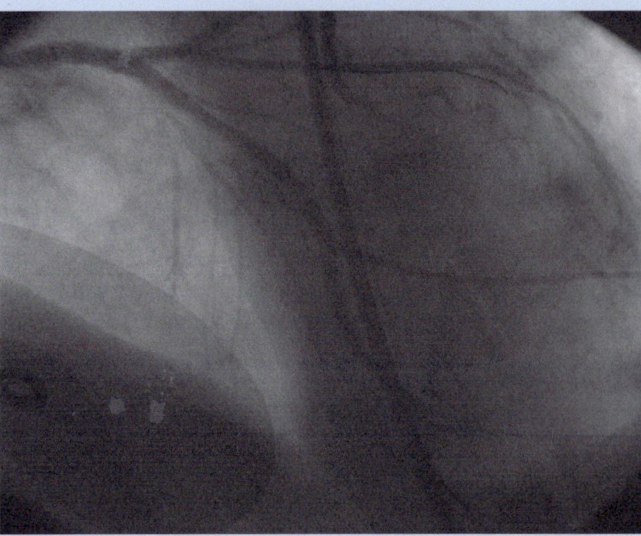

Fig. 38.5 Final results showing patency of all epicardial vessels but persistent slow flow

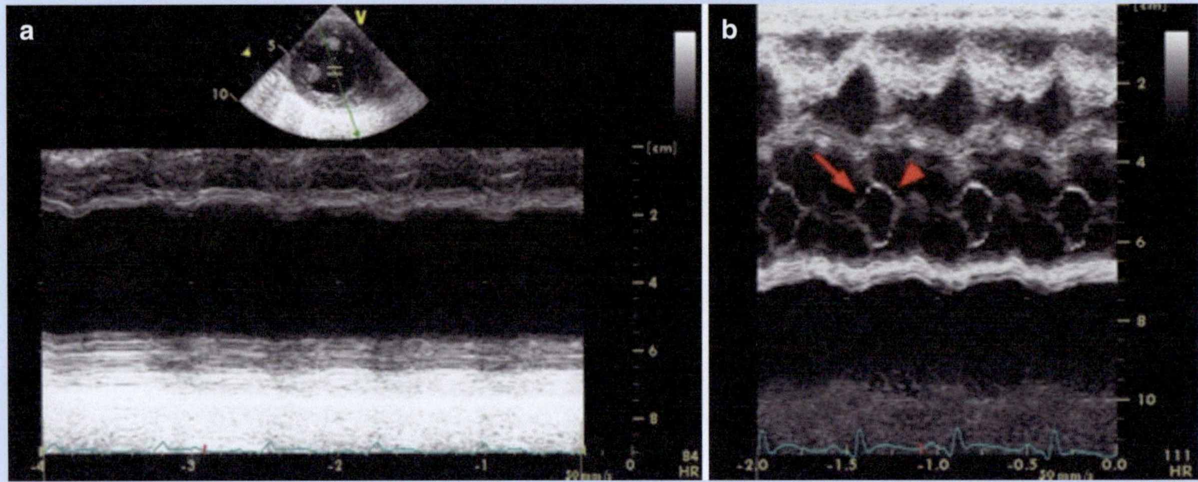

Fig. 38.6 Transthoracic echocardiographic assessment on day 2, with full extracorporeal support. Very poor LV contractility is shown by M-Mode on LV in parasternal short axis view (panel A), as negligible reduction of LV diameter from end-diastole to end-systole (equating to a measured fractional shortening of less than 10%). M-Mode on the aortic valve in the same view (panel B) shows delayed opening (arrow) and premature closure (arrowhead) of the valve, testifying a reduced ejection time and indicating a very small, yet present, LV ejection

Rhythm analysis revealed pulseless electrical activity (PEA). After administration of adrenaline, the patient recovered sinus rhythm with left bundle branch block (at 08:42 pm). An endotracheal tube (ETT) was positioned; duration of cardiopulmonary resuscitation was 35 min.

The patient was admitted to our emergency room and immediately transferred to the Cardiac Catheterization Laboratory. During the procedure, the patient had an episode of ventricular tachycardia (VT) that was successfully treated with direct current shock. Coronary angiography was performed revealing a triple-vessel coronary disease with occlusion of circumflex and right coronary arteries (Fig. 38.7a and b). Percutaneous coronary intervention (PCI) was unsuccessful because of the impossibility of advancing the guidewire (Fig. 38.7c). An intra-aortic balloon pump (IABP) was positioned and the patient was transferred to the intensive care unit (ICU). Chest X-ray showed pulmonary edema and the patient was efficaciously treated with diuretics. After tracheal extubation, he received continuous positive airway pressure (cPAP) treatment. A transthoracic echocardiogram (TTE) revealed a left ventricular systolic dysfunction (ejection fraction 0.38) with inferior wall akinesia.

On June 28 fever appeared. Cultures of blood and bronchial-alveolar lavage (BAL) fluid were positive for *Pseudomonas aeruginosa*; therefore targeted antibiotic therapy was started.

When all cultures became negative, on July 29, the patient underwent coronary artery bypass grafting (CABG) surgery with four grafts (left internal mammary artery to left anterior descending artery, saphenous vein to second diagonal branch, obtuse marginal branch, and posterior descending artery).

Postoperative period was characterized by stable hemodynamics with low dosage of epinephrine (suspended in postoperative day 2) and rapid weaning from mechanical ventilation.

On August 4, 2015, the patient was discharged to a cardiac rehabilitation center.

Case scenario n. 3. A 38-year-old female, after giving birth to a baby, had cardiogenic shock determined by left main coronary artery spontaneous dissection. She underwent ACLS, and after coronary angiography and unsuc-

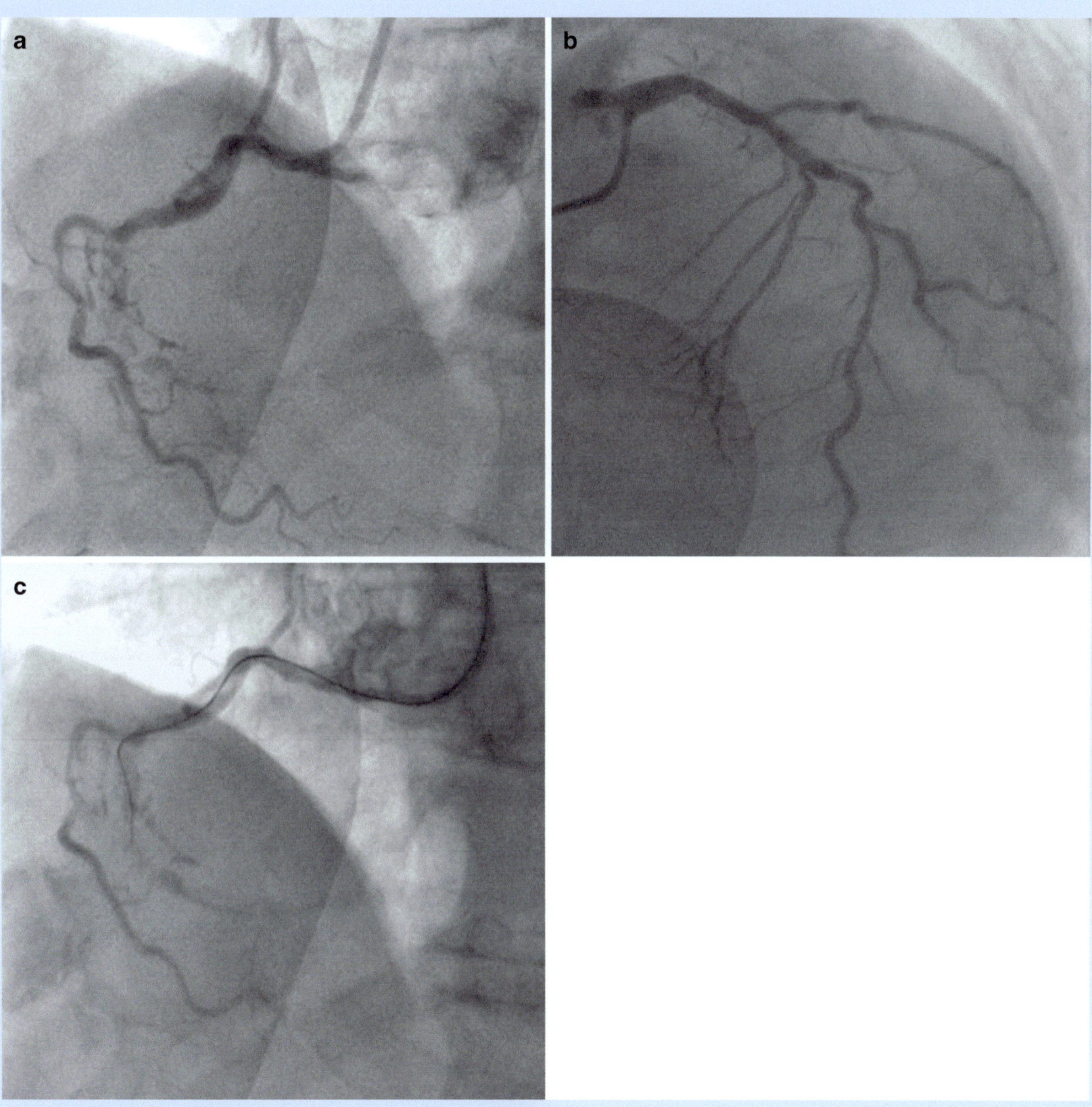

Fig. 38.7 Coronary angiography showing triple-vessel coronary disease, right coronary and circumflex coronary arteries occluded (**a** and **b**), in (**c**) unsucessful PCI

cessful PCI, she was transferred in surgery for coronary bypass. After a double coronary bypass (left internal mammary artery grafted to LAD and saphenous vein to circumflex coronary artery), the patient was unable to wean from extracorporeal circulation despite inotropic support and IAPB positioning [18].

Questions for Case Scenario n. 3

1. What is the therapeutic option for the patient?
   A. Veno-arterial ECMO (VA_ECMO)
   B. Veno-venous ECMO (VV-ECMO)
   C. Left ventricular assist device (LVAD)
2. If ECMO is chosen, which are the cannulation sites and their potential advantages?
   A. Peripheral femorofemoral vein cannulation
   B. Central right atrium-ascending aorta
   C. Peripheral femoral artery-femoral vein

Please see Chap. 58 for the correct answer.

References

1. Hollenberg SM, Kavinsky CJ, Parrillo JE. Cardiogenic shock. Ann Intern Med. 1999;131:47–59.
2. Babaev A, Frederick PD, Pasta DJ, et al. Trends in management and outcomes of patients with acute myocardial infarction complicated by cardiogenic shock. JAMA. 2005;294:448–54.
3. Khalid L, Dhakam SH. A review of cardiogenic shock in acute myocardial infarction. Curr Cardiol Rev. 2008;4(1):34–40.
4. Goldberg RJ, Gore JM, Alpert JS, et al. Cardiogenic shock after acute myocardial infarction. Incidence and mortality from a community-wide perspective, 1975 to 1988. N Engl J Med. 1991;325:1117–22.
5. Holmes DR Jr, Bates ER, Kleiman NS, et al. Contemporary reperfusion therapy for cardiogenic shock: the GUSTO-I trial experience. The GUSTO-I Investigators Global utilization of streptokinase and tissue plasminogen activator for occluded coronary arteries. J Am Coll Cardiol. 1995;26:668–74.
6. Ponikowski P, et al. 2016 ESC Guidelines for the diagnosis and treatment of acute and chronic heart failure: the Task Force for the diagnosis and treatment of acute and chronic heart failure of the European Society of Cardiology (ESC). Developed with the special contribution of the Heart Failure Association (HFA) of the ESC. Eur Heart J. 2016;37(27):2129–200. https://doi.org/10.1093/eurheartj/ehw128.
7. Hochman JS, et al. Early revascularisation in acute myocardial infarction complicated by cardiogenic shock. SHOCK Investigators. Should we emergently revascularize occluded coronaries for cardiogenic shock. N Engl J Med. 1999;341:625–34.
8. Hochman JS, Sleeper LA, White HD, et al. One-year survival following early revascularization for cardiogenic shock. JAMA. 2001;285:190–2.
9. Van Herck JL, Claeys MJ, De Paep R, Van Herck PL, Vrints CJ, Jorens PG. Management of cardiogenic shock complicating acute myocardial infarction. Eur Heart J Acute Cardiovasc Care. 2015;4(3):278–97.
10. Steg PG, James SK, Atar D, et al. ESC Guidelines for the management of acute myocardial infarction in patients presenting with ST-segment elevation. Eur Heart J. 2012;33:2569–619.
11. Hussain F, Philipp RK, Ducas RA, et al. The ability to achieve complete revascularization is associated with improved in-hospital survival in cardiogenic shock due to myocardial infarction: manitoba cardiogenic shock registry investigators. Catheter Cardiovasc Interv. 2011;78:540–8.
12. David S, Wald MD, et al. Randomized trial of preventive angioplasty in myocardial infarction for the PRAMI investigators. N Engl J Med. 2013;369:1115–23.
13. Engstrøm T, et al. Complete revascularisation versus treatment of the culprit lesion only in patients with ST-segment elevation myocardial infarction and multivessel disease (DANAMI-3—PRIMULTI): an open-label, randomised controlled trial. Lancet. 2015;386(9994):665–71.
14. Birnbaum Y, Fishbein MC, Blance C, Siegal R. Ventricular septal rupture after acute myocardial infarction. N Engl J Med. 2002;347:1426–32.
15. Moreyra AE, et al. Trends in incidence and mortality rates of ventricular septal rupture during acute myocardial infarction. Am J Cardiol. 2010;106:1095–100.
16. Westaby S, Kharbanda R, Banning AP. Cardiogenic shock in ACS. Part 1: prediction, presentation and medical therapy. Nat Rev Cardiol. 2012;9:158–71. https://doi.org/10.1038/nrcardio.2011.194. Published online 20 December 2011.
17. Tavakoli R, et al. Results of surgery for irreversible moderate to severe mitral valve regurgitation secondary to myocardial infarction. Eur J Cardiothorac Surg. 2002;21:818–24.
18. Sidebotham D. Troubleshooting adult ECMO. J Extra Corpor Technol. 2011;43:P27–32.

39 Emergency Management of Infective Endocarditis

Antonio Fiore, Alessandro Mazzola, and Antonino M. Grande

Key Points

- Refer patients to expert centers where an "endocarditis team" is present for optimal medical and surgical management.
- In severe aortic regurgitation, do not use beta-blockers: the heart rate decrease will prolong diastolic time worsening aortic regurgitation.
- In acute mitral regurgitation, use positive pressure for respiratory failure, vasodilator drugs to decrease afterload, and dobutamine for its inotropic action.
- Do not delay surgery; there is evidence of good results when surgery is performed during the initial hospitalization period.
- Obtain the best surgical exposure; for example, a superior transseptal approach is indicated for mitral valve surgery in a small left atrium or in case of adhesions from previous cardiac operations or rheumatic activity.

39.1 Introduction

Infective endocarditis (IE) is a life-threatening disease, and despite improvements in its prevention, early diagnosis and treatment remain associated with high mortality (30% at 1 year), severe complications, and its incidence is stable. This situation is attributable to the difficulty of establishing its diagnosis, the emergence of nosocomial virulent microorganisms, and prosthetic valvular or intracardiac device material endocarditis [1].

Endocarditis may affect all native cardiac valves, prostheses valves, or cardiac implantable devices. The infectious lesions affecting the endocardium may be destructive or proliferative. Destructive lesions include leaflet perforation (Fig. 39.1), aorto-mitral separation, or chordae or papillary rupture. Proliferative lesions include vegetation and abscesses of the annulus or the leaflet tissue. The aortic endocarditis is the most frequent followed by mitral, tricuspid, and pulmonary endocarditis. Prosthetic valve endocarditis (PVE) is the most severe form of IE and occurs in 1–6% of patients with valve prostheses. PVE accounts for 10–30% of all cases of IE and affects mechanical and bioprosthetic valves equally [2, 3].

In recent years, different studies and important improvements in imaging procedures have introduced significant advances in the prevention, diagnosis, and treatment of

A. Fiore
Department of Cardiothoracic Surgery, Henri Mondor University Hospital, AP-HP, Paris-Est University, Créteil, France

A. Mazzola
Cardiac Surgery, IRCCS Multimedica, Sesto S. Giovanni, Milano, Italy

A. M. Grande (✉)
Department of Cardiac Surgery, IRCCS Fondazione Policlinico San Matteo, Pavia, Italy
e-mail: amgrande@libero.it

P. Aseni et al. (eds.), *Operative Techniques and Recent Advances in Acute Care and Emergency Surgery*,
https://doi.org/10.1007/978-3-319-95114-0_39

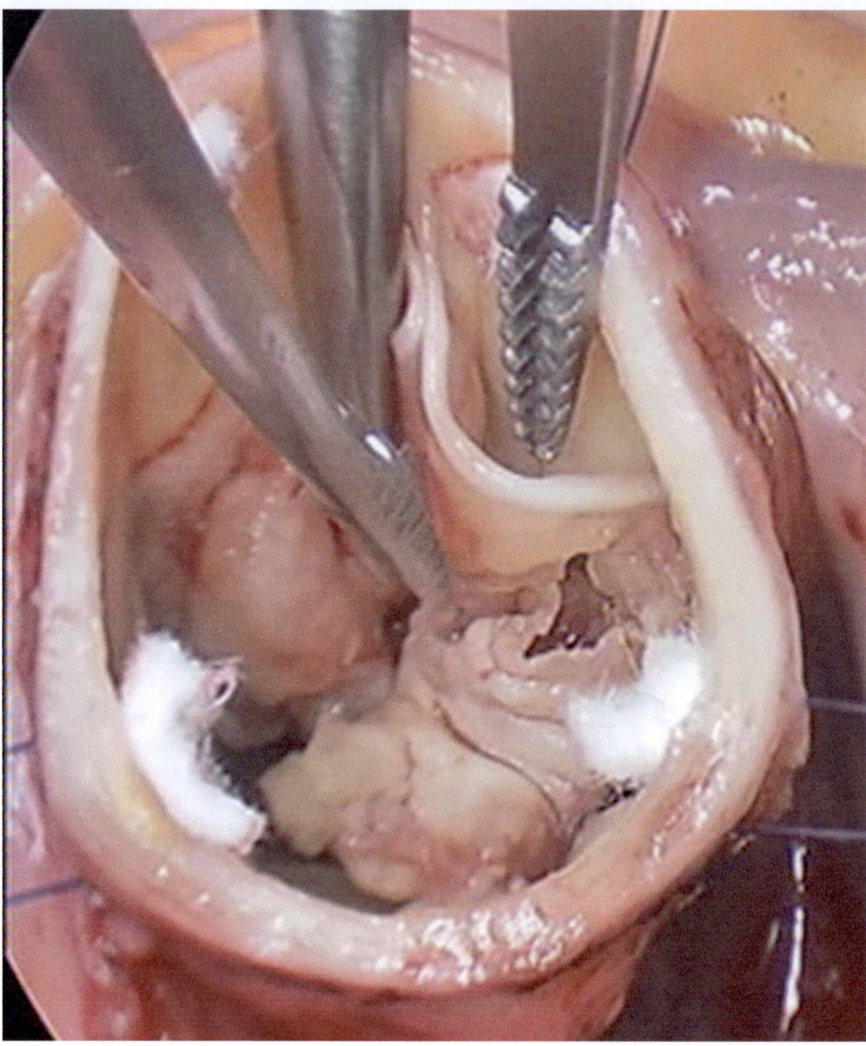

Fig. 39.1 Aortic valve endocarditis with perforation of the non-coronary leaflets, vegetations, and abscess of the annulus

infective endocarditis. For these reasons two major changes were integrated into the updated guidelines of IE [4, 5]: the modification of Duke's criteria [6] (Table 39.1), by integrating nuclear imaging and cardiac computed tomography data in prosthetic valve endocarditis into the major criteria, and setting up the *endocarditis team* where in a reference center, experts in different disciplines collaborate in the care of endocarditis patients for a multidisciplinary emergency management. The reference center must have immediate access to the diagnostic procedure (echocardiography, computed tomography, magnetic resonance imaging, nuclear imaging) and cardiac surgery [7]. A non-reference center can initially manage the noncomplicated cases but must have regular communication with the endocarditis team. Recent studies report an absence of surgery in 25% of patients despite an appropriate indication [8].

Cardiac surgery is required in more than 50% of patients with active infective endocarditis, and this percentage is even higher in left-sided prosthetic valve infections. Early discussion with the surgical team is important and is considered mandatory in all cases of complicated IE (endocarditis with heart failure (HF), abscess or embolic or neurological complications). One major role of the endocarditis team is to define the optimal timing of cardiac surgery.

39.2 Clinical Presentation and Diagnosis

IE may present not only as an acute, rapidly progressive infection, but also as a subacute or chronic disease with low-grade fever and non-specific symptoms that may mislead or confuse initial assessment. IE may present with very different

Table 39.1 Duke's criteria for infective endocarditis diagnosis. For diagnosis, the requirement is two major and one minor criteria or one major and three minor criteria

Major criteria:
• Positive blood culture for infective endocarditis (IE)
– Typical microorganism for IE from two separate blood cultures
– Persistently positive blood cultures
• Evidence of endocardial involvement
– Oscillating intracardiac mass on valve/supporting structures or in the path of regurgitant jet in the absence of an alternative anatomical explanation
– Abscess
– New partial dehiscence of prosthetic valve or new valvular regurgitation
Minor criteria:
• Predisposing heart condition or intravenous drug use
• Fever over 38 °C (>100.4 °F)
• Vascular phenomenon such as major arterial emboli, septic pulmonary infarcts, mycotic aneurysm, intracranial hemorrhage, conjunctival hemorrhage, Janeway lesions
• Immunological phenomenon
– Glomerulonephritis
– Osler nodes
– Roth spots
– Rheumatoid factor
• Microbiological evidence
– Positive blood cultures not meeting major criteria
• Echocardiogram:
– Consistent with IE but not meeting major criterion

aspects depending on the first organ involved, the underlying cardiac disease (if any), the microorganism involved, the presence or absence of complications, and the patient's characteristics [4].

Acute manifestations include *severe sepsis*, *mitral and/or aortic acute regurgitation*, *heart failure*, *or systemic embolization*.

39.2.1 Acute Valvular Regurgitation

Acute severe valvular regurgitation is considered a surgical emergency, and any cardiac valve can be affected although it occurs more often in left-sided valves with the most serious clinical symptoms. Table 39.2 shows the main causes of acute regurgitation for left-sided cardiac valves. Often clinical symptoms are similar to other acute conditions, such as septic shock, pneumonia, or non-valvular heart failure [9].

Up to 90% of patients present with fever, often associated with systemic symptoms. Heart murmurs are found in up to 85% of patients. Up to 25% of patients have embolic complications at the time of diagnosis. Therefore, IE has to be suspected in any patient presenting with fever and embolic phenomena [4].

Positive blood cultures, before antibiotic administration, remain the cornerstone of diagnosis, but in up 31% of all cases of IE, blood cultures are often negative and often pose considerable diagnostic and therapeutic dilemmas. This situation most commonly arises as a consequence of previous antibiotic administration, underlying the need for withdrawing antibiotics and repeating blood cultures but also can be caused by fungi or fastidious bacteria, notably obligatory intracellular bacteria. Isolation of these microorganisms requires culturing them on specialized media, and their growth is relatively slow. According to local epidemiology, systematic serological testing for *Coxiella burnetii*, *Bartonella* spp., *Aspergillus* spp., *Mycoplasma pneumoniae*,

Table 39.2 Causes of acute regurgitation for mitral and aortic valves

Mitral regurgitation	Aortic regurgitation
Spontaneous cordal/papillary muscle rupture	Aortic dissection (type A)
Post-myocardial infarction papillary muscle rupture	Aortic cusp rupture
Blunt chest trauma	Blunt chest trauma
Prosthetic valve dysfunction	Prosthetic valve dysfunction
Endocarditis	Endocarditis
Acute rheumatic carditis	

Brucella spp., and *Legionella pneumophila* should be proposed, followed by specific polymerase chain reaction (PCR) assays for *Tropheryma whipplei*, *Bartonella* spp., and fungi (*Candida* spp., *Aspergillus* spp.) from the blood [4].

In some instances, differential diagnosis of IE may be difficult, for example, in the situations with thrombi, Lambl's excrescences, cusp prolapse, chordal rupture, valve fibroelastoma, degenerative or myxomatous valve disease, strands, systemic lupus (Libman-Sacks) lesions, primary antiphospholipid syndrome, rheumatoid lesions, or marantic vegetations [10].

Echocardiography, either *transthoracic echocardiography* (*TTE*) or *transesophageal echocardiography* (*TOE*), remains the cornerstone of diagnosis (Fig. 39.2), prognostic evaluation, and treatment monitoring of patients with endocarditis (Fig. 39.3a). Recent technological progress has provided three-dimensional TOE (3-DTOE) as a fundamental diagnostic tool in IE (Fig. 39.3b and Fig. 39.9; see Case Scenario). The 3-DTOE improves spatial orientation and allows a more precise and complete examination of intracardiac anatomy [11, 12].

Four major diagnostic criteria are diagnosed by echography: vegetation, valvular perforation, abscess/peri-valvular fistula, and prosthesis dehiscence. TOE is more sensitive than TTE to detect vegetations on the native valve (96% vs. 70%) or prosthesis (92% vs. 50%). The same is true for the diagnosis of peri-valvular abscess (90% vs. 50%) [5].

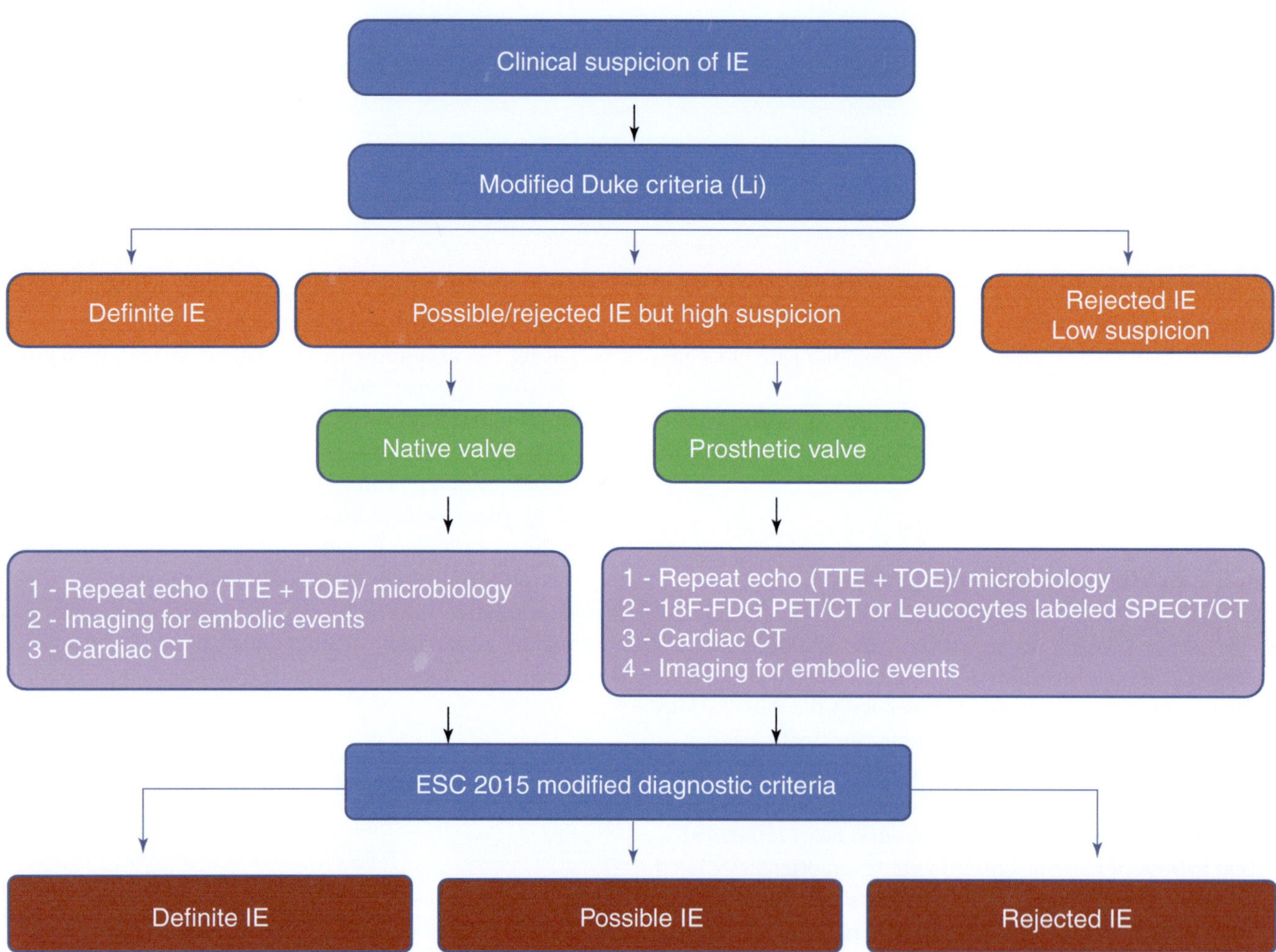

Fig. 39.2 Algorithm for echocardiographic diagnosis in clinical suspicion of infective endocarditis. In case clinical suspicion is still high after a negative TOE, the latter one should be repeated 7–10 days later; *TTE* transthoracic echocardiography, *TOE* transesophageal echocardiography (modified from Habib G et al. [13])

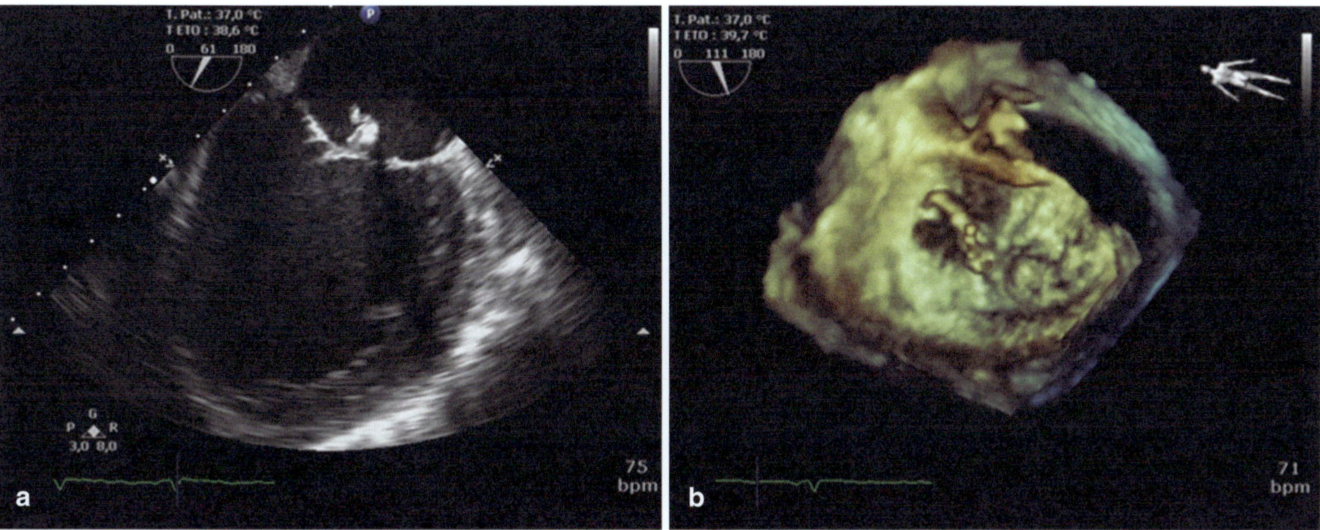

Fig. 39.3 (**a**) Transesophageal echocardiography (TOE), showing a large vegetation of the posterior mitral leaflets. (**b**) Three-dimensional TOE view from the left atrial showing large vegetation and perforation of the posterior mitral leaflet

Therefore, the TTE is performed in all patients suspected of having IE, followed by TOE in case of negative TTE when there is a high index of suspicion for IE, particularly when TTE can lead to suboptimal imaging quality. TOE should also be performed in patients with positive TTE to rule out local complications. In Fig. 39.2 is shown an algorithm for echocardiographic diagnosis in clinical suspicion of IE [11]. Diagnosis may be particularly challenging in IE affecting intracardiac devices, even with the use of TOE. A negative TTE/TOE may occur in about 15% of patients with IE, and it is determined by very small vegetations and by the complexity in identifying vegetations when severe valvular lesions are preexistent or when are atypically located [13].

In cases with an initially negative examination, repeat TTE/TOE must be performed 5–7 days later if the clinical (and biological) level of suspicion is still high or even earlier in the case of *S. aureus* infection.

Multislice computed tomography (CT), positron emission tomography (PET/CT), radiolabeled white blood cell (WBC), and single-photon emission (SPECT/CT) are currently of recognized utility to make IE diagnosis. In particular, in the evaluation of prosthetic valve dysfunction, the CT may be equivalent or superior to echocardiography for the demonstration of prosthesis-related vegetations, abscesses, pseudoaneurysms, and dehiscence [14]. The 18F-fluorodeoxyglucose (18F-FDG) PET/CT allows early diagnosis of endocarditis on the prosthesis by visualizing periprosthetic inflammation at a stage where the TOE and the CT scanner are still negative. Radiolabeled WBC SPECT/CT also detects the periprosthetic infectious processes with a specificity increased compared to the PET scanner. Therefore, the updated guidelines recommend the addition of two major imaging criteria for the diagnosis of endocarditis: the identification of paravalvular lesions by cardiac CT and abnormal activity around the site of implantation detected by 18F-FDG PET/CT (only if the prosthesis was implanted for more than 3 months) or radiolabeled leucocyte SPECT/CT [4].

The most frequent causative microorganisms for IE are *Staphylococcus aureus* and *Streptococcus viridans*, but the incidence of IE by *Staphylococcus epidermidis* is increasing during the last years. Native valve endocarditis is caused by *Streptococcus viridans*, *Streptococcus bovis*, and *Staphylococcus aureus*. The latter *coagulase-negative Staphylococci* and *Enterococci* are the most frequent microorganisms underlying early prosthetic valve infections. The HACEK group (*Haemophilus*, *Actinobacillus*, *Cardiobacterium*, *Eikenella*, *Kingella*) and *Candida* are also potential causes of endocarditis.

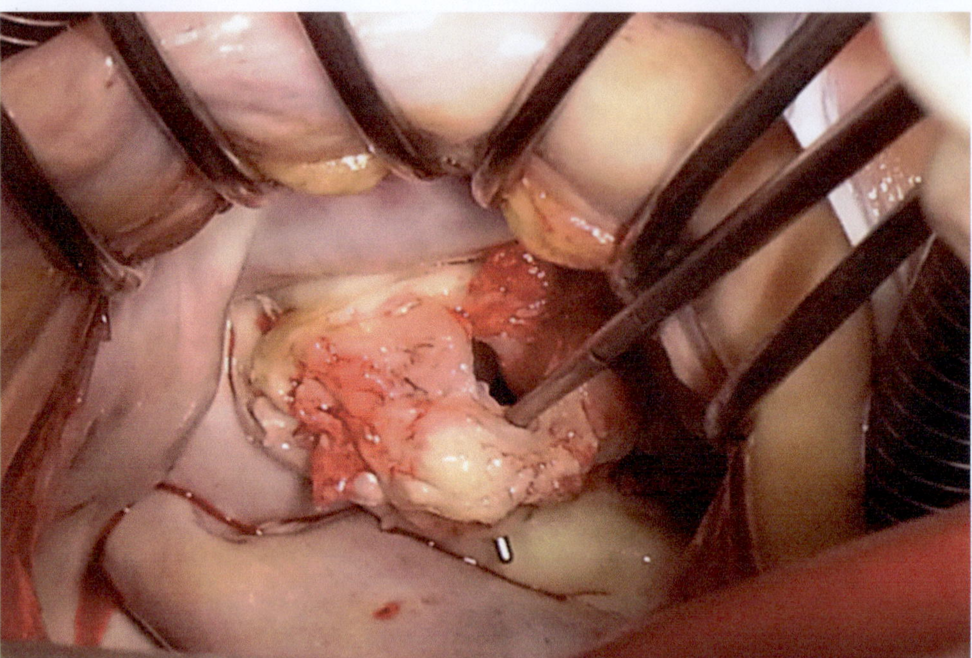

Fig. 39.4 Mitral valve endocarditis with a large vegetation of the anterior mitral leaflet that is perforated

In aortic valve endocarditis, the usual lesions include leaflet vegetations, leaflet destruction, and annular abscess. In the mitral valve endocarditis (Fig. 39.4), we observed the same types of lesion and also chordae or papillary muscle rupture.

The vegetations are clusters of fibrin, leukocytes, macrophages, necrotic tissue, and microorganism; the vegetation is implanted on the valvular tissue and on the prosthetic ring in the PVE. They may be adherent or mobile; with a high variability in size and rate of growth, they can embolize in the coronary artery in the brain, liver, spleen, and kidney. In IE valve structures and neighboring tissues are destroyed by the infection that can cause an abscess extending to the adjacent structures: aorto-mitral curtain, mitral valve, interventricular septum, right ventricle, and right atrium. Abscesses may cause fistula in cardiac chambers. Due to close anatomical relationship between the aortic and the mitral valve, associated mitral and aortic endocarditis can occur in these two valves. The extension of endocarditis from the aortic valve to the mitral valve may be determined by a regurgitant aortic jet or by aortic valve vegetation spread towards the anterior mitral valve. Extension of endocarditis from the mitral valve to the aortic valve may be possible but is rare.

Right-sided IE accounts for 5–10% of IE cases. Although it may occur in patients with a pacemaker, implantable cardioverter-defibrillator (ICD), central venous catheter, or congenital heart disease (CHD), this situation is most frequently observed in intravenous drug abusers (IVDAs), especially in patients with concomitant human immunodeficiency virus (HIV) seropositivity or in immune-suppressed patients. *Staphylococcus aureus* is the predominant infective agent (60–90% of cases) [15, 16].

39.3 Surgical Indication

Cardiac surgery is required in more than 50% of patients with active infective endocarditis during the hospital course. Early surgery is indicated for management of progressive heart failure (HF), to avoid irreversible structural damage caused by severe infection and prevention of embolic events in complicated IE. Although early surgery can avoid death and severe complications, performing surgery during the active phase of IE carries significant risk for these patients. Identification of patients requiring early surgery is frequently difficult and is an important objective of the "endocarditis team." Each case must be individualized and all factors associated with increased risk identified at the time of diagnosis. Early surgery appears particularly beneficial in high-risk patients with heart failure symptoms, large vegetations, and IE caused by *Staphylococcus aureus* [1, 4].

The 2015 guidelines from the European Society of Cardiology (ESC) [5] provide an accurate staging of early surgery according to hemodynamic status: early surgery is graded as "emergency" for surgery performed within 24 h, "urgent" for surgery performed in <7 days, and "elective" when surgery is to be performed after at least 1–2 weeks of antibiotic therapy.

Heart failure is the strongest predictor of poor outcome and the primary cause of early surgery. The acute heart failure observed in 50% of patients with left-sided IE is mainly caused by severe aortic or mitral regurgitation and is rarely related to intracardiac fistulae or to valve obstruction [6]. Cardiac surgery is the only option and should not be delayed. In patients with severe valvular regurgitation without heart failure, the timing of surgery is unclear, but early surgery may be a reasonable option for low-risk patients, especially when subclinical signs of poor hemodynamic tolerance are suspected on echocardiography [4, 17, 18].

Uncontrolled infection is the second cause of early surgery and includes general and local uncontrolled infection. Generally, uncontrolled infection is defined by unexplained persistent bacteremia after 1 week of adequate antibiotic treatment and is mainly caused by virulent microorganisms. Persistent vegetation, abscesses, and increases in vegetation size under antibiotic therapy are considered to be local uncontrolled infections. Urgent surgery is recommended to prevent local and general complications. Antibiotic therapy has limited effect on local complications, and urgent surgery should be performed to prevent the risk of sudden cardiac death or an embolic event [1].

Embolic events are usually asymptomatic and frequent (30–50%) [19] but can be a life-threatening complication of IE related to the migration of cardiac vegetations. The brain and spleen are the most frequent sites of embolism in left-sided IE, while pulmonary embolism is frequent in native right-sided and pacemaker lead IE. The risk of embolism depends mainly on size and mobility of vegetation, and it also depends on other several variables (age, diabetes, atrial fibrillation, previous embolism before therapy, vegetation length, and *S. aureus* infection). The risk of an embolic event is major before the initiation of antibiotics and decreases promptly after initiation of antibiotic therapy, especially after 2 weeks; therefore, the best means to reduce this risk is the prompt institution of appropriate antibiotic therapy [1]. Current guidelines [4] recommend urgent surgery for large isolated vegetation (>15 mm) and vegetation >10 mm with a new embolic event despite adequate antibiotic treatment or in the presence of severe valvular disease.

39.4 Cerebral Complications

The rate of symptomatic cerebral complications ranges between 20% and 50% [19], and they more frequently relate to cerebral infarction than an intracranial hemorrhage (ICH) (Fig. 39.5).

Neurological manifestations occur before or at IE diagnosis in the majority of cases, but new or recurrent events can also take place later in the course of IE. Clinical presentation is variable and may include multiple symptoms or signs in the same patient. Management of these patients may be challenging and requires multidisciplinary expertise to evaluate the risk of cerebral damage related to cardiopulmonary bypass [1, 4].

IE with cerebral infarction requires an aggressive therapy strategy to avoid embolism recurrence. Several consistent studies have demonstrated that early cardiac surgery is superior to delayed surgery, with a low risk of cerebral complications and a good probability of complete neurological recovery. In the absence of coma, cardiac surgery – when required – is best performed without delay in asymptomatic or symptomatic patients with cerebral infarction. When an intracranial hemorrhage (ICH) is present, the indication to surgery is less aggressive and recommends delaying for at least 1 month. However, many patients with ICH have an urgent indication. Therefore, early surgery (before 1 month) – when indicated due to hemodynamic instability – may be performed in patients with ICH after careful evaluation of the sizes and etiologies of hemorrhagic lesions and a multidisciplinary discussion [1, 4].

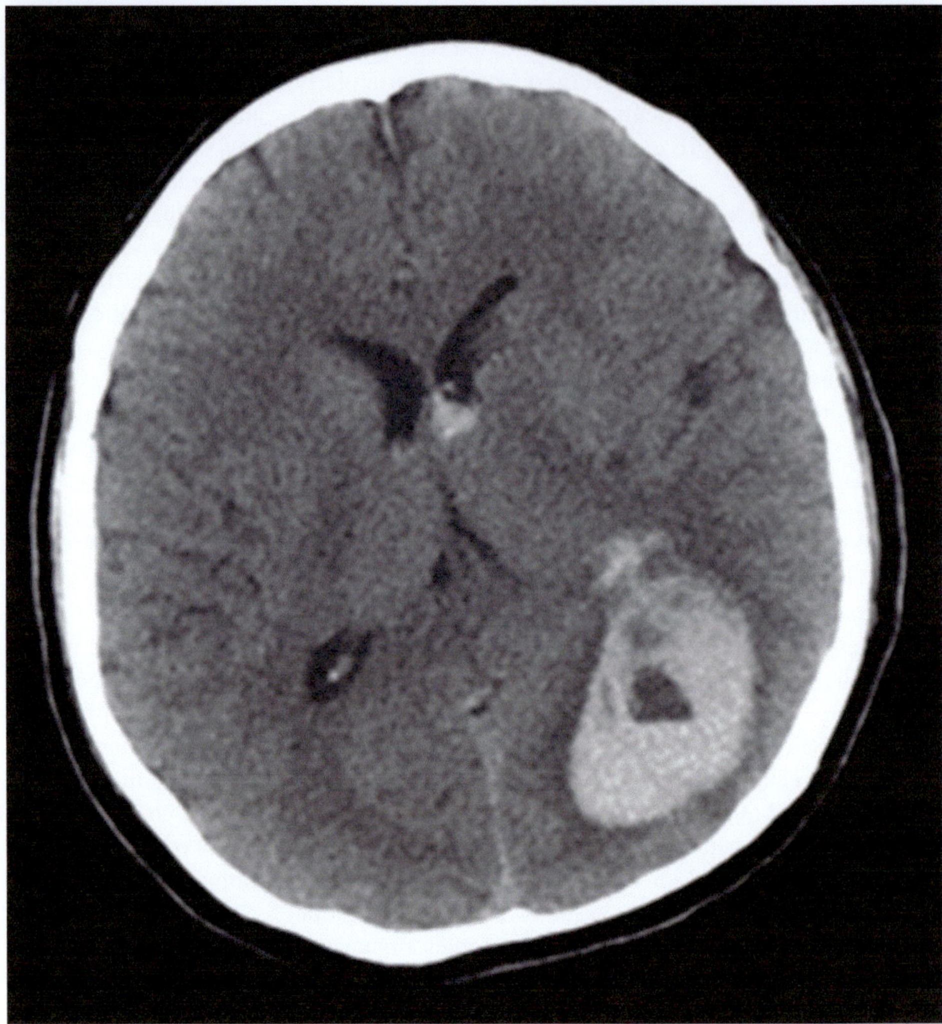

Fig. 39.5 Axial computed tomography scan of the brain showing a large left parieto-occipital intracranial hemorrhage complicated a prosthetic aortic valve endocarditis

39.5 Surgical Management

The advantages of surgery performed during the initial hospitalization period have been confirmed in a large cohort of non-selected patients with IE [20] and confirmed by a recent meta-analysis (of 21 studies) that reported a decrease in 1-year mortality of 20% when surgery was performed within 7 days [9, 21].

The objectives of surgery for infective endocarditis are a complete and extensive excision of infected tissues, allow a bacteriological diagnosis, and perform an anatomical reconstruction of affected structures. The use of foreign material should be kept to a minimum. Where infection is confined to the valve cusps or leaflets, any method to repair or replace the valve may be used. However, valve repair is favored whenever possible, particularly when IE affects the mitral or tricuspid valve without significant destruction. In mitral valve IE, successful valve repair can be achieved by experienced teams in 61–80% of patients. Aortic valve repair in IE can be achieved by experienced teams in up to 33% of patients, but replacement of the aortic valve using a mechanical or biological prosthesis is the technique of choice [4].

Aortic valve endocarditis with concomitant abscess formation needs aggressive diagnostic and therapeutic approaches considering dangerous and ominous complications such as heart block; destruction of mitral, aortic intervalvular fibrosa (see below); extrinsic compression of coronary arteries; fistula to other cardiac chambers; and aortic pseudoaneurysm formation.

Perforations in a single valve cusp or leaflet may be repaired with an untreated or glutaraldehyde-treated autologous or bovine pericardial patch. More extensive destruction of a single leaflet or the presence of an abscess are not necessarily a contraindication for valve repair. The intraoperative assessment of the valve after debridement is of paramount importance in order to evaluate whether the remaining tissue is of sufficient quality to achieve a durable repair. Suturing a patch to achieve a competent valve, whether pericardial, tricuspid autograft or a flipped-over mitral patch, has not been associated with worse results in terms of recurrence of IE or mitral regurgitation when performed by experienced surgeons.

When a durable valve repair is not feasible, that is where the problem arises: the perfect prosthesis does not exist. Therefore, a tailored approach for each patient and the clinical situation should be recommended. Owing to their natural biocompatibility, the use of cryopreserved or sterilized homografts (Fig. 39.6) has been suggested to reduce the risk of persistent or recurrent infection, especially in the presence of annular abscesses.

It is expert opinion and standard strategy in many institutions that the use of a homograft is to be favored over valve prostheses, particularly in the presence of root abscess. Homografts or stentless xenografts or aortic root xenografts (Fig. 39.7) may be preferred in prosthetic valve endocarditis (PVE) or in cases where there is extensive aortic root destruction with aorto-ventricular discontinuity [4].

The most important aspect of the surgical treatment of these patients is radical resection of all infected tissues. The anterior mitral leaflet of the aortic homograft can be effectively used for reconstruction of the outflow tract. A monoblock aorto-mitral homograft has been suggested as a surgical option for extensive bivalvular IE. In experienced hands, the Ross procedure may be used in children or adolescents to facilitate growth and in young adults for extended durability. Cardiac transplantation may be considered in extreme cases where repeated operative procedures have failed to eradicate persistent or recurrent PVE [4].

Patients with PVE have a more serious prognosis than patients with native aortic valve endocarditis, and nosocomial infections are associated with higher mortality than community-acquired infections.

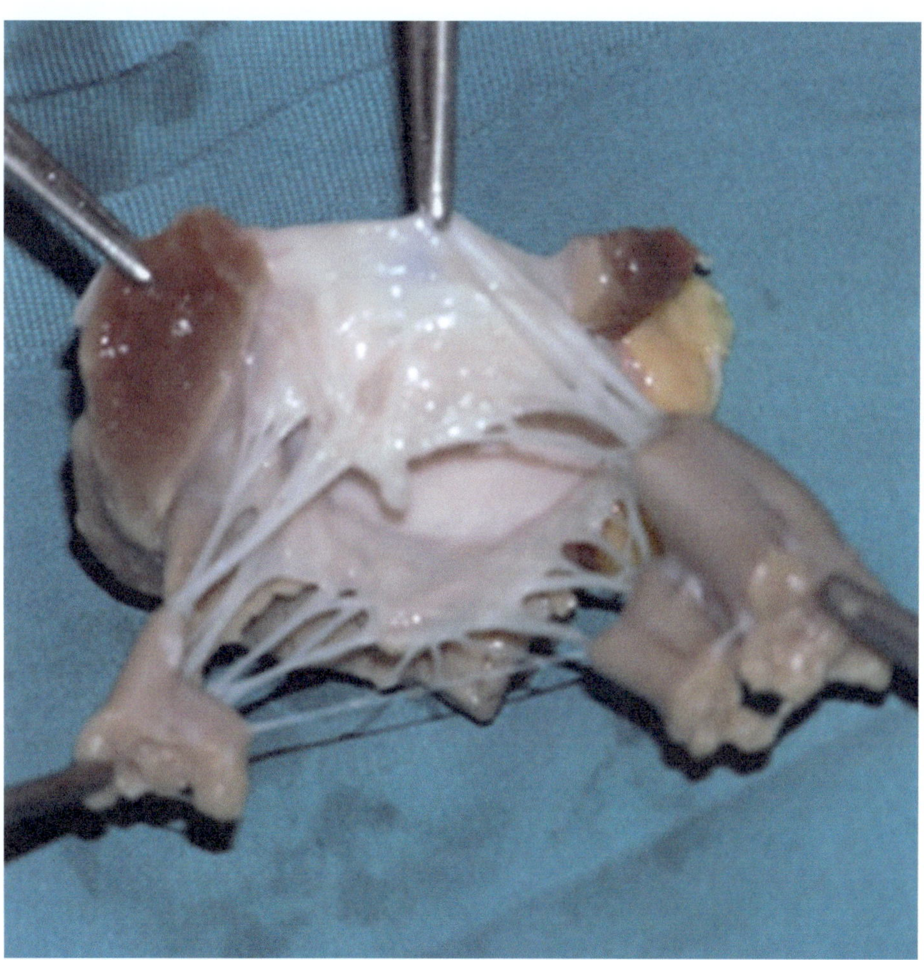

Fig. 39.6 Mitral homograft

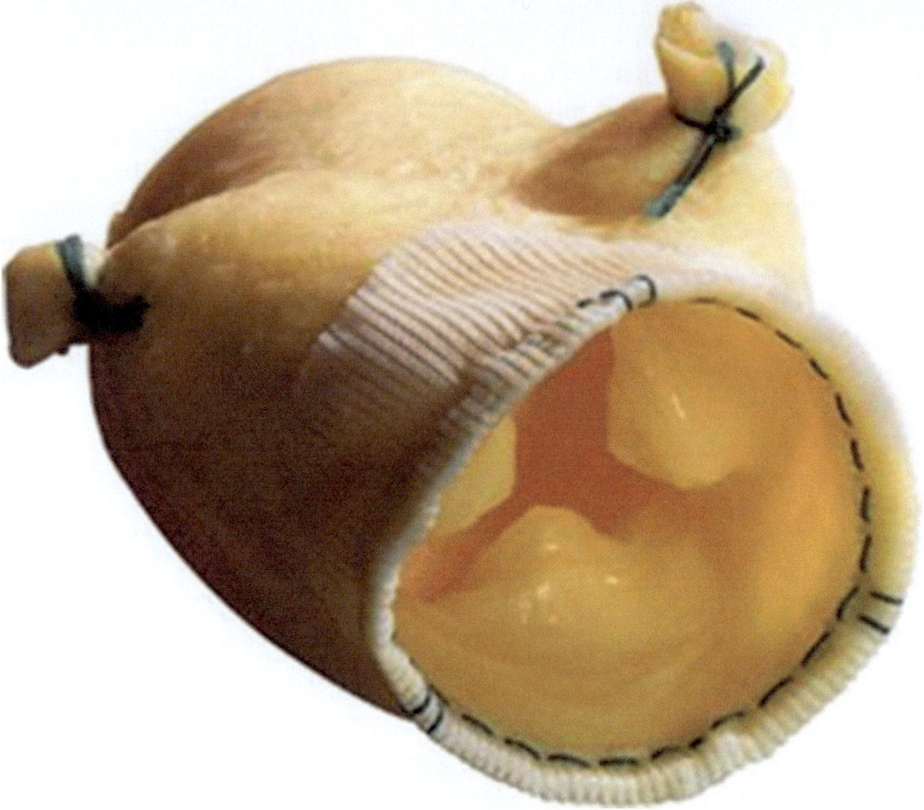

Fig. 39.7 Medtronic Freestyle aortic root xenografts (Courtesy of Medtronic)

Case Scenario

A 66-year-old male, heavy smoker with diabetes mellitus type 1, in May 2015 had fever and chills. He initially responded to empiric antimicrobial treatment, but 1 month later he was hospitalized for heart failure. Combined mitral-aortic valve infective endocarditis was diagnosed, and double valve replacement was done with bioprostheses. Postoperatively, a PET/CT imaging showed L4-L5 hyper-fixation and inflammatory spondylodiscitis. Therefore, in September 2015 he underwent L3-S1 fusion surgery; periradicular tissue cultures were negative. At this time a TTE diagnosed aortic periprosthetic leak with moderate regurgitation.

One month later, the patient was admitted with shortness of breath and early signs of heart failure. A coronary angiography showed a systolic narrowing of the left main trunk (Fig. 39.8).

Questions

1. What has caused left main trunk narrowing?
   A. Left main trunk embolization
   B. Left main trunk spasm
   C. Left main trunk compression
2. Does the patient present angina symptoms?
   A. No
   B. Only after a severe effort
   C. Unstable angina

Comment

3-DTOE showed a large aortic periprosthetic abscess in the mitral-aortic intervalvular fibrosa (MAIVF), a fistulous communication involving both atria, an unexpected systolic compression, and narrowing of the left main trunk, also observed at coronary angiography (Fig. 39.9).

During surgery, a 2.5 × 1.3 cm MAIVF pseudoaneurysm, was visualized in communication with both atria and is located in left aortic sinus underneath left coronary cusp extending below non-coronary cusp; the infective lesion involved mitral valve anterior leaflet thoroughly to the membranous septum. Infected tissues and previously implanted prostheses were removed and replaced with two bioprostheses; the left atrial roof and aortic wall were directly sutured. The postoperative course was favorable, and 30 months later TTE showed normal bioprostheses function [22].

An extrinsic coronary artery compression for pseudoaneurysms of the sinus of Valsalva or pulmonary artery aneurysms is well known [23–25], but only a few sporadic reports showed coronary compression by MAIVF pseudoaneurysm [26, 27]. 3-DTOE allowed to diagnose an asymptomatic but life-threatening compression of the left main trunk, a situation confirmed by coronary angiography.

Mitral-aortic intervalvular fibrosa (MAIVF) is made by fibrous tissue establishing continuity between anterior mitral leaflet and the non-coronary cusp of the aortic valve. Because MAIVF is avascular and thin, it may be more prone to injury and infection. Pseudoaneurysm of this area is a rare complication of infective endocarditis or aortic valve surgery.

Please see Chap. 58 for the correct answer.

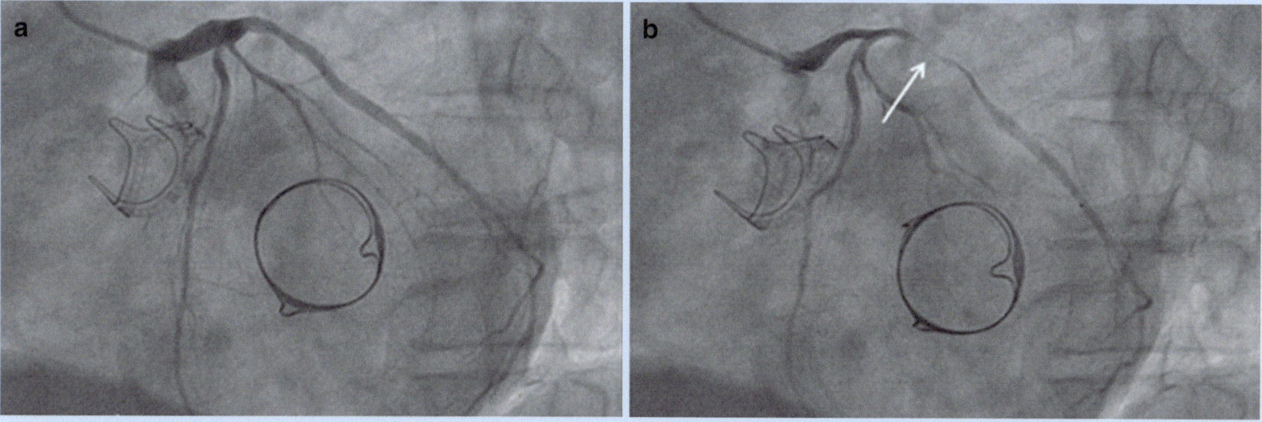

Fig. 39.8 Coronary angiography: (**a**) diastole and (**b**) systole. In **b** the distal left main trunk is narrowed. Reprinted from "Mitral-Aortic Intervalvular Fibrosa Pseudoaneurysm Causing Systolic Compression of Left Main Trunk. Grande AM, et al. Ann Thorac Surg 2017; 103:e461" with permission from Elsevier

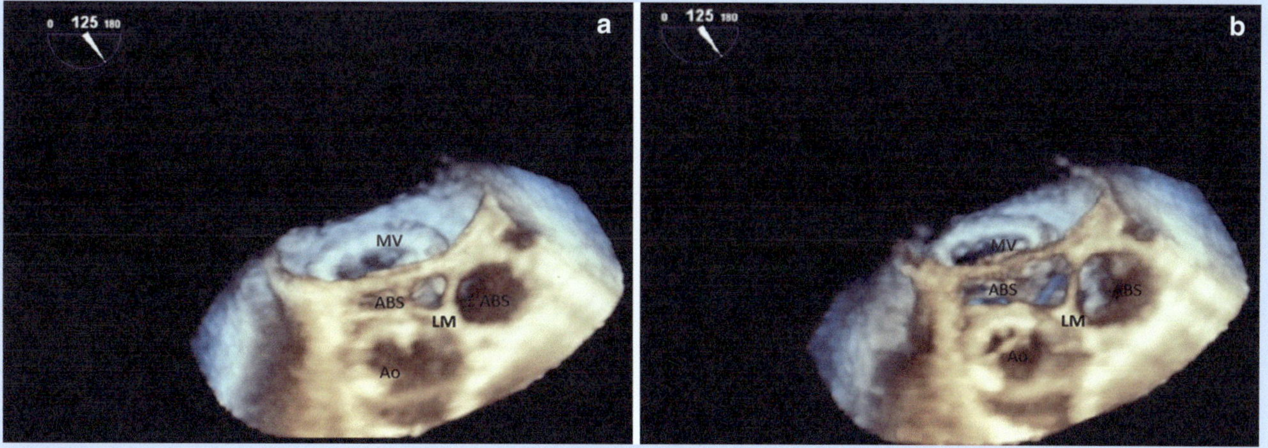

Fig. 39.9 (**a**) Diastole; (**b**) systole. In **b** it is evident the left main trunk compression. *ABS* abscess, *LM* left main trunk, *MV* mitral valve, *Ao* aortic valve. Reprinted from "Mitral-Aortic Intervalvular Fibrosa Pseudoaneurysm Causing Systolic Compression of Left Main Trunk. Grande AM, et al. Ann Thorac Surg 2017; 103:e461" with perssion from Elsevier

References

1. Oliver L, Lepeule R, Moussafeur A, Fiore A, Lim P. Ternacle Early surgery in infective endocarditis: why should we wait? J Arch Cardiovasc Dis. 2016;109(12):651–4.
2. Vongpatanasin W, Hillis LD, Lange RA. Prosthetic heart valves. N Engl J Med. 1996;335:407–16.
3. Habib G, Thuny F, Avierinos JF. Prosthetic valve endocarditis: current approach and therapeutic options. Prog Cardiovasc Dis. 2008;50:274–81.
4. Habib G, Lancellotti P, Antunes MJ, et al. ESC Guidelines for the management of infective endocarditis: the Task Force for the Management of Infective Endocarditis of the European Society of Cardiology (ESC). Endorsed by: European Association for Cardio-Thoracic Surgery (EACTS), the European Association of Nuclear Medicine (EANM). Eur Heart J. 2015;36:3075–128.
5. Nishimura RA, Otto CM, Bonow RO, et al. 2014 AHA/ACC guideline for the management of patients with valvular heart disease: a report of the American College of Cardiology/American Heart Association Task Force on practice guidelines. J Am Coll Cardiol. 2014;63:e57–185.
6. Durak DT, Lukes AS, Bright DK. New criteria for diagnosis of infective endocarditis: utilization of specific echocardiography finding. Duke Endocarditis Service. Am J Med. 1994;96:200–9.
7. The 2015 ESC Guidelines for the management of infective endocarditis. Eur Heart J. 2015;36:3075–23. https://doi.org/10.1093/eurartj/ehv319.
8. Iung B, Doco-Lecompte T, Chocron S, et al. Cardiac surgery during the acute phase of infective endocarditis: discrepancies between European Society of Cardiology guidelines and practices. Eur Heart J. 2016;37:840–8.
9. Stout KK, Verrier ED. Valvular heart disease: changing concepts in disease management. Circulation. 2009;119:3232–41.
10. Sanchez-Enrique C, Vilacosta I, Moreno HG, Delgado-Bolton R, Perez-Alonso P, Martinez A, Vivas D, Ferrera C, Olmos C. Infected marantic endocarditis with leukemoid reaction. Circ J. 2014;78:2325–7.
11. Yong MS, Saxena P, Killu AM, Coffey S, Burkart HM, Wan S-H, Malouf JF. The preoperative evaluation of infective endocarditis via 3-dimensional transesophageal echocardiography. Tex Heart Inst J. 2015;42:372–6.
12. Vrettou AR, Zacharoulis A, Lerakis S, Kremastinos DT. Revealing infective endocarditis complications by echocardiography: the value of real-time 3D transesophageal echocardiography. Hell J Cardiol. 2013;54(2):147–9.
13. Habib G, Badano L, Tribouilloy C, Vilacosta I, Zamorano JL, Galderisi M, Voigt JU, Sicari R, Cosyns B, Fox K, Aakhus S. Recommendations for the practice of echocardiography in infective endocarditis. Eur J Echocardiogr. 2010;11:202–19.
14. Feuchtner GM, Stolzmann P, Dichtl W, Schertler T, Bonatti J, Scheffel H, Mueller S, Plass A, Mueller L, Bartel T, Wolf F, Alkadhi H. Multislice computed tomography in infective endocarditis: comparison with transesophageal echocardiography and intraoperative findings. J Am Coll Cardiol. 2009;53:436–44.
15. Frontera JA, Gradon JD. Right-side endocarditis in injection drug users: review of proposed mechanisms of pathogenesis. Clin Infect Dis. 2000;30:374–9.
16. Wilson LE, Thomas DL, Astemborski J, Freedman TL, Vlahov D. Prospective study of infective endocarditis among injection drug users. J Infect Dis. 2002;185:1761–6.
17. Kang DH. Timing of surgery in infective endocarditis. Heart. 2015;101(22):1786–91.
18. Delahaye F. Is early surgery beneficial in infective endocarditis? A systematic review. Arch Cardiovasc Dis. 2011;104:35–44.
19. Thuny F, Beurtheret S, Mancini J, et al. The timing of surgery influences mortality and morbidity in adults with severe complicated infective endocarditis: a propensity analysis. Eur Heart J. 2011;32:2027–33.
20. Lalani T, Cabell CH, Benjamin DK, et al. Analysis of the impact of early surgery on in-hospital mortality of native valve endocarditis: use of propensity score and instrumental variable methods to adjust for treatment-selection bias. Circulation. 2010;121:1005–13.
21. Anantha Narayanan M, Mahfood Haddad T, Kalil AC, et al. Early versus late surgical intervention or medical management for infective endocarditis: a systematic review and meta-analysis. Heart. 2016;102:950–7.
22. Grande AM, Amoroso F, Crimi G, Ferrario M, Mazzola A. Mitral-aortic intervalvular fibrosa pseudoaneurysm causing systolic compression of left main trunk. Ann Thorac Surg. 2017;103:e461.
23. Chesler E, Korns ME, Porter GE, Reyes CN, Edwards JE. False aneurysm of the left ventricle secondary to bacterial endocarditis with perforation of the mitral-aortic intervalvular fibrosa. Circulation. 1968;37:518–23.
24. Moorthy N, Kumar S, Tewari S, et al. Mitral-aortic intervalvular fibrosa aneurysm with rupture into left atrium: an uncommon cause of acute dyspnea. Heart Views. 2012;13:13–5.
25. Ihdayhid AR, Asrar Ul, Hag M, Dembo L, Yong G. Simultaneous coronary and pulmonary angiography to diagnose critical left main coronary artery stenosis secondary to dilated pulmonary artery. JACC Cardiovascular Interv. 2016;9(11):1193–4.
26. Dahya VJ, Chalasani P. Sinus of Valsalva aneurysm causing extrinsic compression of the left main coronary artery. JACC Cardiovascular Interv. 2015;8(6):e99–100.
27. Kim HW, Chung CH. Mitral-aortic intervalvular fibrosa pseudoaneurysm resulting in the displacement of the left main coronary artery after aortic valve replacement. J Thorac Cardiovasc Surg. 2010;139:e18–20.

Updates in the Management of Esophageal Emergencies (Caustic and Iatrogenic Injuries)

40

Monica Gualtierotti, Elio Treppiedi, Giovanni Ferrari, and Christophe Mariette

Key Points

- Conservative treatment is the most frequent approach after caustic ingestion; respiratory, metabolic, and hemodynamic optimization is the cornerstones of non-operative management.
- Urgent laparotomy is required if clinical or radiologic signs of perforations are present.
- The most common procedure is the esophagogastrectomy with a laparotomy and cervicotomy.
- Esophageal reconstruction should be performed at least 6 months after caustic ingestion.
- Esophageal perforation most frequently occurs secondary to endoscopically induced injury.
- Patients may progress quickly to septic shock, which mandates immediate surgical intervention.
- The time from perforation is vital to determine its management.
- Primary repair and drainage should be used in patients without malignancy.
- Esophageal perforations may be managed non-operatively if patients are not septic and imaging shows a contained perforation.

40.1 Caustic Lesions

Caustic ingestion is an underreported disease in the medical literature; no doubt exists about the clinical relevance of this disease both in the clinical setting and regarding its high economic impact on the health system.

According to the 2013 annual report of the American Association of Poison Control Centers, there were nearly 60,000 cases of exposure to corrosive agents (48,000 to bleach, 7500 to acids, 4000 to alkalis) [1]. Except for data elaborated by the poison control centers and for data published in specialized medical or surgical centers, no other sources are available about the true incidence of this disease and its sequelae. It is well known that this condition needs a high resource-consuming treatment and a significant clinical expertise.

Two age peaks are involved in the esophageal caustic ingestion: children that ingest accidentally such substances and adults with suicidal intent [2].

Concerning the quality of the corrosive agents ingested, the traditional historical division in acids and alkalis is still valid. It is during the first clinical evaluation of the patient that the nature of the corrosive agent should always be identified and the poison control center be contacted.

Several studies have already been published about the different patterns of pathological damages; liquefactive necrosis and saponification with vascular thrombosis are associated

To Monsieur Christophe Mariette (16/11/1969–18/07/2017), the professor who taught me everything about esophageal surgery and I will never forget.

M. Gualtierotti (✉)
Digestive and Oncological Surgery Department, University Hospital C. Huriez, Lille, France

Oncological and Miniinvasive Surgery Department, Niguarda Hospital, Milan, Italy

E. Treppiedi
Digestive and Oncological Surgery Department, University Hospital C. Huriez, Lille, France

Upper Gastrointestinal and General Surgery, University of Verona, Verona, Italy

G. Ferrari
Oncological and Miniinvasive Surgery Department, Niguarda Hospital, Milan, Italy

C. Mariette
Digestive and Oncological Surgery Department, University Hospital C. Huriez, Lille, France

P. Aseni et al. (eds.), *Operative Techniques and Recent Advances in Acute Care and Emergency Surgery*,
https://doi.org/10.1007/978-3-319-95114-0_40

with alkali ingestion in all the gastrointestinal tract; on the other hand, coagulative necrosis is described following acid ingestion [3]. A different kind of major anatomical injury has been advocated which is linked to these different types of pathological damages; alkali damage power is superior to the acid ones, and traditionally alkali ingestion can lead to more damage to the gastrointestinal tract. Traditionally, alkali ingestion is connected to an important esophageal injury as well as to other organ injuries. On the contrary, acid ingestion induces more severe damage to the stomach when compared to alkalis. However, the above historical simplification has not been confirmed by a recent publication in which no significant differences have been found among rates of transmural esophageal necrosis, esophageal stricture formation, failure of endoscopic management of esophageal strictures, and needs for esophageal reconstruction in acid or alkali ingestions [4]. The involvement of the oropharynx and the tracheobronchial tree is an additional risk during caustic ingestion, and the incidence is higher with solid physical form or with the vapor form. As a matter of fact, this involvement should be divided into two main kinds: the direct exposure of the mucosa to the agent (like inhalation of the vapors) and the direct penetration from the digestive tract with a transmural development like in aortoesophageal fistula or esophagus-tracheal fistula.

40.1.1 Clinical Assessment

Clinical scenario ranges from the asymptomatic patient to the unconscious patient in need of an initial reanimation. Thoracic, cervical, and epigastric pain is the most common and unspecific signs; hoarseness and stridor could be linked to a laryngeal injury. Protection of the airway needs to be taken into account in the first evaluation of the caustic ingestion, with the risk of intubation estimated in 10% of all patients [5].

The change of these signs could also be an index of damage progression. If not already present at the first evaluation, esophageal perforation may occur in the first week after the ingestion, with the progression of mucosal ulcerations. A global evaluation of laboratory blood tests is useful to estimate the inflammation level with a dosage of white blood count, inflammation markers, and electrolytic and pH disorders. Metabolic disorders like electrolytic and pH disequilibrium are common, particularly in life-threatening cases.

A radiography of the chest can only evaluate the presence of intra-abdominal air or cervical emphysema as signs of perforation indirectly. Evaluation with water-soluble oral contrast could help identify the site of perforation (like in other cases of esophageal perforation management), but it is useless at this stage of the diagnostic workup.

40.1.2 Diagnosis

The role of the esophagogastroduodenoscopy is to show directly the esophageal mucosa, to stratify the risk of perforation, and to correlate this data with treatment. Although several classifications have been published on this topic, the most useful are the Zargar classification published in 1991 [6].

Grade	Endoscopic features
1	Superficial mucosal edema and erythema
2a	Superficial ulcerations, erosions, exudates
2b	Deep discrete or circumferential ulcerations
3a	Focal necrosis
3b	Extensive necrosis
4	Perforations

An early endoscopic evaluation is mandatory to classify the injury of the esophagus and the stomach. It has been demonstrated that this classification correlates with the early and late complications in the management of patients. The most important limit of the esophagogastroduodenoscopy is the impossibility to evaluate the transmural involvement of the injury. For this reason, many experts have tried to use echoendoscopy as a complementary exam to evaluate the depth of injury into the organ wall; yet, its use has not been validated so far [7].

Computed tomography (CT) scan is the other crucial exam after caustic ingestion, extremely useful in obtaining a clear evaluation of the mediastinum and the abdomen, identifying the presence of a perforation, and evaluating the wall of the esophagus and the stomach with different kinds of CT-based grading system score. A recent study [8] has evaluated the use of the CT for the emergency diagnostic workup of patients with caustic injuries even without endoscopic evaluation; the results show that CT scan accurately predicts the presence of transmural necrosis in emergency decision-making after caustic injuries, even though this approach wasn't confirmed by a review in 2014 [9]. As published by Bonavina et al. in the Consensus Conference of the World Society of Emergency Surgery in 2015, CT is helpful in guiding indications for esophagectomy in patients with grade 3b caustic injury, as it evaluates the presence of transmural esophageal necrosis, which is the cornerstone to decide for an operative or non-operative management [10].

In a recent review published in *The Lancet* by Chirica [11], the management algorithm suggests the use of CT scan to evaluate edema of the gastric or esophageal wall or soft tissues and increased esophageal wall enhancement. In borderline patients with endoscopy or CT scan suspicious for perforation, a surgical approach with laparotomy or laparoscopy is justified. Direct visualization of the stomach could confirm or exclude gastric necrosis and help the surgeon decide whether to resect or not; on the contrary, esophagectomy is a surgical option which can be planned only on preoperative diagnostic workup because no intraoperative findings could help the surgeon in this choice.

40.1.3 End Point-Guided Resuscitation

Medical optimizations, with respiratory and hemodynamic control, are the cornerstones of the non-operative management. If necessary, airway control via tracheal intubation with fiber optic laryngoscopy or tracheotomy should be performed. Gastric lavage is not recommended, and neither is the routine use of a nasogastric tube; the risk to create other lesions or aspiration pneumonia seems superior to the benefits [12]. Proton pump inhibitors or h2 blockers are used; however, no clear data is available. Corticosteroids are controversial and should be reserved for patients with symptoms involving the airway [10]. Broad-spectrum antibiotics should not be administered on a systematic basis; their use should be considered for advanced grades with lung involvement.

40.1.4 Non-operative Management

Conservative treatment is the most frequent approach after caustic ingestion. It could be considered if clinical, biochemical, or radiologic signs of perforations are absent.

According to Zargar's classification, grade 1 and 2a lesions do not usually need an intensive approach; oral feeding is possible, and no specific other measures should be adopted.

Grade 2b and grade 3 lesions should be kept in nil per os and require a medical or surgical intensive care unit (ICU), with monitoring of biochemical and clinical change and evaluation of metabolic and nutritional status; renal failure, metabolic disorders, disseminated intravascular coagulation, or cardiovascular shock could also arise several hours after the ingestion [2]. In this setting, the presence of abdominal symptoms can be a sign of perforation or peritonitis which, together with mediastinitis, are indications for an emergency surgery.

A nutritional support with parenteral nutrition or with enteral nutrition via jejunostomy or nasojejunal tube is mandatory. No clear data is available on the correct timing of subsequent endoscopic or radiologic reevaluation in the non-operative management.

40.1.5 Operative Management

Urgent laparotomy is required if clinical or radiologic signs of perforations are present. The most common procedure is the esophagogastrectomy by a double incision (laparotomy and cervicotomy) with stripping of the esophagus; if a tracheobronchial injury is evident, a transthoracic approach should be used to avoid its enlargement and repair it.

Esophagectomy with gastric preservation and total gastrectomy with esophagojejunostomy can be performed if transmural necrosis is limited to the esophagus or the stomach, respectively [10].

A total gastrectomy is the most common surgical approach if only a gastroresection is needed; partial gastrectomy can be considered even though there are risks linked to the imperfect evaluation of stomach necrosis.

After emergency surgery, immediate reconstruction of the intestinal tract is feasible with an acceptable morbi-mortality, but it should be reserved or referral centers [13]; disadvantages are linked to the necessity of a damage control approach in the emergency context and the theoretical risk of poor tissue quality for the anastomosis. As published by Zerbib [14], a conservative treatment of stage III gastric injury can be feasible, avoiding emergency gastrectomy; if a conservative approach is to be applied to the esophagus, a bipolar exclusion of the esophagus with cervical esophagostomy and abdominal closure of the lumen can be considered in an "organ-sparing context," in order to decrease the morbidity and mortality of an emergency esophagectomy. This approach, however, still hasn't been validated, and complications have been described.

Resection of other abdominal organs, like duodenum or jejunum, is sometimes necessary because of the intraluminal passage of the caustic agent or transmural extension of the necrosis to adjacent organs (e.g., transverse colon, pancreas, etc.). In such context, usually, the extension of necrosis is considered an independent predictor of operative death [15].

Different techniques have been described to manage the pancreatic stump if a duodenopancreatectomy is necessary or to manage the duodenopancreatic tract if it has been preserved [15, 16].

Feeding jejunostomy should be systematically placed at the end of the operation, regardless of the type of surgical procedure performed in the emergency context [10].

40.1.6 Management of Long-Term Sequelae

Late sequelae of caustic ingestion, especially after non-operative management, are common: corrosive strictures and bleeding are the most frequent, but tardive perforations with fistulization to other mediastinal organs have also been described. Esophageal scar retractions with the risk of stricture development, especially in the lower third of the esophagus, seem to shorten the organ and to create an additional risk factor for gastroesophageal reflux, with the danger of aggravating the esophageal stenosis (see Fig. 40.1) [17].

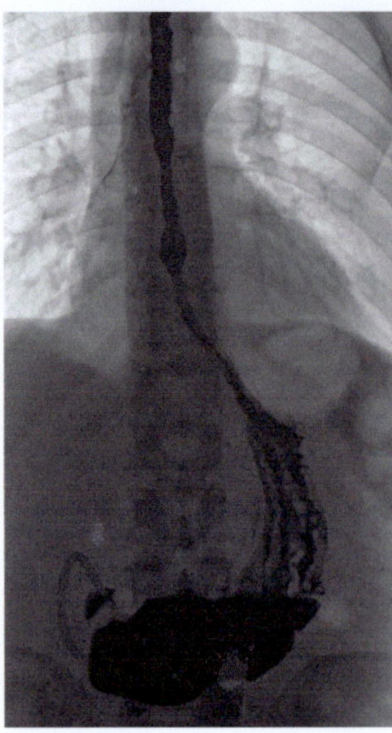

Fig. 40.1 Long-term sequelae with corrosive strictures

Prediction of corrosive strictures is made during the first evaluation; however, an effective preventive treatment does not exist. Medical treatments with local or systemic steroids, NSAIDS or cytotoxic agents, have shown controversial results, and there is no convincing evidence of their efficacy. Early stenting of the esophagus has been evaluated, but its role still needs to be defined.

Endoscopic dilatation carried out with balloon or bougies is the gold standard treatment; no randomized studies specific in caustic, corrosive strictures are available to evaluate these two techniques. During these procedures risk of perforation should not be underestimated, but frequently esophageal perforation in this context is quite contained due to the fibrotic esophageal wall and periesophageal tissues. The usual interval between dilatations varies from less than 1 week to 2–3 weeks, and three or four sessions may provide durable results; the number of dilatations required is unpredictable, and the endoscopic treatment may continue for years [10]. The use of intraluminal stents can be helpful, but the rates of migrations, development of hyperplasic tissue, and recurrence are still the major limits to this technique. In order to solve these problems, a global evaluation of the patient, with nutritional status assessment, symptomatology, and treatment of the psychiatric disease (in case of voluntary ingestion), is mandatory to evaluate a surgical approach. Intraluminal stents are not helpful to treat gastric strictures. Elective surgery represents the treatment of choice for gastric sequelae, usually with partial gastrectomy; gastrocele is also described as a late complication and treated with partial gastric resection [18].

Two main indications of esophageal reconstruction may be identified: failure of endoscopic treatment and restoration of gastrointestinal continuity after emergency esophagectomy. The organ more frequently used as graft is the colon (right, transverse or left colon), with isoperistaltic or anisoperistaltic reconstruction depending on vascular anatomy, previous colonic surgery (elective or during the first stage of resection), and surgeon experience (see Fig. 40.2). The retrosternal route is the standard choice for reconstruction; passage through the posterior mediastinum has also been described, while subcutaneous positioning is no longer utilized.

In the context of elective surgery with the aim to reconstruct the intestinal tract, esophageal reconstruction should be performed at least 6 months after caustic ingestion, and the control of the psychiatric disease should be optimal. The choice to perform an esophagectomy, if not performed before, should also be linked to the risk of developing a malignancy of the esophagus exposed to the caustic agent; this has been described to happen up to 1000 times more frequently than in the general population [19, 20]. As published by Chirica [21], late complications after colon interposition in a high-volume center were recorded in about 55% of patients (stenosis, 36%; reflux, 11%; redundancy 5%); functional failure was recorded in 23% of patients and was associated with a delay in reconstruction inferior to 6 months and emergency tracheotomy.

Pharyngeal reconstruction during esophageal reconstruction for caustic injuries has a negative impact on the functional outcome, but colopharyngoplasty for strictures involving the pharynx is a safe and effective procedure [22]. A temporary tracheostomy is mandatory during the rehabilitation training period after colopharyngoplasty. The use of myocutaneous flaps and free jejunal grafts should be considered for salvage of cervical esophageal reconstruction after previously failed surgical attempts [10].

40.2 Esophageal Perforations

Esophageal perforation(EP) is a life-threatening condition that requires a high index of suspicion and early diagnosis for an optimal outcome [23].

The recent proliferation of using endoscopic procedures in the upper gastrointestinal tract has resulted in an increased incidence of EP.

The diagnosis of EP is established by clinical presentation, computed tomography (CT), contrast esophagogram, and endoscopic evaluation.

The management options vary from primary repair, repair over a drain, esophageal exclusion, esophagectomy, and nonoperative management depending on the location of the perforation, its etiology, the time from its occurrence to the intervention, the overall condition of the patient, and the surgeon experience [24].

Delay in the diagnosis and treatment can significantly influence the overall outcomes of patients sustaining perfora-

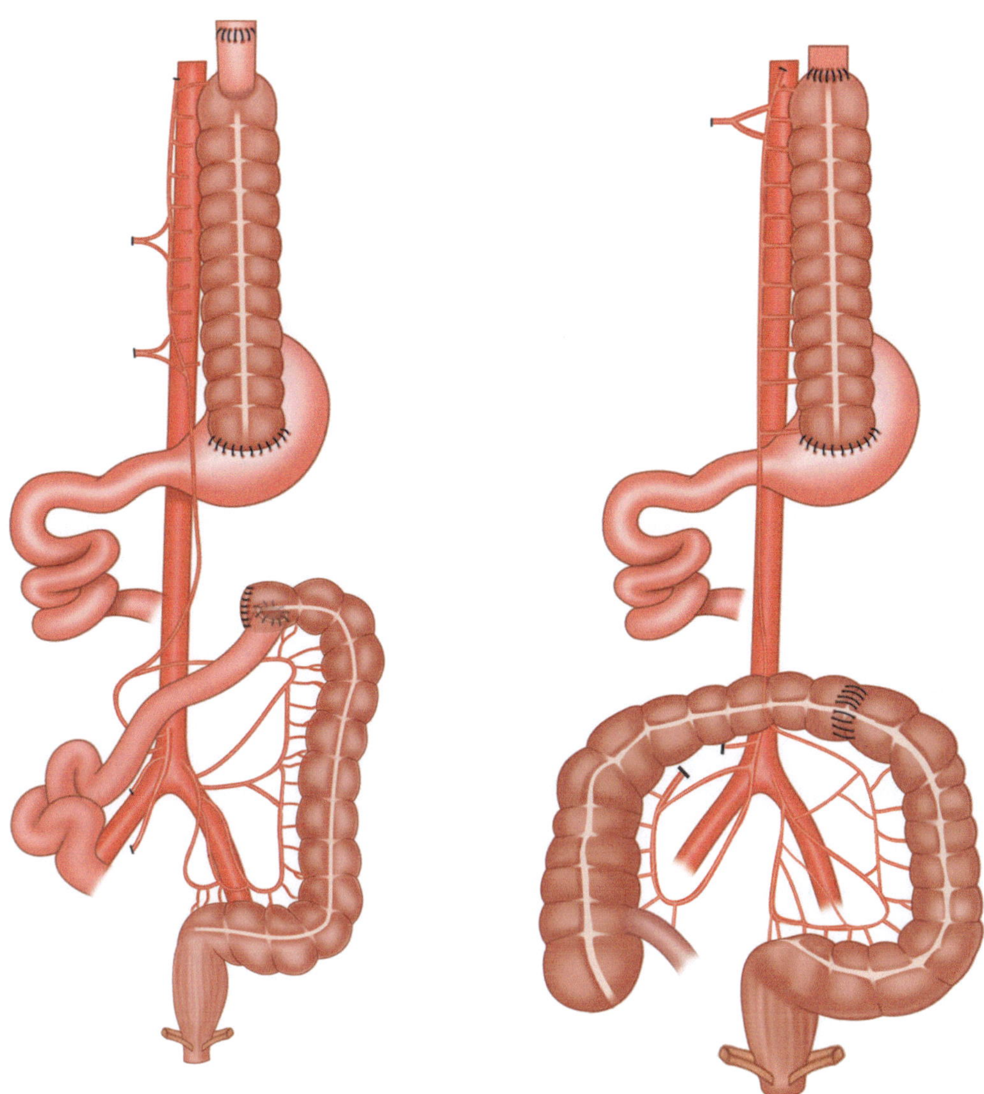

Fig. 40.2 Esophagocoloplasty after esophagectomy with gastric preservation

tions, as can the location of the perforation and the presence of underlying esophageal pathology such as a malignancy.

Published mortality rates have ranged historically between 10% and 40% depending on these multiple factors [25].

40.2.1 Etiology

According to recent reviews of the literature, iatrogenic injuries are the most common types of injury to the esophagus (46–59%), followed by spontaneous perforations (15–37%), foreign body ingestion (6–12%), trauma (9%), tumor, corrosive, and other causes (2%) [26, 27].

40.2.1.1 Iatrogenic Perforations

Endoscopy is the most frequent cause of EP. If the actual risk of EP during diagnostic esophagoscopy is low and is estimated to occur at a frequency of 0.03–0.11% when performed with flexible and rigid fibroscopes, respectively, it increases to 0.1–2% in case of dilation of strictures and between 1 and 5% after sclerotherapy. Coexisting esophageal *diverticula* increase this risk [28].

Forceful pneumatic dilations for achalasia are complicated by perforation in 2–6% of cases, and the risk is increased in women when the achalasia is long-standing and when dilation is performed for the first time [29, 30].

EPs have been reported after difficult endotracheal intubation [31], cardiac endoscopic sonography [32], or insertion of nasogastric or Blakemore tubes [33].

Operative injury to the esophagus can occur during operations on the esophagus or nearby organs. The incidence of EP after anterior osteosynthesis for cervical spine fracture can be as high as 3.4% [34]. These perforations are related to intraoperative injury or migration of osteosynthesis material, sometimes several years later. Thoracic EP has been reported following bronchial artery embolization, pneumonectomy, and pulmonary transplantation [23]. In the lower third of the esophagus, perforation complicates gastroesophageal reflux disease (GERD) and achalasia in, respectively, 3.9 and 7% of cases [35].

40.2.1.2 Spontaneous Perforations

Spontaneous rupture of the esophagus, first described by Boerhaave in 1724 [36], is a spontaneous barotraumatic rupture of the lower third of the esophagus secondary to an abrupt increase in intraesophageal pressure (up to 290 mmHg) during vomiting, associated with the absence of relaxation of the superior sphincter of the esophagus [37].

By extension, most authors regroup under the name of Boerhaave's syndrome, all spontaneous perforations of an otherwise healthy esophagus, whether secondary to vomiting or not. They represent 8–56% of perforations in the recent series. The perforation is located most often (80%) on the left border of the lower third of the thoracic esophagus and measures 3–6 cm on the average and frequently drains into the left pleural or peritoneal cavity. Following the perforation, as a result of negative intrathoracic air pressure, food and fluids are drawn into the mediastinum and pleural cavity leading to a chemical pleuro-mediastinitis. This leads to bacterial mediastinitis, septic shock, and multiorgan failure if adequate drainage is not performed. Despite advances in surgical technique and critical care, spontaneous EP continues to carry a mortality of 20–75% [38].

40.2.1.3 Foreign Bodies

Ingested foreign bodies are responsible for 80% of cervical perforations [23]. The foreign body usually impacts in the esophageal wall at the level of the physiological, narrow portion of the esophagus: Killian's triangle, aortic arch or left bronchial imprint, and esogastric juncture. Prolonged impaction can lead to extra-luminal migration which can perforate nearby organs such as the trachea or the aorta with often fatal outcome. The foreign bodies most often incriminated include dental prostheses and bones. The risk of EP during endoscopic extraction of ingested foreign bodies is estimated at 0.25% [39].

40.2.1.4 Post-trauma Perforations

Traumatic esophageal injury accounts for less than 1% of all admitted trauma patients. The majority of post-trauma esophageal injuries involve cervical esophagus, are due to penetrating trauma, and are rarely isolated. The severity of these lesions is due to associated tracheal lesions (up to 50%) [40]. Blunt cervical esophageal trauma can often be due to direct blows to the neck in a patient with a closed glottis.

Baro-injury has been reported after blunt trauma (road accidents [41], Heimlich maneuver [42]). EP complicates caustic burns mostly when management is delayed.

40.2.1.5 Perforations Occurring on Diseased Esophagus

EP can occur in people with conditions such as esophageal *diverticulum*, Barrett's esophagus, and infective esophagitis even in the absence of instrumental maneuvers [23]. EP complicates 5–8% of esophageal cancers treated with palliative intent; one out of four is fatal. Fistulas between a tumor of the esophagus and the tracheobronchial tree are found in 4.9% of patients with esophageal cancer. These fistulas develop because of tumoral invasion or are secondary to radiation therapy or after insertion of an endoprosthesis [43].

40.2.2 Clinical Presentation

The cause and location of the injury, as well as the interval between perforation and diagnosis, determine the clinical features of esophageal perforation. Diagnosis is often difficult because presentation is inconclusive and often mimics that of other disorders such as myocardial infarction, peptic ulcer perforation, pancreatitis, aortic aneurysm dissection, spontaneous pneumothorax, or pneumonia.

Common clinical manifestations of esophageal perforation include pain, dysphagia, dyspnea, subcutaneous emphysema, fever, tachycardia, and tachypnea.

Any combination of these signs and symptoms following instrumentation of the esophagus or respiratory tract implies perforation until proven otherwise [23].

Clinical examination is directed to assessment of vital signs, which will largely dictate the strategy in the first 24 h of management. A global evaluation of laboratory blood tests is useful to estimate the inflammation level with a dosage of white blood count, inflammation markers, and electrolytic and pH disorders. Metabolic disorders like electrolytic and pH disequilibrium are common, particularly in life-threatening cases.

Cervical perforation of the esophagus is generally less severe and more easily treated than intrathoracic or intra-abdominal perforation because the spread of contamination to the mediastinum through the retro-esophageal space is slow after cervical perforation and attachments of the esophagus to the prevertebral fascia in this region limit lateral dissemination of esophageal flora.

Patients with cervical perforations can present with neck pain, cervical dysphagia, dysphonia, or bloody regurgitation. Subcutaneous emphysema is commonly (up to 60%) found on physical examination and appears radiographically in 95% of patients with cervical esophageal perforation.

Intrathoracic perforations rapidly contaminate the mediastinum. The rupture may immediately extend into the

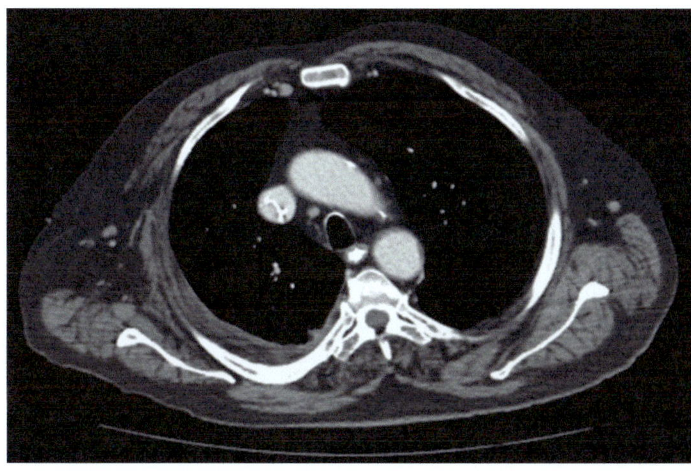
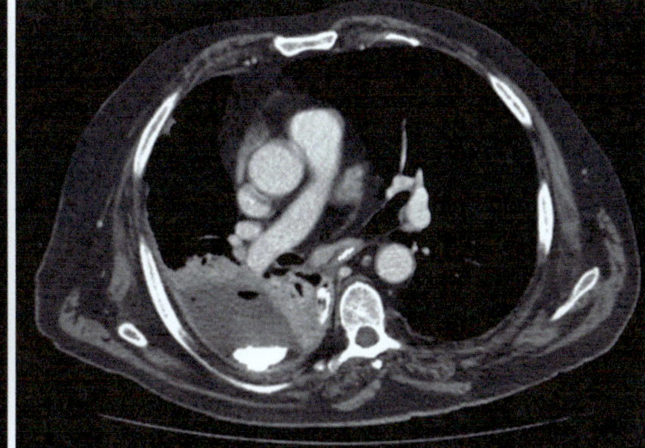

Fig. 40.3 CT scan with gastrografin

pleural cavity, most frequently on the left. As a result of negative intrathoracic pressure, gastric fluids and bacteria are drawn further into the pleural space and pleural effusion results. Contamination disseminates, and sequestration of fluid and hypovolemia results.

In case of spontaneous perforation, the clinical signs most often observed are, in decreasing order of frequency, vomiting (84%), thoracic pain (79%), dyspnea (53%), epigastric pain (47%), or dysphagia (21%). Mackler's triad (thoracic pain, vomiting, and emphysema), although highly suggestive of the diagnosis, is found in less than one-third of cases [44]. In case of delayed diagnosis, sepsis is dominant with tachycardia, tachypnea, fever, and leukocytosis.

Intra-abdominal perforations are uncontained and result in contamination of the peritoneal cavity. Patients complain of epigastric pain irradiated to the shoulders and may present with acute abdomen. As in intrathoracic perforation, the early onset of systemic signs such as tachycardia, tachypnea, and fever with rapid deterioration to systemic sepsis and shock is a characteristic.

40.2.3 Diagnosis

Lateral cervical X-rays can show prevertebral free air in cervical EP; standard lung X-ray is

abnormal in 90% of thoracic perforation showing pleural effusion, pneumothorax or hydropneumothorax, pneumomediastinum, pneumoperitoneum, or retro−pneumoperitoneum but can be normal if taken early [45].

Computed tomography (CT) with gastrografin ingestion is currently the investigation of choice because sensitivity (92–100%) is better than that for esogastroduodenal follow-through (50–75%) (see Fig. 40.3). Moreover, CT can indicate the importance of the extravasation and whether the leak is contained or not, delineate extension to adjacent structures (mediastinitis, pleural effusion, subpleural abscess, intraperitoneal effusion), and thus guide therapy. A non-contained perforation is defined by free extravasation of contrast in the mediastinal or peritoneal cavities. A contained perforation is defined as minimal extravasation of contrast at the perforation site or the presence of pneumomediastinum or pneumoperitoneum without apparent extravasation of contrast [46].

Last, when EP is not confirmed by CT, other diagnoses such as aortic dissection, duodenal ulcer perforation, or pancreatitis can be made.

Flexible, fiber optic esophagoscopy with cautious insufflations is perfectly acceptable for diagnosis of intrathoracic and rarely intra-abdominal and also allows for careful inspection of mucosal viability and underlying disease or malignancy.

In patients who have sustained traumatic injuries, the sensitivity of endoscopy is nearly 100% and the specificity 83% for the detection of EP [47].

40.2.4 End Point-Guided Resuscitation

Medical optimization, with respiratory and hemodynamic control, is the cornerstones of the non-operative management. If necessary, airway control via tracheal intubation with fiber optic laryngoscopy should be performed. Broad-spectrum antibiotics and antifungal and proton pump inhibitors should be administered. With pleural contamination chest drainage is essential.

40.2.5 Non-operative Management

Recently, there has been increasing interest in the non-operative management of esophageal perforation. The term "non-operative management" is misleading because most of these patients will undergo ≥1 the so-called palliative interventions, which include endoscopy, stent placement, drainage gastrostomy, feeding jejunostomy, and/or tube thoracostomy. True non-operative management consists of transfer to intensive care, nil orally, parenteral or enteral nutrition, intravenous antifungals, broad-spectrum antibiotics, and anti-secretory agents. There is no absolute indication or contraindication to the passage of a nasogastric tube because this may help with gastric decompression or may be a source of irritation.

There are no absolute guidelines, but some criteria for non-operative treatment of esophageal perforation have been defined by Cameron et al. and then modified by Altorjay et al. [48, 49]. These criteria consider non-operative management as a possible option in EP with leak contained within the neck or mediastinum, or between mediastinum and visceral lung pleura, without symptoms and signs of septicemia, in absence of underlying neoplastic esophageal disease.

In essence, these are perforations with minimal contamination that freely drain back into the esophagus and in which there is a lack of evidence of systemic toxicity; the most amenable to non-operative management are endoscopic injuries in the hypopharyngeal region. The availability of contrast imaging and expert medical team in esophageal patologies is mandatory.

Patients who are not surgically treated have to be clinically and biologically monitored for 7–10 days without oral alimentation. If the patient's clinical condition remains stable, a CT scan with gastrografin ingestion is used to check whether perforation is closed or not. If there is no leakage, oral alimentation can be started.

If the patient is not stabilized within 24 h, surgical treatment should be considered. The mortality rate for nonsurgical treatment was approximately 22% in the selected cases. A high index of suspicion of failure of non-operative management must be maintained.

40.2.6 Operative Management

EP is a challenging surgical emergency whose operative management includes primary repair, repair over a drain, esophageal exclusion, and esophagostomy.

Primary repair of esophageal perforation, irrespective of delay in diagnosis, is the preferred operative approach. The mortality rate was 3% in primary repair group compared with 18% in patients with esophageal perforation repaired over a drain. Recent literature favors primary repair as the best surgical approach with consistently low mortality ranging from 3% to 13% [50–52]. Esophagectomy is preferred in the setting of obstructive pathology, including cancer, with an associated 11% mortality in our series. Orringer and Sterling reported an overall 88% survival in 24 patients with esophagectomy for esophageal perforation in the setting of obstruction or cancer [53].

40.2.6.1 Primary Repair

Primary repair is the most preferred method for patients with non-contained EP.

Traditionally, primary repair was only appropriate for patients who presented within 24 h of their perforation because of the worse outcomes being reported for those presenting beyond 24 h. In Eroglu study, mortality among patients treated within 24 h of sustaining an injury was substantially reduced compared with those for whom diagnosis and treatment were delayed (respectively, 3 and 36.4%) [25].

An aggressive strategy has prevailed in recent years, making the argument that primary repair is suitable regardless of the time interval after injury for all nonmalignant thoracic perforations and if the esophagus is salvageable. Guided by this aggressive strategy, the survival rate after repair is reported to be about 90% for patients with delayed (>24 h) perforation. However, in those reports, almost all postoperative leaks and mortality occurred in the delayed perforation group [54].

Lin suggests that the effect of primary repair is still a time-dependent issue and recommends that 48 h is the appropriate window for primary repair with a mortality rate of 7%. Beyond this window, primary repair is still the main choice of treatment although its efficacy will be challenged by the increased potential of postoperative leakage even with buttressing suture because the chance of acquiring viable tissue near the perforation site decreases [55].

Primary repair should include esophagomyotomy proximal and distal to the tear, debridement of necrotic tissue, reapproximation of the esophageal mucosa, buttressing of the esophageal musculature over the perforation site, and tissue flaps of pleura or intercostal muscle if in the chest and strap muscles if in the neck. In patients with sepsis, the postoperative leak rate is approximately 40% if the primary repair site of a perforated esophagus is not reinforced. However, if the sutured line is reinforced, the postoperative leak rate decreases to 10% [50, 56, 57].

Surgical treatment of cervical EP consists of left cervicotomy, suturing the perforation in two layers, eventually reinforced by a flap and drainage. The key points of the technique are as follows: the incision is performed along the line of the anterior border of the sternocleidomastoid muscle. The omohyoid muscle is identified and divided. Sharp dissection of the loose areolar tissue medial to the sternocleidomastoid leads to the internal jugular vein. The incision is deepened staying medial to the carotid sheath. Both the middle thyroid vein and inferior thyroid artery may need to be ligated as necessary. At this point, the esophagus can usually be palpated (with nasogastric tube in situ) between the trachea anteriorly and the cervical vertebrae posteriorly. Careful circumferential dissection on the esophageal wall prevents injury to the left recurrent laryngeal nerve. A sling is placed to isolate the esophagus.

Primary repair should include esophagomyotomy proximal and distal to the tear, debridement of necrotic tissue, reapproximation of the esophageal mucosa, and buttressing of the esophageal musculature over the perforation site [50]. In case of delayed diagnosis or loss of tissue, the suture can be reinforced by a muscular flap.

The sternocleidomastoid flap is the most widely used technique. The sternal head is divided as distally as possible near its insertion and separated from the clavicular fascicule, long enough to reach and cover the suture to which it is affixed with individual sutures. The *myocutaneous pectoris maximus* flap is used more rarely. The interposition of a flap between the tracheal suture and the esophageal suture is indispensable when tracheal and esophageal rents are associated.

If an injury is not identified after appropriate dissection and inspection, drainage alone is acceptable.

The best surgical approach to perforations in the middle third of the esophagus is through a right thoracotomy in the sixth intercostal space, and perforations in the lower third are best approached through a left thoracotomy in the seventh intercostal space or through a midline laparotomy. Pleural debridement and decortication have to be performed to allow complete reexpansion of the lung to eliminate potential spaces and the possibility of empyema.

The mediastinum is widely opened and debrided of all necrotic debris and tissue. By eliminating dead space, possible empyema, and localized necrotic tissue, the possibility of secondary breakdown of the esophageal repair is minimized.

Characteristically, the rent in the muscle of the esophagus is smaller than that of the mucosa, so the muscle must be opened to expose the full extent of the mucosal tear. Failure to do so will lead to persistent leaks and disruption of the repair. Esophageal muscle is debrided back to healthy tissue. The esophagus then is closed in two layers (see Fig. 40.4). The repair is tested by injection of air in a nasogastric tube with occlusion of the distal esophagus while under saline solution or by methylene blue injection.

Recognizing that this repair is performed in a contaminated field, buttressing of the repair is prudent. This provides an extra layer of protection to reduce the risk of leak and contain it if a small leak occurs. The intercostal muscle is used preferentially due to its bulk blood supply and large arc of rotation, but it must be anticipated and prepared before placing the intercostal retractor (see Fig. 40.5). Omentum is useful in complicated situations and is probably the most secure means of closure due to its vascularity and resistance to infection. Pleura should not be used in early perforations due to its lack of substance and vascularity. With time and inflammation, pleura can become quite robust and better vascularized; it then can act as a reasonable buttress (see Fig. 40.6). Whichever choice is made, it should be carefully approximated to the esophageal repair with multiple sutures as if doing an anastomosis.

Chest drains are placed in the gutter, next to the repair and along the diaphragm. The chest cavity is thoroughly cleansed before closure. A draining gastrostomy and feeding jejunostomy are performed routinely to avoid reflux of gastric contents on the repair and for an optimal nutritional support.

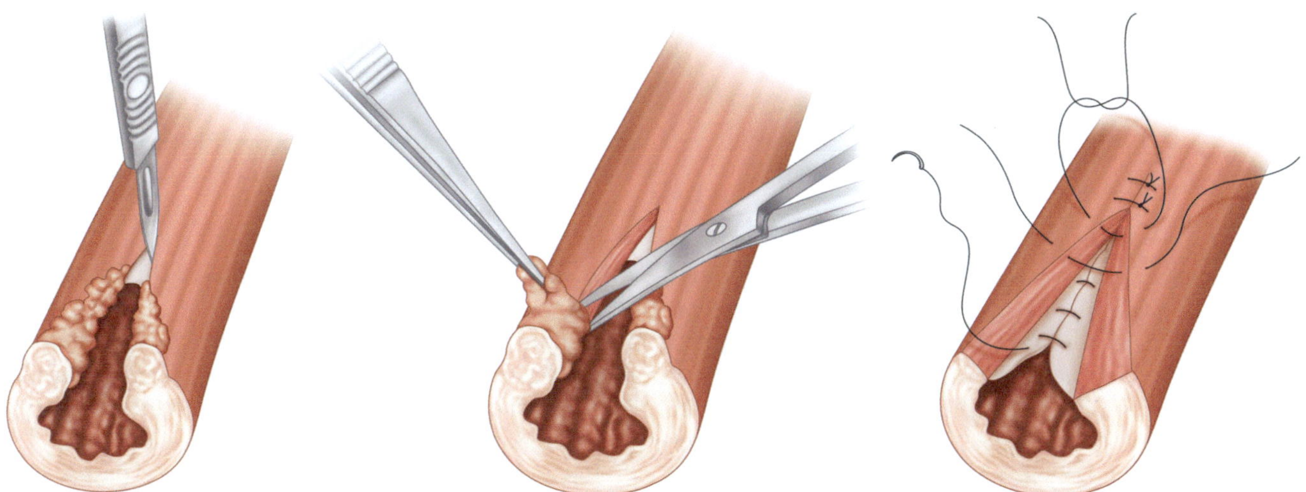

Fig. 40.4 Two layers of suture technique

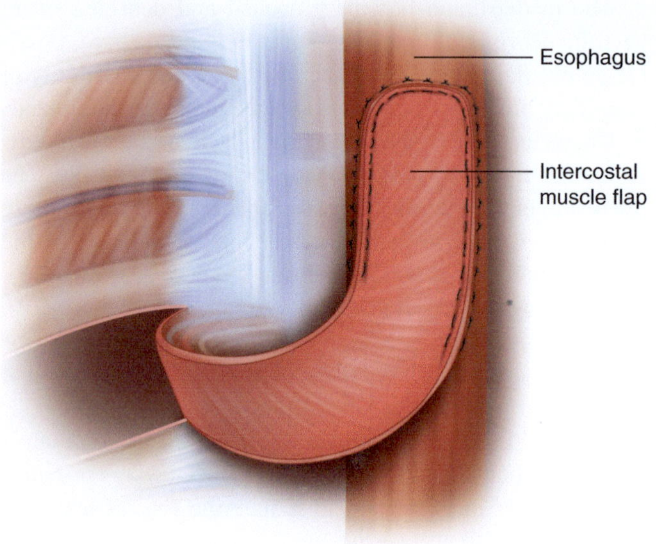

Fig. 40.5 Intercostal muscle flap

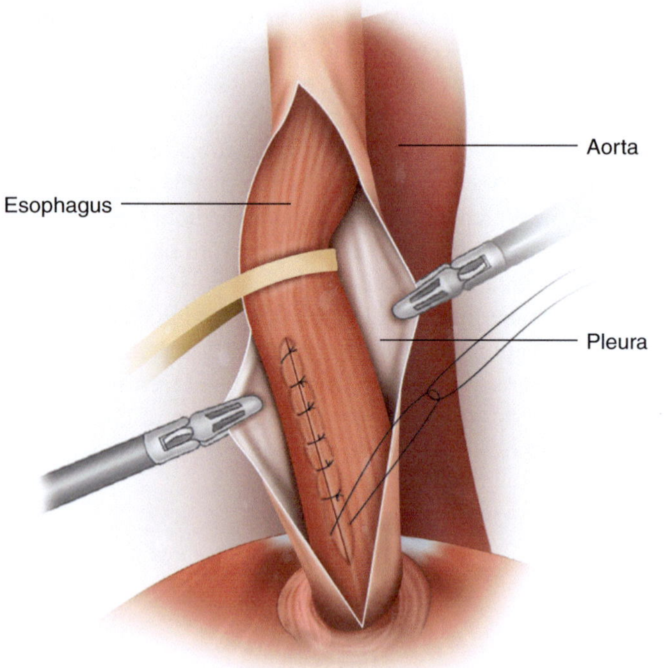

Fig. 40.6 Pleural flap

Treatment of intra-abdominal EP is always surgical and requires an upper midline laparotomy even if laparoscopic approach has been described. The hiatal orifice is enlarged, and the inferior esophagus is widely mobilized. Once localized the perforation and longitudinal myotomy are performed to best expose the mucosal edges, and suture is performed on two layers as previously described. An omental or a fundus flap, easy to perform, should be used as often as possible to reinforce sutures of abdominal EP. In case of EP after dilatation for achalasia, suture should be associated with a seromyotomy controlateral to the perforation and covered with a partial fundoplication wrap.

Pleural, abdominal drainage, gastrostomy, and feeding jejunostomy should be associated.

A CT scan with gastrografin ingestion is obtained routinely on postoperative day 7–10 to check for leaks.

40.2.6.2 Esophagectomy

An esophageal resection is the preferred treatment in cases such as malignancy, scleroderma,

strictures due to caustic burns, strictures not suitable for dilatation, a nonfunctioning esophagus (grade III achalasia), serious mediastinitis, insufficient mediastinal drainage, and dehiscence of primary repair [50, 53].

Esophagectomy has been recommended in this setting because this modality treats the source of contamination and the pathological lesion at the same time.

In cases when there is significant mediastinal/pleural contamination, a transthoracic approach should be undertaken to ensure adequate debridement. But in early iatrogenic cases, the degree of contamination and necrosis is less; therefore, a transhiatal esophagectomy may be performed. Restoration of intestinal continuity should only be undertaken at the first operation if patients are not critically ill and anastomosis has to be performed as far away from the perforation as possible.

A 2004 review of the outcomes of esophageal perforation found that across all published series, resection had a mean mortality of 17% (range, 0–43%) compared with 12% (range, 0–31%) for primary repair.

In a series of 90 patients, Orringer found 30-day mortality rate of 9% among patients with benign disease and of 5% among patients with cancer, showing emergent esophagectomy as a safe procedure when performed at a high-volume center [58].

The value of esophagectomy for cancer perforation was questioned by Di Franco et al. who treated 48 patients with iatrogenic perforation by esophagectomy or non-operatively, most often by stenting, because even if immediate mortality was similar between the two groups (0 vs. 9%), survival was not improved by resection [59].

40.2.6.3 Esophageal Diversion and Delayed Repair

Esophageal exclusion and diversion are the last resort in patients where the ability to tolerate systemic sepsis is impaired due to the initial injury or comorbidities or those "not fit for a esophagectomy" at initial presentation.

It prevents ongoing leakage of salivary and gastric secretions into the thoracic cavity. The role of controlling oral

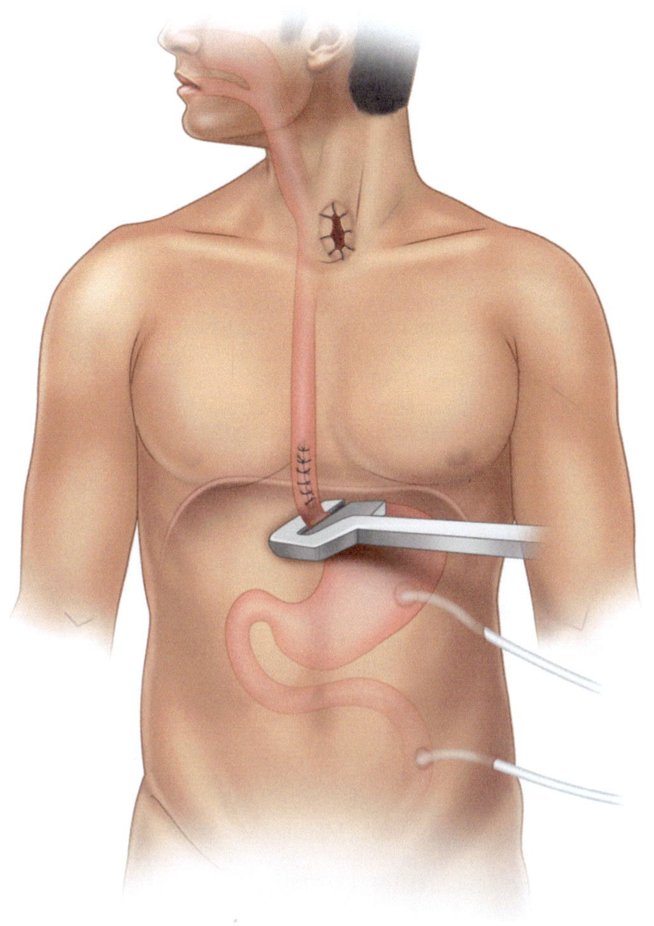

Fig. 40.7 Bipolar exclusion of the esophagus with gastrostomy and jejunostomy

secretions is critical, because undiverted oral secretions have an extremely high concentration of mixed flora.

End stoma or lateral esophagostomy is performed through a left cervicotomy. Following a midline laparotomy, the esophagogastric junction is stapled, and a decompressing gastrostomy and feeding jejunostomy are fashioned (see Fig. 40.7). Several months after resolution of the mediastinal sepsis, reconstruction can be performed with either gastric or colonic interposition [38].

40.2.6.4 T-Tube

T-tube drainage, enhancing direct fistulization of the perforation, has been described essentially in the perforation of thoracic esophagus when all other repair attempts seem to be illusory because of the magnitude of esophageal damage. The perforation is sutured around a large caliber T-tube inserted into the perforation. Opacification of the T-tube is performed before removing the drain 4–6 weeks later.

Linden et al. reported a 9% mortality rate and a 30% reoperation rate in their series of 17 patients [60].

40.2.7 Discussion About New Trends

A combination of minimally invasive techniques, including laparoscopy, thoracoscopy, mediastinoscopy, and endoscopic stenting methods, has been suggested for the treatment of iatrogenic and spontaneous EP.

The use of covered esophageal stents in the management of esophageal perforation has been reported successful in recent series with esophageal leak healed in all patients with no mortality [61]. Stent migration is the main complication (6–35%) [62].

The technique of using hemostatic endoscopic clip has been described and may be used for iatrogenic endoscopic EP diagnosed early [63].

Haveman suggests VATS as an approach effective for adequate surgical debridement and drainage of the mediastinum, in iatrogenic perforation, and in Boerhaave's syndrome minimizing additional surgical trauma these already very ill patients [64].

Kim suggests that primary thoracoscopic esophageal repair is a good surgical alternative for patients with relatively stable vital signs or mild inflammation in Boerhaave's syndrome, regardless of the time interval between the perforation and surgery [65].

Esophageal wall defect of different etiologies (anastomotic leak, iatrogenic perforation, and Boerhaave's syndrome) has been described as treated successfully with endoscopic vacuum therapy in 94% of patients in a recent study [66].

All these procedures need to be validated.

Case Scenario

A 35-year-old man presented himself at the emergency department with a notion of caustic ingestion 1 h before. The patient was in good general conditions without signs of sepsis but with a mild retrosternal and epigastric pain. No cervical emphysema was clinically noted. No other information about nature and quantity of the caustic agent were available. A laryngeal stridor was noted, which worsened over time.

1. Which is your diagnostic algorithm?
   A. Urgent otolaryngology referral, CT scan, and/or upper endoscopy
   B. Only upper endoscopy
   C. Intravenous corticosteroids
   D. Nasogastric tube

Patient's general conditions worsened 3 h after the ingestion with sepsis signs, and he was intubated under fiber optic guide. A CT scan was performed with evidence of important pneumomediastinum and pneumoperitoneum supra- and infra-mesocolic. An upper endoscopy showed extensive esophageal necrosis Zargar 3b from 20 to 35 cm with the impossibility to evaluate the gastric cavity due to the presence of food.

2. Which is your next step?
   A. Surgical exploration by laparotomy and probably esophagogastrectomy with cervicotomy
   B. Esophagectomy by thoracotomy first
   C. Non-operative management using a nasogastric tube and CT scan after 12 h
   D. Only cervical exclusion

Please see Chap. 58 for the correct answer.

References

1. Mowry JB, Spyker DA, Cantilena LR, McMillan N, Ford M. 2013 annual report of the American Association of Poison Control Centers' National Poison Data System (NPDS): 31st annual report. Clin Toxicol. 2014;52(10):1032–283.
2. Contini S, Scarpignato C. Caustic injury of the upper gastrointestinal tract: a comprehensive review. World J Gastroenterol. 2013;19(25):3918–30.
3. Osman M, Russell J, Shukla D, Moghadamfalahi M, Granger DN. Responses of the murine esophageal microcirculation to acute exposure to alkali, acid, or hypochlorite. J Pediatr Surg. 2008;43(9):1672–8.
4. Ducoudray R, Mariani A, Corte H, Kraemer A, Munoz-Bongrand N, Sarfati E, et al. The damage pattern to the gastrointestinal tract depends on the nature of the ingested caustic agent. World J Surg. 2016;40(7):1638–44.
5. Turner A, Robinson P. Respiratory and gastrointestinal complications of caustic ingestion in children. Emerg Med J. 2005;22(5):359–61.
6. Ali Zargar S, Kochhar R, Mehta S, Kumar Mehta S. The role of fiberoptic endoscopy in the management of corrosive ingestion and modified endoscopic classification of burns. Gastrointest Endosc. 1991;37(2):165–9.
7. Kamijo Y, Kondo I, Kokuto M, Kataoka Y, Soma K. Miniprobe ultrasonography for determining prognosis in corrosive esophagitis. Am J Gastroenterol. 2004;99(5):851–4.
8. Chirica M, Resche-Rigon M, Zagdanski AM, Bruzzi M, Bouda D, Roland E, et al. Computed tomography evaluation of esophagogastric necrosis after caustic ingestion. Ann Surg. 2016;264(1):107–13.
9. Bonnici KS, Wood DMDP. Should computerised tomography replace endoscopy in the evaluation of symptomatic ingestion of corrosive substances? Clin Toxicol. 2014;52(9):911–25.
10. Bonavina L, Chirica M, Skrobic O, Kluger Y, Andreollo NA, Contini S, et al. Foregut caustic injuries: results of the world society of emergency surgery consensus conference. World J Emerg Surg. 2015;10(1):44.
11. Chirica M, Bonavina L, Kelly MD, Sarfati E, Cattan P. Caustic ingestion. Lancet. 2017;389(10083):2041–52.
12. Ramasamy K, Gumaste VV. Corrosive ingestion in adults. J Clin Gastroenterol. 2003;37(2):119–24.
13. Chirica M, Kraemer A, Petrascu E, Vuarnesson H, Pariente B, Halimi B, et al. Esophagojejunostomy after total gastrectomy for caustic injuries. Dis Esophagus. 2014;27(2):122–7.
14. Zerbib P, Voisin B, Truant S, Saulnier F, Vinet A, Chambon JP, et al. The conservative management of severe caustic gastric injuries. Ann Surg. 2011;253(4):684–8.
15. Lefrancois M, Gaujoux S, Resche-Rigon M, Chirica M, Munoz-Bongrand N, Sarfati E, et al. Oesophagogastrectomy and pancreatoduodenectomy for caustic injury. Br J Surg. 2011;98(7):983–90.
16. Di Saverio S, Biscardi A, Piccinini A, Mandrioli M, Tugnoli G. Different possible surgical managements of caustic ingestion: diagnostic laparoscopy for Zargar's grade 3a lesions and a new technique of Duodenal Damage Control with 4-tubes ostomy and duodenal wash-out as an option for extensive 3b lesions in unstable patients. Updat Surg. 2015;67(3):313–20.
17. Mutaf O, Genç A, Herek Ö, Demircan M, Özcan C, Arikan A. Gastroesophageal reflux: a determinant in the outcome of caustic esophageal burns. J Pediatr Surg. 1996;31(11):1494–5.
18. Zerbib P, Vinet A, Rogosnitzky M, Truant S, Chambon JP, Pruvot FR. Gastrocele complicates the course of non-operated severe caustic injuries: operative strategies. World J Surg. 2014;38(5):1233–7.
19. Tucker JA, et al. The treatment of caustic ingestion. Otolaryngol Clin N Am. 1979;12(2):343–50.
20. Hugh TB, Kelly MD. Corrosive ingestion and the surgeon. J Am Coll Surg. 1999;189(5):508–22.
21. Chirica M, Veyrie N, Munoz-Bongrand N, Zohar S, Halimi B, Celerier M, et al. Late morbidity after colon interposition for corrosive esophageal injury. Ann Surg. 2010;252(2):271–80.
22. Chirica M, Brette M-D, Faron M, Munoz Bongrand N, Halimi B, Laborde C, et al. Upper digestive tract reconstruction for caustic injuries. Ann Surg. 2015;261(5):894–901.
23. Brinster CJ, Singhal S, Lee L, Marshall MB, Kaiser LR, Kucharczuk JC. Evolving options in the management of esophageal perforation. Ann Thorac Surg. 2004;77(4):1475–83.
24. Kotsis L, Kostic S, Zubovits K. Multimodality treatment of esophageal disruptions. Chest. 1997;112(5):1304–9.
25. Eroglu A, Kurkcuoglu IC, Karaoglanoglu N, Tekinbas C, O.Yimaz. Esophageal perforation: the importance of early diagnosis and primary repair. Dis Esophagus 2004;17(1):91–94.
26. Abbas G, Schuchert MJ, Pettiford BL, Pennathur A, Landreneau J, Landreneau J, et al. Contemporaneous management of esophageal perforation. Surgery. 2009;146(4):749–56.
27. Sdralis E(I)K, Petousis S, Rashid F, Lorenzi B, Charalabopoulos A. Epidemiology, diagnosis, and management of esophageal perforations: systematic review. Dis Esophagus. 2017;30(8):1–6.
28. Kavic S, Basson M. Complications of endoscopy. Am J Surg. 2001;181:319–32.
29. Slater G, Sicular AA. Esophageal perforations after forceful dilatation in achalasia. Ann Surg. 1982;195(2):186–8.
30. Nair LA, Reynolds JC, Parkman HP, Ouyang A, Strom BL, Rosato EFCS. Complications during pneumatic dilation for achalasia or diffuse esophageal spasm, analysis of risk factors, early clinical characteristics, and outcome. Dig Dis Sci. 1993;38(10):1893–904.
31. Jougon J, Cantini O, Delcambre F, Minniti A, Velly J. Esophageal perforation: life threatening complication of endotracheal intubation. Eur J Cardiothorac Surg. 2001;20(1):7–11.
32. Jougon JB, Gallon P, MacBride T, Dubrez J, Velly JF. Esophageal perforation after transesophageal echocardiography. Eur J Cardiothorac Surg. 1999;16(6):686–7.
33. Ahmed A, Aggarwal M, Watson E. Esophageal perforation: a complication of nasogastric tube placement. Am J Emerg Med. 1998;16:64–6.
34. Vrouenraets BC, Been HD, Brouwer-Mladin R, Bruno M, van Lanschot JJ. Esophageal perforation associated with cervical spine surgery: report of two cases and review of the literature. Dig Surg. 2004;21(3):246–9.

35. Campos GM, Vittinghoff E, Rabl C, Takata M, Gadenstatter M, Lin F, et al. Endoscopic and surgical treatments for achalasia: a systematic review and meta-analysis. Ann Surg. 2009;249(1):45–57.
36. Derbes VJ, Mitchell RE Jr. Hermann Boerhaave's atrocis, nec descripti prius, morbi historia: the first translation of the classic case report of rupture of the esophagus, with annotations. Bull Med Libr Assoc. 1955;43:217–40.
37. Korn O, Onate JC, Lopez R. Anatomy of the Boerhaave syndrome. Surgery. 2007;141(2):222–8.
38. Rohtagi A. The role of esophageal diversion and exclusion in management of esophageal perforations. Int J Surg. 2009;7:142–4.
39. Athanassiadi K, Gerazounis M, Metaxas E, Kalantzi N. Management of esophageal foreign bodies: a retrospective review of 400 cases. Eur J Cardiothorac Surg. 2002;21(4):653–6.
40. Weiman DS, Walker WA, Brosnan KM, Pate JW, Fabian TC. Noniatrogenic esophageal trauma. Ann Thorac Surg. 1995;59(4):845–9. discussion 9–50
41. Beal SL, Pottmeyer EW, Spisso JM. Esophageal perforation following external blunt trauma. J Trauma. 1988;28(10):1425–32.
42. Cumberbatch GL, Reichl M. Oesophageal perforation: a rare complication of minor blunt trauma. J Accid Emerg Med. 1996;13(4):295–6.
43. Morgan RA, Ellul JP, Denton ER, Glynos M, Mason RC, Adam A. Malignant esophageal fistulas and perforations: management with plastic-covered metallic endoprostheses. Radiology. 1997;204(2):527–32.
44. Griffiths EA, Yap N, Poulter J, Hendrickse MT, Khurshid M. Thirty-four cases of esophageal perforation: the experience of a district general hospital in the UK. Dis Esophagus. 2009;22(7):616–25.
45. Han SY, McElvein RB, Aldrete JS, Tishler JM. Perforation of the esophagus: correlation of site and cause with plain film findings. Am J Roentgenol. 1985;145(3):537–40.
46. de Lutio di Castelguidone E, Merola S, Pinto A, Raissaki M, Gagliardi N, Romano L. Esophageal injuries: spectrum of multidetector row CT findings. Eur J Radiol. 2006;59(3):344–8.
47. Horwitz B, Krevsky B, Buckman RF Jr, Fisher RS, Dabezies MA. Endoscopic evaluation of penetrating esophageal injuries. Am J Gastroenterol. 1993;88(8):1249–53.
48. Cameron J, Kieffer R, Hendrix T, et al. Selective nonoperative management of contained intrathoracic esophageal disruptions. Ann Thorac Surg. 1979;27:404–8.
49. Altorjay A, Kiss J, Voros A, Bohak A. Nonoperative management of esophageal perforations. Is it justified? Ann Surg. 1997;225:415–21.
50. Wright C. Primary repair for delayed recognition of esophageal perforation in difficult decision in thoracic surgery: an evidence-based approach. New York: Springer; 2008. p. 298–304.
51. Richardson JD. Management of esophageal perforations: the value of aggressive surgical treatment. Am J Surg. 2005;190:161–5.
52. Wu JT, Mattox KL, Wall MJ Jr. Esophageal perforations: new perspectives and treatment paradigms. J Trauma. 2007;63:1173–84.
53. Orringer MB, Stirling MC. Esophagectomy for esophageal disruption. Ann Thorac Surg. 1990;49:35–43.
54. Sung SW, Park JJ, Kim YT, Kim JH. Surgery in thoracic esophageal perforation: primary repair is feasible. Dis Esophagus. 2002;15(3):204–9.
55. Lin Y, Jiang G, Liu L, Jiang JX, Chen L, Zhao Y, Yang J. Management of thoracic esophageal perforation. World J Surg. 2014;38(5):1093–9.
56. Gouge TH, Depan HJ, Spencer FC. Experience with the Grillo pleural flap procedure in 18 patients with perforation of the thoracic esophagus. Ann Surg. 1989;209:612–9.
57. Richardson JD, Tobin GR. Closure of esophageal defects with muscle flaps. Arch Surg. 1994;129:541–8.
58. Seo YD, Orringer MB. Emergent esophagectomy for esophageal perforation: a safe option. Ann Thorac Surg. 2015;100:905–9.
59. Di Franco F, Lamb PJ, Karat D, Hayes N, Griffin SM. Iatrogenic perforation of localized oesophageal cancer. Br J Surg. 2008;95(7):837–9.
60. Linden PA, Bueno R, Mentzer SJ, Zellos L, Lebenthal A, Colson YL, et al. Modified T-tube repair of delayed esophageal perforation results in a low mortality rate similar to that seen with acute perforations. Ann Thorac Surg. 2007;83(3):1129–33.
61. Freeman RK, Van Woerkom JM, Ascioti AJ. Esophageal stent placement for the treatment of iatrogenic intrathoracic esophageal perforation. Ann Thorac Surg. 2007;83:2003–8.
62. Decker P, Lippler J, Decker D, Hirner A. Use of the Polyflex stent in the palliative therapy of esophageal carcinoma: results in 14 cases and review of the literature. Surg Endosc. 2001;15:1444–7.
63. Qadeer MA, Dumot JA, Vargo JJ, Lopez AR, Rice TW. Endoscopic clips for closing esophageal perforations: case report and pooled analysis. Gastrointest Endosc. 2007;66(3):605–11.
64. Haveman JW, Nieuwenhuijs VB, Kobold JPM, van Dam GM, Plukker JT, Hofker HS. Adequate debridement and drainage of the mediastinum using open thoracotomy or video-assisted thoracoscopic surgery for Boerhaave's syndrome. Surg Endosc. 2011;25:2492–7.
65. Cho JS, Kim MS. Thoracoscopic primary esophageal repair in patients with Boerhaave' s syndrome. Ann Thorac Surg. 2011;91:1552–5.
66. Kuhen F, Loske G, Schiffmann L, Gock M, Klar E. Endoscopic vacuum therapy for various defects of the upper gastrointestinal tract. Surg Endosc. 2017; https://doi.org/10.1007/s00464-016-5404-x. [Epub ahead of print]

41 Updates in the Management of Foreign Bodies of the Gastrointestinal Tract

Marta Bini

Key Points

- The majority of ingested FB will spontaneously transit the upper and lower gastrointestinal tract and will be eventually evacuated.
- If a FB has been stuck in the esophagus for more than 24 h the risk of major complications like perforation can increase to more than 14 times.
- Sharp or acuminated objects should be removed as soon as possible.
- Any FB that causes obstruction must be immediately removed.
- In the absence of obstruction symptoms, removal can be postponed not beyond 12–24 h from the presentation as long as the FB isn't a sharp or potentially harmful object.
- Recurrent history of food bolus impaction in a young otherwise healthy male patient should arise the clinical suspicion of eosinophilic esophagitis.
- In some cases, an underlying disease or condition may predispose to FB impaction.
- The risk of major complications due to magnet ingestion becomes actual when two or more magnets are involved.
- Major complications like aortoesophageal fistula (AEF) can occur even 2 weeks after disk battery removal from the esophagus.

Take Home Messages

In the following chapter, you will learn the following:

- How to make an early and correct diagnosis of gastrointestinal foreign body (FB) ingestion or impaction.
- The proper timing and management of patients with gastrointestinal FB.
- The most common endoscopic techniques, essential instruments and devices necessary to perform a safe and effective FB retrieval.
- The management of some specific FB.
- The most common and the most serious complications of FB ingestion.

41.1 Introduction

Foreign bodies (FB) represent a common problem in gastrointestinal emergency endoscopy with an estimated annual incidence in the USA of 11 per 100,000 persons/year and 1,500 deaths/year [1, 2] with an approximate 1.5 ratio between males and females [3].

In most cases, they are located in the upper gastrointestinal tract (UGI) as a consequence of accidental or voluntary ingestion. FB can also be found in lower intestinal tract (LGI) mainly as a result of sexual activity or abuse.

Both American and European Society for Gastrointestinal Endoscopy (ASGE, ESGE) have issued a series of guidelines to help the clinician in the management of GI FB [4, 5].

In this chapter, we will discuss the clinical assessment, the diagnosis and the technical endoscopic approach to gastrointestinal FB.

Electronic Supplementary Material The online version of this chapter (https://doi.org/10.1007/978-3-319-95114-0_41) contains supplementary material, which is available to authorized users.

M. Bini (✉)
Operative Digestive Endoscopy Department, AAST Grande Ospedale Metropolitano Niguarda, Milan, Italy

P. Aseni et al. (eds.), *Operative Techniques and Recent Advances in Acute Care and Emergency Surgery*,
https://doi.org/10.1007/978-3-319-95114-0_41

41.2 Upper GI Foreign Bodies

41.2.1 Clinical Assessment and Symptoms

Ingestion of foreign bodies is mostly accidental, and it's more common in the pediatric population (peak incidence between 6 months and 6 years). More than 85–90% of ingested FB will pass spontaneously through the GI tract and will be eventually evacuated. Medical intervention (endoscopic removal) is required in 10–20% of patients, while less than 1% will need surgical intervention [6]. It should be pointed out that voluntary ingestion leads to a higher percentage of medical and especially surgical intervention, the latter raising to a percentage as high as 16% [7, 8].

Other than children, there are some categories of patients and some clinical conditions which can be considered "at risk" for FB ingestion or impaction (Table 41.1). Patients with previous surgery for congenital atresia can have an increased risk of FB impaction due to a small anastomotic caliber as well as for possible coexisting motility disorders [9]. Multiple FB ingestion is quite common in psychiatric patients in whom voluntary ingestion may be a recurrent event, thus, during clinical assessment of pain and respiratory or obstructive symptoms in these patients, it's important to take into consideration a potential FB ingestion. The most common cause of FB impaction in adults is due to food bolus, while coins are the most common FB in children [1].

Thirty to fifty percent of patients presenting with a FB in the GI tract are asymptomatic, especially when the FB is located in the stomach or in the small bowel. Symptoms are mostly secondary to obstruction and vary depending on the localization, size, and shape of the FB (Table 41.2).

Obstructive symptoms and signs are more common when FB is stuck at the upper esophageal sphincter (UES) level or in the cervical esophagus. Pain, drooling, and dysphagia are the most common symptoms, but the lack of signs or symptoms should not make us rule out the diagnosis.

The lack of verbal communication makes the diagnostic process particularly challenging in infants and small children. In many cases ingestion occurs far from an adult's eye, and for this reason, the kind of FB and the time of ingestion are often uncertain; thus, even in the absence of a positive history, a small child presenting with the above symptoms should lead us to consider a possible FB ingestion [10]. Signs like hematemesis, fever, mediastinitis, subcutaneous crepitus or intoxication symptoms are less frequent but alarming and indicate the onset of major complications like infection, major bleeding or existing perforation. Vomit, pain, or peritonitis may also be the initial clinical presentation of a lower GI tract FB.

Table 41.1 Patients at risk of FB ingestion or impaction

• Children between 6 months and 6 years of age
• Edentulous patients
• Impaired vision patients
• Mentally impaired patients
• Patient with previous GI surgery
• Patients with esophageal motility disorders
• Patient with esophageal stenosis
• Convicts or those who seek secondary gain after access to a medical facility

Table 41.2 Symptoms of FB ingestion

• Epigastric pain
• Dysphagia
• Drooling
• Regurgitation
• Coughing
• Airway obstruction signs
• Hematemesis
• Fever
• Mediastinitis
• Peritonitis
• Intestinal obstruction

41.2.2 Diagnosis

An accurate anamnesis is the first step in the diagnosis of FB ingestion. Pre-existing GI pathologies like esophageal motility disorders or previous esophageal surgery (Table 41.3) can increase the risk of FB impaction. Accurate information about previous dysphagia, previous GI surgery, or reflux esophagitis should be carefully recorded [5, 10]. The presence of dental hardware, type and content of the recent meals (like chicken or fish which may contain bones) as well as a positive history of psychiatric disorders may also provide important information.

After a complete anamnesis has been recorded, the final diagnosis should be estabilished on one or more diagnostic procedures [6, 10, 11].

41.2.2.1 Biplane Radiography

X-ray examination of the neck, chest and abdomen is useful when radiopaque foreign body ingestion is suspected (sensitivity around 80%). Chest X-ray has a sensitivity of 80–90% also in case of aluminum objects when the images are carefully examined. For fish bones and toothpicks, X-ray has a sensitivity that ranges from 2 to 9%, respectively [12]. When it comes to fish bones, it must also be pointed out that

Table 41.3 Pathological conditions at risk of FB impaction

• Esophageal motility disorders
• Esophageal strictures (peptic or neoplastic)
• Achalasia
• Esophageal diverticula
• Patient with previous esophageal and GI surgery

radiography might show some imaging pitfalls in differentiating it from normal anatomical structures and variants [13]. A useful clinical guideine for imaging in suspected or reported GI FB has been published in 2013 by Guelfguat M. et al [53].

41.2.2.2 CT Scan

CT scan provides more accurate information in case of small FB foreign bodies which could not be detected by radiography like plastic FB, fish bones or food bolus, the latter having a rate of false-negative X-ray as high as 87%. It also visualizes the soft tissues surrounding the impacted object and it is recommended in all patients with suspected perforation or other complications [4, 13]. The sensitivity of CT scan in detecting an impacted FB is reported to range from 90 to 100% (sensitivity 97% and accuracy 98%) [6, 13] compared to radiography (respectively, 47% and 52%). The need of IV contrast must be tailored on the kind of FB and on the area where the impaction or complication are suspected. Perforation can be documented by cervical emphysema or pneumomediastinum, while pneumoperitoneum is more rarely seen since the perforation in the abdomen is usually progressive and the intestinal wall tends to seal off preventing the leak of large amounts of air in the peritoneum.

41.2.2.3 Endoscopy

Upper or lower GI endoscopy is the most useful procedure to detect and localize an impacted FB. It also provides accurate information on possible existing damage or lesion of the mucosa or gastrointestinal wall. It's especially useful in case of radiolucent objects where it provides detailed information on their actual size and shape of the FB.

41.2.3 Timing

Once FB body ingestion is confirmed, the first step of management is to decide whether the patient needs medical intervention and if the intervention *is* or *is not* urgent [14, 15]. The indication for urgent endoscopic removal is based not only on patient's clinical conditions and symptoms but also on the *localization*, *shape*, and *content or composition* of the ingested FB (Table 41.4).

Table 41.4 Indications for urgent removal of FB

Any FB that causes obstructive signs or symptoms
Any FB that causes respiratory symptoms
Any FB impacted in the esophagus for more than 24 h
Any FB in the GI tract when the time of ingestion is unknown
Sharp FB
Disk batteries
FB longer than 5–6 cm
Multiple magnets

41.2.3.1 FB Localization

FB impaction occurs most often in areas where GI tract shows physiological narrowing, like upper esophageal sphincter (UES) or pylorus. Angulations, as well as pathological stenosis, may also increase the risk of FB impaction.

Regardless of the shape or size, every impacted FB which causes obstruction, pain, and drooling requires urgent removal. ASGE and ESGE guidelines suggest removal within 2 and 6 h (maximum) [4, 15]. Longer delays may lead to a higher risk of complications [16, 17].

If FB is stuck in the esophagus for more than 24 h, the risk of major complications like perforation or aortoesophageal fistula can increase to more than 14 times [18].

In the absence of obstruction symptoms, removal can be postponed not *beyond 12–24 h* from the presentation as long as the FB isn't a sharp or potentially harmful object.

Stomach FB must be urgently removed only if they are potentially harmful. If the object is not sharp or harmful and if the dimensions are less than 2 cm diameter or 5 cm long, it will most probably spontaneously transit into the duodenum and eventually into the colon [13]. When FB is not retrieved, the patient should be monitored with radiographs and clinical evaluation in order to verify the progression along the GI tract as well as to detect the potential comparison of obstructive signs or symptoms.

Surgical intervention is required if FB fails to progress or complications like hematemesis, melena, GI obstruction, and peritonitis arise.

When a FB stays in the gastric lumen for more than 48–72 h from the time of ingestion, endoscopic removal should be scheduled.

41.2.3.2 FB Shape

Sharp or acuminated objects (Fig. 41.1) should be removed *as soon as possible*.

Radiography will help in localizing the FB and will provide information about exact shape and size. Endoscopy is mandatory in case of radiolucent sharp FB. Sharp objects located in the esophagus should be immediately removed. If a sharp FB reaches the gastric lumen and the size is suitable with the pylorus diameter, it'll most often pass spontaneously. Yet there is an increased risk of complications due to the transit of an acuminated or sharp FB. For this reason, they should always be retrieved if the endoscopic removal can be done safely [19].

41.2.3.3 FB Content

Some FB may not be harmful due to their localization or shape, but the potential dangerousness is due to their content or composition.

This is the case of drugs swallowed by "body packers" [19] for international drug trafficking. Also, disk batteries (DB), as it will be explained in the next paragraphs, are

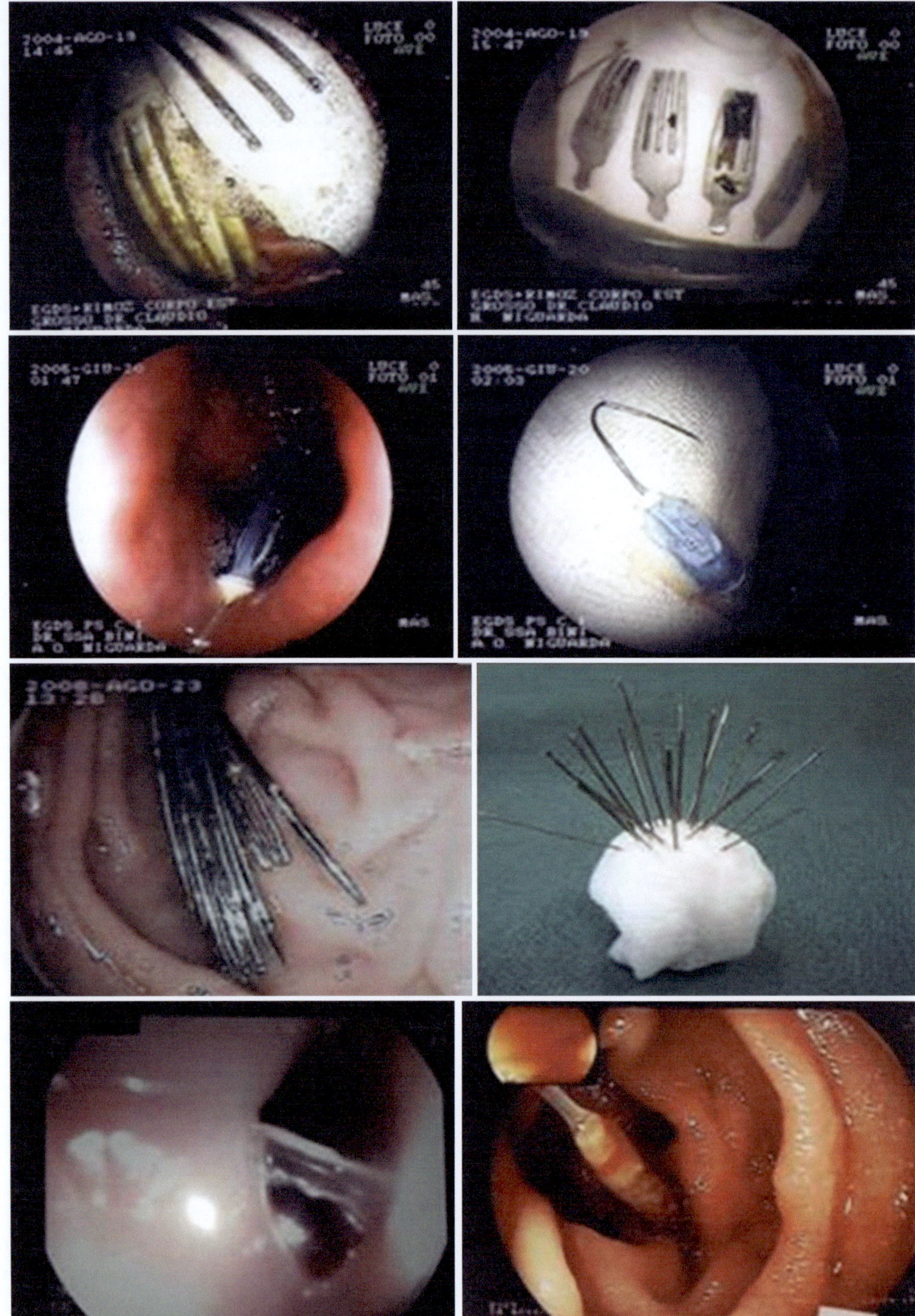

Fig. 41.1 Sharp FB forks, syringe needle, sewing needles, glass fragment, and toothpick duodenal perforation. (Courtesy of Journal of Gastroenterology and Hepatology Research 2015 4: 1524–1532)

extremely dangerous FB, especially when impacted in the esophagus, and they can cause major complications such as perforation, stenosis, and fistulas.

Metallic objects with a possible lead content may cause lead poisoning due to metal absorption [20, 21]. In these cases, lead hematological levels should be monitored, and if they are increased, FB should be urgently retrieved.

41.2.4 Management

Management of FB ingestion varies depending on patients' conditions and FB characteristics.

41.2.4.1 Conservative

As previously stated, the majority of ingested FB will spontaneously transit the upper and lower gastrointestinal tract and will be eventually evacuated. Non-dangerous small FB in asymptomatic patients doesn't need medical intervention [5]. Clinical observation is indicated in order to monitor the progression and the evacuation of the FB.

41.2.4.2 Endoscopic

Ten to twenty percent of ingested foreign bodies will require endoscopic retrieval.

The decision-making process needs a good knowledge of the updated literature and widely accepted international guidelines. The procedure can be challenging and it should be performed by a well-experienced endoscopist.

- A documented expertise in pediatric endoscopy is required [22] when a small child or infant is involved.
- Anesthesiologist assistance is recommended to provide adequate sedation or general anesthesia and guarantee airway protection.
- All the necessary endoscopic instruments and devices, as well as the resuscitation procedure devices, must be available in the endoscopic room or wherever the procedure is performed (emergency room, operatory room).
- Different diameter endoscope availability is also recommended. For FB endoscopic retrieval, the use of wide operative channel scopes is advisable for it will allow us to employ any device. FB in very small children and newborns require the use of small caliber endoscopes and retrieval devices specific for pediatric scopes. It is worth reminding that, under general anesthesia and with an adequate airway protection, it's possible for an experienced endoscopist, when this is the only alternative to surgical intervention, to carefully use a standard endoscope even in children under 12 months of age. Figure 41.1 shows 23 needles extracted from the stomach of a 3-month old child: only the standard endoscope operative channel was wide enough to allow the use of the magnetic probe which was effective in extracting the needles through the endoscopic channel.
- During the endoscopic procedure, the patient should possibly lay on the left side with the head not too flexed on the neck in order to reduce the sharpness of the angle of the upper esophageal sphincter and facilitate the maneuvers.
- Changing patient's position should always be possible in case it gives a better endoscopic access to the ingested object. In case of voluminous FB, a disinflation of the tracheal tube balloon could make the retrieval easier.
- In case of elongated FB, the major diameter of the object should always be kept parallel to the endoscope. Cardias can be a difficult tract to pull the object through. It's advisable not to immediately force the pulling but to maintain a gentle and constant traction and wait until the sphincter pressure diminishes and allows the object to be pulled backward smoothly.
- In small patients a FB located in the upper esophagus can determine a higher risk of airflow obstruction due to the compression of the soft upper airway wall that might be worsened by endoscopic maneuvers which must always be delicate and cautious. Also, hyperinflation should be avoided because it can determine compression of the diaphragm and subsequent respiratory stress [23, 54, 55].

Many retrieval devices (Fig. 41.2) are available for endoscopic grasping of FB; they include different kinds of forceps, rubber cups, snares, Dormia basket and nets. In some occasion handcrafted "homemade" devices have proved more effective than standard devices in extracting peculiar types of FB. The choice should be made on the basis of FB shape and dimensions as well as on the endoscopist personale expertise.

- Testing the grasp on a "twin" or similar object (when available) may be useful to choose the most efficient device [23–25].
- During endoscopic retrieval, special attention must be paid in avoiding devices that might be "trapped or stuck" to the grasped object causing the impossibility to pull out the endoscope.
- Pointed objects must be reoriented, as shown in Fig. 41.3, sometimes also by guiding them into the gastric lumen in order to obtain a better and safer grasp and let the pointed end trail rather than lead [26–28]. The procedure must be particularly careful in case of sharp objects that must always be kept under visual control while the endoscope is pulled out (Video 41.1).
- Flexible endoscopic maneuvers may sometimes be inefficient in extracting a particularly voluminous FB trapped at the upper esophageal sphincter (Fig. 41.4). In these cases, cooperation with the otolaryngologist is advisable. The use of a rigid esophagoscope which allows a better

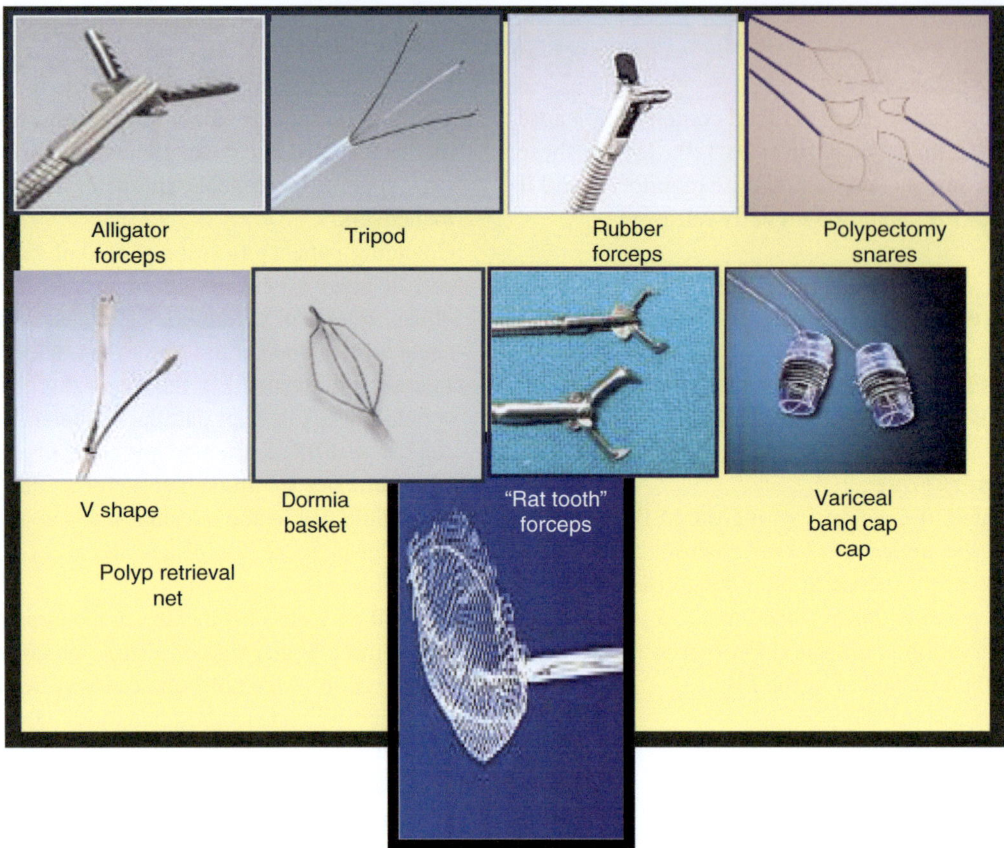

Fig. 41.2 Endoscopic retrieval devices. (Courtesy of Journal of Gastroenterology and Hepatology Research, 2015 4: 1524–1532)

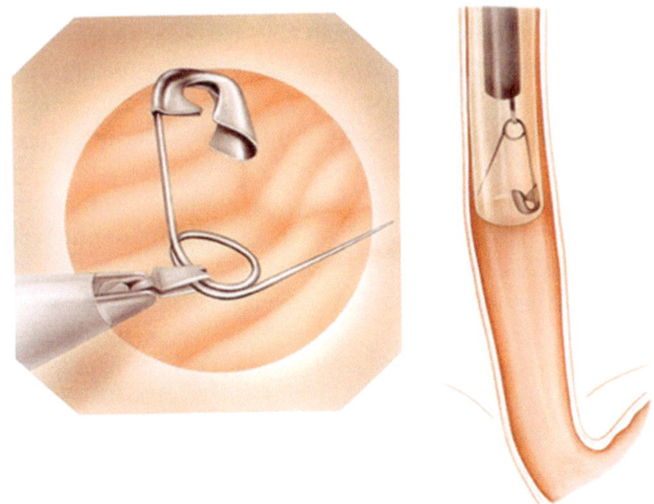

Fig. 41.3 Reorienting a pointed FB. (Courtesy by Area Qualità S.r.l. Milan IT)

dilatation of the sphincter area, as well as the use of bigger and stronger rigid forceps, can be more efficient and effective.

– When possible, it's important to protect the mucosa and the esophageal wall during the extraction. Due to their small diameter, lower and upper esophageal sphincters are areas particularly at risk of iatrogenic lesions. The most common protection devices are shown in Fig. 41.5. Magill forceps can also be a very helpful device during extraction of a FB from the hypopharynx.

41.2.5 Management of Specific FB

The following section will provide information regarding the management of certain types of FB, which, due to their characteristics or to their particular hazardousness, are worth a specific discussion.

41.2.5.1 Food Bolus

Food bolus is the most common type of FB found in adult patients. Usually, it's a meat bolus, but any food can be found especially in patients with an underlying esophageal disease. The following steps are important when dealing with patients with food bolus impaction:

– The presence of bone fragments or denture pieces inside the bolus should always be ruled out with an X-ray before engaging any endoscopic treatment.

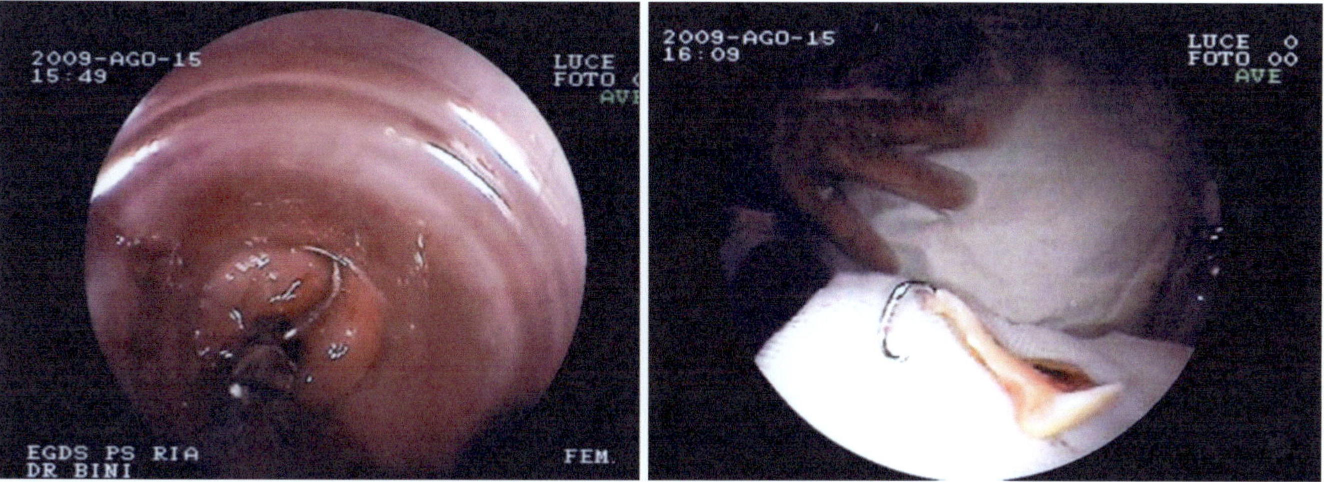

Fig. 41.4 Denture with metal hook that required the use of a rigid esophagoscope to be retrieved. (Courtesy by Area Qualità S.r.l. Milan IT)

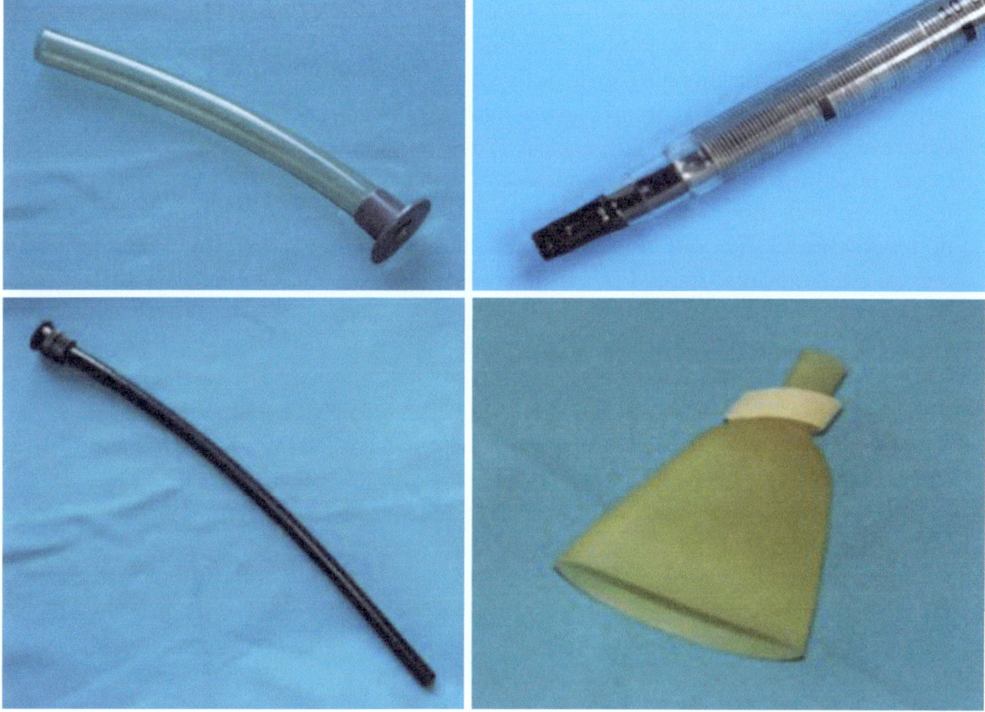

Fig. 41.5 Protection device overtubes, the bell-shaped latex hood, and variceal band ligator cap. (Courtesy of Journal of Gastroenterology and Hepatology Research 2015, 4: 1524–1532)

- When the bolus is impacted at the middle or lower esophagus, a cautious attempt at pushing it forward into the gastric lumen can be made only if no harmful content has been documented, but any forcing or stressing must be avoided especially in case of possible underlying esophageal stricture [4].
- Recurrent history of food bolus impaction in a young otherwise healthy male patient should raise the clinical suspicion of eosinophilic esophagitis [52] which in literature has demonstrated to be involved in almost 33% of food bolus impaction. In these cases, a biopsy specimen will help to make a correct diagnosis and possibly to start an effective medical treatment [11].

41.2.5.2 Coins

Coins are the most frequent FB ingested by children [28, 29] (Fig. 41.6). Children are usually healthy, but in some cases, there might be an underlying disease or condition that may predispose for the FB impaction (esophageal rings, eosinophilic esophagitis, motility disorders).

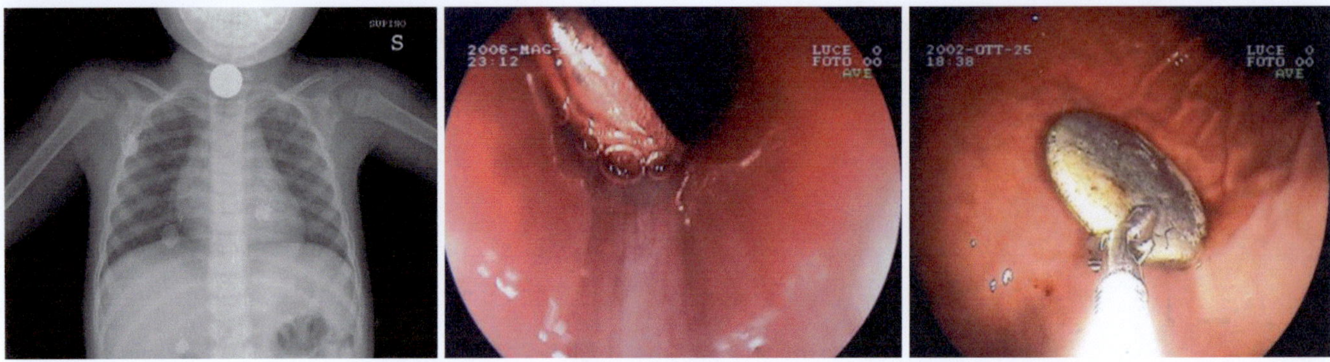

Fig. 41.6 Ingested coins. (Courtesy of Journal of Gastroenterology and Hepatology Research 2015, 4: 1524–1532)

- Around 50% of children with ingested coins are asymptomatic especially if the coin has reached the gastric lumen or the small bowel; when a coin is trapped in the upper esophagus or upper esophageal sphincter inducing total or partial obstruction, the patient presents with pain, drooling, and/or dysphagia.
- The diagnosis must be ruled out or confirmed by a biplane radiography. Lateral views can help to differentiate between ingested and aspirated coins (esophageal or tracheal) as well as to reveal the presence of multiple stacked coins [30].
- It's of uttermost importance that ingested coins are differentiated from disk batteries. The search of "halo" sign or "double ring" sign will help to differentiate between the two radiologically similar FB, as it'll be described further on.
- *Coins impacted in the upper esophagus* should be immediately removed.
- *Coins lodged in the medium or lower esophagus* cause fewer symptoms and have a probability as high as 30% of passing spontaneously [1]. For this reason, most recent guidelines state that patients with coins or similar objects (i.e. buttons) localized in the middle or lower esophagus may be radiologically monitored [5] to verify the FB progression into the gastric lumen. Endoscopic removal should be performed if coin fails to pass into the stomach after 12–24 h.
- If the time of ingestion is unknown or it's suspected to be more >12 h before presentation, urgent removal is indicated no matter what the location in the esophagus is [31].
- *Coins located in the stomach* do not need endoscopic removal since they will most probably transit spontaneously. If coin fails to pass through the pylorus in 48–72 h, an endoscopic removal should be scheduled.
- *Coins in the small bowel* will most probably be evacuated. In this case, watchful waiting is allowed. The progression might be monitored by weekly radiographs, but actually, it's rarely done. Clinical follow-up and evaluation of possible obstructive signs or symptoms as well as stool observation are recommended.

Figure 41.7 displays a simplified algorithm for the treatment of ingested coins proposed by the NASPGHAN Committee in 2015 [31].

41.2.5.3 Magnets

This kind of FB ingestion has become more frequent in recent years as a consequence of the widespread popularity of toys or gadgets containing high-power magnets (rare-earth magnets) (Fig. 41.8).

A recent study of the North Pacific Surgical Association reported more than 22,000 cases of magnet ingestion in the USA from 2201 to 2011 with a fivefold increase in the last 2 years of the study [31, 32].

These kinds of magnets (neodymium magnets) are 10 times stronger than iron magnets, and their voluntary or accidental ingestion can have serious health consequences if not properly managed. In 2007 the US Consumer Product Safety Commission (USCPSC) issued the first warning after the death of a 20-month-old child, as well as 33 other cases of ingestion (https://www.cpsc.gov/content/cpsc-warns-high-powered-magnets-and-children-make-a-deadly-mixthe).

- The risk of major complications due to magnet ingestion becomes actual when *two or more* magnets are involved. The mutual attraction of magnets located in different intestinal loops may lead to compression, necrosis of intestinal wall, and subsequent perforation (Fig. 41.9) [31–33].

In 2012 a NASPGHAN committee of experts developed an algorithm [34] for the management of ingested magnets in children.

- If a solitary magnet is ingested and no other metallic foreign bodies are present in the gastrointestinal tract, it can be managed conservatively with serial radiographs.
- If multiple magnets are ingested, prompt endoscopic removal is indicated if they are in the esophagus or stomach.

Fig. 41.7 A simplified algorithm for management of coin ingestions in children

- Coin ingestion: PA and lateral films, ensure no button battery
  - Esophageal
    - Symptomatic (drooling, dysphagia, respiratory compromise): Urgent endoscopic removal
    - Asymptomatic: Endoscopic removal within 24 hours. Consider glucagon if distal esophageal coin or if endoscopy not readily available
  - Gastric
    - No endoscopy needed: Consider straining stools, laxatives, repeat x-ray at 2 weeks
      - Endoscopic removal if not passed within 2–4 weeks. Repeat x-ray immediately before removal to ensure coin still present
  - Small bowel
    - Clinical observation: Enteroscopy/surgical removal if symptomatic

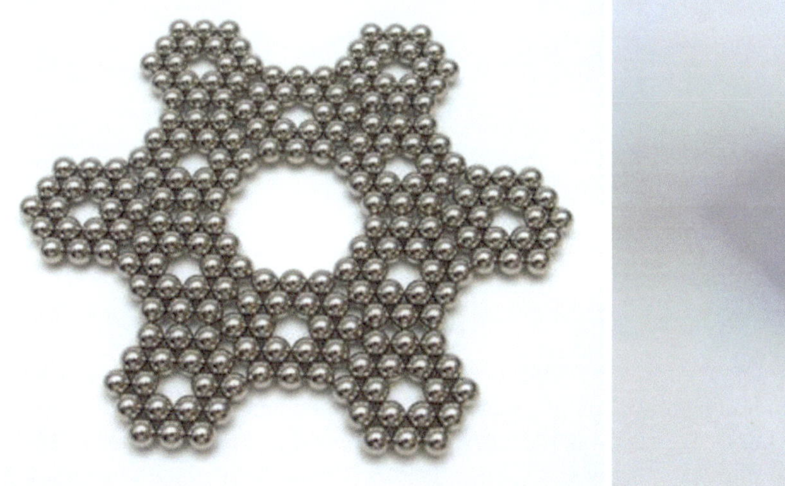

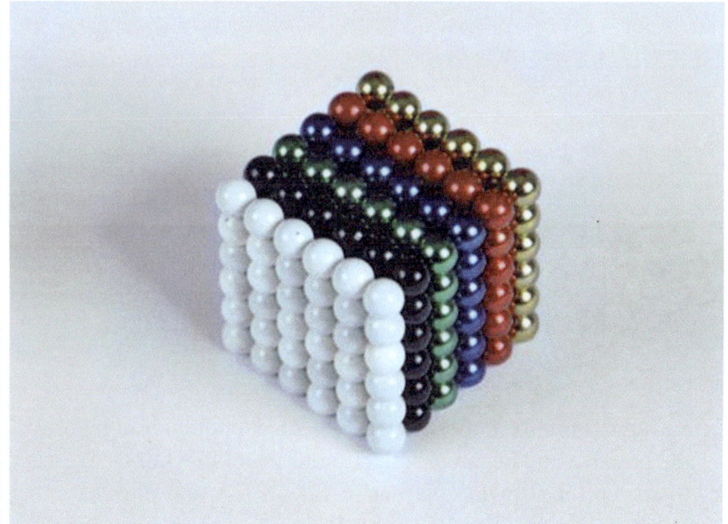

Fig. 41.8 Magnet toys

41.2.5.4 Disk Batteries

Disk batteries (DB) are among the most dangerous FB ingested by children.

The risks and potentially severe consequences of DB ingestion are well known [31, 35, 36]. A short list of major complications is shown in Table 41.5.

Morbidity and mortality have greatly increased in the last years especially after the widespread use of toys, watches, and hearing aids containing larger diameter and higher-voltage lithium batteries [35].

Lithium DB are usually 20–25 mm in diameter which makes impaction more likely in the pediatric esophagus.

– The main pathophysiologic mechanism responsible for the severe and potentially deadly complications of DB esophageal impaction is an electrical mechanism. The

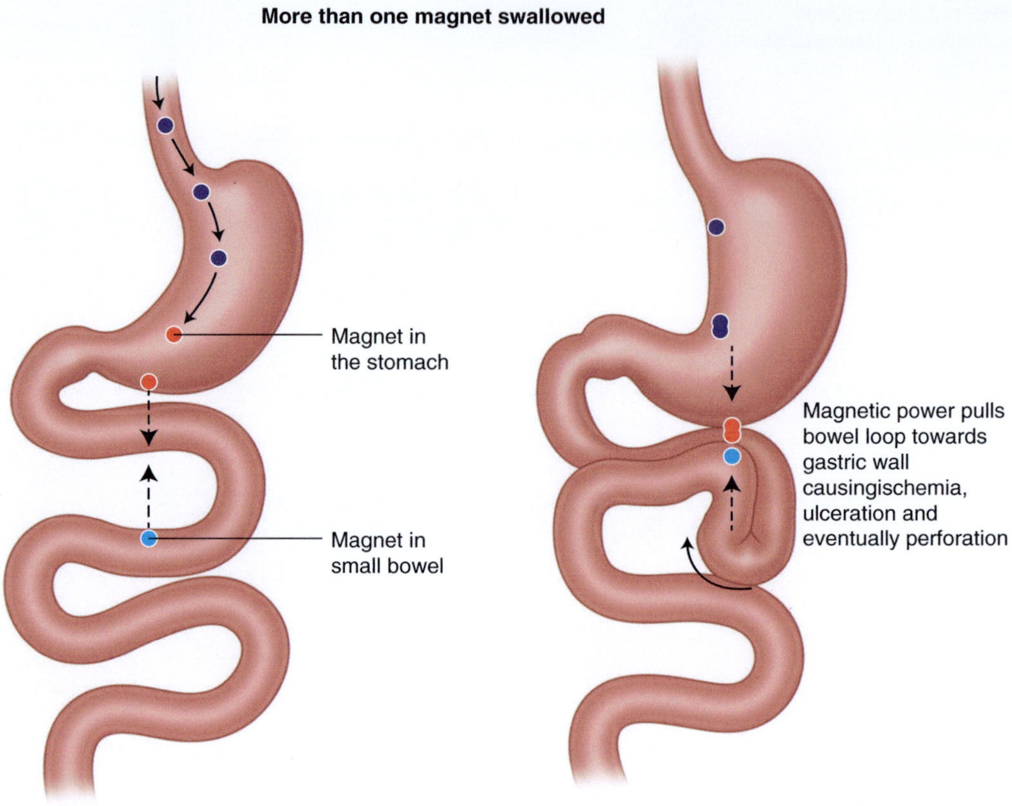

Fig. 41.9 GI lesions due to multiple magnet ingestion

Table 41.5 Complications of DB ingestion

Vocal cord paralysis
Esophageal perforation
Esophageal stricture
Tracheal stenosis
Tracheomalacia
Tracheoesophageal fistula
Hemorrhage from arterial fistula
Infection
Death

Table 41.6 Conditions for a higher risk of complications in DB ingestion

Children younger than 4 years
Large diameter DB >20 mm (high voltage)
Time of ingestion
Location of battery

entrapment of the battery in the esophageal lumen bridges the positive and negative battery poles generating an electrical circuit allowing current to flow. Electrical current from the battery results in the generation of hydroxide radicals in the esophageal tissue leading to a rapid pH tissue increase that causes a caustic injury and coagulative necrosis of the esophageal wall. The necrosis may extend through the adjacent tissue such as the trachea or great thoracic vessels.

- Injury can last for days or weeks after battery removal, because of residual alkali or weakened tissues, which explains the onset of major complications like aorto-esophageal fistula (AEF) even 2 weeks after DB removal.
- It must be pointed out that also "dead" batteries retain enough voltage to generate an external current and cause major tissue damage so they also must be removed promptly.
- Complications are more common in small children (younger than 4 years) when a 20-mm-diameter DB is involved, when the DB is impacted in the esophagus and when the diagnosis is delayed (Table 41.6). Epidemiological studies have demonstrated that the DB ingestion was unwitnessed in 92% of cases of death and 56% of major complications [37]. The majority of lethal complications are due to an aortoesophageal fistula (AOF) with massive uncontrollable bleeding.

As far as January 2017, the National Capital Poison (NCP) Center reported 55 fatalities secondary to DB ingestion (58.1% secondary to AOF) and 215 nonfatal airways or severe esophageal complications (http://www.poison.org/battery/fatalcases) [38].

There have also been concerning reports about deaths occurring as far as 2 weeks after DB removal [3, 35].

These data confirm the importance of a prompt recognition and intervention in the case of DB ingestion in order to decrease and minimize the number and seriousness of complications.

- The diagnostic approach should be multidisciplinary involving the pediatrician, the radiologist, the anesthesiologist, the endoscopist and the cardiothoracic surgeon.
- A neck, chest, and abdominal X-ray must be performed in order to differentiate coins from DB when a round metal object is found in the GI tract. In fact, button batteries have a bilaminar structure and they appear as a double ring or halo ("halo sign") on an anteroposterior plain X-ray, while on the lateral X-ray, DB can be differentiated from coins because of a "step-off" at the separation border between anode and cathode [39].

The National Battery Ingestion Hotline (NBIH) and National Capital Poison Center have issued a guideline for the triage and management of ingested DB which is available on their website (www.poison.org/battery/guideline.asp).

In 2015 NASPGHAN Endoscopy Committee also proposed a management algorithm [31] for the management of ingested DB.

- Prompt endoscopic (within 2 h) removal of DB located in the esophagus is mandatory even in the absence of symptoms.
- An endoscopic evaluation is important also in asymptomatic patients, even if the DB is detected in the stomach as it's been stressed by NASPGHAN [21] Endoscopy Committee. In a recent report, complications have been reported in four cases of DB located in the stomach including one major complication [40].
- Endoscopy is always recommended to reveal potential esophageal lesions due to the previous lodging of the DB in the esophagus especially when the time of ingestion is unknown. If unrecognized, those lesions might lead to major delayed complications independently from battery location in the stomach or beyond at the moment of the X-ray localization.
- In high-risk patients, when possible severe esophageal or vascular lesion is suspected, endoscopic evaluation and removal should be arranged in a *cardiovascular operatory room* where cardiac catheterization and open surgery can be performed.
- When aortic involvement is not suspected, a regular operatory room would be the more appropriate location.
- A well-equipped endoscopic room will be adequate for removing a DB located beyond the esophagus or to evaluate a possible esophageal lesion in low-risk patients.
- Removal should be performed with a 2.8 mm operative channel endoscope to be able to use all the possible necessary grasping devices. When the battery is located in the gastric lumen, endoscopic nets are the most useful retrieval device. When the battery is stuck in the esophagus, grasp forceps (alligator or rat tooth forceps) usually prove more effective in dislodging and retrieving the battery. In rare occasions, particularly when the battery has been trapped at the upper esophageal for more than 2 h, the surrounding mucosa can show marked edema and inflammation, and the battery can be embedded in a deep ulceration; in these cases the dislodging maneuvers can be quite difficult, and the use of a rigid esophagoscope in cooperation with the otolaryngologist can be helpful in obtaining a better dilatation in order to dislodge the battery [41, 42]. Once the battery has been removed from the esophagus, a second look is mandatory to carefully evaluate any possible lesion as well as to rule out the presence of additional FBs in the upper GI tract. Burns and ulcers located in the middle esophagus are at higher risk of AOF. Lesions in the cervical tract are at higher risk of tracheoesophageal fistula or bleeding from inferior thyroid artery. Lesions of the distal esophagus might be less concerning, but serious complications have also been described in these patients.

Unfortunately, due to many different circumstances, the removal can't always be "prompt" as guidelines suggest. Litovitz et al. estimated the time elapse between DB ingestion and the removal in 73 patients with major outcome and the results were (cumulative total) less than 4 h in 7 patients, less than 8 h in 17 patients, less than 12 h in 27 patients, less than 24 h in 36 patients, less than 48 h in 42 patients, less than 3 days in 48 cases, less than 1 week in 60 cases, less than 2 weeks in 67 cases and less than 6 weeks in 72 cases, and 1 case is completely unknown [43]. This highlights that, for different and sometimes inevitable reasons, only a few patients have their DB removed within 6–8 h which increases the risk of fatal complications.

This observation should emphasize that the *most effective management strategy is prevention* and that parents and other child caregivers should be educated about the hazards associated with battery exposure. It should also be stressed the importance that the products containing button batteries are either kept away from children or the batteries are secured safely in the product. Industry changes, including improved packaging, can also contribute in reducing morbidity due to DB ingestion in children.

The management of patients after endoscopic retrieval of the battery is still a controversial topic.

After the retrieval of a FB, if no lesions or symptoms are documented, and the presence of additional objects in the GI tract is ruled out, the patient can be discharged with no need of a follow-up.

In the case of DB even in the case of minor lesions and even if the patient is asymptomatic, a careful clinical follow-up should be scheduled to detect any possible sign of late complications. The onset of fatal late complications reported in recent literature up to 18 days after battery removal [31, 43, 44] suggests extremely careful monitoring and observation of the patient before discharge. Some authors suggest a second endoscopic look at day 4 before reintroducing oral feeding [45].

41.2.5.5 Drug Packages

Concealing illegal substances, mainly heroin or cocaine, for international trafficking is the main reason for drug package ingestion (body packing) [19, 46]. Wrapped in latex condoms or rubber balloons, drugs are swallowed or inserted in the rectum. Packages are usually multiple and radiopaque.

The risk of fatal intoxication due to rupture and leakage during endoscopic retrieval procedure is extremely high and for this reason, there is *no indication* to endoscopic treatment for these FB.

International guidelines advice a conservative treatment with clinical observation and bowel irrigation in asymptomatic patients [3]. Surgical intervention is mandatory in case of signs of bowel obstruction or intoxication [3, 5, 47].

41.3 Lower GI Tract Foreign Bodies

41.3.1 Clinical Assessment

Lower GI FB can be found in patients of all ages, but the majority of reports are about men aged between 30 and 40 [48] as a result of sexual stimulation, body packing (voluntary), or caused by medical practitioners (e.g., broken rectal thermometers or broken enema catheter tips) or by sexual assault (involuntary). They may also be found in abused children and psychiatric patients. Insertion is mostly voluntary, and all rectal FB should be considered as potentially hazardous. The diagnosis can be challenging because patients are often reluctant to seek medical care; often they attend to the emergency room after having received more than one attempt to remove the object by themselves; these maneuvers might also cause rectal lesions. Patients may be embarrassed to reveal the actual reason for their symptoms, and they can complain of abdominal pain, rectal bleeding, or obstructive symptoms (Table 41.7) without being explicit about the FB insertion which sometimes can be days or even weeks before the visit to the emergency room [49]. Otherwise unexplained rectal lesions or bleeding should make us consider a previous insertion of a rectal FB which could have been self-removed.

Table 41.7 Signs and symptoms in presence of Lower GI FB

Pain
Rectal bleeding
Fever
Abscess
Intestinal obstruction

41.3.2 Diagnosis

If the FB body is retained in the lower rectum, a digital exploration will make the diagnosis. If the FB has proceeded in the upper rectum or in the sigmoid colon, an X-ray is necessary to locate the object. X-ray or CT scan evaluation is indicated not only to confirm the diagnosis but also to reveal potential complications like bowel obstruction or perforation. Radiology is also helpful in localizing the FB and will provide accurate information about size and shape which are necessary to plan the proper management.

41.3.3 Management

41.3.3.1 Transanal

Endoscopy can be effective in retrieving a FB from the lower GI tract if:

- The object is close enough to the anus.
- A complete sphincter relaxation is obtained with conscious sedation or general anesthesia.

If the patient is collaborative, a Valsalva maneuver can help to push the object in a position nearer to the anus. Grasping and breaking in pieces fruits or vegetables can also be a useful technique to facilitate the FB body extraction. If the removal is successful, an endoscopic evaluation is recommended to rule out lesions of the rectal mucosa.

41.3.3.2 Endoscopic

Endoscopy can be effective in retrieving a FB from the lower GI tract if:

- The object can be reached by the flexible endoscope, usually in the rectum or distal sigmoid colon.
- The dimensions are suitable for its grasping with the common endoscopic retrieval devices.
- No perforation is documented.
- Polipectomy snares are the most used device used for the removal of large rectal foreign bodies.

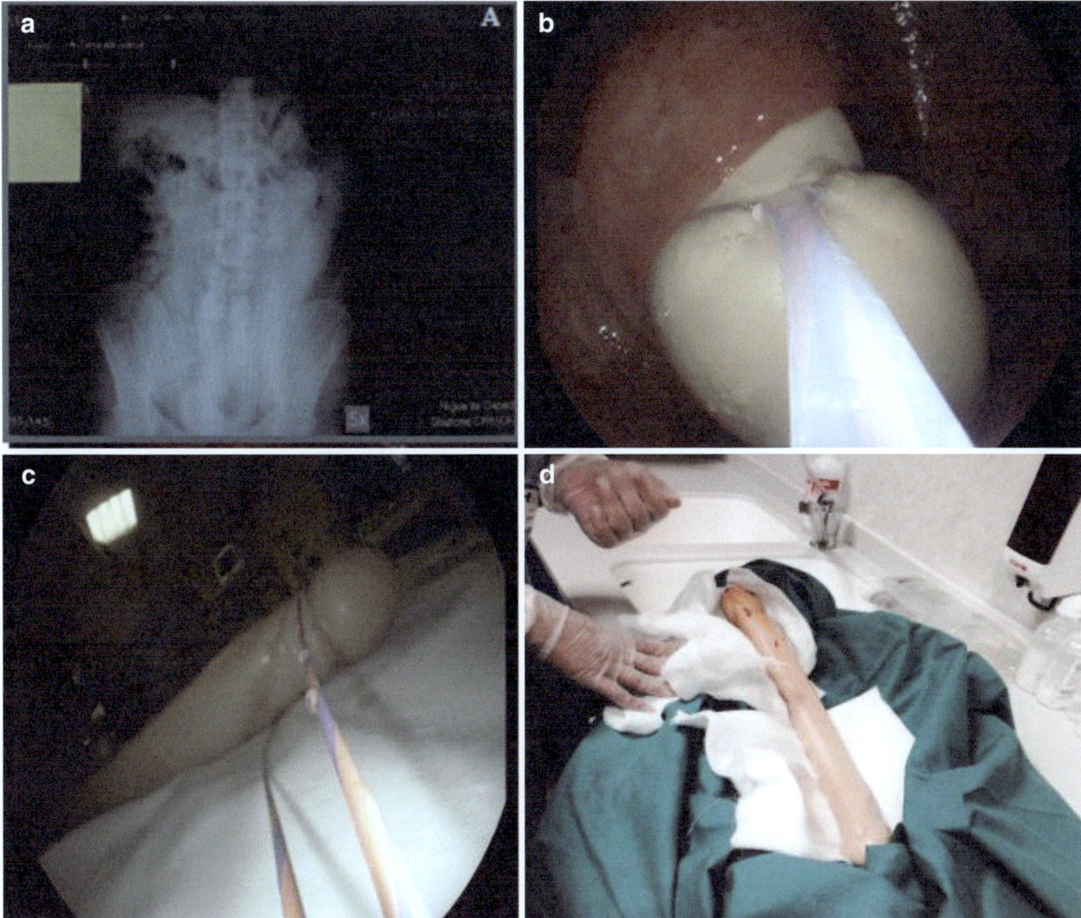

Fig. 41.10 (**a**) Rubber dildo deeply inserted in the sigmoid colon. (**b**–**d**) Polypectomy snare was not wide enough to capture the FB. Thus, a device was "handcrafted" on purpose, inserting an endoscopic guide wire through a pusher catheter to form a wide noose, securely capture the FB, and firmly pull it down

- An abdominal X-ray is advisable after the endoscopic procedure, especially if it was challenging or difficult, to rule out perforation.

Pressure on the left iliac fossa in the downward direction can help to move the FB pushing it into the rectum. The extraction of very large objects (Fig. 41.10a, b, c, d) can be challenging since the usual retrieval devices might prove inefficient. In some cases, a "made-on-purpose" "handcraft" device may be more effective in order to grip and hold the FB and extract it through the anal sphincter.

41.3.3.3 Surgical

When deeply located beyond the rectum, FB may require a surgical approach. Laparoscopic and endoscopic combined technique has been described for removal of deeply inserted foreign bodies [50]. Lake et al. determined that approximately 55% of RFB located in the sigmoid eventually required surgical treatment as opposed to only 24% in cases of rectal objects [51]. The last following section exemplifies, in form of a Case scenario, the practical approach to a patient with upper GI Foreign Body.

Case Scenario

At 7:30 PM a young couple takes their 2-year-old child to the ER because in the last 2 h, the baby has shown a "strange behavior": he seems to feel uncomfortable; he'd been crying for more than half an hour with no apparent reason. No fever or vomiting but in the last hour, he showed some drooling.

They report that he spent the day at home with the baby sitter who said the child was fine until 5 PM. He had his last meal at 12:00 which he regularly ate. He had a nap between 1:30 and 4 PM. After he had woken up, they spent time playing and watching Disney DVD. The babysitter didn't notice anything unusual until 5 PM when the child became querulous and refused his bottle of milk. When the parents came home, the child was crying and apparently had problems in swallowing saliva.

He appears to be a healthy child; his height and weight are normal for his age (erythrocytes 4,200,000, leucocytes 11,000). There was no evidence of pathological signs at the physical examination and oral mucosa inspection. The baby was offered water which he refused to drink.

1. Which would be your first diagnostic step?
   - A. Hospitalize patient for observation and further evaluation.
   - B. Chest X-ray.
   - C. Urgent endoscopic evaluation for possible FB ingestion.

Chest X-ray showed a radiopaque round metallic FB of approximately 2 cm diameter located in the middle esophagus. No signs of perforation or upper airways involvement.

2. What would come next in the management of the FB?
   - A. Cautious waiting for possible spontaneous transit of the FB in the stomach.
   - B. Immediate endoscopy for FB retrieval.
   - C. Further collection of anamnestic data and search for X-ray-specific signs to identify the nature of FB (coin, battery, jewelry).

When specifically asked about the possibility that the child might have swallowed a button battery or a coin, parents told that they might have forgotten a spare battery on the living room bookshelf after they replaced the alarm clock's dead battery. A more accurate evaluation of the FB on the X-ray revealed the halo sign which is typical of DISK battery.

The ultimate diagnosis was "esophageal foreign body (disk battery) due to accidental ingestion".

3. Which are the correct following steps in the management of this patient?
   - A. Endoscopic removal if still in the esophagus after 2–4 h of observation and a second X-ray (dead battery).
   - B. Immediate hospitalization and battery removal in endoscopic room.
   - C. Immediate hospitalization and CT scan to rule out possible transmural lesion of the esophageal wall and/or possible involvement of the aortic wall. Arrange the endoscopic removal in the operating room with the assistance of a cardiothoracic surgeon, availability of all the necessary devices for cardiopulmonary resuscitation, and extracorporeal blood circulation.

The patient was hospitalized. A 23 mm DB was endoscopically removed from the middle esophagus under general anesthesia. The esophageal mucosa showed a superficial 10 mm superficial erosion, no active bleeding.

4. What is the correct follow-up after endoscopic removal?
   - A. If the patient is asymptomatic, dismiss with a 7-day PPI therapy.
   - B. Endoscopic second look to verify the complete healing of the erosion.
   - C. PPI therapy. Possibly a second endoscopic before dismissal. Educate parents to a very careful surveillance of any possible sign of late complication as far as 3 or 4 weeks after the removal (dysphagia, hematemesis).

The patient was dismissed after an endoscopic second look in order to state the complete healing of the mucosa. Parents were educated to a strict surveillance in the following weeks for possible bleeding or GI symptoms. They were also educated about the potential risks of DB ingestion and they were instructed on how to dispose dead batteries and safe storage of any kind of battery keeping it always far from children's reach.

Please see Chap. 58 for the correct answer.

References

1. Crockett SD, Sperry SLW, Brock Miller C, Shaeen NJ, Dellon ES. Emergency care of esophageal foreign body impactions: timing, treatment modalities and resource utilization. Dis Esophagus. 2013;26:105–12.
2. Tenca A. La gestione endoscopica del corpo estraneo nell'adulto. Giornale Italiano di Endoscopia Digestiva. Dicembre 2016:97–100.
3. Bekkerman M, Sachdev AH, Andrade J, Twersky Y, Iqbal S. Endoscopic management of foreign bodies in the gastrointestinal tract: a review of the literature. Gastroenterol Res Pract. 2016;2016:6. Article ID 8520767.
4. Birk M, Bauerfeind P, Deprez PH, Häfner M, Hartmann D, Hassan C, et al. Removal of foreign bodies in upper gastrointestinal tract in adults: European Society of Gastrointestinal Endoscopy (ESGE) Clinical Guideline. Endoscopy. 2016;48:1–8.
5. ASGE Standards of Practice Committee, Ikenberry SO, Jue TL, Anderson MA, Appalaneni V, Banerjee S, Ben-Menachem T, Decker GA, Fanelli RD, Fisher LR, Fukami N, Harrison ME, Jain R, Khan KM, Krinsky ML, Maple JT, Sharaf R, Strohmeyer L, Dominitz JA. Management of ingested foreign bodies and food impactions (ASGE Guideline). Gastrointest Endosc. 2011;73(6):1085–91.
6. Chauvin A, Viala J, Marteau P, Hermann P, Dray X. Management and endoscopic techniques for digestive foreign body and food bolus impaction. Dig Liver Dis. 2013;45(7):529–42.
7. Palta R, Sahota A, Bemarki A, Salama P, Simpson N, Laine L. Foreign-body ingestion: characteristics and outcomes in a lower socioeconomic population with predominantly intentional ingestion. Gastrointest Endosc. 2009;69:426–33.
8. Weiland ST, Schurr MJ. Conservative management of ingested foreign bodies. J Gastrointest Surg. 2002;6:496–500.
9. Jotdar A, Dutta M, Kundua S, Ghosh B, Chatterjee I. Surgically repaired esophagus: an anchor pad for foreign bodies. Egypt J Ear, Nose, Throat Allied Sci. 2016;17:7–10.
10. Gundling F, Seidl H, Stark T, Schneider A, Schepp W. Management of impacted foreign bodies in the upper gastrointestinal tract in adult patients: results of a retrospective case series. Z Gastroenterol. 2012;50(12):1287–91.
11. Kirchner GI, Zuber-Jerger I, Endlicher E, Gelbmann C, et al. Causes of bolus impaction in the esophagus. Surg Endosc. 2011;25:3170–4.
12. Grassi R, Faggian A, Somma F, DeCecco CN, Laghi A, Caseiro-Alves F. Application of imaging guidelines in patients with foreign body ingestion or inhalation: literature review. Semin Ultrasound CT MRI. 2015;36(1):48–56.
13. Liew CJY. Finding nemo: imaging findings, pitfalls, and complications of ingested fish bones in the alimentary canal. Emerg Radiol. 2013;20:311.
14. Hsieh CH, Wang YC, Chen RJ, et al. Comparison of the clinical presentations of ingested foreign bodies requiring operative and nonoperative management. Int Surg. 2005;90(2):99–102.
15. Eisen GM, Baron TH, Dominitz JA, et al. Guideline for the management of ingested foreign bodies. Gastrointest Endosc. 2002;55(7):802–6.
16. Lai AT, Chow TL, Lee DT, Kwok SP. Risk factors predicting the development of complications after foreign body ingestion. Br J Surg. 2003;90(12):1531–5.
17. Jeon SW, Son HS, Kim SK, Jung MK, Cho CM, Tak WY, et al. Factors predictive of risk for complications in patients with oesophageal foreign bodies. Dig Liver Dis. 2011;43(8):632–5.
18. Loh KS, Tan Smith JD, et al. Complications of foreign bodies in the oesophagus. Otolaryngol Hesd Neck Surg. 2000;123:613–6.
19. Wong GCK, Lai KK, Chung CH. Management of body packers in the emergency department. Hong Kong J Emerg Med. 2005;12(2):112–8.
20. Coon T, Miller M, Shirazi F, Sullivan J. Lead toxicity in a 14-year-old female with retained bulled fragments. J Pediatrics. 2006;117(1):227–30.
21. Danialifar TF, Mun-Wah NG, Hunter C, Naon H. Chronic lead toxicity from retained foreign body, Children's Hospital Los Angeles, Keck School of Medicine, University of Southern California. Consult Pediatr. 2012;10:338–9.
22. Rudolph CD, Winter HS, NASPGN Executive Council, NASPGN Training and Education Committee, and Contributing. Requirements for training to ensure competence of endoscopists performing invasive procedures in children. J Pediatr Gastroenterol Nutr. 1999;29:S1–S26.
23. Faiger DO, Stotland BR, et al. Device choice and experience level in endoscopic foreign object retrieval: an in vivo study. Gastrointest Endosc. 1997;45:490–2.
24. Nelson DB, Bosco JJ, Curtis W, Faigel DO, Kelsey PB, Leung JW, et al. Endoscopic retrieval devices. Gastrointest Endosc. 1999;50:932–4.
25. ASGE Technology Committee, Diehl DL, Adler DG, Conway JD, Farraye FA, Kantsevoy SV, Kaul V, Kethu SR, Kwon RS, Mamula P, Rodriguez SA, Tierney WM. Endoscopic retrieval devices. Gastrointest Endosc. 2009;69(6):997. www.giejournal.org.
26. Rossi A, Bini M. Ingestione di corpi estranei in età pediatrica: management e rimozione endoscopica. Il libro bianco dell'endoscopiasta;18.
27. Bini M. Gastrointestinal foreign bodies: clinical aspects and endoscopic management. J Gastroenterol Hepatol Res. 2015;4(3):1524–32.
28. Chinski A, Foltran F, Gregori D, Ballali S, Passali D, Bellussi L. Foreign bodies in the oesophagus: the experience of the buenos aires paediatric ORL clinic. Int J Pediatr. 2010;2010:6. Article ID 490691.
29. Arana A, Hauser B, Hachimi-Idrissi S, Vandenplas Y. Management of ingested foreign bodies in childhood and review of the literature. Eur J Pediatr. 2001;160(8):468–72.
30. Smith MT, Wong RKH. Foreign Bodies. Gastrointest Endosc Clin N Am. 2007;17:361–82.
31. Kramer RE, Lerner DG, Lin T, Manfredi M, Shah M, Stephen TC, et al. Management of ingested foreign bodies in children: a clinical report of the NASPGHAN Endoscopy Committee. J Pediatr Gastroenterol Nutr. 2015;60(4):562–74.
32. Brown J, Otjen JP, Drugas GT. Pediatric magnet ingestion: the dark side of the force. Am J Surg. 2014;207:754–9.
33. Centers for Disease Control and Prevention (CDC). Gastrointestinal injuries from magnet ingestion in children—United States, 2003–2006. MMWR Morb Mortal Wkly Rep. 2006;55:1296–300.
34. Noel RA, Hussain SZ, Bousvaros A, Gilger M, Mamula P, Gupta S, et al. Management of ingested magnets in children. J Pediatr Gastroenterol Nutr. 2012;55(3):239–42.
35. Leinwand K, Brumbaugh DE, Kramer RE. Button battery ingestion in children: a paradigm for management of severe pediatric foreign body ingestions. Gastrointest Endosc Clin. 2016;26(1):99–118.
36. Buttazzoni E, Gregori D, Paoli B, Soriani N, Baldas S, Rodriguez H, et al. Symptoms associated with button batteries injuries in children: an epidemiological review. Int J Pediatr Otorhinolaryngol. 2015;29(15):2200–7.
37. Jatana KR, Litovitz T, Reilly JS, Koltai PJ, Rider G, Jacobs IN. Pediatric button battery injuries: 2013 task force update. Int J Pediatr Otorhinolaryngol. 2013;77(9):1392–9.
38. Center NCP. Fatal button battery ingestions: 41 reported cases. 2015; case data on BBI fatalities to date. http://www.poison.org. Accessed 15 June 2015.
39. Maves MD, Lloyd TV, Carithers JS. Radiographic identification of ingested disk batteries. Pediatr Radiol. 1986;16(2):154–6.
40. Lee JH, Lee JH, Shim JO, Lee JH, Eun B-L, Yoo KH. Foreign body ingestion in children: should button batteries in the stomach be urgently removed? Pediatr Gastroenterol Hepatol Nutr. 2016;19(1):20–8.
41. Snow JB Jr. In: Ballenger's manual of otorhinolaryngology head and neck surgery; 2003.

42. Thabet MH, Basha WM, Askar S. Button battery foreign bodies in children: hazards, management, and recommendations. Biomed Res Int. 2013;2013:7.
43. Litovitz T, Whitaker N, Clark L, White NC, Marsolek M. Emerging battery-ingestion hazard: clinical implications. Pediatrics. 2010;125(6):1168–77.
44. Brumbaugh DE, Colson SB, Sandoval JA, Karrer FM, Bealer JF, Litovitz T, et al. Management of button battery-induced hemorrhage. J Pediatr Gastroenterol Nutr. 2011;52(5):585–9.
45. Ruhl DS, Cable BB, Rieth KK. Emergent treatment of button batteries in the esophagus: evolution of management and need for close second-look esophagoscopy. Ann Otol Rhinol Laryngol. 2014;123(3):206–13.
46. Alfa-Wali M, Atinga A, Tanham M, Iqbal Q, Meng A-Y, Mohsen Y. Assessment of the management outcomes of body packers. ANZ J Surg. 2016;86(10):821–5.
47. Traub SJ, Hoffmann RS, Nelson LS. Body packing- the international concealment of illicit drugs. New Engl J Med. 2003;349:2519.
48. Goldberg JE, Scott RS. Rectal foreign bodies. Surg Clin N Am. 2010;90:173–84.
49. Dl C, Buccimazza I, Anderson FA, et al. Colorectal foreign bodies. Color Dis. 2005;7:98.
50. Berghoff KR, Franklin ME Jr. Laparoscopic-assisted rectal foreign body removal: report of a case. Dis Colon Rectum. 2000;48:1975.
51. Lake JP, Essani R, Petrone P, et al. Management of colorectal retained foreign bodies: predictors of operative intervention. Dis Colon Rectum. 2004;47:1694.
52. Kerlin P, Jones D, Remedios M, Campbell C. Prevalence of eosinophilic esophagitis in adults with food bolus obstruction of the esophagus. J Clin Gastroenterol. 2007;41:356–61.
53. Guelfguat M, Kaplinsky V, Reddy SH, DiPoce J. Clinical guidelines for imaging and reporting ingested foreign bodies. AJR. 2014;203:37–53.
54. Wright CC, Closson FT. Updates in pediatric gastrointestinal foreign bodies. Pediatr Clin N Am. 2013;60:1221–39.
55. Betalli P, Rossi A, Bini M, Bacis G, Borrelli O, Cutrone C, et al. Update on management of caustic and foreign body ingestion in children. Diagn Ther Endosc. 2009;2009:969868.

Updates in the Management of Anorectal Abscess and Inflammatory or Thrombotic Process

42

Andreas Ommer, Markus Noll, and Alois Fürst

Key Points

- The incidence of anal abscess is relatively high. They are most common in young men. The abscess usually originates from the proctodeal glands of the intersphincteric space. A distinction is made between subanodermal, intersphincteric, ischio-anal, and supralevator abscesses.
- The patient history and clinical examination are diagnostically sufficient to establish the indication for surgery. Further examinations (endosonography, MRI) should be considered in case of recurrent abscesses or supralevator abscesses.
- Any anal abscess should be treated surgically. The goal of surgery is thorough drainage of the suppurative focus while preserving the sphincter anatomical structures. Time of surgery depends on clinical symptoms (esp. pain, inflammation).
- Intraoperative fistula exploration demands a surgical team's full attention. Excessive examination to confirm a fistula is not recommended. Primary fistulotomy should only be performed (1) in superficial fistulas and (2) by experienced surgeons. In case of unclear findings or high fistulas, repair should be performed during a second procedure. Overall, the risk of abscess recurrence or secondary fistula formation is low. These conditions may result from insufficient drainage.
- Acne inversa originates from hair follicles. It has a chronic progressive course of disease and usually results in abscess and fistula.
- Currently, radical surgical excision is the only therapy allowing long-term healing.
- Hemorrhoidal thrombosis usually occurs acutely and is usually very painful. Possible causes may be constipation as well as increased straining during bowel movement.
- Anal prolapse with thrombosis should be treated conservatively. Nevertheless, in recent segmental thrombosis, the course of disease can be reduced by excision of thrombosed external hemorrhoids under local anesthetics at an early stage.
- Acute abscess may be a first clinical manifestation of pilonidal sinus. At an acute stage, local limited drainage of the abscess should be performed. Extensive drainage is not indicated.
- After resolution of the acute inflammation of pilonidal sinus long-term healing can be achieved by elective surgery. Plastic procedures with "off-midline" closure should be preferred due to a reduced healing period and the lower rate of recurrence.

Abscess and thrombosis of the hemorrhoidal veins are common causes of anorectal emergencies. Whereas nearly any kind of abscess requires immediate surgical treatment, thrombosis can be managed by conservative treatment in most cases. In this section, we present diagnostics and treatment of different kinds of anorectal suppurations (anal abscess, acne inversa, and abscess in pilonidal sinus) and thrombosis (hemorrhoids, anal veins)

The original version of this chapter was revised. A correction to this chapter can be found at https://doi.org/10.1007/978-3-319-95114-0_59

A. Ommer (✉)
End- und Dickdarm-Zentrum Essen, Essen, Germany

M. Noll · A. Fürst
Caritas-Krankenhaus St. Josef, Regensburg, Germany
e-mail: mnoll@caritasstjosef.de; afuerst@caritasstjosef.de

P. Aseni et al. (eds.), *Operative Techniques and Recent Advances in Acute Care and Emergency Surgery*,
https://doi.org/10.1007/978-3-319-95114-0_42

42.1 Anal Abscess

Anal abscess, together with its chronic form of anal fistula, is a common disease with a relative high incidence of about 2 cases per 10,000 inhabitants per year. It is most likely to occur between the ages of 30 and 50 [1]. Men are more likely to be affected than women [2].

42.1.1 Etiology and Classification

The inner circular muscle of the rectal wall descends into the anal canal, where it becomes the internal sphincter (Fig. 42.1) [3]. This is encircled by an outer funnel of muscular tissue that is composed of the levator, puborectalis, and external sphincter muscles. These two layers are separated by the intersphincteric plane, a fibrous extension of the outer longitudinal muscle layer of the rectum as it extends down into the anal canal. The anal verge is the demarcation between the skin of the anal margin and the anoderm. The anoderm is specialized squamous epithelium, which, although devoid of secondary skin appendages such as hair follicles and sweat glands, has a rich vascular supply and is highly innervated. Midway up the anal canal lies the dentate line (pectinate line). This marks the true mucocutaneous junction between somatically innervated squamous epithelium distally and the viscerally innervated columnar epithelium proximally [3]. Seminal work by Parks and Eisenhammer identified anal glands present at the level of the dentate line and showed that these glands are the etiology of most perirectal abscesses and fistulas [4]. The number of glands varies; they are more frequently found posteriorly [5, 6] and more are found in men than in women [7].

Cryptoglandular abscesses initially originate in the intersphincteric space. From there, they can expand directly toward the perianal region and present as subanodermal or subcutaneous abscesses. An abscess that breaks through the sphincter ani externus muscle results in ischioanal abscess, previously referred to as ischiorectal abscess and the proximal extension into the pelvirectal fossa gives rise to supralevator abscess. A distinction is made between four types of abscess depending on its origin (Fig. 42.2) [9]:

1. Subanodermal abscess
2. Intersphincteric abscess
3. Ischioanal abscess
4. Supralevator abscess

The incidence of the individual types varies, with superficial types being much more common (Table 42.1).

These abscesses contain a mixed flora of intestinal bacteria (especially *E. coli*, Bacteroides) and skin-dwelling bacteria (*Staphylococcus aureus*). However, their differen-

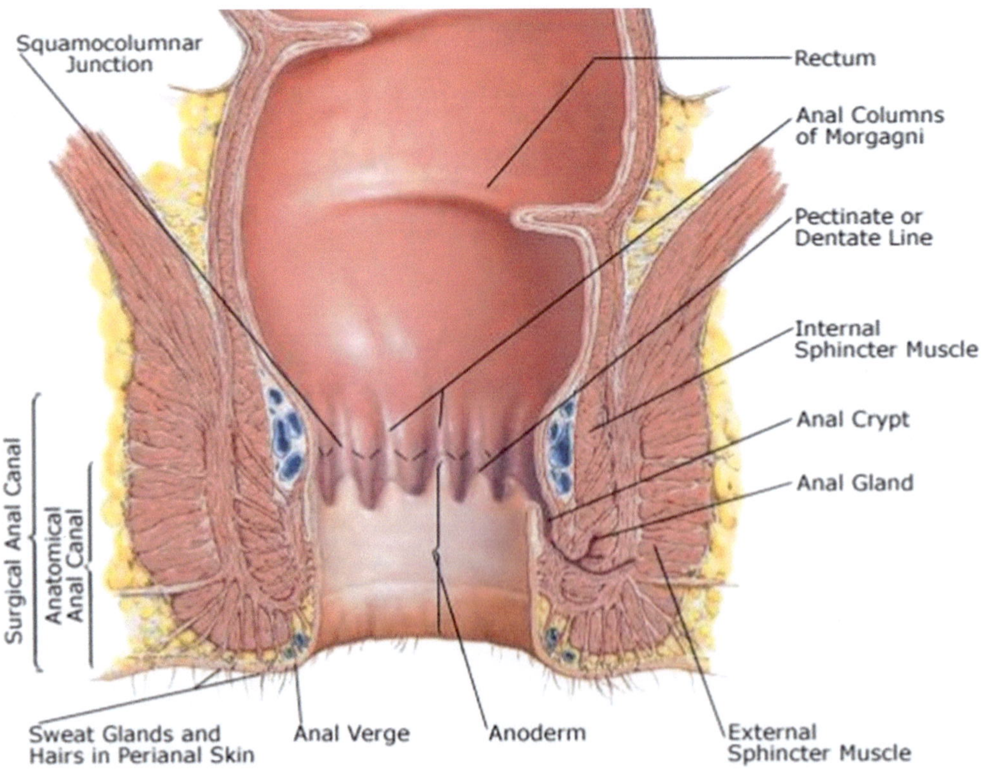

Fig. 42.1 Anatomy of the perianal region

tiation is not relevant for treatment purposes. Special kinds of abscesses are associated with MRSA colonization, tuberculosis, actinomycosis, gonorrhea or caused by foreign body ingestion.

The most relevant different diagnosis is between pilonidal sinus and acne inversa, which may also present in a form of acute abscesses. Abscesses in the course of inflammatory bowel diseases (e.g. Crohn's disease) [16, 17], immunocompromising diseases (e.g. HIV, leukemia) and malignant tumors [18] as well as after pelvic surgery (e.g. laparoscopic anterior resection of the rectum) or injuries [19] constitute special forms.

Smoking, diabetes mellitus, obesity, and alcohol [20, 21] but also some lifestyle factors like spending a large time on sitting, less movement, straining during bowel movement [22] and psychosocial stress [23] are discussed in literature as risk factors for abscess or fistula formation.

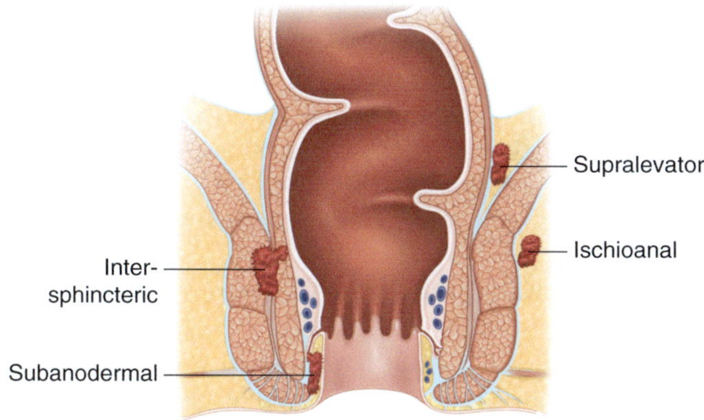

Fig. 42.2 Classification of anal abscesses. Reproduced with permission of Springer Ed. from Ommer A, Herold A, Berg E, Farke S, et al. *S3-Leitlinie Analabszess*. coloproctology (2011) 33: 378–392 [8]

42.1.2 Symptoms and Diagnosis

The symptoms of anal abscess include painful swelling and possible reddening with acute onset within only a few days in the anal region. The diagnosis is mainly based on clinical examination (Fig. 42.3). Perianal redness and warmness are often found in perianal and ischioanal abscesses. Induration can be confirmed by palpation. Especially in intersphincteric abscesses, induration can only be confirmed by bidigital palpation/rectal examination.

Because of the pain involved, rectal examinations should be kept to a minimum. Proctoscopy and rectoscopy supply little additional information and may cause severe pain. Preoperative advanced diagnostics, particularly imaging, is not required in most cases.

Table 42.1 Frequency of the different types of cryptoglandular abscesses

	Abcarian [10] $n = 93$	Ramanujan [11] $n = 1023$	Weber [12] $n = 79$	Athanasiadis [13] $n = 127$	Ommer [14] $n = 323$	Knoefel [15] $n = 323$
Submucosal	4.3%	5.8%	–	–	–	–
Subanodermal (former "perianal")	61%	42.7%	67%	62.3%	39%	1%
Intersphincteric	14%	21.4%	17%	14.7%	35%	71%
Ischioanal (former "ischiorectal")	14%	22.8%	5%	9.1%	19%	22%
Supralevator	2.1%	7.3%	6%	6.5%	7%	6%
Combination	4.5%	–	–	7.4%	–	–

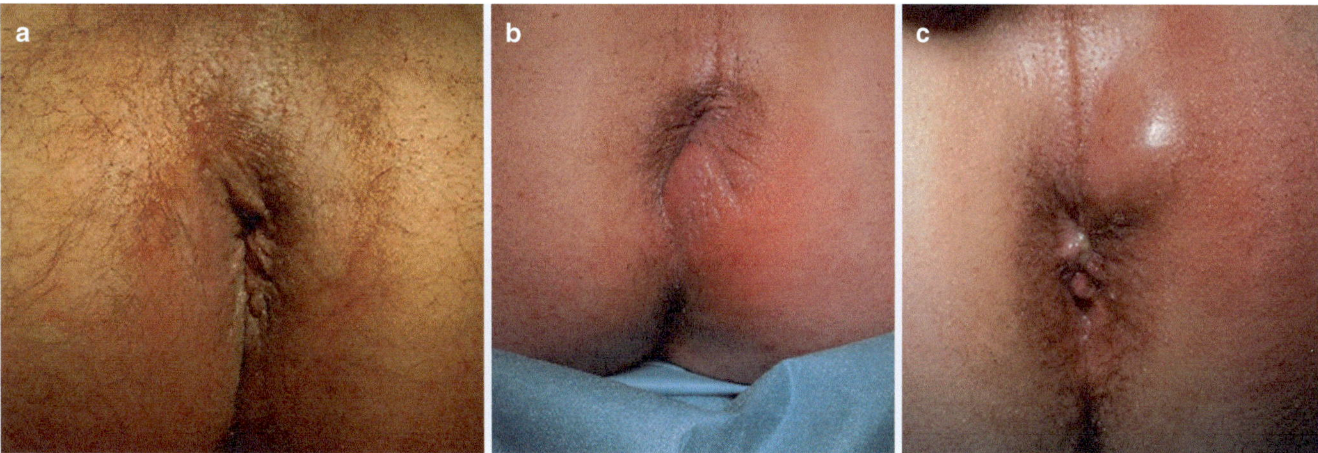

Fig. 42.3 Clinical appearance of anal abscess. (**a**) High intersphincteric abscess at 6.oo, (**b**) intersphincteric abscess at 5.oo, (**c**) ischioanal abscess at 2.oo

Supralevator abscess is a different clinical problem, as inspection does not provide any information. Patients often experience general symptoms such as fever and malaise. In these cases, rectal palpation often reveals an induration or even a fluctuation. Patients typically experience dull pain in the lesser pelvis or back pain [24]. In case of unclear findings, endosonography, computed tomography (CT), or magnetic resonance imaging (MRI) can help localize the abscess (Fig. 42.4) [25–28].

Laboratory diagnostics provides only indirect information for indication of diagnosis. High inflammation parameters (leucocytes, C-reactive protein) in combination with clinical history may indicate a supralevator abscess.

Before surgical intervention, sphincter function should be assessed via an accurate medical history and, if applicable, by evaluating the incontinence score, particularly in view of possible primary fistulotomy. Manometry does not provide additional information and is not diagnostically valuable, particularly in the stage of acute abscess.

In supralevator abscesses, inspection will not provide significant information. Common symptoms are fever and malaise. Palpation will identify indurations or fluctuations. Dull pains in the lesser pelvis or lumbalgia are typical symptoms [29].

Further procedures are performed intraoperatively under anesthesia. They include inspection of the anal canal to confirm or exclude internal fistula opening. The area may be carefully probed using a curved probe, but extensive examination is not recommended. Endosonography allows localization of the abscess, so that the best route of surgical access can be chosen, particularly in case of supralevator abscesses.

In summary, anal abscess is diagnosed using clinical signs and symptoms, inspection, and palpation. Imaging diagnostics should be considered only in case of supralevator abscess or recurrent abscess.

42.1.3 Treatment

42.1.3.1 Surgical Indication

Anal abscess should be treated surgically, with clinical signs and symptoms determining the timing of the surgical intervention. The purpose of the treatment is to decompress the abscess cavity to prevent progressive inflammation with potentially life-threatening complications (e.g. pelvic sepsis or Fournier gangrene [30]) (Fig. 42.5).

While acute abscess is an emergency, surgical intervention is also recommended in case of spontaneous perforation, since insufficient drainage may cause abscess recurrence or fistula formation.

Conservative treatment options, particularly antibiotic treatment, are unlikely to be successful and are not considered appropriate. Abscess smears are unnecessary, as their microbiological results are clinically irrelevant in most cases.

42.1.3.2 Abscess Drainage Technique

The surgical technique depends on the type of abscess. Generally, abscess surgery is performed under general or regional anaesthesia.

In subanodermal and ischioanal abscesses, surgeons should do a perianal excision in order to remove an oval-shaped section of tissue. The incision should run parallel to the fibers of the sphincter ani externus muscle.

Access to intersphincteric abscesses varies according to their location. For abscesses that are entirely intra-anal and feature a connection to the anal canal, transanal drainage, possibly with internal sphincterotomy, is recommended. For subanodermal abscesses, the suitable surgical approach is perianal access with or without fistulotomy.

Drainage of a supralevator abscess can be performed via a transrectal or perianal approach. Endosonography is the most important diagnostic procedure, as it can show whether the muscle plate of the levator ani muscle is intact.

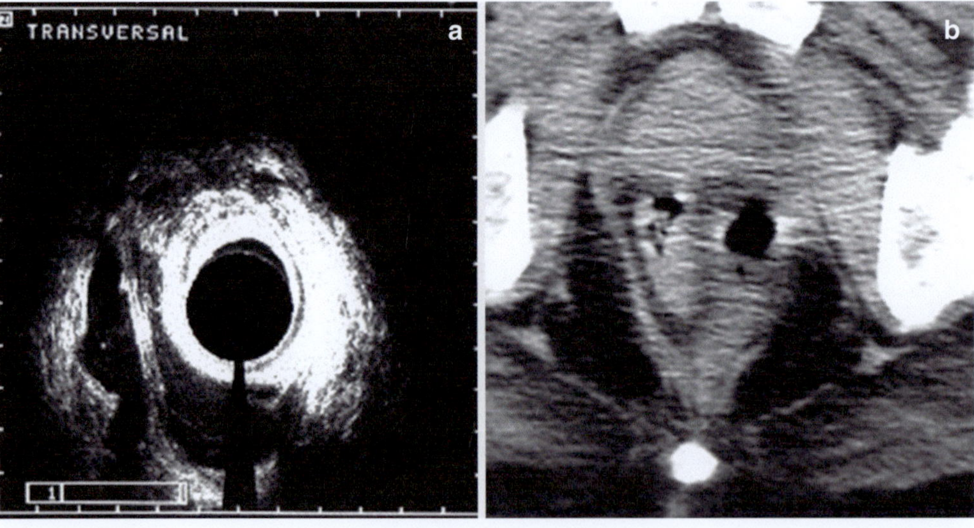

Fig. 42.4 Endosonography (**a**) and computer tomography (**b**) of an anal abscess

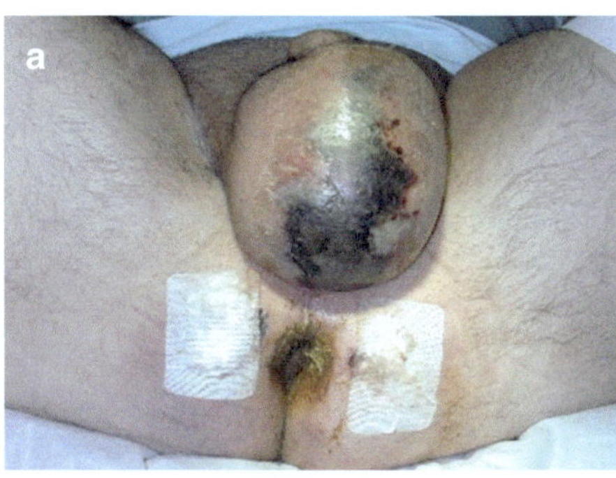

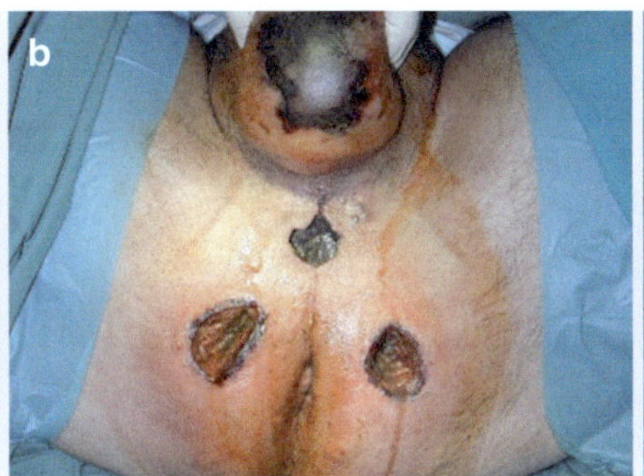

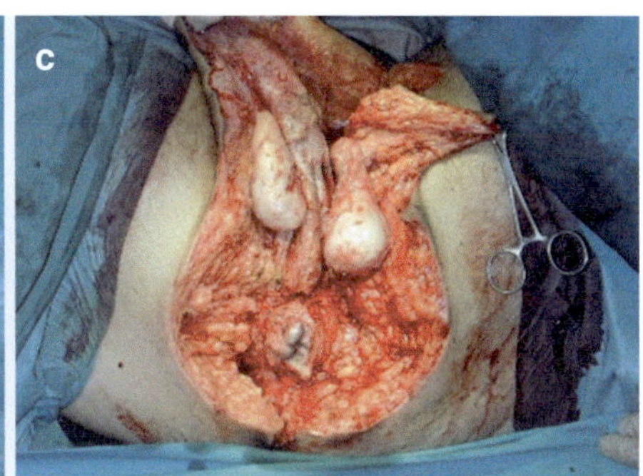

Fig. 42.5 Fournier gangrene. (**a**) Praeop, (**b**) intraop, (**c**) after excision of the necrotic tissue

If the levator ani muscle is intact and the abscess is limited to the pelvirectal fossa, transrectal drainage can be performed to prevent fistula formation.

If the abscess has already broken through the levator ani muscle into the ischioanal fossa, transischioanal drainage is performed. It is important to provide a long-term open route for drainage of the abscess cavity. A drain (e.g. Penrose, Easyflow, or similar) may be put in place for a few days if necessary. Sufficient drainage of anal abscesses is therefore important to prevent recurrence and fistula formation. In case of extensive abscess, generous criteria should be applied when determining the indication for revision under anesthesia. Insufficient drainage [31, 32] and late drainage [33] can cause early recurrence.

Horseshoe abscesses represent a special form of abscess. In most cases, it is located dorsally and involves both ischioanal fossae [34, 35].

The goal of surgical intervention is the thorough drainage of the inflammatory tissue without relevant damage to the adjacent healthy structures, particularly the sphincter apparatus. A flow chart for the treatment of anal abscess and fistula is shown in Fig. 42.6. From that point of view, incontinence following abscess surgery alone is rare, and can be largely prevented by a sphincter-preserving procedure [36].

42.1.3.3 Indications for Primary Fistula Repair

The available literature indicates that fistulas identified in the context of abscess incision do not always require follow-up surgery. Moreover, the fistula may spontaneously close after thorough draining [14, 29, 37].

On the other hand, intraoperative proof of fistula also depends on the localization of the abscess, as the expansion of the infection in the intersphincteric space will determine the layout [8] of the fistula (Table 42.2).

A total of five randomized studies compare excision alone with primary fistulotomy [38–42]. They indicate that primary fistulotomy reduces revision rates but is associated with a higher rate of incontinence. Unfortunately, none of the studies specifies the type of treated fistulas. It seems even more significant, however, that the majority of patients whose fistula was left in place did not undergo another surgical procedure, which suggests that spontaneous healing is possible.

In superficial fistulas, primary fistulotomy appears useful to prevent recurrence and to spare the patients, who are usually young, a second procedure [43]. As described for anal fistula, however, the incontinence rate increases with the amount of sphincter muscle that has been divided and with the number of previous interventions. In this context, it is important to note that abscess excision is often performed as an emergency procedure and by less experienced surgeons, so that the decision about fistulotomy should be left to experienced surgeons in the context of a second procedure. In cases with known complex fistula, insertion of a Seton drain can achieve good drainage and prepare the fistula canal for a second procedure under elective conditions. The placement of a Seton doesn't allow to neglect sufficient surgical drainage (Fig. 42.7). However, the literature indicates that a relevant portion of the confirmed fistulas closes spontaneously. The value of a Seton drain has not been definitively determined. Current publications [44–46], some of which are the subject of lively debate, do not indicate any advantage in favour of the placement of a Seton drain successful closure of the anorectal fistula.

Abscesses based on inflammatory bowel diseases (IBD) (e.g. Crohn's disease) represent a special category. The extents of inflammatory transformations (including rectal mucosa) as well as prior incidents comprising scarring, stenosis or sphincter defects have to be considered. Atypical abscess localizations as well as atypical fistula layouts are common. Especially in cases of intense inflammation and high disease activity, it may be difficult to realize sphincter-preserving fistula therapy. Partial transection of the sphincter muscle should be avoided by all means. Because of the high

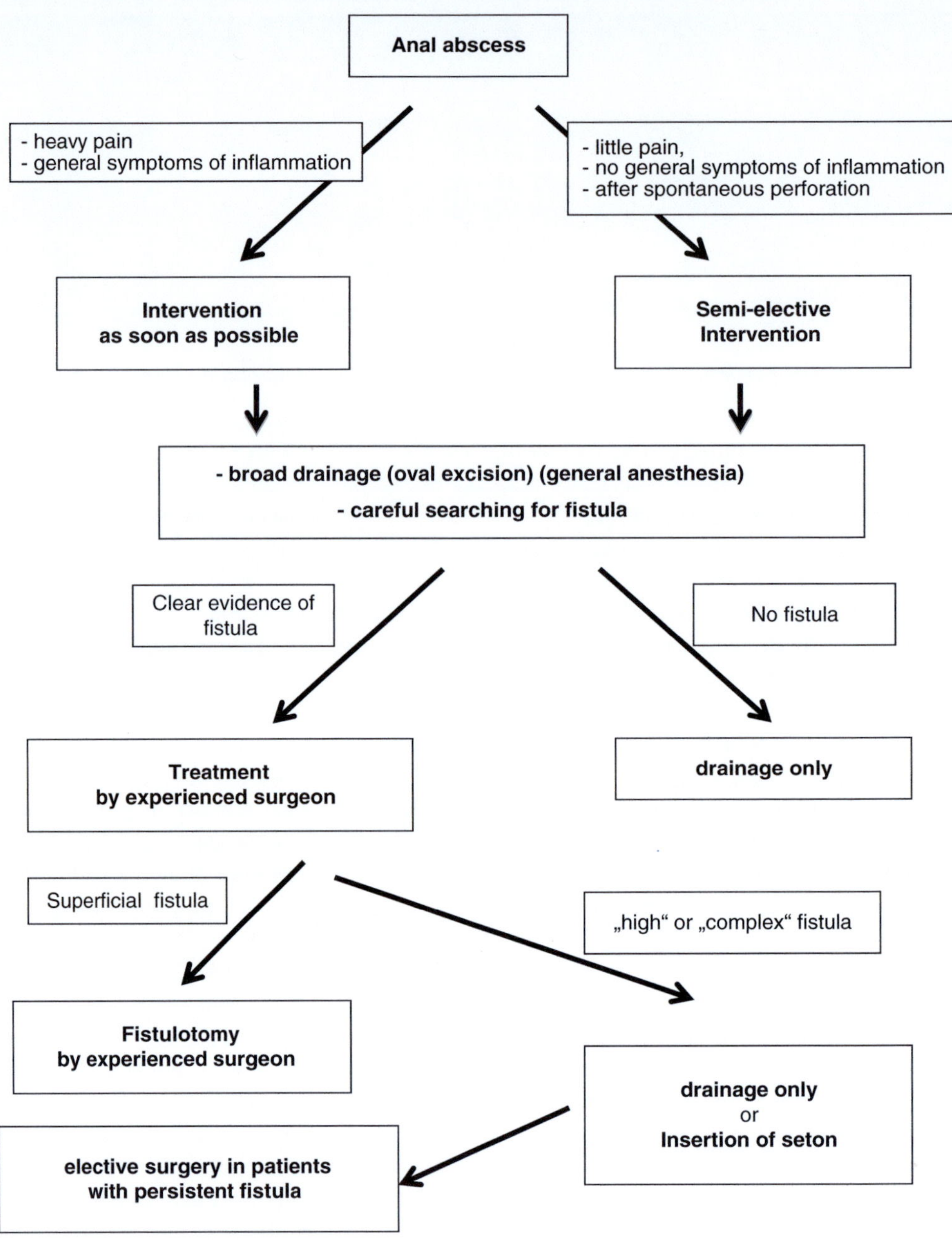

Fig. 42.6 Evidence-based therapies in patients with anal abscess

Table 42.2 Frequency of abscesses and fistulas following surgical therapy of anal abscesses [14]

Localisation of the abscess	Intersphinktere ic fistulas (%)	Transsphincteric fistulas (%)	Suprasphincteric fistulas (%)	Not classificable fistulas (%)	Incidence of fistulas (%)	Recurrent abscess (%)
Subanodermal	2.5	3.4	0	1.7	7.6	7.3
Intersphinkteric	2.9	1.4	1.4	0	5.7	8.0
Ischioanal	0	23.5	0	2.9	26.4	10.9
Supralevator	0	12.5	6.3	0	18.8	25

recurrence rate, placement of Seton drains should be generously considered. It may also serve as long-term therapy.

In summary, superficial fistulas, which perforate only small parts of the anal sphincter, should be treated with primary fistulotomy performed by experienced surgeons. There is no real definition of "experienced surgeon". In our opinion, an experienced surgeon is defined as one who has treated at least 100 fistulas. Nevertheless, every division of parts of

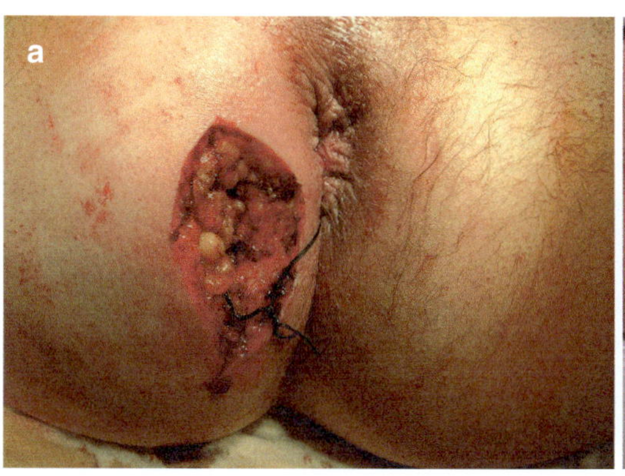

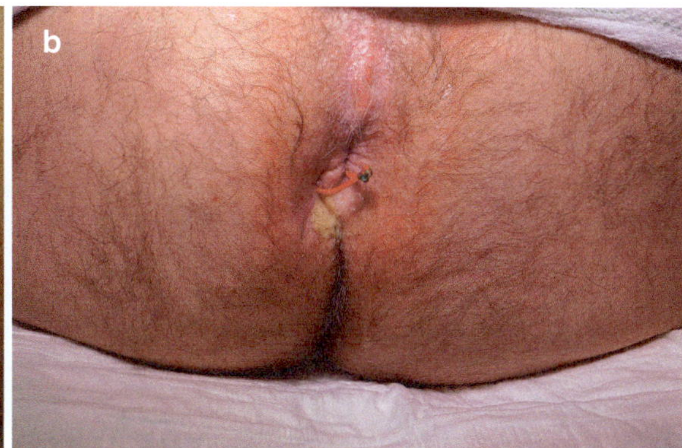

Fig. 42.7 (**a**) Drained large ischioanal abscess with placement of seton through the transsphincteric fistula, (**b**) insufficient drainage of a high ischioanal abscess in spite of seton placement

the anal sphincter bears the risk of fecal incontinence. In case of unclear findings or high and complex fistulas that enclosed large parts of the sphincter or are recurrent, repair should be performed in a second procedure (see Fig. 42.6).

42.1.3.4 Incidence of Confirmed Secondary Fistula

In addition to abscess recurrence, the development of an anal fistula that requires another intervention is the most common sequela to abscess surgery. According to the literature, only some of the abscesses result in development of a chronic fistula [37, 47, 48]. One literature review reports chronic fistulas in 7–66% of cases (median 16%) and abscesses in 4–31% of cases (median 13%) [49].

The rate of confirmed secondary fistulas depends on the location of the abscess. Sözener et al. [48], for instance, found anal fistula following 14% of cases of subanodermal abscess, 35% of intersphincteric abscess and 60% of ischioanal abscess.

In summary, the rate of abscess recurrence and chronic fistulas is relatively low. That means that only a small portion of abscesses leads to chronic fistulas. The probability of fistula development is a function of abscess location. In subanodermal or intersphincteric anal abscesses, fistulas are rare and predominantly superficial, but the rate of complex fistulas is distinctly higher in ischioanal and supralevator abscesses [14]. Incidence depends on the abscess type and can reach up to 40% in ischioanal and supralevator abscesses [15, 40, 42, 50].

Therefore, extensive fistula exploration is not recommended in the initial procedure.

42.1.3.5 Perioperative Management

Specific bowel preparation is not required and would be impossible in most cases because of the patient's pain.

The procedure is usually performed under general or regional anesthesia, in order to enable an adequate excision. Local anesthesia cannot be performed in many cases because of the inflammation. Moreover, general or regional anesthesia enables a pain-free examination of the anal canal when searching for fistulas.

Postoperative care following anal surgery is trouble-free. The external wound should be rinsed regularly and heals by secondary intention. Clear water is best for this purpose, particularly since antiseptic solutions are associated with a risk of cytotoxicity.

Regular wound packing is not required [51]. However, the external opening of the drainage may not be allowed to close prematurely.

The value of accompanying antibiotic treatment has not yet been sufficiently determined [47, 48, 52–55]. In general, however, antibiotic treatment appears to be indicated in exceptional cases only (immune deficiency, serious phlegmonous inflammation,or in patients with prosthetic cardiac valve or valvular disease or recent organ transplantation).

42.2 Acne Inversa

Acne inversa, also called Hidradenitis Suppurativa in English, is a chronic skin disease. It mainly affects the perianal region, but also the axilla and other intertriginous areas. Similar to anal abscesses, it can become manifest as an acute abscess, but chronic inflammations are much more common. Due to its etiology, there is no connection to the anal canal. Persons concerned mainly suffer from pain, secretion, and repeated surgeries; especially in cases of considerable findings [56].

42.2.1 Etiology

Acne inversa is believed to originate from the glands of hair follicles [57]. Occlusion of an excretory duct results in both granulomatous inflammation of the connective tissue as well as formation of subcutaneous nodules, fistulas, fibrosis, and abscesses [56, 58–61]. Nicotine abuse is the most important predisposing factor. Abstention usually results in amelioration of the symptoms. Obesity and genetic factors represent other risk factors [62, 63]. Mechanical irritation of the skin in conjunction with a warm microclimate also promotes acne inversa [64]. The disease can occur at every age, but mostly young adults are affected [56].

42.2.2 Diagnosis

Clinical signs comprise pain and subcutaneous indurations, which are tender on palpation, and may exhibit malodorous purulent secretion (Fig. 42.8). As a sign of chronic course, clinical signs may also comprise scarred lines from prior inflammations. Apart from examination, there are usually no other relevant diagnostic measures. The inflammation can be classified according to Hurley (Table 42.3).

Table 42.3 Hurley's staging system of Acne inversa (based on [58])

Stage I	Solitary or multiple abscesses without fistula and without scarring Prevalence 68%
Stage II	Recurrent isolated abscesses with single or multiple fistulae as well as scarring and strands Prevalence 28%
Stage III	Disseminated affections with multiple scarred strands as well as abscesses in the entire area. Prevalence 4%

42.2.3 Treatment

Without treatment the course of acne inversa is progressive. Therefore, in cases of considerable findings, treatment is strongly recommended. Spontaneous remission is unlikely.

Acute abscesses are mostly located subcutaneously, so that remission following spontaneous perforation is likely to happen. Therefore, emergency surgeries are less common in acne inversa than in perianal abscesses.

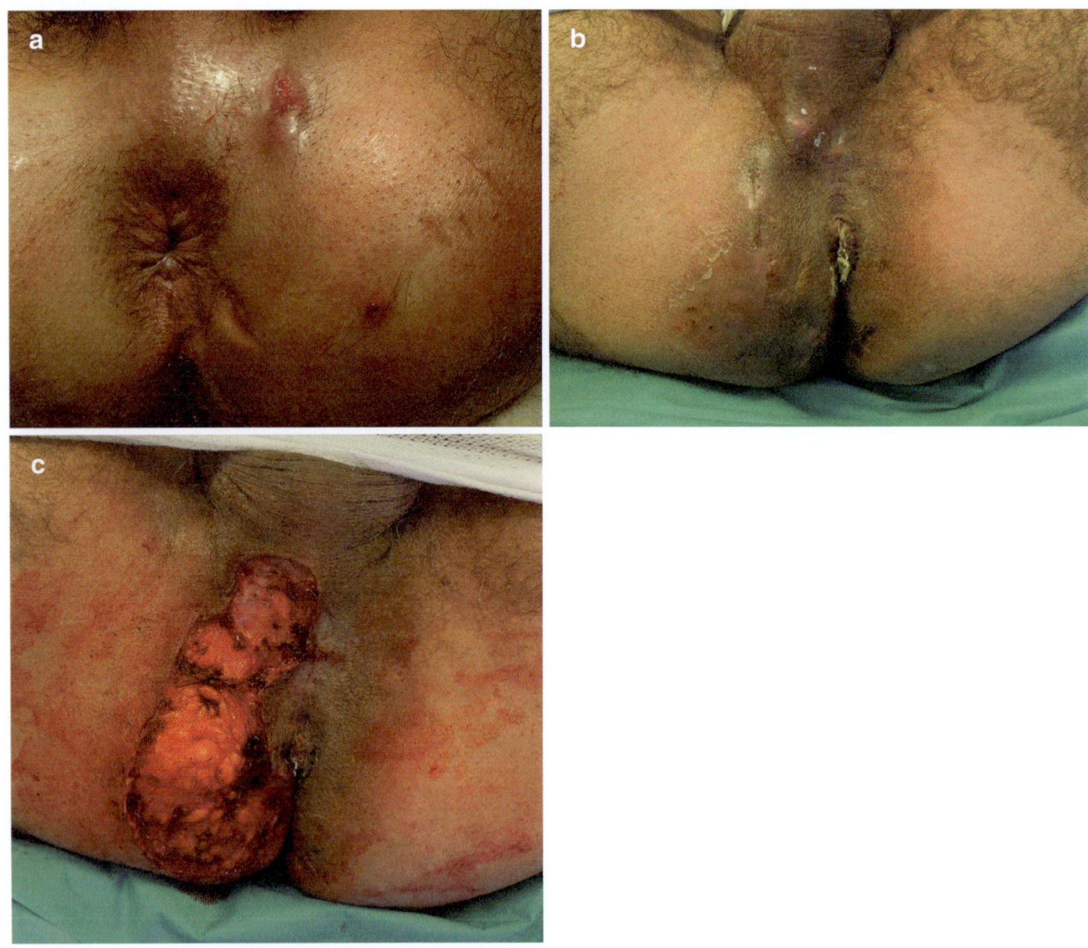

Fig. 42.8 Acne inversa. (**a**) Acne inversa with small area of included tissue, (**b**) wide-spreaded acne inversa, (**c**) after complete resection

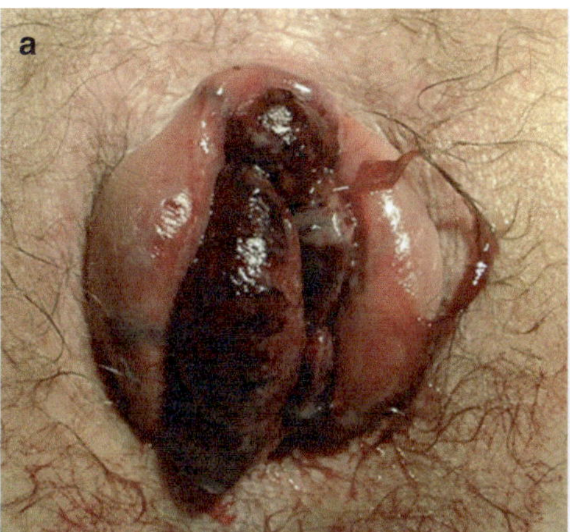

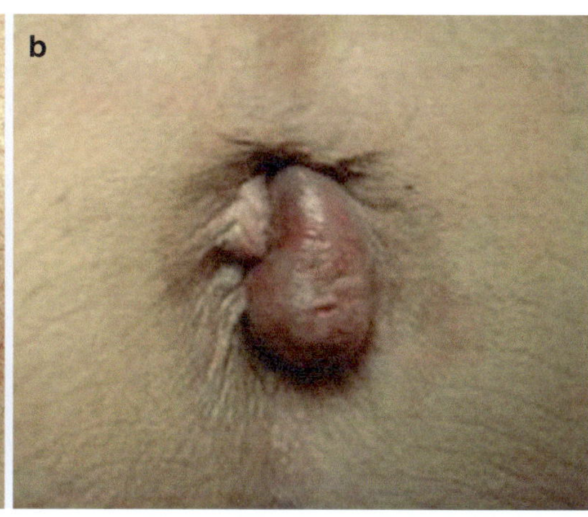

Fig. 42.9 Thrombosed hemorrhoidal prolapse (**a**) and anal vein thrombosis (**b**)

Symptoms can be relieved by different conservative therapy options [65]. In patients antibiotically treated, possible antimicrobial resistances have to be considered [66, 67]. According to current literature, complete remission can only be achieved by radical surgical excision (Fig. 42.8c) [56, 58, 68]. At stage III or higher, radical surgical excision is indicated, even though wound healing might be prolonged. Limited surgical treatment is associated with a higher recurrence rate. Therefore, even small findings should be excised completely. Incision only is not indicated. Especially in the anogenital region, exposure to the air will speed wound healing [68]. Depending on clinical symptoms, the date of surgery can usually be chosen electively. In most cases, radical excision is not reasonable in stages of acute abscess.

42.3 Hemorrhoidal- and Anal Thrombosis

In general common hemorrhoids do not cause pain. Typical discomfort is caused by irritation of the perianal skin by moistening, itching or burning. Enlarged hemorrhoid tissue may cause diffuse rectal pressure pain. Usually, only acute thrombosis is painful. Acute thrombosis is an emergency. Nevertheless, it is only treated marginally in literature and guidelines [69, 70].

42.3.1 Etiology

Thrombosed hemorrhoids are caused by stasis in the hemorrhoidal plexus. It may be caused by increased sphincter tone, as the blood vessels pass through it. Arteries have thicker walls than veins; therefore, veins may be compressed while blood flow in arteries is still active. Blood then starts to retain and to clot. Predisposing factors are constipation in association with squeezing, as well as stress or physical strain.

42.3.2 Diagnosis

Diagnosis is based upon clinical history. Usually, patients complain of acute painful swelling in the anal region (Fig. 42.9). Further diagnosis is done by clinical examination. Broader measures are often limited due to the patient's pain. Endoscopic assessment should be performed by a thin proctoscope in order to exclude a rectal process or inflammation. Two types of thrombosis can be differentiated: thrombosis of the hemorrhoidal tissue (Fig. 42.8a) and thrombosis of the peripheral veins (Fig. 42.8b). Nevertheless, transition between the two categories is usually smooth.

42.3.3 Treatment

While surgical treatment is not indicated in acute thrombosed internal hemorrhoids, surgical treatment (Milligan-Morgan) may be considered in little and segmental thrombosis of single hemorrhoidal node. The aim of the surgical treatment is the excision of the painful tense node. Generally, this can be performed under regional anesthesia [71–73]. The patients benefit from surgical treatment especially in the early phase (first 2–3 days) and in cases of findings of large thrombosed hemorrhoid, as the time until complete remission of the thrombosis as well as the recurrence rate are reduced [70, 72, 74, 75]. It needs to be mentioned that in any case, complete remission can also be achieved without surgery [75]. Therefore, the decision about whether or not to perform surgery needs to be taken according to the patient's individual pain. In case of surgical treatment, complete excision of the prolapsed segment should be performed; not only incision. This can be performed under regional anesthesia [70]. In case of incomplete excision or incision, recurrence rates as well as development of skin folds are significantly increased.

A thrombosed anal prolapse should always be treated conservatively in the first phase. Significant prolapse can be found especially in patients with advanced hemorrhoids [76]. Apart from generous analgesia (especially nonsteroidal anti-inflammatory drugs (NSAIDs)), topical treatments should be used (local anesthetics, cortisone, hip bath) [71]. Nitrates or Diltiazem can be used for relaxation of the sphincter muscle. In most cases, the prolapse cannot be replaced and should therefore not be tried. Complete remission can usually be achieved by conservative measures. Emergency surgical treatment should be avoided, as further swelling may require a larger resection. This may prolong healing and increase the risk of stenosis [77]. Pain can be relieved by surgery. Surgical treatment of the hemorrhoids may be delayed considering possible risks [78] and acute symptoms. Symptoms may also be significantly relieved by fibrosis associated with thrombosis; therefore further treatment can be considered among conservative approaches [71].

42.4 Pilonidal Abscess

Despite the numerous publications during the last eight decades, considerable discrepancies in the treatment of patients with pilonidal disease still exist all around the world. In 2014, German Evidence- and Consensus-based Guidelines have been published for the treatment of pilonidal sinus disease [79, 80].

42.4.1 Etiology

The incidence of pilonidal sinus is 26/100,000 persons [81]. It is assumed to be acquired during adolescence [82], and there might also be a genetical predisposition [83–85]. It seems to be caused by multifactorial events: rubbing movements of the intergluteal cleft are screwing the root side of hairs into the skin, resulting in cavities (so-called sinus or pits) which may contain hair. Hair fragments may penetrate into the skin as barb hook [86], reaching the subcutaneous fat tissue [83]. In this layer, foreign body granuloma develops. They do not heal spontaneously (asymptomatic form), but may result in infection (abscessing and chronic form) [86]. Risk factors are intense hair-growth [81, 87], obesity [88], excessive sweating, and excessive sitting [89–91]. In patients with acute abscess, there can be found fewer sinuses than in patients with a longer duration of illness. This is caused by two factors. Firstly, in acute events, ducts may be closed by swelling. Therefore, they can only be verified in histologic examinations [92]. Secondly, abscessing is less common in pilonidal sinus with fewer sinuses than in pilonidal sinus with multiple sinuses [93]. Prolonged disease does not necessarily result in development of further fistulas and pits [82].

42.4.2 Diagnosis and Classification

Diagnosis of pilonidal sinus is based upon clinical history and clinical examination. Clinical signs are typical, an abscess can usually be identified easily (Fig. 42.10).

In clinical practice, there are three types of manifestation of a pilonidal sinus:

1. Asymptomatic Pilonidal Sinus

   Asymptomatic pilonidal disease is characterized by incidentally detected midline pits causing no complaints to the patient.
2. Acute Pilonidal Abscess

   Acute pilonidal abscess is often a primary manifestation of a pilonidal sinus (Fig. 42.10a). Strong pain might require prompt intervention.
3. Symptomatic Pilonidal Sinus with Fistula

   Chronic pilonidal sinus may exhibit varying numbers of primary or secondary fistulas, which might present purulent secretion (Fig. 42.10b). Patients suffer from pain, secretion and subsequent irritation of the skin.

42.4.3 Treatment

Treatment of an asymptomatic disease does not provide advantages over surgery for symptomatic disease [92] concerning recurrence rate. Also, no spontaneous disease progression had

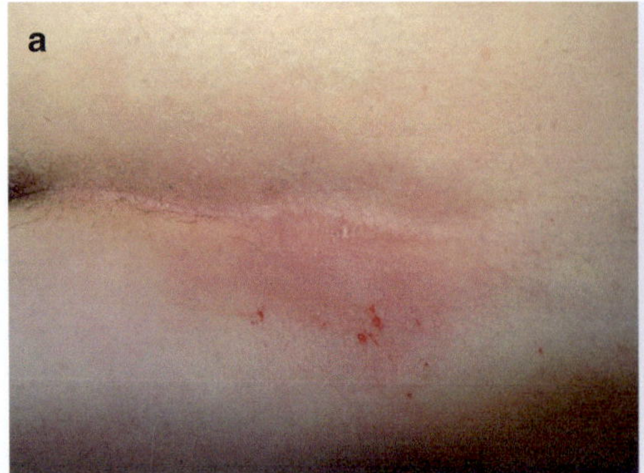

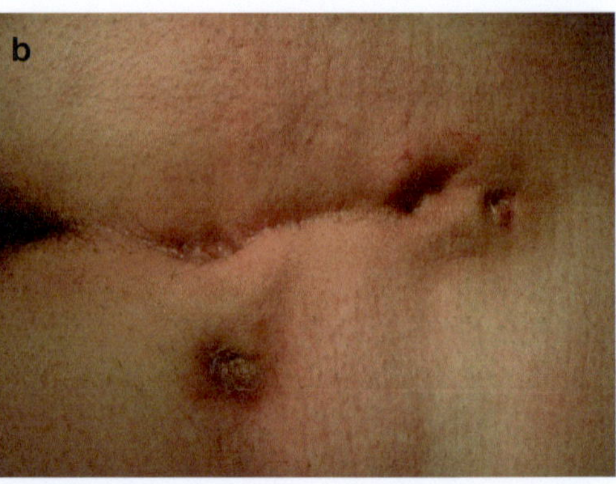

Fig. 42.10 Sinus pilonidalis with acute abscess (**a**) and chronic sinus with fistulization (**b**)

Table 42.4 Summary of recommendations for treatment options in symptomatic pilonidal disease

Subject	Recommendation	Level of evidence	Consensus strength	Grade of recommendation
Treatment of symptomatic and asymptomatic patients	Asymptomatic patients should not undergo any treatment Symptomatic patients should be treated surgically	Low	Strong	
Acute abscess	Incision is preferred for most patients	Low	Strong	
Treatment by phenol	Phenol is not approved for treatment in human beings in Germany due to presumed toxicity	Low	Strong	
Pit picking	Pit picking and similar minimally invasive procedures could be used in patients with limited primary disease	Low	Strong	0
Sinusectomy	A promising minimally invasive procedure, however, the experience is still limited	Low	Strong	
Excision and open wound healing	Prolonged wound healing and delayed return to work as compared to off-midline procedures. The method is simple, and easy reproducible. Thus, open healing should be regarded as standard procedure yet	High	Strong	A
Marsupialisation	Consensus group agreed that marsupialisation should be abandoned due to postoperative pain and unfavorable cosmetic results	Low	Strong	
Midline closure	Midline wound closure should be abandoned due to increased rate of wound dehiscence and high recurrence rate	High	Strong	A
Off-midline procedures	*Off-midline* procedures are associated with lower recurrence rate than midline closure and shorter time to complete wound healing and faster return to work than open healing There are no significant outcome differences between three most frequently used off-midline procedures—Karydakis flap, cleft lift and Limberg flap	High	Strong	A
Rarely used *off-midline* procedures	Results of some rarely used off-midline procedures—V-Y flap, Dufourmentel flap, Z-Plasty—Are comparable to Karydakis flap, cleft lift and Limberg flap	Low	Strong	
Method of anaesthesia	There are no significant differences between surgery under general or regional anaesthesia beyond immediate periprocedural period	Low	Strong	
Antibiotic prophylaxis	A single dose of antibiotic prophylaxis should be given preoperatively	Low	Strong	
Wound drainage	The present data are inconclusive. Hence, no formal recommendation to the use of wound drainage could be made	Low	Strong	0
Postoperative hair removal	Postoperative shaving should not be performed. The use of postoperative laser depilation could not be recommended due to a lack of reliable data	Low	Strong	

been observed in a large-scale observational study [82]. Thus, surgery for asymptomatic disease could not be advocated.

Healing of a perineal sinus can only be archived by surgical intervention. There are several surgical options from minimally invasive treatment (e.g. "Pit picking") to larger interventions with plastic surgery. These options are discussed in actual guidelines [79, 80, 94] (Table 42.4). *Off-midline* procedures are associated with lower recurrence rates than midline closure and shorter time to complete wound healing and faster return to work than open healing. There are no significant outcome differences between three most frequently used off-midline procedures—Karydakis flap, Cleft lift and Limberg flap.

Incision and drainage is indicated in most cases of acute pilonidal abscess, although a needle aspiration followed by antibiotic treatment had been advocated by some authors. As abscesses are often localized subcutaneously, incision using local anesthesia can be performed in many cases. This may lead to immediate relief of pain as well as to reduction of inflammation. Healing does occur in some cases following incision and drainage [95].

In acute stages, radical excision should not be performed in order to avoid large wounds. Only in less extended cases, definitive excision could be performed at the time of primary treatment. Usually, definitive treatment should be conducted after regression of local inflammation, like a chronic pilonidal sinus.

There is a lack of current randomized studies addressing preoperative and/or postoperative antibiotic prophylaxis. A single dose antibiotic prophylaxis is used by most authors and could be recommended empirically.

Case Scenario

A patient reports anal pain since 3 days. This pain is not related to defecation. Examination of the patient exhibits the following clinical signs.

How do you proceed?

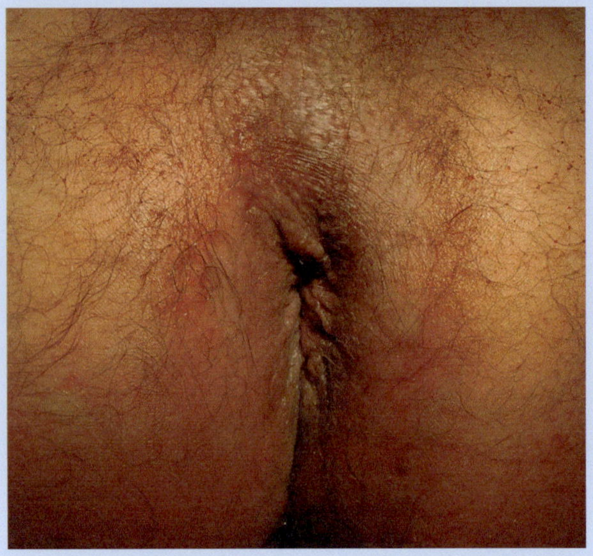

Questions for self-assessment:

1. Which examination is essential?
   A. Rectoskopy
   B. Proctoskoy
   C. Bidigital palpation
   D. Endosonography
2. Which is the treatment of choice in acute anorectal abscess?
   A. Application of local anesthetics
   B. Antibiotic treatment
   C. Regulation of stool consistency
   D. Surgical treatment
3. Which answer is wrong?
   A. Rectoscopy provides only few additional information in anorectal abscesses
   B. Correlation between rectal endosonoghraphy and intraoperative findings are higher than 90%
   C. The abscess should always be treated antibiotically
   D. MRI can provide additional information in recurrent abscesses
4. You are performing an operative treatment of a large ischioanal abscess. Pus is leaking from a fistula in the anal canal. The environment is clearly indurated. The patient is known to have diabetes mellitus. Which treatment may not be performed?
   A. Large drain, no further procedures
   B. Large drain and placement of a Seton drain
   C. It probably is a high anal fistula, therefore primary division with following reconstruction of the sphincter should be performed in order to avoid another surgery
   D. Large drain, antibiotic treatment because of the diabetes mellitus
   E. Drain, placement of a drain in the wound in order to keep the opening unclosed
5. Which is no typical complication following anal abscess surgery?
   A. Local bleeding
   B. Recurrent abscess
   C. Anal incontinence
   D. Urinary retention

Please see Chap. 58 for the correct answer.

References

1. Zanotti C, Martinez-Puente C, Pascual I, Pascual M, et al. An assessment of the incidence of fistula-in-ano in four countries of the European Union. Int J Color Dis. 2007;22:1459–62.
2. Sainio P. Fistula-in-ano in a defined population. Incidence and epidemiological aspects. Ann Chir Gynaecol. 1984;73:219–24.
3. Whiteford MH. Perianal abscess/fistula disease. Clin Colon Rectal Surg. 2007;20:102–9.
4. Klosterhalfen B, Offner F, Vogel P, Kirkpatrick CJ. Anatomic nature and surgical significance of anal sinus and anal intramuscular glands. Dis Colon Rectum. 1991;34:156–60.
5. Abeysuriya V, Salgado LS, Samarasekera DN. The distribution of the anal glands and the variable regional occurrence of fistula-in-ano: is there a relationship? Tech Coloproctol. 2010;14:317–21.
6. Seow-Choen F, Ho JM. Histoanatomy of anal glands. Dis Colon Rectum. 1994;37:1215–8.
7. Lilius HG. Fistula-in-ano, an investigation of human foetal anal ducts and intramuscular glands and a clinical study of 150 patients. Acta Chir Scand Suppl. 1968;383:7–88.
8. Ommer A, Herold A, Berg E, Farke S, et al. S3-Leitlinie Kryptoglanduläre Analfistel. Coloproctology. 2011;33:295–324.
9. Ommer A, Herold A, Berg E, Farke S, et al. S3-leitlinie analabszess. Coloproctology. 2011;33:378–92.
10. Abcarian H. Acute suppurations of the anorectum. Surg Annu. 1976;8:305–33.
11. Ramanujam PS, Prasad ML, Abcarian H, Tan AB. Perianal abscesses and fistulas. A study of 1023 patients. Dis Colon Rectum. 1984;27:593–7.
12. Weber E, Buchmann P. Eröffnung anorectaler Abszesse - mit oder ohne Fistelspaltung. Chirurg. 1982;53:270–2.
13. Athanasiadis S, Fischbach N, Heumuller L, Marla B. Abscessexcision und primare Fistulektomie als Initialtherapie des periproktitischen Abscesses. Eine prospektive Analyse bei 122 Patienten. Chirurg. 1990;61:53–8.
14. Ommer A, Athanasiadis S, Happel M, Köhler A, et al. Die chirurgische Behandlung des anorektalen Abszesses Sinn und Unsinn der primären Fistelsuche. Coloproctology. 1999;21:161–9.

15. Knoefel WT, Hosch SB, Hoyer B, Izbicki JR. The initial approach to anorectal abscesses: fistulotomy is safe and reduces the chance of recurrences. Dig Surg. 2000;17:274–8.
16. Makowiec F, Jehle EC, Becker HD, Starlinger M. Perianal abscess in Crohn's disease. Dis Colon Rectum. 1997;40:443–50.
17. Mardini HE, Schwartz DA. Treatment of perianal fistula and abscess: Crohn's and non-Crohn's. Curr Treat Options Gastroenterol. 2007;10:211–20.
18. Badgwell BD, Chang GJ, Rodriguez-Bigas MA, Smith K, et al. Management and outcomes of anorectal infection in the cancer patient. Ann Surg Oncol. 2009;16:2752–8.
19. Huang WS, Chin CC, Yeh CH, Lin PY, et al. The late onset of an anal abscess caused by a chicken bone that complicated stapled hemorrhoidopexy. Int J Color Dis. 2007;22:1291–2.
20. Devaraj B, Khabassi S, Cosman BC. Recent smoking is a risk factor for anal abscess and fistula. Dis Colon Rectum. 2011;54:681–5.
21. Adamo K, Sandblom G, Brannstrom F, Strigard K. Prevalence and recurrence rate of perianal abscess-a population-based study, Sweden 1997-2009. Int J Color Dis. 2016;31:669–73.
22. Wang D, Yang G, Qiu J, Song Y, et al. Risk factors for anal fistula: a case-control study. Tech Coloproctol. 2014;18:635–9.
23. Cioli VM, Gagliardi G, Pescatori M. Psychological stress in patients with anal fistula. Int J Color Dis. 2015;30:1123–9.
24. Herr CH, Williams JC. Supralevator anorectal abscess presenting as acute low back pain and sciatica. Ann Emerg Med. 1994;23:132–5.
25. Ommer A, Herold A, Berg E, Fürst A, et al. Clinical practice guideline: cryptoglandular anal fistula. Dtsch Arztebl Int. 2011;108:707–13.
26. Ommer A, Herold A, Berg E, Fürst A, et al. German S3 guideline: anal abscess. Int J Color Dis. 2012;27:831–7.
27. Ommer A, Herold A, Berg E, Farke S, et al. S3-Leitlinie Kryptoglanduläre Analfistel - 2. revidierte Fassung. Coloproctology. 2016;39:16–66.
28. Ommer A, Herold A, Berg E, Farke S, et al. S3-Leitlinie Analabszess - 2.revidierte Fassung. Coloproctology. 2016;38:378–98.
29. Hämäläinen KP, Sainio AP. Incidence of fistulas after drainage of acute anorectal abscesses. Dis Colon Rectum. 1998;41:1357–61; discussion 1361–2.
30. Yilmazlar T, Ozturk E, Ozguc H, Ercan I, et al. Fournier's gangrene: an analysis of 80 patients and a novel scoring system. Tech Coloproctol. 2010;14:217–23.
31. Onaca N, Hirshberg A, Adar R. Early reoperation for perirectal abscess: a preventable complication. Dis Colon Rectum. 2001;44:1469–73.
32. Chrabot CM, Prasad ML, Abcarian H. Recurrent anorectal abscesses. Dis Colon Rectum. 1983;26:105–8.
33. Yano T, Asano M, Matsuda Y, Kawakami K, et al. Prognostic factors for recurrence following the initial drainage of an anorectal abscess. Int J Color Dis. 2010;25:1495–8.
34. Tan KK, Liu X, Tsang CB, Koh DC. Identification of the internal anal opening and seton placement improves the outcome of deep postanal space abscess. Color Dis. 2012;15:598–601.
35. Tan KK, Koh DC, Tsang CB. Managing deep postanal space sepsis via an intersphincteric approach: our early experience. Ann Coloproctol. 2013;29:55–9.
36. Ommer A, Wenger FA, Rolfs T, Walz MK. Continence disorders after anal surgery—a relevant problem? Int J Color Dis. 2008;23:1023–31.
37. Rizzo JA, Naig AL, Johnson EK. Anorectal abscess and fistula-in-ano: evidence-based management. Surg Clin North Am. 2010;90:45–68, Table of Contents.
38. Hebjorn M, Olsen O, Haakansson T, Andersen B. A randomized trial of fistulotomy in perianal abscess. Scand J Gastroenterol. 1987;22:174–6.
39. Ho YH, Tan M, Chui CH, Leong A, et al. Randomized controlled trial of primary fistulotomy with drainage alone for perianal abscesses. Dis Colon Rectum. 1997;40:1435–8.
40. Schouten WR, van Vroonhoven TJ. Treatment of anorectal abscess with or without primary fistulectomy. Results of a prospective randomized trial. Dis Colon Rectum. 1991;34:60–3.
41. Tang CL, Chew SP, Seow-Choen F. Prospective randomized trial of drainage alone vs. drainage and fistulotomy for acute perianal abscesses with proven internal opening. Dis Colon Rectum. 1996;39:1415–7.
42. Oliver I, Lacueva FJ, Perez Vicente F, Arroyo A, et al. Randomized clinical trial comparing simple drainage of anorectal abscess with and without fistula track treatment. Int J Color Dis. 2003;18:107–10.
43. Fucini C. One stage treatment of anal abscesses and fistulas. A clinical appraisal on the basis of two different classifications. Int J Color Dis. 1991;6:12–6.
44. Aboulian A, Kaji AH, Kumar RR. Early result of ligation of the intersphincteric fistula tract for fistula-in-Ano. Dis Colon Rectum. 2011;54:289–92.
45. Garg PK, Jain BK. Seton drainage in high anal fistula. Int J Colorectal Dis. 2011;26(11):1495.
46. Mitalas LE, van Wijk JJ, Gosselink MP, Doornebosch P, et al. Seton drainage prior to transanal advancement flap repair: useful or not? Int J Color Dis. 2010;25:1499–502.
47. Lohsiriwat V, Yodying H, Lohsiriwat D. Incidence and factors influencing the development of fistula-in-ano after incision and drainage of perianal abscesses. J Med Assoc Thail. 2011;93:61–5.
48. Sözener U, Gedik E, Kessaf Aslar A, Ergun H, et al. Does adjuvant antibiotic treatment after drainage of anorectal abscess prevent development of anal fistulas? A randomized, placebo-controlled, double-blind, multicenter study. Dis Colon Rectum. 2011;54:923–9.
49. Hamadani A, Haigh PI, Liu IL, Abbas MA. Who is at risk for developing chronic anal fistula or recurrent anal sepsis after initial perianal abscess? Dis Colon Rectum. 2009;52:217–21.
50. Cox SW, Senagore AJ, Luchtefeld MA, Mazier WP. Outcome after incision and drainage with fistulotomy for ischiorectal abscess. Am Surg. 1997;63:686–9.
51. Tonkin DM, Murphy E, Brooke-Smith M, Hollington P, et al. Perianal abscess: a pilot study comparing packing with nonpacking of the abscess cavity. Dis Colon Rectum. 2004;47:1510–4.
52. Llera JL, Levy RC. Treatment of cutaneous abscess: a double-blind clinical study. Ann Emerg Med. 1985;14:15–9.
53. Macfie J, Harvey J. The treatment of acute superficial abscesses: a prospective clinical trial. Br J Surg. 1977;64:264–6.
54. Nunoo-Mensah JW, Balasubramaniam S, Wasserberg N, Artinyan A, et al. Fistula-in-ano: do antibiotics make a difference? Int J Color Dis. 2006;21:441–3.
55. Stewart MP, Laing MR, Krukowski ZH. Treatment of acute abscesses by incision, curettage and primary suture without antibiotics: a controlled clinical trial. Br J Surg. 1985;72:66–7.
56. Bechara FG, Hartschuh W. [Acne inversa]. Hautarzt. 2010;61:39–46.
57. van der Zee HH, Prens EP. Preliminary findings suggest hidradenitis suppurativa may be due to defective follicular support. Br J Dermatol. 2013;168:926–7.
58. Grandel M, Hetzer F. Acne inversa. Coloproctology. 2012;34:57–68.
59. von Laffert M, Stadie V, Wohlrab J, Marsch WC. Hidradenitis suppurativa/acne inversa: bilocated epithelial hyperplasia with very different sequelae. Br J Dermatol. 2011;164:367–71.
60. von Laffert M, Helmbold P, Wohlrab J, Fiedler E, et al. Hidradenitis suppurativa (acne inversa): early inflammatory events at terminal follicles and at interfollicular epidermis. Exp Dermatol. 2010;19:533–7.
61. van der Zee HH, Laman JD, Boer J, Prens EP. Hidradenitis suppurativa: viewpoint on clinical phenotyping, pathogenesis and novel treatments. Exp Dermatol. 2012;21:735–9.

62. Al-Ali FM, Ratnamala U, Mehta TY, Naveed M, et al. Hidradenitis suppurativa (or acne inversa) with autosomal dominant inheritance is not linked to chromosome 1p21.1-1q25.3 region. Exp Dermatol. 2010;19:851–3.
63. Ingram JR. The aetiology of acne inversa: an evolving story. Br J Dermatol. 2011;165:231–2.
64. de Winter K, van der Zee HH, Prens EP. Is mechanical stress an important pathogenic factor in hidradenitis suppurativa? Exp Dermatol. 2012;21:176–7.
65. Blok JL, van Hattem S, Jonkman MF, Horvath B. Systemic therapy with immunosuppressive agents and retinoids in hidradenitis suppurativa: a systematic review. Br J Dermatol. 2013;168:243–52.
66. Fischer AH, Haskin A, Okoye GA. Patterns of antimicrobial resistance in lesions of hidradenitis suppurativa. J Am Acad Dermatol. 2017;76(2):309–313.e2.
67. Ring HC, Riis Mikkelsen P, Miller IM, Jenssen H, et al. The bacteriology of hidradenitis suppurativa: a systematic review. Exp Dermatol. 2015;24:727–31.
68. Wollina U, Tilp M, Meseg A, Schonlebe J, et al. Management of severe anogenital acne inversa (hidradenitis suppurativa). Dermatol Surg. 2011;38:110–7.
69. Halverson A. Hemorrhoids. Clin Colon Rectal Surg. 2007; 20:77–85.
70. Trompetto M, Clerico G, Cocorullo GF, Giordano P, et al. Evaluation and management of hemorrhoids: Italian society of colorectal surgery (SICCR) consensus statement. Tech Coloproctol. 2015;19:567–75.
71. Herold A, Joos A, Bussen D. [Operations for hemorrrhoids: indications and techniques]. Chirurg. 2012;83:1040–8.
72. Jongen J, Bach S, Stubinger SH, Bock JU. Excision of thrombosed external hemorrhoid under local anesthesia: a retrospective evaluation of 340 patients. Dis Colon Rectum. 2003;46:1226–31.
73. Jongen J, Bach S, Stuebinger SH, Bock J-U. Excision einer Perianalvenenthrombose oder eines segmetaeren thrombosierten Anal-/Hämorrhoidalprolapses. Coloproctology. 2002;24:243–52.
74. Greenspon J, Williams SB, Young HA, Orkin BA. Thrombosed external hemorrhoids: outcome after conservative or surgical management. Dis Colon Rectum. 2004;47:1493–8.
75. Jongen J, Dubinskaya A, Peleikis HG, Eberstein A, et al. Konservative und operative Therapie der Analvenenthrombose. Coloproctology. 2009;31:93–8.
76. Jacobs D. Clinical practice. Hemorrhoids. N Engl J Med. 2014;371:944–51.
77. Pillant-Le Moult H, Aubert M, de Parades V. Classical treatment of hemorrhoids. J Visc Surg. 2015;152:S3–9.
78. Kersting S, Herold A, Jung KP, Berg E. [Complication management following hemorrhoid operations]. Chirurg. 2015;86:726–33.
79. Ommer A, Berg E, Breitkopf C, Bussen D, et al. S3-Leitlinie: sinus pilonidalis. Coloproctology. 2014;36:272–322.
80. Iesalnieks I, Ommer A, Petersen S, Doll D, et al. German national guideline on the management of pilonidal disease. Langenbeck's Arch Surg. 2016;401:599–609.
81. Sondenaa K, Andersen E, Nesvik I, Soreide JA. Patient characteristics and symptoms in chronic pilonidal sinus disease. Int J Color Dis. 1995;10:39–42.
82. Doll D, Friederichs J, Dettmann H, Boulesteix A-L, et al. Time and rate of sinus formation in pilonidal sinus disease. Int J Color Dis. 2008;23:359–64.
83. Stelzner F. Die Ursache des Pilonidalsinus und der Pyodermia fistulans sinifica. Langenbecks Arch Chir. 1984;362:105–18.
84. Bascom J. Pilonidal disease: origin from follicles of hairs and results of follicle removal as treatment. Surgery. 1980;87:567–72.
85. Patey DH. A reappraisal of the acquired theory of sacrococcygeal pilonidal sinus and an assessment of its influence on surgical practice. Br J Surg. 1969;56:463–6.
86. Dahl HD, Henrich MH. [Light and scanning electron microscopy study of the pathogenesis of pilonidal sinus and anal fistula]. Langenbecks Arch Chir. 1992;377:118–24.
87. Benedetto AV. Commentary: hair and pilonidal sinus disease. Dermatol Surg. 2010;36:92–3.
88. Arda IS, Guney LH, Sevmis S, Hicsonmez A. High body mass index as a possible risk factor for pilonidal sinus disease in adolescents. World J Surg. 2005;29:469–71.
89. Akinci OF, Bozer M, Uzunkoy A, Duzgun SA, et al. Incidence and aetiological factors in pilonidal sinus among Turkish soldiers. Eur J Surg. 1999;165:339–42.
90. Bolandparvaz S, Moghadam Dizaj P, Salahi R, Paydar S, et al. Evaluation of the risk factors of pilonidal sinus: a single center experience. Turk J Gastroenterol. 2012;23:535–7.
91. Corman M. Classic articles in colonic and rectal surgery. Louis A. Buie, M.D. 1890-1975: jeep disease (pilonidal disease of mechanized warfare). Dis Colon Rectum. 1982;25:384–90.
92. Doll D, Friederichs J, Dusel W, Fend F, et al. Surgery for asymptomatic pilonidal sinus disease. Int J Color Dis. 2008;23:839–44.
93. Doll D, Novotny A, Wietelmann K, Matevossian E, et al. Factors influencing surgical decisions in chronic pilonodal sinus disease. Eur Surg. 2009;41(2):60–5.
94. Steele SR, Perry WB, Mills S, Buie WD. Practice parameters for the management of pilonidal disease. Dis Colon Rectum. 2013;56:1021–7.
95. Jensen SL, Harling H. Prognosis after simple incision and drainage for a first-episode acute pilonidal abscess. Br J Surg. 1988;75:60–1.

Open Abdomen: Indications, Surgical Management, and Critical Care

43

Stefania Cimbanassi and Osvaldo Chiara

Key Points

- Indications for open abdomen (OA) are intra-abdominal complicated infections, trauma, and prevention/treatment of abdominal compartment syndrome (ACS).
- An OA patient is critically ill and requires a multidisciplinary approach.
- The cornerstone in OA management is the prevention of loss of the abdominal domain and the retraction of fascial edges.
- Early primary fascial closure (PFC) should be attempted within 8 days, in order to avoid complications and evolution toward the frozen abdomen.
- Different methods for temporary abdominal closure (TAC) should be tailored on patient needs.
- Entero-atmospheric fistula (EAF) should be converted as soon as possible into a standard enterostomy for a better management.
- A definitive closure requires usually complex surgical reconstruction techniques, with or without the adjunctive use of meshes.

43.1 Introduction

Open abdomen (OA) is a condition in which at the end of laparotomy, performed whether for trauma or for non-trauma surgical emergencies [1, 2], the fascial edges are left purposefully open, in order to avoid the increase of intra-abdominal pressure (IAP) and the onset of intra-abdominal hypertension (IAH) and abdominal compartment syndrome (ACS), to allow abdominal planned re-exploration(s) (PR), or to manage intra-abdominal infections, in a stepwise approach.

Three main indications for OA have been reported: infections, trauma, and prevention/treatment of ACS [2–4]. While the results of randomized non-blinded controlled trial [3] showed that, in case of peritonitis, re-laparotomy on-demand (ROD) strategy offers some advantages in comparison to PR in terms of hospital and ICU length of stay and costs, without differences on mortality, in trauma setting, favorable effects of OA are widely recognized, and OA is considered formally a part of damage control surgery (DCS), to the point that 10–15% of severely injured patients undergo this strategy.

Currently accepted indications to OA in trauma are [1]:

- The need of a second look after DCS, for depacking or assessment of hollow viscus/mesenteric/pancreatic-biliary injuries
- If gross peritoneal contamination is present at the indicative laparotomy
- If trauma induced a significant abdominal wall loss
- Prevention of ACS or treatment of ACS if medical therapy failed

The new classification system [5–7] of OA is depicted in Table 43.1. According to this classification, the severity of open abdomen is increasing through four grades, from a condition of spaced-out fascial edges without complications (grade 1) to worst condition of the frozen abdomen with entero-atmospheric fistula (EAF) (grade 4). It has been demonstrated [8, 9] that the grade of OA has a strong correlation with the possibility of achieving early primary fascial closure (PFC), within 8 days, and consequently with the outcome of patient.

In considering the intrinsic characteristics of OA, and the profound pathophysiological derangements, it's easy to understand how the OA patient is one of the sickest, hypercatabolic surgical patients, for whom a multidisciplinary—surgical and critical care—approach is mandatory.

S. Cimbanassi · O. Chiara (✉)
Trauma Team and Emergency Surgery, Niguarda Trauma Center, AAST Grande Ospedale Metropolitano Niguarda, Milan, Italy
e-mail: stefania.cimbanassi@ospedaleniguarda.it; osvaldo.chiara@ospedaleniguarda.it

P. Aseni et al. (eds.), *Operative Techniques and Recent Advances in Acute Care and Emergency Surgery*,
https://doi.org/10.1007/978-3-319-95114-0_43

Table 43.1 Classification systems of OA [5–7]

Amended classification system	
1A	Clean, no fixation
1B	Contaminated, no fixation
1C	Enteric leak, no fixation
2A	Clean developing fixation
2B	Contaminated, developing fixation
2C	Enteric leak, developing fixation
3A	Clean, frozen abdomen
3B	Contaminated, frozen abdomen
4	Established entero-atmospheric fistula, frozen abdomen

43.2 Surgical Management

The mainstay of OA wound management is represented by the possibility to avoid peritoneal content evisceration and loss of abdominal domain, to actively remove fluid from the peritoneal cavity while improving patient nursing, to prevent EAF onset, to prevent further fascial retraction preserving its integrity, and to make reoperation easy and safe. The ideal method should be also cost-effective. The technique applied for temporary abdominal closure (TAC) may influence survival, complication rate, and time to obtain definitive closure, taking into account that OA closure is best achieved when edema subsides and before the evolution toward the frozen abdomen [5].

Different OA grades warrant different methods for wound coverage, which explains the vast variety of available TAC systems, to be tailored to patient conditions. In grades 1–2, the aim of TAC is to preserve abdominal domain while avoiding adhesion onset and helping PFC [10]. Differently, in complicated grades 3 and 4, the optimal TAC method should help to improve granulation tissue over bowel loops and/or around EAF. A significant improvement of OA management, regardless of grade, has been obtained since the introduction of different methods for the negative-pressure wound therapy (NPWT) [11].

At the right time, several techniques for definitive abdominal wall reconstruction, with or without the use of biological or synthetic meshes, have to be considered [12].

43.2.1 TAC

Several methods for temporary abdominal closure are available. Some are homemade and inexpensive (skin approximation, Bogota bag, Wittmann Patch™, Barker's method) [13–15]; others are commercial (system-based NPWT, synthetic repair materials) [16, 17].

43.2.1.1 Skin Approximation

It is obtained by closing the skin over the fascial defect with running sutures or towel clips. Often used at the end of damage control laparotomy, this system does not allow for the expansion of intra-abdominal content, increasing the risk of IAH. Moreover, it does not prevent fascial edge retraction. It has to be converted into more effective TAC methods as soon as possible.

43.2.1.2 Bogota Bag

A 3-L peritoneal dialysis bag is anchored to the fascial edges or the skin. It does not allow for fluid removal, fascial retraction is not prevented, and loss of the abdominal domain occurs in few days.

43.2.1.3 Fascial Closure Techniques

With these techniques fascial approximation is obtained by progressively folding and reducing in size the absorbable or nonabsorbable mesh sutured to the fascia. Bowel loops are protected by a plastic sheet. Every 2–3 days, the mesh is opened in the midline, the dressing is changed, and the mesh is trimmed or folded to be progressively tightened. NPWT can be used in association.

In Wittman Patch™ (Star Surgical Inc., Burlington, WI), technique re-approximation is allowed by increasing the overlap of two opposite Velcro sheets sutured to the fascia [13].

The three most common methods for NPWT are Barker's, VAC systems, and ABThera™. The main difference among them is the distribution pattern of the preset negative pressure, because of the different mechanical properties of these devices. Using a preset optimal negative pressure of −125 mmHg, a decrease in centrifugal direction from 9 to 2 mmHg in Barker's system, from 43 to 12 mmHg in the VAC Abdominal Dressing, and from 83 to 71 mmHg in ABThera™ has been, respectively, observed [17]. These differences might have repercussions on the effectiveness in cytokine-rich abdominal fluid removal and consequent improvement in systemic inflammatory response, even if comparative studies between commercial devices are lacking.

The favorable effect of NPWT is exerted via the stretching and deformation of the abdominal wall, which promotes neo-angiogenesis [18]. A possible drawback is the increased abdominal wall rigidity induced by NPWT and reduced capacity of peritoneal cavity, with the possibility of IAH and ACS [19]. For this reason, serial measurement of IAP is warranted.

The aim of TAC is to obtain early PFC, within 8 days since the beginning of treatment, in order to avoid the evolution toward the frozen abdomen (grade 3), which precludes any possible surgical procedure with the development of planned ventral hernia. In this case the only way to obtain the coverage of granulation tissue is by native skin flaps or split-thickness skin grafts, delaying a definitive surgical treatment in 6–12 months after full recovery from initial insult.

43.2.2 Management of Entero-Atmospheric Fistulas

The formation of EAF is one of the most dreaded complications of the frozen abdomen, because of local inflammation, sepsis, and metabolic derangement. Risk factors for EAF onset are represented by bowel injuries and repair or anastomosis, colonic resection during DCS, more than 10 L of fluid in 48 h for resuscitation, repeated edematous bowel manipulations and delayed abdominal closure, intra-abdominal sepsis, and the use of nonabsorbable mesh directly over the bowel [1].

EAF should be classified according to the location (deep vs. superficial), anatomy (gastro-atmospheric, entero-atmospheric, colo-atmospheric), number (single, multiple in close proximity, multiple at distance), and daily output (low if <200 mL/day, moderate if 200–500 mL/day, high if >500 mL/day) [20].

A close control of effluent is mandatory to improve granulation of surrounding tissues, in order to rapidly convert an EAF into a standard enterostomy. NPWT is useful and effective in improving granulation and protecting the surrounding tissues from enteric spillage.

If EAF is small and with low output, the granulation tissue is thin, and nutritional status is good, an attempt to directly close the fistula with pledget sutures should be performed. Biological dressing should be used as adjunctive measure to primary closure [21].

Most of the cases need some measure to achieve effluent control and produce granulation of surrounding tissue for skin grafting. The goal is to transform EAF in enterocutaneous fistula, to be controlled with a standard ostomy bag. Different techniques are available (floating stoma, nipple technique, fistula adapter, tube VAC, Silo VAC, VAC chimney, fistula patch) [22–27], which are described in detail elsewhere [21]. In any case, direct intubation of the fistula is not recommended [1].

Surgical reconstruction of gastrointestinal continuity should be attempted only once systemic and local conditions are suitable [21]. The patient must be in good nutritional status (see Sect. 43.3) and free from any septic focus. The anatomy of fistula must be evaluated in advance by fistulography, barium enema, contrast-enhanced computed tomography, magnetic resonance, and endoscopy.

Entry into the peritoneal cavity should first be attempted through the lateral edge of granulation tissue. Once entered, the surgeon must provide complete dissection of the entire bowel; EAF segments are resected, and anastomosis is performed.

A strategy for abdominal wall reconstruction should be planned before surgery. Single-stage and multiple-stage approaches are both effective. Single stage is to be preferred if minimal loss of wall domain is present. If patient's physiological reserve is exhausted after prolonged surgery, multiple-step approach is advisable [21].

In case of larger wall defects, the technique of component separation is useful to obtain additional centimeters of fascial plane, bilaterally [28]. If component separation is not enough to obtain complete fascial closure, meshes should be used as bridges [21]. When a biologic mesh is used for bridging because of contamination or infection, a rate of 70% of recurrent hernia is expected with the need of late reconstruction with synthetic mesh.

43.2.3 Definitive Closure

If fascial closure should not be performed within 8 days, several techniques should be applied in order to improve fascial traction. Simple large sutures or commercial dynamic system (ABRA Canica, Almonte, Ontario, Canada) can be used [29, 30]. The rate of fascial closure can be increased using NPWT combined with mesh-mediated fascial traction.

The aforementioned component separation may be performed as anterior component separation [28], with possible variation as periumbilical perforator sparing (PUPS) method, or as posterior component separation, with transversus abdominis release (TAR) [31]. Fascial plane should be reinforced with a mesh in retromuscular (sublay) space. Usually, non-cross-linked (NCL) biological meshes should be preferred because they facilitate neovascularization and remodeling. They are to be preferred in case of contaminated field, while cross-linked (CL) meshes are valuable options for bridging because of their long-term resistance [21].

Large defect-coverage strategies depend on the presence (type I) or absence (type II) of intact skin. Type I defects should be repaired with component separation plus synthetic mesh, eventually improved by previous injection of botulinum toxin A. Type II defects can be treated by microvascular flaps [32].

43.3 Critical Care

OA represents a big challenge for intensivists, since the pathophysiological changes into the abdominal cavity have dramatic repercussions on cardiorespiratory function, metabolic state, and nutritional asset. An OA patient is also prone to infection inside and outside abdominal cavity, which may impair and delay the possibility of early PFC, with consequent increased risk for EAF onset, which may enhance a vicious cycle with increased morbidity and mortality rates.

Some strategies have to be applied correctly in order to achieve favorable targets (Table 43.2), a close hemodynamic monitoring, in association with contemporaneous resuscitation and correction of metabolic derangement, which man-

Table 43.2 ICU management of the open abdomen patient [33]

• Sedation, anxiolysis, and systemic neuromuscular blockade (NMB) RASS-4, paralytics with BIS monitor
• Resuscitation, normalization of acidosis pH > 7.2
• Correction of coagulopathy: blood product resuscitation INR < 1.5
• Correction of hypothermia: passive and active rewarming methods Ideal core temperature > 37°
• Monitoring for abdominal compartment syndrome (ACS) IAH < 12 mmHg
• Ventilation strategy Low volume 5–6 mL/kg body weight
• NPWT of OA
• Nutritional support Supplement protein 2 g/kg

dates careful fluid management; adequate ventilation strategy, resorting to appropriate sedation, paralysis, and analgesia; nutritional support; and antibiotic therapy [33].

Hemodynamic monitoring is best achieved via an indwelling catheter for repeated intra-arterial pressure measurements and recording of other dynamic parameters, such as stroke volume variation (SVV) or the pulse pressure differential, which are more accurate than static ones (central venous pressure, left atrial pressure) [34]. If further clarifications about patient hemodynamic status are needed, a selected use of Swan-Ganz catheter may be useful.

Vasopressors are not substitutive of fluids, and they should be used only in a fully resuscitated patient to maintain mean arterial pressure higher than 65 mmHg.

Taking into account that an increasing IAP >10 mmHg induces an increase in afterload; a decrease in preload, with consistent reduction of cardiac output (CO); and an increase of systemic vascular resistances (SVR), serial measurement—every 6 h—of IAP is warranted, according to the WSACS guidelines [6]. This can be performed via a urinary bladder catheter [35] or via commercially available transducer kits [36].

A goal-directed fluid resuscitation, in order to avoid fluid overload which worsens bowel edema, is best achieved by infusion of isotonic crystalloids, preferring Ringer's lactate (RL) over normal saline (NS), to avoid hyperchloremic acidosis if large amounts of fluid are required [37].

It has been also demonstrated [38] that a multimodal strategy (small-volume resuscitation, forced diuresis, hemofiltration, open-lung ventilation with high level of positive end-expiratory pressure—PEEP) to obtain fluid mobilization from the interstitium, achieving a net negative fluid balance, may improve early PFC.

During fluid resuscitation great attention must be paid to avoid hypothermia, keeping core temperature >36 °C, to correct intercurrent coagulopathy, assessing coagulation state by traditional laboratory tests (PT, APTT, PLT, fibrinogen) and/or by viscoelastic method (TEG, ROTEM®) [39, 40]. Hypoperfusion and metabolic disturbances have to be avoided. Targets are PT and APTT<1.5, PLT > 50 × 10^9/L, fibrinogen >2.0 g/L, Hb 7–9 g/dL and pH > 7.2, and lactate <2 mEq/L.

Mechanical ventilation is challenging; thus close interaction between the thoracic cavity and the abdominal compartment exists. In an OA patient, a lung-protective ventilation strategy should be adopted, applying low tidal volumes (5–6 mL/kg) and a target plateau pressure below 30–35 cmH_2O [41]. The best PEEP is that which avoids alveolar derecruitment and contrasts IAP, without cardiopulmonary impairment and fascial edge retraction. If this strategy fails, prone positioning should be considered [42].

Adequate neuromuscular blockade is mandatory to avoid abdominal wall rigidity and fascial retraction.

An OA patient must receive preemptive pain relief and then sedated if necessary (analgo-sedation) [43]. Intravenous opiates are the drug of first-line class of choice to treat non-neuropathic pain [44] although non-opiates should be considered to decrease the amount of opiates administered, decreasing their side effects [45].

Sedatives are to be titrated to maintain a light rather than deep level of sedation, preferring non-benzodiazepines (propofol, dexmedetomidine) in order to attempt a daily spontaneous breathing trial [46]. There are no recommendations for use of pharmacologic prevention strategy [47]. To treat delirium atypical antipsychotic should be administered.

Patients with OA are in hypercatabolic state, associated with muscle proteolysis and protein malnutrition due to significant protein losses from exposed viscera. This situation may lead rapidly to nitrogen imbalance, while a positive nitrogen balance is considered to be a primary goal of nutritional support. An estimate of 2 g of nitrogen per liter of abdominal fluid loss is constant, and it can be used for calculating daily nitrogen balance. A recent revision of nitrogen balance formula has been proposed [48]:

$$\text{Nitrogen balance} = \text{nitrogen intake} - (\text{UUN} + 4) + 2 \times \text{abdominal fluid output (in liters)}$$

where 4 represents the grams of daily cutaneous and gastrointestinal nitrogen losses.

An early nutritional plan is the cornerstone, and the enteral route (EN) must be preferred if feasible. Only contraindication to EN is a residual viable bowel shorter than 75 cm [48]. If gastrointestinal tract is intact, post-pyloric feeding tube should be used. If EAF is present, the anatomy and location of EAF should be assessed to tailor the best route of feeding.

Daily intake of 20–30 kcal/kg of nonprotein calories has to be supplied with standard polymeric formula, enriched with 1.5–2.5 g/kg of proteins. Immune nutrition may help decrease inflammatory response. Oral solid intake should be favored once the critical phase is over [48].

Table 43.3 Antimicrobial regimen according to type of infections (CA-IAIs vs. IH-IAIs) and patient physiological characteristics [33]

	Stable, noncritical no ESBL risk factor	Stable, noncritical with ESBL risk factors	Critically ill no ESBL risk factors	Critically ill with ESBL risk factors
CA-IAIs	Amoxicillin/ clavulanate 2.2g/6 h OR Ciprofloxacin 400 mg/8 h + Metronidazole 500 mg/6 h	Ertapenem 1 g/24 h OR Tigecycline 100 mg LD then 50 mg/12 h	Piperacillin/tazo-bactam 8/2 g LD then 16/4/day (continuous infusion or every 6 h)	Meropenem 500 mg/6 h OR Imipenem 500 mg/4 h ± Fluconazole 600 mg LD then 400 mg/24 h
IHA-IAs		Piperacillin 8 g LD than 16 g (continuous infusion or 6 g/4 h) + Tigecycline 100 mg LD than 50 mg/12 h + Fluconazole 600 mg LD than 400 mg/24 h		Piperacillin 8 g LD than 16 g (continuous infusion or 4 g/6 h) + Tigecycline 100 mg LD than 50 mg/12 h + Echinocandin (– caspofungin 70 mg, than 50 mg/die – anidulafungin200 mgLD, than 100 mg/die – micafungin 100 mg/die) or Meropenem 500 mg/6 h Imipenem 500 mg/4 h + Teicoplanin LD 12 mg/kg/12 h for 3 doses then 6 mg/kg/12 h (PD target 20–30 mg/L) + Echinocandin (– caspofungin 70 mg, than 50 mg/die – anidulafungin200 mgLD, than 100 mg/die – micafungin 100 mg/die)

Notwithstanding the OA patient is prone to both intra-abdominal and extra-abdominal infections; OA condition per se does not warrant any additional period of antibiotic coverage that should be directed toward the underlying disease that culminates in the OA. In case of community-acquired intra-abdominal infections (CA-IAIs), a short-term therapy using narrow spectrum of activity drugs is preferred, while a coverage against extended-spectrum beta-lactamase (ESBL) producers is advised if risk factors exist. In contrast, in case of intrahospital-acquired infections (HA-IAIs), a combined regimen with a broad-spectrum antibiotic coverage is preferred, lasting 3–5 days. De-escalation to the most appropriate single agent should be performed as soon as possible as the susceptibility profile is available. The duration of therapy should be 7–10 days. Empirical fungal coverage with echinocandin regimen for *Candida* spp. is recommended for patients with HA-IAIs and for critically ill patients with CA-IAIs [49]. Suggested drugs according to type of infections are depicted in Table 43.3.

References

1. Chiara O, Cimbanassi S, Biffl W, et al. International consensus conference on open abdomen in trauma. J Trauma Acute Care Surg. 2016;80:173–83.
2. Rotondo MF, Schwab CW. Damage control: an approach for improved survival in exsanguinating penetrating abdominal trauma. J Trauma. 1993;45:914–21.
3. Van Ruler O, Mahler CV, Boer KR, et al. Comparison of on-demand *vs* planned relaparotomy in patients with severe peritonitis. A randomized trial. JAMA. 2007;298:865–72.
4. Cheatham ML, Malbrain MNG, Kirkpatrick A, et al. Results from international conference of experts on intra-abdominal hypertension and abdominal compartment syndrome. II recommendations. Intensive Care Med. 2007;33:951–62.
5. Bjorck M, Bruhin A, Cheatham M, et al. Classification important step to improve management of patients with an open abdomen. World J Surg. 2009;33:1154–7.
6. Kirkpatrick AW, Roberts DJ, De Waele JD, et al. Intra-abdominal hypertension and the abdominal compartment syndrome: updated consensus definitions and clinical practice guidelines from the World Society of the Abdominal Compartment Syndrome. Intensive Care Med. 2013;39:1190–206.

7. Bjorck M, Kirkpatrick AW, Cheatham M, et al. Amended classification of the open abdomen. Scand J Surg. 2016;105:5–10.
8. Bjarnason T, Montgomery A, Acosta S, et al. Evaluation of the open abdomen classification system: a validity and reliability analysis. World J Surg. 2014;38:3112–24.
9. Kafka-Ritsch R, Zitt M, Schorn N, et al. Open abdomen treatment with dynamic sutures and topical negative pressure resulting in a high primary fascial closure rate. World J Surg. 2012;36:1765–71.
10. Chiara O, Cimbanassi S, Negreanu J. Methods for temporary abdominal closure. In: Chiara O, Cimbanassi S, editors. Atlas of open abdomen in trauma-how I do it. Minerva Medica; 2017. p. 11–8.
11. Ryczerc AM, Slack P, McNulty AK. Distribution assessment comparing continuous and periodic wound instillation in conjunction with negative pressure wound therapy using an agar-based model. Int Wound J. 2013;10:214–20.
12. Roberts DJ, Zygun DA, Grendar J, et al. Negative pressure wound therapy for critically ill adults with open abdominal wound: a systematic review. J Trauma Acute Care Surg. 2012;73:629–39.
13. Vargo D, Richardson D, et al. Management of the open abdomen: from initial operation to definitive closure. Am Surg. 2009;75:S1–S22.
14. Keramati M, Srivastava A, Sakabu S, et al. The Wittmann patch™ as a temporary abdominal closure device after decompressive celiotomy for abdominal compartment syndrome following burns. Burns. 2008;34:493–7.
15. Barker DE, Kaufman HJ, Smith LA, et al. Vacuum pack technique of temporary abdominal closure: a 7-years experience with 112 patients. J Trauma. 2000;48:201–6.
16. Rasilainen SK, Mentula PJ, Leppaniemi AK. Vacuum and mesh-mediated fascial traction for primary closure of the open abdomen in critically ill surgical patients. Br J Surg. 2012;99:1725–32.
17. Lindstedt S, Malmsjo M, Helbowicz J, et al. Comparative study of microvascular blood flow in the intestinal wall, wound contraction and fluid evacuation during negative pressure therapy in laparostomy using V.A.C abdominal dressing and ABThera™ open abdomen negative pressure therapy system. Int Wound J. 2013;10:411–7.
18. Patel NY, Cogbill TH, Kallies KJ, et al. Temporary abdominal wall closure: long term outcomes. J Trauma. 2011;65:337–42.
19. Ouellet JF, Ball CG. Recurrent abdominal compartment syndrome induced by high negative pressure abdominal closure dressing. J Trauma. 2011;71:785–6.
20. Wainstein DE, Tungler V, Ravazzola C, et al. Management of external small bowel fistulae. Challenges and controversies confronting the general surgeon. Int J Surg. 2011;9:198–203.
21. Chiara O, Cimbanassi S. Entero-atmospheric fistula(s). In: Chiara O, Cimbanassi S, editors. Atlas of open abdomen in trauma-how I do it. Minerva Medica; 2017. p. 26–40.
22. Subramanian MH, Liscum KR, Hirshberg A. The floating stoma: a new technique for controlling exposed fistula in abdominal trauma. J Trauma. 2005;53:386–8.
23. Layton B, DuBose J, Nichols S, et al. Pacifying the open abdomen with concomitant intestinal fistula: a novel approach. Am J Surg. 2010;190:e48–50.
24. Jannasch O, Chiapponi C, Tautenhahn J, et al. The fistula adapter, an evolving device in treatment of entero-atmospheric fistulae. Negat Pressure Wound Ther. 2014;1:112–4.
25. Goverman J, Yelon JA, Platz JJ, et al. The "Fistula VAC", a technique for management of enterocutaneous fistula arising within the open abdomen: a report of 5 cases. J Trauma. 2006;60:428–31.
26. Ramsay PT, Mejia VA. Management of entero-atmospheric in the open abdomen. Am Surg. 2010;76:637–9.
27. Verhaalen A, Walkins B, Brasel K. Techniques and cost effectiveness of enteroatmospheric fistula isolation. Wounds. 2010;22:212–7.
28. Ramirez OA, Ruas E, Dellon AL. "Component separation" method for closure of abdominal wall defects: an anatomic and clinical study. Plast Reconstruct Surg. 1990;86:519–26.
29. Burlew CC, Moore EE, Biffl WL, et al. One hundred percent fascial approximation can be achieved in the postinjury open abdomen with a sequential closure protocol. J Trauma. 2012;72:235–41.
30. Salman AE, Yetisir F, Aksoy M, et al. Use of dynamic closure system in conjunction with vacuum assisted closure therapy in delayed closure of open abdomen. Hernia. 2014;18:99–104.
31. Pauli EM, Rosen MJ. Open ventral hernia repair with component separation. Surg Clin North Am. 2013;93:1111–3.
32. Tukiainen E, Leppaniemi A. Reconstruction of extensive abdominal wall defects with microvascular tensore fascia latae flap. Br J Surg. 2011;98:880–4.
33. Cimbanassi S, Lippi, M, Chiara O. Intensive care management of the open abdomen patient. In: Chiara O, Cimbanassi S, editors. Atlas of open abdomen in trauma-how I do it. Minerva Medica; 2017. p. 50–66.
34. Malbrain M, De Laet E. Intra-abdominal hypertension: evolving concepts. Clin Chest Med. 2009;30:45–70.
35. Koehl R. Intra-abdominal hypertension and abdominal compartment syndrome. Crit Care Nurse. 2012;32:19–32.
36. De Waele JJ, De L, De Keulenaer B, et al. The effect of different reference transducer positions on intra-abdominal pressure measurement. A multicenter analysis. Intensive Care Med. 2008;34:1299–303.
37. Finfer S, Bellomo R, Boyce N, et al. A comparison of albumin and saline for fluid resuscitation in intensive care unit. N Engl J Med. 2004;350:2247–56.
38. Rossaint R, Bouillon B, Cerny V, et al. The European guideline on management of major bleeding and coagulopathy following trauma: fourth edition. Crit Care. 2016;20:100–55.
39. Veigas PV, Callum J, Rizoli S, et al. A sustematic review on the rotational thromboelastometry (ROTEM®) values for the diagnosis of coagulopathy, prediction and guidance of blood transfusion and prediction of mortality in trauma patients. Scand J Trauma Resusc Emerg Med. 2016;24:114–28.
40. Cortes-Puentes GA, Gard KE, Adams AB, et al. Value and limitations of transpulmonary pressure calculations during intra-abdominal hypertension. Crit Care Med. 2013;41:1632–7.
41. Guerrero M, Cannizzo F, Falta E, et al. Prone ventilation in a United State Marine with acute respiratory distress syndrome and open abdominal injury. South Med J. 2009;102:637–9.
42. Mehta S, Burry L, Martinez-Motta JC, et al. A randomized trial of daily awakening in critically ill patients managed with a sedation protocol: a pilot trial. Crit Care Med. 2008;36:2092–9.
43. Payen JF, Chanques G, Mantz J, et al. Current practices in sedation and analgesia for mechanical ventilated critically ill patients: a prospective multicenter patient-based study. Anesthesiology. 2007;107:858–60.
44. Memis D, Inal MT, Kavalci G, et al. Intravenous paracetamol reduced the use of opioids, extubation time, and opioid-related adverse effects after major surgery in intensive care unit. J Crit Care. 2010;25:458–62.
45. Barr J, Fraser GL, Puntillo KL, et al. Clinical practice guidelines for the management of pain, agitation and delirium in adult patients in the intensive care unit. Crit Care Med. 2013;41:263–306.
46. Girard TD, Pandharipande PP, Carson SS, et al. Feasibility, efficacy, and safety of antipsychotic for intensive care unit delirium: the MIND randomized, placebo-controlled trial. Crit Care Med. 2010;38:428–37.
47. Cheatham ML, Safsak K, Brzezinski SJ, et al. Nitrogen balance, protein loss and the open abdomen. Crit Care Med. 2007;35:127–31.
48. Majercik S, Kinikini M, White T. Enteroatmospheric fistula: from soup to n uts. Nutr Clin Pract. 2012;27:507–12.
49. Dutton WD, Diaz JJ Jr, Miller RS. Critical care issues in managing complex open abdominal wound. J Intensive Care Med. 2012;27:161–7.

Necrotizing Soft Tissue Infections (NSTI)

44

Stefania Cimbanassi and Osvaldo Chiara

Key Points

- NSTIs are characterized by progressive and often fatal evolution.
- "Hard signs" of NSTIs are represented by hemorrhagic bullae, subcutaneous crepitus, and skin necrosis.
- Surgical debridement must be timely and extensively performed, and it represents the mainstay of treatment.
- Broad-spectrum antibiotic therapy should be started as soon as possible and then narrowed on the basis of bacterial isolation.
- HBO should be considered as an adjunctive therapy, but it should not jeopardize surgical debridement.

44.1 Introduction

Necrotizing soft tissue infections (NSTIs) represent a particular variety of complicated soft tissue infections (Table 44.1), which warrant a prompt and aggressive treatment, because they are limb- and life-threatening. They are rare conditions characterized by rapid but subtle onset of spreading inflammation and necrosis starting from the fascia, involving muscles and subcutaneous fat, with subsequent necrosis of the overlying skin. The most common sites of infection are extremities, particularly upper limbs (10–48%), and lower extremities (28%). The perineum (21%), trunk (18%), and head or neck (5%) represent other body regions frequently involved (Fig. 44.1) [1].

S. Cimbanassi (✉) · O. Chiara
Trauma Team and Emergency Surgery, Niguarda Trauma Center, AAST Grande Ospedale Metropolitano Niguarda, Milan, Italy
e-mail: stefania.cimbanassi@ospedaleniguarda.it; osvaldo.chiara@ospedaleniguarda.it

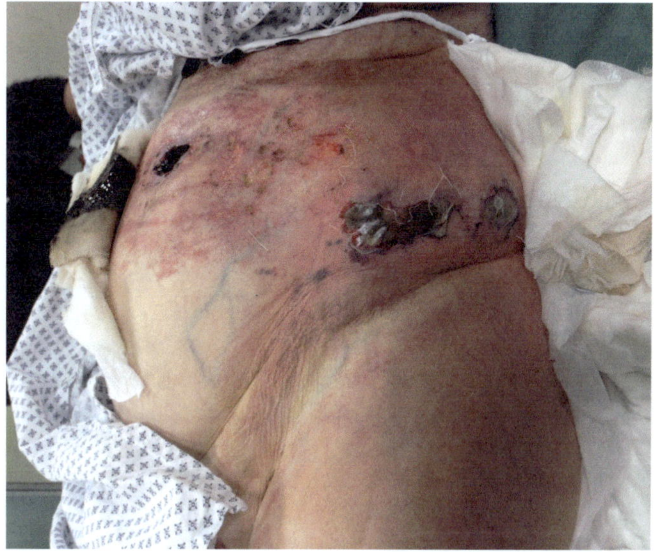

Fig. 44.1 Clinical pathway for NSTIs management

Table 44.1 Classification of severe skin and soft tissue infections by the US Food and Drug Administration [1]

Uncomplicated **Can be treated by surgical incision alone**
Superficial infections, such as: – Simple abscesses – Impetiginous lesions – Furuncles – Cellulitis – Infections associated with bites or animal contact
Complicated **Significant underlying disease state that complicates response to treatment**
Deep soft tissue requires significant surgical debridement. – Infected deep ulcers – Infected burns – Major abscesses – NSTIs – Surgical site infections (SSI) – Infections in the immunocompromised host

P. Aseni et al. (eds.), *Operative Techniques and Recent Advances in Acute Care and Emergency Surgery*, https://doi.org/10.1007/978-3-319-95114-0_44

Table 44.2 Bacterial toxins and their effects

Bacteria	Toxins	Effects
Clostridium spp.	α-toxin	Tissue necrosis Cardiocirculatory failure
Streptococci and staphylococci	M1–M3 proteins A,B,C exotoxins, streptolysin O, superantigens	Increased endothelial adhesion and resistance to phagocytosis Endothelial damage, edema, reduced microcirculatory flow Increased TNF-α, IL-1, and IL-6 release Inflammatory response amplification Vomiting

Table 44.3 Necrotizing fasciitis classification (modified from Low and Greer [9])

Type	Species	Localization
Type I	Polymicrobial: at least one anaerobic ± facultative anaerobes (*Enterobacteriaceae*, non-group A streptococci)	The trunk, abdomen, and perineum
Type II	Monomicrobial: group A β-hemolytic streptococci and/or other streptococci ± staphylococci	Extremities
Type III	Marine *Vibrio* or *Bacillus*	Extremities

Some comorbidities are recognized as independent risk factors for NSTIs, such as diabetes mellitus (30%), immunosuppression (17%), end-stage renal failure, liver cirrhosis, pulmonary diseases (6%), malignancies (5%), and use of injection drugs [2]. The wide spread of the disease process is enabled by bacterial toxins, collagenase, peptidase, streptokinase, and hyaluronidase [3], which induce a local tissue damage, enhanced by ischemia and colliquative necrosis (Table 44.2). This local response mirrors a broad systemic inflammatory response syndrome (SIRS), worsening toward sepsis, septic shock, multiorgan failure (MOF), and death. Even with optimal treatment, NSTIs portend significant morbidity and have mortality rates of 25–35%. Significant associations with negative outcomes have been detected for a large number of factors, such as extremes of age (>60 years <1 year), immunologic compromise, and systemic disease. The main factor associated with negative outcome is the late surgical debridement [1].

44.2 Microbiological Classification

NSTIs are categorized into three specific types based on the microbiologic etiology of infection (Table 44.3). In general, polymicrobial infections tend to have longer incubation period than monomicrobial infections.

Type I Type I NSTIs are classically polymicrobial with various species of gram-positive cocci, gram-negative rods, and anaerobes—including clostridial species—typically being isolated [1, 4–6]. They are usually located at the trunk, abdominal wall, perianal, and groin areas. Patients are typically older, with several comorbidities, such as diabetes, and often have no history of trauma. Clostridial infections—gas gangrene—represent a subtype of type I NSTIs, which deserve special attention, because they present with a rapid onset and evolution (few hours after inoculation), whereas most bacterial species require 2 or more days to become symptomatic. Once the patient manifests shock, mortality exceeds 50% [4].

Type II Type II NSTIs are monomicrobial, most commonly caused by group A *Streptococcus pyogenes* (GAS), less frequently by other streptococci or staphylococci. Type II are less invasive and typically affect healthy, immune-competent patients. Predominant isolation occurs at the head/neck and extremities. GAS may present together or complicate streptococcal toxic shock syndrome (STSS) in 30% of cases. The invasive characteristic of group A β-streptococci is due to the secretion of a wide range of exotoxins, such as streptolysin O and streptolysin S, streptokinases, streptodornase, M protein superantigens, and hyaluronidases, which act in combination inducing neutrophil/macrophage degranulation, breakdown of hyaluronic acid, digestion of fibrin and clots, and decrease of pus viscosity, facilitating its transmission along the fascial planes [3].

Type III Type III NSTIs are monomicrobial caused by gram-negative marine *Vibrio* species, usually *Vulnificus* or *Bacillus.* It is associated with fulminant course, with development of MOF within 24 h, if not treated, even in the absence of any localized cutaneous evidence of infection [7–9].

44.3 Clinical Presentation and Diagnosis

44.3.1 Signs and Symptoms

Signs and symptoms are essentially identical for all types of NSTIs. The most constant initial clinical feature is pain out of proportion to physical findings, in which case NSTI should be considered in differential diagnosis. Some authors have proposed a three-step progression of NSTIs, whereby blisters or bulla formation is a sign of progression to disease-intermediate severity, and hemorrhagic bullae, skin necrosis, and crepitus represent "hard signs" of NSTIs (Table 44.4). It is important to emphasize that these "hard signs," although typical and specific, are present in only 10–40% of patients, with potential progression in 24–48 h, especially when NSTIs are sustained by *Streptococcus* species. Signs and symptoms of systemic toxicity, such as fever or shock, are

Table 44.4 Necrotizing soft tissue infection signs and symptoms

Early	Late
Local	
Skin puncture or injury	Hematic/gas bullae
Erythema	Necrosis
Warmness	Crepitus
Tenderness	Purple/blue skin color
Myalgia	Hypoesthesia
Hypersensitive skin	Sensory/motor deficit
Systemic	
Pain out of proportion	Fever (sometime hypothermia)
Swelling	Hypotension
Fever	Mental confusion
	Multiorgan failure

Table 44.5 Laboratory Risk Indicator for Necrotizing Fasciitis (LRINEC) score system [15]

Variable	Value	LRINEC score points
C-reactive protein (mg/dL)	<150	0
	>150	4
WBC (cells/mm^3)	<15	0
	15–25	1
	>25	2
Hemoglobin (g/dL)	>13.5	0
	11–13.5	1
	<11	2
Sodium (mmol/L)	≥135	0
	<135	2
Creatinine (mg/dL)	≤1.6	0
	>1.6	2
Glucose (mg/dL)	≤180	0
	>180	1
LRINEC score point, sum	**Risk category**	**NSTI probability**
≤5	Low	<50%
6–7	Intermediate	50–75%
≥8	High	≥75%

less frequent than expected. Particularly, in immunocompromised patients fever is present at the admission in 32–53% of cases and hypotension in 11–18% of cases.

44.3.2 Laboratory

Laboratory signs are not specific. Usually, increase in white blood cell count (WBC), creatine phosphokinase, prothrombin time, and activated partial thromboplastin time and decrease in albumin and sodium (Na+) concentrations are observed. Some authors [10–14] found that WBC >15,000 cells/mm^3 and a serum sodium level greater than 135 mmol/L had a negative predictive value of 99% and a 90% sensitivity for detecting NSTIs. The most widely adopted score is the Laboratory Risk Indicator for Necrotizing Fasciitis (LRINEC) (Table 44.5) [15]. Among LRINEC parameters, glucose and C-reactive protein are considered predictors of mortality in critically ill patients, in relation to sepsis hyperglycemia and end-stage renal failure. A LRINEC score ≥6 was found to have a 92% positive predictive value and a 96% negative predictive value in diagnosing NSTIs. A creatine phosphokinase value >600 IU/L may help to differentiate NSTIs due to GAS from other etiologies.

44.3.3 Imaging Evaluation

There is a limited role for imaging in the evaluation of NSTIs. Plain film radiography can show subcutaneous emphysema, but although it is considered fairly specific finding for *Clostridium* infection, it is rare and nonspecific. Computed tomography (CT) scan has 100% sensitivity and 81% specificity in diagnosing NSTIs. Positive predictive value is 76% and negative predictive value 100%. CT scan may demonstrate fascial thickening, edema, subcutaneous gas, and abscess formation. A CT scan score has been proposed (Table 44.6), and a score value >6 has 86% sensitivity and 91% specificity for NSTIs [16]. Fascial thickening on T2-weighted magnetic resonance imaging (MRI) has a sensitivity of 90–100% but a specificity of 50–85% for NSTIs [17]. Peripheral enhancement within muscles on T1-weighted MRI is more specific. MRI offers a limited use in critically ill patient, and the delay in treatment is probably inappropriate in any setting of suspected NSTIs. Ultrasound examination should consider the bedside point-of-care imaging tool for those patients who are too sick to undergo CT scan or MRI [18]. Ultrasound has 88.2% sensitivity and 93.3% specificity for NSTIs, although its positive predictive value, negative predictive value, and accuracy are 95.4%, 95.4%, and 91.9%, respectively. Diffuse subcutaneous swelling and free fluid >4 mm along the fascial plane are considered positive sonographic signs for NSTIs.

In questionable cases, notwithstanding that the clinical suspicion for NSTIs is high, a bedside 2-cm skin incision can be made with dissection carried down to the fascia, allowing the surgeon to assess the adherence of the fascia to the other soft tissue layers (finger test) [19, 20]. If the subcutaneous tissue can be dissected off the deep fascia with minimal resistance, the finger test is positive. A pasty gray necrotic tissue, thin purulent fluid with gray-brown "dishwater" appearance, a generalized lack of bleeding, and visibly thrombosed vessels and/or muscle that does not contract to electrocautery stimulation confirm the diagnosis of NSTIs, mandating extensive surgical debridement.

Table 44.6 CT scan score for NSTIs [16]

Sign	Score
Subcutaneous emphysema	5
Muscular/fascial edema	4
Fluid collections/abscesses	3
Lymphadenopathy	2
Subcutaneous edema	1

44.4 Therapy

Initial treatment of patients with NSTIs requires a multimodal approach, consisting of aggressive surgical debridement, antibiotic therapy, metabolic support, and adjunctive measures [4].

44.4.1 Surgery

Surgical debridement is a mandatory life-saving procedure and should be performed as soon as possible, since a ninefold increase in mortality if the procedure is delayed more than 24 h after hospital admission has been reported [21]. Another important determinant of mortality is the adequacy of debridement. Surgical debridement must be done until brisk bleeding occurs from adjacent tissue [2]. All necrotic tissues, including fascia, must be removed to reduce bacterial load and inflammatory stimuli and facilitate recovery. The wound must be bluntly probed in all directions, especially in highly suspected areas such as any pockets or subcutaneous or submuscular extension of infection. Intraoperative biopsy should include the interface between living and dead tissue [22]. Skin blisters are not caused by infection but by thrombosis of penetrating deeper vessels, and thus there is no role for culture of superficial bullae. Deep intraoperative cultures may allow for appropriate narrowing of antibiotics. Usually, repeated debridements are necessary every 12–36 h (as dictated by conditions of the wound), until the infection is controlled.

In case of perineal NSTIs, a temporary diverting colostomy is reasonable for protection of perineal/perianal wound. Otherwise, although the patient remains intubated, stooling can be managed by the use of a fecal management system and maintaining liquid stools [23]. NSTIs of the extremities often require amputation, especially if joints are involved or because loss of muscle is extensive enough to leave the limb defunctionalized.

Since tissues are edematous and highly secreting, the best option is to leave the wound open after debridement. Sterile dressings with normal saline-soaked gauzes once or twice daily may be used to cover the wounds in the interim. Negative-pressure wound therapy (NPWT) may be used to promote healing and wound closure, particularly in case of large defects [24]. Wound coverage, when not possible by direct closure, can be achieved by split-thickness skin grafts or flaps.

44.4.2 Antibiotic Therapy

Broad-spectrum antibiotic should be administered for coverage of gram-positive, gram-negative bacteria, aerobes, and anaerobes [3]. The possibility of MRSA infection should be considered. Several multidrug regimens have been proposed, including high-dose penicillin, high-dose clindamycin, and fluoroquinolone or aminoglycoside [25]. Liberal use of clindamycin is justified for several reasons, taking into account the number of different organisms commonly implicated in NSTIs. Clindamycin inhibits expression of M protein superantigen, which is one of the key factors in the pathophysiology of NSTIs. Clindamycin also suppresses the production of α-toxin by *C. perfringens*. Clindamycin shows general immunomodulatory effect, such as dose-dependent suppression of *E. coli* lipopolysaccharide (LPS)-induced production of proinflammatory cytokine TNF-α by monocytes. De-escalation of antibiotic therapy, with an attempt to decrease to monotherapy if possible, should be performed as early as possible, once culture results returned. The suggested therapeutic scheme is reported in Table 44.7.

Table 44.7 Therapeutic scheme for NSTIs [25]

Necrotizing fasciitis
Linezolid 600 mg bid + Piperacillin/tazobactam 4/0.5 g LD in 30 min, then 16/2 g qd or Daptomycin 6 mg/kg qd + Piperacillin/tazobactam 4/0.5 g LD in 30 min, then 16/2 g qd + Clindamycin 600–900 mg qd
Fournier's gangrene
• **Without signs of sepsis** Piperacillin/tazobactam 4/0.5 g LD in 30 min, then 16/2 g qd + Clindamycin 600–900 mg qd
• **With signs of sepsis** Meropenem 1 g LD in 30 min, then 1 g qd drip infusion + Linezolid 600 mg bid

LD loading dose

44.4.3 Critical Care

In patients with NSTIs, metabolic and hemodynamic support should be started as soon as possible, in order to minimize the systemic inflammatory response. Vast fluid losses should be observed, such as the inflammatory mediator-induced relative hypovolemia. Crystalloids are indicated during the initial phase of volemic resuscitation. Hemodynamic targets are [26]:

- Mean arterial pressure (MAP) ≥65 mmHg
- Central venous pressure (CVP) of 8–12 mmHg
- Central venous oxygen saturation ($ScvO_2$) >70%
- Urine output >0.5 mL/kg/h

Nutritional support should be optimized, and the enteral route should be preferred. During the initial phase, suggested caloric intake should be of 25 Kcal/kg/daily, to be increased to 30 kcal/kg/daily in the following weeks [25].

Analgesia should be optimized in order to facilitate wound care. Pain can be divided into three types: background pain, breakthrough pain, and procedural pain. Different drugs should be used to address the different types of pain. Background pain is preexisting to the diagnosis and should be treated with a long-acting narcotic, such as methadone. Breakthrough pain is a transient worsening of background pain provoked by movement; it should be addressed with the addition of a short-acting narcotics, such as morphine or oxycodone. Procedural pain is treated with a combination of narcotic, morphine or oxycodone, and short-term anxiolytics, such as midazolam or lorazepam [4]. In case of neuropathic pain, gabapentin can be useful [27].

44.4.4 Other Therapies

In cases of staphylococcal and streptococcal infections, intravenous immunoglobulin (IVIg) administration should be beneficial, in order to bind exotoxins produced by bacterial and to reduce systemic inflammatory response. The available studies on immunoglobulin therapy are underpowered and nonrandomized [28, 29]; thus IVIg therapy should be limited to a critically ill patient with only staphylococcal or streptococcal NSTIs or both.

Postsurgery hyperbaric oxygen (HBO) therapy is a generally accepted possibility [30]. Experimental studies proved that exposure at 2.5 ATA pressure increased subcutaneous tissue oxygen tension levels fivefold compared to initial levels [31]. In contrast, other studies examining HBO and NSTIs have reported that the use of HBO provided no benefits and may be associated with increased mortality [32]. Taking into account the controversial results of HBO in NSTIs, it should be considered as an adjunctive treatment only in stable patients who have already been surgically debrided, treated with broad-spectrum antibiotics, and medically optimized. Certainly, HBO therapy should not jeopardize the standard therapy for NSTIs, specifically, adequate and timely debridement.

Case Scenario

An 82-year-old female with a radiologically inserted gastrostomy (RIG) and several comorbidities (severe aortic valve insufficiency, ischemic cardiac disease, pacemaker implant, polymyositis, lower limb vascular insufficiency, respiratory insufficiency) was admitted to the hospital because of RIG displacement. The patient was hypothermic (core T 35 °C) and hypotensive (90/70 mmHg). Surgical evaluation has been performed revealing output of dark fluid of unknown origin from RIG orifice and truncal skin compromise (Fig. 44.2) with edema, erythema, and dark bullae. Laboratory findings were WBC 22.85 × 10^9, C-reactive protein 28 mg/dL, hemoglobin 11.1 g/L, creatinine 1.7 mg/dL, glucose 107 mg/dL, and sodium 140 mmol/L.

1. Is this a complicated soft tissue infection?
   A. No.
   B. Yes.
   C. Microbiological tests are necessary to determine if complicated or not.
   D. The available elements are insufficient to answer.

This is a complicated soft tissue infection as demonstrated by the presence of cutaneous and systemic compromise.

2. Does CT scan (Fig. 44.3) represent the optimal diagnostic tool in this patient?
   A. Yes.
   B. No.
   C. MRI should be preferred.
   D. Plain films would be enough.

CT scan is the optimal diagnostic tool because it may demonstrate fascial thickening, edema, subcutaneous gas, and abscess formation, with a sensitivity of 100% and a specificity of 81%, respectively. It can be promptly performed in acute setting, allowing for rapid surgical debridement.

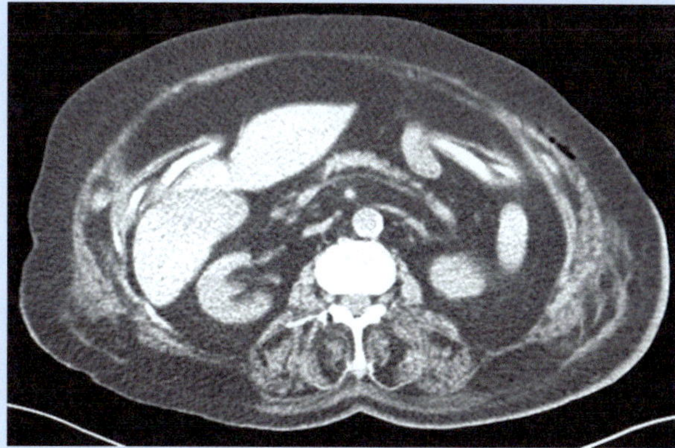

Fig. 44.2 CT scan of torso NSTI demonstrating free air into abdominal wall

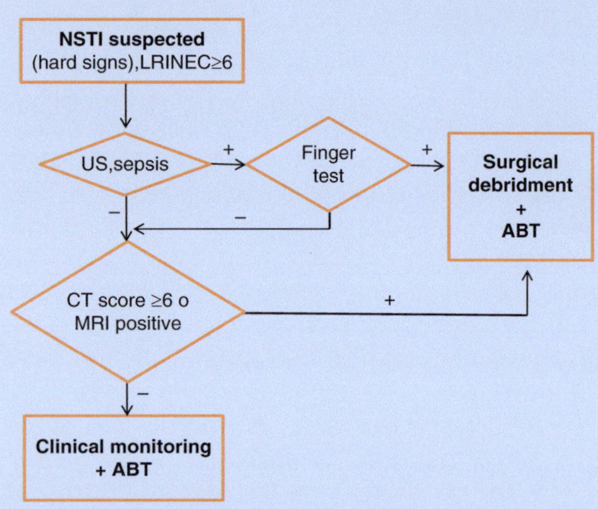

Fig. 44.3 Flow-chart for diagnosis of NSTI

3. Are there laboratory findings of systemic compromise, suggesting NSTIs?
   A. Yes.
   B. No.
   C. The available elements are insufficient to answer.
   D. The evaluation should be done after an appropriate period of resuscitation.

The main laboratory signs of systemic compromise are represented by leukocytosis, increase of C-reactive protein, increased creatinine levels, and hypernatremia. Particularly, leukocytosis $>15 \times 10^9$ and hypernatremia >135 mmol/L have a negative predictive value of 99% and a 90% sensitivity for detecting NSTIs.

4. Which type of infection is suspected in this kind of patient?
   A. Type I polymicrobial
   B. Type II monomicrobial
   C. Fournier's gangrene
   D. Type III

This is an old patient suffering from several comorbidities. Moreover cutaneous alterations are located at the trunk. This is a condition typically sustained by various species of gram-positive cocci, gram-negative rods, and anaerobes—including clostridial species.

5. Which is the treatment of choice for this patient?
   A. Surgical debridement alone
   B. Broad-spectrum antibiotic therapy alone
   C. Surgical debridement plus antibiotic therapy
   D. HBO

An early and aggressive surgical debridement is necessary, in association with initial empiric antibiotic therapy in order to improve patient survival. All nonviable tissues must be extensively removed, and repeated surgical procedures must be planned every 12–36 h (as dictated by conditions of the wound), until the infection is controlled.

Please see Chap. 58 for the correct answer.

References

1. Lancerotto L, Tocco I, Salmaso R, Vindigni V, Bassetto F. Necrotizing fasciitis: classification, diagnosis, and management. J Trauma. 2012;72:560–6.
2. Sarani B, Strong M, pascual J, Schwab CW. Necrotizing fasciitis: current concepts and review of the literature. J Am Coll Surg. 2009;208:279–88.
3. Shiroff AM, Herlitz GN, Gracias VH. Necrotizing soft tissue infections. J Int Care Med. 2014;29:138–44.
4. Hakkarainen TW, Kopari NM, Pham TN, Evans HL. Necrotizing soft tissue infections: review and current concepts in treatment, systems of care, and outcomes. Curr Probl Surg. 2014;51:344–62.
5. Salcido R. Necrotizing fasciitis: reviewing the causes and treatment strategies. Adv Skin Wound Care. 2007;20:288–93.
6. Liu YM, Chi CY, Ho MW. Microbiology and factors affecting mortality in necrotizing fasciitis. J Microbiol Immunol Infect. 2005;38:430–5.
7. Tsai YH, Huang TJ, Hsu RW. Necrotizing soft tissue infections and primary sepsis caused by Vibrio vulnificus and Vibrio cholerae no-O1. J Trauma. 2009;66:899–905.
8. Kao LS, Lew DF, Arab SN, et al. Local variation in the epidemiology, microbiology, and outcome of necrotizing soft tissue infections: a multicenter study. Am J Surg. 2011;202:139–45.
9. Low DE, McGeer A. Skin and soft tissue infections: necrotizing fasciitis. Curr Opin Infect Dis. 1998;11:119–23.
10. Wong CH, Wang YS. The diagnosis of necrotizing fasciitis. Curr Opin Infect Dis. 2005;18:101–6.

11. Seal DV. Necrotizing fasciitis. Curr Opin Infect Dis. 2001;142: 127–32.
12. Seal DV, hay RJ, Middleton KR. Skin and wound infection: investigation and treatment in practice. London, UK: Martin Dunitz; 2000.
13. Wall D, Kleain S, Black S, de Virgilio C. A simple model to help distinguish necrotizing from non-necrotizing soft-tissue infections. Am J Surg. 2000;191:227–31.
14. Wall D, de Virgilio C, Black S, Klein S. Objective criteria may assist in distinguishing necrotizing fasciitis from non-necrotizing soft-tissue infections. Am J Surg. 2000;179:17–21.
15. Wong C, Khin L, Heng K, Tan K, Low C. The LRINEC (laboratory risk indicator for necrotizing fasciitis) score: a tool for distinguishing necrotizing fasciitis from other soft-tissue infections. Crit Care Med. 2004;32:1535–41.
16. Zacharias N, Velmahos GC, Salama A, et al. Diagnosis of necrotizing soft tissue infections by computed tomography. Arch Surg. 2010;145:452–5.
17. Kim KT, Kim YJ, Lee W, et al. Can necrotizing infectious fasciitis be differentiated from nonnecrotizing infectios fasciitis with MR imaging? Radiology. 2011;259:816–24.
18. Yen ZS, Wang HP, Ma HM, Chen SC, Chen WJ. Ultrasonographic screening of clinically-suspected necrotizing fasciitis. Acad Emerg Med. 2002;9:1448–51.
19. Childers BJ, Potyondy LD, Nachreiner R, et al. Necrotizing fasciitis: a fourteen-year retrospective study of 163 consecutive patients. Am Surg. 2002;68:109–16.
20. Anaya DA, Dellinger EP. Necrotizing soft-tissue infection: diagnosis and management. Clin Infect Dis. 2007;44:705–10.
21. Wong CH, Chang HC, Pasupathy S, Khin LW, Tan JL, Low CO. Necrotizing fasciitis: clinical presentation, microbiology, and determinants of mortality. J Bone Joint Surg Am. 2003;85: 1454–60.
22. Majeski JA, Majeski E. Necrotizing fasciitis: improved survival with early recognition by tissue biopsy and aggressive surgical treatment. South Med J. 1997;90:1065–8.
23. Estrada O, Martinez I, Del Bas M, Salvans S, Hidalgo LA. Rectal diversion without colostomy in Fournier's gangrene. Tech Coloproctol. 2009;13:157–9.
24. Ozturk E, Ozquc H, Ylmazlar T. The use of vacuum-assisted closure therapy in the management of Fournier's gangrene. Am J Surg. 2009;197:660–5.
25. Sartelli M, Malangoni MA, May KA, et al. World Society of Emergency Surgery (WSES) guidelines for management of skin and soft tissue infections. World J Emerg Surg. 2014;9:57–74.
26. Angus DC, Van der Poll T. Severe sepsis and septic shock. N Engl J Med. 2013;369:840–51.
27. Tiipana EM, hamunen K, Kontinen VK, kalso E. Do surgical patients benefit from perioperative gabapentin/pregabalin? A systematic review of efficacy and safety. Anesth Analg. 2007;104:1545–56.
28. Darabi K, Abdel-Wahab O, Dzik WH. Current usage of intravenous immunoglobulin and the rationale behind it: the Massachusetts General Hospital data and the review of the literature. Transfusion. 2006;46:741–53.
29. Schrage B, Duan G, Yang LP, Fraser JD, Proft T. Different preparations of intravenous immunoglobulin vary their efficacy to neutralize streptococcal superantigens: implications for treatment of streptococcal toxic shock syndrome. Clin Infect Dis. 2006;43:743–6.
30. Mulla ZD. Hyperbaric oxygen in necrotizing fasciitis. Plast Reconstr Surg. 2008;122:1984–5.
31. Hassan Z, Mullins RF, Friedman BC, et al. Treating necrotizing fasciitis with or without hyperbaric oxygen therapy. Undersea Hyperb Med. 2010;37:115–23.
32. George ME, Rueth NM, Skarda DE, et al. Hyperbaric oxygen does not improve outcome in patients with necrotizing soft tissue infections. Surg Infect. 2009;10:21–3.

Part IV

Surgical Critical Care and Special Topics

45 Advances in Sepsis Management

Daniele Coen

Key Points

- Sepsis is a time-dependent condition that should be carefully looked for in all acute patients. The use of scores like MEWS and NEWS may help recognize patients at high risk of mortality or ICU transfer. The recently proposed qSOFA score is probably less sensitive than MEWS and NEWS.
- Focused ultrasonography may assist in early differential diagnosis and helps in the identification of septic sources that should be removed.
- Early and appropriate antibiotic therapy is the intervention more clearly associated with a positive prognosis. Wide-spectrum antimicrobials should be started as soon as the diagnosis of sepsis has been suspected and samples have been collected for microbiology.
- Aggressive fluid therapy is indicated in the resuscitative phase of patients in shock. Patients who are not hypotensive should be treated with a personalized approach, regularly reevaluating individual fluid responsiveness. Whenever possible, a prolonged positive fluid balance should be avoided, and euvolemia should be aimed at within the first 24 h.
- Vasopressors have useful hemodynamic effects but are not devoid of adverse reactions (mainly increased myocardial oxygen consumption and arrhythmias). When indicated, these drugs should not be used too early nor too late. Patients with persisting shock would probably benefit more when vasopressors are started between 1 and 2 h from diagnosis after adequate fluid replacement has been initiated.

D. Coen (✉)
Grande Ospedale Metropolitano Niguarda, Milan, Italy
e-mail: daniele.coen@ospedaleniguarda.it

45.1 Introduction

Sepsis has been known since ancient times. For decades the instruments used in modern medicine to treat this condition have not changed. Source removal, antibiotics, fluids, vasopressors, and inotropes have been the mainstay of therapy. Oxygen, ventilation, and transfusions have also an important role in supporting vital functions in septic patients. Unfortunately, new therapies based on growing knowledge of the pathophysiology of this syndrome (e.g., PCR, steroids, immunoglobulins, nitric oxide synthetase inhibitors) have proven of doubtful or only marginal efficacy [1–3].

Nevertheless, in most recent years, the choice, the timing, and the modality of administration of available treatments have changed. Moreover, epidemiological data, large clinical trials, and consensus conference statements have helped physicians to better stratify the population of septic patients, favoring a more individualized therapeutic approach.

Today, despite persisting areas of uncertainty, one point is clear to all emergency clinicians: sepsis must be considered a time-dependent condition, just like MI, stroke, or major trauma. It is thus necessary that septic patients are identified as early as possible and that a timely and appropriate treatment is started far before they can find their way to an intensive care unit (ICU). At the same time, doctors should be aware that sepsis is often the fatal event in the clinical history of a chronic and fragile patient. If an aggressive approach is not likely to help their patients, physicians should be able to avoid futility and be willing to offer adequate palliation [4].

45.2 Definitions and Diagnostic Criteria

It is important to consider that definitions in medicine may pursue different goals, like describing the epidemiology of a disease, stating the criteria for inclusion in clinical trials, and helping doctors in their day-to-day clinical work. From a

P. Aseni et al. (eds.), *Operative Techniques and Recent Advances in Acute Care and Emergency Surgery*,
https://doi.org/10.1007/978-3-319-95114-0_45

clinical point of view, sepsis can be defined as a severe infection that produces organ dysfunction, thus increasing morbidity and mortality. The presence of organ dysfunction, due to an aberrant or dysregulated host response, is indeed what differentiates sepsis from infection.

Sepsis is a syndrome, not a single disease, and it is shaped by pathogen factors (type and virulence of the responsible microorganisms) and host factors (e.g., genetic determinants, age, comorbidities, site of the infection) with characteristics that evolve over time.

The history of sepsis definitions [5–7] is summarized in Table 45.1, and it has been well-discussed in a recent contribution from the literature [8]. The most recent definitions proposed by the Third International Consensus Definitions for Sepsis and Septic Shock (Sepsis-3) [7] have been endorsed by most, but not all, scientific societies; notably, the American College of Chest Physicians (ACCP) published a statement disputing the new proposal [9]. Further refinements are to be expected, as the proponents themselves acknowledge, when writing "Aspects of the new definitions do indeed rely on expert opinion; further understanding of the biology of sepsis, the availability of new diagnostic approaches, and enhanced collection of data will fuel their continued reevaluation and revision." Yet, the current Sepsis-3 definition, which is based on a huge amount of epidemiological data, will help for sure in the planning of new epidemiological studies and clinical trials and might facilitate the early recognition and more timely management of patients with sepsis.

Table 45.1 A synthetic history of sepsis definitions

Consensus conference	Criteria
Consensus Conference ACCP/SCCM 1992	Sepsis is defined as the presence or presumed presence of an infection accompanied by evidence of a systemic response called the systemic inflammatory response syndrome. Systemic inflammatory response syndrome is defined as the presence of 2 or more of the following: (1) temperature greater than 38 °C (100.4 °F) or less than 36 °C (96.8 °F); (2) pulse rate greater than 90 beats/min; (3) respiratory rate greater than 20 breaths/min (or PaCO2 less than 32 torr); and (4) WBC count greater than 12,000/mm^3 or less than 4000/mm^3, or greater than 10% immature band forms. Severe sepsis is defined as the presence of sepsis and 1 or more organ dysfunctions. Septic shock is defined as the presence of sepsis and refractory hypotension
International Sepsis Definition Conference 2001	Sepsis is defined more broadly but also more vaguely than infection plus systemic inflammatory response syndrome. It requires the presence of *some* of a long list of clinical and laboratory findings (general variables, inflammatory variables, hemodynamic variables, organ dysfunction variables, tissue perfusion variables). The definition of severe sepsis and septic shock is invariate
Third International Consensus Definitions for Sepsis and Septic Shock 2016	Sepsis is defined as life-threatening organ dysfunction caused by a dysregulated host response to infection. For clinical practice, organ dysfunction is represented by an increase in the Sequential Organ Failure Assessment (SOFA) score of 2 points or more. With this definition, sepsis takes the place of what was formerly defined as severe sepsis. Septic shock is defined as a subset of sepsis in which particularly profound circulatory, cellular, and metabolic abnormalities are associated with a greater risk of mortality than with sepsis alone. Patients with septic shock are clinically identified by a vasopressor requirement to maintain a mean arterial pressure of 65 mmHg or greater and serum lactate level greater than 2 mmol/L (>18 mg/dL)

Table 45.2 reports the SOFA score, which has been proposed by Sepsis-3 as the instrument to evaluate the number and severity of organ failures. Although the SOFA score was not born as a mortality score, it is useful to know that values of 0–6 are associated with a mortality rate lower than 10%, while values >12 predict a mortality higher than 50%.

From the point of view of the practicing physician, it is probably more important to diagnose sepsis rather than to define it. So it may be useful to reaffirm that in order to suspect sepsis, it is necessary that two elements are contemporarily present: infection (diagnosed or suspected) and organ dysfunction.

Organ dysfunction may manifest itself as a clinical sign (e.g., altered consciousness, hypotension, dyspnea, etc.) or as an altered laboratory result (e.g., renal or hepatic failure, disseminated coagulation, hypoxemia, etc.). A septic shock should be diagnosed when organ dysfunction manifests itself as hypotension not responsive to adequate volume replacement and requiring the use of vasopressors.

Sepsis-induced organ dysfunction may be occult; therefore, it is necessary to investigate its presence in any patient presenting with infection. Conversely, an unrecognized infection may cause new-onset organ dysfunction. Any unexplained organ dysfunction should then raise the possibility of an underlying infection.

Early detection of sepsis requires that staff caring for patients in acute hospital settings is competent in monitoring, measuring, interpreting, and promptly responding to clinical changes in the acutely ill patient.

Point of care ultrasound is emerging as an effective and reliable tool for the identification of the septic source. It is likely that its growing use among emergency physicians will help in the early recognition of the site of infection, leading to more appropriate and prompt antimicrobial therapy and source control strategies [10].

Table 45.2 Sequential (sepsis-related) organ failure assessment score

System	Score 0	1	2	3	4
Respiration					
PaO_2/FiO_2 (mm Hg)	≥400	<400	<300	<200[a]	<100[a]
Coagulation					
Platelets (×10³/μL)	≥150	<150	<100	<50	<150
Hepatic					
Bilirubin (mg/dL)	<1.2	1.2–1.9	2.0–5.9	6.0–11.9	≥12.0
Cardiovascular					
Blood pressure	MAP ≥70 mmHg	MAP <70 mmHg	Dopamine ≤5 or dobutamine any dose[b]	Dopamine 5.1–15 or epinephrine ≤0.1 or norepinephrine ≤0.1[b]	Dopamine >15 or epinephrine >0.1 or norepinephrine >0.1[b]
CNS					
Glasgow coma score	15	13–14	10–12	6–9	<6
Renal					
Creatinine (mg/dL)	<1.2	1.2–2.9	3.0–3.4	3.5–5.0	≥5.0
Urine output (mL/24 h)				<500	<200

[a]With respiratory support
[b]Cathecolamine doses expressed as μg/kg/min for at least 1 h

45.3 Pathophysiology

Mechanisms that determine the evolution of sepsis are complex and multifaceted. While research on the pathogenesis of this syndrome unceasingly produces new knowledge, it is not yet clear why severe infections may induce normal inflammatory reaction in some patients and a dysregulated, self-destructive process in other ones. During septic shock, the mechanisms that usually occur as a normal physiologic response to localized infection (activation of neutrophils and monocytes, release of inflammatory mediators, local vasodilation, increased endothelial permeability, and activation of coagulation pathways) take place on a systemic scale. This leads to diffuse endothelial disruption, vascular permeability, vasodilation, and thrombosis of end-organ capillaries. Endothelial damage itself further activates inflammatory and coagulation cascades, creating a positive feedback loop which leads to further endothelial and end-organ damage.

Among the mechanisms that play a role in the evolution of sepsis, the following are being actively investigated:

- *Host response* (anti-inflammatory and pro-inflammatory reactions, nitric oxide). Both pro-inflammatory and anti-inflammatory mechanisms can act to clear the infection and help tissue recovery or cause organ injury and favor secondary infections. Hyperproduction of nitric oxide in the endothelium may contribute to hypotension, cardiodepression, and vascular hyporeactivity in septic shock.
- *Immunity* (pathogen-associated molecular patterns, PAMPs, and damage-associated molecular patterns—DAMPs or alarmins). Depending on the target cell and the cellular context, the interaction between PAMPs and DAMPs can lead to cell differentiation or cell death, and either inflammation or inhibition of inflammation.
- *Coagulation* (excess fibrin deposition, impaired anticoagulant mechanisms, thrombin activation of protease-activated receptors). Sepsis is almost invariably associated with altered coagulation which may lead to disseminated intravascular coagulation.
- *Microcirculation* (lesions to glycocalyces, increased endothelial permeability, microvascular thrombosis, reduced red cell deformability). Endothelial lesions are critical in the development of vascular leak, edema, and subsequent shock. The accumulation of parenchymal and interstitial fluid increases the distance required for the diffusion of oxygen and further compromises microvascular perfusion increasing interstitial pressure.

All of the previous, which shall not be discussed here in detail, have been extensively reviewed in the literature [11–14]. These mechanisms play a role in the development of organ failure determining in the end impaired tissue oxygenation. When sustained, mitochondrial damage ensues, starting a vicious circle that heralds the irreversibility of septic shock.

Among the relevant macrovascular aspects in the pathophysiology of septic shock, cardiac impairment is of particular relevance. Up to 50% of patients with septic shock have systolic LV dysfunction, and almost as many have features of diastolic dysfunction [15, 16]. Potential candidates responsible for septic cardiomyopathy include PAMPs, cytokines, and nitric oxide.

45.4 Prognosis

Severe sepsis is one of the top ten causes of death in the United States, affecting one out of three ICU patients. Reports using administrative data show a declining trend in hospital mortality rates for patients with severe sepsis [17–19]. However, changing trends in coding patterns or hospital discharge patterns could affect them, resulting in biased mortality estimates. In contrast with this often held hypothesis, a meta-analysis of clinical studies has shown that administrative data do not differ from data derived from clinical trials that show a decrease in mortality of about 3.0% annually, from 46% during years 1991–1995 to 29% during years 2006–2009 [20].

Prognosis of septic patients is influenced by age, co-pathologies, site of infection, number of failing organs, and development of shock. Biomarkers and scores have been developed to help clinicians in the early identification of patients at risk of major complications and higher mortality.

Lactate is a well-known marker of severity, being, for the most part, a direct expression of tissue hypoperfusion [21–24]. A lactate value >4 mmol/L has been addressed as "cryptic shock" by some authors, being considered as negative an indicator as persisting hypotension [25]. Lactate reduction during the first hours of treatment (lactate clearance) was shown to be a positive prognostic indicator [26]. Procalcitonin is also directly related to increasing severity of infections. It has been demonstrated that among intensive care patients with sepsis, failure to decrease procalcitonin by more than 80% is a significant independent predictor of mortality.

Sepsis-3 proposes to use a new simple bedside criteria (qSOFA) to identify septic patients at high risk of an adverse outcome. This new measure incorporates altered mentation, systolic blood pressure of 100 mm Hg or less, and respiratory rate of 22/min or greater. In the proponents' view, qSOFA should be easier to calculate (although less robust) than SOFA and much more specific than the time-honored SIRS criteria, since 90% of intensive care unit patients and 50% of general ward patients meet the SIRS criteria at some point during their hospitalization [27]. Although this is certainly true, the results of the first studies on qSOFA are not encouraging. Indeed qSOFA seems to be a late indicator of severity among infected patients, and its sensibility is inferior both to SIRS and to the NEWS and MEWS, which are already monitored in many countries [28].

Less than one every five patients who will die or be transferred to the ICU will have met >2 qSOFA criteria when infection is first suspected. For this reason, qSOFA, if used at all, should be recalculated after the initiation of therapy. At the moment there seems to be no reason for hospitals already using the NEWS or MEWS for switching to qSOFA.

45.5 Timing of Treatment

Sepsis is now indisputably considered a time-dependent condition. This is due on the one hand to the aforementioned pathophysiological knowledge that inversely links the reversibility of organ damage to the duration of septic shock [1], and on the other to the results of clinical studies, mainly in the field of antimicrobial therapy. At variance with MI and stroke though, in the case of sepsis there are no silver bullets, like revascularization, at our disposal, but rather, an array of interventions (often addressed to as "bundles"), difficult to disentangle as to their time dependency.

Moreover, evidence from the literature comes mainly in the form of epidemiological or observational studies, and there is a lack of randomized clinical trials, which would be ethically not acceptable.

For these reasons, with the noticeable exception of early antibiotic therapy (which has a strong level of recommendation and moderate evidence), the Surviving Sepsis Campaign 2016 guidelines [29] consider the precocity of most treatments as a best practice statement (BPS), that is, the recommendation of a treatment which is thought to be highly beneficial in the absence of a methodologically formal evidence (Table 45.3).

Interestingly, a recent meta-analysis, though stressing the indication to start adequate antimicrobial therapy as soon as possible, was not able to demonstrate a significant mortality benefit of administering antibiotics within 3 h of emergency department triage or 1 h of shock recognition [30]. This is at variance with single clinical trials that have shown a mortality increase for each hour of delay in treatment.

Similarly, a multicenter prospective observational analysis, while confirming that mortality was lower in septic patients who underwent source control than in those who did not, could not link the time to source control to survival [31].

Table 45.3 SSC 2016 guidelines statements on the timing of treatment [29]

• Sepsis and septic shock are medical emergencies, and we recommend that treatment and resuscitation begin immediately (BPS)
• We recommend that a specific anatomic diagnosis of infection requiring emergent source control be identified or excluded as rapidly as possible in patients with sepsis or septic shock and that any required source control intervention be implemented as soon as medically and logistically practical after the diagnosis is made (BPS)
• We recommend prompt removal of intravascular access devices that are a possible source of sepsis or septic shock after other vascular access has been established (BPS)
• We recommend that administration of IV antimicrobials be initiated as soon as possible after recognition and within 1 h for both sepsis and septic shock (strong recommendation, moderate quality of evidence; grade applies to both conditions)

The timing of fluid administration poses particular and complex problems which will be discussed in the appropriate section.

We can conclude that, although the indication to approach septic patients as early as possible is here to stay, the recommendation of specific timing metrics in international guidelines is not always supported by the currently available evidence.

It is appropriate to end this section reporting the words from a recent statement from SSC Leadership on Time Zero in the Emergency Department [32], where we are reminded that a timely diagnosis is the inescapable prerequisite of early treatment:

"The importance of close monitoring in the sepsis patient population cannot be underestimated. Later development of hypotension in patients who were normotensive at ED triage is not the only indication of severe sepsis. Awareness of organ dysfunction other than hypotension is equally important. Frequent observations for changes in vital signs will lead to early recognition and improved outcomes, despite the occasional inability to achieve all of the time-sensitive indicators".

45.6 Antibiotics

A frequently cited paper from Kumar et al. [33] reported a 7.6% increase in mortality for each hourly delay after the onset of septic shock. Several other studies have reported increased mortality associated with delays in antibiotic administration either from shock recognition or time from ED triage [34, 35], although less clear results have also been documented [30, 36]. Recently a delay in the administration of the second dose of antibiotics has also been related to a worse outcome [37]. So, while it is recognized that a delay to administer an appropriate antimicrobial therapy will have a negative effect on patient outcomes, it is yet a matter of debate the exact time frame when this may happen.

Of note, a paper comparing randomized versus observational studies on EGDT has demonstrated that the only intervention associated with EGDT better survival, in 31 observational studies with historical controls, was faster and more appropriate antibiotic co-intervention. Randomized trials, which did not show any advantage for EGDT had, on the contrary, short and similar time to antibiotics in the two groups [38].

With these premises, it is unfortunate that many emergency department patients with sepsis still do not receive antibiotics until they arrive on the inpatient unit [39].

In practice, the management of a patient with severe sepsis requires that cultures are collected right after the diagnosis is suspected and that broad-spectrum antibiotics are started promptly thereafter. The choice of empirical antimicrobial therapy should be based on site of infection, local ecology, patient characteristics, and the pharmacokinetics and pharmacodynamics of the antibiotics [40]. Inappropriate initial antimicrobial therapy, defined as an antimicrobial regimen that lacks in vitro activity against the isolated organism(s) responsible for the infection, has been associated with excess mortality in critically ill patients [41, 42]. It has also been demonstrated that when antibiotics are used among septic emergency department patients, drug-resistant bacteria are infrequently covered [39, 43]. Recent analyses suggest that improved targeting of empiric antimicrobials for multidrug-resistant bacteria, *Candida* species, methicillin-resistant *S. aureus*, and *P. aeruginosa* would have the greatest impact in reducing mortality from inappropriate antimicrobial treatment in patients with severe sepsis and septic shock [30, 44, 45].

In severe infection, guidelines recommend the use of a combination of antibiotics [46]. Although the evidence is scanty, it is commonly accepted that antimicrobial therapy of the critically ill patient should be based on written protocols because when the selection of antibiotics is left solely to the discretion of the attending physician, the rate of appropriate use may be very low [47].

When the results of cultures become available, treatment should be reevaluated to either de-escalate or escalate the antibiotics. This is associated with decreased incidence of superinfection and reduced development of antimicrobial resistance [48]. Yet no advantages for patients with sepsis have been clearly demonstrated [49, 50]. Increasing attention has been given in recent years to the dosing and modality of administration of antibiotics that may best prevent the development of resistant pathogens. Given for granted that pharmacokinetics and pharmacodynamics should drive the modality of administration of antibiotics, based on their time-dependent or concentration dependent action, the debate centers on the opportunity to administer higher doses of concentration-dependent antibiotics. This would allow reaching the so-called mutant prevention concentration (MPC), avoiding concentrations in the mutant selection window (MSW), that is, an above MIC critical range of antibiotic concentrations where drug-resistant bacterial mutants could be selectively enriched and amplified (Fig. 45.1) [40, 51]. A shorter period of treatment is also a way to prevent antibiotic resistance. Clinical improvement and possibly the reduction in the values of the biomarker procalcitonin should guide the duration of therapy [52, 53]. Yet, the advantage of a procalcitonin-guided antibiotic stewardship has been recently disputed by a retrospective cohort study enrolling more than 20,000 patients in 107 US intensive care units,

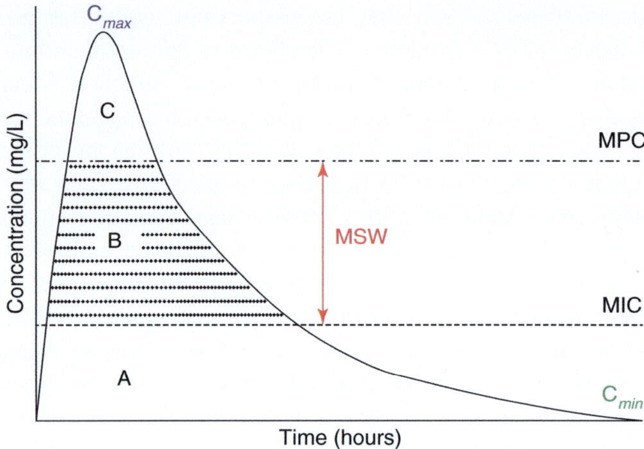

Fig. 45.1 The mutant selection window (MSW). When time-dependent antibiotics reach a concentration that is above the minimum inhibitory concentration (MIC) but below the mutant prevention concentration (MPC), resistant mutants may be selectively amplified. The longer the time spent by an antibiotic in this concentration zone, the greater the opportunity for resistant mutants to be selected and amplified. C_{max} maximum drug concentration, C_{min} minimum drug concentration. (Adapted from Abdul Aziz, et al. [40])

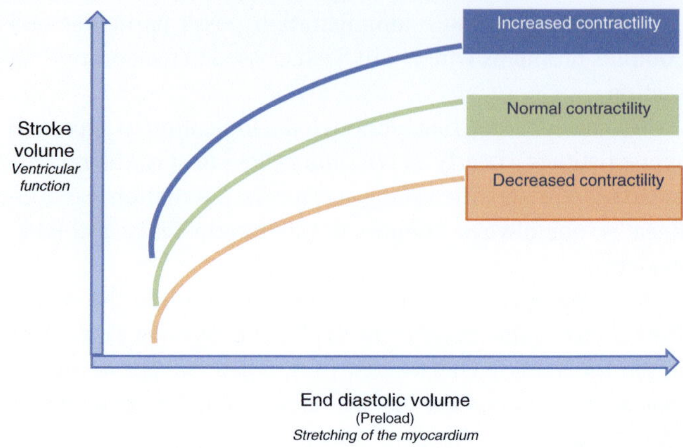

Fig. 45.2 The Frank-Starling curves in the hyperactive, normal, and diseased heart. In a normal heart, an augmented preload increases stroke volume until a plateau phase is reached. In a failing heart, response to increasing preload is negligible, the plateau is reached much sooner, and further fluid administration may prove detrimental for the development of interstitial and alveolar edema

showing that procalcitonin use was not associated with improved antibiotic use or other clinical outcomes in real-world settings [54].

45.7 Fluids

The administration of fluids is for sure one of the most important means that doctors have to control septic shock in its early phases when peripheral vasodilation is the main cause of the reduction in precharge and cardiac output. It is also clear that to achieve their goal, fluids should be administered as boluses, so to guarantee that a sufficient volume remains in the intravascular space in spite of the physiological drive that forces most of them to move to the interstitium within tens of minutes [55].

A word of caution comes from physiology as well as from studies that have investigated fluid balance beyond the very first hours of fluid resuscitation. The messages from physiopathology come from the Frank-Starling curve in normal and failing hearts. As it can be seen in Fig. 45.2, normal hearts respond briskly and efficiently to fluid administration at low cardiac volumes, reaching a plateau progressively at higher volumes, when the effect of fluids becomes negligible. In the failing heart though, this level is reached much more quickly until further fluid administration can paradoxically result in a lower CO [56].

Clinical studies, on their side, have not yet come to a conclusion as to how much fluid is adequate for good management of septic patients. It is indeed clear that "excessive" fluid administration may increase the risk of mortality, but the definition of how much fluid is excessive is still a matter of debate.

In the EGDT trial by Rivers et al. [57], fluid administration was one of the interventions that differentiated treated versus control patients (approximately 5 ± 3 L vs. 3.5 ± 2.5 L in the first 6 h). This was not true in the three trials that disputed the efficacy of EGDT some 15 years later [58–60]. Nevertheless, early fluid administration was relevant also in these studies, since patients in both arms received approximately 2 L of fluids before randomization and 2 more within the following 6 h of treatment. A recent cohort study on a US database suggests that mortality increases when higher than 5 L of fluids is given in the first day of treatment [61], but although this association is well-proved, causality may not be inferred from this data. Finally, many studies document a strong association between positive fluid balance and mortality in ICU patients at times varying between 12 and 96 h [62–65].

At this point, one might conclude that there is no "one fits all" recipe in fluid administration and that volume replacement should be guided by clinical and instrumental assessment of every individual patient.

One should also recognize that fluid replacement pursues different goals during the different phases of treatment and that fluid administration should be progressively reduced moving from resuscitation to stabilization. A de-escalation phase should be entered as soon as possible, with the aim of reaching euvolemia within the first 24 h [66, 67].

As to the choice of fluids, it is now established that colloids offer no advantage over crystalloids and are associated with more frequent adverse events [68–70]. Among crystalloids, balanced solutions may have some advantage over saline when high volumes are infused [71, 72]. Lastly, the level of evidence for the routine use of albumin is low, although some advantage has been documented for patients with septic shock who need high volumes of crystalloids [73, 74].

45.8 Vasoactive Agents

Vasopressor and inotrope medications are vasoactive agents used in shock states to assist in the restoration of impaired perfusion. These drugs have diverse and often overlapping physiologic effects.

The use of vasoactive agents in septic shock has not been extensively addressed by clinical trials. Studies have mostly compared different agents, without coming to conclusions as to the optimal agents and the optimal timing. Thus, this element of care is mainly guided by expert opinion [75–77].

Nevertheless, available data is sufficient to consider norepinephrine as superior to dopamine in the treatment of septic shock [78], and as such norepinephrine has been advised as the first-line vasopressor by the Surviving Sepsis Campaign guidelines [29].

Among possible reasons for inconsistent findings in the existing literature is that vasoactive agents are often used simultaneously with fluids for the same indications of hypotension and hypoperfusion. A recent multicenter study has investigated the interaction between fluids and vasoactive agents on mortality in septic shock, concluding that it may be detrimental to start vasoactive agents within the first hour after shock onset and suggesting to delay them for at least 1 h while the fluid resuscitation is begun. Mortality was lowest when vasoactive agents were started 1–6 h after access, with more than 1 L of fluids in the first hour and more than 2.5 L from hours 1–6 [79]. Other studies seem to confirm that, when indicated, vasoactivity should be started early when hypotension persists after the initial fluid resuscitation [76, 80].

Considering the possible difficulty and risks of obtaining a central vein access during the immediate resuscitation phase of septic shock in the ED or in the general ward, it comes as good news a recent systematic review concluding that the peripheral administration of vasopressors is safe for short durations (<2 h) via large bore catheters that are placed proximal to the antecubital and popliteal fossae [81]. At least one more study has shown that vasopressors may be safely infused peripherally for a longer time when a protocol of peripheral venous access and treatment of extravasation is strictly adhered to [82].

Conclusions

Sepsis is a leading cause of morbidity and mortality which affects one in three ICU patients. Over the last two decades, prompter and more targeted interventions have improved prognosis, but the toll that patients pay to this syndrome is still very high. Early recognition through frequent monitoring of acute patients, timely and appropriate antibiotics, and a judicious use of fluids and vasopressors is, at the moment, the fundamental of successful treatment.

Case Scenario

A 42-year-old man with a history of hypertension underwent an elective hernia repair. Although the case went well, 12 h postoperatively, the patient complained of abdominal pain and became unstable. His blood pressure dropped to 85/45 mm Hg, heart rate was 120, and severe hypoxemia developed. His temperature was 37.2 °C. The surgeon in charge ordered a computed tomography (CT) angiogram to exclude pulmonary embolism (PE). Although no PE was found, the CT revealed changes consistent with early ARDS and images from the abdomen demonstrated significant peritoneal fluid.

1. Could this patient be septic?
   A. Yes, because he could have peritonitis and has signs of organ dysfunction.
   B. No, it is more likely that he bled in his abdomen.
   C. No, because he has not a fever, nor other clear signs of infection.
   D. Yes, because he has a low blood pressure.

2. How would you first approach fluid therapy?
   A. Colloids 500 mL to be repeated as needed
   B. Ringer lactate 250–500 mL boluses to a maximum of 20 mL/kg in 30 min
   C. Saline 1000 mL + albumin 20% 300 mL in 30 min
   D. Ringer lactate infusion 300 mL/h

3. Would you administer antibiotics?
   A. Yes, I would administer a third-generation cephalosporin with extended spectrum on *Pseudomonas aeruginosa*.
   B. No, I would rather perform a laparoscopy first.
   C. Yes, I would definitely administer a combination therapy of antibiotics aiming at wide-spectrum coverage.
   D. No; antibiotics induce resistant strains, and I think there is time to wait for the result of cultures.

4. Would you go back to the OR?
   A. Yes, there is definitely the possibility of a removable source, and the patient should be brought back to the OR within 12 h.
   B. Yes, a laparoscopy or laparotomy is urgent and necessary both to establish the diagnosis and to proceed to surgical therapy if needed.
   C. No, antibiotics and fluids will probably suffice to take care of a possible abdominal infection. Watchful waiting is a suitable alternative.
   D. No, the patient should first be transferred to ICU to take care of his ARDS.

5. Would you consider using vasopressors in this patient?
   A. No, his heart is running too fast, and the risk of arrhythmia is definitely too high.
   B. Yes, I would start dopamine at low doses, to favor renal perfusion without increasing oxygen consumption by the heart.
   C. Yes, I would start high-dose epinephrine and then quickly titrate down when an acceptable PA value is reached.
   D. Yes, I would consider low-dose norepinephrine and then titrate up if low blood pressure persists, after administration of at least 20 mL/kg of crystalloids.

Please see Chap. 58 for the correct answer.

References

1. Duran-Bedolla J, Montes de Oca-Sandoval MA, Saldaña-Navor V, et al. Sepsis, mitochondrial failure and multiple organ dysfunction. Clin Invest Med. 2014;37(2):E58–69.
2. Seymour CW, Rosengart MR. Septic Shock. Advances in diagnosis and treatment. JAMA. 2015;314(7):708–17.
3. Perner A, Gordon AC, De Backer D. Sepsis: frontiers in diagnosis, resuscitation and antibiotic therapy. Intensive Care Med. 2016;42:1958–69.
4. Nelson JE, Mathews KS, Weissman DE, et al. Integration of palliative care in the context of rapid response. A report from the Improving Palliative Care in the ICU Advisory Board. Chest. 2015;147(2):560–9.
5. American College of Chest Physicians/Society of Critical Care Medicine Consensus Conference. Definitions for sepsis and organ failure and guidelines for the use of innovative therapies in sepsis. Crit Care Med. 1992;20:864–74.
6. Levy MM, Fink MP, Marshall JC, et al. 2001 SCCM/ESICM/ACCP/ATS/SIS international sepsis definitions conference. Intensive Care Med. 2003;29:530–8.
7. Singer M, Deutschman CS, Seymour CW, et al. The Third International Consensus Definitions for Sepsis and Septic Shock (Sepsis-3). JAMA. 2016;315(8):801–10.
8. Scott MC. Defining and diagnosing sepsis. Emerg Med Clin N Am. 2017;35:1–9.
9. Simpson SQ. New sepsis criteria: a change we should not make. Chest. 2016;149(5):117–8.
10. Cortellaro F, Ferrari L, Molteni F, et al. Accuracy of point of care ultrasound to identify the source of infection in septic patients: a prospective study. Intern Emerg Med. 2017;12:371–8.
11. Angus DC, van der Poll T. Severe Sepsis and Septic Shock. New Engl J Med. 2013;369:840–51.
12. Boomer JS, To K, Chang KC, et al. Immunosuppression in patients who die of sepsis and multiple organ failure. JAMA. 2011;306:2594–605.
13. Lee WL, Slutsky AS. Sepsis and endothelial permeability. New Engl J Med. 2010;363:689–91.
14. Mira JC, Gentile LF, Mathias BJ. Sepsis pathophysiology, chronic critical illness, and persistent inflammation-immunosuppression and catabolism syndrome. Crit Care Med. 2017;45:253–62.
15. Romero-Bermejo FJ, Ruiz-Bailen M, Gil-Cebrian J, Huertos-Ranchal MJ. Sepsis-induced cardiomyopathy. Curr Cardiol Rev. 2011;7:163–83.
16. Sato R, Nasu M. A review of sepsis-induced cardiomyopathy. J Intensive Care. 2015;3:48.
17. Kumar G, Kumar N, Taneja A, et al. Nationwide trends of severe sepsis in the 21st century (2000-2007). Chest. 2011;140:1223–31.
18. Lagu T, Rothberg MB, Shieh MS, et al. Hospitalizations, costs, and outcomes of severe sepsis in the United States 2003 to 2007. Crit Care Med. 2012;40:754–61.
19. Kaukonen KM, Bailey M, Suzuki S, et al. Mortality related to severe sepsis and septic shock among critically ill patients in Australia and New Zealand, 2000-2012. JAMA. 2014;311:1308–16.
20. Stevenson EK, Rubenstein AR, Radin GT, et al. Two decades of mortality trends among patients with severe sepsis: a comparative meta-analysis. Crit Care Med. 2014;42:625–31.
21. Vernon C, Letourneau JL. Lactic acidosis: recognition, kinetics, and associated prognosis. Crit Care Clin. 2010;26:255–83.
22. Revelly JP, Tappy L, Martinez A, et al. Lactate and glucose metabolism in severe sepsis and cardiogenic shock. Crit Care Med. 2005;33:2235–40.
23. Puskarich MA, Trzeciak S, Shapiro NI, et al. Outcomes of patients undergoing early sepsis resuscitation for cryptic shock compared with overt shock. Resuscitation. 2011;82(10):1289–93.
24. Zhang Z, Xu X. Lactate clearance is a useful biomarker for the prediction of all-cause mortality in critically ill patients: a systematic review and meta-analysis. Crit Care Med. 2014;42:2118–25.
25. Mikkelsen ME, Miltiades AN, Gaieski DF, et al. Serum lactate is associated with mortality in severe sepsis independent of organ failure and shock. Crit Care Med. 2009;37:1670–7.
26. Jones AE, Shapiro NI, Trzeciak S, et al. Lactate clearance vs central venous oxygen saturation as goals of early sepsis therapy: a randomized clinical trial. JAMA. 2010;303:739–46.
27. Schuetz P, Birkhahn R, Sherwin R, et al. Serial procalcitonin predicts mortality in severe sepsis patients: results from the Multicenter

Procalcitonin MOnitoring SEpsis (MOSES) study. Crit Care Med. 2017;45:781–9.
28. Churpek MM, Snyder A, Han X, et al. Quick Sepsis-related Organ Failure Assessment, Systemic Inflammatory Response Syndrome, and Early Warning Scores for detecting clinical deterioration in infected patients outside the intensive care unit. Am J Respir Crit Care Med. 2017;195(7):906–11.
29. Rhodes A, Evans LE, Alhazzani W, et al. Surviving Sepsis Campaign: International Guidelines for Management of Sepsis and Septic Shock: 2016. Crit Care Med. 2017;45:1–67.
30. Sterling SA, Miller WR, Pryor J, et al. The impact of timing of antibiotics on outcomes in severe sepsis and septic shock: a systematic review and meta-analysis. Crit Care Med. 2015;43:1907–15.
31. Martínez ML, Ferrer R, Torrents E, et al. Impact of source control in patients with severe sepsis and septic shock. Crit Care Med. 2017;45:11–9.
32. The Surviving Sepsis Campaign. Statement from SSC Leadership on Time Zero in the Emergency Department. www.survivingsepsis.org/SiteCollectionDocuments/Time-Zero.pdf
33. Kumar A, Roberts D, Wood KE, et al. Duration of hypotension before initiation of effective antimicrobial therapy is the critical determinant of survival in human septic shock. Crit Care Med. 2006;34:1589–96.
34. Ferrer R, Martin-Loeches I, Phillips G, et al. Empiric antibiotic treatment reduces mortality in severe sepsis and septic shock from the first hour: results from a guideline-based performance improvement program. Crit Care Med. 2014;42:1749–55.
35. Whiles BB, Deis AS, Simpson SQ. Increased time to initial antimicrobial administration is associated with progression to septic shock in severe sepsis patients. Crit Care Med. 2017;45(4):623–9.
36. Puskarich MA, Trzeciak S, Shapiro NI, et al. Association between timing of antibiotic administration and mortality from septic shock in patients treated with a quantitative resuscitation protocol. Crit Care Med. 2011;39:2066–71.
37. Leisman D, Huang V, Zhou Q, et al. Delayed second dose antibiotics for patients admitted from the emergency department with sepsis: prevalence, risk factors, and outcomes. Crit Care Med. 2017;45(6):956–65.
38. Kalil AC, Johnson DW, Lisco SJ, Sun J. Early goal-directed therapy for sepsis: a novel solution for discordant survival outcomes in clinical trials. Crit Care Med. 2017;45:607–14.
39. Filbin MR, Arias SA, Camargo CA Jr, et al. Sepsis visits and antibiotic utilization in U.S. Emergency Departments. Crit Care Med. 2014;42:528–35.
40. Abdul-Aziz MH, Lipman J, Mouton JW, et al. Applying pharmacokinetic/pharmacodynamic principles in critically ill patients: optimizing efficacy and reducing resistance development. Semin Respir Crit Care Med. 2015;36:136–53.
41. Kollef MH, Sherman G, Ward S, et al. Inadequate antimicrobial treatment of infections: a risk factor for hospital mortality among critically ill patients. Chest. 1999;115:462–74.
42. Shorr AF, Micek ST, Welch EC, et al. Inappropriate antibiotic therapy in Gram-negative sepsis increases hospital length of stay. Crit Care Med. 2011;39:46–51.
43. Ferrer R, Artigas A, Suarez D, et al. Effectiveness of treatments for severe sepsis: a prospective, multicenter, observational study. Am J Respir Crit Care Med. 2009;180:861–6.
44. Burnham JP, Lane MA, Kollef MH. Impact of sepsis classification and multidrug-resistance status on outcome among patients treated with appropriate therapy. Crit Care Med. 2015;43:1580–6.
45. Vazquez-Guillamet C, Scolari M, Zilberberg MD, et al. Using the number needed to treat to assess appropriate antimicrobial therapy as a determinant of outcome in severe sepsis and septic shock. Crit Care Med. 2014;42:2342–9.
46. Vazquez-Grande G, Kumar A. Optimizing antimicrobial therapy of sepsis and septic shock: focus on antibiotic combination therapy. Semin Respir Crit Care Med. 2015;36:154–66.
47. Dupont H, Mentec H, Sollet J, et al. Impact of the appropriateness of initial antibiotic treatment on the outcome of ventilator-associated pneumonia. Intensive Care Med. 2001;27:355–62.
48. Textoris J, Wiramus S, Martin C, Leone M. Antibiotic therapy in patients with septic shock. Eur J Anaesthesiol. 2011;28:318–24.
49. Schuts EC, Hulscher MEJL, W Mouton JW, et al. Current evidence on hospital antimicrobial stewardship objectives: a systematic review and meta-analysis. Lancet Inf Dis. 2016;16:847–56.
50. Silva BNG, Andriolo RB, Atallah ÁN, Salomão R. De-escalation of antimicrobial treatment for adults with sepsis, severe sepsis or septic shock. Cochrane Database Syst Rev. 2013;(3):CD007934.
51. Landelle C, Marimuthu K, Harbarth S. Infection control measures to decrease the burden of antimicrobial resistance in the critical care setting. Curr Opin Crit Care. 2014;20:499–506.
52. de Jong E, van Oers JA, Beishuizen A, et al. Efficacy and safety of procalcitonin guidance in reducing the duration of antibiotic treatment in critically ill patients: a randomised, controlled, open-label trial. Lancet Infect Dis. 2016;16:819–27.
53. Barlam TF, Cosgrove SE, Abbo LM, et al. Implementing an antibiotic stewardship program: guidelines by the Infectious Diseases Society of America and the Society for Healthcare Epidemiology of America. Clin Infect Dis. 2016;62:e51–77.
54. Chu DC, Mehta AB, Walkey AJ. Practice patterns and outcomes associated with procalcitonin use in critically ill patients with sepsis. Clin Infect Dis. 2017;64(11):1509–15.
55. Loflin R, Winters ME. Fluid resuscitation in severe sepsis. Emerg Med Clin N Am. 2017;35:60–74.
56. Marik PE, Lemson J. Fluid responsiveness: an evolution of our understanding. P Br J Anaesth. 2014;12:217–20.
57. Rivers E, Nguyen B, Havstad S, et al. Early goal-directed therapy in the treatment of severe sepsis and septic shock. N Engl J Med. 2001;345:1368–77.
58. Mouncey PR, Osborn TM, Power GS, et al. Trial of early, goal-directed resuscitation for septic shock. N Engl J Med. 2015;372:1301–11.
59. Yealy DM, Kellum JA, Huang DT, et al. A randomized trial of protocol-based care for early septic shock. N Engl J Med. 2014;370:1683–93.
60. Peake SL, Delaney A, Bailey M, et al. Goal-directed resuscitation for patients with early septic shock. N Engl J Med. 2014;371:1496–506.
61. Marik PE, Linde-Zwirble WT, Bittner EA, Sahatjian J, Hansell D. Fluid administration in severe sepsis and septic shock, patterns and outcomes: an analysis of a large national database. Intensive Care Med. 2017;43(5):625–32.
62. Sakr Y, Rubatto Birri PN, Kotfis K, et al. Higher fluid balance increases the risk of death from sepsis: results from a large international audit. Crit Care Med. 2017;45:386–94.
63. Acheampong A, Vincent JL. A positive fluid balance is an independent prognostic factor in patients with sepsis. Crit Care. 2015;19:251.
64. de Oliveira FS, Freitas FG, Ferreira EM, et al. Positive fluid balance as a prognostic factor for mortality and acute kidney injury in severe sepsis and septic shock. J Crit Care. 2015;30:97–101.
65. Boyd JH, Forbes J, Nakada TA, et al. Fluid resuscitation in septic shock: a positive fluid balance and elevated central venous pressure are associated with increased mortality. Crit Care Med. 2011;39:259–65.
66. Hoste EA, Maitland K, Brudney CS, et al. Four phases of intravenous fluid therapy: a conceptual model. Br J Anaesth. 2014;113(5):740–7.
67. Leone M. Septic shock resuscitation: assembling the puzzle. Crit Care Med. 2014;42:2294–5.
68. Annane D, Siami S, Jaber S, et al. Effects of fluid resuscitation with colloids vs crystalloids on mortality in critically ill patients presenting with hypovolemic shock: the CRISTAL randomized trial. JAMA. 2013;310(17):1809–17.

69. Perner A, Haase N, Guttormsen AB, et al. Hydroxyethyl starch 130/0.4 versus Ringers Acetate in severe sepsis. N Engl J Med. 2012;367:124–34.
70. Haase N, Perner A, Hennings LI, et al. Hydroxyethyl starch 130/0.38–0.45 versus crystalloid or albumin in patients with sepsis: systematic review with meta-analysis and trial sequential analysis. Br Med J. 2013;346:f839.
71. Mohd Yunos N, Bellomo R, Hegarty C, et al. Association between a chloride-liberal vs chloride-restrictive intravenous fluid administration strategy and kidney injury in critically ill adults. JAMA. 2012;308:1566–72.
72. Raghunathan K, Shaw A, Nathanson B, et al. Association between the choice of IV crystalloid and in-hospital mortality among critically ill adults with sepsis. Crit Care Med. 2014;42:1585–91.
73. Finfer S, McEvoy S, Bellomo R, et al. Impact of albumin compared to saline on organ function and mortality of patients with severe sepsis. Intensive Care Med. 2011;37(1):86–96.
74. Caironi P, Tognoni G, Masson S, et al. Albumin replacement in patients with severe sepsis or septic shock. N Engl J Med. 2014;370(15):1412–21.
75. Jentzer JC, Coons JC, Link CB, et al. Pharmacotherapy update on the use of vasopressors and inotropes in the intensive care unit. J Cardiovasc Pharmacol Ther. 2015;20(3):249–60.
76. Marik P, Bellomo S. A rational approach to fluid therapy in sepsis. Br J Anaesth. 2016;116(3):339–49.
77. Avni T, Lador A, Lev S, et al. Vasopressors for the treatment of septic shock: systematic review and meta-analysis. PLoS One. 2015;10(8):e0129305. http://www.ncbi.nlm.nih.gov/pmc/articles/PMC4523170/?report5reader. Accessed 10 Mar 2016.
78. De Backer D, Aldecoa C, Nijmi H, et al. Dopamine versus norepinephrine in the treatment of septic shock: a meta-analysis. Crit Care Med. 2012;40(3):725–30.
79. Jason Waechter J, Kumar A, Lapinsky SE, et al. Interaction between fluids and vasoactive agents on mortality in septic shock: a multicenter, observational study. Crit Care Med. 2014;42:2158–68.
80. Bai X, Yu W, Ji W. Early versus delayed administration of norepinephrine in patients with septic shock. Crit Care. 2014;18:532.
81. Loubani OM, Green RS. A systematic review of extravasation and local tissue injury from administration of vasopressors through peripheral intravenous catheters and central venous catheters. J Crit Care. 2015;30(3):653.e9–17.
82. Cardenas-Garcia J, Schaub KF, Belchikov YG, et al. Safety of peripheral intravenous administration of vasoactive medication. J Hosp Med. 2015;10(9):581–5.

Initial Resuscitation of Hemorrhagic Shock and Massive Transfusion Protocol

46

Lucio Bucci

Key Points

- In a substantial bleeding patient, especially in severely injured trauma, clinicians have to correlate the deranged physiology with clinical signs with caution and an appropriate grade of suspicion.
- In life-threatening blood loss, coagulation derangements, metabolic disorders, and complex microcirculation both with tissue disorders have constantly to be considered: hemodynamic-driven resuscitation aims to maintain hemodynamic coherence in the macrocirculation and the microvasculature as well.
- Less than prior fluids' administration during damage control resuscitation seeks to minimize overloads resulting in tissue edema and organ failure, dilutional coagulopathy, and coagulation interferences; moreover, endothelial damage plays a role in inducing an increased permeability, interstitial edema, activation of both inflammatory, and coagulation systems with very similar consequences like those observed in sepsis state.
- Rapid identification of patients who are actively bleeding and need early activation and treatment adopting a massive transfusion protocol in the first hours represents the main objective of the entire working team.
- Early identification of hypoperfusion, acidosis, and the risk of coagulopathy using base deficit and lactate may usually help predict the development of coagulopathy in trauma patients and direct therapy.
- Hypothermia, associated with acidosis, hypotension, and coagulopathy in severely injured patients, remains one of the most preventable causes of morbidity and mortality among severely injured patients.
- The first mandatory goal is "to save the ship"; once hemostasis is achieved both with hemostatic competence, refining objectives in a "listen to the cell needs" fashion becomes a priority, with tailored assessments and well-defined end points.
- Consider two main aspects within the same entity: the "trauma injury" *and* the "trauma disease" as well.
- Next generation of hemodynamic monitoring could include microcirculation monitoring systems, as well as hemostatic support monitoring with Point of Care (POC) Viscoelastic Hemostatic Assays.

46.1 Introduction

Hemorrhage is considered the most preventable cause of in-hospital deaths worldwide, especially in massive injured exsanguinating trauma, being trauma itself the top cause of death in the population aged less than 45 years old [1, 2]. Patients suffering from a substantial bleeding, apart from the sites and the several involved causes, represent a major challenge for all the clinicians involved in taking care of these critical ills. The modern approach refers to a multidisciplinary working team, provided with technical and nontechnical skills (i.e., behaviors, leadership, communication) [3, 4], aiming to the treatment of the bleeding: in a few words, "to stop the bleeding" as soon as possible. Every day in their clinical activity, anesthesiologists and intensivists, both with

L. Bucci (✉)
Intensive Care Unit "G. Bozza" I Service of Anesthesia and Intensive Care, ASST Grande Ospedale Metropolitano Niguarda, Milan, Italy
e-mail: lucio.bucci@ospedaleniguarda.it

P. Aseni et al. (eds.), *Operative Techniques and Recent Advances in Acute Care and Emergency Surgery*, https://doi.org/10.1007/978-3-319-95114-0_46

surgeons, endoscopy specialists, interventional radiologists, and more recently, blood bankers are challenged in various scenarios such as trauma, major surgery, gastrointestinal (GI) tract hemorrhage, aortic aneurysm rupture, and postpartum hemorrhage (PPH) with possible life-threatening blood loss. Moreover, the paradigm shift in the last two decades' treatment options takes into account more recent aspects, focusing on coagulation derangements, metabolic disorders, and, ultimate, complex, profound microcirculation and tissue disorders. The management of bleeding in these patients involves outstanding clinical aspects, requiring a pathophysiological and, possibly, a clinicopathological approach.

The damage control (DC) approach is widely defined as "first of all, a surgeon's mindset," especially in severe trauma patients. In particular, the term damage control, borrowed from the US Navy, refers to a series of techniques adopted to save a wrecked ship, without restoring it to its pre-damage state [5]. DC represents an attitude that goes beyond the purely technical and practical skills in critical situations with severe blood loss; surgical or interventional radiological techniques have the goal to stop the bleeding as soon as possible, when rapid diagnostic tools have oriented trauma surgeon on where the source(s) is (are) and how better to control it/them.

In recent years, damage control resuscitation (DCR) has been proposed as the preferred strategy to manage severe bleeding trauma patients, aiming to minimize blood loss until definitive hemostasis is achieved [6]. The main principles were first applied in military environment in combat casualty care [7, 8] and thereafter successfully translated in civilian trauma setting as well, with the goal of "stop the bleeding" and two fundamental targets: first, to restore intravascular volume to assure tissue perfusion and O2 delivery and, second, to achieve rapid hemostatic competence focusing on the imbalanced coagulation system with early-goal coagulation therapy, based on massive transfusion (or "hemorrhage" as several authors termed) protocol (MTP) and less than prior fluids' administration and/or coagulation factor strategy, based on point-of-care (POC) viscoelastic assays to guide treatment options (i.e., coagulation factor concentrates, fibrinogen concentrate, blood derivatives). As a part of primary care of the hemorrhagic patient, POC diagnostic tool such as thromboelastography/metry (TEG™/TEM™) has become more and more employed by anesthesiologists, intensivists, in some cases blood bank specialists, and trauma surgeons, beyond the well-known use for many years in cardiac surgery and liver transplantation, to ensure a rapid, appropriate, and correct diagnosis such as in a *theranostic approach* (a term derived from the fusion of two words: *thera*peutic and diag*nostic*), in order to administer the appropriate and goal-directed treatment(s) [9, 10]. However, there is a lack of data in the literature regarding a comparison between fixed ratio and goal-directed POC-guided product strategies; nevertheless, some authors argue that the two strategies are not mutually exclusive "per se" [11–13].

In this chapter four topics are focused:

- An overlook of the pathophysiology of hemorrhagic shock: the main aspects of physiology we have to remember and how to link to the patient's clinical signs, for a correct understanding of "what is happening and what I have to do."
- The updated concept of *hemodynamic coherence* regarding the intimate connections between the macrocirculation and the microcirculation: what we observe, what we look for, and what we should keep in mind about the maintenance of the hemodynamic coherence, for the expected microcirculation restoration would not be achieved in any case by the hemodynamic resuscitation strategies.
- The types of fluids as a part of the hemorrhagic shock resuscitation from the beginning of blood loss and hemodynamic derangement: the paradigm shift of what to use and, moreover, how much and when to treat especially the seeker patients, in particular those with severe bleeding injuries, focusing on the vascular endothelial damage and its consequences.
- The massive transfusion protocol (MTP) approach, as a part of the damage control resuscitation (DCR) strategy, actually employed in many high-level trauma centers; a brief overview of the main characteristics, including when to activate, when to start, and when to stop it will be discussed.

46.2 The Pathophysiology of Hemorrhagic Shock: Remembering Physiology with Links to the Clinical Signs

Shock is defined as a clinical condition of insufficient oxygen delivery with inadequate tissue perfusion. Hypovolemic shock due to hemorrhage is considered worldwide the most common in-hospital preventable cause of death after a severe trauma; therefore, in this section the pathophysiology of hemorrhagic shock as a consequence of blood loss after major traumatic injuries will be focused. When hemorrhage occurs, the human body starts to attempt for compensating blood losses. The goal is to maintain oxygen delivery (DO2) to vital organs in order to keep their main functions [14]. Principle compensatory mechanisms are represented by (a) an increase in heart rate, due to the aortic arch and the carotid body baroreceptor stimulation via a decrease in their inhibition of the sympathetic nervous system, (b) vasoconstriction that attempts to maintain blood pressure, and (c) neuroendocrine stimulation, via activation on one side of the renin-angiotensin-aldosterone system with the goal of restoring the circulating volume and, on the other side, stimulation of the HPA (hypothalamus-pituitary-adrenal) axis, with an increase in cortisol release, which acts in an osmotically way to maintain circulating volume. The tissues themselves attempt to a major fraction of oxygen extraction, trying to maintain their metabolic needs and functions as well. However, during acute hemorrhage, venous return is one of the main components of body's attempts to compensate blood loss. It is well known how venous return constitutes a major determinant of cardiac output (CO) in terms of preload. During substantial acute bleeding, the "tank" system tries to maintain venous pressure within the venous system itself. Two main factors are considered in promoting the venous system to compensate during acute hemorrhage: first, a modification in venous elastance and, second, the mobilization of unstressed blood volume into stressed blood volume as well [15]. The main goal is to preserve the mean circulatory filling pressure to sustain venous return and thus CO during major hemorrhage. How does the cell respond to this state of hypovolemic shock? Decreased oxygen and nutrient supply delivery due to hemorrhage are the principally observed results; rapid blood loss decreases CO and DO2, with oxygenation sustained by a shift in O2 dissociation curve and a local metabolic vasodilation. Hypoxia enhances capillary recruitment with an O2 diffusion increase due to a reduced diffusion distance. When all these attempts, both with adaptive modifications in the microvasculature, are not sufficient and are overwhelmed, a metabolic shift toward an anaerobic metabolic state is observed, in which the rate of DO2 that occurs is defined as the "critical" DO2 (DO2crit) [16]. Moving from aerobic to anaerobic metabolism *below* the DO2crit characterizes the state of "compensated" shock. The production of cellular ATP is maintained, along with the main cellular goals such as protein synthesis and contractile functions. When ATP supplies are unable to fit with cellular needs, the "uncompensated" shock condition occurs, up to irreversible cellular damage comprehending failure of membrane ion movements, swelling, increased free radical species, acidosis, and ultimate loss of adenosine nucleotides from the cell as well. All these derangements are clinical expressed by an increase in plasmatic lactate levels.

How vital signs correlate with physiology alterations during hemorrhage and shock state? Does the clinical picture truly reflect the real patient condition and his compensatory attempts in response to increasing amount of blood loss? Looking at the classical four classes of shock proposed by the American College of Surgeons in the ATLS classification, it is possible to identify a first phase of blood loss up to 30%; within this class and the clinical features observed, mainly increased heart rate and vasoconstriction, the classical autonomic response by activated sympathetic system is the physiological platform, with clinical signs such as mild tachycardia and maintained blood pressure with vital organ perfusion as well [17, 18]. Moving on a second, more severe phase with an increase in blood loss beyond 30%, the physiological response dramatically changes, and the body works to save needs in the face of very poor supplies. The sequence gets involved with sympatho-inhibitory effects, activation of the C-fibers in the left cardiac ventricle with signals to parasympathetic system, and finally, inhibition of the sympathetic system. The resulting clinical features observed are a normal or decreased heart rate, with blood pressure trends going downward. In this phase, DO2crit appears: DO2 decreases; consumption rate in terms of VO2 is not sustained by increased extraction rate from tissues anymore. This represents a very delicate and harmful phase, where clinical evidence markedly contrasts with ATLS signs in the classical classification of shock classes (marked tachycardia related to an increasing degree of a severe hemorrhage) [19]. In this view, caution is appropriate in evaluating clinical signs of a severe trauma patient with an ongoing blood loss, maintaining a high index of suspicion and avoiding false sense of security, whereby a low or normal heart rate is observed, especially in the absence of tissue injury.

46.3 The Hemodynamic Coherence: What We Look and What We Should Keep in Mind

During hemorrhagic shock, an intact relationship between the macrocirculation and the microcirculation should be preserved; this is termed "hemodynamic coherence," to figure out that hemodynamic-driven resuscitation effects on macrocirculatory system spread out to the microvasculature, then assuring tissue perfusion [20, 21]. However, hemorrhage, trauma injuries, reperfusion, and activation of inflammation system can damage both macro- *and* microcirculation, threatening compensatory mechanisms with loss of hemodynamic coherence: the more severe the shock, the reperfusion, and the inflammation, the more impaired the compensatory response of microcirculation to an acute DO2 failure. In critical situations, restoring macrovasculature damages and derangements could be ineffective on microcirculation and tissue oxygenation [22]. It becomes fundamental to keep in mind that several other factors can induce microvasculature abnormalities in bleeding patients such as in severe trauma settings. The degree and severity of tissue injuries both with the shock intensity can activate the inflammatory system via release of several endogenous factors named DAMPs (damage-associated molecular patterns) from activated immune cells and/or from necrotic cells, then enhancing microcirculation damage. Several of these molecules are passively released from the dying cells (and not from those cells dying with an apoptotic program); others are actively secreted. DAMPs link with inflammatory cell membrane receptors (e.g., Toll-like receptor-4: TLR-4), triggering the transcription of genes aiming to the production of many pro-inflammatory cytokines. The final result appears to be a

SIRS (systemic inflammatory response syndrome) clinical condition, with activation and a possible derangement of the coagulation system in the more critical patients.

HMGB1 (high-mobility group box 1) is a DAMP that correlates with the severity of hypoperfusion (*cause* of its release), with the inflammatory cytokine levels (*effect* of its widespread release) and the final outcome of the more injured patients (the final effect of the SIRS condition and the coagulopathy derived from the coagulation system derangement) [23–25].

From a clinical and practical point of view, it appears reasonable that a real-time monitoring of microcirculation could become a cornerstone of hemodynamic evaluation during hemorrhage resuscitation protocol, focusing both on hemostatic competence and becoming a "gold standard" issue in the next future generation of the resuscitation strategy itself.

46.4 Types of Fluids in Hemorrhagic Shock Resuscitation: New Insights with a Paradigm Shift for Improving Treatment Strategies

The correction of a shock state and a deranged physiology are the main goals of a severe bleeding trauma patient resuscitation, having a relevant impact on the outcome as much as overall surgical procedures of the injured tissues. In the last two decades, trauma community reviewed and developed new approaches focusing on resuscitation strategies, moving from military experiences (e.g., from last Iraq and Afghanistan campaigns) and promptly translating into civilian settings, with increased attention to the type, amounts, and timing of fluid treatment. This paradigm shift nowadays is of paramount relevance for any clinician taking care of severely traumatized patient arriving in hospital emergency room with a profound hemorrhage and a shock state [26]. Fluids are the most employed treatment worldwide for hypovolemic-hemorrhagic shock, aiming to refill intravascular volume and increase cardiac preload and ultimately trying to improve tissue perfusion. But fluid therapy represents only one element of a complex resuscitative algorithm, the well-known DCR approach for the substantial bleeding injured patient in which fundamental principles include less than prior crystalloids, permissive hypotension, balanced ratio transfusion of blood components, and possibly a goal-directed management and correction of coagulopathy. Types of fluids for resuscitation purposes are broadly characterized into crystalloid and colloid solutions. In particular, *crystalloids* are solutions of ions freely permeable, containing concentrations of sodium and chloride that identify the grade of tonicity of the solution. *Colloids* are a suspension of molecules within a carrier solution relatively unable to cross the healthy semipermeable capillary membrane owing to the molecular weight of the molecules [27]. In the early phase of in-hospital resuscitation of the massively injured patients, damage control surgery (DC) and damage control resuscitation (DCR) with early hemostatic control are applied. DCR strategies address rapid control of the source(s) of surgical bleeding, avoiding hypothermia, acidosis, and hypocalcemia both with the very early provision of packed red blood cells (PRBCs), coagulation factors (FFP and/or factor concentrates), and platelets in a balanced ratio. A careful administration with limitation of excessive fluids like crystalloids and colloids to decrease hemodilution can prevent the adverse effects on coagulation factor activity and, finally, most likely on endothelial glycocalyx layer (EGL) of the vascular barrier integrity, especially in intravascular hypervolemia situations, via the release of atrial natriuretic peptides with activation of several metalloproteinases [28]. Crystalloids are cheaper than other types of fluids, being widely available and representing the first-line solution of resuscitative therapy. However, large amounts of this fluid are involved in a well-recognized role as a primary cause of cellular and tissue edema with clinically significant relevances: interstitial edema, organ dysfunction/failure, increase in abdominal pressure with possible compartment syndrome, difficult ventilation, and inability to abdominal wall closure. Several concerns are raised with an excessive amount of saline resuscitation in terms of hyperchloremic acidosis; in that view balanced solutions are increasingly suggested as the first-line resuscitation fluids in patients with trauma [29]. Colloids like HES solutions are produced by hydroxyethyl substitution of amylopectin obtained from sorghum, maize, or potatoes. A high degree of substitution on glucose molecules protects against hydrolysis by nonspecific amylases in the blood, thereby prolonging intravascular expansion, but this action increases the potential for HES to accumulate in tissues, such as the skin, liver, and most of all the kidney, hesitating in organ failure. The use of HES, particularly high-molecular-weight preparations, has been associated with coagulation derangements, such as changes in viscoelastic measurements and fibrinolysis.

46.5 The Massive Transfusion Protocol: Build It, Activate It, Use It, and Stop It

In the early phase of blood loss and shock state in a clinical condition like aortic aneurysmal rupture, GI tract severe bleeding, and postpartum hemorrhage (PPH) and especially in the trauma patient, DCR and the turn on of a massive transfusion protocol (MTP) constitute the paramount treatments. The classical and widely accepted definition of a massive transfusion as ten or more RBC units in 24 h rely on retrospective data; in more recent definition based on provided data matched with real-life, pragmatic settings refer to transfusion of RBCs units in the first 4–6 h [30, 31].

In their very recent review, White and coworkers describe blood speculating about a unique unit based on biological and pragmatical point of views, considering the *liquid* blood and its cellular and enzymatic components as existing and functioning in concert with the bathed endothelium, with all the close and intimate regulations derived. The *blood-endothelial unit*, which they referred to in their paper, is more simply named as "*blood*," approached as a single *organ system*; the single components are thoughts to be inextricably linked, closely supporting each other's function [32]. The authors consider the *blood failure* during hemorrhage "an emergent state of blood occurring during accumulation of a critical level of oxygen debt": in a single word, a *shock* condition. To meet the definition of blood failure, a low tissue DO2 critical, both with endotheliopathy, platelet dysfunction and coagulopathy should all be present. However, it is useful to consider them together given their intimate interconnections. In this view, to treat hemorrhagic blood failure appropriately, a comprehensive approach should consider all the possible treatments that simultaneously address its multiple components. Repayment of O2-debt must be achieved in addition to contemporaneous treatment of both endothelial damage and coagulopathy. This is the main reason why, *in the end*, the treatment of hemorrhagic shock is based on transfusions with:

- Packed red blood cells (PRBCs), addressing O2 debt by increasing the oxygen carrying (O2-content), cardiac output, and ultimately oxygen delivery (DO2).
- Fresh frozen plasma (FFP), in order to support cardiac output via intravascular volume filling both with providing coagulation factors to support the hemostatic competence. A major focusing aspect of plasma transfusion is that it may have also an additional benefit, providing endothelial protection by restoring several protective enzymes that can contribute to sealing the endothelial barrier and increasing the glycocalyx recovery [33–35]. Plasma has also been independently linked to multi-organ failure and lacks the cellular elements required to fully restore clot formation [36].
- Early platelet transfusion is associated with improved outcome in the acutely bleeding trauma patients. Platelet concentrates contribute to hemostasis by increasing thrombin formation, increasing clot stiffness, and increasing resistance to clot lysis [37].
- Cryoprecipitate provides a rich source of fibrinogen, factor VIII and von Willebrand factor and is primarily used to sustain hemostasis, while also possibly offering benefit to endothelium. Early fibrinogen support can recover viscoelastic clot strength when given in concentrated fashions, and cryoprecipitate may provide grams of fibrinogen per dose [38–41].

A ratio-based massive transfusion protocol contains the inner reasons abovementioned to treat the more severely injured patients. The main goals of a MTP are summarized hereby:

- An institutional system for delivering blood products from the blood bank to the patient's point of care [42]
- To address the organizational issues able to respond to a massive hemorrhage [43]
- To reduce provider's variability, facilitating team communication, simplifying administration of pre-defined blood component ratios [31]

Early treatment goals in the bleeding trauma patient have changed based on recent findings. The severely injured patients requiring a MTP have shown a decrease in mortality based on a more aggressive and balanced approach regarding treatment with blood products. Moreover, recent data suggested a combined approach of early balanced ratio-based blood products; point-of-care (POC) viscoelastic hemostatic assays (VHA) for a rapid, bedside diagnostic phase, hemostatic resuscitation even with coagulation adjunctives; and finally, a goal-directed therapy to complete resuscitation [44].

There is evidence to support the early use of a 1:1:1 ratio (or almost a 1:2 ratio of FFP, PRBCs) blood product transfusion protocol to restore the amount of losses, to improve oxygen delivery, and to refill clotting factors in those substantially bleeding trauma patients [45]. In the PROMMTT study, a multicenter prospective observational trial data were analyzed in more than 900 trauma patients with hemorrhage who received at least 1 RBC unit within the first 6 h, at least 3 RBC units within 24 h, and survived for at least half an hour after hospital arrival [46]. The authors demonstrated a statistically significant decrease in in-hospital mortality when early treatment with higher ratios of fresh frozen plasma (FFP) and platelets to RBCs was employed. Moreover, each unit increases both in plasma and platelets to RBCs ratio within the first 6 h, in which hemorrhage is the first cause of death, was associated with an adjusted hazard ratio (HR) of 0.31 (95%CI 0.16–0.58) and 0.55 (95%CI 0.31–0.98) of in-hospital mortality, respectively.

Regarding FFP administration, beyond the actually well-known possible side effects and complications, in particular TRALI and ARDS [47], data from experimental models of hemorrhagic shock and analysis of EGL degradation and derangement, both with pilot studies in humans, evidenced that FFP administration may play a protective and restorative role on a previously damaged glycocalyx, more likely showing to blood-borne protein activity and glycosaminoglycans (GAGs) in physiologic plasma concentrations. This is one of the main reasons why several authors are considering the protection or restoration of the damaged glycocalyx, such as in severe traumatic hemorrhagic patients, a potential therapeutic option, as FFP administration in this acute care setting [34, 48–50].

In victims of severe trauma with early imbalance of the coagulation system, recent data suggest to consider the trauma-induced coagulopathy (TIC) as an "endogenous disturb" of the coagulation itself, in which major triggers are represented by the shock itself, in terms of hypoperfusion (expressed by negative base deficit in a blood gas analysis and lactate values) and the endothelial damage, the last correlating with the severity of the injury as injury severity score (ISS) value [51]. Recent data suggest that in the pathophysiology of TIC, one of the main aspects may be related to endothelial damage, in particular with its glycocalyx layer (endothelial glycocalyx layer, EGL). This structure is located on the surface of endothelial cells as a negative-charged thin layer, with antiadhesive and anticoagulant functions; these properties allow the maintenance of vascular barrier integrity and at the same time a protective role of the same endothelial cells [52–54]. All these causes, tissue and vascular injuries, hypoperfusion conditions, the activation of the neurohormonal hypothalamic-adrenal axis both with the inflammatory system, and the endogenous catecholamines released from adrenal glands, act as a boost for endothelial systemic activation and damage, with consequent increase in permeability (loss of endothelial intercellular junctions) and derangement of the coagulation system with evidence of early coagulopathy [55]. In systemic circulation it has been observed the release of molecules indicating the damage and the degradation of the glycocalyx (a phenomenon termed "shedding") such as syndecan-1, both with markers of endothelial derangements like soluble thrombomodulin (sTM), the vascular endothelial growth factor (VEGF), and the Weibel-Palade body degranulation (containing tissue plasminogen activator (TPA) and angiopoietin-2) [53]. Johansson and his group found that in more severe trauma patients with massive hemorrhage and major glycocalyx degradation, an elevated auto-heparinization due to increase of heparan sulfate was observed, both with an increase of the burden of the types of injuries in those patients with elevated circulating levels of syndecan-1. These observations are associated with a more severe coagulopathy, with a reduction of plasmatic levels of activated protein C (aPC), increased fibrinolysis, increased soluble thrombomodulin (sTM), a prolongation of standard coagulation test such as aPTT, and definitively a worse outcome with increased mortality [56].

Furthermore, in their very recent review, Johansson and coworkers, focusing on their data regarding more than 3000 patients suffering from apparently different types of diseases such trauma, sepsis, myocardial infarction, and post-cardiac arrest syndrome, propose that shock itself, with its effect on the sympathoadrenal system, both with the endothelial glycocalyx and the hemostatic cells in the circulating blood, results in phenotypic modifications that characterize the clinical condition of acute critical illness, despite the different types of primary "hit" [57]. The catecholamine-induced damage to the endothelium acts with an endothelial breakdown resulting in glycocalyx shedding, disruption of tight junctions with capillary leakage, and a procoagulant feature in the microcirculation, responsible for the further reduction of oxygen delivery (due to increased tissue pressure) and microvascular thrombosis, creating a vicious circle with ultimate organ failure. The early genetic responses to severe trauma, burn injury, and sepsis endotoxemia are similar; the body response in various *acute* critical conditions characterized by a shock state is relatively homogenous and most likely adapted from an evolutionary point of view.

All the clinicians involved in the primary care of a critically bleeding patient with a severe trauma have long identified that *time* plays against the ongoing blood loss and that earlier initiation of resuscitation in view of DCR and hemostatic support improves the outcome. In this view, logistic difficulties and hurdles have to be overcome to release and expedite massive transfusion components.

To activate a MTP in trauma setting in a timely fashion, good practices suggested are:

- Alert blood bank since prehospital report.
- In ER: clinical signs, injury complexity, rapid diagnostic tools, monitoring, lab exams, and compromised physiology analysis.
- Scoring systems to stratify the risk of severe bleeding could be applied, for example, TASH and ABC.
- Activation of code-red MTP to blood bank via a dedicated phone line, starting to release a pre-defined blood component ratio.

To turn off the MTP, several clinical and biochemical conditions have to be considered:

- Once the bleeding source control is achieved: in a word, hemostasis.
- A decrease in transfusion rate and patients needs.
- A decrease in vasopressors requirement if any used.
- Hemodynamic stability observed.
- Urine output.
- An improvement in base deficit (BD) and acidosis, lab coagulation tests, VHA, and lactate.

In summary, MTP is adopted for an early identification of critical bleeding patients, an anticipation of coagulopathy, and an immediate "empiric" treatment with higher-ratio blood component therapy. Its development and updating in each institutional reality and the therapeutic adoption aim to predict patients who are actively bleeding and *not* to predict massive transfusion, both with earlier treatment of coagulopathy. MTP has the goal to anticipate coagulopathy and does not require routine coagulation tests for blood component delivery [58].

46.6 Conclusion and Highlights

In the last two decades, a development of new treatment strategies for critical bleeding patients has occurred, particularly for trauma patients with severe hemorrhage.

All the substantial bleeding patients in acute scenarios including trauma as well, major surgery, gastrointestinal (GI) tract hemorrhage, aortic aneurismal rupture, and postpartum hemorrhage (PPH) represent a major challenge of the daily practical activity of anesthesiologists and intensivists, both with surgeons, interventional radiologists, and blood banker too, taking care of a possible life-threatening blood loss, with consequences on coagulation derangements, metabolic disorders, and finally, complex profound microcirculation and tissue disorders. Fewer volumes of fluid resuscitation seek to minimize overloads resulting in tissue edema and organ failure, dilutional coagulopathy, and coagulation interferences. In particular, new insights both from preclinical and clinical data are better characterizing the relationships between the damaged endothelium and the glycocalyx shedding, with consequences on the aforementioned increased permeability and interstitial edema and even more on inflammatory system activation and coagulation imbalance.

Rapid identification of patients who are actively bleeding and for whom early activation and administration of a massive transfusion protocol in the first hours represent the main objectives of the entire working team, with a well-known correlation regarding mortality and an improved patients' outcome.

To restore physiology and homeostasis, in parallel with hemostatic control as soon as possible, represent the primary care project of all the involved specialists managing a critical bleeding patient, in order to ameliorate the entire trauma team work as well and to manage such a precious resource as blood and blood components. Finally, the amplitude of the acute inflammatory response and its profound relationships with the coagulation system and cellular elements, namely platelets and innate immunity cells, correlate with the outcome of the major trauma patients. However, with the better understandings of the very complicated biology of this *trauma disease* entity, both with the involved mechanisms in activation of the innate immunity secondary to trauma injury, it will be possible to obtain, in the next future, molecules with *biomarker* features. This would be adopted by clinicians to better characterize a more precise clinical time course both with new therapeutical strategies and options, in order to act in a timely and more targeted fashion to improve the outcome of the most seriously bleeding patients, especially those with severe *trauma injuries*.

Case Scenario: Woman, 64 Years Old, Cyclist vs. Truck

2014, February. Traffic road accident 12.30 h: cyclist woman crashed and got stuck in the truck wheels (Fig. 46.1)

12.45 h: Helicopter rescue team on site, alert, BP 85/45, HR 115, GCS 15, sat 99%

Rapid breathing shallow but bilateral murmur normal

Degloving injury to the pelvis and right limb, instability of the pelvis

2 IV lines

Crystalloids 500 mL

Colloid 300 mL

Rapid sequence intubation

Helicopter transfer to Niguarda Trauma Center Hospital, Milan

ER 13:30 h:

Transfusion 2 0've PRBCs

Crystalloids 1000 mL

Colloid 500 mL

Activation of MT protocol

Pelvic binder

Central line 12 F

Pelvic X-ray (Fig. 46.2)

Trauma surgeon: extraperitoneal pelvic packing; temporary closure of the femoral vein

Start with massive transfusion protocol 1:1:1 ratio

OR 14:15 h: Lac 5.7; BE −7.5; T 34.5 °C

I MTP pack adopting a level-1 high-flow transfusion system,

TXA 1 g bolus, TXA 1 g/8 h (Fig. 46.3)

In Fig. 46.4 a flow diagram of the in-hospital patient route is depicted.

At ICU admission the total amount of blood products transfused during the first 8 h treatment was (Fig. 46.4):

- 34 PRBCs
- 34 FFPs
- 30 Cryos
- 32 PLTs

Question n. 1

In this type of trauma injuries, which would be the ideal target of blood pressure in patient without traumatic brain injury?

A. 70–85 mm Hg.
B. 90–100 mm Hg ("permissive hypotension").
C. 120–80 mm Hg.
D. Any pressure value would be acceptable if >75.

Question n. 2

An early activation of a massive transfusion protocol is indicated in this type of patient due to:

A. The type of trauma itself
B. Rapidly addressing the coagulopathy looking at hemostatic resuscitation
C. Lower fluid infusion
D. A-B-C together

Please see Chap. 58 for the correct answer.

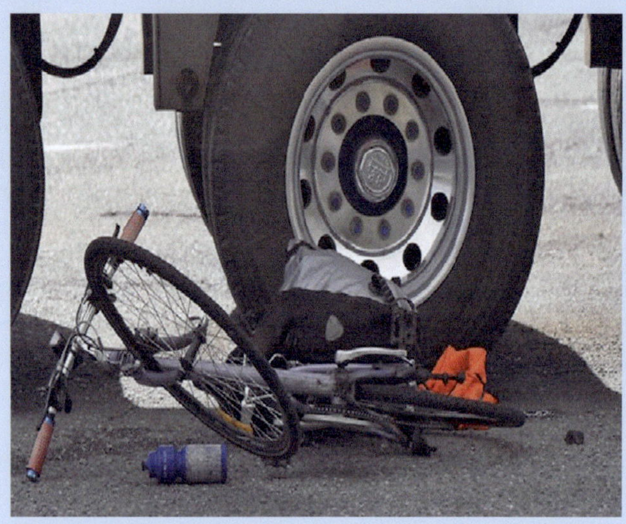

Fig. 46.1 Traffic road accident, bicycle vs. truck

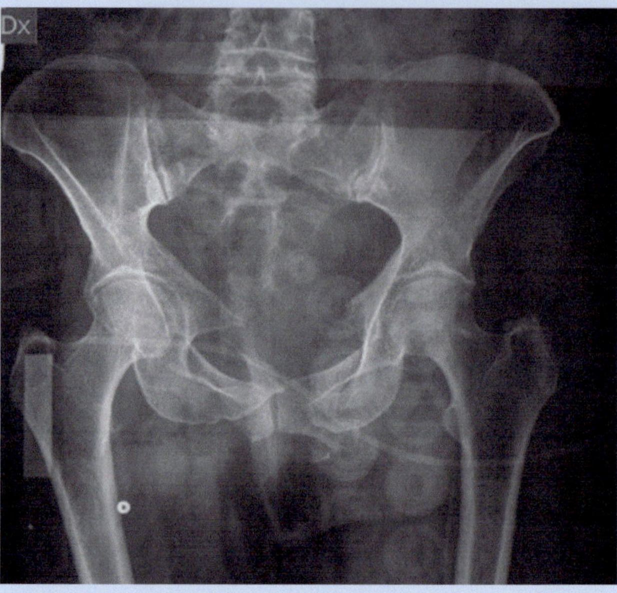

Fig. 46.2 Pelvic X-rays showing multiple fractures (vertical shear type fracture) of the pelvis. Pelvic binder in site

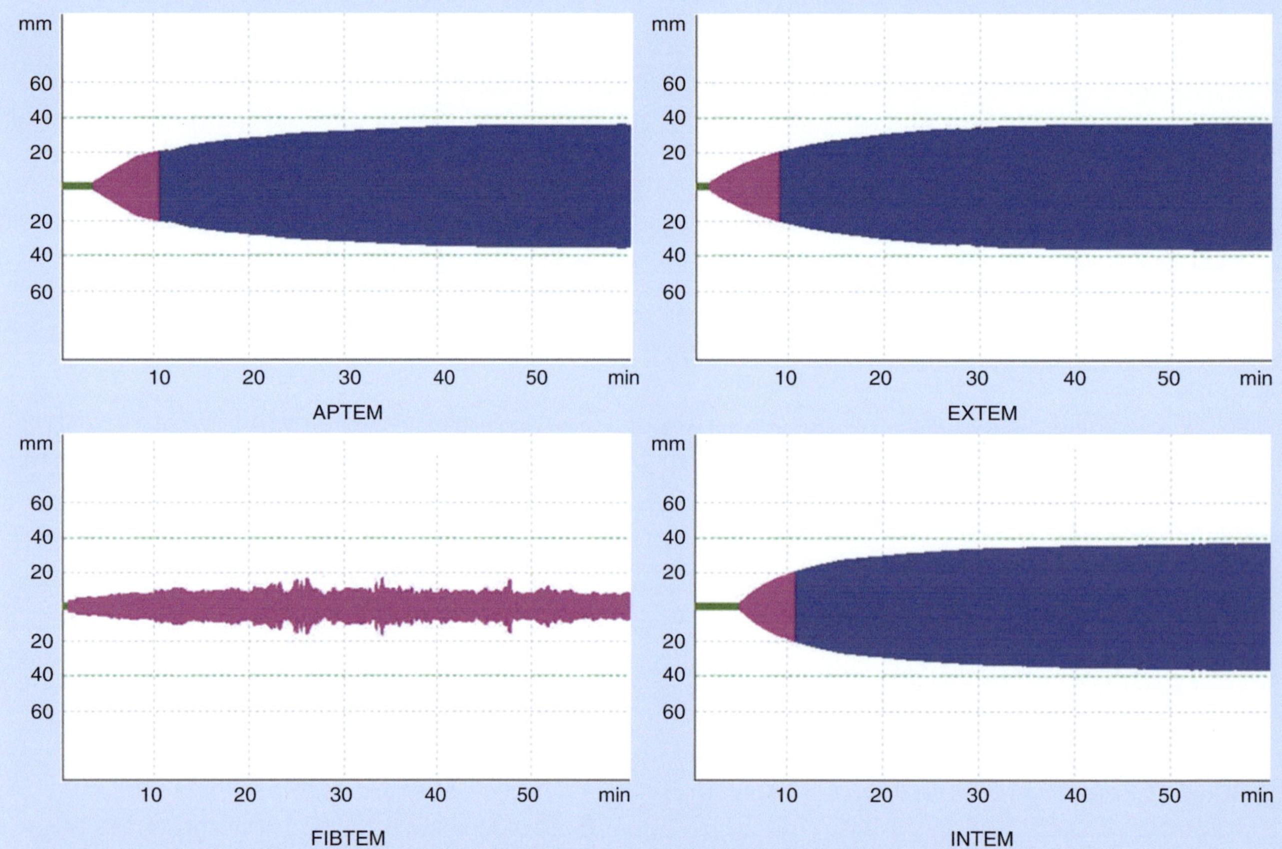

Fig. 46.3 ROTEM™ runned at first arrival in the OR. A platelet and fibrinogen deficit is showed. Patient transfused with PLTs and cryoprecipitated

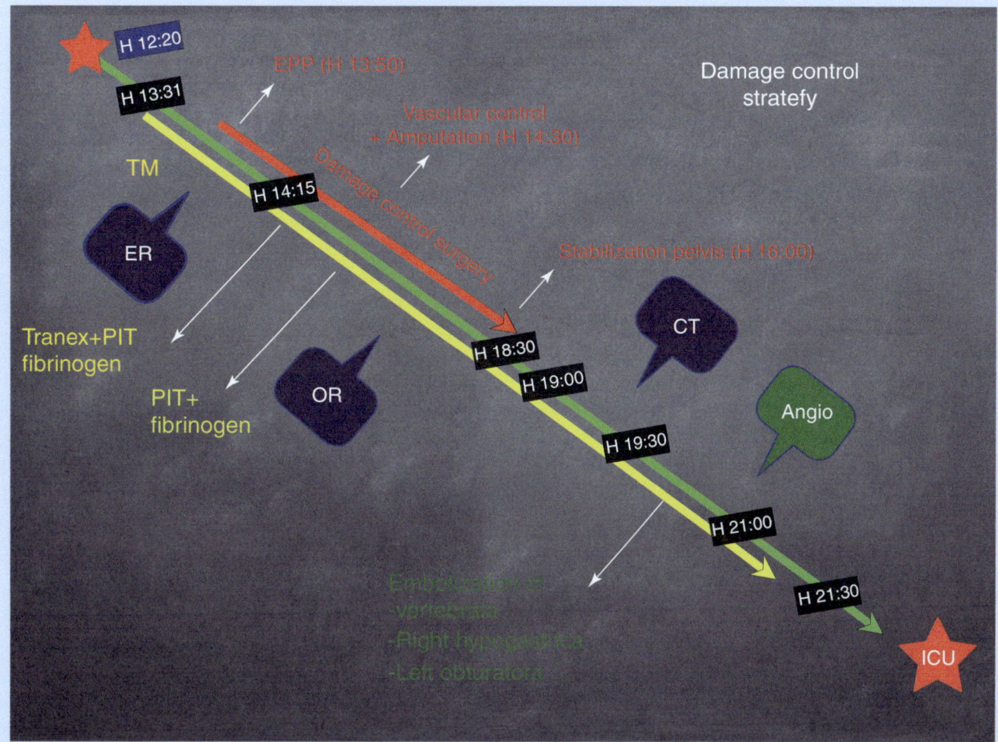

Fig. 46.4 A summary flow diagram of the trauma patient. From ER arrival to definitive ICU admission 8 h passed; first CT scan at 19:30 h followed by vascular embolizations in angio-suite

References

1. Cothren CC, Moore EE, Hedegaard HB, et al. Epidemiology of urban trauma deaths: a comprehensive reassessment 10 years later. World J Surg. 2007;31(7):1507–11.
2. Murray CJ, Lopez AD. Mortality by cause for eight regions of the world: Global Burden of Disease Study. Lancet. 1997;349:1269–76.
3. Hargestam M, Hultin M, Brulin C, et al. Trauma team leaders' nonverbal communication: video registration during trauma team training. Scand J Trauma Resusc Emerg Med. 2016;24:37–49.
4. Leenstra NF, Jung OC, Johnson A, et al. Taxonomy of trauma leadership skills: a framework for leadership training and assessment. Acad Med. 2016;91:272–81.
5. Shapiro MB, Jenkins DH, Schwab CW, et al. Damage control: collective review. J Trauma. 2000;49(5):969–78.
6. Bogert JN, Harvin JA, Cotton BA. Damage control resuscitation. J Intensive Care Med. 2016;31(3):177–86.
7. Simmons RL, Collins JA, Heisterkamp CA, et al. Coagulation disorders in combat casualties I. Acute changes after wounding. II. Effects of massive transfusion. 3. Post-resuscitative changes. Ann Surg. 1969;169(4):455–82.
8. McLaughlin DF, Niles SE, Salinas J, et al. A predictive model for massive transfusion in combat casualty patients. J Trauma. 2008;64(2 Suppl):S57–63.
9. Levy JH, Faraoni D, Sniecinski RM. Perioperative coagulation management in the intensive care unit. Curr Opin Anesthesiol. 2013;26:65–70.
10. Kozek-Langenecker SA. Coagulation and transfusion in the postoperative bleeding patient. Curr Opin Crit Care. 2014;20:460–6.
11. Nascimento B, Callum J, Tien H, et al. Effect of a fixed-ratio (1:1:1) transfusion protocol versus laboratory-results-guided transfusion in patients with severe trauma: a randomized feasibility trial. CMAJ. 2013;185(12):583–9.
12. Tapia NM, Chang A, Norman M, et al. TEG-guided resuscitation is superior to standardized MTP resuscitation in massively transfused penetrating trauma patients. J Trauma Acute Care Surg. 2013;74(2):378–85.
13. Ho AM, Holcomb JB, Ng CS, et al. The traditional vs "1:1:1" approach debate on massive transfusion in trauma should not be treated as a dichotomy. Am J Emerg Med. 2015;33(10):1501–4.
14. Schultz W, McConachie I. Vital signs after haemorrhage—caution is appropriate. Trends Anaesth Crit Care. 2015;5:89–92.
15. Shen T, Baker K. Venous return and clinical hemodynamics: how the body works during acute hemorrhage. Adv Physiol Educ. 2015;39:267–71.
16. Kalla M, Herring N. Physiology of shock and volume resuscitation. Surgery. 2013;31(11):545–51.
17. Rady MY, Kirkman E, Cranley J, et al. Nociceptive somatic nerve stimulation and skeletal muscle injury modify hemodynamics and oxygen transport and utilization after resuscitation from haemorrhage. Crit Care Med. 1996;24(4):623–30.
18. Jacobsen J, Secher NH. Heart rate during haemorrhagic shock. Clin Physiol. 1992;12(6):659–66.
19. Kirkman E, Watts S. Haemodynamic changes in trauma. Br J Anaesth. 2014;113(2):266–75.

20. Tachon G, Harrois A, Tanaka S, et al. Microcirculatory alterations in traumatic hemorrhagic shock. Crit Care Med. 2014;42:1433–41.
21. Dubin A, Pozo MO, Ferrara G, et al. Systemic and microcirculatory responses to progressive hemorrhage. Intensive Care Med. 2009;35:556–64.
22. Libert N, Harrois A, Duranteau J. Haemodynamic coherence in haemorrhagic shock. Best Pract Res Clin Anaesthesiol. 2016;30:429–35.
23. Cohen MJ, Brohi K, Calfee CS, et al. Early release of high mobility group box nuclear protein 1 after severe trauma in humans: role of injury severity and tissue hypoperfusion. Crit Care. 2009;13:R174.
24. Manson J, Thiemermann C, Brohi K. Trauma alarmins as activators of damage-induced inflammation. Br J Surg. 2012;99(S1):12–20.
25. Bianchi ME. DAMPs, PAMPs and alarmins: all we need to know about danger. J Leukoc Biol. 2007;81:1–5.
26. Chang R, Holcomb JB. Optimal fluid therapy for traumatic hemorrhagic shock. Crit Care Clin. 2017;33:15–36.
27. Myburgh JA, Mythen MG. Resuscitation fluids. N Engl J Med. 2013;369:1243–51.
28. Chappell D, Jacob M. Role of the glycocalyx in fluid management: small things matter. Best Pract Res Clin Anaesthesiol. 2014;28:227–34.
29. Advanced Trauma Life Support (ATLS) for doctors. Chicago: American College of Surgeons Committee on Trauma; 2012. http://www.facs.org/trauma/atls/index.html.
30. Shafi S, Collinsworth AW, Richter KM, et al. Bundles of care for resuscitation from hemorrhagic shock and severe brain injury in trauma patients—translating knowledge into practice. J Trauma Acute Care Surg. 2016;81(4):780–94.
31. Stephens CT, Gumbert S, Holcomb JB. Trauma-associated bleeding: management of massive transfusion. Curr Opin Anesthesiol. 2016;29:250–5.
32. White NJ, Ward KR, Pati S, et al. Hemorrhagic blood failure: oxygen debt, coagulopathy, and endothelial damage. J Trauma Acute Care Surg. 2017;82(6S Suppl 1):S41–9.
33. Emerson CP, Ebert RV. A study of shock in battle casualties: measurements of the blood volume changes occurring in response to therapy. Ann Surg. 1945;122(5):745–72.
34. Kozar RA, Peng Z, Zhang R, et al. Plasma restoration of endothelial glycocalyx in a rodent model of hemorrhagic shock. Anesth Analg. 2011;112(6):1289–95.
35. Pati S, Wataha K, Menge T, et al. Spray-dried plasma and fresh frozen plasma modulate permeability and inflammation in vitro in vascular endothelial cells. Transfusion. 2013;53(Suppl 1):80S–90S.
36. Johnson JL, Moore EE, Kashuk JL, et al. Effect of blood products transfusion on the development of postinjury multiple organ failure. Arch Surg. 2010;145(10):973–7.
37. Moore HB, Moore EE, Chapman MP, et al. Viscoelastic measurements of platelet function, not fibrinogen function, predicts sensitivity to tissue-type plasminogen activator in trauma patients. J Thromb Haemost. 2015;13(10):1878–87.
38. Fries D, Martini WZ. Role of fibrinogen in trauma-induced coagulopathy. Br J Anaesth. 2010;105(2):116–21.
39. Morrison JJ, Ross JD, Dubose JJ, et al. Association of cryoprecipitate and tranexamic acid with improved survival following wartime injury: findings from the MATTERs II Study. JAMA Surg. 2013;148(3):218–25.
40. Curry N, Rourke C, Davenport R, et al. Early cryoprecipitate for major haemorrhage in trauma: a randomised controlled feasibility trial. Br J Anaesth. 2015;115(1):76–83.
41. Rourke C, Curry N, Khan S, et al. Fibrinogen levels during trauma hemorrhage, response to replacement therapy, and association with patient outcomes. J Thromb Haemost. 2012;10(7):1342–51.
42. Nunez TC, Young PP, Holcomb JB. Creation, implementation, and maturation of a massive transfusion protocol for the exsanguinating trauma patient. J Trauma. 2010;68:1498–505.
43. Shaz BH, Dante CJ, Harris FIS, et al. Transfusion management of trauma patients. Anesth Analg. 2009;108:1760–8.
44. Johansson PI, Stensballe J, Rosenberg I, et al. Proactive administration of platelets and plasma for patients with a ruptured abdominal aortic aneurysm: evaluating a change in transfusion practice. Transfusion. 2007;47(4):593–8.
45. Rossaint R, Bouillon B, Cerny V, et al. The European guideline on management of major bleeding and coagulopathy following trauma: fourth edition. Crit Care. 2016;20(1):100.
46. Holcomb JB, del Junco DJ, Fox EE, et al. The prospective, observational, multi-center, major trauma transfusion (PROMMTT) study: comparative effectiveness of a time-varying treatment with competing risks. JAMA Surg. 2013;148:127–36.
47. Pandey S, Vyas GN. Adverse effects of plasma transfusion. Transfusion. 2012;52(suppl 1):65S–79S.
48. Torres LN, Sondeen JL, Ji L, et al. Evaluation of resuscitation fluids on endothelial glycocalyx, venular blood flow and coagulation function after hemorrhagic shock in rats. J Trauma Acute Care Surg. 2013;75(5):759–66.
49. Pati S, Matijevic N, Doursout M-F, et al. Protective effects of Fresh Frozen Plasma on vascular endothelial permeability, coagulation and resuscitation after hemorrhagic shock are time dependent and diminish between days 0 and 5 after thaw. J Trauma. 2010;69:S55–63.
50. Haywood-Watson RJ, Holcomb JB, Gonzales EA, et al. Modulation of Syndecan-1 shedding after hemorrhagic shock and resuscitation. PLoS One. 2011;6(8):e23530.
51. Maegele M, Schochl H, Cohen MJ. An update on the coagulopathy of trauma. Shock. 2014;41:S1, 21–5.
52. Weinbaum S, Tarbell JM, Damiano ER. The structure and function of the endothelial glycocalyx layer. Annu Rev Biomed Eng. 2007;9:121–67.
53. Noel P, Cashen S, Patel B. Trauma-induced coagulopathy: from biology to therapy. Semin Hematol. 2013;50:259–69.
54. Ostrowski SR, Johannson P. Endothelial glycocalyx degradation induces endogenous heparinization in patients with severe injury and early traumatic coagulopathy. J Trauma Acute Care Surg. 2012;73:60–6.
55. Pierce A, Pittet J-F. Inflammatory response to trauma: implications for coagulation and resuscitation. Curr Opin Anesthesiol. 2014;27(2):246–52.
56. Johannson P, Stensballe J, Rasmussen LS, et al. A high admission syndecan-1 level, marker of endothelial glycocalyx degradation, is associated with inflammation, protein C depletion, fibrinolysis, and increased mortality in trauma patients. Ann Surg. 2011;254:194–200.
57. Johansson PI, Stensballe J, Ostrowski SR. Shock induced endotheliopathy (SHINE) in acute critical illness—a unifying pathophysiologic mechanism. Crit Care. 2017;21:25.
58. Khan S, Allard S, Weaver A, et al. A major haemorrhage protocol improves the delivery of blood component therapy and reduces waste in trauma massive transfusion. Injury. 2013;44(5):587–92.

Nutrition Support in Critically Ill Surgical Patients

47

Lee-anne Chapple and Marianne Chapman

Key Points

- Nutrition risk screening should occur prior to elective surgery or within 48 h of admission following emergency surgery.
- If possible, enteral nutrition should commence within 24 h after elective surgery, or within 24 h of ICU admission for emergency surgery.
- Calorie and protein delivery should be provided to meet estimated targets, with adequacy monitored regularly and implementation of strategies to minimise interruptions.
- Immunonutrition is indicated pre- and post-operatively in certain surgical groups.
- Enteral nutrition should be provided when oral intake is not sufficient to meet nutritional needs.
- If oral or enteral nutrition is inadequate for 7 days or longer, supplemental or full parenteral nutrition should be commenced.

47.1 Introduction

The nutritional needs of critically ill surgical patients differ to other critically ill populations. Unlike patients admitted to ICU following the exacerbation of a chronic medical condition, surgical patients are admitted following an acute trauma or elective or emergency surgical procedure so may be less likely to have poor nutritional status at baseline.

Optimal nutrition support has the potential to improve survival, clinical outcomes, functional status, and quality of life in critically ill patients. Adequate nutrition is important to enhance wound healing and prevent muscle wasting and infective complications. However, inappropriate delivery of nutrition support may also cause harm.

Many critically ill patients, particularly those receiving mechanical ventilation, cannot take nutrition orally, and it is therefore provided through artificial means, either enterally (into the stomach or duodenum) or parenterally (into the veins). Elevated nutritional needs and factors that impede the delivery of adequate nutrition support mean that alternative delivery methods and focused nutrition therapy may be required for these patients. There are also a number of conditions, such as open abdomen, pancreatitis, and fistulae that require specific feeding strategies to optimise outcomes.

Generally, the surgeon plays an integral role in the initiation of nutrition support and minimisation of disruptions to feeding and should therefore have a good understanding of the nutritional needs of critically ill surgical patients. The aim of this chapter is to provide evidence-based guidance for nutrition support to improve the outcomes of critically ill surgical patients including those classified as 'injured' such as trauma and burns or 'post-operative' such as gastrointestinal and thoracic surgery. This chapter will cover aspects of nutrition support including the delivery route, amount, type, and monitoring of nutrition support.

47.2 Physiological Response to Surgery and Injury

Both elective surgery and acute injury are followed by a period of elevated metabolism in response to 'stress'. The effect size and duration of this stress response are related to the severity of the injury or surgery. In elective surgical

L.-a. Chapple · M. Chapman (✉)
Discipline of Acute Care Medicine, School of Medicine, University of Adelaide, Adelaide, SA, Australia

National Health and Medical Research Council of Australia Centre for Clinical Research Excellence in Nutritional Physiology and Outcomes, Adelaide, SA, Australia

Intensive Care Research Unit, Royal Adelaide Hospital, Adelaide, SA, Australia
e-mail: lee-anne.chapple@adelaide.edu.au; Marianne.chapman@sa.gov.au

P. Aseni et al. (eds.), *Operative Techniques and Recent Advances in Acute Care and Emergency Surgery*, https://doi.org/10.1007/978-3-319-95114-0_47

patients, the increase in metabolic rate may be small, whereas in major trauma such as a severe head injury or burns, the hypermetabolic phase is profound and can persist for over a month post-injury [1].

Post-injury, a number of metabolic changes occur, which result in protein catabolism, reduced glucose utilisation, fat oxidisation, and fluid retention, as shown in Fig. 47.1. If not managed with appropriate nutrition support, these changes result in muscle degradation, hyperglycaemia, and poor wound healing.

47.3 Nutrition Requirements

Despite demonstrated elevation in energy expenditure and protein breakdown, one of the greatest areas of debate in the field of critical care nutrition is around the amount of calories and protein to deliver in order to optimise patient outcomes. The first part of this dilemma is how we determine the energy expenditure of individual patients in a clinical setting? And secondly, if we deliver nutrition to meet these needs, will that positively affect the patient's outcome?

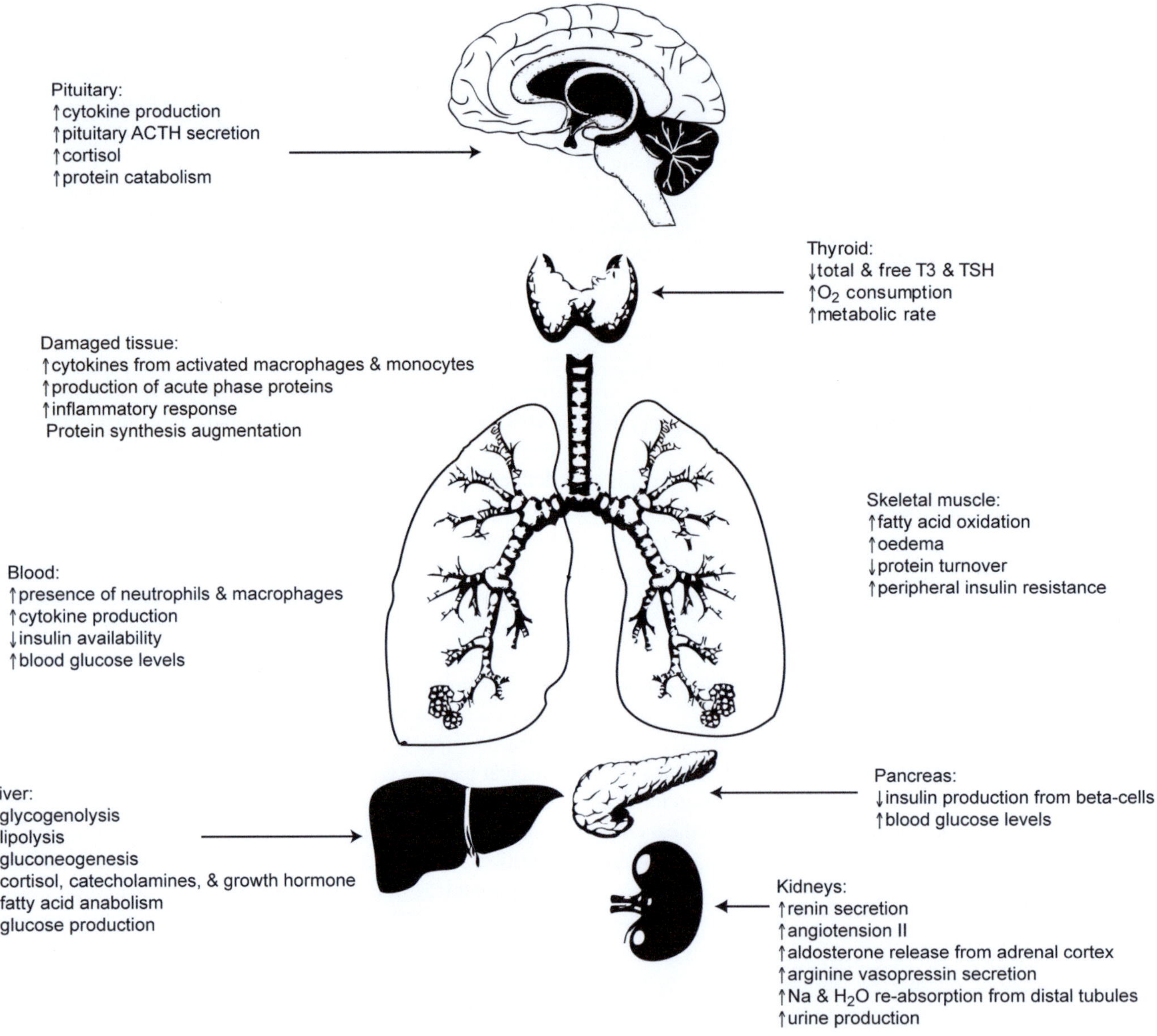

Fig. 47.1 Metabolic changes in response to trauma and injury. *ACTH* adrenocorticotropic hormone, *TSH* thyroid-stimulating hormone, O_2 oxygen, *Na* sodium, H_2O water

47.3.1 Calorie Requirements

Caloric prescriptions are usually determined by estimating energy expenditure with the idea that calorie delivery should match energy expenditure. In a clinical setting, the most accurate way to do this is with indirect calorimetry (IC) to measure oxygen and carbon dioxide gas exchange. However, the routine use of IC is time-consuming and impractical. Each measure takes approximately 30 min to conduct, requires expensive equipment, and can be affected by factors such as air leaks and patient movement and hence should be conducted by practitioners with extensive training and experience in its use. Accordingly, it may be best restrict IC to research purposes or to patients in whom energy prescription is unpredictable such as those with burns, head injury, and obesity [2, 3].

A common alternative to IC is the use of a predictive equation to estimate energy expenditure. A large number of equations exist, and while these are easy and efficient to conduct at the bedside, the majority has been developed using data from healthy volunteers and hence over- or underestimates nutritional needs in critical illness [4]. The most frequently used predictive equations and their comparison to IC are listed in Table 47.1. Of these the Penn State equation has the greatest correlation with IC in critical illness. Alternatively, it is also an accepted practice in ICU to prescribe energy delivery using a simple weight-based prescription, typically 25–30 kcal/kg body weight/day for mechanically ventilated patients, recognising that energy utilisation in patients varies substantially both between patients and over time meaning this prescription is likely to be frequently inaccurate as an indication of energy expenditure.

Additionally the calculations used to determine energy expenditure are weight based. While there are inherent errors in the use of actual, premorbid, adjusted, and ideal body weight, there is no evidence to support the use of any particular weight. Ideal body weight accounts, to some degree, for differences in body composition and metabolically active tissues and hence may be preferred.

It is not known whether matching energy delivery to energy expenditure is important for optimal clinical outcomes, particularly in the post-operative or post-trauma period in the patient who has normal nutritional status at baseline.

In a heterogeneous critically ill population, there is current controversy regarding how many calories should be delivered early in the ICU admission to optimise outcomes. While a number of observational studies in heterogeneous critically ill patients have reported an association between greater energy delivery and improved outcomes, including mortality, increased ventilator-free days, and expedited physical recovery [5, 6], a number of randomised controlled trials (RCTs) have failed to support this finding. A meta-analysis of eight RCTs reported that more energy delivery does not improve mortality [7]. In surgical patients, there are limited data available on the effect of target versus trophic nutrition (minimal amount of enteral nutrition) delivered early post-operatively, and hence full feeding is recommended.

Table 47.1 List of predictive equations used and comparison to indirect calorimetry

Equation	Year developed	Variables	Population developed	Accuracy with IC in critical illness
Harris-Benedict	1919	Age Weight Height +Stress/activity factor	239 healthy subjects	Without added factors: 15% different from IC
Swinamer	1990	Body surface area Body temp Respiratory rate Tidal volume	112 ICU pts	55% of estimates within 10%
Ireton-Jones	1992	Age Sex Weight Trauma/burn factor	65 ICU pts	28–52% of estimates within 10% in nonobese 72% of estimates within 10% in obese
Mifflin-St Jeor	1990	Age Sex Weight Height	498 healthy subjects	Correlation with IC $R^2 = 0.69$
Penn State	1998/2003	Harris-Benedict equation Body temperature Minute ventilation	169 ICU pts	79% of estimates within 10% in nonobese 61% of estimates within 10% in obese

47.3.2 Protein Requirements

In health, recommended protein requirements are ~0.75–0.8 g/kg body weight/day. Nitrogen balance and protein tracer studies in critical illness demonstrate an increase in both protein breakdown and synthesis, with an overall negative nitrogen balance [8, 9], yet data on the effect of varying protein doses on clinical or functional outcomes is sparse. A number of small clinical studies of protein doses have been conducted with the primary outcome of nitrogen balance [10] or total body protein determined using in vivo neutron activation [11], yet the relationship between these outcomes and clinical improvements has not been demonstrated.

Observational data suggest that increased protein delivery is associated with improved outcomes [12–14], yet a recent meta-analysis reported no relationship between incidental lower or higher protein delivery and mortality, length of stay, or incidence of infections [15]. A small RCT in 119 predominantly surgical patients receiving parenteral nutrition compared protein doses of 0.8–1.2 g/kg [16]. While the actual protein dose received varied marginally between the two groups (0.9 vs. 1.1 g/kg/day), patients receiving more protein had less fatigue and greater ultrasound-derived forearm muscle thickness by day 7, highlighting the potential for adequate protein to improve patient-centred outcomes.

Despite a sparsity of data, it is generally accepted that greater protein delivery is likely to be beneficial during critical illness, with potential benefits in terms of wound healing, improved immune function, and prevention of muscle atrophy. Expert opinion is that 1.2–2.0 g protein/kg body weight/day should be provided [17]. In the absence of high-quality data, protein targets for planned surgical patients should aim towards the lower end of this range, while the higher target should be used in patients with extensive burns or severe head injuries.

47.4 Nutrition Screening and Assessment

With a large number of patients admitted to ICU, and many staying for short periods of time only, it is important to identify those patients that are most likely to benefit from nutrition support. There are over 70 nutrition risk screening and assessment tools available; however, the majority of these are not feasible to conduct in critically ill patients, as they require patient co-operation or have not been validated for use in an ICU population. Table 47.2 shows nutritional risk screening and assessment tools commonly used in the ICU setting and their application to ICU.

In elective surgical patients, nutrition risk screening should be performed preoperatively. In patients identified as high risk, nutrition intervention should be implemented at this time and a delay in surgery considered in severely malnourished patients in order to reduce post-operative complications [18]. For unplanned surgical admissions, it is recommended that patients be screened for nutritional risk within 48 h of ICU admission, regardless of the specific tool used.

For patients identified to be at high risk for malnutrition, a clinical diagnostic assessment, preferably conducted by a trained dietitian, should include a thorough examination of the patients' current nutritional intake, weight status, and factors that may influence post-operative nutrition status. Traditionally, measures of weight, or body mass index, have been used to assess nutritional status, however, these may be misleading due to substantial fluid shifts that occur during critical illness. In other clinical areas, biochemical parameters such as albumin, prealbumin, and transferrin are used to assess nutritional status, yet interpretation of these measures in ICU is unreliable as they can be influenced dramatically by the acute-phase inflammatory response [19–21].

There have been recent improvements in more sophisticated assessment of anthropometry to assess nutritional status in critically ill patients including ultrasonography of muscle size and bioelectrical impedance that uses an electric current to estimate body composition [22]. These techniques show promise in enabling objective measurement of muscle mass over time but require refinement before being introduced as standard clinical care.

47.5 Preoperative Nutrition

For patients deemed at high nutritional risk, a preoperative intervention incorporating nutrition, exercise, improved glycaemic control, and smoking cessation is recommended in an effort to reduce major complications and hospital length of stay [24].

Immediately prior to surgery requiring anaesthesia, a period of fasting is required to minimise the risk of perioperative aspiration. However, the age-old 'fast from midnight' is now obsolete, with fasting guidelines commonly recommending abstaining from solid food for 6 h and clear fluids for 2 h [18, 25]. There is no reason to hold PN during surgery. Given the deleterious effects of extended fasting periods in critically ill patients, it has been suggested that patients with a protected airway (the presence of a cuffed endotracheal tube for ventilatory support), who are not having a surgical procedure on the gastrointestinal tract or airway, can receive enteral nutrition (EN) up until surgery [26, 27].

As highlighted previously, hyperglycaemia is common following surgical stress, yet managing this using intensive

Table 47.2 Common nutrition risk screening and assessment tools and their application to critically ill patients

Tool/measure	Description	Developed for	Positives	Corresponding outcomes
Nutrition risk screening tools				
MUST	BMI Weight loss (%) last 3–6 months Acute disease effect score (intake last 5 days)	Community	Good reliability Good content validity	Hospital LOS Mortality in elderly pts Discharge location in ortho pts
NRS-2002	BMI <20.5 kg/m^2 Recent weight loss (%) Intake in last week Disease severity Age	Hospital setting	Good reliability Includes disease severity	Reduced hospital LOS
MNA-SF	Intake last 3 months Weight loss (%) last 3–6 months Anthropometry (BMI, CC) Mobility Recent acute disease Neuropsychological issues	Elderly: hospital and community	Good reliability	
NUTRIC score	Age, injury severity, co-morbidities, days in hospital prior to ICU admission	ICU	External validity	28-day and 6-month mortality Ventilator-free days in 28 days
Nutrition assessment tools				
SGA	Medical history (weight, intake, GI symptoms, functional capacity) and physical assessment	General surgical inpatients ICU	Good intra- and inter-reliability [23]	Incidence of infection Hospital LOS Mortality
MNA	18 items: diet intake, weight loss, mobility, BMI, functional capacity, pressure sores, medications, level of independence, self-reported health status, physical assessment	Elderly patients		

BMI body mass index, *CC* calf circumference, *LOS* length of stay, *MNA* mini nutritional assessment, *MNA-SF* Mini Nutrition Assessment-Short Form, *MUST* Malnutrition Universal Screening Tool, *NRS* nutrition risk screening tool, *PG-SGA* patient-guided subjective global assessment, *SGA* subjective global assessment

insulin therapy can result in reduced organ function and mortality [28]. Preoperative carbohydrate loading has been suggested as one strategy to ameliorate these effects by minimising the depletion of glycogen stores that occur during surgery [29]. A carbohydrate-based drink of 800 mL the night before, and 400 mL 2 h prior to, surgery has been shown to improve insulin resistance, enhance return of bowel function, and improve post-operative nutritional intake, with no adverse effects on aspiration or anaesthesia-related complications [30].

47.6 Post-operative Nutrition

47.6.1 Route

In some critically ill patients, particularly those receiving mechanical ventilation, nutrition support cannot be taken orally, while in other groups, nutritional needs cannot be met through oral nutrition alone. Therefore, nutrition may be delivered enterally, via a thin tube into the stomach or duodenum. Further, particular surgical procedures may prevent patients being fed via the gastrointestinal tract, in which case parenteral nutrition (PN), directly into the veins, may be required.

For patients that are unable to meet their prescribed nutritional requirements orally, EN should be commenced in preference to PN given the additional benefits of EN, such as maintaining gut integrity and reduced costs [31]. Clear contraindications to EN include intestinal obstruction, bowel ischaemia, and the presence of fistulae [32], in which case PN can be considered. However, there is no benefit in commencing PN early, particularly if there is a likelihood that the patient will be able to commence oral or EN within 7–10 days [33, 34].

In patients who have demonstrated the inability to tolerate gastric feeding, evidenced by large gastric residual volumes, or are at high risk of aspiration, postpyloric feeding may be more effective.

Finally, some critically ill surgical patients will require more permanent feeding options, such as insertion of a percutaneous endoscopic gastrostomy (PEG) tube. There are limited studies that explore the appropriate timing of insertion or provide guidance on how this decision should be made. A small study in head-injured and stroke patients demonstrated a reduced risk of ventilator-acquired pneumonia with early gastrostomy placement [35], and the ESPEN surgical guidelines recommend PEG insertion be considered if enteral feeding for greater than 4 weeks is required [29].

47.6.2 Timing

While once controversial, there is now a demonstrated clear benefit to initiating EN early after surgery [36, 37]. Historically, delays occurred in the initiation of nutrition support until bowel sounds were present, or due to concerns of complications of aspiration or ischaemic bowel. Recent evidence negates these concerns, with evidence to suggest that bowel sounds do not represent mucosal integrity, barrier function, or absorptive capacity [17]. While practitioners have previously held concerns regarding the safety of delivery of EN through anastomoses, recent studies have demonstrated that this practice is both safe and associated with improved outcomes. A meta-analysis looking at studies on the timing of initiation of feeding after surgery that involved bowel anastomosis showed no differences in complication rates and a trend towards reduced mortality and length of stay with early EN [36]. In patients following GI surgery, early EN has been shown to reduce post-operative complications by 45% with no increase in anastomotic leak [38].

In ventilated surgical patients, two meta-analyses of RCTs have demonstrated the benefit of early EN (within 24 h) over delayed EN in relation to survival, hospital length of stay, and incidence of pneumonia and infections [39, 40].

47.6.3 Immunonutrition

Surgery is associated with immune impairment and oxidative stress, increasing the risk of subsequent infection. The provision of immune-modulating nutrients, commonly encompassing arginine, glutamine, omega-3 fatty acids, and nucleotides, is thought to improve the immune response to stress.

Immunonutrition, delivered for 5–7 days preoperatively, has been shown to significantly reduce post-operative infectious and non-infectious complications and hospital length of stay compared to standard EN [41, 42], particularly in patients undergoing major gastrointestinal and high-risk surgery [43–45]. While there are promising results in other surgical patient groups, the evidence is not yet conclusive enough to change routine clinical practice across the board [46].

Post-operatively, the major benefits of immunonutrition have been seen when delivered for 5–7 days after surgery in specific patient populations including those at severe nutritional risk, trauma patients, and those undergoing major surgery of the neck and abdomen [29].

The optimal dose, profile, timing, and duration are yet to be confirmed; however, studies of single immunonutrients, including arginine and omega-3 fatty acids, have been unable to replicate the results of studies utilising a combination of nutrients. Therefore, the provision of at least 1 L/day of a commercially available, immunonutrition-containing oral or enteral formula is recommended [29, 47].

In contrast to surgical patients, the safety of immunonutrition has not been demonstrated in other critically ill populations, particularly patients with multi-organ failure or sepsis where the outcomes are worse with this intervention [48].

47.7 Barriers to Adequate Nutrition and Monitoring

Regardless of the energy and protein targets prescribed, delivery of nutrition support in the ICU is usually well below ordered amounts. A number of observational studies report critically ill patients receive around 50% of their estimated energy requirements [49, 50]. Observational data from an international cohort of critically ill patients showed that when compared to medical patients, patients post-surgery had greater nutritional deficits, had longer delays in the initiation of nutrition, and were less likely to receive EN [51]. There are a number of factors that may contribute to 'underfeeding' in a critically ill population.

47.7.1 Interruptions

A major cause of inadequate nutrition support is the interruption to feed delivery for fasting for surgical or diagnostic procedures. In trauma patients 42% of interruptions were shown to be due to surgical or diagnostic procedures [52]. While these are often unavoidable, it has been demonstrated that the length of fasting may be inappropriate. A small retrospective study showed EN was ceased for 6.5 (SD, 6.2) h prior to a planned procedure and took 1.9 (SD, 3.0) h to recommence on procedure completion [53]. When compared to the institution's guidelines, 23% of these episodes were deemed unnecessary. In addition, compared to medical patients, surgical patients are more likely to have a delay in the initiation of nutrition support [51]. Strategies to reduce interruptions to nutrition support could include volume-based feeding (a daily target volume rather than hourly rate), appropriate fasting periods, and minimisation of theatre cancellations.

47.7.2 Refeeding

During extended periods of negligible nutritional intake, adaptive responses result in the utilisation of free fatty acids as the primary energy source in place of glucose. The rapid reintroduction of nutrient, in particular carbohydrates, results in a return to carbohydrate metabolism, leading to increased insulin production, hypophosphataemia, hypokalaemia, hypomagnesaemia, thiamine deficiency, and sodium and fluid retention. These collective metabolic consequences are termed refeeding, which, when unmanaged, can place the patient at risk of arrhythmias, fluid overload, and cardiac failure [54]. Screening of patients to identify those at higher risk of refeeding should occur according to the NICE guidelines [55], with a focus on patients who are underweight and have recent unintentional weight loss or a history of alcohol abuse. For those deemed at high risk, nutrition should be introduced slowly starting at 10 kcal/kg/day and progressing towards goal rate over 4–7 days, with daily monitoring and correction of electrolyte disturbances [55]. A RCT has demonstrated that protocolised caloric restriction in critically ill adults with hypophosphataemia is associated with improved survival [56].

47.7.3 Blood Glucose Control

Surgical stress results in insulin resistance and hyperglycaemia, leading to increased risk of infectious complications, impaired wound healing, and increased risk of mortality. A protocol incorporating intravenous insulin delivery can be used to optimise blood glucose control, even in patients who were not previously diabetic. It is important not only to avoid hyperglycaemia but also hypoglycaemia and glucose variability. Following the publication of the NICE-SUGAR trial, most ICUs aim for a blood glucose concentration of 4–10 mmol/L (72–180 mg/dL) [57].

47.8 Specific Considerations

47.8.1 Burns

It is well known that a major burn is associated with a significant increase in metabolic rate of 150–200% of usual values [58, 59], and this hypermetabolic state can persist for up to 2 years post-injury. It has been suggested that the metabolic state is proportional to the total body surface area (TBSA) of the burn [60]. Indirect calorimetry can be used to direct caloric goals where available, yet in the absence of this, the best predictive equation is the Toronto equation that incorporates the percent TBSA [60].

In addition, the significant fluid resuscitation required to maintain blood pressure in burns leads to oedema, which may result in paralytic ileus. Early EN, delivered in the first 6–12 h following injury, reduces the risk of ileus and attenuates the inflammatory response [17, 60]. In addition, protein delivery should be provided to meet 1.5–2 g/kg body weight/day to counteract the catabolic state [17, 60]. Burned patients also benefit from trace element supplementation to replace exudative losses, promote wound healing, and enhance immune response. Supplementation with selenium, zinc, and copper has also been shown to reduce rates of pneumonia [61].

Unfortunately, the ability to meet these elevated demands is challenging. Patients have substantial calorie and protein deficits, and these are associated with increased mortality [62]. Delayed gastric emptying is prevalent in up to 80% of patients, impeding tolerance of enteral nutrition [63]. Patients are also fasted frequently for procedures such as wound debridement and skin grafting further impeding nutritional delivery [62], and consideration of continuing EN through these procedures is warranted. Close monitoring of nutritional adequacy and strategies to improve delivery, such as early placement of postpyloric feeding tubes, should be implemented to ensure estimated requirements are met. Observational data suggest that energy delivery affects outcomes, including survival, in this group [62].

47.8.2 Head Injury

In patients with a severe head injury, metabolic rate has been shown to be elevated up to 200% of usual values and remains elevated even 30 days post-injury [1]. EN should be commenced within 24 h of injury, with benefits in terms of mortality and infectious complications [64]. Calorie and protein targets should be met by at least day 5 of admission [65, 66] with nutritional adequacy shown to reduce duration of mechanical ventilation and time to discharge alive from both ICU and hospital [67]. Similar to patients with burns, patients with head injury often stay in hospital for extended periods of time, and factors such as dysphagia and post-traumatic amnesia—resulting in frequent tube removal and food refusal—lead to substantial calorie and protein deficits throughout the hospital admission [68].

47.8.3 Open Abdomen

In the critically ill surgical/trauma patient, leaving the abdomen open for a period is sometimes necessary in order to manage infection and prevent post-operative complications

[69]. While there are concerns of paralytic ileus, bowel dilation, and poor haemodynamics with early EN in patients with open abdomen, these concerns are not justified in the literature [70]. Two observational studies of nutrition support in patients with an open abdomen reported that early EN was associated with a trend to faster closure and significant reduction in pneumonia [71, 72]. The American Society of Parenteral and Enteral Nutrition recommends early EN be instigated in patients with an open abdomen, provided there is no bowel injury present [17]. In addition, protein demands are higher in patients with an open abdomen, with a significant loss of nitrogen from the exposed surface of the abdominal viscera [73]. It has been recommended that an additional 15–30 g of protein be provided per litre of exudate lost; however, this is based on observed protein levels in exudate, rather than on defined clinical benefit [17].

47.8.4 Pancreatitis

Previously, PN was given preference over EN in order to avoid pancreatic stimulation and hence inflammation [74]. However, EN has since been shown to be safe and is actually associated with a reduction in pancreatitis-associated inflammation [75]. EN commenced within 24–48 h has been shown to reduce incidence of multiple organ dysfunction syndrome, systemic inflammatory response syndrome, infection, hyperglycaemia, and ICU length of stay [76, 77]. The nasogastric route can be used safely in the first instance although gastric emptying is frequently slow which may result in gastric feeding intolerance [78]. Prokinetic agents or postpyloric feeding can then be used as needed. In severe pancreatitis, American Society of Parenteral and Enteral Nutrition guidelines recommend commencing EN at a trophic rate and advancing to target rate once pulse and blood pressure have stabilised [17], yet this is not echoed in the equivalent European guidelines [79]. Despite some initial promising results, the routine use of glutamine, probiotics, or omega-3 fatty acids in this population is not recommended [80].

47.8.5 Anastomoses

Historically, PN has been used in preference to EN in patients with gastrointestinal anastomoses due to a concern with the EN leading to anastomotic dehiscence. However, a meta-analysis of 1240 patients with GI anastomoses demonstrated that early post-operative EN significantly reduced complications, with no increase in anastomotic dehiscence [38]. Therefore, EN should be commenced early when oral intake is insufficient to meet nutritional needs.

47.8.6 Fistulae

Fistula severity can be classified according to exudate output: low output (200 mL/24 h), moderate output (200–500 mL/24 h), and high output (>500 mL/24 h) [81]. High-output fistulae are associated with higher mortality and morbidity and a lower chance of spontaneous closure [82, 83]. For high-output fistulae, the initial aim is to correct acid-base and electrolyte abnormalities [84]. Fluid and electrolyte replacement should aim to meet that lost from exudate, with replacement using an electrolyte solution containing around 90 mmol of sodium and 30 mmol potassium per litre solution [82]. In some cases, achieving fluid replacement orally may be unachievable, and intravenous fluids and supplemental PN will be required. Patients should limit ordinary (hypotonic, sodium-free) fluids to no more than 500 mL/24 h [82].

In low- or moderate-output fistulae, early EN is associated with earlier fistula closure and lower rate of fistula recurrence [84]. However, the provision of a standard EN formula may increase fistulae output, and in cases of short bowel length, the absorptive capacity of EN by the gut will be reduced [84]. The use of an elemental formula may be better tolerated by some patients; however, in most high-output fistulae, or those that are located higher anatomically, PN should be used [84, 85].

For high-output fistulae, nutritional requirements are elevated due to ongoing losses. Protein delivery should aim to meet 1.5–2.5 g/kg/day [85], and caloric needs should be 1.5–2 times above energy expenditure [84]. Malnutrition is common, and lower calorie delivery has been shown to be associated with higher mortality [86]. Therefore, priority should be placed on adequate delivery of calories to these patients.

47.9 Team Involvement

The nutritional management of critically ill surgical patients is complex. The heterogeneous population means nutritional needs are often difficult to predict, and multiple challenges exist that impede the delivery of adequate nutrition. Decisions around the type, amount, and route of nutrition support are usually multifactorial, and one solution may come at the expense of another. Therefore, it is particularly important that decisions around nutrition support involve a multidisciplinary team, including a dietitian, surgeon, intensivist, nurse practitioner, speech pathologist, and the patient/family member. Clear communication between all members of the team is required in order to form a consensus nutrition plan.

Conclusion

In surgical and critically ill patients, nutritional needs can be complex, and increased and nutrition therapy has the potential to improve clinical outcomes including survival. Focus should be placed on the preoperative identification of patients at nutritional risk and the provision of early and adequate nutrition support, usually via the enteral route.

References

1. Foley N, Marshall S, Pikul J, Salter K, Teasell R. Hypermetabolism following moderate to severe traumatic acute brain injury: a systematic review. J Neurotrauma. 2008;25(12):1415–31.
2. Schlein KM, Coulter SP. Best practices for determining resting energy expenditure in critically ill adults. Nutr Clin Pract. 2014;29(1):44–55.
3. Compher C, Frankenfield D, Keim N, Roth-Yousey L, Evidence Analysis Working Group. Best practice methods to apply to measurement of resting metabolic rate in adults: a systematic review. J Am Diet Assoc. 2006;106(6):881–903.
4. Frankenfield DC, Coleman A, Alam S, Cooney RN. Analysis of estimation methods for resting metabolic rate in critically ill adults. JPEN. 2009;33(1):27–36.
5. Alberda C, Gramlich L, Jones N, et al. The relationship between nutritional intake and clinical outcomes in critically ill patients: results of an international multi-center observational study. Intensive Care Med. 2009;35:1728–37.
6. Wei X, Day AG, Ouellette-Kuntz H, Heyland DK. The association between nutritional adequacy and long-term outcomes in critically ill patients requiring prolonged mechanical ventilation: a multicenter cohort study. Crit Care Med. 2015;43(8):1569–79.
7. Tian F, Wang X, Gao X, et al. Effect of initial calorie intake via enteral nutrition in critical illness: a meta-analysis of randomised controlled trials. Crit Care. 2015;19:180.
8. Rooyackers O, Kouchek-Zadeh R, Tjader I, Norberg A, Klaude M, Wernerman J. Whole body protein turnover in critically ill patients with multiple organ failure. Clin Nutr. 2015;34(1):95–100.
9. Plank LD, Hill GL. Sequential metabolic changes following induction of systemic inflammatory response in patients with severe sepsis or major blunt trauma. World J Surg. 2000;24(6):630–8.
10. Clifton GL, Robertson CS, Grossman RG, Hodge S, Foltz R, Garza C. The metabolic response to severe head injury. J Neurosurg. 1984;60(4):687–96.
11. Ishibashi N, Plank LD, Sando K, Hill GL. Optimal protein requirements during the first 2 weeks after the onset of critical illness. Crit Care Med. 1998;26(9):1529–35.
12. Nicolo M, Heyland DK, Chittams J, Sammarco T, Compher C. Clinical outcomes related to protein delivery in a critically ill population: a multicenter, multinational observation study. JPEN. 2016;40(1):45–51.
13. Weijs PJ, Stapel SN, de Groot SD, et al. Optimal protein and energy nutrition decreases mortality in mechanically ventilated, critically ill patients: a prospective observational cohort study. JPEN. 2012;36(1):60–8.
14. Allingstrup MJ, Esmailzadeh N, Wilkens Knudsen A, et al. Provision of protein and energy in relation to measured requirements in intensive care patients. Clin Nutr. 2012;31(4):462–8.
15. Davies M, Chapple L, Chapman M, Moran J, Peake S. Protein delivery and clinical outcomes in the critically ill: a systematic review and meta-analysis. Crit Care Resusc. 2017;19(2):117–27.
16. Ferrie S, Allman-Farinelli M, Daley M, Smith K. Protein requirements in the critically ill: a randomized controlled trial using parenteral nutrition. JPEN. 2016;40(6):795–805.
17. McClave SA, Taylor BE, Martindale RG, et al. Guidelines for the provision and assessment of nutrition support therapy in the adult critically ill patient: Society of Critical Care Medicine (SCCM) and American Society for Parenteral and Enteral Nutrition (A.S.P.E.N.). JPEN. 2016;40(2):159–211.
18. Lassen K, Soop M, Nygren J, et al. Consensus review of optimal perioperative care in colorectal surgery: Enhanced Recovery After Surgery (ERAS) Group recommendations. Arch Surg. 2009;144(10):961–9.
19. Vincent JL, Dubois MJ, Navickis RJ, Wilkes MM. Hypoalbuminemia in acute illness: is there a rationale for intervention? A meta-analysis of cohort studies and controlled trials. Ann Surg. 2003;237(3):319–34.
20. Raguso CA, Dupertuis YM, Pichard C. The role of visceral proteins in the nutritional assessment of intensive care unit patients. Curr Opin Clin Nutr Metab Care. 2003;6(2):211–6.
21. Davis CJ, Sowa D, Keim KS, Kinnare K, Peterson S. The use of prealbumin and C-reactive protein for monitoring nutrition support in adult patients receiving enteral nutrition in an urban medical center. JPEN. 2012;36(2):197–204.
22. Earthman CP. Body composition tools for assessment of adult malnutrition at the bedside: a tutorial on research considerations and clinical applications. JPEN. 2015;39(7):787–822.
23. Sheean PM, Peterson SJ, Gurka DP, Braunschweig CA. Nutrition assessment: the reproducibility of subjective global assessment in patients requiring mechanical ventilation. Eur J Clin Nutr. 2010;64(11):1358–64.
24. Jie B, Jiang ZM, Nolan MT, Zhu SN, Yu K, Kondrup J. Impact of preoperative nutritional support on clinical outcome in abdominal surgical patients at nutritional risk. Nutrition. 2012;28(10):1022–7.
25. Australian and New Zealand College of Anaesthetists. Guidelines on pre-anaesthesia consultation and patient preparation. 2016. www.anzca.edu.au. Accessed 11 Apr 2017.
26. Segaran E, Barker I, Hartle A. Optimising enteral nutrition in critically ill patients by reducing fasting times. J Intensive Care Soc. 2016;17(1):38–43.
27. Pousman RM, Pepper C, Pandharipande P, et al. Feasibility of implementing a reduced fasting protocol for critically ill trauma patients undergoing operative and nonoperative procedures. JPEN. 2009;33(2):176–80.
28. Krinsley JS. Effect of an intensive glucose management protocol on the mortality of critically ill adult patients. Mayo Clin Proc. 2004;79(8):992–1000.
29. Weimann A, Braga M, Harsanyi L, et al. ESPEN guidelines on enteral nutrition: surgery including organ transplantation. Clin Nutr. 2006;25(2):224–44.
30. Awad S, Varadhan KK, Ljungqvist O, Lobo DN. A meta-analysis of randomised controlled trials on preoperative oral carbohydrate treatment in elective surgery. Clin Nutr. 2013;32(1):34–44.
31. Hadfield RJ, Sinclair DG, Houldsworth PE, Evans TW. Effects of enteral and parenteral nutrition on gut mucosal permeability in the critically ill. Am J Respir Crit Care Med. 1995;152:1545–8.
32. Braga M, Ljungqvist O, Soeters P, et al. ESPEN guidelines on parenteral nutrition: surgery. Clin Nutr. 2009;28(4):378–86.
33. Casaer MP, Hermans G, Wilmer A, Van den Berghe G. Impact of early parenteral nutrition completing enteral nutrition in adult critically ill patients (EPaNIC trial): a study protocol and statistical analysis plan for a randomized controlled trial. Trials. 2011;12:21.

34. Doig GS, Simpson F, Sweetman EA, et al. Early parenteral nutrition in critically ill patients with short-term relative contraindications to early enteral nutrition: a randomized controlled trial. JAMA. 2013;309(20):2130–8.
35. Kostadima E, Kaditis AG, Alexopoulos EI, Zakynthinos E, Sfyras D. Early gastrostomy reduces the rate of ventilator-associated pneumonia in stroke or head injury patients. Eur Respir J. 2005;26(1):106–11.
36. Lewis SJ, Andersen HK, Thomas S. Early enteral nutrition within 24 h of intestinal surgery versus later commencement of feeding: a systematic review and meta-analysis. J Gastrointest Surg. 2009;13(3):569–75.
37. Doig GS, Heighes PT, Simpson F, Sweetman EA. Early enteral nutrition reduces mortality in trauma patients requiring intensive care: a meta-analysis of randomised controlled trials. Injury. 2011;42(1):50–6.
38. Osland E, Yunus RM, Khan S, Memon MA. Early versus traditional postoperative feeding in patients undergoing resectional gastrointestinal surgery: a meta-analysis. JPEN. 2011;35(4):473–87.
39. Doig GS, Heighes PT, Simpson F, Sweetman EA, Davies AR. Early enteral nutrition, provided within 24 h of injury or intensive care unit admission, significantly reduces mortality in critically ill patients: a meta-analysis of randomised controlled trials. Intensive Care Med. 2009;35(12):2018–27.
40. Marik PE, Zaloga GP. Early enteral nutrition in acutely ill patients: a systematic review. Crit Care Med. 2001;29(12):2264–70.
41. Burden S, Todd C, Hill J, Lal S. Pre-operative nutrition support in patients undergoing gastrointestinal surgery. Cochrane Database Syst Rev. 2012;11:CD008879.
42. Braga M, Wischmeyer PE, Drover J, Heyland DK. Clinical evidence for pharmaconutrition in major elective surgery. JPEN. 2013;37(5 Suppl):66S–72S.
43. Marik PE, Zaloga GP. Immunonutrition in high-risk surgical patients: a systematic review and analysis of the literature. JPEN. 2010;34(4):378–86.
44. Cerantola Y, Hubner M, Grass F, Demartines N, Schafer M. Immunonutrition in gastrointestinal surgery. Br J Surg. 2011;98(1):37–48.
45. Marimuthu K, Varadhan KK, Ljungqvist O, Lobo DN. A meta-analysis of the effect of combinations of immune modulating nutrients on outcome in patients undergoing major open gastrointestinal surgery. Ann Surg. 2012;255(6):1060–8.
46. Drover JW, Dhaliwal R, Weitzel L, Wischmeyer PE, Ochoa JB, Heyland DK. Perioperative use of arginine-supplemented diets: a systematic review of the evidence. J Am Coll Surg. 2011;212(3):385–99.
47. Kudsk KA. Immunonutrition in surgery and critical care. Annu Rev Nutr. 2006;26:463–79.
48. Heyland DK, Novak F, Drover JW, Jain M, Su X, Suchner U. Should immunonutrition become routine in critically ill patients? A systematic review of the evidence. JAMA. 2001;286(8):944–53.
49. De Beaux I, Chapman M, Fraser R, et al. Enteral nutrition in the critically ill: a prospective survey in an Australian intensive care unit. Anaesth Intensive Care. 2001;29:619–22.
50. De Jonghe B, Appere-De-Vechi C, Fournier M, et al. A prospective survey of nutritional support practices in intensive care unit patients: what is prescribed? What is delivered? Crit Care Med. 2001;29:8–12.
51. Drover JW, Cahill NE, Kutsogiannis J, et al. Nutrition therapy for the critically ill surgical patient: we need to do better! JPEN. 2010;34(6):644–52.
52. Morgan LM, Dickerson RN, Alexander KH, Brown RO, Minard G. Factors causing interrupted delivery of enteral nutrition in trauma intensive care unit patients. Nutr Clin Pract. 2004;19(5):511–7.
53. Passier RH, Davies AR, Ridley E, McClure J, Murphy D, Scheinkestel CD. Periprocedural cessation of nutrition in the intensive care unit: opportunities for improvement. Intensive Care Med. 2013;39(7):1221–6.
54. Stanga Z, Brunner A, Leuenberger M, et al. Nutrition in clinical practice-the refeeding syndrome: illustrative cases and guidelines for prevention and treatment. Eur J Clin Nutr. 2008;62(6):687–94.
55. National Collaborating Centre for Acute Care. Nutrition support in adults: Oral nutrition support, enteral tube feeding and parenteral nutrition. 2006. www.rcsend.ac.uk. Accessed 18 Apr 2017.
56. Doig GS, Simpson F, Heighes PT, et al. Restricted versus continued standard caloric intake during the management of refeeding syndrome in critically ill adults: a randomised, parallel-group, multicentre, single-blind controlled trial. Lancet Respir Med. 2015;3(12):943–52.
57. Finfer S, Chittock DR, Su SY, et al. Intensive versus conventional glucose control in critically ill patients. NEJM. 2009;360(13):1283–97.
58. Curreri PW, Richmond D, Marvin J, Baxter CR. Dietary requirements of patients with major burns. J Am Diet Assoc. 1974;65(4):415–7.
59. Saffle JR, Medina E, Raymond J, Westenskow D, Kravitz M, Warden GD. Use of indirect calorimetry in the nutritional management of burned patients. J Trauma. 1985;25(1):32–9.
60. Rousseau AF, Losser MR, Ichai C, Berger MM. ESPEN endorsed recommendations: nutritional therapy in major burns. Clin Nutr. 2013;32(4):497–502.
61. Berger MM, Eggimann P, Heyland DK, et al. Reduction of nosocomial pneumonia after major burns by trace element supplementation: aggregation of two randomised trials. Crit Care. 2006;10(6):R153.
62. Czapran A, Headdon W, Deane AM, Lange K, Chapman MJ, Heyland DK. International observational study of nutritional support in mechanically ventilated patients following burn injury. Burns. 2015;41(3):510–8.
63. Nguyen NQ, Ng MP, Chapman M, Fraser RJ, Holloway RH. The impact of admission diagnosis on gastric emptying in critically ill patients. Crit Care. 2007;11(1):R16.
64. Wang X, Dong Y, Han X, Qi XQ, Huang CG, Hou LJ. Nutritional support for patients sustaining traumatic brain injury: a systematic review and meta-analysis of prospective studies. PLoS One. 2013;8(3):e58838.
65. Bratton S, Chestnut R, Ghajar J, et al. Guidelines for the management of severe traumatic brain injury. XII. Nutrition. J Neurotrauma. 2007;24(Suppl 1):S77–82.
66. Chourdakis M, Kraus M, Tzellos T, et al. Effect of early compared with delayed enteral nutrition on endocrine function in patients with traumatic brain injury: an open-labeled randomized trial. JPEN. 2012;36(1):108–16.
67. Chapple LS, Chapman MJ, Lange K, Deane AM, Heyland DK. Nutrition support practices in critically ill head-injured patients: a global perspective. Crit Care. 2016;20:6.
68. Chapple LS, Deane AM, Heyland DK, et al. Energy and protein deficits throughout hospitalization in patients admitted with a traumatic brain injury. Clin Nutr. 2016;35:1315–22.
69. Regner JL, Kobayashi L, Coimbra R. Surgical strategies for management of the open abdomen. World J Surg. 2012;36(3):497–510.
70. Moore SM, Burlew CC. Nutrition support in the open abdomen. Nutr Clin Pract. 2016;31(1):9–13.
71. Dissanaike S, Pham T, Shalhub S, et al. Effect of immediate enteral feeding on trauma patients with an open abdomen: protection from nosocomial infections. J Am Coll Surg. 2008;207(5):690–7.
72. Powell NJ, Collier B. Nutrition and the open abdomen. Nutr Clin Pract. 2012;27(4):499–506.

73. Cheatham ML, Safcsak K, Brzezinski SJ, Lube MW. Nitrogen balance, protein loss, and the open abdomen. Crit Care Med. 2007;35(1):127–31.
74. Fallis LS. Results of conservative treatment of acute pancreatitis. Ann Surg. 1941;113(6):1070–1.
75. Windsor AC, Kanwar S, Li AG, et al. Compared with parenteral nutrition, enteral feeding attenuates the acute phase response and improves disease severity in acute pancreatitis. Gut. 1998;42(3):431–5.
76. Sun JK, Mu XW, Li WQ, Tong ZH, Li J, Zheng SY. Effects of early enteral nutrition on immune function of severe acute pancreatitis patients. World J Gastroenterol. 2013;19(6):917–22.
77. Olah A, Romics L Jr. Enteral nutrition in acute pancreatitis: a review of the current evidence. World J Gastroenterol. 2014;20(43):16123–31.
78. Eatock FC, Chong P, Menezes N, et al. A randomized study of early nasogastric versus nasojejunal feeding in severe acute pancreatitis. Am J Gastroenterol. 2005;100(2):432–9.
79. Meier R, Ockenga J, Pertkiewicz M, et al. ESPEN guidelines on enteral nutrition: pancreas. Clin Nutr. 2006;25(2):275–84.
80. Lodewijkx PJ, Besselink MG, Witteman BJ, et al. Nutrition in acute pancreatitis: a critical review. Expert Rev Gastroenterol Hepatol. 2016;10(5):571–80.
81. Yanar F, Yanar H. Nutritional support in patients with gastrointestinal fistula. Eur J Trauma Emerg Surg. 2011;37(3):227.
82. Arebi N, Forbes A. High-output fistula. Clin Colon Rectal Surg. 2004;17(2):89–98.
83. Campos AC, Andrade DF, Campos GM, Matias JE, Coelho JC. A multivariate model to determine prognostic factors in gastrointestinal fistulas. J Am Coll Surg. 1999;188(5):483–90.
84. Dudrick SJ, Panait L. Metabolic consequences of patients with gastrointestinal fistulas. Eur J Trauma Emerg Surg. 2011;37(3):215–25.
85. Polk TM, Schwab CW. Metabolic and nutritional support of the enterocutaneous fistula patient: a three-phase approach. World J Surg. 2012;36(3):524–33.
86. Chapman R, Foran R, Dunphy JE. Management of intestinal fistulas. Am J Surg. 1964;108:157–64.

Management Strategies in Geriatric Trauma Care

48

Maurice F. Joyce, Justin Benoit, and Ruben J. Azocar

Abbreviations

CSE	Combined spinal-epidural
GCS	Glasgow coma scale
ISS	Injury severity score
NOAC	Novel oral anticoagulant
TBI	Traumatic brain injury
TLS	Advanced Trauma Life Support

Key Points

- Geriatric-specific triage and evaluation tools allow for more appropriate disposition and better management of geriatric trauma patients.
- Assessment of frailty is a useful adjunct in the initial trauma evaluation and can be used by physicians to help guide patients and their families.
- The most effective and cost-efficient techniques to manage orthopedic and neurologic traumatic injuries are still unclear, and further research must focus on the effects of various techniques on outcomes.
- Orthogeriatrics emphasizes a multidisciplinary approach to the care of elderly trauma patients with traumatic orthopedic injuries and ultimately may lead to better outcomes.
- Early recognition of clinical momentum in the management of traumatic injuries in geriatric patients may prevent futile and potentially unwanted care.

M. F. Joyce
Department of Anesthesiology, The Warren Alpert Medical School of Brown University, Providence, RI, USA
e-mail: Maurice.Joyce1@lifespan.org

J. Benoit · R. J. Azocar (✉)
Department of Anesthesiology, Tufts Medical Center, Boston, MA, USA
e-mail: JBenoit@tuftsmedicalcenter.org; RAzocar@tuftsmedicalcenter.org

48.1 Introduction

Over the last several decades, there has been a significant shift in population demographics, leading to a so-called silver tsunami that has had a major impact on the healthcare industry. According to the 2010 United States census, the elderly population, defined as age 65 years old and older, is the fastest-growing segment of the population [1]. This change has led to a concurrent shift in trauma demographics from young male patients to elderly male and female patients, often injuring themselves via a fall from standing or motor vehicle collision. The National Trauma Data Bank indicates that traumatic injuries in people age 55 years old and older have increased from 32 to 43% since 2010 [2, 3]. This demographic shift is especially troublesome as geriatric trauma patients have higher mortality rates and worse long-term outcomes when compared to younger patients [4, 5]. Just as pediatric patients are not "little adults," geriatric patients are not simply adults with gray hair and thus require a specialized approach to their care. This chapter will review a systematic and tailored approach to the management of geriatric trauma patients with a focus on orthopedic trauma and neurologic trauma.

48.2 Physiologic Alterations of the Geriatric Patient

Physiologic changes associated with aging are not pathologic per se, but one's ability to respond to stressful stimuli becomes compromised [6]. The organ systems that are most affected by aging include the central nervous, cardiovascular, respiratory, and renal systems. Additionally, geriatric patients have altered pharmacokinetic and pharmacodynamic responses to medications.

As individuals get older, there are reductions in the mass of the brain, cerebral blood flow, and neurotransmitter activity, all of which are vital for safe daily functioning [7, 8].

P. Aseni et al. (eds.), *Operative Techniques and Recent Advances in Acute Care and Emergency Surgery*,
https://doi.org/10.1007/978-3-319-95114-0_48

These changes can lead to diminished proprioception and subsequent gait instability, ultimately leading to an increased frequency of falls. Cardiovascular changes in the elderly population include an increased incidence of diastolic dysfunction, leading to pulmonary hypertension and diastolic heart failure [9]. Arrhythmias such as atrial fibrillation and other conduction defects are pervasive with progressive fibrosis of regions of the cardiac conduction system [9, 10]. Respiratory considerations include loss of pharyngeal reflexes, changes in compliance of the lung and chest wall, increased A-a gradient with shunting, and increased closing capacity causing hypoxia [11]. Renal dysfunction increases significantly with aging. Renal blood flow decreases by half in addition to loss of renal tubular mass, leading to variable elimination times of medications [12, 13]. Glomerular filtration rate consistently decreases, as well as one's ability to concentrate urine [14–16]. Taken together, these physiologic alterations demonstrate why a specialized approach is needed in the care of geriatric trauma patients.

48.3 Triage and Evaluation of Geriatric Trauma Patients

As described previously, elderly trauma patients have higher mortality rates, worse long-term outcomes, and higher complication rates when compared to younger trauma patients [4, 5]. In fact, Grossman et al. demonstrated that there was a mortality rate increase of 6.8% for each year over age 65 [17]. Further, elderly trauma patients have significantly higher incidences of hospital-acquired complications such as post-traumatic pneumonia [18]. This outcome inconsistency is largely explained by the higher rate of pre-existing conditions in the geriatric population. However, there is considerable room for improving these unsettling statistics through a tailored approach to the triaging, evaluation, and management of this patient population.

Geriatric patient volume. There is a clear relationship between patient volume and outcomes including mortality in the healthcare industry [19]. This relationship is also found when analyzing the outcomes of geriatric trauma patients. In a single-state retrospective cohort study, Matsushima et al. demonstrated that trauma centers that cared for a larger volume of geriatric trauma patients were more likely to have lower rates of in-hospital mortality and major complications when caring for this population [20]. Interestingly, those centers that cared for a larger volume of younger trauma patients had higher rates of major complications for geriatric trauma patients. These findings have led some to advocate for triage of these patients to trauma centers with geriatric-specific emergency departments or integrated geriatric consults [21, 22]. More research on the effectiveness of these strategies must be done though, as current studies have failed to show a mortality benefit [23].

Geriatric-specific trauma triage criteria. Due to the high mortality and complication rates (and thus large financial burden) observed in elderly trauma patients, there is intense interest in early identification of patients in the field that will require advanced trauma care. Many trauma centers use mechanism of injury and vital signs as a means of triage and criteria for trauma team activation. However, this protocol may be insufficient for this special patient population. Demetriades et al. demonstrated that despite having high injury severity scores (ISS), patients aged 70 years and older often had normal vital signs [24]. Thus, some have advocated for a lower threshold for trauma team activation in geriatric trauma patients, including simply using age as a criterion [25–27]. Hammer et al. demonstrated that an age threshold of 70 years for full trauma team activation, regardless of mechanism of injury or presenting vital signs, improved outcomes and was cost-effective (i.e., low rate of over-triaging) [28].

Geriatric-specific trauma evaluation. While the systematic "ABCDE" approach to trauma evaluation and resuscitation as taught in Advanced Trauma Life Support (ATLS) is important for the care of geriatric trauma patients, it is insufficient [29]. A tailored approach using the ATLS algorithm as a framework is a necessary step in improving overall outcomes [30].

The initial step of the ATLS approach to trauma patient evaluation is assessment of the *airway*. Ensuring a patent airway with the ability to phonate meaningfully suggests that the patient can adequately protect their airway [31]. The integrity of the lower esophageal sphincter decreases with age which results in an increased susceptibility to aspiration events, requiring increased vigilance and the consideration of early intubation [30, 31]. Elderly trauma patients may also have macroglossia or cervical spine changes related to arthritis, leading to airway obstruction and mobility problems in the neck, respectively [31, 32].

The trauma evaluation is continued with assessment of *breathing*. As discussed previously, with aging there are multiple changes to the chest wall and lung parenchyma which ultimately lead to ventilation-perfusion mismatching and reduced compliance. Taken together, these changes result in an increased risk of hypoxia, requiring careful attention to pulse oximetry and early application of supplemental oxygen [31, 32]. Importantly, due to this baseline susceptibility to hypoxia, one must be extremely judicious in the use of systemic opioids or sedatives in this population. Further, any additional insult to respiratory effort such as rib fractures may prove fatal [33].

A thorough evaluation of hemodynamics is then undertaken while assessing *circulation*. Remodeling of the heart due to chronic hypertension, a frequently encountered comorbidity in the elderly, leads to progressive diastolic dysfunction and heart failure. Additionally, arrhythmias such as atrial fibrillation are prevalent due to alterations in the cardiac conduction system [30, 34]. Common medications such as beta-blockers increase the risk of inadequate sympathetic nervous system response to trauma [30, 31]. Importantly, due to the use of these agents, a geriatric trauma patient may present with deceivingly normal vital signs [24].

Of utmost importance in the evaluation of the elderly trauma patient is the assessment of trauma-related neurological *deficits* [32, 34, 35]. There is a high likelihood of atherosclerosis leading to an increased incidence of strokes and acute neurological deficits. Additionally, elderly trauma patients are especially susceptible to falls, often resulting in the tearing of bridging veins in the dura and subsequent subdural hematomas, potentially requiring urgent surgical intervention [32, 34, 35]. An emerging concern in this patient population is the increasing utilization of novel oral anticoagulants (NOACs) for conditions such as atrial fibrillation [36]. While use of an anticoagulant did not formerly present a clinical dilemma as reversal agents were readily available, the anticoagulant effects of NOACs are not always readily reversible. The effects of these agents on trauma outcomes in this population and the development of reversal agents for NOACs will certainly remain an area of intense interest [37, 38].

The final portion of the trauma evaluation is assessment of environmental *exposure*. Thermoregulatory changes and alterations in the integumentary system in the geriatric population lead to rapid-onset hypothermia, resulting in altered drug metabolism, coagulopathy, altered acid-base homeostasis, electrolyte imbalances, and decreased wound healing [30]. It is vital to monitor temperature and maintain normothermia by keeping elderly trauma patients covered and potentially using adjuncts such as forced air warming devices.

In addition to the standard components of the ATLS "ABCDE" approach to trauma patient evaluation, these authors advocate for the addition of an "F"—an assessment of patient *frailty* [39]. While there is universal decline in baseline physiologic parameters among geriatric patients, there is considerable heterogeneity in the degree of this decline. Frailty provides a means of assessing this heterogeneity [40]. Currently, there is no universally accepted definition of frailty, though there are multiple published "frailty indices" [41, 42]. There is literature within the trauma community that suggests that frailty is an independent predictor of adverse discharge disposition and in-hospital complications [43–45]. An immediate assessment of frailty during the initial trauma evaluation may allow more appropriate disposition of elderly trauma patients in addition to providing more context when discussing potential outcomes with elderly trauma patients and their families.

48.4 Orthopedic Injuries in Geriatric Trauma Patients

One of the most devastating and disabling injuries in geriatric trauma patients is hip fractures. Katsoulis et al. demonstrated that all-cause mortality was increased in American and European patients after suffering a hip fracture and remained elevated for up to 4 years [46]. Due to the complexities associated with the management of these patients, the field of orthogeriatrics was created. The field aims to improve the care and coordination of geriatric patients suffering orthopedic trauma with a particular focus on hip fractures [47]. A recent study showed that even with an integrated orthogeriatric team, nearly half of geriatric patients with orthopedic injury experienced an in-hospital complication such as delirium, anemia, urinary tract infection, or pneumonia [48]. In a separate study, Folbert et al. demonstrated that recovery to preoperative functional status post-fracture was limited even for those individuals who had high functional status prior to their injury [49]. However, this same team also found that a collaborative approach between multiple disciplines helped to decrease 1-year mortality rate to 23.2% compared to a control of 35.1% ($p < 0.001$) [49]. The enormous public health and financial burden of these injuries make it vitally important to find the most effective way to care for this patient population.

There is significant debate about the most appropriate and effective treatment modality for an elderly patient suffering from a hip fracture. Tan et al. examined 2756 elderly patients with hip fractures with 74% undergoing surgical management and 26% undergoing medical management. They found that the complication rate in the group that underwent surgical management was approximately half that of the group that underwent medical management (6.6% vs. 12.5%) [50]. Additionally, hospital length of stay was 15.7 days in the surgical group and 22.4 days in the nonsurgical group [50]. In a separate study, delay of surgery was found to be associated with an increased mortality risk, especially in males and patients with a higher ASA status classification [51]. Similarly, Moja et al. looked at 190,000 patients with hip fractures from 1948 through 2011 and found that a surgical delay of greater than 1–2 days was associated with an increased mortality risk [52]. There is conflicting literature, however, as a study by Choi et al. found no statistically significant impact of time to surgery on 30-day mortality, 60-day mortality, or in-hospital complications [53]. More research is clearly needed to help guide management decisions. One current study, the HIP Fracture Accelerated Surgical Treatment and Care Track (HIP ATTACK) trial, is an international randomized controlled trial of 1200 patients with hip fractures that require a surgical intervention. This study is assessing accelerated medical clearance and accelerated surgical intervention as compared to the current standard of care and their impact on 30-day risk of major perioperative complications.

The two primary anesthetic modalities for hip fracture surgery are general anesthesia and regional anesthesia. In 2004, a Cochrane review showed an equivocal decrease in 1-month mortality and deep vein thrombosis incidence in patients with hip fractures who received regional anesthesia [54]. However, many subsequent studies have not shown any morbidity or mortality differences between these two anesthetic approaches [55–57]. While the lack of a mortality benefit has been shown to be reproducible, there is evidence of a modestly shorter hospital length of stay with regional anesthesia [58]. A recent study investigated the type of anesthesia that was chosen for total hip prosthesis, partial hip prosthesis, and proximal femoral nail placement. They determined that length of surgery is an important variable, and with a total hip replacement, a combined spinal-epidural (CSE) should be the anesthetic of choice given that there are no contraindications to regional anesthesia [59]. Elderly patients with more comorbidities were suggested to be less tolerant of general anesthesia [59]. MacDonald et al. showed that patients that underwent general anesthesia were in the operating room longer with a longer operative time when compared to patients who received a spinal [60]. A decrease in blood loss with spinal anesthesia compared to general anesthesia has also been demonstrated [58, 59]. Most recently, regional anesthesia has been shown to be superior in terms of quicker time to mobilization and decreased requirement for opioids [61].

48.5 Neurologic Injuries in Geriatric Trauma Patients

In 2013, according to the Centers for Disease Control and Prevention, traumatic brain injuries (TBI) contributed to approximately 2.8 million emergency department visits, including a rapid increase in those resulting from falls in older adults [62]. Traumatic brain injuries can lead to intracranial hematomas and can be stratified by initial Glasgow coma scale (GCS). Intracranial hematomas are seen in 24–45% of patients with a severe TBI (GCS 3–8) and 3–12% of patients with a moderate TBI (GCS 9–12) [63].

Two major types of intracranial hemorrhage are acute subdural hematoma and chronic subdural hematoma. Acute subdural hematomas occur most often from low-velocity mechanical falls in the elderly population. Diagnosis of this condition is based on imaging studies such as CT scan. Evans et al. investigated what radiological factors were most suggestive of the need for surgical intervention for an acute subdural hematoma. The strongest predictors were hematoma thickness greater than 10 mm and midline shift greater than 1 mm [64]. These two factors showed a 100% sensitivity and 83% specificity [64].

Surgical versus medical management of acute subdural hematomas remains a controversial topic. Herou et al. analyzed prognostic factors in elderly patients who were managed either medically or surgically after a closed TBI. They found that the highest risk of mortality was associated with lower levels of consciousness, high-energy trauma, one fixed and dilated pupil, and more extensive intracranial pathology [65]. Factors that were not found to be associated with a poor outcome included use of warfarin, advanced age, and degree of midline shift [65]. In contrast, a single-center observational study found that age and GCS scores were the most significant predictors of clinical outcome for patients with acute subdural hematomas that were managed surgically [66]. Patients over the age of 70 who had surgical management of their acute subdural hematoma tended to have worse outcomes [66]. In terms of medical management, Morris et al. found that patients with conservatively managed traumatic acute subdural hematomas were less likely to require eventual surgical hematoma evacuation when compared to those patients with nontraumatic acute subdural hematomas [67]. Notably, those patients that required hematoma evacuation following initial surgical management had higher mortality.

Chronic subdural hematomas are commonly found in the elderly with increased morbidity and mortality approaching that of hip fractures at the 1-year mark [68]. There has been a rise in the incidence of chronic subdural hematomas over the last decade that can be most likely attributed to increased imaging on the elderly after falls and the increased use of anticoagulants [68]. Surgical intervention on this patient population is based on deteriorating clinical presentation and decreased GCS score [69]. However, Stippler et al. found that there is no difference in the disposition of patients over 90 years old who receive either surgical or medical management of their chronic subdural hematoma [70]. Remarkably, only 24% of these patients return home, regardless of presenting GCS score [70].

Not surprisingly, the cost associated with neurocritical care and neurosurgery in the geriatric population is immense. Concurrently, prognosis has been shown to be poor in this population (and overall) after intracranial hemorrhage. Weimer et al. found that up to 50% of patients were either dead or moderately to severely disabled at 3 months after a subdural hematoma [71]. Older age was an independent risk factor for poor outcome. Further research needs to clarify how to care for these patients in the most judicious, safe, and cost-efficient manner.

48.6 Clinical Momentum

A full discussion of trauma in the geriatric population would be incomplete without mention of clinical momentum in the setting of futile and potentially unwanted intensive medical care. Clinical momentum is a recently recognized systems-level characteristic that is especially prevalent in the intensive care unit [72]. Similarly, it is easy to recognize in the management of geriatric trauma patients. As discussed, the literature is clear that overall outcomes for elderly patients after traumatic injury are poor. It is imperative that physicians explain this information frankly to patients and their families in the context of the patient's wishes in addition to their pre-existing frailty. A procedure generally begets another procedure in the management of traumatic injuries in the geriatric population; thus it is important to clarify goals of care early.

Conclusion

The incidence of traumatic injury in the geriatric population continues to rise at a rapid rate and presents a significant challenge to the healthcare system. There has been a shift from young, previously healthy trauma patients to patients that are older and frailer. While this shift would be expected to be associated with poorer outcomes, it is clear that a more tailored approach to the care of these patients will help ameliorate the currently unsettling outcome statistics. Modified ATLS trauma evaluations and the field of orthogeriatrics are two examples of improved approaches. In addition, there must be earlier recognition of potential clinical momentum and early candid discussions regarding likely outcomes and goals of care with patients and their families. Further research should focus on current and new tailored approaches to the care of geriatric trauma patients and their effects on outcomes.

Acknowledgement *Disclosure*: No.

References

1. Howden LM, Meyer JA. Age and sex composition: 2010. 2010 Census Briefs, US Department of Commerce, Economics and Statistics Administration. U.S. Census Bureau; 2010.
2. American College of Surgeons Committee on Trauma. National Trauma Data Bank 2010 Annual Report; 2010. p. 1–93.
3. American College of Surgeons Committee on Trauma. National Trauma Data Bank 2016 Annual Report; 2016. p. 1–147.
4. Bonne S, Schuerer DJ. Trauma in the older adult: epidemiology and evolving geriatric trauma principles. Clin Geriatr Med. 2013;29(1):137–50.
5. Hashmi A, Ibrahim-Zada I, Rhee P, Aziz H, Fain MJ, Friese RS, Joseph B. Predictors of mortality in geriatric trauma patients: a systematic review and meta-analysis. J Trauma Acute Care Surg. 2014;76(3):894–901.
6. Cook DJ, Rooke GA. Priorities in perioperative geriatrics. Anesth Analg. 2003;96(6):1823–36.
7. Inouye SK, Westendorp RG, Saczynski JS. Delirium in elderly people. Lancet. 2014;383(9920):911–22.
8. Yankner BA, Lu T, Loerch P. The aging brain. Annu Rev Pathol. 2008;3:41–66.
9. Lakatta EG. Arterial and cardiac aging: major shareholders in cardiovascular disease enterprises. Circulation. 2003;107(3):490–7.
10. Cheitlin MD. Cardiovascular physiology—changes with aging. Am J Geriatr Cardiol. 2003;12(1):9–13.
11. Lalley PM. The aging respiratory system—pulmonary structure, function and neural control. Respir Physiol Neurobiol. 2013;187(3):199–210.
12. Lindeman RD. Overview: renal physiology and pathophysiology of aging. Am J Kidney Dis. 1990;16(4):275–82.
13. Weinstein JR, Anderson S. The aging kidney: physiological changes. Adv Chronic Kidney Dis. 2010;17(4):302–7.
14. McLean AJ, Le Couteur DG. Aging biology and geriatric clinical pharmacology. Pharmacol Rev. 2004;56(2):163–84.
15. Vestal RE. Aging and pharmacology. Cancer. 1997;80(7):1302–10.
16. Hämmerlein A, Derendorf H, Lowenthal DT. Pharmacokinetic and pharmacodynamic changes in the elderly. Clin Pharmacokinet. 1998;35(1):49–64.
17. Grossman MD, Miller D, Scaff DW, Arcona S. When is an elder old? Effect of preexisting conditions on mortality in geriatric trauma. J Trauma Acute Care Surg. 2002;52(2):242–6.
18. Aitken LM, Burmeister E, Lang J, Chaboyer W, Richmond TS. Characteristics and outcomes of injured older adults after hospital admission. J Am Geriatr Soc. 2010;58(3):442–9.
19. Spaliviero M, Eastham JA. Relationship between surgical volume and patient outcomes. Trends Urol Men's Health. 2015;6(2):7–12.
20. Matsushima K, Schaefer EW, Won EJ, Armen SB, Indeck MC, Soybel DI. Positive and negative volume-outcome relationships in the geriatric trauma population. JAMA Surg. 2014;149(4):319–26.
21. Carpenter CR, Platts-Mills TF. Evolving prehospital, emergency department, and "inpatient" management models for geriatric emergencies. Clin Geriatr Med. 2013;29(1):31–47.
22. Moseley MG, Hawley MP, Caterino JM. Emergency department observation units and the older patient. Clin Geriatr Med. 2013;29(1):71–89.
23. Olufajo OA, Tulebaev S, Javedan H, Gates J, Wang J, Duarte M, Kelly E, Lilley E, Salim A, Cooper Z. Integrating geriatric consults into routine care of older trauma patients: one-year experience of a level I trauma center. J Am Coll Surg. 2016;222(6):1029–35.
24. Demetriades D, Sava J, Alo K, Newton E, Velmahos GC, Murray JA, Belzberg H, Asensio JA, Berne TV. Old age as a criterion for trauma team activation. J Trauma Acute Care Surg. 2001;51(4):754–7.
25. Calland JF, Ingraham AM, Martin N, Marshall GT, Schulman CI, Stapleton T, Barraco RD. Evaluation and management of geriatric trauma: an Eastern Association for the Surgery of Trauma practice management guideline. J Trauma Acute Care Surg. 2012;73(5):S345–50.
26. Werman HA, Erskine T, Caterino J, Riebe JF, Valasek T. Development of statewide geriatric patients trauma triage criteria. Prehosp Disaster Med. 2011;26(3):170–9.
27. Ichwan B, Darbha S, Shah MN, Thompson L, Evans DC, Boulger CT, Caterino JM. Geriatric-specific triage criteria are more sensitive than standard adult criteria in identifying need for trauma center care in injured older adults. Ann Emerg Med. 2015;65(1):92–100.
28. Hammer PM, Storey AC, Bell T, Bayt D, Hockaday MS, Zarzaur BL Jr, Feliciano DV, Rozycki GS. Improving geriatric trauma outcomes: a small step toward a big problem. J Trauma Acute Care Surg. 2016;81(1):162–7.

29. Kortbeek JB, Al Turki SA, Ali J, Antoine JA, Bouillon B, Brasel K, Brenneman F, Brink PR, Brohi K, Burris D, Burton RA. Advanced trauma life support, the evidence for change. J Trauma Acute Care Surg. 2008;64(6):1638–50.
30. Agarwal S, Azocar RJ. Trauma and the geriatric patient. In: Barnett SR, editor. Manual of geriatric anesthesia. New York: Springer; 2013. p. 193–200.
31. Deiner S, Silverstein JH, Abrams KJ. Management of trauma in the geriatric patient. Curr Opin Anesthesiol. 2004;17(2):165–70.
32. Aschkenasy MT, Rothenhaus TC. Trauma and falls in the elderly. Emerg Med Clin. 2006;24(2):413–32.
33. Vana PG, Mayberry J, Luchette FA. Management and complications of rib fractures in older adults. Curr Geriatr Rep. 2016;5(1):25–30.
34. Gillies D. Elderly trauma: they are different. Aust Crit Care. 1999;12(1):24–30.
35. Pudelek B. Geriatric trauma: special needs for a special population. AACN Adv Crit Care. 2002;13(1):61–72.
36. Desai NR, Krumme AA, Schneeweiss S, Shrank WH, Brill G, Pezalla EJ, Spettell CM, Brennan TA, Matlin OS, Avorn J, Choudhry NK. Patterns of initiation of oral anticoagulants in patients with atrial fibrillation—quality and cost implications. Am J Med. 2014;127(11):1075–82.
37. Marano G, Vaglio S, Pupella S, Liumbruno GM, Franchini M. How we treat bleeding associated with direct oral anticoagulants. Blood Transfus. 2016;14(5):465.
38. Hoffman M, Monroe DM. Reversing targeted oral anticoagulants. ASH Educ Program Book. 2014;2014(1):518–23.
39. Joyce MF, Gupta A, Azocar RJ. Acute trauma and multiple injuries in the elderly population. Curr Opin Anaesthesiol. 2015;28(2):145–50.
40. Joseph B, Pandit V, Sadoun M, Zangbar B, Fain MJ, Friese RS, Rhee P. Frailty in surgery. J Trauma Acute Care Surg. 2014;76(4):1151–6.
41. Kim SW, Han HS, Jung HW, Kim KI, Hwang DW, Kang SB, Kim CH. Multidimensional frailty score for the prediction of postoperative mortality risk. JAMA Surg. 2014;149(7):633–40.
42. Theou O, Brothers TD, Mitnitski A, Rockwood K. Operationalization of frailty using eight commonly used scales and comparison of their ability to predict all-cause mortality. J Am Geriatr Soc. 2013;61(9):1537–51.
43. Joseph B, Pandit V, Rhee P, Aziz H, Sadoun M, Wynne J, Tang A, Kulvatunyou N, O'Keeffe T, Fain MJ, Friese RS. Predicting hospital discharge disposition in geriatric trauma patients: is frailty the answer? J Trauma Acute Care Surg. 2014;76(1):196–200.
44. Joseph B, Pandit V, Zangbar B, Kulvatunyou N, Hashmi A, Green DJ, O'Keeffe T, Tang A, Vercruysse G, Fain MJ, Friese RS. Superiority of frailty over age in predicting outcomes among geriatric trauma patients: a prospective analysis. JAMA Surg. 2014;149(8):766–72.
45. Joseph B, Pandit V, Zangbar B, Kulvatunyou N, Tang A, O'Keeffe T, Green DJ, Vercruysse G, Fain MJ, Friese RS, Rhee P. Validating trauma-specific frailty index for geriatric trauma patients: a prospective analysis. J Am Coll Surg. 2014;219(1):10–7.
46. Katsoulis M, Benetou V, Karapetyan T, Feskanich D, Grodstein F, Pettersson-Kymmer U, Eriksson S, Wilsgaard T, Jørgensen L, Ahmed LA, Schöttker B. Excess mortality after hip fracture in elderly persons from Europe and the USA: the CHANCES project. J Intern Med. 2017;281(3):300–10.
47. Tarazona-Santabalbina FJ, Belenguer-Varea Á, Rovira E, Cuesta-Peredó D. Orthogeriatric care: improving patient outcomes. Clin Interv Aging. 2016;11:843.
48. Folbert EC, Hegeman JH, Gierveld R, van Netten JJ, Van Der Velde D, Ten Duis HJ, Slaets JP. Complications during hospitalization and risk factors in elderly patients with hip fracture following integrated orthogeriatric treatment. Arch Orthop Trauma Surg. 2017;137(4):507–15.
49. Folbert EC, Hegeman JH, Vermeer M, Regtuijt EM, van der Velde D, Ten Duis HJ, Slaets JP. Improved 1-year mortality in elderly patients with a hip fracture following integrated orthogeriatric treatment. Osteoporos Int. 2017;28(1):269–77.
50. Tan ST, Tan WP, Jaipaul J, Chan SP, Sathappan SS. Clinical outcomes and hospital length of stay in 2,756 elderly patients with hip fractures: a comparison of surgical and non-surgical management. Singap Med J. 2017;58(5):253.
51. Ricci WM, Brandt A, McAndrew C, Gardner MJ. Factors effecting delay to surgery and length of stay for hip fracture patients. J Orthop Trauma. 2015;29(3):e109.
52. Moja L, Piatti A, Pecoraro V, Ricci C, Virgili G, Salanti G, Germagnoli L, Liberati A, Banfi G. Timing matters in hip fracture surgery: patients operated within 48 hours have better outcomes. A meta-analysis and meta-regression of over 190,000 patients. PLoS One. 2012;7(10):e46175.
53. Choi HJ, Kim E, Shin YJ, Choi BY, Kim YH, Lim TH. The timing of surgery and mortality in elderly hip fractures: a retrospective, multicenteric cohort study. Indian J Orthop. 2014;48(6):599.
54. Parker MJ, Handoll HH, Griffiths R. Anaesthesia for hip fracture surgery in adults. Cochrane Database Syst Rev. 2004;4(4):CD000521.
55. Davis FM, Woolner DF, Frampton C, Wilkinson A, Grant A, Harrison RT, Roberts MT, Thadaka R. Prospective, multi-centre trial of mortality following general or spinal anaesthesia for hip fracture surgery in the elderly. Br J Anaesth. 1987;59(9):1080–8.
56. Brox WT, Chan PH, Cafri G, Inacio MC. Similar mortality with general or regional anesthesia in elderly hip fracture patients. Acta Orthop. 2016;87(2):152–7.
57. Zuo D, Jin C, Shan M, Zhou L, Li Y. A comparison of general versus regional anesthesia for hip fracture surgery: a meta-analysis. Int J Clin Exp Med. 2015;8(11):20295.
58. Neuman MD, Rosenbaum PR, Ludwig JM, Zubizarreta JR, Silber JH. Anesthesia technique, mortality, and length of stay after hip fracture surgery. JAMA. 2014;311(24):2508–17.
59. Esenyel AE, Esenyel CZ, Ervatan Z, Yakar N, Cakirgoz M, Kalkar I, Seyran M. Comparison of anesthetic administration according to method of hip surgery. Eur J Med. 2017;49(1):26.
60. MacDonald SJ, Somerville L, Howard J, Naudie DD, McAuley J, McCalden R, Bourne R. Spinal vs general anesthesia in THA: an analysis using prospectively collected clinical patient data. Orthop Proc. 2012;94(Suppl XXXVIII):115.
61. Greimel F, Maderbacher G, Zeman F, Grifka J, Meissner W, Benditz A. No clinical difference comparing general, regional and combination anesthesia in hip arthroplasty: a multicenter cohort-study regarding perioperative pain management and patient satisfaction. J Arthroplast. 2017;32(11):3429–33.
62. Taylor CA. Traumatic brain injury–related emergency department visits, hospitalizations, and deaths—United States, 2007 and 2013. MMWR Surveill Summ. 2017;66(9):1–16.
63. Thurman D, Guerrero J. Trends in hospitalization associated with traumatic brain injury. JAMA. 1999;282(10):954–7.
64. Evans JA, Bailey M, Vail A, Tyrrell PJ, Parry-Jones AR, Patel HC. A simple tool to identify elderly patients with a surgically important acute subdural haematoma. Injury. 2015;46(1):76–9.

65. Herou E, Romner B, Tomasevic G. Acute traumatic brain injury: mortality in the elderly. World Neurosurg. 2015;83(6):996–1001.
66. Benedetto N, Gambacciani C, Montemurro N, Morganti R, Perrini P. Surgical management of acute subdural haematomas in elderly: report of a single center experience. Br J Neurosurg. 2017;31(2):244–8.
67. Morris NA, Merkler AE, Parker WE, Claassen J, Connolly ES, Sheth KN, Kamel H. Adverse outcomes after initial non-surgical management of subdural hematoma: a population-based study. Neurocrit Care. 2016;24(2):226–32.
68. Adhiyaman V, Asghar M, Ganeshram KN, Bhowmick BK. Chronic subdural haematoma in the elderly. Postgrad Med J. 2002;78(916):71–5.
69. Shapey J, Glancz LJ, Brennan PM. Chronic subdural haematoma in the elderly: is it time for a new paradigm in management? Curr Geriatr Rep. 2016;5(2):71–7.
70. Stippler M, Ramirez P, Berti A, MacIndoe C, Villalobos N, Murray-Krezan C. Chronic subdural hematoma patients aged 90 years and older. Neurol Res. 2013;35(3):243–6.
71. Weimer JM, Gordon E, Frontera JA. Predictors of functional outcome after subdural hematoma: a prospective study. Neurocrit Care. 2017;26(1):70–9.
72. Kruser JM, Cox CE, Schwarze ML. Clinical Momentum in the Intensive Care Unit. A Latent Contributor to Unwanted Care. Ann Am Thorac Soc. 2017;14(3):426–31.

Acute Compartment Syndrome

49

Fabio Ferla, Arianna Ciravegna, Anna Mariani, Vincenzo Buscemi, Riccardo De Carlis, and Paolo Aseni

Key Points

- Compartment syndrome is defined as an elevation of the interstitial pressure in a closed osseo-fascial compartment that results in microvascular compromise.
- High suspicion is mandatory when risk factors are present: missing the diagnosis could be lethal.
- In the case of abdominal compartment syndrome, bladder pressure measurement is considered the diagnostic gold standard.
- In the case of acute compartment syndrome of extremities, clinical exam is sufficient to make the diagnosis.
- Surgical decompression is the main treatment for acute compartment syndrome (both abdominal and of the extremities).
- Compartment syndrome could happen in every compartment of the body.

49.1 Introduction

The first report of a syndrome that could be called "compartmental" is by Dr. Richard von Volkmann in 1881 [1]. The Volkmann's syndrome occurred after the application of splints or bandages to the upper extremity and was characterized by an initial paralysis and a subsequent flexion contracture of the hand and forearm. Volkmann believed the syndrome was the result of an ischemic process due to impaired arterial perfusion leading to muscle cell death.

In the early twentieth century, Jepsen reproduced the observations by Volkmann on animal models: he showed that limb fractures acted like splints or bandages rising compartment (defined as a closed space surrounded by muscular aponeurosis) pressure. When the compartment pressure reached the perfusion pressure, blood flow stopped, tissue death occurred, and the syndrome appeared [2].

With time, authors described many syndromes sharing the pathogenesis reported by Jepsen, and nowadays, thanks to Matsen [3], any disorder characterized by "an elevation of the interstitial pressure in a closed osseo-fascial compartment that results in microvascular compromise" is classified as compartmental.

In the present chapter, we aim to face syndromes that may be faced by emergency surgeons: the abdominal compartment syndrome and the acute compartment syndrome of the limbs.

49.2 Abdominal Compartment Syndrome

49.2.1 Definition

The abdominal compartment syndrome is defined according to the Cartagena 2013 WCACS (World Congress of the Abdominal Compartment Society) [4] reported in Table 49.1. Specifically, ACS (abdominal compartment

F. Ferla (✉) · A. Mariani
Department of General Surgery and Transplantation, ASST Grande Ospedale Metropolitano, Niguarda Ca' Granda Hospital, Milan, Italy

A. Ciravegna
Department of General Surgery and Transplantation, ASST Grande Ospedale Metropolitano, Niguarda Ca' Granda Hospital, Milan, Italy

Department of Surgery, University of Milano-Bicocca, San Gerardo Hospital, Monza, Italy

V. Buscemi · R. De Carlis
Department of General Surgery and Transplantation, ASST Grande Ospedale Metropolitano, Niguarda Ca' Granda Hospital, Milan, Italy

Department of Surgical Sciences, University of Pavia, Pavia, Italy

P. Aseni
Dipartimento di Emergenza Urgenza, ASST Grande Ospedale Metropolitano Niguarda, Milan, Italy

P. Aseni et al. (eds.), *Operative Techniques and Recent Advances in Acute Care and Emergency Surgery*, https://doi.org/10.1007/978-3-319-95114-0_49

Table 49.1 Abdominal compartment syndrome definitions according to the Cartagena WCACS 2013

Definition 1	IAP is the steady-state pressure concealed within the abdominal cavity
Definition 2	The reference standard for intermittent IAP measurements is via the bladder with a maximal instillation volume of 25 mL of sterile saline
Definition 3	IAP should be expressed in mmHg and measured at endexpiration in the supine position after ensuring that abdominal muscle contractions are absent and with the transducer zeroed at the level of the midaxillary line
Definition 4	IAP is approximately 5–7 mmHg in critically ill adults
Definition 5	IAH is defined by a sustained or repeated pathological elevation in IAP C 12 mmHg
Definition 6	ACS is defined as a sustained IAP > 20 mmHg (with or without an APP < 60 mmHg) that is associated with new organ dysfunction/failure
Definition 7	IAH is graded as follows: Grade I IAP 12–15 mmHg; Grade II IAP 16–20 mmHg; Grade III IAP 21–25 mmHg; Grade IV IAP > 25 mmHg
Definition 8	Primary IAH or ACS is a condition associated with injury or disease in the abdominopelvic region that frequently requires early surgical or interventional radiological intervention
Definition 9	Secondary IAH or ACS refers to conditions that do not originate from the abdominopelvic region
Definition 10	Recurrent IAH or ACS refers to the condition in which IAH or ACS redevelops following previous surgical or medical treatment of primary or secondary IAH or ACS
Definition 11	APP = MAP – IAP
Definition 12	A polycompartment syndrome is a condition where two or more anatomical compartments have elevated compartmental pressures
Definition 13	Abdominal compliance is a measure of the ease of abdominal expansion, which is determined by the elasticity of the abdominal wall and diaphragm. It should be expressed as the change in intra-abdominal volume per change in IAP
Definition 14	The open abdomen is one that requires a temporary abdominal closure due to the skin and fascia not being closed after laparotomy
Definition 15	Lateralization of the abdominal wall is the phenomenon where the musculature and fascia of the abdominal wall, most exemplified by the rectus abdominus muscles and their enveloping fascia, move laterally away from the midline with time

ACS abdominal compartment syndrome, *APP* abdominal perfusion pressure, *IAH* intra-abdominal hypertension, *IAP* intra-abdominal pressure, *MAP* mean arterial pressure

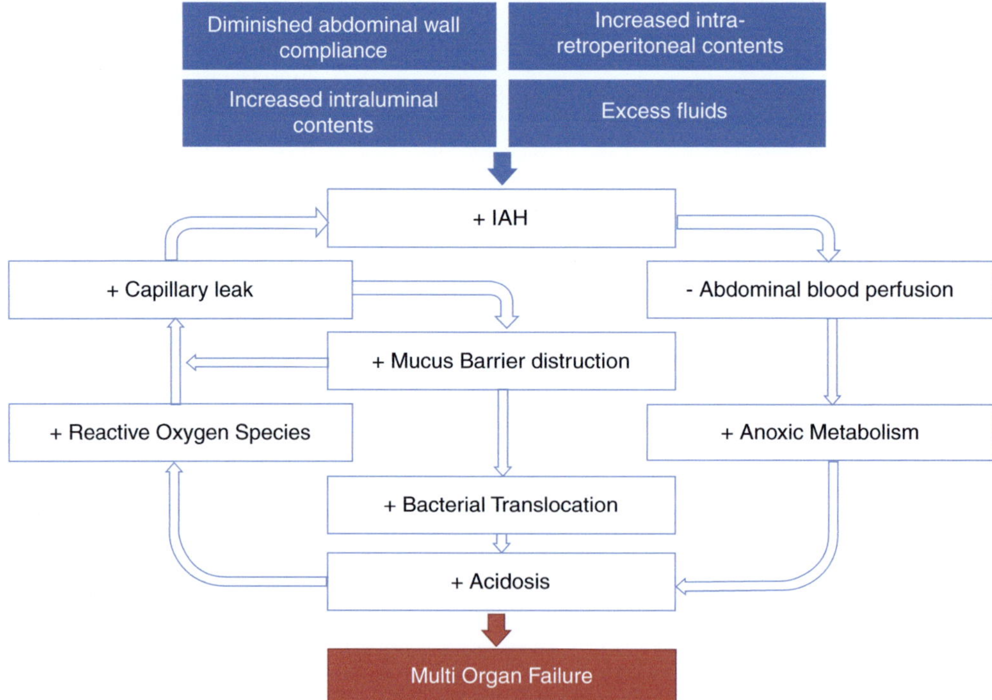

Fig. 49.1 Pathophysiology of the abdominal compartment syndrome

syndrome) is defined as a sustained IAP (intra-abdominal pressure) >20 mmHg (with or without an abdominal perfusion pressure (APP) <60 mmHg) that is associated with new organ dysfunction/failure. Figure 49.1 summarizes the pathophysiology of the abdominal compartment syndrome.

49.2.2 Common Etiology and Risk Factors

On a general basis, IAH (intra-abdominal hypertension) and ACS develop if one of four main conditions occurs abruptly: (1) diminished abdominal wall compliance, (2) increased intraluminal contents, (3) increased intra-retroperitoneal

Table 49.2 Abdominal compartment syndrome risk factors according to the Cartagena WCACS 2013

Diminished abdominal wall compliance	*Increased intra-luminal contents*	*Others/miscellaneous*
Abdominal surgery	Gastroparesis/gastric distention/ileus	Age
Major trauma	Ileus	Bacteremia
Major burns	Colonic pseudo-obstruction	Coagulopathy
Prone positioning	Volvulus	Increased head of bed angle
		Massive incisional hernia repair
Increased intra-abdominal contents	*Capillary leak/fluid resuscitation*	Mechanical ventilation
Acute pancreatitis	Acidosis	Obesity or increased body mass index
Distended abdomen	Damage control laparotomy	PEEP
Hemoperitoneum/pneumoperitoneum or intra-peritoneal fluid collections	Hypothermia	Peritonitis
Intra-abdominal infection/abscess	Increased APACHE-II or SOFA score	Pneumonia
Intra-abdominal or retroperitoneal tumors	Massive fluid resuscitation or positive fluid balance	Sepsis
Laparoscopy with excessive insufflation pressures	Polytransfusion	Shock or hypotension
Liver dysfunction/cirrhosis with ascites		
Peritoneal dialysis		

contents, and (4) capillary leak and/or massive fluid/blood infusion.

Diminished abdominal wall compliance is typical in obese patients undergoing massive ventral hernia repair and in burned patients with skin retraction. Increased intraluminal contents occur in bowel obstruction and pseudo-obstruction. Increased intra-retroperitoneal contents typically happen when hemoperitoneum, retro-hemoperitoneum (typically caused by aorta aneurysm rupture), and intra- or extraperitoneal packing are present. Capillary leak and/or massive fluid/blood infusion can happen when shock gut is present or when more than 5 L of crystalloids or more than ten packed red blood cells units are administered in less than 24 h.

The complete list of risk factors for ACS developed by the WCACS 2013 [4] is reported in Table 49.2.

49.2.3 Diagnosis

To make the diagnosis of ACS, a high index of suspicion is necessary: in patients presenting one or more risk factors, IAP should be assessed at least every 8 h.

Clinical exam alone has a poor diagnostic power [5, 6], and the bladder pressure measurement is considered the diagnostic gold standard by many authors. The measurement should be performed with the patient in a supine position: after complete voiding of the bladder, 50–100 mL of saline solution should be instilled through the catheter to fill it partially. The goal is to have the bladder not collapsed or distended (and contracting) either. The column of liquid in the catheter should be connected with a transducer previously zeroed at the level of the pubic symphysis: the revealed pressure is a close approximation of the IAP.

49.2.4 Effects of IAH on Individual Systems

Respiratory system: Increasing IAP determines progressive diaphragm elevation; this results in decreased chest and lung compliance, reduced tidal volumes, and increased airway pressure. In these settings, the pulmonary function could be impaired, and the patient could suffer from hypercapnia (determining acidosis) and hypoxia and could develop respiratory failure.

Cardiovascular system: On one hand, blood return from inferior vena cava diminishes if IAP increases; on the other, elevated intrathoracic pressure and augmented intra-abdominal resistances increase the cardiac post-load; the result is a reduction in stroke volume. The heart compensates increasing its rate at first, but eventual dropping in cardiac output is likely. The concomitant hypercapnia and the subsequent acidosis could aggravate the cardiac failure by inhibiting the whole cardiovascular system.

In these settings, CVP and pulmonary artery wedge pressure are elevated and don't reflect the intravascular volume status anymore.

Renal system: IAH affects renal system by a mechanism which is not completely clear: probably multiple events occur resulting in glomerular filtration rate (GFR) reduction. IAH seems to reduce blood flow in renal veins; the resulting renal congestion seems to be responsible for renal edema, increased intracapsular pressure, and increased microcirculation resistance; these conditions justify the decrease in urinary output that could progress from oliguria to anuria and eventual kidney failure. Interestingly increased pressure on ureters doesn't seem to affect the renal function: ureteral stenting, while IAP is rising, doesn't impact on renal impairment.

Gastrointestinal system: As well as for kidneys, IAH results in gastrointestinal blood stream slowing down.

Low mesenteric flow could be demonstrated by gastric pH and tonometry variation. A recent study on laparoscopy showed that 15 mmHg intra-abdominal pressure is sufficient to reduce gut perfusion of 11–54%; that is why untreated ACS could easily lead to bowel ischemia and eventual death. In this setting, liver could suffer too: reduced portal flow from the gastrointestinal tract seems to be the main reason for liver impairment; no secure demonstration of this phenomenon has been made in animal or human model though.

CNS: IAH can cause a marked increase in intracranial pressure.

49.2.5 Treatment

Facing the rise of IAP could be challenging: the first goal of the treatment is to identify and correct any possible cause of ACS; this goal could be achieved by "non-operative management" and "surgical intervention.

Non-operative management pivots on four main elements [7]:

1. Decrease intraluminal gastrointestinal contents. The use of nasogastric/rectal tube or the use of gastro/colon prokinetic agents could be very helpful in these settings. Minimization of enteral nutrition and colonscopic decompression could be necessary as well.
2. Evacuation of the intra-abdominal space-occupying lesions. This goal could be achieved by percutaneous drainage of intra-abdominal collections.
3. Improve abdominal wall compliance. To achieve this goal, it is necessary to ensure adequate analgesia and sedation, to remove constrictive dressings and abdominal eschars, to avoid prone position (paying attention to maintain the head of bed >20°), and to consider neuromuscular blockade.
4. Optimize fluid management and perfusion. To achieve this goal, it is necessary to avoid excessive fluid administration aiming for negative balance, to use hypertonic fluids and colloids and to increase diuresis, to consider hemodialysis/ultrafiltration, and to maintain APP > 60 mmHg (with vasoactive medications when needed).

When non-operative management fails, IAH should be addressed by surgical intervention.

Common indications for surgery are:

1. IAP > 35 mmHg in repeated measurements
2. IAP 25–35 mmHg and progressive organ failure
3. Renal and pulmonary dysfunction
4. APP < 50 mmHg

Many techniques have been described to decompress the abdomen [8]; every technique has its own advantages and disadvantages as listed below. If IAH is following previous abdominal surgery, choosing the same incision is generally the best option.

1. Laparostomy: could be performed by midline incision (Fig. 49.2) (it is relatively safe, easy to perform, and nearly always effective; entero-atmospheric fistulas and high risk of persistent open abdomen are the main disadvantages) or by transverse subcostal incision (Fig. 49.3) (it is effective and has a higher rate of fascial closure; the major disadvantages are it is more time-consuming, and if fascial closure can't be achieved, complex reconstructions with loss of abdominal muscle function are nearly always unavoidable).

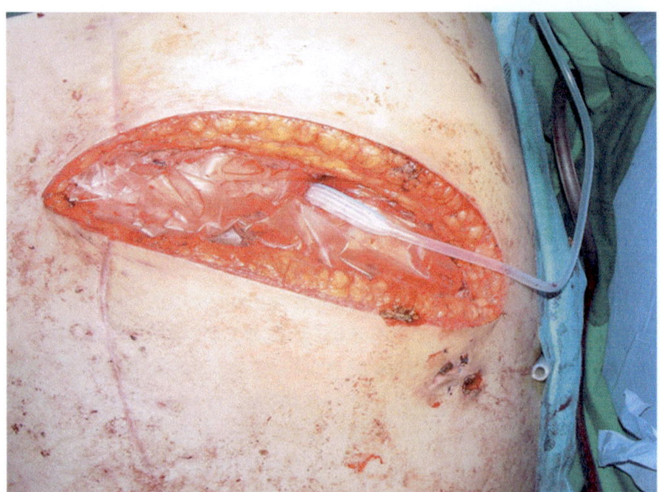

Fig. 49.2 Midline incision

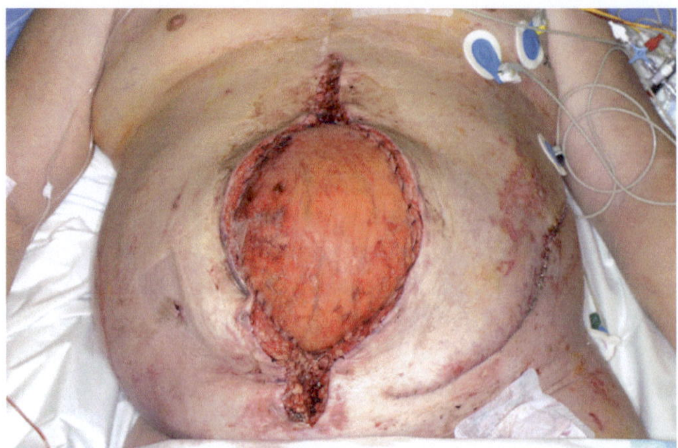

Fig. 49.3 Transverse subcostal incision

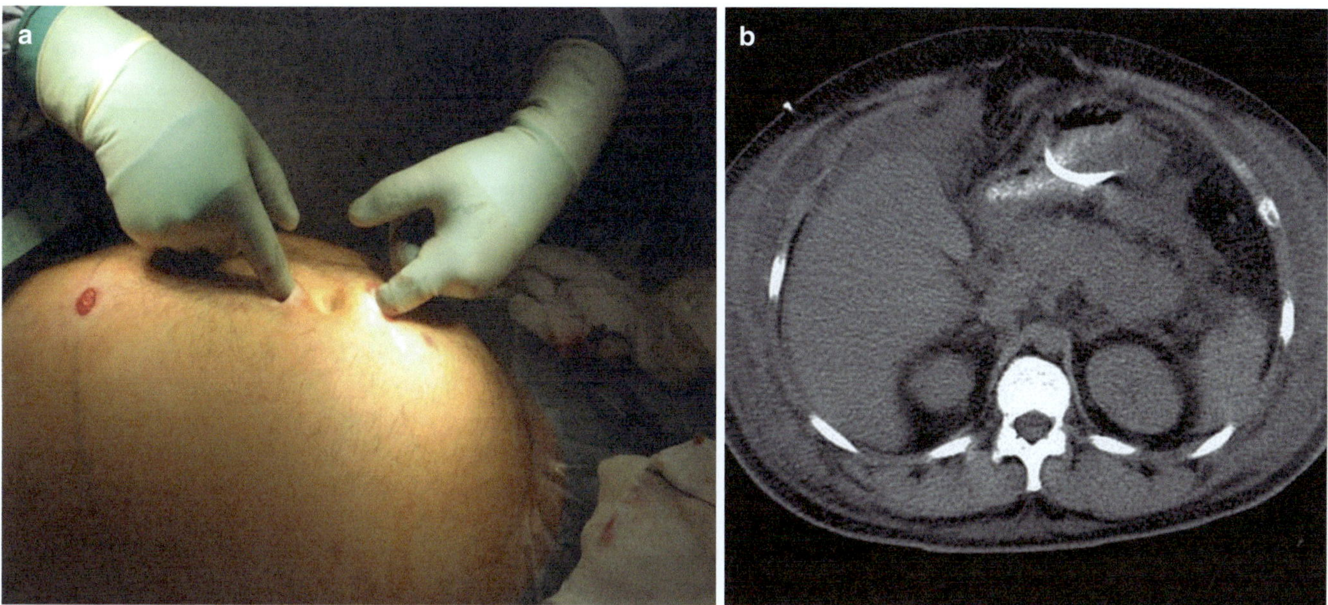

Fig. 49.4 Subcutaneous linea alba fasciotomy: performing the procedure (**a**), CT scan after the procedure (**b**)

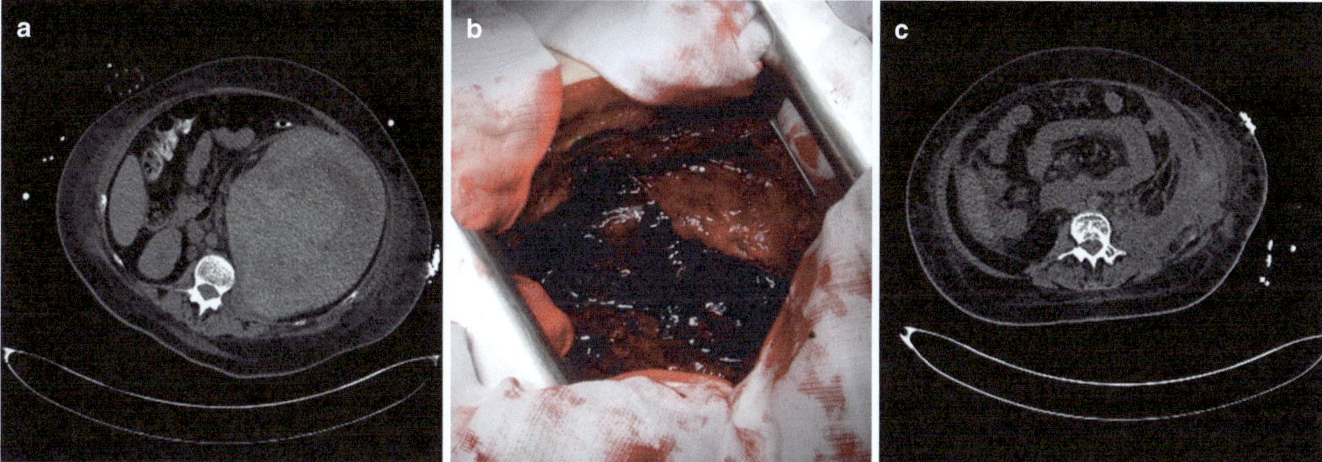

Fig. 49.5 Extraperitoneal posterior decompression: huge extraperitoneal hematoma at the CT scan (**a**); the surgical field (**b**); CT scan after decompression (**c**)

2. Subcutaneous linea alba fasciotomy (SLAF) (Fig. 49.4): through two or three short horizontal skin incisions, subcutaneous anterior abdominal fasciotomy at the linea alba is performed. The peritoneum is left intact. SLAF is effective in about 50–70%; it prevents open abdomen and its related complications, but it is always associated with a subsequent hernia. The cost-effectiveness (due to the lesser need of nursing care) is an advantage.
3. Extraperitoneal posterior decompression (Fig. 49.5): it is performed to evacuate a retroperitoneum mass (generally a hematoma) compressing the abdomen. It is effective and prevents open abdomen. The main disadvantage is it can be performed only if an extraperitoneal mass is causing IAH.

Independently from the chosen technical approach, the surgery could result in three physiological changes:

1. A sudden drop in systemic vascular resistance
2. A fall in intrathoracic pressure
3. A washout of toxic products (lactic acid and potassium)

These changes could lead to the potentially dangerous "abdominal decompression syndrome." This syndrome is characterized by arrhythmias, myocardial depression, hypotension, and possibly barotrauma/volutrauma (due to the administration of a suddenly inadequate tidal volume).

To avoid this syndrome, a careful anesthesiologic conduct and effective communication between surgeon and anesthetist are mandatory during every phase of the decompressive operation.

49.3 Acute Compartment Syndrome of the Limbs

49.3.1 Definition

With the understanding of the pathophysiology underneath the Volkmann's syndrome, the definition of acute compartment syndrome (ACS) evolved, and the two classical signs (paralysis and a subsequent flexion contracture of the hand and forearm) have been replaced by the presence of a compartment pressure equal or bigger than the blood perfusion pressure.

49.3.2 Common Etiology and Risk Factors

The most common cause of ACS is trauma of the limbs. In a Scottish study on 164 patients presenting ACS, they found that 69% of them had fractures (being diaphyseal tibial fractures the most frequent (36%) followed by fractures of the distal radius (9.8%)) [9].

In the absence of fracture, older age, vascular injuries, and ischemia/reperfusion episodes are at higher risk for acute compartment syndrome development.

Elderly individuals found lying down on the ground with several hours of immobility should raise suspicion for compartment syndrome: the low blood flow determined by the prolonged contact with a hard surface could lead to swelling of a limb and trigger the pathological process. Similarly, vascular injuries and ischemia/reperfusion episodes trigger ACS in about 50% of the cases [10], and high suspicion is mandatory [11].

49.3.3 Diagnosis

The diagnosis of acute compartment syndrome of the limb is based on physical exam. The hallmark symptoms of the syndrome are the 6 P's: pain with passive stretch, pulselessness, pallor, poikilothermia, paresthesias, and paralysis.

Extreme pain (more than expected) seems to be the most reliable symptoms in early stages of ACS and should raise suspicion. Comparison with a contralateral limb is important too: extremities with impending or active compartment syndrome are often swollen and shiny compared to the uninjured extremity.

The instrumental diagnosis of acute compartment syndrome of the limb is not mandatory but could be achieved by needle manometer (using an 18-g straight needle, side-port needle, slit catheter, or wick catheter). The measurement should be taken with the patient in a supine position; the measured extremity should be at the heart level; the needle should be placed perpendicular to muscle belly, near to the fracture site or the area of maximum tension. Needle measurement is contraindicated when underlying neurovascular structures are at risk; the patient suffers from coagulopathy or local diffuse cellulitis.

In a paper from 1979 [12], Hargens showed that intracompartmental pressures of 120 mmHg could lead to complete nerve blockage in less than 2 h; pressures around 30–40 mmHg could determine partial nerve blockage in 6–8 h; pressures lower than 20 mmHg didn't determine nerve conduction impairment in any conditions. On the basis of these observations, the authors suggested that 30 mmHg should be considered the critical compartment pressure to start the treatment.

49.3.4 Treatment

Treatment for acute compartment syndrome starts with removal of any cast, splint, or bandage from the affected limb. Then fasciotomies should be performed to decompress any compartment affected by the syndrome. Table 49.3 shows the compartments of the upper limb and Table 49.4 the compartments of the lower limb.

Table 49.3 Compartments of the upper limb

Region	Compartments	
Arm	Anterior	
	Posterior	
	Deltoid[a]	
Forearm	Volar	Superficial deep
	Dorsal	Mobile wad
	Hand	Extensor anconeus
Hypothenar	Thenar	
	Adductor pollicis	
	Dorsal interossei	
	Volar interossei	
	Finger (x5)	

[a]Deltoid doesn't lie in a real compartment, but its fascia is thick and may need decompression

Table 49.4 Compartments of the lower limb

Region	Compartments	
Thight	Anterior	
	Medial	
	Posterior	
Leg	Anterior	
	Lateral	
	Poterior	Superficial Deep
Foot	Medial	
	Lateral	
	Interosseus (×4)	
	Central	Superficial Central Deep

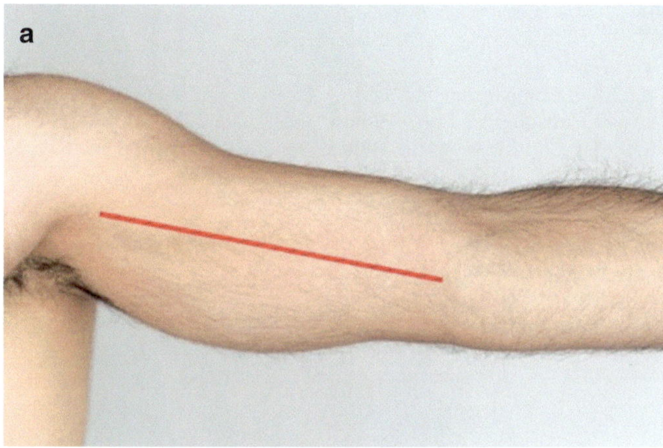

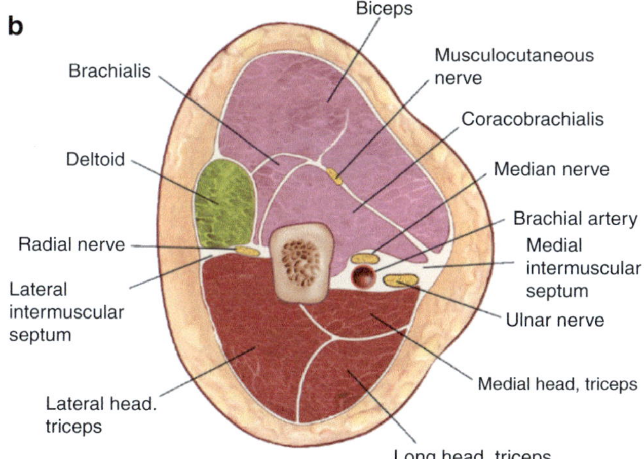

Fig. 49.6 Arm decompression. The anterior and posterior compartments could be decompressed by a single median incision (**a**). Compartments of the arm (**b**): in red the posterior compartment, in purple the anterior compartment, in green the deltoid compartment. With permission of Springer Nature; from Patel K., Major N. (2009) Compartmental Anatomy. In: Davies A., Sundaram M., James S. (eds) Imaging of Bone Tumors and Tumor-Like Lesions. Medical Radiology. Springer, Berlin, Heidelberg

The anterior and posterior compartments of the arm can be decompressed by a single median incision (Fig. 49.6). Once the fascia and the lateral intermuscular septum are identified, two longitudinal incisions in the fascia overlying the anterior and posterior compartments are made.

The forearm can be decompressed by two incisions as shown in Fig. 49.7. On the volar aspect of the forearm, the incision is curvilinear, starts at the antecubital fossa, and goes down toward the mid-palm. If necessary, the incision is carried further distally to release the carpal tunnel as well. The second incision decompresses the dorsal compartment: it starts from the lateral epicondyle, goes straight down at the center of the forearm, and ends at the center of the wrist.

Hand compartment decompression lines are shown in Fig. 49.8.

Decompressing the anterior and posterior compartments by a single incision is sufficient most of the time since the medial compartment is rarely affected by the ACS. The incision is shown in Fig. 49.9. Once the fascia lata is opened, the anterior compartment is decompressed. Dissection and elevation of the vastus lateralis give access to the intermuscular septum. The incision of this septum decompresses the posterior compartment.

Leg decompression can be obtained by two different techniques. The first is based on a single incision: it is made directly over the fibula; the anterior and lateral compartments are accessed elevating a skin flap anteriorly; and the superficial and deep posterior compartments are accessed by elevating a posterior flap.

The second technique is based on two incisions (Fig. 49.10). The medial incision is 3 cm posterior to the tibia and allows access to the superficial and deep posterior compartments. The lateral incision is centered between the tibial crest and fibular shaft and allows access to the anterior and lateral compartments. Care should be taken while making this access to preserve the superficial peroneal nerve.

The decompression of the foot is controversial since the burden of long-term procedure complications could overcome the attended benefit from the surgery. The procedure is performed through two dorsal incisions and a single medial incision. The dorsal incisions are made over the second and fourth metatarsals allowing for decompression of the interosseous, central, medial, and lateral compartments. The third incision is made on the medial aspect of the foot, inferior to the first metatarsal allowing better decompression of the central compartment.

A delay in treating an acute compartment syndrome could be dramatic and lead to permanent disability, amputation, or even death [3]. That is why prompt recognition and treatment (possibly within 6 h) of the ACS should be considered a priority.

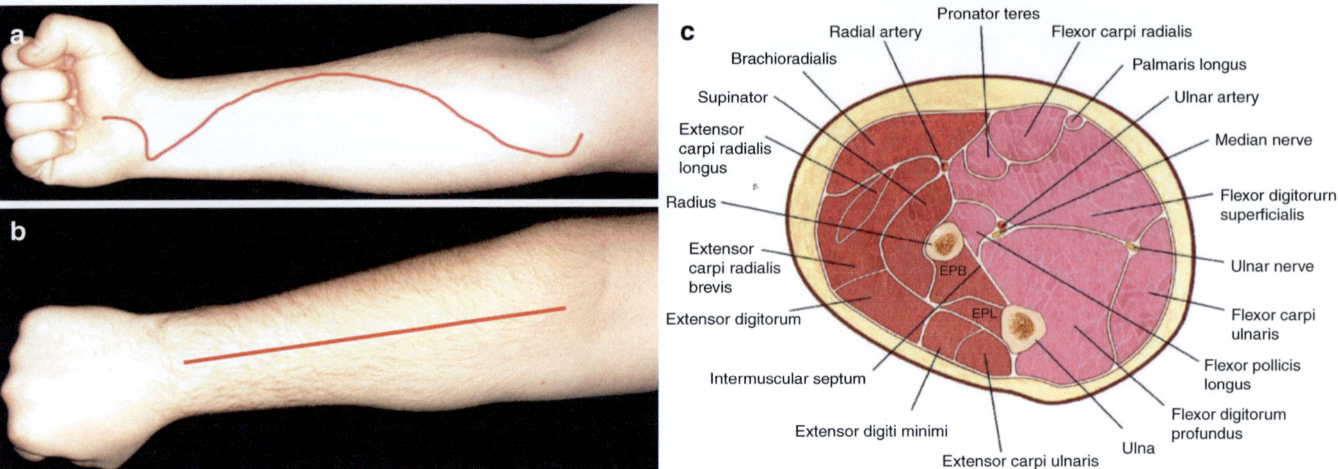

Fig. 49.7 Forearm decompression: volar incision (**a**), dorsal incision (**b**), compartments (**c**): in purple the volar compartment, in red the dorsal compartment. With permission of Springer Nature; from Patel K., Major N. (2009) Compartmental Anatomy. In: Davies A., Sundaram M., James S. (eds) Imaging of Bone Tumors and Tumor-Like Lesions. Medical Radiology. Springer, Berlin, Heidelberg

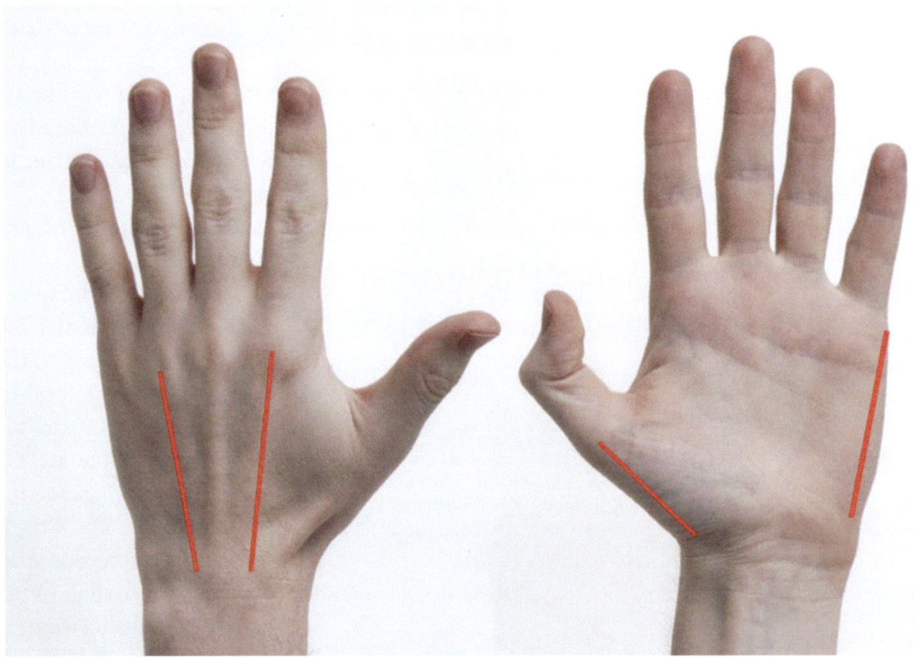

Fig. 49.8 Incision lines to decompress the hand compartments

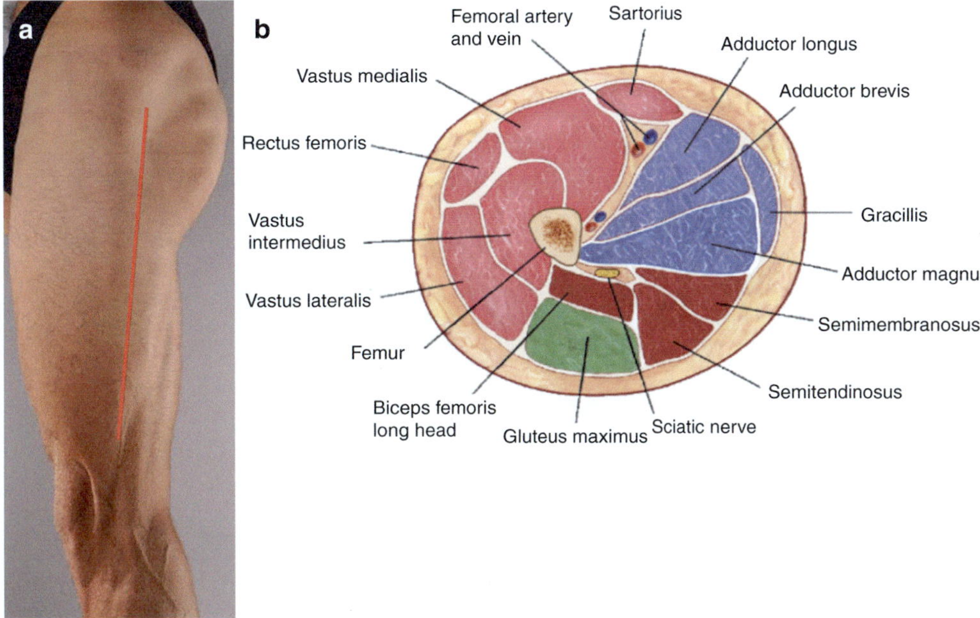

Fig. 49.9 Tight incision line (**a**); tight compartments (**b**): in purple the anterior compartment, in blue the medial compartment, in red the posterior compartment. With permission of Springer Nature; from Patel K., Major N. (2009) Compartmental Anatomy. In: Davies A., Sundaram M., James S. (eds) Imaging of Bone Tumors and Tumor-Like Lesions. Medical Radiology. Springer, Berlin, Heidelberg

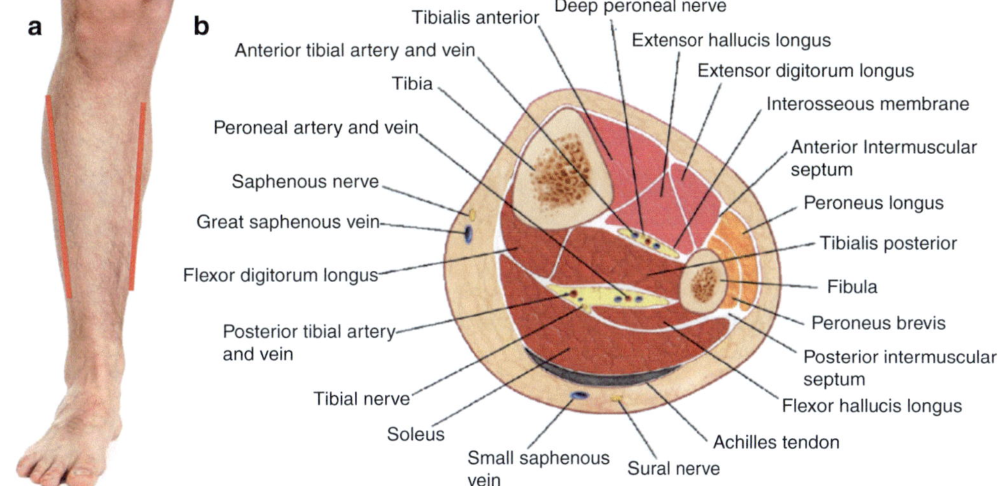

Fig. 49.10 Leg incision lines (**a**); leg compartments (**b**): in purple the anterior compartment, in orange the lateral compartment, in red the posterior compartment. With permission of Springer Nature; from Patel K., Major N. (2009) Compartmental Anatomy. In: Davies A., Sundaram M., James S. (eds) Imaging of Bone Tumors and Tumor-Like Lesions. Medical Radiology. Springer, Berlin, Heidelberg

Case Scenario

We present the case of a 56-year-old male undergoing liver transplant for HCC on HCV cirrhosis. The hepatectomy and implantation were uneventful; vitals were stable during the whole procedure, and blood loss was minimal (300 mL). After the reperfusion, the graft swelled up making the abdomen closure tricky because of a slight tension of the wound. Within 6 h after the surgery, the abdomen became distended, and the respiratory and kidney functions got impaired. Systolic tension was stable at 100 mmHg while diastolic was 85 mmHg. Lactates were stably 4.5 mmol/L. IAP (measured by transurethral probe) was increasing: when it reached 26 mmHg, we performed a CT scan showing intra-abdominal clots with no sign of active bleeding. The patient was taken to the operatory room: after clot removal (Fig. 49.11) and accurate hemostasis, a Bogota bag was placed and an open treatment performed. After 48 h, the liver, kidney, and respiratory functions were normal, and the wound could be closed without any other complications.

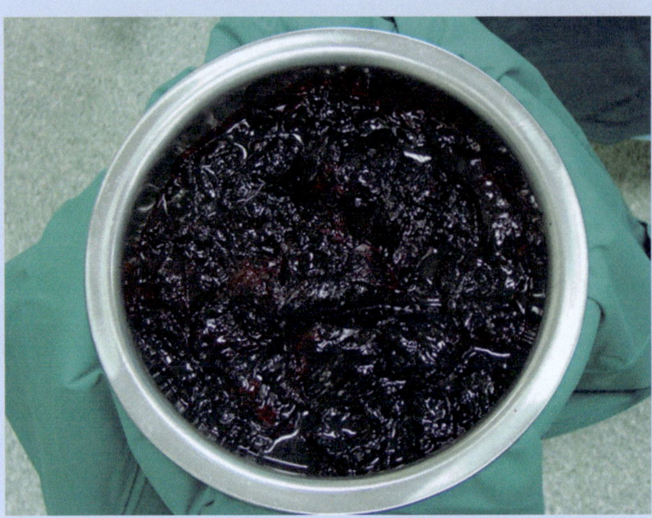

Fig. 49.11 Case scenario: clots removed during open treatment for ACS

Questions:

1. What are the clinical signs that could have raised the suspicion of ACS?
   A. The distended abdomen
   B. Respiratory and kidney function impairment
   C. Low blood tension and reduced lactate clearance
   D. All of the above
2. The impaired kidney function is caused by:
   A. Decreased blood flow in renal veins and kidney congestion
   B. Compression on the ureters
   C. Increased blood catabolite concentration
   D. All of the above
3. The impaired respiratory function is caused by:
   A. Diaphragm elevation
   B. Reduced chest and lung capacity
   C. Increased airway pressure
   D. All of the above
4. In the present case, the most important element to confirm the ACS was:
   A. The clinical sign
   B. The increased bladder pressure
   C. The CT scan
   D. The lactate level
5. What was the main goal of the surgery in the present case?
   A. Check the anastomosis
   B. Reduce the IAP
   C. Avoid early incisional hernia
   D. All of the above

Please see Chap. 58 for the correct answer.

References

1. von Volkmann R. The classic: ischaemic muscle paralyses and contractures. Clin Orthop Relat Res. 2007;456:20–1. https://doi.org/10.1097/BLO.0b013e318032561f.
2. Jepson PN. Ischaemic contracture: experimental study. Ann Surg. 1926;84:785–95.
3. Rorabeck CH. The treatment of compartment syndromes of the leg. J Bone Joint Surg Br. 1984;66:93–7.
4. Kirkpatrick AW, Roberts DJ, De Waele J, et al. Intra-abdominal hypertension and the abdominal compartment syndrome: updated consensus definitions and clinical practice guidelines from the World Society of the Abdominal Compartment Syndrome. Intensive Care Med. 2013;39:1190–206. https://doi.org/10.1007/s00134-013-2906-z.
5. Sugrue M, Bauman A, Jones F, et al. Clinical examination is an inaccurate predictor of intraabdominal pressure. World J Surg. 2002;26:1428–31. https://doi.org/10.1007/s00268-002-6411-8.
6. Kirkpatrick AW, Brenneman FD, McLean RF, et al. Is clinical examination an accurate indicator of raised intra-abdominal pressure in critically injured patients? Can J Surg. 2000;43:207–11.
7. Cheatham ML. Nonoperative management of intraabdominal hypertension and abdominal compartment syndrome. World J Surg. 2009;33:1116–22. https://doi.org/10.1007/s00268-009-0003-9.
8. Leppäniemi A. Surgical management of abdominal compartment syndrome; indications and techniques. Scand J Trauma Resusc Emerg Med. 2009;17:17. https://doi.org/10.1186/1757-7241-17-17.
9. McQueen MM, Gaston P, Court-Brown CM. Acute compartment syndrome. Who is at risk? J Bone Joint Surg Br. 2000;82:200–3.
10. Branco BC, Inaba K, Barmparas G, et al. Incidence and predictors for the need for fasciotomy after extremity trauma: a 10-year review in a mature level I trauma centre. Injury. 2011;42:1157–63. https://doi.org/10.1016/j.injury.2010.07.243.
11. Blaisdell FW. The pathophysiology of skeletal muscle ischemia and the reperfusion syndrome: a review. Cardiovasc Surg. 2002;10:620–30.
12. Hargens AR, Romine JS, Sipe JC, et al. Peripheral nerve-conduction block by high muscle-compartment pressure. J Bone Joint Surg Am. 1979;61:192–200.

Multiple Organ Dysfunction Syndrome After Trauma: Update 2017

50

Andrea DeGasperi, Lucio Bucci, and Bianca M. Wahlen

It is important to remember that SIRS, MODS, MOF[…] are terms with arbitrary definitions that cannot be treated as such. The specific underlying diseases causing these conditions must be identified and treated while organ function is supported……. The whole problem of organ failure continues to perplex clinicians and scientists, and it contributes to fatal outcomes for patients with illnesses, infections, and injuries after operations. We know a lot about these problems but frequently can do little. The best approach remains patient and organ support to prevent failure

Arthur E Baue

Key Points

- In spite of the incidence when multiple organ failure (MOF) is decreasing, MOF remains one of the major causes of morbidity, mortality, and critical resource utilization.
- The definition of MOF is still a matter of debate: scores are used to grade its severity (MODS, SOFA, Denver score): results may be of course different according to scores' sensibility and specificity, making harmonization of the scores and shared definitions mandatory.
- The development of organ dysfunction (OD) is related to the intensity of the trauma and from the balance between trauma-induced simultaneous inflammatory and anti-inflammatory responses.
- Prevention of major dysfunctions of the cardiovascular, respiratory, and renal systems remains the mainstay strategy, mainly based on early, adequate, aggressive supportive measures.

A. DeGasperi (✉)
2° Servizio Anestesia e Rianimazione, Ospedale Niguarda Ca' Granda, Milan, Italy
e-mail: andrea.degasperi@ospedaleniguarda.it

L. Bucci
1° Servizio Anestesia e Rianimazione, Ospedale Niguarda Ca' Granda, Milan, Italy
e-mail: lucio.bucci@ospedaleniguarda.it

B. M. Wahlen
Department of Trauma Surgery, Hamad General Hospital, Doha, Qatar

50.1 Introduction

Irrespective of the type (blunt, penetrating, thermal, or chemical), any trauma creates an anatomical injury to tissues: in the vast majority of cases, a systemic inflammatory response syndrome (SIRS) is boosted since the early phase and is present during the first 72 h. As recently reported by several authors [1–3], severe trauma promotes a hyperinflammatory state able to lead to a condition of organ(s) dysfunction known as *multiple organ dysfunction syndrome* (MODS), which in a continuum might end to multiple organ failure (MOF) and in the worst cases to death. MOF and MODS following major trauma are still associated with relevant morbidity (respiratory, cardiovascular, and renal failure) and high mortality (close to 40%). As assessed by Offner and Moore, MODS and MOF reflect the progress of both the patient and the organ dysfunctioning condition(s) over time [2]: in spite of the reported decrease of MOF incidence over time, mortality is still high.

The term "multiple organ failure" was proposed by Eiseman et al. in 1977 describing in a group of patients the progressive organ failure [4, 5]. According to Fry, MOF is the result of a nonspecific response to the activation of inflammation after an ischemia-reperfusion injury, secondary to tissue disruption, release of factors from the injured tissue, and counter-regulation mechanisms [3]. Initially considered as the consequence of a "one-hit" model (organ dysfunction generated by an intense SIRS after the injury, able to overwhelm the resuscitation procedures), MODS was then described as the result of a "two-hit" model. A less severely traumatized patient develops a "moderate" SIRS after resuscitation but becomes vulnerable to otherwise less severe inflammatory insults (among them transfusions, surgical aggression, postsurgical complications, infection) able to amplify SIRS and evolve to MODS [4]. In this latter condi-

P. Aseni et al. (eds.), *Operative Techniques and Recent Advances in Acute Care and Emergency Surgery*,
https://doi.org/10.1007/978-3-319-95114-0_50

tion, the degree of organ dysfunction dictates the use of artificial support(s) to failing organ(s) available in the ICUs [4–6]. According to the most updated hypotheses [6–8], *organ dysfunction* (OD) after trauma is now considered the result of the balance between two opposite, differently intense but simultaneous, responses, triggered by the first injury: (a) the SIRS, whose intensity is dependent on the magnitude of injury, severity of shock, and coexisting conditions, and (b) its opposite, formerly defined "compensatory anti-inflammatory responsive syndrome" (CARS), now renamed SARS (*systemic anti-inflammatory response syndrome*). Early OD or, in the most severe cases, early MOF, is the result of the intense proinflammatory response (SIRS) triggered by the innate immune system and the simultaneously present early anti-inflammatory response (SARS) due to the inhibition of the adaptive immune system (leading in extreme cases to apoptosis). According to the results coming from the GLUEGRANT project [7], the limitation of the proinflammatory status should create a protective setting against the consequences of a second hit. However, a persistent severe anti-inflammatory condition could lead to immunoparalysis, impaired healing, and infections, thus opening up to a late OD or late MOF. Very recently, Hazeldyne et al. were able to confirm that the dynamic nature of the immune response to trauma is evident very early (within 1 h after trauma) as a simultaneous activation and suppression: SIRS and CARS are then concomitantly and immediately induced [8]. Studying the genomic expression of SIRS and SARS, the GLUEGRANT project researchers were able to confirm the simultaneity of inflammatory and anti-inflammatory responses [7].

50.2 The Definition of Multiple Organ Failure (MOF): An Open Problem

In spite of the huge number of studies (840 hits for clinical trials and 3739 hits for review articles in PubMed), the definition of MOF remains a debated item. According to recent reviews and studies [6, 9–11], scores are commonly used to define (or better, to "grade") MOF after trauma. This issue is not without relevance, since MOF scoring systems, able to impact on incidence, duration, organ dysfunction patterns, and mortality prediction, might eventually change the way to define the epidemiology and/or to manage trauma patients. Only in the presence of a shared definition of MOF will incidence, duration, and mortality after trauma not be biased by wide variations in reporting [9, 10]. SOFA (Sequential Organ Failure Assessment) score, MODS (Multiple Organ Dysfunction Score, four grades for six organ systems), and Denver score (four grades for four organ systems) (Table 50.1) are the most commonly used scores. While every score performs well in terms of predictivity, SOFA and MODS scores seem to be more sensitive (meaning more MOFs but lower mortality rate) than Denver score (meaning fewer MOFs but higher mortality rate), making this latter score more specific. Frohlich et al. [9] compared the three scores to "quantify" posttraumatic multiple organ failure (MODS, Denver, SOFA). Discussing their results, the authors underlined the more relevant differences among the three scores. Interestingly enough, Denver score does not consider central nervous system and coagulation items, which could have a relevant impact on the outcome prediction and possibly on resource utilization. The authors came to the following conclusions: (a) comparable ability of the three scores in predicting the outcome of severely injured patients (including subjects with severe brain injury), (b) Denver and SOFA best predictors of resource utilization, and (c) better performance of MODS score in predicting mortality. Into their vision, MOF incidence relied almost entirely on the applied score [9]. In the most recent epidemiological study performed on 491 severe trauma patients (median ISS 25.3), Hutching et al. [10] were able to conclude that Denver score might be more accurate in identifying true "high-risk" patients. As a matter of fact, while MODS and SOFA scores were too much sensitive (too many MOFs but with low mortality rate), Denver score at day 3 identified less MOF patients (45% of the entire cohort), but with significantly higher MOF-associated mortality, supporting its better performance in terms of specificity. According to Hutching et al. [10], while a lower sensibility of Denver score might increase the risk of a potential miss of "at-risk" trauma patients, the higher the specificity targets, the most severe the trauma patients, thus truly defining the high-risk patient. Eagerly awaiting for a "definitive" word on this extremely debated item [11], harmonization of the "competing" scores and definitions appears not only advisable but mandatory [9–11].

According to the GLUEGRANT study results, respiratory and cardiovascular failures were the most commonly observed ODs (close to half of the patients), renal and liver failures being less frequent (less than 20%). Early MOF (within less than 3 days from trauma) had high early mortality (up to 60%), mainly due to cardiovascular dysfunction (40%), followed by kidney (38%), liver (19%), and lung (12%) dysfunction/failure. According to Sauaia et al. [6], MOF survivors still represent an enormous burden for the health-care systems worldwide, being responsible for prolonged ICU stay and a relevant need for sophisticated technological resources , closely correlated with the artificial support of vital functions. A new scenario is now emerging with the "persistent inflammation-immunosuppression catabolism syndrome" (PICS): associated with the aggressive treatment of the first injury to prevent MODS (and in fact, the incidence of MODS is now reducing), a new OD phenotype is on the rise, being now evident in patients discharged from long ICU periods to rehabilitation facilities [7].

Table 50.1 Postinjury MOF scores (Frohlich M et al. Which score should be used for posttraumatic multiple organ failure? Comparison of the MODS, DENVER and SOFA scores. Scand J Trauma, Resusc, Emerg Med, 2016; 24: 130)

Summary of the Denver score, SOFA score and MOD score					
Dysfunction	Grade 0	Grade 1	Grade 2	Grade 3	Grade 4
Denver score					
Pulmonary, PaO_2/FIO_2 (mmHg)	>208	208–165	165–83	<8i	
Hepatic, bilirubin, (mmHg)	<34	34–58	69–137	>137	
Renal creatinine, (μmol/L)	<159	160–210	211–420	>420	
Cardiac inotropes[a]	No inotropes	Only one inotrope at a small dose	Any inotrope at moderate dose or >1 agent at small dose	Any inotrope at large dose or >2 agents at moderate dose	
SOFA score					
Pulmonary, PaO_2/FIO_2, (mmHg)	>400	≤400	≤300	≤200	≤100
Coagulation, platelet count, ($\times 10^3/\mu L$)	>150	≤150	≤100	≤50	≤20
Hepatic, bilirubin, (μmol/L)	<20	20–32	33–101	102–204	>204
Cardiovascular, inotropes[b] in μg/kg/min	No hypo tension	Mean arterial pressure <70 mmHg	Dopa ≤5 or any Dobu dose	Dopa > 5 or Epi ≤ 0.1 or Nor ≤ 0.1	Dopa > 15 or Epi > 0.1 or Nor > 0.1
Renal, creatinine, (μmol/L)	<110	110–170	171–299	300–440	>440
Central nervous system, GCS	15	13–14	10–12	5–9	<6
MODS					
Pulmonary, PaO_2/FIO_2, (mmHg)	>300	226–300	151–225	76–150	≤51
Renal, creatinine, (μmol/L)	≤100	101–200	201–350	351–500	>500
Hepatic, bilirubin, (μmol/L)	≤20	21–60	61–120	121–240	>240
Cardiovascular, PAR[c]	≤10.0	10.1–15.0	15.1–20.0	20.1–30.0	>300
Coagulatten, platelet count, $\times 10^3/\mu L$	>120	81–120	51–80	21–50	≤20
Central nervous system, GCS	15	13–14	10–12	5–9	<6

[a]Inotrope doses (in μg/kg/min): vasopressin: small <0.3, moderate 0.03–0.07, large >0.07; dopamine: small <6, moderate 6–10, large >10; dobutamine: small <0.6, moderate 6–10, large >10; epinephrine: small <0.06, moderate 0.06–0.15, large >0.15; norepinephrine: small <0.11, moderate 0.11–05, large >0.5

[b]*Dopo* dopamine, *Dobu* dobutamine, *Epi* epinephrine, *Nor* norepinephrine

[c]PAR = Heart rate × central venous pressure/mean arterial blood pressure

50.3 MOF and Risk Factors

Risk factors definition is another point of debate. Generally speaking, frequently reported risk factors for MOF after trauma are massive transfusion, major abdominal trauma, and multiple fractures [5]. According to Sauaia et al. [6], risk factors for MOF are male sex, age, obesity, severity of injury, units of red blood cells (RBCs) transfused within the first 12 h, and acidosis, as specific "markers" associated with the altered physiologic profile. Instead, risk factors for MOF-related death are female sex, severity of injury, and entity of early transfused RBCs.

50.4 Pathophysiology Keynotes

According to the very recent review by Sauaia et al. on MOF pathophysiology in injured patients [6], cell apoptosis is different in healthy individuals and traumatized or septic patients. Healthy undamaged cells are scavenged without triggering immune responses. On the contrary, after trauma or infection, innate and adaptive immune responses are triggered by the release from the damaged cells of alarmins and damage-associated molecular patterns (DAMPs, the latter very similar to pathogen-associated molecular patterns, PAMPs). In particular, the severity of tissue injuries together with profound shock conditions can activate an inflammatory response via release of DAMPs from activated immune cells and/or from necrotic cells, resulting in enhanced microcirculation damage. DAMPs react with inflammatory cell receptors (e.g., Toll-like receptor 4, TLR-4), triggering gene transcription involved in the production of proinflammatory cytokines. The final result is a SIRS state, including activation and a possible derangement of the coagulation system in the more severe patients [12]. In fact, DAMPs (which include HMGB1 [high mobility group box protein-1], heat shock proteins, uric acid, and DNA) are recognized by components of innate and acquired immunity (mainly TLR-4) able to transduce signals in response to DAMPs after ischemia-reperfusion injury and to activate several signal pathways (mainly nuclear factor kappa-B [NF-kB]). A large part of the proteins identified in plasma of traumatized patients and released into circulation behave as DAMPS, triggering pattern recognition receptors and creating, according to Zhang et al. [13], a sepsis-like state: these molecules might become the link between SIRS, inflammation, and trauma [13]. HMGB1 correlates with (a) the severity of hypoperfusion (the *cause* of its release), (b) the inflammatory cytokine levels (the *effect* of its widespread release), and (c) the final outcome of the more injured patients (the final effect of the SIRS condition and the coagulopathy derived from the coagulation system derangement) [14, 15]. Recent data suggest that, in the complex pathophysiology of the so-called trauma-induced coagulopathy (TIC), one of the main aspects may be related to endothelial damage, in particular its glycocalyx layer (endothelial glycocalyx layer, EGL), located on the surface of endothelial cells as a negative-charged thin layer with anti-adhesive and anticoagulant functions [16–18]. Tissue and vascular injuries, hypoperfusion conditions, the activation of the neurohormonal hypothalamic-adrenal axis together with the inflammatory system, and the endogenous catecholamines released from the adrenal glands all act as a boost for endothelial systemic activation and damage, with consequent increase in permeability and coagulation derangement with evidence of early coagulopathy [19]. Johansson and his group, exploring data regarding more than 3000 patients with apparently different diseases such as trauma, sepsis, myocardial infarction, and post-cardiac arrest syndrome, found that shock itself, with its effect on the sympatho-adrenal system, together with the endothelial glycocalyx and the hemostatic cells, results in modifications of the phenotype response which characterize the clinical condition of acute critical illness, despite the different types of the primary "hit." The endothelial damage induced by an over-release of catecholamine results in glycocalyx shedding, disruption of tight junctions with capillary leakage, and a procoagulant state in the microcirculation, responsible for a further reduction of oxygen delivery (due to increased tissue pressure) and microvascular thrombosis: this vicious circle is responsible for a final condition of organ failure. In the end, the early genetic responses to severe trauma, burn injury, and sepsis endotoxemia are similar: the body attempts and responses in various *acute* critical conditions characterized by a shock state are all relatively homogenous and most likely adapted from an evolutionary point of view [20]. Interestingly enough, patients with long-standing PICS had persistent neutrophilia with lymphopenia, recurrent infections, progressive sarcopenia in spite of nutrition support and poor wound healing, and classic markers of a severe catabolic state leading to very poor outcome. Beyond the scope of the paper is to go deeper into the definition of the role of gut, platelets, complement, TLRs, neutrophils, macrophages, and cytokines in the specific setting of trauma: interested readers are referred to the very recent and exhaustive Sauaia's review [6].

50.5 Early Trauma Management and Interventions Aiming at Prevention of MOF

To treat an established MOF is largely supportive and sometimes frustrating: more practical could be to start early treatments (in some sense "preventive" if possible) able to impact on the balance between SIRS and SARS. Very recently a research agenda for trauma critical care has been proposed by an international experts' network: their attention has been addressed on major factors leading to death and possible relevant priority areas of research [21]. Head injury is still the first cause of major disability, while hemorrhage and bleeding complications are the leading causes of preventable deaths. As underlined by the expert panel, the level of evidence for many of the procedures or treatments proposed for the care of trauma patients is low, whether or not traumatic brain injury (TBI) is present [TBI is not considered in this article]. Damage control resuscitation (DCR) and damage control surgery (DCS) lead in the recent past to a sensible reduction of major complications (included reduced MODS/MOF): however, in spite of these improvements, mortality and utilization of critical care supports are still relevant [21]. According to Asehnoune et al. [21], contemporary DCR strategy relies, in spite a low level of evidence, upon the following:

(a) Restricted fluid replacement therapy, with reduced use of crystalloids and colloids (no difference according to the most recent Cochrane review in trauma between colloids and crystalloids) [22] and limitation of the use of vasopressors in the hypovolemic patient [22, 23].
(b) Permissive hypotension to reduce hemorrhage from bleeding sites and to avoid dilutional coagulopathy, only

exception to permissive hypotension being TBI, a condition in which hypotension has to be avoided [4, 13].

(c) (c) Reconstitution of hemostatic competence in traumatic coagulopathy since the early phases of treatment with the administration of fresh frozen plasma (FFP)/platelets/RBCs in 1:1:1 ratio. This strategy is associated in the most recent literature with better hemostatic profile in major bleeding trauma patients and with decreased early mortality [13, 15, 16, 19]. In this specific setting, restrictive transfusion policies, now the rule in many clinical settings, were proposed by some authorities in the recent past [6, 24, 25].

(d) Coagulopathy in the severe trauma patient recognizes a complex interplay between endothelial dysfunction and enhanced fibrinolysis together with a possible role for resuscitation component-induced coagulopathy [25].

(e) Early use of cryoprecipitate or fibrinogen concentrates and of tranexamic acid to treat hyperfibrinolysis is now considered a relevant aspect of standard care [26–33]. Viscoelastic tests (mainly thromboelastography/thromboelastometry) are gaining in this setting considerable interest, even if evidence is lacking so far [21, 26, 30–33].

Due to the relevant impact acute respiratory failure has in MOF after trauma (present in >50% of the cases), strategies to avoid artificial ventilation-induced lung injury (barotrauma, volutrauma, atelectrauma) and the consequent inflammatory "parenchymal" reactions are more and more implemented [34–36]. Protective lung strategy in artificial ventilation is now standard of care in every clinical setting where mechanical ventilation is used: such strategy should avoid pulmonary (local) and extrapulmonary (systemic) effects mediated by inflammatory cytokines, thus potentially preventing or reducing ODs [6, 21].

Compromised adrenal function might be a hallmark in severe trauma patients and could be associated with poor outcome. Even if debated, because based on clinical criteria and not on solid evidence, stress doses of hydrocortisone (200–300 mg/day) have been associated with improved survival in trauma patients unresponsive to fluids and pressors: the dose should be enough to downregulate the proinflammatory response, but not too large to induce a condition of excessive immunomodulation/immunodepression able to impair healing [6, 21, 37, 38].

As a matter of fact, positive immunomodulation is reported to be achieved with dedicated, "aggressive" early enteral nutrition ("immunonutrition"), able to impact on the incidence of nosocomial infections: however rigorous studies are needed for a solid demonstration of the reverse of the shock-induced mucosal injuries and the attenuated consequences of the increased gut permeability and bacterial translocation. Caution is mandatory when discussing immunomodulatory or "immune-enhancing" products. Even if in the presence of appealing experimental support, few phase 1 trials have been concluded (safety studies), and no phase 2 studies are available so far.

Conclusions

MODS and MOF after trauma are still a major problem worldwide: in spite of the improved outcomes, morbidity, resource allocation, disabilities, and mortality which are still high and able to heavily impact on every national health system. Shared and standardized definitions together with harmonized scores are needed for a better description of MOF incidence, still reported in ranges too wide to be reliable.

In the next few years, improvements in this challenging field should come from big data sharing and new treatment paradigms, developed from innovative diagnostics (including new appropriate biomarkers) and advanced therapeutic interventions.

References

1. Offner PJ, Moore EE. Risk factors for MOF and patter of organ failure following severe trauma, Chap 4. In: Baue AE, Faist E, Fry DE, editors. Multiple organ failure. New York: Springer; 2000. p. 30–43.
2. Baue AE. Hystory of MOF and definition of organ failure, Chap 1. In: Baue AE, Faist E, Fry DE, editors. Multiple organ failure. New York: Springer; 2000. p. 3–13.
3. Fry DE. MODS: an introduction, Chap 3. In: Deitch EA, Vincent J-L, Windsor A, editors. Sepsis and multiple organ dysfunction. Philadelphia: WB Saunders; 2002. p. 19–25.
4. Moore FA, Moore EE. MODS following trauma, Chap 4. In: Deitch EA, Vincent J-L, Windsor A, editors. Sepsis and multiple organ dysfunction. Philadelphia: WB Saunders; 2002. p. 26–33.
5. Baue AE. MOF, MODS, and SIRS: what is in a name or an acronym? Shock. 2006;25:438–49.
6. Sauaia A, Moore FA, Moore EE. Postinjury inflammation and organ dysfunction. Crit Care Clin. 2017;33:167–91.
7. Xiao W, Mindrinos MN, Seok J, Cuschieri J, Cuenca AG, Gao H, et al. A genomic storm in critically injured humans. J Exp Med. 2011;208:2581–90.
8. Hezeldine J, Naumann DN, Toman E, Davies D, Bishop JRB, Su Z, et al. Prehospital immune response and development of multiple organ dysfunction syndrome following traumatic injury: a prospective cohort study. PLOS Med. 2017; https://doi.org/10.1371/journal.pmed.1002338.
9. Frohlich M, Wafaisade A, Mansuri A, Koenen P, Probst C Maegele M, et al. Which score should be used for posttraumatic multiple organ failure? Comparison of the MODS, DENVER and SOFA scores. Scand J Trauma Resusc Emerg Med. 2016;24:130. https://doi.org/10.1186/s13049-016-0321-5.
10. Hutchings L, Watkinson P, Young JD, Willett K. Defining multiple organ failure after major trauma: a comparison of the Denver, Sequential Organ Failure Assessment, and Marshall scoring systems. J Trauma Acute Care Surg. 2017;82:534–41.
11. Rendy L, Sapan HB, Kalesaran LTB. Multiple organ dysfunction syndrome prediction score in multi trauma patients. Int J Surg Open. 2017;8:1–6.

12. Bianchi ME. DAMPs, PAMPs and alarmins: all we need to know about danger. J Leukoc Biol. 2007;81:1–5.
13. Zhang Q, Raoof M, Chen Y, et al. Circulating mitochondrial DAMPs cause inflammatory responses to injury. Nature. 2010;464(7285):104–7.
14. Cohen MJ, Brohi K, Calfee CS, et al. Early release of high mobility group box nuclear protein 1 after severe trauma in humans: role of injury severity and tissue hypoperfusion. Crit Care. 2009;13:R174.
15. Manson J, Thiemermann C, Brohi K. Trauma alarmins as activators of damage-induced inflammation. Br J Surg. 2012;99(S1):12–20.
16. Weinbaum S, Tarbell JM, Damiano ER. The structure and function of the endothelial glycocalyx layer. Annu Rev Biomed Eng. 2007;9:121–67.
17. Noel P, Cashen S, Patel B. Trauma-induced coagulopathy: from biology to therapy. Semin Hematol. 2013;50:259–69.
18. Ostrowski SR, Johannson P. Endothelial glycocalyx degradation induces endogenous heparinization in patients with severe injury and early traumatic coagulopathy. J Trauma Acute Care Surg. 2012;73:60–6.
19. Pierce A, Pittet J-F. Inflammatory response to trauma: implications for coagulation and resuscitation. Curr Opin Anesthesiol. 2014;27(2):246–52.
20. Johansson PI, Stensballe J, Ostrowski SR. Shock induced endotheliopathy (SHINE) in acute critical illness – a unifying pathophysiologic mechanism. Crit Care. 2017;21:25.
21. Asenhnoune K, Balogh Z, Citerio G, Cap A, Billiar T, Stocchetti N, et al. The research agenda for trauma critical care. Intens Care Med. https://doi.org/10.1007/s00134-017-4895-9.
22. Perel P, Roberts I, Ker K. Colloids versus crystalloids for fluid resuscitation in critically ill patients. Cochrane Database Syst Rev. 2013;(2):CD000567.
23. Brinck T, Handolin L, Lefering R. The effect of evolving fluid resuscitation on the outcome of severely injured patients: an 8-year experience at a tertiary trauma center. Scand J Surg. 2016;105:109–16. https://doi.org/10.1177/1457496915586650.
24. Simmons JW, Powell MF. Acute traumatic coagulopathy: pathophysiology and resuscitation. Br J Anaesth. 2016;117:iii31–43. https://doi.org/10.1093/bja/aew328.
25. Napolitano LM, Kurek S, Luchette FA, et al. Clinical practice guideline: red blood cell transfusion in adult trauma and critical care. Crit Care Med. 2009;37(12):3124–57.
26. Rossaint R, Bouillon B, Cerny V, et al. The European guideline on management of major bleeding and coagulopathy following trauma: fourth edition. Crit Care. 2016;20:100. https://doi.org/10.1186/s13054-016-1265-x.
27. Shakur H, Roberts I, CRASH-2 trial Collaborators, et al. Effects of tranexamic acid on death, vascular occlusive events, and blood transfusion in trauma patients with significant haemorrhage (CRASH-2): a randomised, placebo-controlled trial. Lancet. 2010;376:23–32. https://doi.org/10.1016/S0140-6736(10)60835-5.
28. Moore EE, Moore HB, Gonzalez E, et al. Rationale for the selective administration of tranexamic acid to inhibit fibrinolysis in the severely injured patient. Transfusion. 2016;56(Suppl 2):S110–4. https://doi.org/10.1111/trf.13486.
29. Curry N, Rourke C, Davenport R, et al. Early cryoprecipitate for major haemorrhage in trauma: a randomised controlled feasibility trial. Br J Anaesth. 2015;115:76–83. https://doi.org/10.1093/bja/aev134.
30. Gonzalez E, Moore EE, Moore HB, et al. Goal-directed hemostatic resuscitation of trauma-induced coagulopathy: a pragmatic randomized clinical trial comparing a viscoelastic assay to conventional coagulation assays. Ann Surg. 2016;263:1051–9. https://doi.org/10.1097/SLA.0000000000001608.
31. Oyeniyi BT, Fox EE, Scerbo M, et al. Trends in 1029 trauma deaths at a level 1 trauma center: impact of a bleeding control bundle of care. Injury. 2017;48:5–12.
32. National Institute for Clinical Excellence (NICE). Major trauma assessment and initial management guidelines. 2016. https://www.nice.org.uk/guidance/.
33. Holcomb JB, Tilley BC, Baraniuk S, et al. Transfusion of plasma, platelets, and red blood cells in a 1:1:1 vs a 1:1:2 ratio and mortality in patients with severe trauma: the PROPPR randomized clinical trial. JAMA. 2015;313:471–82. https://doi.org/10.1001/jama.2015.12.
34. ARDS network Ventilation with lower tidal volumes as compared with traditional tidal volumes for acute lung injury and the acute respiratory distress syndrome. the acute respiratory distress syndrome network. N Engl J Med. 2000;342:1301–8.
35. Petrucci N, De Feo C. Lung protective ventilation strategy for the acute respiratory distress syndrome. Cochrane Database Syst Rev. 2013;(2):CD003844.
36. Roquilly A, Cinotti R, Jaber S, et al. Implementation of an evidence based extubation readiness bundle in 499 brain-injured patients. A before-after evaluation of a quality improvement project. Am J Respir Crit Care Med. 2013;188:958–66. https://doi.org/10.1164/rccm.201301-0116OC.
37. Offner PJ, Moore EE, Ciesla D. The adrenal response after severe trauma. Am J Surg. 2002;184(6):649–53.
38. Islam NM, Bradley BA, Ceredig R. Sterile post-traumatic immunosuppression. Clin Transl Immunol. 2016;5:e77. https://doi.org/10.1038/cti.2016.13.

Acute Respiratory Failure: Ventilatory Support and Extracorporeal Membrane Oxygenation (ECMO)

51

Riccardo Pinciroli, Alfio Bronco, Alberto Lucchini, and Giuseppe Foti

Key Points

- Acute respiratory failure (ARF) is defined as the impaired capacity of the lungs to either maintain a normal oxygen delivery to the tissues or a sufficient removal of carbon dioxide from the periphery. Based on arterial blood gas (ABG) analysis, ARF can be categorized as hypoxemic (PaO_2 lower than 60 mmHg) or hypercapnic ($PaCO_2$ higher than 50 mmHg). The evaluation of an ARF patient should always take into account the history of the patient, as well as the pathophysiology of the underlying acute disease.
- Hypoxemia can be mainly caused by conditions leading to ventilation/perfusion (*V*/*Q*) mismatch, due to reduced ventilation despite adequate blood flow. This can be due to impaired airflow dynamics, like in obstructive lung diseases, or to the presence of fluid in the alveoli. Taking *V*/*Q* mismatch to the extreme, shunt occurs whenever perfusion is not at all matched by ventilation. An impaired diffusion across the alveolar membrane, a decreased venous content, and the inspiration of hypoxic gas mixtures are other possible causes of low arterial oxygenation.
- Hypercapnic respiratory failure, also known as "pump" failure, is mainly due to a reduced clearance of the gas from the lungs associated with an impaired alveolar ventilation. Hypercarbia develops whenever a patient is unable to generate the work of breathing required by the organism to compensate physiologic derangements due to the underlying disease process. Disease states leading to neuromuscular dysfunction or decreased neural respiratory drive may cause or precipitate $PaCO_2$ elevation.
- The purpose of mechanical ventilation is that of assisting (or replacing) lung function until resolution of the primary disease leading to ARF. The clinical assessment of the patient's work of breathing (tachypnea, use of accessory muscles, fatigue) and an altered ABG analysis, in the context of a global evaluation of the patient's history, are the main tools guiding the physician whenever the choice to ventilate is being considered.
- In selected cases, noninvasive ventilation (NIV) might be indicated as the first line of treatment. Hypercapnic respiratory failure is a common scenario. Particularly, NIV is the standard of care for patients affected by chronic obstructive pulmonary disease (COPD) presenting with an acute exacerbation of their chronic condition. Noninvasive CPAP has become the first-line therapy of choice to treat hypoxemia in cardiogenic pulmonary edema. Helmets are a reliable interface for the noninvasive delivery of CPAP.

R. Pinciroli (✉)
University of Milan-Bicocca Medical School, Monza, MB, Italy

Anesthesia and Intensive Care 1, ASST Grande Ospedale Metropolitano Niguarda, Milan, Italy

A. Bronco
Department of Anesthesia and Critical Care, Ospedale San Gerardo, ASST Monza, Monza, MB, Italy
e-mail: a.bronco@asst-monza.it

A. Lucchini
Department of Anesthesia and Critical Care, Ospedale San Gerardo, ASST Monza, Monza, MB, Italy

Dipartimento di emergenza e urgenza, Terapia intensiva generale, ASST Monza, Ospedale S. Gerardo, Università Milano-Bicocca, Monza, MB, Italy
e-mail: a.lucchini@asst-monza.it

G. Foti
University of Milan-Bicocca Medical School, Monza, MB, Italy

Department of Anesthesia and Critical Care, Ospedale San Gerardo, ASST Monza, Monza, MB, Italy
e-mail: g.foti@asst-monza.it

P. Aseni et al. (eds.), *Operative Techniques and Recent Advances in Acute Care and Emergency Surgery*,
https://doi.org/10.1007/978-3-319-95114-0_51

- Mechanical ventilation aims at maintaining an adequate alveolar ventilation and oxygen delivery, thus restoring acid-base balance and reducing the patient's work of breathing. The risk of ventilator-induced lung injury (VILI) demands the adoption of a lung-protective ventilatory strategy. That includes a low tidal volume of 6–8 mL/kg, a plateau pressure <30 cmH_2O, a driving pressure <15 cmH_2O, and appropriate and stable PEEP levels.
- A mechanical ventilator can be set to deliver either full or partial respiratory support. In order to accordingly set and regulate the ventilatory settings, among the several available options, the operator must consider three main variables: (1) trigger (how the ventilator determines when a breath is initiated), (2) control (what aspect of inspiration is primarily controlled by the ventilator at inspiration), and (3) cycling (what signals the ventilator to terminate inspiration and start expiration).
- Complications of mechanical ventilation include a wide array of adverse conditions, among the most frequent are (1) ventilator-induced lung injury (VILI), (2) ventilator-associated pneumonia (VAP), (3) hemodynamic instability, and (4) ventilator-induced diaphragmatic dysfunction (VIDD).
- Extracorporeal membrane oxygenation (ECMO) is a lifesaving technique in which the patient's venous blood is drained toward an artificial gas exchanger, through which it is oxygenated and decarboxylated. Arterialized blood can then be returned to the patient. Blood can be reinfused either to the arterial (veno-arterial, VA-ECMO) or to the venous circulation (veno-venous, VV-ECMO), more frequently adopted for the sole purpose of respiratory support.
- The continuous contact between blood and the surface biomaterials the ECMO circuit is made of inevitably results in an increased risk of thrombotic complications. Unfractionated heparin (UFH) is the most frequently used anticoagulant. UFH is given both as a bolus (50–100 units per kilogram) at the time of cannulation and by continuous infusion (10 UI/kg/h) during ECMO. A strict monitoring of the patient's coagulation status is always conducted, including standard laboratory data, activated clotting time (ACT), and thromboelastography (TEG).

51.1 Acute Respiratory Failure

Acute respiratory failure (ARF) is defined as the impaired capacity of the lungs to either maintain a normal oxygen (O_2) delivery to the tissues or a sufficient removal of carbon dioxide (CO_2) from the periphery [1]. Physicians, as well as several other healthcare providers, often come upon this clinical entity, particularly if involved in the acute and critical care setting. A failing respiratory function potentially leads to inadequate gas exchange, inevitably associated with life-threatening imbalances in arterial oxygenation and acid-base status.

Respiratory failure generally is the consequence of a discrepancy between the respiratory workload required by the organism and the ability of the patient's respiratory system to actually meet such requirements with the necessary strength and endurance [2]. In clinical practice, based on arterial blood gas (ABG) analysis, ARF can be categorized as hypoxemic, or type I (PaO_2 lower than 60 mmHg), and hypercapnic, or type II ($PaCO_2$ higher than 50 mmHg) [3]. However, while ABG analysis should always be carefully evaluated, the rapid development of both hypoxemia and hypercapnia often occurs. Moreover, the possibility of preexisting derangements of gas exchange due to chronic conditions should always be considered.

The evaluation of an ARF patient should always take into account the history of the patient, as well as the pathophysiology of the underlying acute disease.

ARF can result from diseases impacting the proper function of any part of the respiratory system. This includes the upper and lower respiratory tract, pulmonary circulation, central and peripheral nervous systems, respiratory muscles, and the chest wall. Furthermore, ARF can result whenever the lung responds to systemic acute disease processes leading to tissue hypoperfusion, like shock.

51.1.1 Hypoxemic Respiratory Failure

Hypoxemia can be mainly caused by conditions leading to:

(a) *Ventilation/perfusion (V/Q) mismatch or shunt*
(b) *Diffusion impairment*
(c) *Decreased mixed venous oxygen content*
(d) *Inspiration of hypoxic gas mixtures*

(a) *Ventilation/Perfusion (V/Q) Mismatch or Shunt*

V/Q mismatch is the most common pathophysiology of hypoxemia. Healthy lungs regularly show areas of discrepancy between ventilation (higher at the apex) and perfusion (higher at the bases). However, pathologic *V/Q* mismatch leads to a decrease in PaO_2, generally due to reduced ventilation despite adequate blood flow. This can be due to impaired airflow dynamics, like in obstructive lung diseases, or to the presence of fluid in the alveoli. *V/Q* mismatch responds to supplemental O_2 administration.

Taking *V/Q* mismatch to the extreme, shunt occurs whenever perfusion is not at all matched by ventilation ($V/Q = 0$). Shunt occurs when the alveoli collapse (atelectasis), or the alveolar space is completely occupied by fluid or exudate, like in pulmonary edema or pneumonia, respectively. In the case of a true shunt, little or no increase in arterial oxygenation occurs even with a high fraction of inspired oxygen (FiO_2) [2].

(b) *Diffusion Impairment*

Impaired diffusion of gas across the alveolar membrane typically occurs in interstitial lung diseases (e.g., idiopathic pulmonary fibrosis, sarcoidosis). Due to an abnormal interstitium, even with a physiologic pressure gradient, the alveolar-capillary membrane is unable to regularly exchange gases at the air-blood interface [4].

(c) *Decreased Mixed Venous Oxygen Content*

The oxygen venous admixture within the pulmonary artery represents the end product of O_2 delivery and consumption. Mixed venous oxygen saturation (SvO_2), measured through a pulmonary artery catheter, and its surrogate, central venous oxygen saturation ($ScvO_2$), are routinely used in the ICU as markers of tissue O_2 extraction, particularly in the setting of heart failure and sepsis. A low SvO_2 might be associated with a decreased O_2 delivery (reduced tissue perfusion, hypoxemia, low hemoglobin concentration) and/or increased O_2 consumption (e.g., fever, burns, hyperthyroidism, increased muscular activity). As a result, a low mixed venous O_2 inevitably increases the gradient that needs to be leveled by the lungs, possibly leading to arterial hypoxia. Furthermore, it is not unusual for disease states leading to a low SvO_2, like congestive heart failure, to concomitantly impact lung function, thus the possibility to ultimately reach an adequate arterial O_2 tension [5].

(d) *Inspiration of Hypoxic Gas Mixtures*

While a rare instance, hypoxemia may develop when inspired O_2 is lower than the minimum physiologic requirement (21% at sea level). The decrease in barometric pressure, like in high altitude, results in a lower partial pressure of O_2, thereby leading to hypoxemia.

51.1.2 Hypercapnic Respiratory Failure

Hypercapnic respiratory failure is also known as ventilatory or "pump" failure. A reduced minute ventilation (MV) rate is, in fact, the main factor leading to an increase in $PaCO_2$ due to a reduced clearance of the gas from the alveoli.

However, ventilatory dead space and the carbon dioxide produced by the body (VCO_2) are also part of the equation determining arterial CO_2. Increased dead space is a known issue in obstructive diseases, like chronic obstructive pulmonary disease (COPD) [6]. Furthermore, in patients undergoing invasive mechanical ventilation, the presence of the endotracheal tube and the ventilator circuits, connecting the patient to the ventilator machine, must be taken into account as additional dead space. On the other hand, systemic conditions, like fever, muscular effort, shivering, or a high caloric intake, can result in an increased VCO_2. Finally, a reduced *V/Q* ratio, while primarily leading to hypoxia, might also affect the availability to the pulmonary circulation of alveolar space within which to discharge CO_2, thereby leading to hypercapnia.

Whatever its origin, an increased $PaCO_2$ can be promptly corrected by an increase in MV, triggered by our feedback respiratory control systems. However, hypercarbia may arise due to an impaired CO_2 clearance capability. Particularly:

(a) *Decreased ventilatory drive*
(b) *Neuromuscular dysfunction*
(c) *Respiratory overload*

(a) *Decreased Ventilatory Drive*

A reduction of MV, possibly up to complete apnea, may arise a consequence of a reduced neural ventilatory drive. Any impairment of the function of the medullary respiratory centers, as well as the aortic and carotid bodies, might, therefore, lead to hypercapnic respiratory failure. This can be caused by several different conditions, such as drug overdose or sedative medications, central nervous system (CNS) diseases or injuries, and metabolic derangements. The patient always presents with an altered level of consciousness [7].

(b) *Neuromuscular Dysfunction*

Despite a normal central neural drive, patients might also fail to achieve an effective CO_2 clearance in case of underlying conditions leading to neuromuscular dysfunction. Spinal cord injury, motor neuron (e.g., amyotrophic lateral sclerosis) [8] or nerve disorders (e.g., Guillain-Barré syndrome) [9], neuromuscular junction (e.g., myasthenia gravis) [10], and primary muscular diseases (e.g., muscular dystrophy) [11] are the main categories. A variable degree of muscular weakness, up to complete paralysis, is the outcome of such disorders. The involvement of respiratory muscles is common and often life-threatening [12].

(c) *Respiratory Overload*

Generally speaking, whatever the culprit of ARF, assuming a preserved neural drive and an intact neuromuscular respiratory effector system, hypercapnic ventilatory failure may develop whenever a patient is unable to meet the work of breathing (WOB) required to compensate physiologic derangements due to the underlying disease process. The primary insult can be diverse. In case of severe alterations of respiratory mechanics, typical of obstructive diseases, the patient might not be able to adequately compensate the development of excessive airway resistance and intrinsic positive end-expiratory pressure (auto-PEEP), thereby showing CO_2 retention. As well, any condition affecting the integrity of the chest wall and pleural space (hemo-/pneumothorax, pleural effusion, rib fractures) might impose the patient an abnormal effort. An excessive respiratory workload can be demanded by hypermetabolic states, like major burns. Finally, hypercapnia may also develop in a primarily hypoxic ARF, as soon as the patient shows signs of exhaustion.

51.1.3 Acute Respiratory Failure in Trauma Patients

Trauma is the leading cause of death and disability in adults up to the middle of the fifth decade of life. In the trauma population, chest injury accounts for a significant portion of the resulting morbidity and mortality [13]. Thoracic trauma caused by blunt mechanisms is most frequently associated with motor vehicle accidents (MVAs). However, falls, interpersonal violence, or blasts also are likely scenarios [14]. The chest wall is typically affected, with potentially multiple fractures of its bones (ribs, clavicle, scapulae, sternum), leading to a pain-induced reduction of the inspiratory excursion. Traumatic disruption of the pleural integrity might lead to pneumothorax and/or hemothorax. Pulmonary contusions may arise due to direct lung trauma, with the accumulation of blood and fluids within the parenchyma, leading to shunt and hypoxia [15] (Fig. 51.1). Additionally, evidence suggests further injury might be associated with the liberation of lung inflammatory mediators secondary to blunt chest trauma.

Generally speaking, the development of atelectasis, both due to direct pulmonary contusion and pain-related hypoventilation, is a known consequence of blunt thoracic trauma and the most frequent pathophysiology underlying the development of posttraumatic acute respiratory failure [16].

However, in the trauma setting, intubation and mechanical ventilatory support may often be required also due to non-primarily pulmonary critical conditions, such as CNS depression and/or systemic hypoperfusion [17].

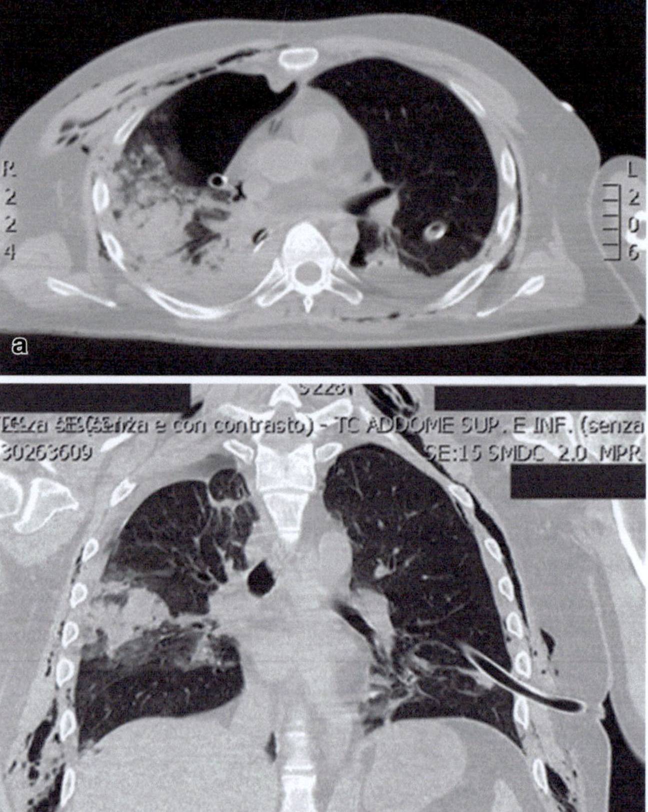

Fig. 51.1 Transverse (**a**) and coronal (**b**) plane views of a computed tomography scan performed in a trauma victim with severe blunt thoracic trauma due to a fall. Bilateral pneumothorax and a significant right lung contusion are visible, with a large subcutaneous emphysema. The patient suffered multiple rib fractures. The left scapula, right clavicle, and the sternum were also fractured (not showed)

51.2 The Choice to Ventilate in the Acute Setting

Once ARF has been identified, the need for ventilatory support might have to be established. Mechanical ventilation does not save lives per se. Its aim is that of assisting (or replacing) lung function until resolution of the underlying disease. The original reason leading to ARF, and then ventilatory support, must, therefore, always be taken into account. Particularly, the prospective consideration of the short-term reversibility of the acute disease might significantly influence the choice of the right support strategy, most importantly the use of noninvasive vs. invasive ventilation.

Clinically, however, the choice to ventilate can rely on the assessment of essentially two broad categories of physiological indicators [18]:

(a) *Clinical assessment of the patient's work of breathing*
(b) *Arterial blood gas analysis*

(a) *Clinical Assessment of the Patient's Work of Breathing*
The clinical presentation of ARF involves the presence of respiratory muscle fatigue. Severe tachypnea (respiratory rate >35/min) is an early sign, due to the increased demand for alveolar ventilation. Bradypnea can follow with the development of exhaustion. The use of accessory inspiratory muscles or abdominal breathing indicates the presence of an excessive respiratory workload.

(b) *Arterial Blood Gas Analysis*
Hypoxemia not responding to supplemental oxygen is a strong indicator for ventilation. The value of PaO_2 must always be normalized to the administered FiO_2 to determine the PaO_2/FiO_2 (*P*/*F*) ratio.
On the other hand, hypercapnia must be evaluated together with a pH assessment, in order to precisely identify the possible presence of a preexisting $PaCO_2$ elevation, chronically compensated by renal bicarbonate retention.
However, generally speaking, a *P*/*F* ratio of 200 and/or a pH <7.2 with a $PaCO_2$ >55 mmHg prompts the implementation of ventilatory support.

51.2.1 The Noninvasive Option

The gold standard for restoring normal gas exchange in ARF is endotracheal intubation and mechanical ventilation. However, in selected cases, a noninvasive ventilatory support strategy might be indicated as the first line of treatment. The aim is to improve gas exchange while avoiding the burden of endotracheal intubation [19].

The term "noninvasive ventilation" (NIV) refers to a broad category of essentially any mode of positive-pressure ventilation which can be delivered without the need for an endotracheal tube. Continuous positive airway pressure (CPAP) alone can also be administered through noninvasive systems. While often grouped together, an important physiologic differentiation between intermittent-positive-pressure NIV and noninvasive CPAP needs to be emphasized. The rationale for the application of mechanical breaths is that of replacing, to a variable extent, the impaired function of respiratory muscles, therefore correcting alveolar hypoventilation. Differently, CPAP is an entirely spontaneous breathing mode, with no mechanical positive-pressure breaths ever being delivered. The only variable set by the operator is the level of PEEP. For this reason, technically, CPAP should not even be classified as a "ventilation" strategy. Patients with *V*/*Q* mismatch, or shunt, due to a decreased volume of the aerated lung (edema or atelectasis), benefit from the alveolar recruitment caused by the continuously increased baseline airway pressure [20].

Thus, as a general rule of thumb, patients with hypercapnic respiratory failure are those most likely to benefit from mechanical NIV, whereas subjects with hypoxemic ARF might not need any more support than that provided by the right PEEP setting with CPAP [21]. The different indication between the two is important, particularly when choosing the best noninvasive interface to be used for a given patient.

The choice to treat a patient noninvasively, before considering endotracheal intubation, is very well supported by the literature in several different clinical scenarios [22]. Both the pathophysiology of the underlying condition and how rapidly that is expected to resolve are the two main factors to be considered.

In the acute setting, probably the most frequent and strongly supported indication for NIV is hypercapnic respiratory failure [23]. Particularly, NIV is the standard of care for COPD patients presenting with an acute exacerbation of their chronic condition [24]. Early NIV administration may prevent endotracheal intubation. In this particular population, whenever feasible, limiting invasiveness is of paramount importance, and the use of NIV significantly impacts clinical outcome [25]. Higher mortality and longer hospital length of stay would be associated with the extremely difficult weaning of COPD patients, should they all be intubated and invasively ventilated. Other acute care settings where NIV has proven beneficial also include (1) ventilatory support in immunocompromised patients, due to the lower risk of nosocomial respiratory tract infections [26], and (2) post-extubation respiratory failure [27].

On the other hand, noninvasive CPAP has become the first-line therapy of choice to treat hypoxemia in cardiogenic pulmonary edema [18, 28]. While the use of face masks is

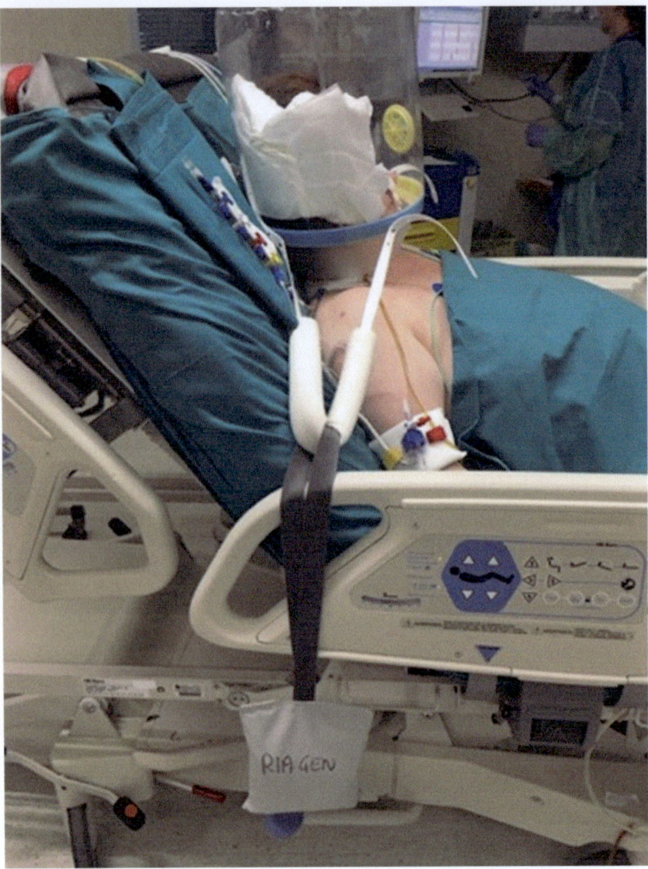

Fig. 51.2 Noninvasive CPAP with a helmet interface in the ICU

the most often reported technique, helmets were shown to be a reliable interface for the noninvasive delivery of CPAP (Fig. 51.2) [29–31]. NIV should be implemented only if hypercapnia is present.

Conversely, there is conflicting evidence supporting the use of noninvasive strategies to correct severe hypoxemia due to pneumonia and acute respiratory distress syndrome (ARDS), with a reported high failure rate. In general, particular attention should be paid to an arterial oxygenation not improving within 1 or 2 h after the introduction of any form of noninvasive support. Compared to the face mask, patients undergoing noninvasive CPAP show an increased tolerance to the helmet interface, thus leading to a longer time of application. The possibility to use any noninvasive modality for a prolonged period is a crucial factor in correctly determining the patient's response [32, 33]. Nonetheless, delaying intubation in these patients and exposing them to an inadequate form of ventilatory assistance might not only be useless but potentially harmful [34].

Additionally, absolute exclusion criteria for the use of noninvasive ventilatory support strategies are (1) the risk of aspiration, (2) complete apnea, (3) hemodynamic instability, (4) lack of cooperation by the patient, and (5) craniofacial injuries or malformations preventing the placement of a noninvasive interface [18].

51.3 Principles of Invasive Ventilatory Support

Patients with severe ARF due to a condition which is not expected to readily resolve require invasive mechanical ventilation following appropriate sedation and endotracheal intubation.

The following section will briefly summarize the main features of invasive ventilatory support. Due to the extremely complex nature of the topic, only the basic principles will be reviewed. The dedicated literature and textbooks of artificial mechanical ventilation should be used as a reference for a more detailed description.

51.3.1 Targets of Mechanical Ventilation

The goals of mechanical ventilation in ARF are (1) to maintain adequate alveolar ventilation and oxygen delivery, (2) to restore acid-base balance, and (3) to reduce WOB. In case of alveolar collapse with loss of lung volume, reinstating and maintaining an adequate lung volume are also a target [35].

The benefits of mechanical ventilation, however, come at a price.

The risk of ventilator-induced lung injury (VILI) demands the adoption of a lung-protective ventilatory strategy. Lung protection during mechanical ventilation consists of four essential principles:

(a) *Low tidal volume (TV)*
(b) *Safe transpulmonary pressure (TPP)*
(c) *Driving pressure <15 cmH$_2$O*
(d) *Appropriate and stable PEEP levels*

(a) *Low Tidal Volume (TV)*

The use of small tidal volumes of 6–8 mL/kg of ideal body weight (IBW) is the mainstay of therapy for protective lung ventilation due to evidence of a significant survival benefit in ARDS patients. However, the concept of lung protection with low TV ventilation is now extended to all ARF patients requiring mechanical ventilation [36].

(b) *Safe Transpulmonary Pressure (TPP)*

TPP is the difference between alveolar and pleural pressure. It represents the actual distending energy applied in the lungs in order to reach alveolar expansion.

Evidence suggests that setting PEEP in order to obtain an end-expiratory TPP greater than 0 [37], and an end-inspiratory TPP below 26 cmH$_2$O [38], may improve gas exchange, respiratory mechanics, and outcome. Clinically, the estimation of pleural pressure can only be obtained measuring the pressure within an esophageal balloon. In postsurgical ARDS patients, an impaired chest wall compliance can influence the pressure-volume relationship during ventilation. This can be detected by an abnormally elevated esophageal pressure (P_{es}). However, routine P_{es} monitoring is currently not widely adopted [39].

Plateau pressure (P_{plat}) is the airway pressure measured at zero flow during an inspiratory hold and the most commonly adopted surrogate of TPP in clinical practice. The bedside assessment of P_{plat} allows the detection of how injurious our ventilatory settings might be due to overdistension. As a general principle, P_{plat} should be maintained as low as possible, with 28 cmH_2O commonly accepted as the upper safety limit, provided a normal chest wall compliance [36].

(c) *Driving Pressure <15 cmH_2O*

Driving pressure (ΔP), calculated as P_{plat}-PEEP, has been recently proposed by Amato et al. as a useful tool for the optimization of protective ventilation in ARDS patients. The ΔP measure is easy to obtain, and, compared to the 6–8 mL/kg tidal volume rule, it might provide the clinician a more accurate index of how appropriately the ventilator is being set for a particular patient. According to the proposed evidence, a value of ΔP 15 cmH_2O or higher is associated with a higher mortality rate [40]. However, further studies are needed in order to establish its definitive clinical relevance.

(d) *Appropriate and Stable PEEP Levels*

PEEP must be set to treat alveolar derecruitment and carefully adjusted in order to avoid the cyclic opening and closing of diseased lung units. No consensus exists on the best strategy for PEEP setting and modulation. However, evidence suggests that, in ARDS patients, a high-PEEP/low-TV ventilation strategy is associated with a reduced mortality rate [41, 42].

51.3.2 Ventilatory Modes

A detailed distinction among the several different available ventilatory modes is further complicated due to the use, by each different manufacturer, of unique brand names, with no official taxonomy available. However, in the following section, we will try to concisely describe a general rule to identify the main features of the most often used modes of mechanical ventilation [18].

Whenever trying to understand the features of every ventilatory mode, three main variables must be taken into account (Table 51.1):

1. *Trigger*: how the ventilator determines when a breath is initiated (time vs. patient)
2. *Control variable*: what aspect of inspiration is primarily controlled by the ventilator at inspiration (pressure vs. flow)
3. *Cycling*: what signals the ventilator to terminate inspiration and start expiration (time, volume, or flow)

Broadly speaking, a ventilator can be set to deliver either full respiratory support, whenever the whole energy needed to ensure alveolar ventilation is provided by the machine, or partial respiratory support, in case only a fraction of the WOB is supplied by the ventilator. Full respiratory support generally implies either [1] the complete absence of patient's triggering (e.g., general anesthesia, CNS disorders) or [2] a severe disease, whose management might be eased by the absence of spontaneous breathing, obtained through deep sedation, with or without muscle paralysis.

51.3.2.1 Continuous Mandatory Ventilation (CMV)

Both pressure-controlled and volume-controlled continuous mandatory ventilation modes allow for the complete support of ventilation, with total respiratory muscle rest. This is the most often selected mode for the initiation of ventilatory support. Sedation is often necessary, and care should be

Table 51.1 Trigger control variable and cycling features of the most frequently adopted ventilatory modes

Ventilator/Mode	Trigger	Control variable	Cycling
Continuous Mandatory Ventilation (CMV)			
Volume-Controlled (CMV-VC)	Time	Flow	Time
Pressure-Controlled (CMV-PC)		Pressure	
Assist/Control Ventilation (A/C)			
Volume-Controlled (A/C-VC)	Time or Patient	Flow	Time
Pressure Controlled (A/C-PC)		Pressure	
Synchronized Intermittent Mandatory Ventilation (SIMV)			
Mandatory breaths	Time	Flow (SIMV-VC) or	Time
Synchronized breaths	Patient	Pressure (SIMV-PC)	
Spontaneous breaths	Patient	Pressure	Flow
Pressure Support Ventilation	Patient	Pressure	Flow

directed at avoiding barotrauma, or low MV, in volumetric or pressometric modes, respectively.

51.3.2.2 Assist/Control Ventilation (ACV)

Assist/control ventilation has a mix of mandatory and fully supported assisted breaths. A baseline respiratory rate is set, but all breaths, once triggered, are equally controlled, either by volume or pressure. The patient can still set his or her own respiratory rate, while allowing, at the same time, to provide respiratory muscle rest and adequate ventilatory support for most clinical indications.

51.3.2.3 Synchronized Intermittent Mandatory Ventilation (SIMV)

A mix of mandatory and assisted breaths, some of which are synchronized with spontaneous breaths. It might be used as a mean of providing partial or full ventilatory support. Disadvantages include the potential development of respiratory muscle dysfunction and delayed weaning.

51.3.2.4 Pressure Support Ventilation (PSV)

In PSV, no mandatory breaths are delivered by the ventilator. Every breath is triggered by the patients. Probably the most comfortable mode for the awake, conscious patient. However, minimum minute volume ventilation is not guaranteed. PSV is typically initiated upon resolution of the early acute phase of ARF.

51.3.3 Adverse Effects of Invasive Ventilatory Support

Complications of mechanical ventilation include a wide array of adverse conditions, among the most frequent:

(a) *Ventilator-induced lung injury*
(b) *Ventilator-associated pneumonia (VAP)*
(c) *Hemodynamic instability*
(d) *Ventilator-induced diaphragmatic dysfunction (VIDD)*

(a) *Ventilator-Induced Lung Injury*

Barotrauma

Pneumothorax or pneumomediastinum may arise due to excessive alveolar pressure during mechanical ventilation, particularly in ARDS patients. Attention must be paid to monitoring peak (<45 cmH_2O) and, more importantly, plateau airway pressures that should be kept <30 cmH_2O [43].

Volutrauma

ARDS infiltrates typically present as consolidated lung areas interposed with healthy normal parenchyma. The very low compliance of more diseased units leads to overdistention of the remaining lung whenever positive-pressure ventilation is initiated. Alveolar inflammation may follow. The concept of lung-protective ventilation was developed to prevent overdistention of the healthy lung parenchyma [44].

(b) *Ventilator-Associated Pneumonia (VAP)*

Ventilator-associated pneumonia (VAP) is one of the most frequent hospital-acquired infections occurring in intubated patients. It is defined as a lung parenchyma infection developing within 48 h from endotracheal intubation. VAP is associated with higher mortality, morbidity, and costs [45].

(c) *Hemodynamic Instability*

Positive-pressure ventilation affects preload, afterload, and ventricular compliance. The net effect in most situations is a decrease in cardiac output [46].

(d) *Ventilator-Induced Diaphragmatic Dysfunction (VIDD)*

The diaphragm is the main inspiratory muscle. A preserved diaphragmatic function is an essential requirement for the liberation of patients from mechanical ventilation. Evidence suggests that a prolonged time of ventilation leads to a significant reduction of diaphragmatic force-generating capacity, together with structural injury and muscle atrophy. In recent years, significant progress has been made in the identification of the pathophysiology underlying diaphragmatic dysfunction [47]. This led to an increased awareness of the fact that mechanical ventilation by itself, while lifesaving, causes severe weakness of the one inspiratory muscle which might allow for the patient to be eventually weaned from it. VIDD is associated with worse outcomes, including a higher mortality rate [48].

51.4 Extracorporeal Membrane Oxygenation (ECMO)

In case of refractory impairment of gas exchange despite an optimized ventilatory strategy, extracorporeal membrane oxygenation (ECMO) represents the only possibility to rescue patients with otherwise fatal respiratory failure [49, 50].

ECMO is a lifesaving technique in which patient's venous blood is drained toward an artificial gas exchanger, through which it is oxygenated and decarboxylated. Arterialized blood can then be returned to the patient. Blood can be reinfused either to the arterial (veno-arterial ECMO) or to the venous circulation (veno-venous ECMO). Nowadays veno-arterial ECMO (VA-ECMO) is applied mainly for circulatory support, since it can replace both the heart and lung functions, whereas veno-venous ECMO (VV-ECMO) usually is the technique of choice for the sole purpose of respiratory support [51].

The first reported successful use of ECMO in a trauma patient was performed by Hill in 1972 [52]. More recently, VV-ECMO has become a treatment option to restore adequate oxygenation, allow protective ventilation, and reduce the risk of multiorgan failure in posttraumatic ARDS patients [53].

In general, according to the Extracorporeal Life Support Organization (ELSO) guidelines, there are no absolute contraindications to ECMO [54]. Each patient should be considered individually with respect to risks and benefits. However, the ELSO guidelines highlight some conditions associated with poor outcome, even if ECMO is initiated, particularly:

(a) Mechanical ventilation with maximal oxygen requirement and injurious airway pressure (FiO_2 >0.9, P_{plat} >30 cmH_2O) for 7 days or more
(b) Significant immunosuppression (absolute neutrophil count <400/mm^3)
(c) Not recoverable comorbidity (e.g., major CNS damage or terminal malignancy)
(d) Cerebral hemorrhage that is recent or expanding

Age is not an absolute contraindication; however, the risk of both treatment failure and complications increases.

In the trauma population, no specific guidelines are currently available. Thus, ECMO may be considered for pulmonary injuries not responding to mechanical ventilation. Particularly, VV-ECMO can be a very attractive option in patients with associated stable non-evolving traumatic brain injury, where the brain damage would be worsened by the elevated intrathoracic pressure and permissive hypercapnia, which might be needed in case of concomitant posttraumatic ARDS. However, ECMO should be considered only after a careful risk-benefit assessment, due to the need of anticoagulation and the subsequent hazards of a pro-hemorrhagic status, particularly in the trauma setting. A section dedicated to the management of coagulation during ECMO has been added accordingly.

Technical and physiological aspects of VV-ECMO as well as the current management of mechanical ventilation while on ECMO will be discussed here. A brief review of the complications associated with this extracorporeal treatment is also proposed. A representative image of a typical VV-ECMO setup in adult patients is provided in Fig. 51.3.

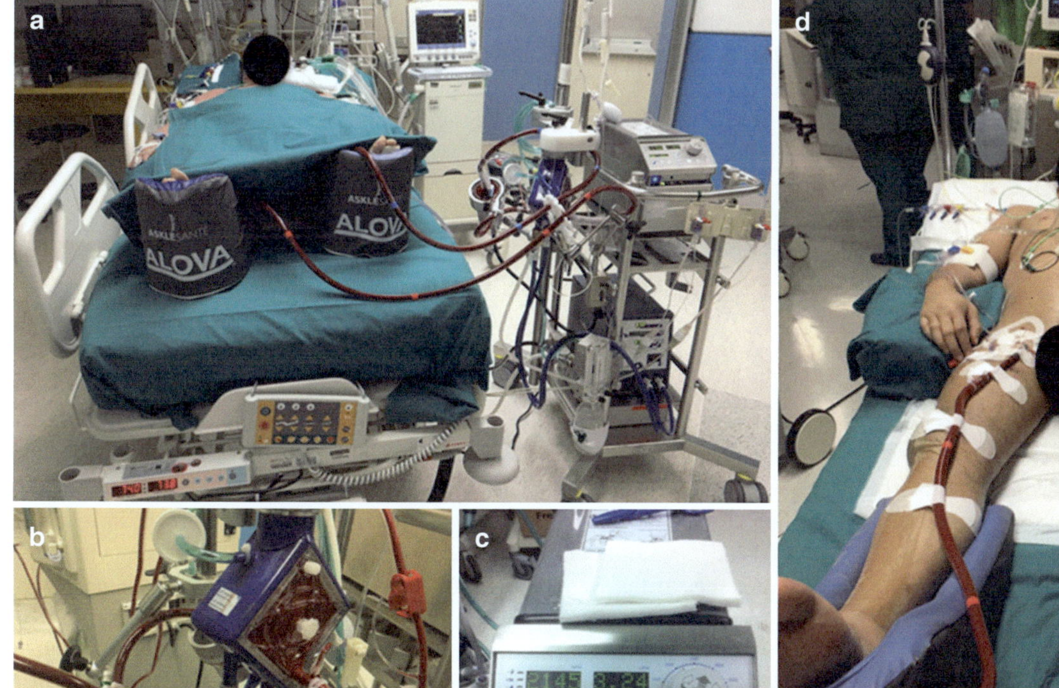

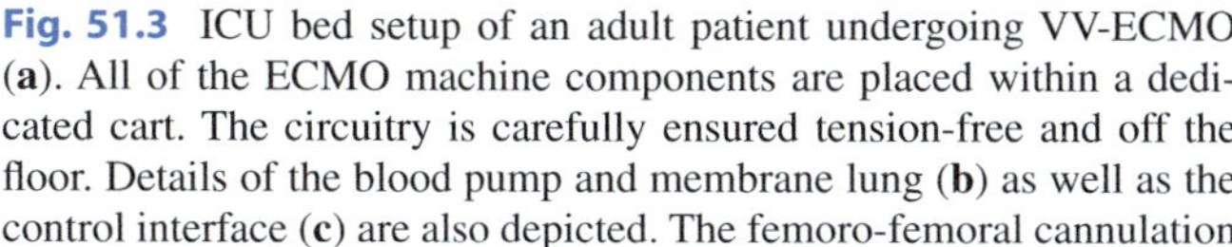

Fig. 51.3 ICU bed setup of an adult patient undergoing VV-ECMO (**a**). All of the ECMO machine components are placed within a dedicated cart. The circuitry is carefully ensured tension-free and off the floor. Details of the blood pump and membrane lung (**b**) as well as the control interface (**c**) are also depicted. The femoro-femoral cannulation approach (**d**) is often adopted. The reinfusion cannula (red marks) can be identified, carrying highly oxygenated blood pumped through the membrane lung from the drainage cannula (blue marks). Highly skilled and extensively trained ICU staff is required in order to provide a safe and effective care in such context

51.4.1 Technical Aspects

The VV-ECMO circuit mainly consists of a drainage venous cannula; a blood pump (BP); an oxygenator called membrane lung (ML), connected to a source of air and oxygen through a blender; and a return cannula, reinfusing artificially oxygenated blood back into the patient's venous system.

The first step to perform ECMO is to obtain adequate vascular access. Percutaneous cannulation is preferred to surgical cannulation in almost all cases, mostly because it requires a shorter time to be performed, while being safer in terms of bleeding, infection, and risk of decannulation. Cannulas can be placed in femoral veins, jugular veins, and, less frequently, subclavian veins. A few different approaches have been described in the literature to perform VV-ECMO support. The most frequently adopted are (1) the femoro-femoral approach, (2) the femoral-jugular approach, and (3) the single vessel approach, with the use of a double-lumen cannula (Avalon Elite®, Maquet, Rastatt, Germany) [55–60].

The position of the cannulas within the vena cava is crucial, due to the possibility of blood recirculation, which clearly reduces the performance of the ECMO system, mostly in terms of oxygenation. In case the femoro-femoral approach is adopted, the tip of the drainage cannula should be placed at the level of L1-L2 vertebrae, while the reinfusion cannula should be placed at the cavo-atrial junction. With a femoral-jugular approach, the risk of blood recirculation still exists, but it is certainly lower. The femoral drainage cannula should be positioned, again, at the L1-L2 level, while the reinfusion cannula, entering the internal jugular vein, should be positioned proximal to the right atrium. The double-lumen cannula allows for both drainage and reinfusion through the same jugular vein. In this case, the cannula must be positioned through the right atrium, with the distal tip of the cannula (drainage) opening into the inferior vena cava, while reinfusion is guaranteed through a second separate lumen opening into the right atrium, at the level of the tricuspid valve [61–63]. Ultrasound and fluoroscopy are generally required at the bedside during the cannulation process, in order to facilitate correct positioning.

Another extremely important technical aspect of cannulation is the choice of cannula's size. A small-sized cannula might lead to insufficient oxygenation capabilities of the extracorporeal system. On the other hand, a careful assessment of the vein diameter should be conducted to limit the likelihood of complications at cannulation. A preliminary ultrasound study of available vascular access might help the clinician to choose the most appropriate and safe diameter.

51.4.2 Physiology of VV-ECMO

VV-ECMO is indicated mainly when the natural lung cannot ensure adequate oxygenation, even after optimization of ventilation at 100% FiO_2. At the same time, carbon dioxide (CO_2) is removed by the membrane lung. However, oxygen delivery and carbon dioxide removal are two very distinct features of VV-ECMO [17]. Simply put, oxygenation mainly relies on the amount of blood flowing through the membrane lung and the machine FiO_2, whereas the total sweep gas flow rate determines blood decarboxylation. Adequate CO_2 removal is much easier to achieve than oxygenation. The whole CO_2 excess produced by a critically ill-sedated patient can be completely removed by VV-ECMO, even with a low flow of blood passing through the membrane lung (1–1.5 L/min). On the other hand, for the same subject, adequate oxygen delivery requires a higher ECMO blood flow (3–5 L/min). Several less invasive low-flow devices are available to achieve extracorporeal CO_2 removal. However, high-flow ECMO remains the only available support for extracorporeal oxygenation.

During VV-ECMO, deoxygenated blood from the tissues is drained by the negative pressure generated by the blood pump. Transfer of oxygen through the artificial lung is determined by the partial pressure gradient of oxygen and significantly influenced by the extracorporeal blood flow. Blood oxygenated by the artificial lung returns to the right heart, thus mixing with deoxygenated venous blood coming from the periphery. Essentially, VV-ECMO improves arterial oxygenation increasing the oxygen content of mixed venous blood.

VV-ECMO is an in-series circuit with the normal circulation. For this reason, besides the respective performances of the natural and the artificial lung, oxygen delivery and CO_2 removal are strictly influenced by the cardiac output of the patient. Patient undergoing VV-ECMO support should maintain an adequate cardiac output (CO) to ensure adequate oxygen delivery. VV-ECMO does not directly affect hemodynamics. Elevated pulmonary vascular resistances, which are often present in ARDS, on the other hand, can benefit from the well-oxygenated blood entering in the pulmonary circulation, partially reducing hypoxic vasoconstriction. What needs to be clear is that VV-ECMO does not provide any form of circulatory support of a worsening of cardiac function. In such cases, the potential benefit of setting up (or converting to) VA-ECMO should be considered.

The use of VA-ECMO in ARDS, although not strictly contraindicated, prompts consideration of two potentially relevant side effects, which can be spared by the use of VV-ECMO:

(a) Limb ischemia on the side of arterial femoral cannulation. The positioning of a small reperfusion cannula distal to the femoral artery cannulation point is often required.

(b) *Harlequin syndrome*, i.e., hypoxia of the upper body due to the preserved function of the natural heart pumping deoxygenated blood through the aortic arch [64].

51.4.3 Mechanical Ventilation During VV-ECMO

No consensus exists about the optimal ventilation strategy for a patient undergoing VV-ECMO. However, like for every patient with ARDS, the aim of mechanical ventilation is to support respiratory function while treating the underlying disease, possibly causing the least possible harm to the patient's lung. Therefore, the general indications regarding the use of protective lung ventilation also apply. In practice, referral to an ECMO center is usually considered whenever the patient's pulmonary function is so compromised that adequate gas exchange cannot be achieved with the support of mechanical ventilation only. The patient keeps deteriorating with positive ventilatory pressures often already beyond the upper safety limits. In this context, once on ECMO, the need for the natural lung to provide for gas exchange is reduced, potentially even up to complete lung bypass. The lungs can be unburdened, thus minimizing VILI [65, 66]. A lung-protective strategy with low tidal volumes and high PEEP was shown to decrease mortality in ARDS patients [67, 68]. However, according to a recent survey, ventilation practices on ECMO widely vary among different centers [69]. Most likely, the lack of compelling evidence leads clinicians to base decisions about how to ventilate an ECMO patient based on experience and institutional habits. The ELSO guidelines themselves leave this decision to the individual ECMO center [54].

Once the patient is cannulated and on ECMO, the FiO_2 should be reduced to <0.4, and ventilator settings should lead to a P_{plat} <25 cmH_2O and TV reduced to 6 mL/kg or less with a respiratory rate around 10 bpm. Patients can be heavily sedated during the first 24–48 h, and pCO_2 should be corrected with great caution. Extubation, or early tracheostomy, should be pursued if feasible. Jenks et al. showed, in an international survey, that extubation practices are increasing among ECMO centers, with 27% of patients being extubated while on ECMO in pediatric hospitals, 41% in adult-pediatric mixed centers, and 52% in adult hospitals.

51.4.4 Management of Coagulation During VV-ECMO

The continuous contact between the blood and the surface biomaterials the ECMO circuit is made of inevitably results in an inflammatory and coagulation response, thereby increasing the risk of bleeding and thrombotic complications [70, 71]. Significant progress on the biocompatibility of ECMO components has been made by manufacturers. Nevertheless, the management and monitoring of coagulation still are a cornerstone of treatment in ECMO patients. Their hemostatic balance is shifted toward a hypercoagulable state, determining an increased risk of thrombosis. On the other hand, the necessary antithrombotic therapy can cause bleeding. In other words, platelets and the coagulation cascade should be inhibited enough to reduce the risk of clot formation while patient should maintain an effective coagulation capacity, in order to avoid bleeding.

In ECMO candidates, a baseline coagulation laboratory workup is obtained, namely, complete blood count (CBC), prothrombin time (PT)/international normalized ratio (INR), activated partial thromboplastin time (aPTT), fibrinogen, D-dimer, activated clotting time (ACT), antithrombin III (ATIII), and thromboelastography (TEG). Preexisting significant coagulopathy should be corrected by administering blood components (fresh frozen plasma, platelets, cryoprecipitate, etc.) and/or vitamin K.

Unfractionated heparin (UFH) is the antithrombotic agent most widely used during ECMO. UFH is given as a bolus (50–100 units per kilogram) at the time of cannulation and by continuous infusion (10 units of heparin per kilogram per hour) during ECMO. UFH infusion dosage should be titrated with regular ACT monitoring. ACT should be maintained 1.5 times higher than the baseline value. APTT is another useful test to monitor coagulation. However, since multiple variables influence the coagulation cascade in ECMO patients, no indication about a standard UFH dose currently exists.

In our experience, TEG is a useful bedside test to discriminate the several different possible coagulation derangements. A "flat line" on the kaolin-activated TEG test, associated with a normal kaolin + heparinase TEG, should be avoided, prompting a decrease in UFH infusion. ATIII concentration is also very important during ECMO support. Heparin acts, in fact, by activating ATIII. In case of low ATIII levels, clotting occurs even while a high dose of heparin is being administered. Thus, ATIII should be maintained in the normal range (80–120% of control). If inadequate, ATIII can be supplied by transfusing fresh frozen plasma or by ATIII concentrate. Concomitantly, the platelet count should be maintained higher than $80{,}000 \times 10^6$/L, transfusing platelets if needed [54].

51.4.5 Complication, Morbidity, and Mortality During VV-ECMO

As of today, the ECMO treatment still shows a significant rate of complications. That is due to its technical complexity and the severity of the conditions of patients for whom it becomes the only lifesaving opportunity. Although complications associated with VV-ECMO are common (40% of patients), a small impact has been reported on overall mortality, accounting for only 7% of fatal outcome cases [72]. Bleeding has always been considered the most significant risk during ECMO, potentially impacting mortality. Intracerebral hemorrhage is always a particular concern for ICU physicians involved with ECMO support. However, a recent meta-analysis showed that, while frequent (30% of complications), the overall mortality attributable to bleeding events is actually low (3.3%) [64].

Additional reported ECMO complications are (1) pneumothorax, related to cannulation, (2) limb ischemia (VA-ECMO), (3) diffuse intravascular coagulopathy, (4) heparin-induced thrombocytopenia, (5) intravascular hemolysis, (6) deep venous thrombosis, (7) pulmonary embolism, and (8) bloodstream infection. The possibility of complications associated with the ECMO circuit must also be carefully considered (e.g., clot formation, thrombotic or gas embolism) [29, 66, 73–77].

The estimation of overall mortality rates in patients undergoing ECMO treatment must always be carefully considered. VA- and VV-ECMO are often pooled together, like in a recent analysis reporting a 35–40% overall mortality rate [78]. However, mortality in patients with VA-ECMO is often higher due to the possibility of an underlying cardiac nonreversible illness. Mortality up to 60–80% is reported in adult patients treated with VA-ECMO for a refractory post-cardiotomy cardiogenic shock [79]. Conversely, the mortality rate was 20–30% in a recent study analyzing patients treated with VV-ECMO for respiratory failure [80]. Due to difficulties in appropriately selecting ECMO candidates, the severity and evolving character of the disease, the complexity of the technique, and the associated risks and costs, it is preferable for ECMO to be implemented only in a limited number of highly specialized referral centers.

Case Scenario

Part 1

R.F., male, 33 years old, 75 kg, 180 cm, is taken to the emergency department after suffering a high-speed motorcycle accident. He was intubated with a 7.5 mm tube at the scene for hypoxemia and Glasgow Coma Scale 7. Vital signs at admission were heart rate 130 bpm, blood pressure 90/50 mmHg, and O_2 saturation 99% at 100% O_2. The CT scan showed multiple rib fractures, with a 1 cm right anterior-superior pneumothorax and a right lower lobe contusion. The patient also suffered (1) a severe head trauma, as confirmed by CT evidence of areas of subarachnoid hemorrhage within the right frontal lobe and Sylvian fissure; (2) abdominal trauma, with a 3 cm subcapsular inactive hepatic hematoma; and (3) an unstable pelvic ring fracture with arterial blushing at contrast CT. Therefore, the patient required a combined emergent procedure including superselective transcatheter iliac embolization and temporary pelvic stabilization by means of an external fixator. A cerebral intraparenchymal fiberoptic catheter was also placed for intracranial pressure monitoring (first value: 8 mmHg). He was then admitted to the ICU postoperatively. Due to the altered mental status, the lung contusions, and the potentially evolving hemorrhagic lesions, the patient stayed intubated and mechanically ventilated. At day 3, the patient develops a 39 °C fever with purulent sputum, and the *P*/*F* ratio drops from 280 to 120. A chest X-ray shows worsening infiltrates, while the most recent laboratory results report white blood cell count of 16×10^9/L.

Questions

1. What is the most likely diagnosis leading to respiratory failure?
   A. Posttraumatic ventilator-associated pneumonia and moderate ARDS
   B. Septic shock
   C. Diffuse axonal injury
2. How would you manage the patient in the ICU?
   A. Seek transfer to a neuro-ICU for the management of intracranial bleeding.
   B. Early extubation and noninvasive ventilation.
   C. Continued mechanical ventilation, microbial cultures, antibiotics, sedation, advance hemodynamic monitoring, vasopressors if needed.
3. Which would be the most appropriate ventilatory settings?
   A. PS 8 cmH_2O, PEEP 10 cmH_2O, FiO_2 0.8
   B. CMV-VC at 6 mL/kg tidal volume, RR 22/min, PEEP 15 cmH_2O, FiO_2 0.5
   C. CMV-PC at 10 mL/kg tidal volume and RR 30/min (to prevent hypercapnia), PEEP 5, FiO_2 0.3

Comments to Case Scenario: Part 1

The patient likely developed an early-onset ventilator-associated pneumonia over the highly predisposing substrate of a severely traumatized lung parenchyma. Moderate acute respiratory distress syndrome (ARDS) is developing due to both trauma and the overlying infection.

Empirical antibiotic therapy is readily started, awaiting the results of bacterial cultures for a possible microbiological diagnosis of the likely causative agent. Meanwhile, the ventilator is initially set in order to deliver a 450 mL tidal volume (TV), approximately 6 mL/kg, in a volume-controlled continuous mandatory mode. A positive end-expiratory pressure (PEEP) of 15 cmH_2O is selected, based on an improved oxygenation (*P*/*F*: 180) and the evidence of a respiratory system compliance allowing a plateau pressure (P_{plat}) of 25 cmH_2O. The resulting driving pressure (ΔP) is 10 cmH_2O. Respiratory rate (RR) is set at 22–24 bpm, leading to a $PaCO_2$ of 44 mmHg with a 7.35 pH. The intracranial pressure (ICP) constantly stays in a safe range (<15 mmHg). Slight hypercapnia may be allowed, in order to persevere with the protective ventilation, provided no ICP increments are seen. The hemodynamic status may be an issue. The necessarily increased intrathoracic pressure may cause hypotension in a subject who likely suffered a recent significant posttraumatic hemorrhage. Concomitant hypoxic pulmonary vasoconstriction may also arise. Advanced hemodynamic monitoring with a pulmonary artery catheter is implemented, revealing a slight mean pulmonary artery pressure elevation (28 mmHg), with a wedge pressure constantly lower than 15 mmHg. Volume infusion and/or vasoactive drugs may be deemed necessary. Intravenous sedation and analgesia are continued, together with the administration of a muscle relaxant.

Part 2

Through the following days, a progressive worsening of oxygenation, lung mechanics, and imaging is observed, leading to a critical *P*/*F* value of 80. Protective ventilation settings cannot be effectively maintained anymore at day 6. ΔP increases to 17 cmH_2O, for a P_{plat} of 32 cmH_2O. Diffuse consolidation can be seen on the chest X-ray. No response to recruitment maneuvers and increasing PEEP levels can be observed. Arterial pH progressively decreases, alongside a $PaCO_2$ >50 mmHg.

1. What's the most likely mechanism underlying the patient's conditions?
   A. ARDS worsening with refractory impairment of gas exchange and impossibility to effectively maintain protective ventilatory settings
   B. Hemorrhage from an uncontrolled traumatic bleeding source
   C. Multiorgan failure due to shock and systemic hypoperfusion
2. Were VV-ECMO started, how would you set the ventilator?
   A. PS 15 cmH_2O, PEEP 5 cmH_2O.
   B. A ventilator is not needed; the membrane lung takes care of gas exchange.
   C. CMV-VC 380 mL, RR 10/min, PEEP 13 cmH_2O.
3. During VV-ECMO support, which anticoagulation strategy would you use, and how would you monitor its appropriateness?
   A. Unfractionated intravenous heparin (bolus 50/kg at cannulation, infusion 100/kg/h) may be even considering slightly reduced dosages due to the history of traumatic hemorrhage. ACT, aPTT, ATIII, platelet count, TEG.
   B. Oral anticoagulants with daily INR monitoring.
   C. I would use no anticoagulation in the trauma setting, thus only monitoring D-dimer and signs of clotting within the ECMO circuit.

<u>Comments to Case Scenario: Part 2</u>

High-flow (4 L/min) VV-ECMO is started after bilateral percutaneous cannulation of the femoral veins. Ventilator settings are subsequently modified as follows: TV 280 mL, RR 10/min, and PEEP 13 cmH_2O. The ΔP and a P_{plat} dropped to 10 and 23 cmH_2O, respectively. The ABG analysis shows a *P*/*F* of 160, a $PaCO_2$ of 38 mmHg, and a pH of 7.3.

As this example of multiple traumatic injuries (including the brain, abdominal, and pelvic lesions) clearly represents, extreme caution must be taken while considering the pros and cons of ECMO. Particular care should be directed toward the risks of systemic anticoagulation. A small bolus of UFH 2000 UI at cannulation is administered. A continuous maintenance infusion of UFH 700 UI/h plus antithrombin III (ATIII) 1000 UI/day is also planned. The resulting aPTT ratio is 1.3. ATIII is 90%. Thromboelastography is performed, clearly showing heparin-associated anticoagulation: R-time is 2.5-fold increased at the kaolin-activated test, whereas a normal value results if the sample is mixed with a heparinase-containing solution. Blood clotting within the circuitry, elevated D-dimer, and/or an impaired artificial lung function are signs to be closely monitored in order to avoid ECMO-related thrombotic complications.

The patient eventually recovered. After 12 days of ECMO, he was successfully disconnected from the extracorporeal support and decannulated. Weaning from mechanical ventilation was completed at day 35, and the patient was extubated. Due to the need of NIV post-extubation and some degree of cognitive impairment due to brain injury, the patient was discharged to the ward a week later, after a total of 42 ICU days.

Please see Chap. 58 for the correct answer.

References

1. Vasilyev S, Schaap RN, Mortensen JD. Hospital survival rates of patients with acute respiratory failure in modern respiratory intensive care units. An international, multicenter, prospective survey. Chest J. 1995;107(4):1083–8.
2. West JB. Respiratory physiology—the essentials. 8th ed. Philadelphia: Lippincott Williams & Wilkins; 2008.
3. Campbell EJ. Respiratory failure. Br Med J. 1965;1(5448):1451–60.
4. American Thoracic Society. Idiopathic pulmonary fibrosis: diagnosis and treatment. International consensus statement. American Thoracic Society (ATS), and the European Respiratory Society (ERS). Am J Respir Crit Care Med. 2000;161(2 Pt 1):646–64.
5. Greene KE, Peters JI. Pathophysiology of acute respiratory failure. Clin Chest Med. 1994;15(1):1–12.
6. Nunn JF. Nunns applied respiratory physiology. 4th ed. Woburn, MA: Butterworth-Heinemann Medical; 1993.
7. Caruana-Montaldo B, Gleeson K, Zwillich CW. The control of breathing in clinical practice. Chest J. 2000;117(1):205–25.
8. Howell BN, Newman DS. Dysfunction of central control of breathing in amyotrophic lateral sclerosis. Muscle Nerve. 2017;56(2):197–201.
9. Orlikowski D, Prigent H, Sharshar T, Lofaso F, Raphael JC. Respiratory dysfunction in Guillain-Barré syndrome. Neurocrit Care. 2004;1(4):415–22.
10. Blichfeldt-Lauridsen L, Hansen BD. Anesthesia and myasthenia gravis. Acta Anaesthesiol Scand. 2012;56(1):17–22.
11. Bach J, Goncalves M, Chiou M, Hart N, Toussaint M. Noninvasive respiratory care received by individuals with duchenne muscular dystrophy since 1979. Respir Care. 2017;62(8):1120–1.
12. Aboussouan LS. Respiratory disorders in neurologic diseases. Cleve Clin J Med. 2005;72(6):511–20.
13. Battle C, Hutchings H, Lovett S, Bouamra O, Jones S, Sen A, et al. Predicting outcomes after blunt chest wall trauma: development and external validation of a new prognostic model. Crit Care. 2014;18(3):R98.
14. Centers for Disease Control and P. FastStats: accidents or unintentional injuries. FastStats: Accidents or unintentional injuries; 2017.
15. Ziegler DW, Agarwal NN. The morbidity and mortality of rib fractures. J Trauma. 1994;37(6):975–9.
16. Simon B, Ebert J, Bokhari F, Capella J, Emhoff T, Hayward T, et al. Management of pulmonary contusion and flail chest: an Eastern Association for the Surgery of Trauma practice management guideline. J Trauma Acute Care Surg. 2012;73(5 Suppl 4):61.
17. Karmy-Jones R, Jurkovich GJ, Shatz DV, Brundage S, Wall MJ, Engelhardt S, et al. Management of traumatic lung injury: a Western Trauma Association Multicenter review. J Trauma. 2001;51(6):1049–53.
18. Kacmarek RM, Stoller JK, Heuer A. Egan's fundamentals of respiratory care-E-Book. 11th ed. Philadelphia: Elseiver; 2016.
19. Organized jointly by the American Thoracic Society the European Respiratory Society, the European Society of Intensive Care Medicine Sociétè de Rèanimation de Langue Française, and approved by ATS Board of Directors, December 2000, editors. International Consensus Conferences in Intensive Care Medicine: noninvasive positive pressure ventilation in acute Respiratory failure. Am J Respir Crit Care Med. 2001;163(1):283–91.
20. Tobin MJ. Principles and practice of mechanical ventilation. New York: McGraw-Hill; 2006.
21. Mehta S, Hill NS. Noninvasive ventilation. Am J Respir Crit Care Med. 2001;163(2):540–77.
22. Garpestad E, Brennan J, Hill NS. Noninvasive ventilation for critical care. Chest J. 2007;132(2):711–20.
23. Lightowler JV, Wedzicha JA, Elliott MW, Ram FSF. Noninvasive positive pressure ventilation to treat respiratory failure resulting from exacerbations of chronic obstructive pulmonary disease: cochrane systematic review and meta-analysis. BMJ. 2003;326(7382):185.
24. Brochard L, Mancebo J, Wysocki M, Lofaso F, Conti G, Rauss A, et al. Noninvasive ventilation for acute exacerbations of chronic obstructive pulmonary disease. N Engl J Med. 1995;333(13):817–22.
25. Osadnik CR, Tee VS. Non-invasive ventilation for the management of acute hypercapnic respiratory failure due to exacerbation of chronic obstructive pulmonary disease. Cochrane Database Syst Rev. 2017;(7):CD004104.
26. Huang HB, Xu B, Liu GY, Lin JD, Du B. Use of noninvasive ventilation in immunocompromised patients with acute respiratory failure: a systematic review and meta-analysis. Crit Care. 2017;21:4.
27. Ferrer M, Valencia M, Nicolas JM, Bernadich O, Badia JR, Torres A. Early noninvasive ventilation averts extubation failure in patients at risk: a randomized trial. Am J Respir Crit Care Med. 2006;173(2):164–70.
28. Bersten AD, Holt AW, Vedig AE, Skowronski GA, Baggoley CJ. Treatment of severe cardiogenic pulmonary edema with continuous positive airway pressure delivered by face mask. N Engl J Med. 1991;325(26):1825–30.
29. Patroniti N, Zangrillo A, Pappalardo F, Peris A, Cianchi G, Braschi A, et al. The Italian ECMO network experience during the 2009 influenza A(H1N1) pandemic: preparation for severe respiratory emergency outbreaks. Intensive Care Med. 2011;37(9):1447–57.
30. Chiumello D, Pelosi P, Carlesso E, Severgnini P, Aspesi M, Gamberoni C, et al. Noninvasive positive pressure ventilation delivered by helmet vs. standard face mask. Intensive Care Med. 2003;29(10):1671–9.
31. Bellani G, Patroniti N, Greco M, Foti G, Pesenti A. The use of helmets to deliver non-invasive continuous positive airway pressure in hypoxemic acute respiratory failure. Minerva Anestesiol. 2008;74(11):651–6.
32. Principi T, Pantanetti S, Catani F, Elisei D, Gabbanelli V, Pelaia P, et al. Noninvasive continuous positive airway pressure delivered by helmet in hematological malignancy patients with hypoxemic acute respiratory failure. Intensive Care Med. 2004;30(1):147–50.
33. Patel BK, Wolfe KS, Pohlman AS, Hall JB, Kress JP. Effect of noninvasive ventilation delivered by helmet vs face mask on the rate of endotracheal intubation in patients with acute respiratory distress syndrome: a randomized clinical trial. JAMA. 2016;315(22):2435–41.
34. Brochard L, Slutsky A, Pesenti A. Mechanical ventilation to minimize progression of lung injury in acute respiratory failure. Am J Respir Crit Care Med. 2017;195(4):438–42.
35. Hess RD, Kacmarek RM. Essentials of mechanical ventilation. New York: McGraw-Hill; 2003.
36. Acute Respiratory Distress Syndrome Network, Brower RG, Matthay MA, Morris A, Schoenfeld D, Thompson BT, et al. Ventilation with lower tidal volumes as compared with traditional tidal volumes for acute lung injury and the acute respiratory distress syndrome. N Engl J Med. 2000;342(18):1301–8.
37. Talmor D, Sarge T, Malhotra A, O'Donnell CR, Ritz R, Lisbon A, et al. Mechanical ventilation guided by esophageal pressure in acute lung injury. N Engl J Med. 2008;359(20):2095–104.
38. Grasso S, Mascia L, Del Turco M, Malacarne P, Giunta F, Brochard L, et al. Effects of recruiting maneuvers in patients with acute respiratory distress syndrome ventilated with protective ventilatory strategy. Anesthesiology. 2002;96(4):795–802.

39. Akoumianaki E, Maggiore SM, Valenza F, Bellani G, Jubran A, Loring SH, et al. The application of esophageal pressure measurement in patients with respiratory failure. Am J Respir Crit Care Med. 2014;189(5):520–31.
40. Amato MBP, Meade MO, Slutsky AS, Brochard L, Costa ELV, Schoenfeld DA, et al. Driving pressure and survival in the acute respiratory distress syndrome. N Engl J Med. 2015;372(8):747–55.
41. Briel M, Meade M, Mercat A, Brower RG, Talmor D, Walter SD, et al. Higher vs lower positive end-expiratory pressure in patients with acute lung injury and acute respiratory distress syndrome: systematic review and meta-analysis. JAMA. 2010;303(9):865–73.
42. Fan E, Del Sorbo L, Goligher EC, Hodgson CL, Munshi L, Walkey AJ, et al. An Official American Thoracic Society/European Society of Intensive Care Medicine/Society of Critical Care Medicine Clinical Practice Guideline: mechanical ventilation in adult patients with acute respiratory distress syndrome. Am J Respir Crit Care Med. 2017;195(9):1253–63.
43. Anzueto A, Frutos-Vivar F, Esteban A, Alía I, Brochard L, Stewart T, et al. Incidence, risk factors and outcome of barotrauma in mechanically ventilated patients. Intensive Care Med. 2004;30(4):612–9.
44. Gattinoni L, Carlesso E, Cadringher P, Valenza F, Vagginelli F, Chiumello D. Physical and biological triggers of ventilator-induced lung injury and its prevention. Eur Respir J Suppl. 2003;47:15s–25s.
45. Mietto C, Pinciroli R, Patel N, Berra L. Ventilator associated pneumonia: evolving definitions and preventive strategies. Respir Care. 2013;58(6):990–1007.
46. Vieillard-Baron A, Matthay M, Teboul JL, Bein T, Schultz M, Magder S, et al. Experts' opinion on management of hemodynamics in ARDS patients: focus on the effects of mechanical ventilation. Intensive Care Med. 2016;42(5):739–49.
47. Bellani G, Pesenti A. Assessing effort and work of breathing. Curr Opin Crit Care. 2014;20(3):352–8.
48. Petrof BJ, Hussain SN. Ventilator-induced diaphragmatic dysfunction: what have we learned? Curr Opin Crit Care. 2016;22(1):67–72.
49. Del Sorbo L, Cypel M, Fan E. Extracorporeal life support for adults with severe acute respiratory failure. Lancet Respir Med. 2014;2(2):154–64.
50. Combes A, Leprince P, Luyt C-E, Bonnet N, Trouillet J-L, Léger P, et al. Outcomes and long-term quality-of-life of patients supported by extracorporeal membrane oxygenation for refractory cardiogenic shock. Crit Care Med. 2008;36(5):1404–11.
51. Brodie D, Bacchetta M. Extracorporeal membrane oxygenation for ARDS in adults. N Engl J Med. 2011;365(20):1905–14.
52. Hill JD, O'Brien TG, Murray JJ, Dontigny L, Bramson ML, Osborn JJ, et al. Prolonged extracorporeal oxygenation for acute post-traumatic respiratory failure (shock-lung syndrome). Use of the Bramson membrane lung. N Engl J Med. 1972;286(12):629–34.
53. Morris AH, Wallace CJ, Menlove RL, Clemmer TP, Orme JF, Weaver LK, et al. Randomized clinical trial of pressure-controlled inverse ratio ventilation and extracorporeal CO2 removal for adult respiratory distress syndrome. Am J Respir Crit Care Med. 1994;149(2 Pt 1):295–305.
54. ELSO, editor. Guidelines for cardiopulmonary extracorporeal life support, version 1.3. Ann Arbor. 2013. http://www.elso.org/.
55. Field ML, Al-Alao B, Mediratta N. Open and closed chest extrathoracic cannulation for cardiopulmonary bypass and extracorporeal life support: methods, indications, and outcomes. Postgrad Med J. 2006;82(967):323–31.
56. Stulak JM, Dearani JA, Burkhart HM, Barnes RD, Scott PD, Schears GJ. ECMO cannulation controversies and complications. Semin Cardiothorac Vasc Anesth. 2009;13(3):176–82.
57. Sidebotham D, McGeorge A, McGuinness S, Edwards M, Willcox T, Beca J. Extracorporeal membrane oxygenation for treating severe cardiac and respiratory failure in adults: part 2-technical considerations. J Cardiothorac Vasc Anesth. 2010;24(1):164–72.
58. Sidebotham D, Allen SJ, McGeorge A, Ibbott N, Willcox T. Venovenous extracorporeal membrane oxygenation in adults: practical aspects of circuits, cannulae, and procedures. J Cardiothorac Vasc Anesth. 2012;26(5):893–909.
59. Ganslmeier P, Philipp A, Rupprecht L, Diez C, Arlt M, Mueller T, et al. Percutaneous cannulation for extracorporeal life support. Thorac Cardiovasc Surg. 2011;59(2):103–7.
60. Wang D, Zhou X, Liu X, Sidor B, Lynch J, Zwischenberger JB. Wang-Zwische double lumen cannula-toward a percutaneous and ambulatory paracorporeal artificial lung. ASAIO J. 2008;54(6):606–11.
61. Javidfar J, Brodie D, Wang D, Ibrahimiye AN, Yang J, Zwischenberger JB, et al. Use of bicaval dual-lumen catheter for adult venovenous extracorporeal membrane oxygenation. Ann Thorac Surg. 2011;91(6):1763–8; discussion 9.
62. Camboni D, Philipp A, Lubnow M, Bein T, Zausig Y, Hilker M, et al. Extracorporeal membrane oxygenation by single-vessel access in adults: advantages and limitations. ASAIO J. 2012;58(6):616–21.
63. Dolch ME, Frey L, Buerkle MA, Weig T, Wassilowsky D, Irlbeck M. Transesophageal echocardiography-guided technique for extracorporeal membrane oxygenation dual-lumen catheter placement. ASAIO J. 2011;57(4):341–3.
64. Sangalli F, Patroniti N, Pesenti A. ECMO-extracorporeal life support in adults. Mailand: Springer; 2014.
65. Davies SW, Leonard KL, Falls RK, Mageau RP, Efird JT, Hollowell JP, et al. Lung protective ventilation (ARDSNet) versus airway pressure release ventilation: ventilatory management in a combined model of acute lung and brain injury. J Trauma Acute Care Surg. 2015;78(2):240–9; discussion 9–51.
66. Schmidt M, Stewart C, Bailey M, Nieszkowska A, Kelly J, Murphy L, et al. Mechanical ventilation management during extracorporeal membrane oxygenation for acute respiratory distress syndrome: a retrospective international multicenter study. Crit Care Med. 2015;43(3):654–64.
67. Slutsky AS, Ranieri VM. Mechanical ventilation: lessons from the ARDSNet trial. Respir Res. 2000;1(2):73–7.
68. Deutschman CS, Neligan PJ. Evidence-based practice of critical care. 2nd ed. Philadelphia: Elsevier; 2016.
69. Jenks CL, Tweed J, Gigli KH, Venkataraman R. An international survey on ventilator practices among extracorporeal membrane oxygenation centers. ASAIO J. 2017;63(6):787–92.
70. Peek GJ, Firmin RK. The inflammatory and coagulative response to prolonged extracorporeal membrane oxygenation. ASAIO J. 1998;45(4):250–63.
71. Ranucci M. The conundrum of anticoagulation and hemostatic management in ECMO patients. Minerva Anestesiol. 2016;82(2):147–8.
72. Vaquer S, de Haro C, Peruga P, Oliva JC, Artigas A. Systematic review and meta-analysis of complications and mortality of venovenous extracorporeal membrane oxygenation for refractory acute respiratory distress syndrome. Ann Intensive Care. 2017;7(1):51.
73. Mols G, Loop T, Geiger K, Farthmann E, Benzing A. Extracorporeal membrane oxygenation: a ten-year experience. Am J Surg. 2000;180(2):144–54.
74. Müller T, Philipp A, Luchner A, Karagiannidis C, Bein T, Hilker M, et al. A new miniaturized system for extracorporeal membrane oxygenation in adult respiratory failure. Crit Care (London England). 2009;13(6):R205.

75. Noah MA, Peek GJ, Finney SJ, Griffiths MJ, Harrison DA, Grieve R, et al. Referral to an extracorporeal membrane oxygenation center and mortality among patients with severe 2009 influenza A(H1N1). JAMA. 2011;306(15):1659–68.
76. Roch A, Hraiech S, Masson E, Grisoli D, Forel JM, Boucekine M, et al. Outcome of acute respiratory distress syndrome patients treated with extracorporeal membrane oxygenation and brought to a referral center. Intensive Care Med. 2014;40(1):74–83.
77. Haneya A, Diez C, Philipp A, Bein T, Mueller T, Schmid C, et al. Impact of acute kidney injury on outcome in patients with severe acute respiratory failure receiving extracorporeal membrane oxygenation. Crit Care Med. 2015;43(9):1898–906.
78. Aubron C, Cheng AC, Pilcher D, Leong T, Magrin G, Cooper DJ, et al. Factors associated with outcomes of patients on extracorporeal membrane oxygenation support: a 5-year cohort study. Crit Care (London, England). 2013;17(2):R73.
79. Beiras-Fernandez A, Deutsch M-A, Kainzinger S, Kaczmarek I, Sodian R, Ueberfuhr P, et al. Extracorporeal membrane oxygenation in 108 patients with low cardiac output—a single-center experience. Int J Artif Organs. 2011;34(4):365–73.
80. Australia and New Zealand Extracorporeal Membrane Oxygenation Influenza Investigators, Davies A, Jones D, Bailey M, Beca J, Bellomo R, et al. Extracorporeal membrane oxygenation for 2009 influenza A(H1N1) acute respiratory distress syndrome. JAMA. 2009;302(17):1888–95.

Mechanical Circulatory Support: LVAD in Heart Failure

52

Aldo Cannata and Claudio Francesco Russo

Key Points

- LVAD supports only the left ventricle. Therefore right ventricular function must be thoroughly assessed before LVAD implantation.
- Clinical use of LVAD must be integrated with heart transplantation. LVAD strategies are bridge to transplantation, bridge to candidacy, and destination therapy.
- Because of donor shortage, in the United States, less than 50% of LVAD patients bridged to heart transplantation are transplanted at 2 years from device implantation. In other countries that proportion could be even inferior.
- The most frequent reasons for bridge to candidacy and destination therapy are reversible severe pulmonary hypertension and advanced age, respectively.
- Bleeding and driveline infection are the most frequently observed complications during LVAD support.

52.1 Introduction

Advanced heart failure (AHF) is a medical condition associated with a poor prognosis. The definition of AHF is different among clinical trials [1]. Nevertheless, it is usually applied to patients with dyspnea during mild exercise or even at rest (IIIb and IV NYHA classes), with a severely depressed left ventricular ejection fraction (<25%) and cardiac index <2.0 L/min/m^2 in spite of optimal medical management and cardiac resynchronization. The gold standard treatment for AHF remains heart transplantation. Long-term survival following transplantation is excellent, approaching 60% at 10 years [2]. However, heart transplantation is severely limited by the number of suitable donors. In fact, at the end of the year 2014, in Eurotransplant database, 1140 patients were on the active waiting list for heart transplantation [3]. During the following 12 months, only 605 transplantations were performed in countries participating to Eurotransplant. Therefore, a significant proportion of patients affected by AHF cannot benefit from heart transplantation because of donor shortage with consequent dismal prognosis. Moreover, a similar outcome is experienced by patients older than 65 years, who are usually excluded from heart transplantation.

A. Cannata (✉) · C. F. Russo
Department of Cardiac Surgery, Niguarda Hospital, Milan, Italy

Department of Cardiac and Thoraco-Vascular Surgery, ASST Grande Ospedale Metropolitano Niguarda, Milan, Italy
e-mail: aldo.cannata@ospedaleniguarda.it; claudiofrances.russo@ospedaleniguarda.it

52.2 Purpose and Clinical Strategy of Current Intracorporeal LVAD

Intracorporeal left ventricular assist device (LVAD) is an implantable device designed for long-term support of the left ventricle. Significant differences between LVAD and heart transplantation are shown in Table 52.1. It is important to recognize that *LVAD is not a replacement therapy* because *it supports only the left ventricle*. Moreover, it is promptly available when needed, whereas the availability of a suitable donor depends on chance and competition. This is a significant difference, particularly for patients experiencing a worsening of the clinical conditions. Finally, hemodynamic performance of LVAD, expressed in terms of flow, is standardized and reliable during the perioperative period. However, graft function is quite variable, depending on the conditions of the donor and the recipient and the duration of ischemia. In fact, acute graft failure remains the first cause of death during the first month following heart transplantation [2].

Due to improved long-term outcomes of the device and chronic donor shortage, intracorporeal LVAD is currently

P. Aseni et al. (eds.), *Operative Techniques and Recent Advances in Acute Care and Emergency Surgery*,
https://doi.org/10.1007/978-3-319-95114-0_52

Table 52.1 Differences between intracorporeal LVAD and heart transplantation

	LVAD	HTx
Function	LV support only	Heart replacement
Availability	Prompt	Unpredictable
Hemodynamic performance	Standardized	Depends on donor/recipient features
Cost	≈80,000€	Donation act

seen as an alternative to heart transplantation in very selected patients [4]. Nevertheless, the long-term prognosis is still better following transplantation than after LVAD implantation. Therefore, best outcomes are obtained using an integrated use of transplantation and LVAD, adopting different strategies.

52.2.1 LVAD as Bridge to Transplantation (BTT)

Intracorporeal LVAD is implanted in patients in active waiting list for heart transplantation, experiencing a deterioration of clinical conditions (e.g., inotrope dependence) and/or for whom a long wait for a suitable donor is foreseen because of large body size or AB0 group. Patients return in active waiting list following an adequate period of recovery after LVAD implantation (usually 6 months). In the most recent era of INTERMACS Registry, BTT as initial strategy involved 30% of patients [5].

52.2.2 LVAD as Bridge to Candidacy (BTC)

Intracorporeal LVAD is implanted in patients affected by AHF, with reversible conditions that contraindicate heart transplantation. The most frequent indication for BTC is severe pulmonary hypertension with pulmonary vascular resistance >4–5 Wood Units. Eligibility for heart transplantation is re-evaluated after 6–12 months after LVAD implantation. In the most recent era of INTERMACS Registry, BTC as initial strategy involved 23% of patients [5].

52.2.3 LVAD as Destination Therapy (DT)

Intracorporeal LVAD is implanted in patients affected by AHF, who are not eligible for heart transplantation because of irreversible conditions that contraindicate heart transplantation. The most frequent indication to DT is an age older than 65 years. Other conditions mandating DT are listed in Table 52.2 [6]. In the most recent era of INTERMACS Registry, BTT as initial strategy involved nearly 46% of patients [5].

Table 52.2 Conditions contraindicating heart transplantation and mandating destination therapy [6]

Modifiable condition	%
Renal dysfunction	22
High body mass index	16
Pulmonary hypertension	12
Still smoking	7
Limited social support	5
Severe diabetes	5
Repeated non-compliance	4
Illicit drug use	4
Alcohol abuse	3
Patient refuses transplant	3
Limited cognition/understanding	2
Contraindication to immunotherapy	2
Risk of recurrent infection	1
Severe depression	1
Current infection	1
Malnutrition/cachexia	1
Musculoskeletal limitations	1
Non-modifiable condition	**%**
Advanced age	33
Other comorbidity	9
Peripheral vascular disease	8
Pulmonary disease	8
Frailty	5
Fixed pulmonary hypertension	5
History of solid-organ cancer	5
History of lymphoma, leukemia	3
Multiple sternotomies	3
Other major psychiatric diagnoses	2
Heparin-induced thrombocytopenia	1
Major stroke	1
Allosensitization	1
Recent pulmonary embolus	1

The initial strategy could evolve in different ways according to patient conditions and donor availability. The lack of improvement of pulmonary hypertension after an adequate period of LVAD support mandates the change of BTC strategy in *de facto permanent LVAD support*. Similarly, patients bridged to transplantation may develop contraindications to transplantation during LVAD support (e.g., disabling stroke, renal failure, age > 65 years) that transform the initial strategy in *de facto permanent LVAD support.*

52.3 Selection of Patients for LVAD Implantation

Indications. Current indications of LVAD implantations are the following [7, 8]:

- Heart failure symptoms (NYHA IIIb–IV) during at least 45 of the last 60 days

- Heart failure symptoms refractory to optimal medical management
- Frequent rehospitalizations for heart failure symptoms
- Left ventricle ejection fraction <25%
- Peak V_{O_2} < 14 mL/kg/min
- Non-responder to cardiac resynchronization therapy
- Increasing diuretic requirement
- Continued need for inotropic drugs because of systemic hypotension, renal and/or liver injury, or worsening pulmonary congestion
- Intravenous inotropic drugs for ≥14 days
- Intra-aortic balloon pump for ≥7 days

According to the INTERMACS classification, candidates to LVAD are stratified in seven classes with worsening prognosis (Table 52.3). This classification allows a more detailed description of patients in NYHA classes III and IV. In the INTERMACS Registry, 95% of LVAD implants were performed in INTERMACS levels 1–4 and 80% in levels 2–4 [5]. Owing to increased risk of perioperative mortality among patients in INTERMACS level 1, it is current practice to proceed promptly to LVAD implantation in patients that are deteriorating, before the occurrence of cardiogenic shock.

52.4 Evaluation of Right Ventricular Function

Because the LVAD unloads only the left ventricle, it is crucial that the right ventricle is able to cope with the increased systemic venous return afforded by the artificial pump. A severe dysfunction of the right ventricle is an absolute contraindication to LVAD. Therefore, a thorough evaluation of right ventricular function is mandatory before the implant. Such evaluation is performed using echocardiography and cardiac catheterization [9].

Table 52.3 INTERMACS levels

	Official shorthand	Further description	NYHA class	Inotrope
Level 1	*Crash and burn*	Refractory cardiogenic shock	IV	Yes
Level 2	*Sliding on inotropes*	Deterioration despite inotropes	IV	Yes
Level 3	*Stable inotrope dependent*		IV	Yes
Level 4	*Resting symptoms*		IV	No
Level 5	*Housebound*	Symptoms for minimal activity	IV	No
Level 6	*Walking wounded*	Symptoms for mild activity	IIIb	No
Level 7	*Advanced NYHA III*		III	No

52.4.1 Echocardiography

Besides routine gross evaluation of right ventricle dimensions and contractility, echocardiography allows a more precise quantification of right heart function according to several parameters:

- Tricuspid annular plane systolic excursion (TAPSE): a parameter investigating the longitudinal shortening of the right ventricle (normal value: ≥16 mm); it is noteworthy that the interpretation of TAPSE may be confounded by the presence of significant tricuspid regurgitation (overestimation of the right ventricle function) and postsurgical adhesions in patients with a history of previous cardiac surgery (underestimation of right ventricle function).
- RV fractional area change (RVFAC): a two-dimensional parameter describing the right ventricle function (normal value: >35%).
- Tissue Doppler imaging (TDI): tricuspid annular plane velocity (*S′*, normal value: ≥10 cm/s).
- Right ventricle longitudinal strain: evaluation of the cyclic deformity of right ventricle during cardiac cycle.

Severe tricuspid regurgitation could be associated with a severe dysfunction of the right ventricle, particularly if there are tethering of leaflets and chordate and significant dilatation of the valve annulus. However, severe tricuspid regurgitation could be secondary also to functional interference or organic lesions on the leaflets from pacemaker and defibrillator leads, even in the absence of significant right ventricle dysfunction.

52.4.2 Cardiac Catheterization

The evidence of pulmonary hypertension at cardiac catheterization is usually associated with a right ventricle still able to withstand high pulmonary vascular resistance (PVR). Therefore, in such scenario the risk of perioperative right heart failure is negligible. On the other side, the observation of pulmonary artery pressure (PAP) that is slightly increased, or even within the normal range, must raise suspicion of significant right ventricle dysfunction in a patient candidate to LVAD. A small difference (<10 mmHg) between mean PAP and mean right atrial pressure strongly suggests a severe dysfunction of the right ventricle. In such scenario, the right ventricle behaves like a passive conduit more than like a pump, and the implant of a LVAD is contraindicated; other options should be considered, like heart transplantation or total artificial heart.

52.5 Technical Specifications of Current Intracorporeal LVAD

General features of current intracorporeal LVAD. Current intracorporeal LVAD shares the same general structure (Fig. 52.1). They are implanted inside the chest cavity and are composed by the inflow cannula, fixed to the left ventricular apex held in position by a sewing ring; the pump, receiving the blood coming from the inflow cannula; and the outflow cannula, anastomosed to the ascending aorta and delivering the blood coming from the pump. The pump is connected to an external controller and an electric energy source through a percutaneous driveline. The pump can also be connected to a fixed external monitor that allows detailed examination of pump parameters and alarms and fine regulation of pump speed and functions.

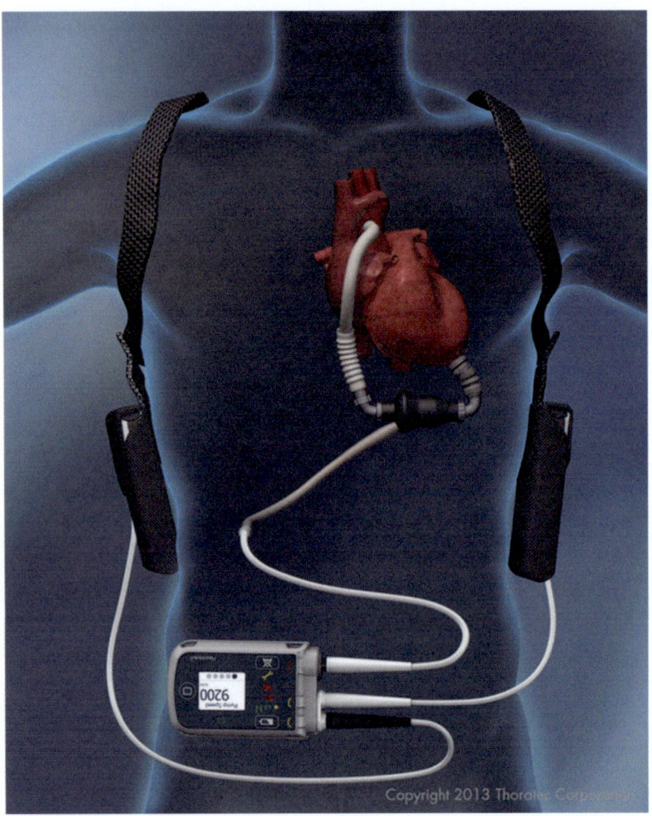

Fig. 52.1 HeartMate II system is shown as an example of the arrangement of current intracorporeal LVAD. The pump receives blood from the left ventricular cavity through the inflow cannula. Blood is pumped to the ascending aorta through the outflow cannula. The pump is connected to an external wearable controller using the percutaneous driveline. A pair of wearable batteries is connected to the controller (reproduced with the permission of *Thoratec Corporation*)

52.5.1 HeartMate II (Thoratec Inc., Pleasanton, CA, USA)

First implanted in man in 2001, HeartMate II is considered an axial flow pump because the blood flow is parallel to the long axis of the pump. It generates a continuous flow (Fig. 52.2). Therefore, in the absence of left ventricular ejection, the arterial pressure is pulseless. It weighs 290 g and it is 7 cm long with an external diameter measuring 4 cm. The volume of the implanted pump is about 90 mL. The smallest patient who received HeartMate II pump had 1.33 m^2 body surface area. The pump is implanted into the chest outside the pericardial cavity, just in front of the anterior aspect of the left hemidiaphragm. The mechanism of the pump is based on an internal rotor which is rotated by an electromagnetic field generated by the motor. The rotor is the only moving part inside the pump, and it is pivoted to two fixed stators. The blood is propelled by the rotor from the left ventricular cavity to the outflow cannula that is usually anastomosed to the lateral aspect of the ascending aorta. HeartMate

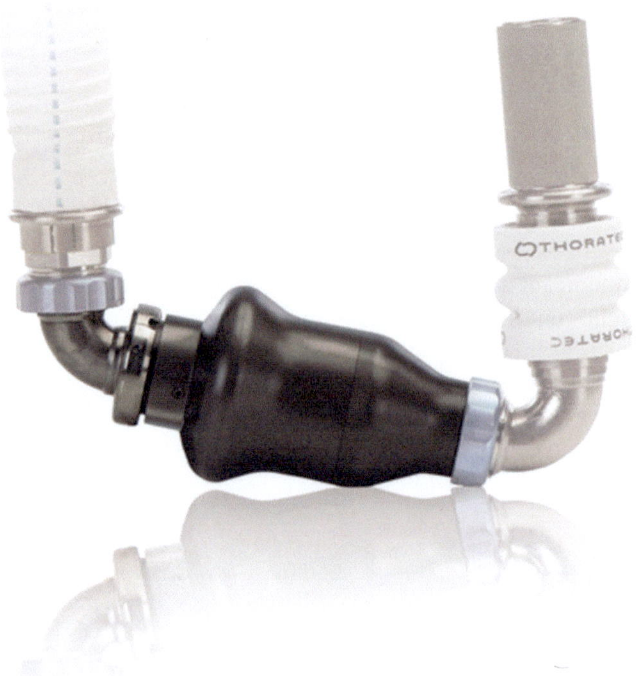

Fig. 52.2 Thoratec HeartMate II, comprising the inflow cannula (on the right side), the pump body (center), and the outflow cannula (on the left) (reproduced with the permission of *Thoratec Corporation*)

II is capable of generating blood flow up to 10 L/min. Pump speed ranges from 8000 to 15,000 rpm during operation. The system comprises the wearable system controller, the power base unit, and batteries (Fig. 52.1). The pump can be operated by AC power or by a pair of batteries, which are worn around the patient's waist and may last up to 12 h before needing to be recharged. Electrical power and data are delivered through a percutaneous driveline. Data about pump function and alarms are displayed on the system driver. HeartMate II received FDA approval for bridge to transplantation in April 2010 and destination therapy in January 2010. It has been implanted in more than 20,000 patients worldwide (source: Thoratec official website).

52.5.2 HVAD

First implanted in man in 2006, HVAD centrifugal pump (HeartWare International, Framingham, MA, USA) is designed for an intrapericardial implantation because of its small size (Fig. 52.3). In fact, it weighs 160 g, and its external diameter and volume are 53 mm and 50 mL, respectively. Because of its small size, HVAD can be implanted in patients with a body surface ≥1.2 m^2. It has one internal impeller suspended by magnetic/hydrodynamic forces. Because of impeller suspension, the mechanism is devoid of points of mechanical contact. The inflow cannula is integrated with the pump body. The blood is pumped to the ascending aorta through a 10 mm outflow graft. Operating range is from 1800 to 4000 rpm. Maximum obtainable flow is 10 L/min. The system comprises an external controller, an external monitor, and batteries. Data about pump flow and speed, battery status, and alarms are shown on the external controller. The pump can be operated by AC power or wearable batteries. Each battery provides up to 6 h of power before needing to be recharged. Electrical power and data are delivered through a 4.8 mm diameter percutaneous driveline. In 2012 FDA granted approval for bridge to transplantation to HeartWare HVAD. It has been implanted in more than 13,000 patients worldwide (source: HeartWare official website).

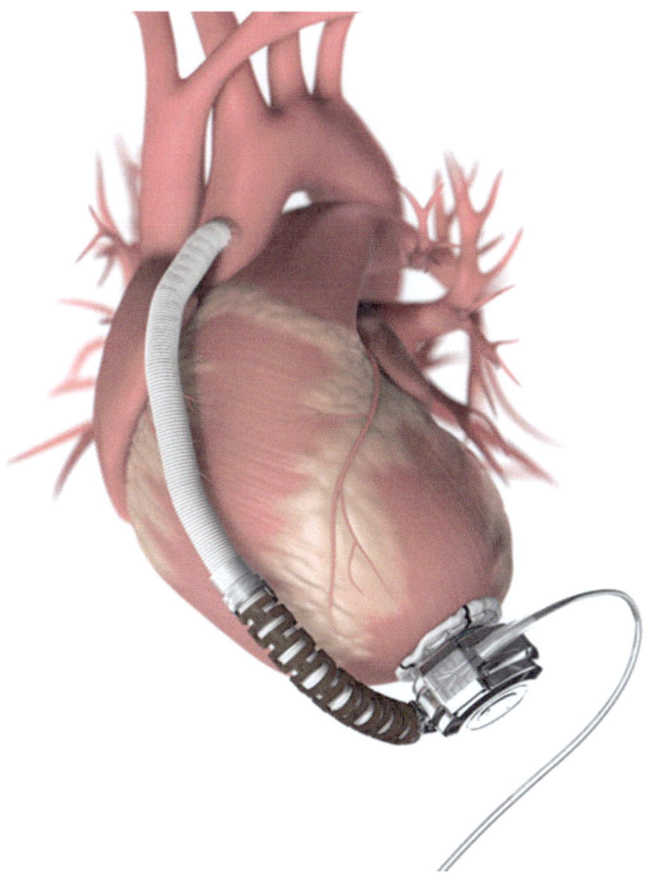

Fig. 52.3 HeartWare HVAD system (reproduced with the permission of *HeartWare International*)

52.5.3 HeartMate III

The centrifugal-flow LVAS (Left Ventricular Assist System—Thoratec Inc., Pleasanton, CA, USA) has been recently introduced into the clinical practice (Fig. 52.4). It weighs 200 g. The diameter and the height (excluding the inflow cannula) of pump body are 50 and 56 mm, respectively; pump volume is 80 mL. The manufacturer does not provide a minimum body surface area compatible for HeartMate III implantation. Its design allows an intrapericardial placement. The pump is acted by a fully magnetically levitated

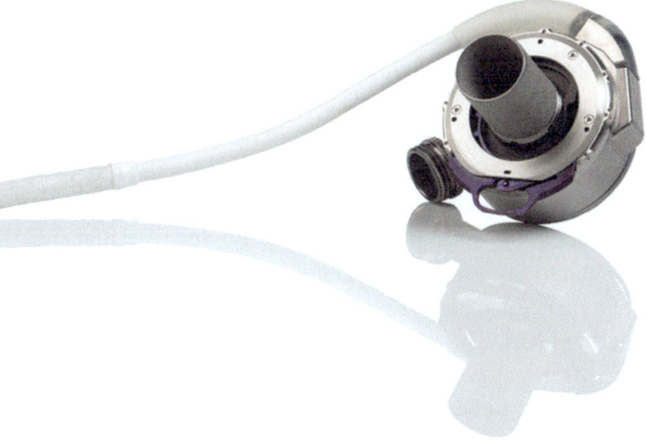

Fig. 52.4 Thoratec HeartMate III: the inflow cannula (center of the image) is integrated with the pump body (reproduced with the permission of *Thoratec Corporation*)

rotor. Such mechanism, devoid of mechanical bearings, allows the minimization of wear of pump components. Moreover, also shear forces and heat generation are kept at a minimum level, to reduce damage to blood components. Thrombogenicity is also decreased by the texturing of the internal surfaces of the pump with titanium microspheres. Operating range is from 3000 to 9000 rpm, and the achievable maximum pump flow is 10 L/min. A pulsatile flow is obtained by periodic decrease of rpm (every 2 s). The blood is pumped from the left ventricular cavity to the 14 mm outflow cannula that is usually anastomosed to the lateral aspect of the ascending aorta. HeartMate III can be operated using AC power or charged wearable batteries. A pair of charged batteries provides up to 17 h of support under nominal operating conditions. The pump is connected to external wearable system controller (or to the power unit) and batteries through a percutaneous driveline. Data about pump parameters (flow, power, pulsatility index), battery charge status, and alarms are shown on the system controller.

52.6 Standard Technique: Median Sternotomy

LVAD implantation is performed through a median sternotomy in most of the cases. Intrathoracic pocket for the device is needed only for HeartMate II, whereas HeartWare HVAD and HeartMate II are designed to be implanted inside the pericardial cavity. Driveline is tunneled through the abdominal wall before systemic heparinization in order to reduce the risk of bleeding along the driveline course. Normothermic cardiopulmonary bypass is started after cannulation of the proximal aortic arch and the right atrium. A two-stage venous cannula is adopted in case of isolated LVAD implantation. However, bicaval venous cannulation is mandatory in case of combined procedures requiring opening of the atria (suture of patent foramen ovale, tricuspid annuloplasty, mitral valve replacement for valve stenosis). The surgical field is routinely flooded with CO_2 in order to decrease the risk of complications secondary to gaseous embolization. An aortic vent is placed on mild suction. Usually, for isolated LVAD implantation, aortic cross-clamping and cardioplegic arrest are not needed, and the implantation is performed on the beating heart. The apex of the left ventricle is elevated using wet warm gauzes placed into the pericardial cavity. The site for the inflow cannula is on the anterolateral wall of the apex, within the angle between distal left anterior descending artery and its more distal diagonal branch. The correct orientation of the inflow cannula is toward the mitral orifice, with an intraventricular course parallel to the interventricular septum. The sewing ring is anchored to the left ventricle apex using 12 pledgeted mattress 2-0 polypropylene (or braided polyester) sutures. A coring tool is inserted into the ventricular cavity through an incision inside the sewing ring, and a full-thickness circular piece of myocardium is removed. The ventricular cavity is carefully inspected; thrombus, scar, or chordae are removed in order to avoid obstruction of the inflow cannula or stroke. The inflow cannula is inserted into the sewing ring and firmly secured to it. Left ventricle, pump, and outflow graft are de-aired. Outflow graft is anastomosed to the ascending aorta on a side-biting clamp using a continuous 4-0 polypropylene suture. A needle is placed on the outflow graft, and the LVAD is started at low flow in order to complete de-airing. Then, the site-biting clamp on the ascending aorta is released, and the aortic vent is placed on strong suction. De-airing and weaning from cardiopulmonary bypass are conducted as usual. Before chest closure, several measures should be adopted in order to decrease the amount of postsurgical mediastinal adhesions and to prevent direct adherence between the sternum, heart, and great vessels. Such measures decrease the risk associated with resternotomy and mediastinal dissection at the time of heart transplantation or LVAD replacement for device failure. A sealant could be applied on the epicardium in order to prevent the formation of intrapericardial adhesions [10, 11]. The outflow graft is enveloped into a sheet of ePTFE. Moreover, a further sheet of ePTFE is sutured to the edges of pericardiotomy in order to form a physical barrier between the heart, great vessels, outflow graft, and sternum [12]. Finally, the skin around the driveline is approximated using fine sutures in order to eliminate dead space around the cable and to promote healing of the driveline exit site.

52.7 Outcomes

Survival. In the current era, following the implantation of an intracorporeal LVAD, the 1-year survival is 80%, and the 2-year survival is 70% [5]. Such results seem to be satisfactory in comparison to the 2-year survival following heart transplantation, ranging from 80 to 90% [2]. However, a clearer picture is offered from an analysis of outcomes according to the strategy of LVAD implantation and to the clinical conditions at the time of implant. In fact, the 2-year survival is 80% and 65% among implants performed as bridge to transplantation and destination therapy, respectively [5]. Patients implanted in cardiogenic shock (INTERMACS level 1) or in worsening clinical conditions despite inotropic therapy (INTERMACS level 2) have a significantly increased risk of early death when compared to less critical clinical profiles. However, it should be underscored that INTERMACS levels 1 and 2 are not predictors of late mortality. Other predictors of early death following LVAD implantation are older age, female gender, higher body mass index, history of stroke, destination therapy strategy, right heart failure, liver and renal failure, and previous cardiac surgery. Most frequent causes of death are neurological complications, multiorgan failure, withdrawal of support, and major infection.

52.7.1 Quality of Life

Quality of life improves significantly following the implantation of an intracorporeal LVAD. Starling and colleagues [13] reported that in a nonrandomized observational study, the functional status was significantly better after LVAD implantation. By 2 years, 69% of implanted patients were in NYHA class I or II, versus 37% of patients treated using optimal medical management. Moreover, quality of life, as evaluated by EuroEuroQol 5 dimensions, a 5-level questionnaire, and a depression screening questionnaire (Patient Health Questionnaire), was significantly improved among LVAD patients as compared to patients medically managed. Similar observations have been made by several groups [14, 15]. Nevertheless, it is well recognized that quality of life after LVAD implant is significantly worse as compared to heart transplantation [14, 15]. Poor outcomes in terms of quality of life are observed in 7.3% of patients surviving more than 1 year following LVAD implantation [16]. Risk factors for poor outcome were higher body mass index, lower hemoglobin levels, history of previous cardiac surgery, history of cancer, and severe diabetes mellitus. Particularly, adverse events occurring during the first 6 months after implant seem to have a major detrimental effect on quality of life [17].

52.7.2 Reversal of Pulmonary Hypertension

The unloading of the left ventricle achieved by the LVAD pump allows a significant decrease of pressure inside the left atrium and pulmonary veins. After several months of LVAD support, a decrease of PAP and PVR is observed in most of the patients. The improvement in pulmonary circulation is crucial in order to achieve the eligibility to heart transplantation as a bridge to candidacy patients and to decrease the risk of graft failure as a bridge to transplant patients. Gupta and colleagues [18] reported that, after several months of LVAD support, mean PAP and PVR decreased from 38.8 to 22.9 mmHg and from 3.7 to 2.2, respectively. Both changes were statistically significant. Mikus and colleagues [19] observed a significant decrease of mean PAP, PVR, and trans-pulmonary gradient (mean PAP—mean left atrial pressure) in LVAD patients affected by fixed (i.e., pharmacologically not reversible) pulmonary hypertension. However, the reversal of pulmonary hypertension occurred during the first 6 months from the implant, and longer support did not add any further beneficial effect.

52.7.3 Bridge to Heart Transplantation

For patients implanted according to a bridge to transplant strategy, the rate of heart transplantation depends on survival during LVAD support as well as the access to a suitable donor. It is noteworthy that the access to a donor depends on rules for organ allocation and patient priority status. This could be increased by development of complications (thromboembolism, device infection, etc.) during support. Moreover, in the United States, the United Network for Organ Sharing (UNOS) granted a 30-day period (also known as *grace period*) of highest priority (Status 1A) to all LVAD patients independently from the occurrence of complications. The grace period has been conceived in order to be exploited during periods of clinical stability, increasing the chance of transplantation before the onset of complications. In INTERMACS Registry (i.e., in the United States), the proportion of patients transplanted is 31% and 45% at 1 and 2 years following LVAD implant, respectively [5]. In other countries this rate may be significantly lower. The outcomes of heart transplantations seem to be significantly worse among patients with an infected LVAD, whereas other LVAD-related complications do not have an appreciable influence on survival [20].

52.7.4 Complications During LVAD Support

Despite a good survival rate, the incidence of major complications is relevant during LVAD support. In the current era, the most frequent complications occurring during LVAD support are bleeding (7.79 events/100 patient months) and infection (7.28 events/100 patient months). The rate of stroke and right heart failure is significantly lower, being 1.61 and 0.49 events/100 patient months, respectively [5]. Two thirds of patients experienced a major event (infection, bleeding, stroke, device malfunction, death) within 12 months since the start of support. The incidence of rehospitalization is high, being 75% at 1 year from LVAD implantation. The rate of isolated mechanical or electrical failure of LVAD is exceedingly rare.

The incidence of driveline infection varies greatly according to the definitions adopted for the studies, ranging from 10 to 48% [21]. It is an early complication in 20% of cases [22]. Trauma to the skin surrounding the driveline seems to be a major risk factor for the development of infection. Patient information and education is mandatory in order to avoid inadvertent injury to the exit site of the driveline during normal daily activities. When infection occurs, it is very difficult to eradicate without the removal of the LVAD. Driveline dressings, wound care performed by surgeons, and antibiotics could limit the spread of infection. Therefore, heart transplantation is the therapeutic option with the highest potential of cure of the infection. Unfortunately, in most of cases, the patient gains access to transplantation only when the infection is very advanced and localized even into the mediastinum and/or extended to the bloodstream. This explains the poorer outcomes of urgent heart transplantation for an infected device [20].

It is noteworthy that a significant increase in the incidence of HeartMate II thrombosis has been observed since 2011, even if the absolute incidence remained low (6% at 6 months from implantation) [23]. The risk of thrombosis peaks during the first 6 months of support, with a gradually increasing risk during late follow-up. The management of such complication is not yet standardized. Nevertheless, in the current practice, thrombolytic therapy is suggested in cases of early diagnosis of thrombosis and when the surgical risk of a pump exchange is judged to be prohibitive. However, pump exchange is recommended when the thrombosis is subacute or chronic, because it is very likely that at this stage the thrombus is becoming organized and fibrous. It has been reported that the procedure of pump exchange is associated with a decreased survival and an increased incidence of device infection and neurological events [23]. Finally, urgent heart transplantation is an alternative option in patients in active list.

52.8 Future Developments

Current complication rate during LVAD support mandates continuous technological progress of the devices. Bleeding and driveline infection are today the more frequent complications observed among patients, and commonsense suggests that technological progress should first fix such issues. Current standard medical treatment for LVAD patients is represented by the association of warfarin and one or two antiplatelet drugs (e.g., low-dose aspirin ± clopidogrel). Improvements in biocompatibility of LVAD, in terms of decreased activation of coagulation and inflammatory system, could reduce the need for antithrombotic therapies. Damage to blood components could be minimized by pump mechanisms that are frictionless and don't generate heat. Also an improved texturing of the internal surfaces of the device could reduce thrombogenicity. In the future, a LVAD managed only with antiplatelet drugs could lead to a lower incidence of bleeding during support, prolonging the survival rate. Transcutaneous energy transfer (also known as TET) between the batteries and the pump could eliminate the need for a percutaneous driveline, which remains the Achilles' heel of current LVAD systems because of infection rate and compromised quality of life. TET was first introduced into the clinical practice with LionHeart LVAD more than 15 years ago, but unfortunately it did not gain wide acceptance because of controversial results in terms of infections [24], and finally, the system was abandoned. Nevertheless, TET is still hampered by formidable technical issues related to the high power required by LVAD, the degradation of power transfer and efficiency according to environmental conditions and tissue composition, and chronic heat generation into the skin layer [25].

Case Scenario

A 47-year-old male (height 190 cm, weight 100 kg; blood group 0) affected by idiopathic dilated cardiomyopathy was urgently admitted to the intensive care unit because of low cardiac output syndrome. He underwent mitral valve replacement with a mechanical prosthesis 5 years ago because of severe mitral regurgitation. During the last 2 years, he was listed for heart transplantation with a low priority because of good clinical conditions. At admission, an intra-aortic balloon pump was promptly placed, and intravenous infusion of epinephrine was started. Despite intensive treatment, a significant improvement of cardiac output did not occur. Therefore, an intracorporeal LVAD has been urgently implanted as a bridge to heart transplantation.

1. Why the priority for heart transplantation was not increased to urgent?
   - A. Mechanical mitral valve prosthesis is a relative contraindication for urgent heart transplantation.
   - B. The chance to obtain a suitable donor in a short time was judged very low because of the large body size and ABO group (many competitors in 0 group).
   - C. Because of the intra-aortic balloon pump.
2. In the presence of mechanical mitral valve prosthesis:
   - A. The INR must be higher than 3.5 during LVAD support.
   - B. The mechanical prosthesis must be replaced with a bioprosthesis at the time of LVAD implantation.
   - C. The aortic valve should be also replaced at the time of LVAD implantation.
3. The *conditio sine qua non* for LVAD implantation is:
   - A. Preserved right ventricular function
   - B. Body surface area >1.7 m^2
   - C. The absence of mitral valve regurgitation

Please see Chap. 58 for the correct answer.

References

1. Bjork JB, Alton KK, Georgiopoulou VV, Butler J, Kalogeropoulos AP. Defining advanced heart failure: a systematic review of criteria used in clinical trials. J Card Fail. 2016;22(7):569–77.
2. Lund LH, Edwards LB, Dipchand AI, Goldfarb S, Kucheryavaya AY, Levvey BJ, et al.; International Society for Heart and Lung Transplantation. The Registry of the International Society for Heart and Lung Transplantation: thirty-third adult heart transplantation Report-2016; focus theme: primary diagnostic indications for transplant. J Heart Lung Transplant. 2016;35(10):1158–69.
3. Eurotransplant International Foundation. Annual Report 2015. https://www.eurotransplant.org/cms/mediaobject.php?file=AR_ET_20153.pdf.
4. Ponikowski P, Voors AA, Anker SD, Bueno H, Cleland JG, Coats AJ, et al.; Authors/Task Force Members. 2016 ESC Guidelines for the diagnosis and treatment of acute and chronic heart failure: The Task Force for the diagnosis and treatment of acute and chronic heart failure of the European Society of Cardiology (ESC)Developed with the special contribution of the Heart Failure Association (HFA) of the ESC. Eur Heart J. 2016;37(27):2129–200.
5. Kirklin JK, Naftel DC, Pagani FD, Kormos RL, Stevenson LW, Blume ED, et al. Seventh INTERMACS annual report: 15,000 patients and counting. J Heart Lung Transplant. 2015;34(12):1495–504.
6. Kirklin JK, Naftel DC, Kormos RL, Stevenson LW, Pagani FD, Miller MA, et al. Third INTERMACS annual report: the evolution of destination therapy in the United States. J Heart Lung Transplant. 2011;30(2):115–23.
7. Gustafsson F, Rogers JG. Left ventricular assist device therapy in advanced heart failure: patient selection and outcomes. Eur J Heart Fail. 2017;19(5):595–602.
8. Peura JL, Colvin-Adams M, Francis GS, Grady KL, Hoffman TM, Jessup M, et al.; American Heart Association Heart Failure and Transplantation Committee of the Council on Clinical Cardiology; Council on Cardiopulmonary, Critical Care, Perioperative and Resuscitation; Council on Cardiovascular Disease in the Young; Council on Cardiovascular Nursing; Council on Cardiovascular Radiology and Intervention, and Council on Cardiovascular Surgery and Anesthesia. Recommendations for the use of mechanical circulatory support: device strategies and patient selection: a scientific statement from the American Heart Association. Circulation. 2012;126(22):2648–67.
9. Hayek S, Sims DB, Markham DW, Butler J, Kalogeropoulos AP. Assessment of right ventricular function in left ventricular assist device candidates. Circ Cardiovasc Imaging. 2014;7(2):379–89.
10. Cannata A, Petrella D, Russo CF, Bruschi G, Fratto P, Gambacorta M, et al. Postsurgical intrapericardial adhesions: mechanisms of formation and prevention. Ann Thorac Surg. 2013;95(5):1818–26.
11. Cannata A, Petrella D, Gambacorta M, Russo CF, Bruschi G, Martinelli L. Histological findings following use of CoSeal in a patient with a left ventricular assist device. Surg Innov. 2013;20(6):NP35–7.
12. Vitali E, Russo C, Tiziano C, Lanfranconi M, Bruschi G. Modified pericardial closure technique in patients with ventricular assist device. Ann Thorac Surg. 2000;69(4):1278–9.
13. Starling RC, Estep JD, Horstmanshof DA, Milano CA, Stehlik J, Shah KB, et al.; ROADMAP Study Investigators. Risk assessment and comparative effectiveness of left ventricular assist device and medical management in ambulatory heart failure patients: the ROADMAP Study 2-Year Results. JACC Heart Fail. 2017. pii:S2213-1779(17)30164-6.
14. Emin A, Rogers CA, Banner NR, Steering Group, UK Cardiothoracic Transplant Audit. Quality of life of advanced chronic heart failure: medical care, mechanical circulatory support and transplantation. Eur J Cardiothorac Surg. 2016;50(2):269–73.
15. Jakovljevic DG, McDiarmid A, Hallsworth K, Seferovic PM, Ninkovic VM, Parry G, et al. Effect of left ventricular assist device implantation and heart transplantation on habitual physical activity and quality of life. Am J Cardiol. 2014;114(1):88–93.
16. Arnold SV, Jones PG, Allen LA, Cohen DJ, Fendler TJ, Holtz JE, et al. Frequency of poor outcome (death or poor quality of life) after left ventricular assist device for destination therapy: results from the INTERMACS Registry. Circ Heart Fail. 2016;9(8). pii: e002800.
17. Grady KL, Wissman S, Naftel DC, Myers S, Gelijins A, Moskowitz A, et al. Age and gender differences and factors related to change in health-related quality of life from before to 6 months after left ventricular assist device implantation: Findings from Interagency Registry for Mechanically Assisted Circulatory Support. J Heart Lung Transplant. 2016;35(6):777–88.
18. Gupta S, Woldendorp K, Muthiah K, Robson D, Prichard R, Macdonald PS, et al. Normalisation of haemodynamics in patients with end-stage heart failure with continuous-flow left ventricular assist device therapy. Heart Lung Circ. 2014;23(10):963–9.
19. Mikus E, Stepanenko A, Krabatsch T, Loforte A, Dandel M, Lehmkuhl HB, Hetzer R, Potapov EV. Reversibility of fixed pulmonary hypertension in left ventricular assist device support recipients. Eur J Cardiothorac Surg. 2011;40(4):971–7.
20. Healy AH, Baird BC, Drakos SG, Stehlik J, Selzman CH. Impact of ventricular assist device complications on posttransplant survival: an analysis of the United network of organ sharing database. Ann Thorac Surg. 2013;95(3):870–5.
21. Pereda D, Conte JV. Left ventricular assist device driveline infections. Cardiol Clin. 2011;29:515–27.
22. Goldstein DJ, Naftel D, Holman W, Bellumkonda L, Pamboukian SV, Pagani FD, et al. Continuous-flow devices and percutaneous site infections: clinical outcomes. J Heart Lung Transplant. 2012;31(11):1151–7.
23. Kirklin JK, Naftel DC, Kormos RL, Pagani FD, Myers SL, Stevenson LW, et al. Interagency Registry for Mechanically Assisted Circulatory Support (INTERMACS) analysis of pump thrombosis in the HeartMate II left ventricular assist device. J Heart Lung Transplant. 2014;33(1):12–22.
24. Pae WE, Connell JM, Adelowo A, Boehmer JP, Korfer R, El-Banayosy A, et al.; Clinical Utility Baseline Study (CUBS) Group. Does total implantability reduce infection with the use of a left ventricular assist device? The LionHeart experience in Europe. J Heart Lung Transplant. 2007;26(3):219–29.
25. Bocan KN, Sejdić E. Adaptive transcutaneous power transfer to implantable devices: a state of the art review. Sensors (Basel). 2016;16(3). pii:E393.

Extracorporeal Membrane Oxygenation (ECMO) in Trauma

53

Antonino M. Grande, Antonella Degani, Antonio Fiore, and Paolo Aseni

Key Points

- Do not hesitate to use ECMO when respiratory and circulatory parameters are irreversibly worsened.
- Use a circuit as short as possible; the relationship between resistance and circuit length is directly proportional: flow resistance within the circuit increases when the circuit is longer. Moreover, longer circuit lengths have a greater contact surface for flowing blood inside it, a greater need for priming solution, and greater heat loss. The circuit should only be long enough to go safely from the patient to the pump and facilitate patient transport.
- It is better to use fewer connectors as possible. Each connector within the circuit causes the creation of a turbulent flow area. In these areas, clots may form more easily.
- Check for the absence of kinks, twists, and the right connections of the fluid tubing in the entire circuit.
- Use only what is essential for the good performance of the circuit as it makes it in such a way that it is possible to deal with unforeseeable situations.
- Dual lumen cannula insertion in the jugular vein should be done under transesophageal echocardiographic control for the risk of myocardial perforation.
- In VA (veno-arterial)-ECMO, avoid limb ischemia by using end-to-side chimney graft or by positioning a distal perfusion cannula.

53.1 Introduction

Polytrauma patients in most cases succumb to severe head and/or thoracoabdominal injuries. The trimodal mortality model in trauma, introduced in the 1980s [1, 2], refers to immediate deaths, early deaths, and late deaths. According to this model, there is a first mortality peak where death is immediate or occurs within minutes of the trauma or 1 h of arrival to the hospital; the reported mortality rate was up to 64%. The second mortality peak shows death occurring within 24 h of hospital arrival, determining up to 30% mortality [2]; once again, mortality is a consequence of massive lesions that may be effectively treated. Finally, the late death, which in Trunkey's description [2] accounts for about 20% mortality, is defined as deaths occurring days or weeks after the trauma. The subsequent development of regionalized trauma networks with rapid transportation of patients from the scene to specialized trauma centers [3], along with improved imaging modalities and surgical techniques, has determined a significative mortality reduction. Therefore, in traumatic lung injuries that do not respond to conventional mechanical ventilation, other treatments may help: chemical paralysis [4], prone positioning, inhaled prostacyclins, and pressure-controlled inverse ratio ventilation [5]. When all these treatment provisions are not adequate, and lung compliance becomes worse, the increased inspiratory pressures may cause barotrauma and further impaired lung function. Furthermore, ECMO should be used in case of traumatic bronchopleural fistula that is associated with very high mortality up to 67% with important morbidity [6, 7] and as a bridge to surgery in trauma

A. M. Grande (✉) · A. Degani
Department of Cardiac Surgery, IRCCS Fondazione Policlinico San Matteo, Pavia, Italy
e-mail: amgrande@libero.it; degani.a@smatteo.pv.it

A. Fiore
Department of Cardiothoracic Surgery, Henri Mondor University Hospital, AP-HP, Paris-Est University, Créteil, France

P. Aseni
Dipartimento di Emergenza Urgenza, ASST Grande Ospedale Metropolitano Niguarda, Milano, Italy

P. Aseni et al. (eds.), *Operative Techniques and Recent Advances in Acute Care and Emergency Surgery*,
https://doi.org/10.1007/978-3-319-95114-0_53

patients with low tracheal lacerations or transections that cause respiratory failure by inadequate alveolar ventilation due to V/Q (ventilation/perfusion) mismatch from severe air leak [8–11]. If trauma affects only one lung, ECMO allows a selective ventilation of the healthy lung, while the injured one, collapsing, has time to heal [6, 8].

Nevertheless, trauma patients may present acute heart failure, e.g., due to a serious bleeding, to stunned heart following direct trauma (severe contusion and hematoma), or to depression determined by acidosis and hypothermia.

In these cases ECMO has been proven to be an adequate therapeutic tool that may grant patient's tissue perfusion supporting cardiac and respiratory functions. Therefore, the clinical use of ECMO is becoming increasingly frequent showing a dramatic improvement in survival rate [8].

53.2 ECMO System

A standard ECMO circuit consists essentially of the following components (Figs. 53.1 and 53.2):

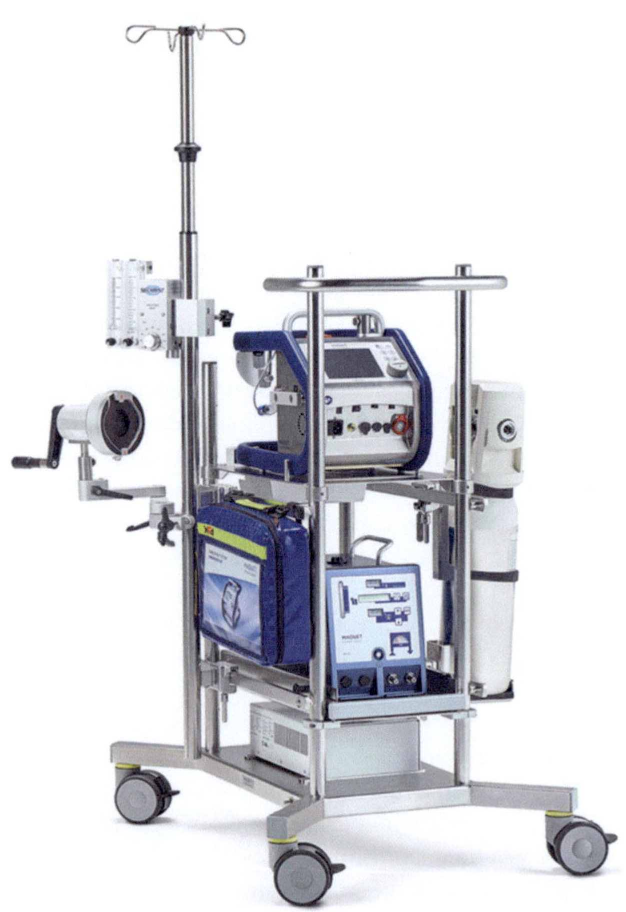

Fig. 53.1 ECMO system (with permission from Getinge, Germany)

(a) Blood pump. Semiocclusive roller pumps have been substituted by centrifugal pump where a spinning rotor generates flow and pressure. The pump must supply a flow rate of 75–150 mL/kg/min (patients <10 kg; <18 months) and 2400 $mL/m^2/min$ for others. One widely used pump is the Rotaflow centrifugal pump (Maquet Cardiopulmonary AG, Hirrlingen, Germany) that is employed in combination with the Maquet® Rotaflow console [12]. This device has high durability, lower hemolysis, less blood pressure, and a reduced chance of forming a microemulsion. Several other ECMO blood pump systems are now available and placed on the market: Medtronic Affinity Centrifugal Blood Pump (Medtronic, Minneapolis, MN), Medos Deltastream pump system (Medos Medizintechnik AG, Stolberg, Germany), Sorin (Mirandola, Modena, Italy), and Thoratec (Pleasanton, California, USA).

(b) Oxygenators. These are devices that provide O_2 and eliminate CO_2 from the venous blood. One of the most widely used is Quadrox Maquet®, polymethylpentene (PMP) with Bioline Coating that has an approval for 14 days continuous use, and consequently the need for oxygenator replacement is significantly reduced [13]. It has the following technical characteristics:
   - Blood flow ratio: 0.5–7 L/min.
   - Priming volume: 335 mL.
   - Effective gas exchange surface: 1.8 m^2.
   - Effective heat exchange surface: 0.4 m^2.

   Another oxygenator is Eurosets (Medolla, Italy) validated for 14 days of use (Europe only), providing both cardiac and respiratory support. The gas exchanger is coated with lipid-based phosphorylcholine coating, and it contains an integral heat exchanger.

(c) Air/oxygen blender and gas lines. The blender is utilized to mix air and oxygen into a gas source ranging from 21 to 100% oxygen. The blender is connected to the oxygenator via a simple tubing (Fig. 53.2).

(d) Heat exchanger. This device is positioned distal to the oxygenator to replace ambient heat loss and maintain patient temperature.

(e) Circuit tubing (cannulas and related lines) between the vascular accesses.

   The ECMO circuit tubing consists of polyvinyl chloride (PVC) conduits treated with a biocompatible coating. Because blood is exposed to the non-biologic surfaces of the circuit, complex reactions may involve either the coagulation pathway or the inflammatory response pathway with activation of the coagulant complement and cascade. Anyway, the biocompatible coating does not eliminate these hematological reactions completely [14].

   Cannulas used in extracorporeal circulation are tubes of polymeric material, designed to circulate the blood with

Fig. 53.2 Schematic standard ECMO circuit. (1) Venous cannula, (2) Blood centrifugal pump, (3) Oxygenator, (4) Arterial cannula, (5) Control system, (6) Heat exchanger

the lowest degree of turbulence [15]. Cannulas must also be "robust" enough to avoid bending or collapse, but, at the same time, they must be flexible and easily handled. Their gauge and length are the main determinants of the ECMO flow. The size of the cannulas must be sufficient to allow the optimum theoretical flow for each patient. The cannulas are tailored to peripheral use with a fine and durable wall that is wire reinforced in order to avoid bending and kinking.

The venous cannula presents an end hole and side holes to maximize drainage; furthermore side holes allow flow if the end is occluded.

There are *single lumen* (Fig. 53.3) and *dual lumen* (Fig. 53.4) cannulas. The first ones are utilized to provide venous (V) and arterial (A) access in patients who undergo VA-ECMO or in case of multiple site venous access in patients getting a VV-ECMO. For instance, the common site in the VV-ECMO is the femoral/jugular vein. A large cannula (23–25F) should be placed for drainage and somewhat smaller cannula (19–21F) for venous reinfusion.

There are several types of cannula with respect to design and size, ranging from 6F (2 mm diameter) to 51F (17 mm), and most of them are manufactured with wire-reinforced bodies to prevent occlusion [16].

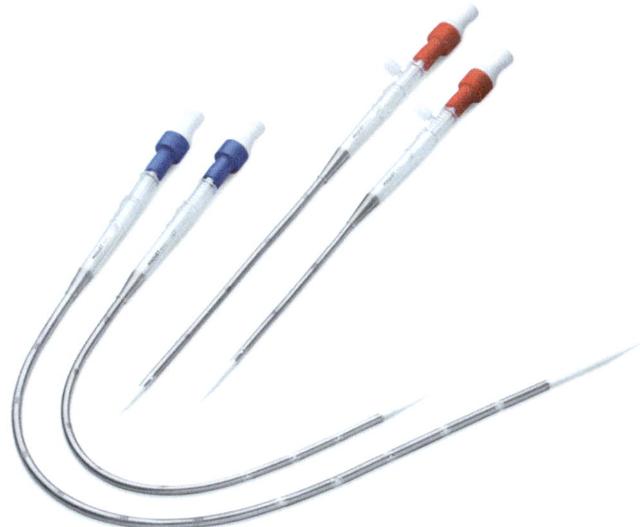

Fig. 53.3 Single lumen cannula (with permission from Getinge, Germany)

The dual lumen cannula is available for VV-ECMO using a single-vessel approach in the internal jugular vein: the blood is drained from one lumen and then is returned to the patient via the smaller one; for the

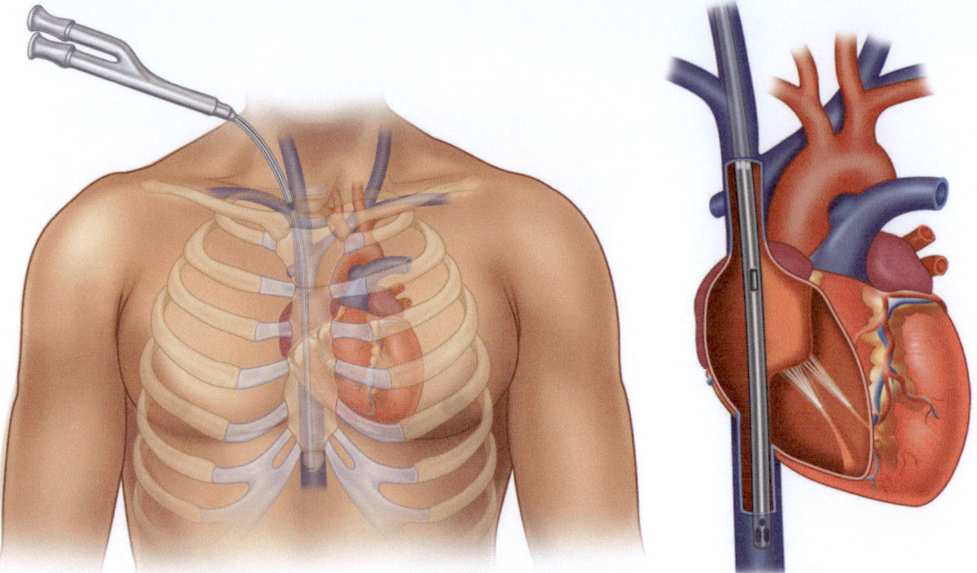

Fig. 53.4 Dual lumen cannula. Dual lumen cannula (with permission from Getinge, Germany)

Avalon dual lumen cannula, sizes range from 13 to 31F; other small cannulas are the OriGen (Austin, TX) dual lumen cannula that is available in 12, 15, and 18F sizes; it is manufactured from non-wire-reinforced polyurethane and may be subject to structural deformation after insertion; the Covidien ECMO (Mansfield, MA) cannula is also manufactured from non-wire-reinforced polyurethane. It is only available in 14F overall diameter [14]. For smaller sizes, it is recommended to position this type of cannula under transesophageal echocardiographic control for the risk of cardiac perforation [8, 17].

(f) Interhospital transport circuit. The Maquet Cardiohelp System is the smallest portable heart-lung support system designed to treat and to transport patients needing extended respiratory and/or circulatory support (Fig. 53.5). The Maquet Cardiohelp HLS modules integrate three major Extracorporeal Life Support (ECLS) circuit components (oxygenator, pump, and heat exchanger) into a single product. The system is coated with the Maquet Bioline thromboresistant surface [18].

(g) ECMO circuit. The ECMO circuit includes an outflow cannula connected to an outflow line linked in turn to a centrifugal pump. The pump injects the blood through an oxygenator and the heat exchanger in the inflow line. The arterial blood is reinjected to the patient by an inflow cannula.

In the acronym VA-ECMO, the drainage site is positioned prior the injection site, venoarterial ECMO; VV-ECMO means venovenous ECMO that can be femoro-right internal jugular veins (drainage from femoral vein and inflow in the jugular vein).

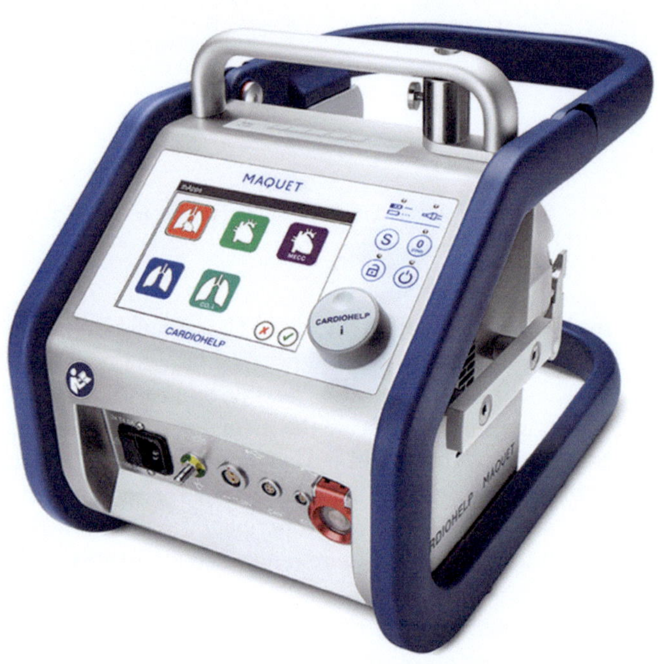

Fig. 53.5 The Getinge Cardiohelp System is a small and lightweight heart-lung support system (with permission from Getinge, Germany)

53.2.1 Venovenous ECMO (VV-ECMO)

– Double-site VV-ECMO is the most efficient technique for respiratory support, especially in case of high level of O_2 requirement [19]. The right internal jugular and the right or the left femoral veins are cannulated percutaneously. The right or "ideal" position of the outflow and the inflow cannulas are the junction between the right atrium and the inferior vena cava and the superior vena cava, respectively. The outflow cannula insertion length corresponds roughly to the length between the skin insertion point and the

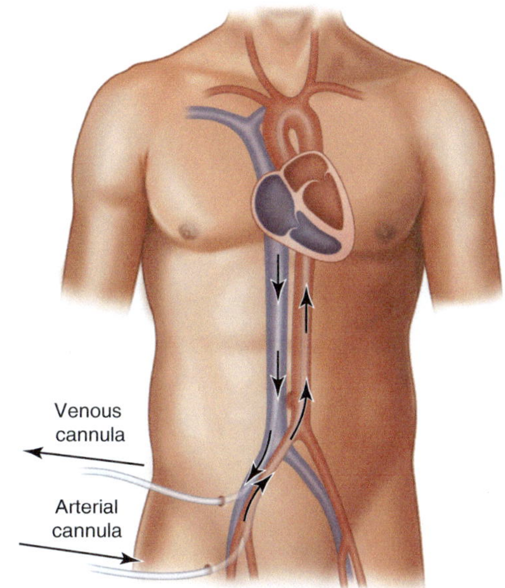

Fig. 53.6 On the left, schematic drawing showing venovenous ECMO: the venous blood is drained from the right femoral vein, and inflow is in the right jugular vein. On the right, schematic drawing showing venoarterial ECMO: the blood is drained from the right femoral vein, and inflow is in the right femoral artery

xiphoid process. The cannula is positioned under echocardiographic control.

- It is very important to utilize large cannulas (e.g., 25 Fr femoral cannula and 24 Fr right internal jugular cannula); in this way the VV-ECMO flow may reach 8 L/min.
- Single-site VV-ECMO. It is obtained by a single-site dual lumen cannula, the Avalon elite™ (Avalon elite™, Maquet cardiopulmonary GmbH, Rastatt, Germany). The cannula is routinely positioned in the right internal jugular vein: the outflow lumen drains from both the superior vena cava and the inferior vena cava; the inflow port is placed directly in the right atrium, in front of the tricuspid valve (Fig. 53.6).

53.2.2 Venoarterial ECMO (VA-ECMO)

VA-ECMO is indicated in trauma patients that present circulatory collapse and cardiogenic shock: in most of the cases it is positioned with a femoro-femoral access. Arterial and venous cannulas are positioned in the femoral vessels using the Seldinger technique with a completely percutaneous approach or after surgical cutdown. In the latter we cannulate the femoral vessels from the same side; surgical exposure allows to introduce under direct vision the cannula: a double purse-string suture around the insertion point will prevent air embolisms and hemorrhagic leaks and tie the cannula in place. Limb ischemia, the most frequent complication, is avoided by using end-to-side chimney graft or supplying blood by positioning a distal perfusion cannula (Fig. 53.7). If it is planned a percutaneous procedure (e.g., heart catheterization), it is better to utilize the femoral artery from one side and the femoral vein from the other side. The size of the venous cannula should be as large as possible (e.g., 25 Fr).

The size of the injection cannula depends on the caliber of the femoral artery and constitutes a balance between the risk of the inferior limb ischemia and the maximal flow available. It seems that a 21F inflow cannula is an optimal size in this configuration.

53.2.3 Anticoagulation

Chen and al [20]. describes minimal or none systemic heparinization reaching the target activated coagulation time (ACT) at 170 s. Ahmad [5] suggests, if not contraindicated in the patient, to maintain anticoagulation using heparin with ACT 160–180 s. Arlt and colleagues [21] (University Hospital Regensburg, Germany) reported initially heparin-free ECMO in severe trauma patients with resistant cardiopulmonary failure and coexisting bleeding; they found an improvement in therapy and outcome even in disastrous trauma patients. These findings were confirmed by Bonacchi et al. [22]

53.3 ECMO Support in Potential Organ Donors After Brain Death Determination

An increasing number of trauma patients, despite appropriate and immediate control of life-threatening injuries, may progress to brain death. In an attempt to counteract the

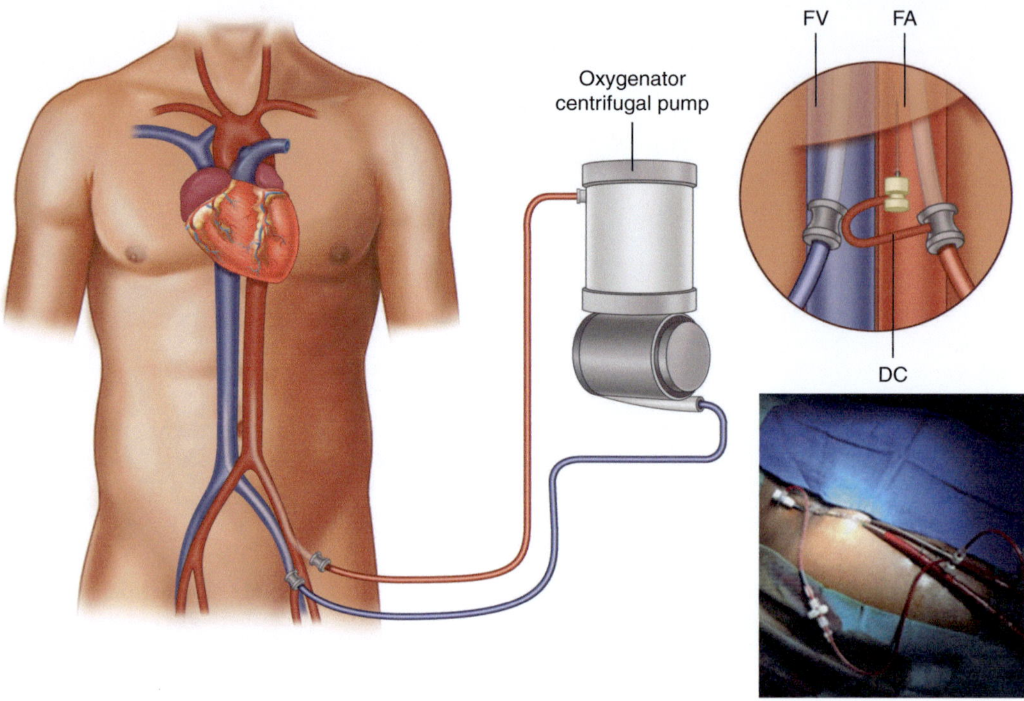

Fig. 53.7 Surgical approach to femoral vessels (*FV* femoral vein, *FA* femoral artery); in the enlarged circle, there is the distal perfusion cannula (DC), inserted distally the inflow arterial cannula. On the right, a surgical view: the two femoral, cannulas and and the DC that allows distal perfusion of the limb

worldwide organ shortage, in potential donors requiring aggressive vasoactive drugs, ECMO support should be considered in order to prevent damage and organ failure in case of transplantation. In this respect, there is an implementation of protocols that accept donation after cardiac death (DCD) and this measure has created a donor group that is frequently referred to as non-heart-beating donors (NHBDs). In brain dead potential donors organ perfusion must be optimized, endocrine homeostasis stabilized, and organs safeguarded; therefore, it is paramount to assure organ perfusion utilizing the least support of vasoactive drugs. Timing of ECMO support depends on several factors such as unstable hemodynamic (systolic blood pressure <90 mmHg) despite vasoactive drugs or a low oxygen saturation ($SaO_2 < 90\%$) despite ventilation support with high levels of positive end-expiratory pressure and high fractions of inspired oxygen ($FiO_2 > 80\%$). Therefore, A-V ECMO should be applied in early stages after brain death to perfuse abdominal organs before their retrieval; this practice has increased the organ supply for transplantation by approximately 20% in several countries. Furthermore, during the ECMO period the next of kin have the time to accept the death and to consider donation.

Another dilemma is: how long does the heart have to stop beating before you can declare a person dead? The time required to define the irreversibility of death varies widely among different countries. There is a no-touch period, defined as the time between the cessation of circulation and respiration and the determination of death, which ranges from 5 to 20 min. In Italy, the time interval to diagnose death is 20 min of cardiac arrest, demonstrated by continuous electrocardiographic recording. As matter of fact an interval time longer than that adopted in the United States and other European countries may negatively impact on organ viability, prolonging the warm ischemia time. ECMO support provides extra-circulatory support to patients with cardiorespiratory failure who would otherwise be expected to die. However, it should be remembered that in some studies, brain death has been reported as a complication of ECMO support. In this scenario, severe trauma patients with resistant cardiopulmonary failure and coexisting bleeding, the initial experience with heparin-free ECMO reported by Bonacchi [22] seems remarkable.

Finally it should be remembered that patients who are on ECMO support pose unique challenges to confirm the diagnosis of brain death. Brain death testing has been differently reported in the limited literature available with the majority of reports without information whether or not the patient remained on the ventilator with pressure support settings or he was taken off the ventilator. Due to the substantial continuous increase in ECMO utilization and the more frequent ethical and legal implications involved in brain death declaration, it is imperative that consensus guidelines should be developed in order to guide clinicians to the brain death diagnosis in ECMO patients.

53.4 Results

ECMO circuit needs systemic heparinization, therefore its use in trauma is controversial because patients often present with intracranial lesions and acute coagulopathy and may require multiple surgical procedures. Moreover, trauma surgeons and intensivists are concerned about the high risk of possible lethal bleeding, and they hesitate to position ECMO in a trauma patient. Anyway, there are more and more studies showing that ECMO improves survival in trauma patients [22–25].

A recent study, from the Department of Surgery, University of Maryland School of Medicine (USA), showed the results with the use of ECMO from January 2006 to November 2015 [5]. During this period 46 patients were treated with ECMO, 39 (85%) received a VV-ECMO and of these, 17 (44%) patients survived to discharge. There were no survivors among VA-ECMO patients. Survivors had a lower BMI (median, 25.4 vs. 27.3 kg/m^2; $p = 0.046$), a higher arterial pH (7.4 vs. 7.2, $p = 0.02$), and a lower $PaCO_2$ (44 vs. 57, $p = 0.02$). Anyway, survivors and non-survivors were not significantly different with regard to sex (62% vs. 82% male, $p = 0.27$) and CCI (Charlson Comorbidity Index) (94% vs. 86% with CCI 0, $p = 1.00$); there was no difference in admission GCS (Glasgow Coma Scale), systolic blood pressure, serum creatinine, white blood cell count, hematocrit, platelet count, PaO_2 level, arterial pH base deficit, or vasoactive drip requirement between the two groups. Mortality is undoubtedly high, but it is important to underline that all the patients, before ECMO, had failed maximal medical therapy, and a 44% survival represents a significant improvement vs. a fatal situation. In this context, ECMO can play a role both as a hemodynamic (for myocardial contusion) and ventilatory (for pulmonary contractions, tracheobronchial fistulas) support. The presence of a pelvic hematoma caused by trauma is not a contraindication to femoral-femoral ECMO [26–29]. When immediate surgery is not appropriate in a patient with profound physiologic depletion, hypercarbia, hypoxia, and shock requiring vasoactive medication, a damage control approach by ECMO support should be strongly considered. In this way it may be possible to have an early control of hemorrhage and contamination, resuscitation in the intensive care unit, and delayed definitive surgery after normalization of patient's hemodynamics. However, since the current knowledge of ECMO support is based on observational experience and retrospective studies, prospective controlled trials are needed to gather more evidence on safety and efficacy of ECMO support in different clinical settings.

Case Scenario

A 65-year-old male, polytrauma patient, developed a severe ARDS (Acute respiratory distress syndrome); his FO_2/PO_2 ratio was 50 mmHg, and his peripheral O_2 saturation was 80% despite maximal mechanical ventilation. Blood pressure was 105/70 mmHg with minimal inotropic support and heart rate 118/min. He was connected on VV-ECMO: a return cannula was inserted into the right atrium via the right internal jugular vein (19F), and a drainage cannula was inserted into the right femoral vein and positioned in the inferior vena cava. Thirty minutes after ECMO started, the patient remained severely hypoxic despite a circuit flow of 5.5 L/min and a post-oxygenator saturation in O_2 of 100%. Increasing pump speed to 4.500 rpm and circuit flow to 6.5 L/min did not ameliorate respiratory data. Arterial O_2 saturation is 83, while O_2 saturation in drainage line is 79%.

1. What is the most probable reason for the persistent hypoxemia?
   A. An oxygenator defect.
   B. Recirculation of blood between the return and drainage cannulas.
   C. Bilateral massive pneumothorax.
2. What would you suggest to do to improve hypoxemia?
   A. Change oxygenator.
   B. Adjust the cannula position: the return cannula tip should be positioned in the right atrium toward the tricuspid valve.
   C. Arrange for a VA-ECMO.

Please see Chap. 58 for the correct answer.

References

1. Baker CC, Oppenheimer L, Stephens B, Lewis FR, Trunkey DD. Epidemiology of trauma deaths. Am J Surg. 1980;140:144–50.
2. Trunkey DD. Trauma. Accidental and intentional injuries account for more years of life lost in the U.S. than cancer and heart disease. Among the prescribed remedies are improved preventive efforts, speedier surgery and further research. Sci Am. 1983;249:28–35.
3. Sobrino J, Shafi S. Timing and causes of death after injuries. Proc (Bayl Univ Med Cent). 2013;26:120–3.
4. Barton RG, Craft WB, Mone MC, Saffle JR. Chemical paralysis reduces energy expenditure in patients with burns and severe respiratory failure treated with mechanical ventilation. J Burn Care Rehabil. 1997;18:455–60.
5. Ahmad SB, Menaker J, Kufera J, O'Connor J, Scalea TM, Stein DM. Extracorporeal membrane oxygenation after traumatic injury. J Trauma Acute Care Surg. 2017;82:587–91.
6. Garlick J, Maxson T, Imamura M, Green J, Prodhan P. Differential lung ventilation and venovenous extracorporeal membrane oxygenation for traumatic bronchopleural fistula. Ann Thorac Surg. 2013;96:1859–60.

7. Pierson DJ, Horton CA, Bates PW. Persistent bronchopleural air leak during mechanical ventilation. A review of 39 cases. Chest J. 1986;90:321–3.
8. Dreizin D. Extracorporeal membrane oxygenation in plytrauma : what the radiologist needs to know. Emerg Radiol. 2015;22:565–76.
9. Enomoto Y, Watanabe H, Nakao S, Matsuoka T. Complete thoracic tracheal transection caused by blunt trauma. J Trauma Acute Care Surg. 2011;71:1478.
10. Daoud O, Augustin P, Mordant P, et al. Extracorporeal membrane oxygenation in 5 patients with bronchial fistula with severe acute lung injury. Ann Thorac Surg. 2011;92:327–30.
11. Sian K, McAllister B, Brady P. The use of extracorporeal membrane oxygenation therapy in the delayed surgical repair of a tracheal injury. Ann Thorac Surg. 2014;97:338–40.
12. Brogan TV, Lequier L, Lorusso R, MacLaren G, Peek G. Extracorporeal life support: the ELSO Red Book. 5th ed: Red Book; 2017. p. 61.
13. Yu K, Long C, Hei F, Li J, Liu J, Ji B, et al. Clinical evaluation of two different extracorporeal membrane oxygenation systems: a single center report. Artif Organs. 2011;7:733–7.
14. McMullan DM, Emmert JA, Permut LC, et al. The inflammatory and coagulative response to prolonged extracorporeal membrane oxygenation. Eur J Cardiothorac Surg. 2011;39:392–7.
15. Hill JG, Bruhn PS, Cohen SE, Gallagher MW, Manart F, Moore CA, Seifert PE, Askari P, Banchieri C. Emergent applications of cardiopulmonary support: a multiinstitutional experience. Ann Thorac Surg. 1992;54:699–704.
16. Lequier L, Horton SB, McMulla DM, Bartlett RH. Extracorporeal membrane oxygenation circuitry. Pediatr Crit Care Med. 2013;14:S7–12.
17. Hirose H, Yamane K, Marhefka G, Cavarocchi N. Right ventricular rupture and tamponade caused by malposition of the Avalon cannula for venovenous extracorporeal membrane oxygenation. J Cardiothorac Surg. 2012;7:36. https://doi.org/10.1186/1749-8090-7-36.
18. Brogan TV, Lequier L, Lorusso R, MacLaren G, Peek G. Extracorporeal life support: the ELSO Red Book. 5th ed. Red Book;2017. p. 69.
19. Reeb J, Olland A, Renaud S, Lejay A, Massard G, Falcoz P-E. Vascular access for extracorporeal life support: tips and tricks. J Thorac Dis. 2016;8:S353–63.
20. Chen TH, Shih JY, Shih JJ. Early percutaneous heparin-free venovenous extra corporeal life support (ECLS) is a safe and effective means of salvaging hypoxemic patients with complicated chest trauma. Acta Cardiol Sin. 2016;32:96–102.
21. Arlt M, Philipp A, Voelkel S, Rupprecht L, Mueller T, Hilker M, Graf B, Schmid C. Extracorporeal membrane oxygenation in severe trauma patients with bleeding shock. Resuscitation. 2010;81:804–9.
22. Bonacchi M, Spina R, Torracchi L, harmelin G, Sani G, Peris A. Extracorporeal life support in patients with severe trauma: an advanced treatment strategy for refractory clinical settings. J Thorac Cardiovasc Surg. 2013;145:1617–26.
23. Ried M, Bein T, Philipp A, Müller T, Graf B, Schmid C, Zonies D, Diez C, Hofmann HS. Extracorporeal lung support in trauma patients with severe chest injury and acute lung failure: a 10-year institutional experience. Crit Care. 2013;17(3):R110.
24. Madershahian N, Wittwer T, Strauch J, Franke UF, Wippermann J, Kaluza M, Wahlers T. Application of ECMO in multitrauma patients with ARDS as rescue therapy. J Card Surg. 2007;22:180–4.
25. Guirand DM, Okoye OT, Schmidt BS, Mansfield NJ, Aden JK, Martin RS, Cestero RF, Hines MH, Pranikoff T, Inaba K, et al. Venovenous extracorporeal life support improves survival in adult trauma patients with acute hypoxemic respiratory failure: a multicenter retrospective cohort study. J Trauma Acute Care Surg. 2014;76(5):1275–81.
26. Schupp M, Swanedelder JL, Peek GJ, Sonoswxki AW, Spyt TJ. Postoperative extracorporeal membrane oxygenation for severe intraoperative SRS 10 h after multiple trauma. Br J Anaesth. 2003;90:91–4.
27. Masiakos PT, Hirsch EF, Millham FH. Management of severe combined pulmonary and myocardial contusion with extracorporeal membrane oxygenation. J Trauma. 2003;54:1012–5.
28. Michaels AJ, Schriener RJ, Kolla S, Awad SS, Rich PB, Reickert CR, Ypunger J, Hirschl RB, Bartlett RH. Extracorporeal life support in pulmonary failure after trauma. J Trauma. 1999;46:638–45.
29. Perchinsky MJ, Long WB, Hill JG, Parson JA, Bennet JB. Extracorporeal cardiopulmonary life support with heparin-bonded circuitry in the resuscitation of massively injured trauma patients. Am J Surg. 1995;168:488–91.

Hyper-Urgent Liver Transplantation for Posttraumatic and Surgical Iatrogenic Acute Liver Failure

54

Andrea Lauterio, Stefano Di Sandro, Riccardo De Carlis, Arianna Ciravegna, Paolo Aseni, and Luciano De Carlis

Abbreviations

ACLF	Acute-on-chronic liver failure
ALF	Acute liver failure
BDI	Bile duct injury
ELS	Extracorporeal liver support
HPB	Hepato-pancreato-biliary
hu-LT	Hyper-urgent liver transplantation
IVC	Inferior vena cava
LT	Liver transplantation
MOF	Multiple organ failure
PNF	Primary nonfunction
PV	Portal vein
TLS	Toxic liver syndrome
TPCS	Temporary portocaval shunt

A. Lauterio (✉) · S. Di Sandro · A. Ciravegna
Department of General Surgery and Transplantation, ASST Grande Ospedale Metropolitano Niguarda, Milan, Italy
e-mail: andrea.lauterio@ospedaleniguarda.it

R. De Carlis
Department of General Surgery and Transplantation, ASST Grande Ospedale Metropolitano Niguarda, Milan, Italy

Department of Surgical Sciences, University of Pavia, Pavia, Italy

P. Aseni
Department of Emergency, ASST Grande Ospedale Metropolitano Niguarda, Milan, Italy

L. De Carlis
Department of General Surgery and Transplantation, ASST Grande Ospedale Metropolitano Niguarda, Milan, Italy

University of Milano-Bicocca, School of Medicine, Milan, Italy
e-mail: LUCIANOGREGORI.DECARLIS@ospedaleniguarda.it

Key Points

- Liver transplantation may ultimately represent the only lifesaving option to manage acute liver failure after trauma or fatal iatrogenic liver injuries.
- The success rate of nonoperative management of hepatic trauma—defined as a no surgical procedure required—generally exceeds 90%.
- Clinicians are constantly reminded about the importance of early referral for patients with hepatic trauma or severe iatrogenic liver injuries to a tertiary center with experienced HPB and transplant surgery.
- Patients initially and repeatedly treated in nonspecialist hospitals and referred for LT in the ALF setting have been reported to have worse outcomes.
- Liver resection could be a surgical option only when the hepatic infarction and necrosis are limited, and liver function preserved because any surgical or infectious complication after a major hepatectomy could represent a contraindication to proceed to LT.
- Hu-LT for the management of severe liver injury and ALF may represent a surgical challenge requiring technically difficult and time-consuming procedures such as total hepatectomy and LT as a two-stage procedure, temporary portocaval shunt (TPCS), venovenous extracorporeal circulation, and complex vascular reconstructions.
- In the era of organ shortage, when an hu-LT is indicated for worsening ALF, the patient's clinical conditions, signs associated with irreversible neurologic injuries, and near-certain intraoperative mortality should be taken into account to avoid wasting of liver grafts.

P. Aseni et al. (eds.), *Operative Techniques and Recent Advances in Acute Care and Emergency Surgery*,
https://doi.org/10.1007/978-3-319-95114-0_54

54.1 Introduction

Liver transplantation (LT) may ultimately represent the only lifesaving option to manage acute liver failure (ALF) after trauma or fatal iatrogenic liver injuries. The operative and nonoperative strategies involved in the management of high-grade traumatic liver injuries have been addressed in a different dedicated chapter. However, the medical conditions related to ALF, primary nonfunction (PNF) after primary LT, acute-on-chronic liver failure (ACLF), and all other causes of ALF not strictly related to emergency surgery will be not discussed in this chapter.

Severe iatrogenic liver injuries, e.g., massive otherwise unsalvageable liver trauma, exsanguinating hemorrhage, or significant hepatic necrosis, may represent causes of hyper-urgent LT (hu-LT). This chapter summarizes the traumatic causes of hu-LT and discusses our own experience along with surgical advances in this uncommon transplant setting.

In the era of organ shortage, the indication for hu-LT for a worsening ALF should be carefully evaluated in consideration of the rapidly changing clinical conditions of the single patient. Clinical signs clearly associated with irreversible neurologic damage with near-certain intraoperative or perioperative mortality should be taken into account to avoid wasting of a liver graft.

54.2 Acute Liver Failure: Definition and Background

Regardless of etiology, ALF (acute liver failure) is defined as severe liver injury with a rapid onset (<26 weeks' duration) that results in hepatic encephalopathy and coagulopathy (INR $\geq$ 1.5) in patients without the pre-existing liver disease. The clinical picture can be a rapid-onset encephalopathy, with marked cerebral edema, systemic inflammation, and multiorgan dysfunction (MODS) [1] with elevated transaminases, hyperbilirubinemia, and severe coagulopathy. MODS is preceded by oliguria, hypotension, impaired gas exchange, hypoglycemia, and pancytopenia with a sudden and marked drop in platelet count. Referral to a dedicated liver unit for evaluation of urgent LT is mandatory. The King's College Criteria, developed in the early 1980s, remain the most widely used and accepted criteria for LT in patients with ALF [1, 2].

54.2.1 Toxic Liver Syndrome

In 1993, Ringe et al. first described the so-called toxic liver syndrome (TLS) in the setting of ALF in patients with nonfunctioning grafts, hemodynamic and renal instability caused by acute hepatic necrosis [3]. TLS usually occurs following liver graft failure or acute rejection after LT, but can also be associated with traumatic or postoperative causes. The full-blown picture is characterized by cardiovascular shock and renal and respiratory failure requiring resuscitation efforts such as vasopressor support, hemodialysis, and mechanical ventilation. The pathophysiologic mechanism of TLS remains unclear but seems to be related to toxic metabolites (cytokines and cardio-suppressive factors) released from devitalized liver parenchyma as described in liver graft ischemia-reperfusion injury.

54.2.2 Extracorporeal Liver Support

The use of extracorporeal liver support (ELS), including single-pass albumin dialysis, molecular adsorbent recirculating system (MARS) and Prometheus®, has been reported and reviewed in the recent years [4, 5] with encouraging results both in the treatment of ALF as a bridge to LT for patients with hepatic necrosis resulting from the management of traumatic liver injury. Ginsberg et al. recently reported on MARS application to restore hepatic function and avoid hu-LT in three patients with traumatic liver injuries developing high-grade hepatic necrosis [5] suggesting a possible novel therapeutic application; the study was insufficiently powered to demonstrate a clear benefit, and the authors concluded that the procedure might be considered provided it will not delay consultation for consideration of LT.

54.3 Technical Aspects of Hyper-Urgent Liver Transplantation

Hu-LT liver for the management of severe liver injury and ALF may represent a surgical challenge requiring technically difficult and time-consuming procedures such as pre-transplant total hepatectomy, temporary portocaval shunt (TPCS) or venovenous extracorporeal circulation, urgent liver procurement from a deceased donor, and LT as a second-stage procedure with vascular and biliary reconstructions.

Since TPCS was first introduced in the early 1990s as a surgical option to improve hemodynamic stability during LT in recipients with portal hypertension, its role has remained controversial, and its use is now still limited in the current surgical practice of LT [6]. On the other hand, a two-stage LT intended as total hepatectomy, TPCS, and subsequent LT could be a useful strategy for patients presenting exsanguinating hepatic injuries with uncontrollable vascular or parenchymal bleeding [3, 7]. TLS secondary to massive hepatic necrosis requires urgent total hepatectomy, and TPCS is the only possibility to bridge patients to wait for a compatible deceased liver donor without inducing splanchnic congestion and hemodynamic instability. Total hepatectomy might also improve the metabolic, coagulation and hemodynamic profiles of these patients while waiting for a suitable liver donor [3].

Urgent total hepatectomy may represent the ultimate life-saving option in exceptional situations of grade V and VI liver trauma with an impending risk of death from exsanguination or ALF. Two different clinical scenarios can be described for indication to immediate total hepatectomy: massive bleeding due to liver damage only controllable with full hepatectomy and ALF with progressive clinical deterioration in the days following the trauma; in this case the purpose of urgent total hepatectomy is to clean the patient of the toxic effects sustained by a necrotic organ. The anhepatic phase should be kept to a minimum despite anecdotal reports of anhepatic times exceeding 48 h [8]. The potential risks and benefits of this drastic maneuver should be carefully evaluated by the clinicians involved.

Before performing TPCS careful hemostasis should be attempted during the hepatectomy because of the impaired coagulation during the anhepatic phase. Anhepatic patients are at high risk of fatal hypothermia, acidosis, and coagulation profile impairment. For these reasons anhepatic patients should be observed in the operating room by a dedicated team of intensivists from the liver unit or transferred to the ICU until a liver graft becomes available.

Different surgical procedures have been described to perform TPCS. From the technical point of view, two basic options can be applied to shunt the portal flow to the systemic circulation: an end-to-side anastomosis between the main portal vein (PV) and the anterior wall of the suprarenal inferior vena cava (IVC) or a porto-suprahepatic anastomosis [9]. Rarely, if a vena cava preserving hepatectomy is possible, an extracorporeal portocaval shunt with a heparinized catheter can be inserted to connect the PV to the femoral vein without any anticoagulation therapy or additional pump supply [10]. A venovenous bypass by a centrifugal pump without systemic heparinization may represent the only possible option in patients requiring total liver vascular exclusion or resection of the IVC to overcome massive bleeding, as previously reported by our institution [11].

Extra-anatomical vascular reconstruction in patients with severe iatrogenic injuries of the hepatic hilum elements remains an important tool in the surgeon's armamentarium. The use of vascular allografts was first described by Starzl and colleagues and is still a common surgical practice in LT [12]. Cryopreserved and banked or freshly procured vascular grafts from deceased donors should be considered for supraceliac or infrarenal aortohepatic conduits. Vascular reconstruction using deceased donor iliac artery as an interposition graft in LT has already been investigated and reviewed in transplant surgery together with the use of cryopreserved arterial grafts more recently reported in living donor LT [13, 14]. Excellent long-term results recently proved the longevity of the PV conduits using the donor's iliac vein in LT [15]. The reported results may also apply to other complex surgical settings such as severe vascular injuries requiring hu-LT.

Resection and replacement of the IVC could occasionally be required during LT for severe iatrogenic injury of the liver or IVC. Different reconstruction strategies using biological materials (autologous and heterologous) and synthetic grafts such as polytetrafluoroethylene (PTFE) and polypropylene (Dacron) have been described to replace the vena cava [11, 16]. The use of glutaraldehyde-treated bovine pericardium or an autogenous peritoneal-fascial graft from a flap of parietal peritoneum backed by the posterior rectus sheath has recently been advocated as alternative to prosthetic IVC reconstruction showing long-term patency without permanent anticoagulation treatment [17].

54.4 Indications for Hyper-Urgent Liver Transplantation

Hu-LT has seldom been reported in the treatment of other severe iatrogenic liver injuries after abdominal and hepato-pancreato-biliary (HPB) surgery, whereas hu-LT for hepatic trauma was first reported 30 years ago and recently reviewed [18, 19].

54.4.1 Hepatic Trauma

The liver is one of the most commonly injured parenchymal organs due to its size and position in the abdomen. Most traumatic hepatic injuries are related to blunt trauma during motor vehicle accidents.

A wide spectrum of vascular or parenchymal injuries may occur after hepatic trauma with severity varying from limited subcapsular hematoma to massive intrahepatic infarction and capsular lacerations with severe vascular damage and complete liver avulsion. A trauma organ injury scale was devised by the American Association for the Surgery of Trauma in 2008 and is currently adopted to classify hepatic trauma into six grades [20].

Since the introduction of so-called damage control strategies in the management of hepatic trauma, and the widespread application of nonsurgical management options mainly based on interventional radiology procedures (angioembolization), high-risk surgical operations have been performed in a specific and limited setting. Generally speaking, the success rate of nonoperative management—defined as a no surgical procedure required—generally exceeds 90% [21, 22]. Hepatic necrosis may represent an acceptable complication after angioembolization in high-grade liver injuries, requiring specific interventions such as drainage, debridement, or liver resection.

LT may represent the last chance when conservative procedures fail to overcome massive hemorrhage requiring total hepatectomy or when a patient develops ALF secondary to angioembolization-induced major hepatic necrosis [23].

Although the first LT for the management of patients with hepatic trauma was first reported in 1987 [18], the medical literature lacks large studies supporting its use. A recently published study from the European Liver Transplant Registry (ELTR) reported the outcome of LT for hepatic trauma in 73 recipients over a period of 25 years across 37 centers in Europe [19]. The postoperative mortality and graft loss rates at 3 months after LT were 42.5% (31/73) and 46%, respectively, while the overall 5-year rates were 50.7% and 44.9%, respectively. From the standpoint of transplant surgery, the study reported superior outcomes in patients transplanted with IVC preservation using the piggyback technique and avoiding the standard technique without the use of the venovenous bypass. The results of this large study indicate that LT seems justified in patients with severe liver trauma not exceeding grade IV with an injury severity score below 33 and when all other treatment options have failed. In the emergency setting, LT has also been described in rare cases of liver avulsion or total crush injury, when a total hepatectomy is required. In these cases, different types of shunting procedures have been described, most of them anecdotally. The venovenous bypass by a centrifugal pump without systemic heparinization (femoral vein and portal vein to axillary vein by pass) is the most frequent type of shunt used by surgeons familiar with its use [24, 25].

54.4.2 Severe Iatrogenic Liver Injuries After Cholecystectomy

Regardless of the entity of the injury, the incidence of cholecystectomy-induced bile duct injury (s) ranges from 0.1 to 0.3%, rising to 0.6% when considering the laparoscopic approach [26, 27]. A small number of LT procedures to treat cholecystectomy-induced severe bile duct or vascular injuries have been reported in the literature, and a few were performed for ALF. Some recently described series provide important insights.

In 2011, data from a national retrospective survey performed in Argentina over 20 years reported 19 (0.7%) LT secondary to BDI [28] among a total of 2766 LT performed from 1990 to 2009. The indication for LT was liver cirrhosis in 18 cases and ALF in the remaining patient. No intraoperative mortality was reported, but four patients died during the first month after LT, and another four died in the late postoperative period.

In 2013, the Spanish Liver Transplantation Study Group reviewed the outcomes of 27 patients transplanted after cholecystectomy-induced BDI over a 24-year period [29]. Results after hu-LT for ALF were discouraging. LT for ALF was indicated after laparoscopic cholecystectomy in 7 patients, while the other 20 underwent LT for secondary cirrhosis. Two of the acute recipients died while on the waiting list, one from MODS, and the other remained anhepatic after a total hepatectomy required for massive liver necrosis and TLS. Four of the five recipients who underwent LT for ALF died within 30 days after transplant. In 2012, Strasberg and colleagues addressed the pathogenesis and management of "extreme" vasculobiliary injuries during cholecystectomy, reporting outcomes after cholecystectomy for severely inflamed gallbladders in eight patients [30]. Unfortunately, one patient developed infarction of the bile ducts after injury to the proper hepatic artery and died of sepsis in the postoperative period after urgent LT. The authors claimed that fundus-down cholecystectomy should be avoided in the presence of inflammation to prevent extreme vasculobiliary injuries.

Another two cases of LT for iatrogenic injuries among 12 patients referred for the management of complicated cholecystectomy were recently reported [31]. One of those patients was listed for an emergency LT after a complicated laparoscopic cholecystectomy with angioembolization to overcome an intrahepatic right lobe hematoma and bleeding resulting from a complicated endoscopic biliary stent placement. The patient required emergency surgical exploration, a total hepatectomy with TPCS and a two-stage LT after a 2-day anhepatic period.

54.4.3 Other Causes of Severe Iatrogenic Liver Injuries

Indications for hu-LT to manage severe iatrogenic liver injuries after abdominal surgery and HPB surgery or causes other than injuries during cholecystectomy are rare, and very few cases have been reported.

Three lethal complications resulting from severe iatrogenic injury of the PV during bariatric surgery [32] were described in 2006. The authors claimed that PV ligation with immediate patient referral to an LT center for emergency transplant might improve the outcome in case of severe PV injury.

Another two cases of iatrogenic porta hepatis transection requiring an urgent two-stage liver LT [33] were reported in 2009. In the first case, severe porta hepatis transection occurred during an open adrenalectomy, and a primary PV repair attempted to transfer the patient to an LT unit.

Due to progression of the hepatic dysfunction and worsening hemodynamics, the patient underwent a two-stage LT. In the other case, severe iatrogenic injury occurred during a laparoscopic cholecystectomy converted to an open operation to control a massive bleeding before emergency transfer of the patient to a tertiary center. The extent of the PV injury precluded successful reconstruction of the PV flow, and a two-stage LT was performed 20 h later. Patients presenting with severe portal transection cannot be treated expectantly, and prompt radiological evaluation and surgical intervention are mandatory to attempt to restore hepatic flow.

Hepatic resections should not be the only options entertained, and LT should be promptly evaluated on a case-by-case basis.

Di Benedetto et al. [34] reported in 2010 details of their experience in the treatment of severe hepatic injuries after transjugular intrahepatic portosystemic shunt placements in two cirrhotic patients where surgical and radiological attempts had failed to stop the bleeding after parenchymal and vascular rupture. Although the indications for LT were ALF after artery embolization and uncontrollable hemobilia, this experience highlights the importance of a prompt referral to a tertiary center to offer LT as the only curative option.

Case Scenarios

We recently reviewed our experience as a tertiary referral center offering both a specialist HPB referral service and an abdominal organ transplantation service with hu-LT to manage severe iatrogenic liver injuries occurring during HPB surgery [35].

Case n. 1: the first lifesaving LT performed by our institution has been described in detail elsewhere and highlights some important technical features of the surgical technique adopted [11]. A total hepatectomy with retrohepatic IVC resection after a venovenous bypass was carried out to overcome the hemodynamic instability and an uncontrollable bleeding from the confluence of the suprahepatic veins during liver resection for a giant symptomatic hepatic hemangioma arising from the caudate lobe with compression of the retrohepatic IVC. The extensive liver congestion excluded any attempt to proceed to an ex vivo major hepatectomy, and a request for hu-LT was launched. A Dacron interposition prosthesis replaced the retrohepatic vena cava, and an end-to-side TPCS was performed between the recipient PV and the Dacron prosthesis. The patient was successfully transplanted with a long-term follow-up. LT was carried out as a two-stage procedure. Temporary venovenous bypass was employed during the anhepatic phase but was disconnected due to severe fibrinolysis and hypothermia. A portocaval shunt was performed, and the inferior vena cava outflow was restored by a Dacron interposition prosthesis. A side-to-side cavo-caval anastomosis between the graft retrohepatic vena cava and the Dacron interposition graft was performed, whereas the portal vein, hepatic arterial, and biliary tract were reconstructed by the conventional technique.

Case n. 2: a 52-year-old woman was referred to our center from another HPB tertiary center without an LT program. Before referral, the patient had ALF resulting from a radiologically assisted hepatic artery embolization to overcome a massive intrahepatic bleeding with rapid deterioration of clinical status due to hemorrhagic shock in a patient initially affected by bi-lobar intrahepatic lithiasis treated by bile-duct exploration and a Roux-en-Y hepatico-jejunal anastomosis. After the patient's referral, a conservative liver resection such as right extended hepatectomy was excluded because of the liver failure and the massive hepatic infarction extending to the left lobe. Liver resection could be a surgical option only before the hepatic infarction and when necrosis was limited with preserved liver function. An urgent LT was planned, and a liver graft became available 16 h later. The patient was successfully transplanted. Despite the massive right lobe hematoma extending to segment IV with signs of extrahepatic rupture, the hepatectomy was carried out with hemodynamic stability, and TPCS and venovenous bypass were not required. The liver implant was performed in a piggyback fashion and a Roux-en-Y reconstruction carried out using the same intestinal loop created during the first surgery.

Questions

1. The clinical picture of ALF acute liver failure is defined as deterioration of liver function with:
   A. Rapid onset hepatic encephalopathy (<26 weeks) and coagulopathy (INR ≥ 1.5) in a patient without the pre-existing liver disease
   B. Severe liver injury and ALT > 3.000 IU/L
   C. Severe liver injury with ALT > 3.000 and bilirubin >10 mg/dL
   D. Severe liver Injury in a patient with GCS < 9
2. Toxic liver syndrome (TLS) in the setting of ALF was first described by Ringe as:
   A. Nonfunctioning liver grafts, impaired hemodynamics, and renal instability caused by acute hepatic necrosis after liver transplantation
   B. Nonfunctioning liver grafts, impaired hemodynamics, and renal instability caused by acute hepatic necrosis after high-grade liver trauma
   C. Impaired hemodynamics and renal instability caused by acute hepatic necrosis after hepatic artery angioembolization
   D. Hyperammonemia and high-grade liver injury
3. Indications for hyper-urgent liver transplantation are:
   A. Patients with liver trauma who develop ALF secondary to angioembolization-induced major hepatic necrosis
   B. Patients with ALF and iatrogenic major hepatic necrosis following hepatobiliary procedures
   C. Liver avulsion or total crush injury, when a total hepatic resection must be done to control massive hemorrhage for unsalvageable liver trauma
   D. A, B, and C

Please see Chap. 58 for the correct answer.

References

1. De Gasperi A, Findlay JY, Klinck JR. Critical care of the patient with liver disease. In: Oxford textbook of transplant anaeshesia and critical care. https://doi.org/10.1093/med/9780199651429.003.0021.
2. O'Grady JC, Alexander GJ, Hayllar KM, Williams R. Early indicators of prognosis in fulminant hepatic failure. Gastroenterology. 1989;97(2):439–45.
3. Ringe B, Lübbe N, Kuse E, et al. Total hepatectomy and liver transplantation as two-stage procedure. Ann Surg. 1993;218:3–9.
4. Nevens F, Laleman W. Artificial liver support devices as treatment option for liver failure. Best Pract Clin Gastroenterol. 2012;26(1):17–26.
5. Ginsberg Z, Thurman P, Scalea T, Stein D. Extracorporeal liver support for trauma-induced hepatic disfunction. J Trauma Acute Care Surg. 2016;80(6):1039–44.
6. Tzakis AG, Reyes J, Nour B, Marino IR, Todo S, Starzl TE. Temporary end-to-side portacaval shunt in orthotopic hepatic transplantation in humans. Surg Gynecol Obstet. 1993;176(2):180–2. PMID: 8421808.
7. Ringe B, Pichlmayr R, Ziegler H, et al. Management of severe hepatic trauma by two-stage total hepatectomy and subsequent liver transplantation. Surgery. 1991;109:792–5.
8. Arora H, Thekkekandam J, Tesche L, et al. Long-term survival after 67 hours of anhepatic state due to primary liver allograft nonfunction. Liver Transpl. 2010;16:1428–33.
9. Robles R, Parrilla P, Acosta F, Bueno FS, Ramirez P, Lujan JA, et al. Portosuprahepatic shunt as an alternative to portocaval shunt in an hepatic patients waiting for an orthotopic liver transplant. Transplant Proc. 1999;31(6):2400–1. PMID: 10500639.
10. Pratschke S, Meimarakis G, Bruns CJ, Kaspar M, Prix N, Zachoval R, et al. Temporary intraoperative porto-caval shunt: useless or beneficial in piggy back liver transplantation? Transpl Int. 2013;26(1):90–8. https://doi.org/10.1111/tri.12007. PMID: 23237579.
11. Aseni P, Lauterio A, Slim AO, Giacomoni A, Lamperti L, De Carlis L. Life-saving super-urgent liver transplantation with replacement of retrohepatic vena cava by Dacron graft. HPB Surg. 2010;2010. pii: 828326. https://doi.org/10.1155/2010/828326. PMID: 20811479.
12. Starzl TE, Halgrimson CG, Koep LG, Weil R, Taylor PD, et al. Vascular homograft from cadaveric organ donors. Surg Gynecol Obstet. 1979;149:737.
13. Chatzizacharias NA, Aly M, Praseedom RK. The role of arterial conduits for revascularisation in adult orthotopic liver transplantation. Transplant Rev (Orlando). 2016. pii: S0955-470X(16)30067-2. https://doi.org/10.1016/j.trre.2016.10.008. [Epub ahead of print] Review. PMID: 27884502.
14. Ali MA, Yong CC, Eng HL, Wang CC, Lin TL, Li WF, et al. Cryopreserved arterial grafts as a conduit in outflow reconstruction in living donor liver transplantation. J Hepatobiliary Pancreat Sci. 2015;22(6):498–504. https://doi.org/10.1002/jhbp.240. PMID: 25783415.
15. Nikitin D, Jennings LW, Khan T, Vasani S, Ruiz R, Sanchez EQ, Chinnakotla S, Levy MF, Goldstein RM, Klintmalm GB. Twenty years' follow-up of portal vein conduits in liver transplantation. Liver Transpl. 2009;15(4):400–6. https://doi.org/10.1002/lt.21698. PMID: 19326411.
16. Palma AF, Oberkofler CE, Raptis DA, Eshmuminov D, de Rougemont O, Schnyder A, et al. Novel rescue procedure for inferior vena cava reconstruction in living-donor liver transplantation using a vascular graft recovered 25 h after donors' circulatory death and systematic review. Transpl Int. 2014;27(2):204–10. https://doi.org/10.1111/tri.12238. Review.
17. Pulitanó C, Crawford M, Ho P, Gallagher J, Joseph D, Stephen M, et al. The use of biological grafts for reconstruction of the inferior vena cava is a safe and valid alternative: results in 32 patients in a single institution. HPB (Oxford). 2013;15(8):628–32. https://doi.org/10.1111/hpb.12029. PMID: 23458108.
18. Esquivel CO, Bernardos A, Makowka L, Iwatsuki S, Gordon RD, Starzl TE. Liver replacement after massive hepatic trauma. J Trauma. 1987;27:800–2.
19. Krawczyk M, Grat M, Adam R, Polak WG, klempnauer J, Pinna A, et al. Liver transplantation for hepatic trauma: a study from the European Liver Transplant Registry. Transplantation. 2016;100(11):2372–81.
20. Tinkoof G, Esposito TJ, Reed J, et al. American Association for the Surgery of Trauma Organ Injury Scale I: spleen, liver, and kidney, validation based on the National Trauma Data Bank. J Am Coll Surg. 2008;207:646–55.
21. Hurtuk M, Reed RL, Esposito TJ, Davis KA, Luchette FA. Trauma surgeons practice what they preach: the NTDB story on solid organ injury management. J Trauma. 2006;61(2):243–54.
22. Green CS, Bulger EM, Kwan SW. Outcomes and complication of angioembolization for hepatic trauma: a systematic review of the literature. J Trauma Acute Care Surg. 2016;80(3):529–35.
23. Dabbs DN, Stein DM, Scalea TM. Major hepatic necrosis: a common compliction after angioembolization for treatment of high-grade liver injuries. J Trauma. 2009;66:621–9.
24. Peitzman AB, Marsh JW. Advanced operative techniques in management of complex liver injury. J Trauma Acute Care Surg. 2012;73(3):765–70.
25. Coccolini F, Catena F, Moore EE, Ivatury R, Biffl W, Peitzman A, et al. WSES Classification and guidelines for liver trauma. World J Emerg Surg. 2016;11:50.
26. Roslyn JJ, Binns GS, Hughes EF, Saunders-Kirkwood K, Zinner MJ, Cates JA. Open cholecystectomy. A contemporary analysis of 42,474 patients. Ann Surg. 1993;218(2):129–37. PMID: 8342992.
27. Richardson MC, Bell G, Fullarton GM. Incidence and nature of bile duct injuries following laparoscopic cholecystectomy: an audit of 5913 cases. West of Scotland Laparoscopic Cholecystectomy Audit Group. Br J Surg. 1996;83(10):1356–60. PMID: 8944450.
28. Ardiles V, McCormack L, Quinonez E, Goldaracena N, Mattera J, Ciardullo M, et al. Experience using liver transplantation for the treatment of severe bile duct injuries over 20 years in Argentina: results from a National Survey. HPB (Oxford). 2011;13(8):544–50. https://doi.org/10.1111/j.1477-2574.2011.00322.x. PMID: 21762297.
29. Parrilla P, Robles R, Varo E, Jiménez C, Sánchez-Cabús S, Pareja E, Spanish Liver Transplantation Study Group. Liver transplantation for bile duct injury after open and laparoscopic cholecystectomy. Br J Surg. 2014;101(2):63–8. https://doi.org/10.1002/bjs.9349. PMID: 24318962.
30. Strasberg SM, Gouma DJ. Extreme vasculobiliary injuries: association with fundus-down cholecystectomy in severely inflamed gallbladders. HPB (Oxford). 2012;14(1):1–8. https://doi.org/10.1111/j.1477-2574.2011.00393.x. PMID: 22151444.
31. Leale I, Moraglia E, Bottino G, Rachef M, Dova L, Cariati A, et al. Role of liver transplantation in bilio-vascular liver injury after cholecystectomy. Transplant Proc. 2016;48(2):370–6. https://doi.org/10.1016/j.transproceed.2015.12.035. PMID: 27109958.
32. Huerta S, Li Z, Livingston EH. Outcome of portal injuries following bariatric operations. Obes Surg. 2006;16(1):105–9. PMID: 16417768.
33. Zaydfudim V, Wright JK, Pinson CW. Liver transplantation for iatrogenic porta hepatis transection. Am Surg. 2009;75(4):313–6. PMID: 19385291.
34. Di Benedetto F, Mimmo A, D'Amico G, De Ruvo N, Cautero N, Montalti R, et al. Liver transplantation due to iatrogenic injuries: two case reports. Transplant Proc. 2010;42(4):1375–7. https://doi.org/10.1016/j.transproceed.2010.03.077. PMID: 20534306.
35. Lauterio A, De Carlis R, Di Sandro S, Ferla F, Buscemi V, De Carlis L. Liver transplantation in the treatment of severe iatrogenic liver injuries. World J Hepatol. 2017;9(24):1022–9. https://doi.org/10.4254/wjh.v9.i24.1022.

The Potential Organ Donor: Current Trends and Management

55

Riccardo De Carlis, Marinella Zanierato, Giorgio Antonio Iotti, Paolo Aseni, and Luciano De Carlis

Key Points

- Establishing the best therapeutic strategies for patients with major trauma has led to significant improvement in donor conversion rates and utilization of deceased donors.
- Optimizing donor management is fundamental to increase the numbers of organs available for transplantation.
- Declaration of death on the basis of neurologic criteria preserves transplantable organs from the detrimental warm ischemia that limits donation after cardiac death (DCD).
- Brain death causes numerous physiological derangements, which make brain-dead donors fragile and essentially unstable.
- Many countries worldwide have explored the option of DCD to expand the organ donor pool.
- Normothermic regional perfusion (NRP) is a very effective method for preservation and functional assessment of DCD abdominal organs.
- NRP permits unhurried warm organ dissection and cold flash directly through the femoral cannulae, minimizing the risk of graft injury.
- The combination of NRP followed by machine perfusion can be considered a promising new frontier for organ recovery from DCD.

55.1 Introduction

Treatment of the trauma patient has improved enormously over the last few decades, achieving better results and survival rates. Although increasing numbers of trauma patients receive immediate and appropriate control of life-threatening injuries, some eventually progress to brain death. Establishment of the best therapeutic strategies for patients with extensive and major trauma, such as damage control surgery—a new emerging discipline with the aim of preventing patients progressing to an unsalvageable metabolic state—has led to significant improvements also in donor conversion rates and increased the utilization of deceased donors. Approximately 30% of all deceased organ donors come from trauma patients who have suffered devastating neurologic injury and have progressed to brain death.

Though donation rates have increased over the past decade, many patients still die on the waiting list for organ transplantation. Many individuals who satisfy the criteria for becoming organ donors eventually fail to donate because of lack of consent. But even when consent is given, organs may be deemed unsuitable for donation because of their condition, or the donor may develop cardiac arrest (CA) before organs can be recovered. Medical failures prior to organ procurement in brain-dead patients may be preventable in many cases, and optimizing donor selection and management has thus become a priority [1, 2]. Early recognition and physiological maintenance of the potential organ donor, and

R. De Carlis (✉)
Department of General Surgery and Transplantation, ASST Grande Ospedale Metropolitano Niguarda, Milan, Italy

Department of Surgical Sciences, University of Pavia, Pavia, Italy
e-mail: riccardo.decarlis@ospedaleniguarda.it

M. Zanierato · G. A. Iotti
Intensive Medicine Department, IRCCS Policlinico San Matteo, Pavia, Italy

P. Aseni
Department of General Surgery and Transplantation, ASST Grande Ospedale Metropolitano Niguarda, Milan, Italy

L. De Carlis
Department of General Surgery and Transplantation, ASST Grande Ospedale Metropolitano Niguarda, Milan, Italy

School of Medicine, University of Milano-Bicocca, Milan, Italy

P. Aseni et al. (eds.), *Operative Techniques and Recent Advances in Acute Care and Emergency Surgery*,
https://doi.org/10.1007/978-3-319-95114-0_55

close coordination with the local organ procurement organization, are all important aspects of this process.

In the late 1990s, Jenkins et al. estimated that only 15–20% of potential donors actually become donors in the United States [1]. In 2012, brain deaths eligible for organ donation amounted to 8944 in the United States, with a donor conversion rate of 72.5 eligible donors per 100 eligible deaths [3]. In Italy, 2341 brain deaths were reported in 2015, and just under half were utilized as donors (1163, 49.8%) with lack of consent to donation 30.5% [4].

Since the definition of brain death diagnosis criteria in the 1960s, most organs have been procured from patients who have progressed to brain death. In recent years, however, donation after cardiac death (DCD) has grown substantially in the effort to expand the donor pool, and programs involving new perfusion methods have been developed to allow maintenance of organ function in spite of warm ischemia [2, 5–7].

This chapter discusses organ donation from deceased donors, highlighting the margins of improvement in their management from declaration of death to organ recovery and defining the possible applications of the new perfusion technologies. Living donation is another possibility to expand the donor poll, but it will be not analyzed here.

55.2 Donation After Brain Death (DBD)

The possibility of certifying death based on neurologic criteria in individuals who have lost all neurologic function, but continue to sustain a heartbeat and have their respiration supported, allows a flash of cold preservation solution simultaneously with CA during the donor operation, thus preserving the organs from detrimental warm ischemia [8, 9]. The most common causes of death in this group are cerebrovascular accident, traumatic brain injury, and anoxia. Traumatic brain injury, once the most common cause of brain death, has now been overtaken by cerebrovascular accident. Trauma donors are generally younger and healthier than stroke donors [10].

55.2.1 Death Declaration Based on Neurologic Criteria

Death was defined by the ad hoc committee of the Harvard Medical School in 1968 as the irreversible cessation of whole brain function [8, 11]. The diagnosis of death by neurologic criteria requires clinical and instrumental evidence of complete and irreversible absence of brain function, and the exclusion of confounding factors [8]. Confounding factors that must be ruled out include hypothermia, circulatory shock, drug intoxication, endogenous metabolic intoxication states such as renal or hepatic failure, and the prolonged effects of neuromuscular blocking agents and sedatives [11].

Different brain death criteria have been adopted in different countries. In the United States and in Italy, declaring death on the basis of neurologic criteria uses the concept of whole brain death, according to which loss of cortical function and brainstem reflexes has to be demonstrated. In the United Kingdom, only the loss of brainstem function is required [8]. According to Italian law, brain death is diagnosed according to the following criteria: (1) deep coma, (2) absence of brainstem reflexes and positive apnea testing (no breathing effort is observed at a partial arterial pressure of carbon dioxide more than 60 mmHg and pH more than 7.4 after discontinuation of mechanical ventilation), (3) flat electroencephalogram, and (4) absence of cerebral blood flow at imaging (e.g., cerebral angiography) for children younger than 1 year of age and when there are factors affecting clinical evaluation or electroencephalography. There must be an observation period lasting at least 6 h [12].

55.2.2 Authorization for Organ Donation

From a legal point of view, organ donation is an anatomical gifting and not a healthcare decision for the donor. For this reason it does not involve standard informed consent [13, 14]. The approach to authorization for organ donation internationally adheres to a model of either explicit or presumed consent. An explicit consent system requires the consent of the individual or family. Mechanisms for designating oneself as an organ donor include signing a donor card or registering through a donor state registry. In a presumed consent system, consent is instead presumed unless the individual has exercised the right to refuse donation. The presumed consent model still follows voluntary gift law principles [14].

An interview study in the United States has shown that, among families that deny donation, 53% did not receive an adequate explanation of brain death, and those who decide against donation generally have less understanding of brain death than those who agree to it [15]. Several recent studies have shown that in-house transplant coordinators at various trauma centers, in the form of a dedicated physician or other specially trained healthcare providers, were able to significantly increase family consent rates [10, 16]. The discussion with the potential donor's family needs to be caring but unambiguous and direct in stating that the individual is dead, and the distinction should always be clear between the event of death and organ donation [8].

55.2.3 Physiological Maintenance of the Brain-Dead Donor

Once the established neurologic criteria have been fulfilled, the patient is declared dead. Physicians are under no moral or legal obligation to continue medical support for a cadaver, except when they are dealing with an organ donor [8]. In this case, every effort must be made to maintain homeostasis of the brain-dead donor until the procurement, thus preserving the organs to be transplanted.

55.2.3.1 Brain Death Physiopathology

Brain death causes numerous physiological derangements, producing profound hemodynamic and metabolic abnormalities (Table 55.1). The two main mechanisms responsible for these changes are the loss of integrated neurologic regulation and the sustained release of pro-inflammatory cytokines, which have negative effects on the function of numerous systems [11]. This makes the brain-dead donor physiologically fragile and unstable. Thus, organ recovery must proceed promptly to avoid potential donor loss.

Cardiovascular effects of brain death result first from the so-called autonomic storm and later from profound reductions in sympathetic outflow [11]. When ischemia reaches the vagal nuclei in the lower medulla, unopposed sympathetic stimulation occurs, and this autonomic storm causes a significant increase in vascular resistance. Subsequently, loss of spinal sympathetic pathways causes total sympathectomy, with consequent systemic vasodilatation, bradycardia, and hemodynamic instability. Restoration of blood pressure typically requires volume replacement and vasopressors. High doses of vasopressors may lead to organ ischemia and worsen the transplant outcome, but clinical data are conflicting. Nevertheless, combination therapy may avoid excessively high doses of a single agent with strong vasoconstrictor effects [2].

Table 55.1 Common physiological derangements in brain-dead donors

Type	Complication
Cardiac	– Hypotension
	– Arrhythmias
Pulmonary	– Neurogenic pulmonary edema
	– Aspiration pneumonia
	– Ventilator-associated pneumonia
Hematologic	– Thrombosis
	– DIC and coagulopathy
Neuroendocrine	– Diabetes insipidus
	– SIADH
	– Hypothyroidism
	– Adrenal insufficiency
	– Insulin resistance and hyperglycemia
Electrolytes	– Hyponatremia
	– Hypomagnesemia
	– Hypokalemia
	– Hypocalcemia
	– Hypophosphatemia
Thermoregulation	– Hypothermia

DIC disseminated intravascular coagulation; *SIADH* syndrome of inappropriate antidiuretic hormone secretion

The pulmonary capillaries may be subjected to excessive hydrostatic pressure when left atrial pressure exceeds pulmonary artery pressure because of vasoconstriction. This results in capillary wall disruption and leakage of protein-rich fluid into the pulmonary interstitium, explaining what is termed neurogenic pulmonary edema [11]. Other potential donor respiratory complications include ventilator-associated and aspiration pneumonia [10].

The hematologic system is adversely affected as the high catecholamine and cortisol levels create a temporary hypercoagulable state. The passage of cerebral gangliosides into the systemic circulation and the consequent release of fibrinolytic factors can lead to significant coagulopathy and spontaneous hemorrhage [2, 11].

Neuroendocrine changes occur in relation to hypothalamic-pituitary axis dysfunction. The most commonly reported manifestation is diabetes insipidus due to antidiuretic hormone deficiency, which can further exacerbate low vascular resistance hypovolemia. It can be treated with desmopressin or vasopressin, if vasopressors are otherwise required. The syndrome of inappropriate antidiuretic hormone secretion (SIADH) may also be observed. Anterior pituitary deregulation frequently translates into significant reduction of thyroid hormone and cortisol levels [11].

Hormone therapy to the donor has been a topic of controversy. There are data suggesting that thyroid hormone may relieve hemodynamic instability in brain-dead donors. Its use has been associated with complete reversal of anaerobic metabolism, reducing the need for vasopressor support, preventing cardiovascular collapse, and stabilizing the hemodynamically unstable donor [10, 11, 16].

Different electrolyte derangements can occur in the brain-dead donor, secondary to the altered cellular membrane permeability and diabetes insipidus. Wide variations in body temperature and hypothermia are the result of central dysregulation, thyroid dysfunction, and exposure and infusion of large volumes of crystalloids and blood products and can exacerbate coagulopathy or precipitate arrhythmia and CA.

55.2.3.2 Optimizing the Management of the Brain-Dead Donor

Even with aggressive treatment, more than 25% of potential donors may be lost due to hemodynamic instability [11]. The American Society of Transplantation and American Society of Transplant Surgeons advocate the use of standardized donor management protocols [16]. Early admission to the intensive care unit with an aggressive donor management protocol has reduced the incidence of cardiovascular collapse in donors and improved organ recovery and function in recipients [10]. A protocol of aggressive donor management should include the following: (1) pulmonary artery catheterization to monitor hemodynamic status and tissue perfusion; (2) maintenance of an adequate systemic perfusion pressure with aggressive infusion of fluids and vasopressors; (3) hormonal therapy, consisting of thyroid hormone; and (4) identification of brain death-related complications and prompt intervention [11, 16].

55.2.4 Donor Evaluation and Risk Assessment

Exclusion criteria for a potential organ donor are essentially based on the history, clinical examination, and blood tests; specific tests and imaging may serve to complete the evaluation of individual organs (e.g., coronary angiography). Donors are consequently stratified according to specific classes of risk, as shown in Table 55.2. If the evaluation does not allow a clear definition of the class of risk, the opinion of some expert consultants (second opinion) is needed.

Age is not an absolute exclusion criterion for organ donation, and in fact the percentage of liver transplants from octogenarian donors has risen steadily in Western countries in the last few years [17]. Absolute exclusion criteria are human immunodeficiency virus (HIV) infection; active malignant neoplasms with risk of metastases; untreatable, generalized infections; and documented prion disease. However, some HIV-positive to HIV-positive transplants have been recently reported in the literature [18]. Relative and organ-specific contraindications may vary from center to center and in relation to the recipient's conditions and urgency. A specific discussion of these aspects is beyond the scope of this chapter [19].

55.2.5 General Principles of Surgical Technique for DBD Organ Recovery

The guiding principle of organ procurement in DBD is the avoidance of warm ischemia. This can be achieved during procurement with in situ organ cooling by intravascular infusion of the cold preservation solution at the time of circulatory arrest. For abdominal organ recovery in stable donors, we recommend first gaining access to the retroperitoneal space and checking the abdominal aorta, with subsequent accurate dissection of the hepatic hilum, splenic artery, and left gastric artery and recognition of any vascular abnormalities before in situ cooling. A rapid en bloc retrieval technique should be used only if the donor becomes unstable. This procedure minimizes warm ischemia times during hemodynamic instability and can be safely applied in critical situations even by non-expert surgeons, but the risk of vascular and graft injury is significantly higher [9].

55.3 Donation After Cardiac Death (DCD)

Many countries worldwide have explored the option of donation after circulatory death (DCD) to expand the organ donor pool [20]. The DCD procedure seeks to obtain transplantable organs from patients previously declared dead following cessation of their circulatory and respiratory functions. DCD are classified, in accordance with the Maastricht criteria [21], in the following four categories (Table 55.3): donors who are declared dead outside the hospital and are brought into hospital without any attempt at resuscitation (Type 1); donors in whom CA occurs unexpectedly, and for whom resuscitation attempts are unsuccessful (Type 2); donors for whom CA is expected after withdrawal of treatment (Type 3); and donors in whom CA occurs during or after brain death diagnostic procedures (Type 4).

The original Maastricht classification was modified during the International DCD Conference in Paris in 2013, to define the exact circumstances of the circulatory arrest and consequent warm ischemic organ damage better [22]. The two main discriminant factors are maintained in the modified Maastricht classification: the circumstances of CA (sudden or planned) and the initial therapeutic procedure (resuscitation or not). The "location" has been added: where the sudden CA occurs (outside or inside the hospital).

DCD donors can be considered either uncontrolled (uDCD) or controlled (cDCD). Types 1 and 2 are defined as uncontrolled donors on the basis of unexpected CA and

Table 55.2 Class of risk in organ donor evaluation

Class of risk	Description
Standard	Evaluation did not identify a transmissible disease
Calculated risk	Despite the presence of transmissible diseases, transplantation is allowed for recipients with the same disease or with a protective serological status
	Donors with documented bacteremia and/or bacterial meningitis if the donor received target antimicrobial treatment for a minimum of 24–48 h
Increased but acceptable	Transmissible diseases are identified during donor evaluation but organ utilization is justified by the specific health situation of the recipient or the severity of his clinical condition
Unacceptable	Absolute contraindication
Not assessable	Evaluation does not allow appropriate risk assessment for transmissible diseases

Table 55.3 Maastricht DCD categories

Category	Description
I	Dead on arrival
II	Unsuccessful resuscitation
III	Awaiting cardiac arrest
IV	Cardiac arrest while brain dead

unsuccessful resuscitation. uDCD are considered to be very marginal donors because of the deleterious effect of warm ischemia. There is also the risk of being unable to obtain all necessary medical data within the short time frame provided by uDCD procedures. Donation in this setting should be designed to minimize the duration of warm ischemia and its impact on organ viability, to ensure the greatest possible safety for the donated organ.

Type 3 is defined as controlled donors, when death occurs in an ICU patient who is deemed to have a catastrophic and non-recoverable brain injury. In these patients, after the decision that any additional care is futile, life-sustaining treatment can be withdrawn. In cDCD the CA is expected, allowing the organ recovery to be planned [23].

DCD remains an activity restricted to a limited number of countries, and there are also considerable differences in its practice between countries. In Australia, Belgium, the Netherlands, the United Kingdom, and the United States, DCD donors are predominantly controlled, whereas in Spain, France, and Italy, DCD donors are most commonly uncontrolled (although these countries too have recently embarked on cDCD programs). The different approaches may be related to different legislations, ethical concerns, practices at the end of life, and organizational approaches to the treatment of out-of-hospital CA [24]. In Belgium and the Netherlands, cDCD is also possible after euthanasia.

The main impediment to DCD is the higher incidence of complications or of impaired graft function as a result of extended periods of warm ischemia. Organs from these donors sustain appreciable warm ischemic injury, and graft function must be carefully assessed for their potential use for transplantation. The unpredictable consequences of warm ischemic injury during low-flow or no-flow prior to death, together with the no-touch period required for death declaration according to national laws, result in extensive ischemia-reperfusion injury (IRI). IRI is the main factor causing graft dysfunction after transplantation [23, 25].

During ischemia transport mechanisms involving Na^+/K^+ and Ca^{2+}/Mg^{2+} ATPase are inhibited, resulting in entry of water and cell swelling. Ischemia also causes rapid accumulation of toxic products such as lactate and hypoxanthine produced by anaerobic metabolism. These processes are exacerbated by reperfusion, resulting in an inflammatory response with subsequent release of free radicals.

There is still no univocal definition of warm ischemia time (WIT) [26]. In controlled DCD, WIT can be defined as the interval between support withdrawal and the start of cold perfusion [20]. Research has shown that agonal periods of more than 2 h duration are not acceptable for transplantation purposes. Currently there is a tendency to define and record the warm ischemia at the onset of hemodynamic instability (referred to as "functional warm ischemia"). It involves sustained hypotension and may have a substantial impact on warm ischemic damage to DCD organs.

In uncontrolled DCD, WIT can have an even more significant impact, since the exact period of circulatory arrest is usually not known [27]. Furthermore, between CA and the start of organ perfusion, there is a period of cardiopulmonary resuscitation (CPR), varying in duration and efficacy.

The time required to define the irreversibility of death varies widely between different countries. The no-touch period, defined as the time between the cessation of circulation and respiration and the determination of death, ranges from 5 to 20 min [28]. In Italy, the interval to diagnosis of death is 20 min of CA, demonstrated by a continuous electrocardiography recording. This is clearly longer than the interval adopted in the United States and other European countries and may negatively affect organ viability, prolonging the WIT.

55.3.1 Warm Ischemia Time and Organ Preservation in DCD

The key for the recovery of most DCD grafts has been the implementation of cytoprotective mechanisms in preservation techniques in order to stop or even reverse cellular injury [29]. By the end of 2000, there was already a fair amount of data, showing that the use of normothermic recirculation, namely, abdominal regional perfusion (ARP), could avoid and reverse warm ischemia injury. ARP can restore a warm, oxygenated blood flow through the organs and thus ensure adequate tissue perfusion between the donor's death and organ procurement [30]. ARP has proved to be the most effective method for preservation and functional assessment of abdominal organs. It reverses ischemic injury and at the same time allows an evaluation of the quality of potential grafts.

ARP has been applied clinically using both hypo- and normothermic strategies. With hypothermic perfusion, metabolic processes are suppressed; with normothermic regional perfusion (NRP), cell metabolism is fully restored [31]. A period of postischemic NRP in DCD donors is useful to restore cellular energy substrates, lower the levels of nucleotide degradation products, and improve the concentrations of endogenous antioxidants prior to graft recovery. Like ARP, NRP has proved to be the most effective method for preservation and functional assessment of abdominal DCD organs. It reverses ischemic injury and at the same time allows evaluation of the quality of potential grafts. NRP allows organs to recover in situ from warm ischemic damage [32] providing oxygen and nutrients to restore metabolic processes, which in turn enable repair of damaged cells, correct the acidosis, restore the depleted adenosine triphosphate (ATP), regulate calcium homeostasis, and remove free radicals. Hypothermic perfusion has been mainly limited to DCD kidney transplantation, and NRP has been used to improve and assess the quality of DCD kidneys, livers, and even pancreas for transplantation.

NRP has marked a significant advance in organ recovery and has the potential to increase organ recovery rates, with its applicability in both controlled and uncontrolled DCD donors. Furthermore, its ability to restore ATP supplies and permit dynamic assessment of organ function prior to transplantation may allow more precise graft selection and achieve better long-term outcomes in comparison with kidneys or livers that were flushed in situ directly after the declaration of death [33].

55.3.2 Uncontrolled Donation After Circulatory Death

Although this type of donation can substantially boost the potential donor pool, it is still restricted to a few countries. Spain and France have the most experience with uDCD. It has also been developed in other countries such as Italy and Belgium and recently in Portugal, Russia, and Poland [7, 32, 33, 34].

Patients with witnessed in- or out-of-hospital refractory cardiac arrest (CA) are considered eligible. In the out-of-hospital scenario, the emergency medical service is mobilized to the scene of witnessed CA, where it starts advanced life support in accordance with international standard guidelines, using an automated chest compression system. If the CA is refractory, the patient is maintained on an automated chest compression system and transferred to a hospital. In the hospital, if the asystolic period persists and no reversible cause is identified, the CA is considered irreversible and further attempts at resuscitation futile. The declaration of death is formalized in the hospital, based on the absence of ECG and spontaneous respiratory activity, in accordance with local law. Heparin may be administered before death is declared (in countries where this is allowed by law).

After declaration of death, external cardiac massage is restarted with automated chest compression; the femoral artery and veins are cannulated, and ARP or NRP is set in motion, with the aim of preserving organ function while the family may express non-opposition to donation [34]. A Fogarty balloon catheter is inserted through the contralateral femoral artery and inflated in the supraceliac aorta, to reduce the total perfused volume and prevent cardiac and brain perfusion. Cannulae are connected to an extracorporeal circuit incorporating a membrane oxygenator, a centrifugal pump, and a heat exchanger (Fig. 55.1). The circuit is primed with 100–800 mL of Ringer's acetate solution, sometimes buffered with sodium bicarbonate.

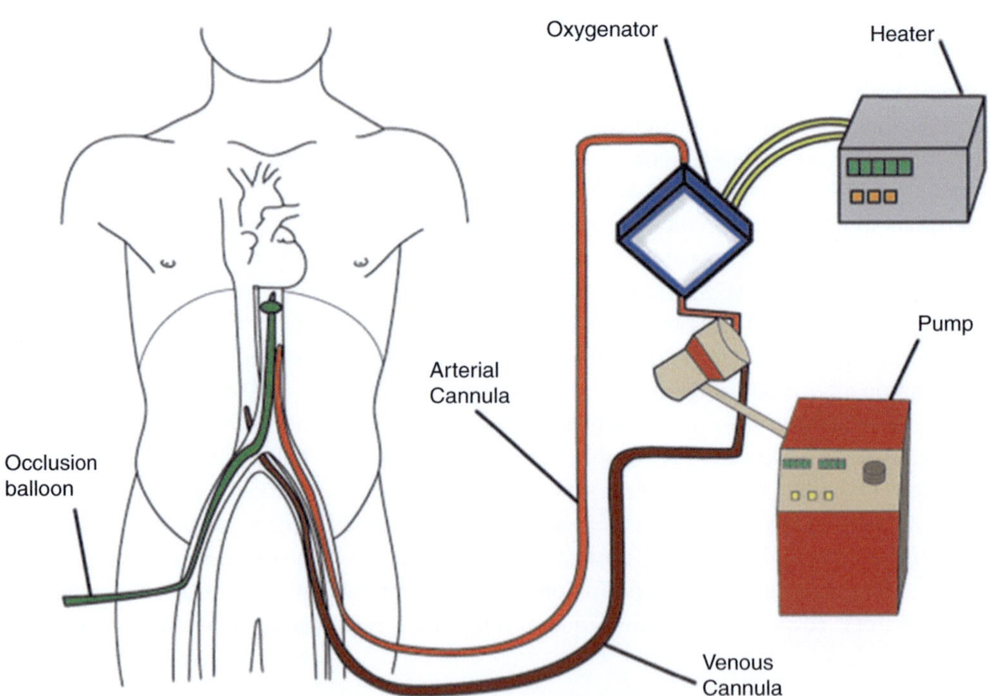

Fig. 55.1 Scheme of the normothermic regional perfusion circuit

Pump flow is maintained in the 1.7–3.0 L/min range, temperature at 35.5–37.5 °C, and pH 7.0–7.4. The circuit sweep gas flow and FiO_2 are adjusted to keep $PaCO_2$ in the 30–45 mmHg range and SaO_2 98% or more. Full heparinization is warranted, and autologous blood perfusate from the donor cadaver is used. During the period of NRP, blood samples are collected for biochemical and gasometric parameters, and the donor is assessed for possible contraindications to donation [35]. Indicative criteria for donation include witnessed arrest, age less than 65 years for kidneys and livers, 50–55 for lungs, cause of death known or presumed, and non-bleeding abdominal injuries. Total WIT (time from CA to start of NRP) should be less than 150 min.

55.3.3 Controlled Donation After Circulatory Death

In the case of cDCD, CA occurs following planned withdrawal of life-sustaining support (WLST) after it has been demonstrated that further intensive treatment is "futile" and inappropriate, in the best interest of a critically ill patient, according to the patient's personal rights. DCD donation accounts for over 40% of deceased donation in the United Kingdom, and similar percentages are seen in other Northern European countries. Unlike other types of DCD, in the controlled scenario, the CA is expected [36]. Although the majority of actual cDCD donors die from catastrophic nonrecoverable brain injury, data from the Netherlands, Spain, the United Kingdom, and the United States suggest that up to 15% of cDCD die from other conditions such as end-stage respiratory failure or neuromuscular disease [37]. When the planned WLST is discussed with the relatives of patients who have a nonreversible disease, organ donation can be an appropriate consideration. Currently, in countries where such programs are implemented, there are useful guidelines to assist physicians in therapy withdrawal.

After WLST in cDCD, a variable period of progressive hypoxia and hypotension develops until the onset of CA and determination of death, known as the agonal phase. Most transplant programs will limit this phase to 60–90 min to exclude potential harmful effects. However, data are still very limited.

Following the Spanish experience with uDCD, several countries have explored the feasibility of NRP in cDCD using similar technology (heat exchanger, oxygenator, and pump). Few studies have described the use of regional perfusion in controlled DCD donation in normothermic as well as hypothermic conditions [5]. These studies reported an increase in organ recovery rates compared with standard preservation procedures. However, the essential prerequisite in these studies was the possibility of using heparin and vascular cannulation prior to the patient's death. Interestingly, in different countries, different interventions are allowed antemortem: heparin and vessel cannulation are allowed in Spanish and French guidelines, and specific informed consent must be obtained.

55.3.4 General Principles of Surgical Technique for DCD Organ Recovery

For controlled DCD donors, a super-rapid recovery technique is generally adopted. Prior to withdrawal of support, the donor is draped, and the surgical instruments, preservation solution, and tubing are prepared. Once death has been formally declared, the surgeons return to the operating room. Speedy access to the abdomen is gained through a midline laparotomy, the distal aorta is cannulated, and perfusion with cold preservation solution is started. Then the sternum is split, the thoracic aorta is cross-clamped, and the inferior vena cava is vented into the right chest. The inferior mesenteric vein may be cannulated to perfuse the portal system [9, 38, 39]. Because visceral dissection is performed in the cold without the possibility of taking pulses, the risk of graft and vessel injury is higher than in DBD donors [9, 40].

Conversely, NRP in DCD donors permits an unhurried donor operation, which can be conducted in the same way as for DBD donors, drastically minimizing the risk of graft injury. Cannulation of the aorta is generally not necessary, and cold preservation solution can be flushed directly through the previously inserted femoral arterial cannula [5–7, 34]. Simultaneous portal perfusion is always advisable.

55.3.5 Ex Situ Machine Perfusion of the DCD Grafts

Static cold storage (SCS) is a suboptimal means of maintaining the viability of grafts from DCD. Increasing importance has been paid in recent years to machine perfusion (MP) for the ex situ phase of DCD organ preservation. MP preserves the organs dynamically, providing continuous circulation of preservation solution or blood at various temperatures. Experimental data suggest either hypothermic or normothermic MP as superior to SCS [41]. Vascular resistance during kidney MP correlates with delayed graft function and survival. Although the predictive value is low, this information could be used as an extra parameter for pretransplant evaluation of DCD kidneys [42, 43].

Hypothermic oxygenated perfusion (HOPE) has shown a protective effect in DCD livers against hepatocyte injury and Kupffer cell activation, but we still lack reliable markers and cutoffs predicting liver function posttransplant [44]. The Zurich group first reported that HOPE offered important benefits in preserving high-risk DCD livers and increasing graft survival [45, 46]. The combination of NRP with subsequent MP could offer the best way to improve the viability and transplantability of livers and kidneys from DCD, drawing on the recognized advantages of these two technologies [6].

55.3.6 The Italian Scenario in DCD

In Italy, the main, limiting obstacle to the development of DCD programs so far has been the legal framework for the determination of death: using the cardiocirculatory criteria necessary for DCDs, death can be legally declared only after a 20-min period in which no cardiac electrical activity and a flat ECG have been recorded.

The first program on DCD donor management in Italy, the Alba Program, started in 2007 at the Policlinico San Matteo in Pavia [47]. Three different scenarios are now under consideration for enrollment in this DCD protocol:

1. Subjects who undergo witnessed CA, without restoration of spontaneous circulation with advanced life support in accordance with international guidelines (refractory CA), and are transferred to the hospital under automated chest compression. If there is no indication for extracorporeal life support (ECLS), these subjects are enrolled in the DCD program. The declaration of "cardiac" death is formalized in the hospital, based on the absence of ECG for 20 min, according to Italian law.
2. Subjects under ECLS, in whom the extracorporeal support is withdrawn because of futility according to current criteria. The death declaration will be formalized according to recent Italian National Transplant Center guidelines.
3. Subjects with catastrophic non-recoverable brain injury, who undergo CA and no attempt at resuscitation is made.

Organ preservation was based on NRP and started immediately after death had been declared using the circulatory criteria. For the first experimental years, the program focused only on kidney DCDs, considered more resilient to ischemic damage. The results so far are encouraging on many accounts such as organ function and recovery rates.

More recently, the procedure has been redefined to include liver recovery, which was first done in September 2015 by the transplant team of Niguarda Hospital (Milan) [5]. The results of the DCD liver transplant series originating from this experience, which subsequently included cases from a few other regional and extra-regional donor hospitals, show that DCD liver transplantation is possible in Italy with good results despite the exceptionally long WIT [7, 48, 49]. The use of NRP followed by MP – first introduced by the group of Niguarda – can be considered a new, promising frontier for liver recovery from DCD in clinical practice [6, 7].

References

1. Jenkins DH, Reilly PM, McMahon DJ, Hawthorne RV. Minimizing charges associated with the determination of brain death. Crit Care. 1997;1:65–70.
2. Keegan MT, Wood KE, Coursin DB. An update on ICU management of the potential organ donor. In: Vincent JL, editor. Intensive care medicine. Annual update 2010. Heidelberg: Springer; 2011. p. 547–59.
3. Israni AK, Zaun D, Bolch C, Rosendale JD, Snyder JJ, Kasiske BL. Deceased organ donation. Am J Transplant. 2016;16:195–215.
4. Trapianti—Statistiche. http://www.trapianti.salute.gov.it/cnt/cnt-Statistiche.jsp. Accessed 26 Mar 2017.
5. De Carlis L, Lauterio A, De Carlis R, Ferla F, Di Sandro S. Donation after cardiac death liver transplantation after more than 20 minutes of circulatory arrest and Normothermic regional perfusion. Transplantation. 2016;100:e21–2.
6. De Carlis L, De Carlis R, Lauterio A, Di Sandro S, Ferla F, Zanierato M. Sequential use of normothermic regional perfusion and hypothermic machine perfusion in donation after cardiac death liver transplantation with extended warm ischemia time. Transplantation. 2016;100:e101–2.
7. De Carlis R, Di Sandro S, Lauterio A, Ferla F, Dell'Acqua A, Zanierato M, De Carlis L. Successful donation after cardiac death liver transplants with prolonged warm ischemia time using normothermic regional perfusion. Liver Transpl. 2017;23:166–73.
8. Manno EM, Wijdicks EFM. The declaration of death and the withdrawal of care in the neurologic patient. Neurol Clin. 2006;24:159–69.
9. De Carlis R, Sguinzi R, Grande AM, Aseni P. Multiple organ retrieval: general principles, organ preservation, and new strategies. In: Aseni P, Grande AM, De Carlis L, editors. Multiorgan procurement for transplantation. A guide to surgical technique and management. Heidelberg: Springer; 2016. p. 79–90.
10. Ley EJ, Salim A. Organ donation. In: Velmahos GC, Degiannis E, Doll D, editors. Penetrating trauma: a practical guide on operative technique and peri-operative management. 2nd ed. Heidelberg: Springer; 2017. p. 623–8.
11. Jenkins DH, Reilly PM, Schwab CW. Improving the approach to organ donation: a review. World J Surg. 1999;23:644–9.
12. Gazzetta Ufficiale—Decreto 11 aprile. 2008. http://www.gazzettaufficiale.it/atto/serie_generale/caricaDettaglioAtto/originario?atto.dataPubblicazioneGazzetta=2008-06-12&atto.codiceRedazionale=08A04067&elenco30giorni=false. Accessed 26 Mar 2017.
13. Abt PL, Marsh CL, Dunn TB, Hewitt WR, Rodrigue JR, Ham JM, Feng S. Challenges to research and innovation to optimize deceased donor organ quality and quantity. Am J Transplant. 2013;13:1400–4.
14. Glazier AK. The principles of gift law and the regulation of organ donation. Transpl Int. 2011;24:368–72.
15. Franz HG, DeJong W, Wolfe SM, Nathan H, Payne D, Reitsma W, Beasley C. Explaining brain death: a critical feature of the donation process. J Transpl Coord. 1997;7:14–21.
16. Salim A, Velmahos GC, Brown C, Belzberg H, Demetriades D. Aggressive organ donor management significantly increases the number of organs available for transplantation. J Trauma. 2005;58:991–4.
17. Ferla F, De Carlis R, Mariani A, De Carlis L. Liver transplant using octogenarian donors. Liver Transpl. 2016;22:1040–1.
18. Lauterio A, Moioli MC, Di Sandro S, Travi G, De Carlis R, Merli M, Ferla F, Puoti M, De Carlis L. HIV-positive to HIV-positive liver transplantation: To be continued. J Hepatol. 2018;S0168-8278:32180–9.
19. Grande AM, Aseni P. Preoperative evaluation and arrangements for multiorgan donation: general principles and contraindications. In: Aseni P, Grande AM, De Carlis L, editors. Multiorgan procurement

for transplantation: a guide to surgical technique and management. Heidelberg: Springer; 2016. p. 19–34.
20. Neyrinck A, Raemdonck D, Van Monbaliud D. Donation after circulatory death: current status. Curr Opin Anaesthesiol. 2013;26:382–90.
21. Kootstra G, Daemen JH, Oomen AP. Categories of non-heart-beating donors. Transplant Proc. 1995;27:2893–4.
22. Thuong M, Ruiz A, Evrard P, Kuiper M, Boffa C, Akhtar MZ, Neuberger J, Ploeg R. New classification of donation after circulatory death donors definitions and terminology. Transpl Int. 2016;29:749–59.
23. Balibrea JM, Núñez-Peña JR, García-Martín MC, Olmedilla Y, Martín-Antona E, Berthuin J, Rancan L, Vara E, Balibrea JL. The differential tissue expression of inflammatory, oxidative stress, and apoptosis markers in human uncontrolled non-heart-beating donors. Transplantation. 2013;95:1346–53.
24. Monbaliu D, Pirenne J, Talbot D. Liver transplantation using donation after cardiac death donors. J Hepatol. 2012;56:474–85.
25. Domínguez-Gil B, Haase-Kromwijk B, Van Leiden H, et al. Current situation of donation after circulatory death in European countries. Transpl Int. 2011;24:676–86.
26. Manara AR, Murphy PG, O'Callaghan G. Donation after circulatory death. Br J Anaesth. 2012;108:i108–21.
27. Rodríguez-Arias D, Deballon IO. Protocols for uncontrolled donation after circulatory death. Lancet. 2012;379:1275–6.
28. Morrissey PE, Monaco AP. Donation after circulatory death: current practices, ongoing challenges, and potential improvements. Transplantation. 2014;97:258–64.
29. Net M, Valero R, Almenara R, et al. The effect of normothermic recirculation is mediated by ischemic preconditioning in NHBD liver transplantation. Am J Transplant. 2005;5:2385–92.
30. Valero R, Cabrer C, Oppenheimer F, et al. Normothermic recirculation reduces primary graft dysfunction of kidneys obtained from non-heart-beating donors. Transpl Int. 2000;13:303–10.
31. Hessheimer AJ, Billault C, Barrou B, Fondevila C. Hypothermic or normothermic abdominal regional perfusion in high-risk donors with extended warm ischemia times: impact on outcomes? Transpl Int. 2015;28:700–7.
32. Hessheimer AJ, García-Valdecasas JC, Fondevila C. Abdominal regional in-situ perfusion in donation after circulatory determination of death donors. Curr Opin Organ Transplant. 2016;21:322–8.
33. Fondevila C, Hessheimer AJ, Flores E, et al. Applicability and results of Maastricht type 2 donation after cardiac death liver transplantation. Am J Transplant. 2012;12:162–70.
34. Fondevila C, Hessheimer AJ, Ruiz A, et al. Liver transplant using donors after unexpected cardiac death: novel preservation protocol and acceptance criteria. Am J Transplant. 2007;7:1849–55.
35. Savier E, Dondero F, Vibert E, et al. First experience of liver transplantation with type 2 donation after cardiac death in France. Liver Transpl. 2015;21:631–43.
36. Oniscu GC, Randle LV, Muiesan P, Butler AJ, Currie IS, Perera MTPR, Forsythe JL, Watson CJE. In situ normothermic regional perfusion for controlled donation after circulatory death—the United Kingdom experience. Am J Transplant. 2014;14:2846–54.
37. Magliocca JF, Magee JC, Rowe SA, Gravel MT, Chenault RH, Merion RM, Punch JD, Bartlett RH, Hemmila MR. Extracorporeal support for organ donation after cardiac death effectively expands the donor pool. J Trauma. 2005;58:1095–101.
38. Casavilla A, Ramirez C, Shapiro R, Nghiem D, Miracle K, Bronsther O, Randhawa P, Broznick B, Fung JJ, Starzl T. Experience with liver and kidney allografts from non-heart-beating donors. Transplantation. 1995;59:197–203.
39. Reich DJ, Mulligan DC, Abt PL, et al. ASTS recommended practice guidelines for controlled donation after cardiac death organ procurement and transplantation. Am J Transplant. 2009;9:2004–11.
40. Ausania F, White SA, Pocock P, Manas DM. Kidney damage during organ recovery in donation after circulatory death donors: data from UK National Transplant Database. Am J Transplant. 2012;12:932–6.
41. Shapey IM, Muiesan P. Regional perfusion by extracorporeal membrane oxygenation of abdominal organs from donors after circulatory death: a systematic review. Liver Transpl. 2013;19: 1292–303.
42. Moers C, Smits JM, M-HJ M, et al. Machine perfusion or cold storage in deceased-donor kidney transplantation. N Engl J Med. 2009;360:7–19.
43. Jochmans I, Moers C, Smits JM, et al. The prognostic value of renal resistance during hypothermic machine perfusion of deceased donor kidneys. Am J Transplant. 2011;11:2214–20.
44. Schlegel A, de Rougemont O, Graf R, Clavien P-A, Dutkowski P. Protective mechanisms of end-ischemic cold machine perfusion in DCD liver grafts. J Hepatol. 2013;58:278–86.
45. Dutkowski P, Schlegel A, De Oliveira M, Müllhaupt B, Neff F, Clavien PA. HOPE for human liver grafts obtained from donors after cardiac death. J Hepatol. 2014;60:765–72.
46. Dutkowski P, Polak WG, Muiesan P, Schlegel A, Verhoeven CJ, Scalera I, DeOliveira ML, Kron P, Clavien P-A. First comparison of hypothermic oxygenated PErfusion versus static cold storage of human donation after cardiac death liver transplants: an international-matched case analysis. Ann Surg. 2015;262:764–71.
47. Geraci P, Sepe V. Non-heart-beating organ donation in Italy. Minerva Anestesiol. 2011;77:613–23.
48. Vergano M, Magavern E, Baroncelli F, et al. Making a case for controlled organ donation after cardiac death: the story of Italy's first experience. J Crit Care. 2017;38:129–31.
49. De Carlis R, Di Sandro S, Lauterio A, Botta F, Ferla F, Andorno E, Bagnardi V, De Carlis L. Liver grafts from donors after cardiac death on regional perfusion with extended warm ischemia compared with donors after brain death. Liver Transpl. 2018 [Epub ahead of print].

Periprocedural Iatrogenic Injuries and Death in Emergency and Trauma Surgery: A Forensic Perspective

56

Antonio Osculati, Silvia D. Visonà, and Matteo Moretti

56.1 Introduction

The present leading-edge medical and surgical science has turned into a victim of its own achievements, and the masses, aware of the enormous advances in medical technology via media interest and wide publicity, always expect the best outcome, thanks to the latest techniques with regard to health problems. This gives rise to the widespread interest in the issue of medical liability and leads every health professional to feel the need to develop an understanding of basic substantive and procedural law. In acute care and emergency surgery, the medical doctor has to deal with a critically ill subset of patients, including trauma, which has a greater potential for permanent disability or death. For this reason, the fear of being sued is particularly felt in this field of medicine. Moreover, the setting in which the emergency physicians practice has been defined as an information-poor, high-risk, technology-rich environment, which may lend itself to defensive practice [1]. In a Massachusetts survey, emergency physicians estimated that 30% of computed tomography (CT) and 19% of magnetic resonance imaging (MRI) ordered were for "defensive purposes" [2]. The emergency medicine and surgery is a unique setting, where the peculiar characteristics and dynamics contribute to making this healthcare environment conducive to potential error. The decision-making process in this clinical setting is urgent as well as complex and often based on incomplete information. In addition, clinicians must deal with families and surrogates, which add a further level of interaction, communication, and expectations since the patient is not able to participate in the decision-making regarding his or her treatment.

A. Osculati (✉) · S. D. Visonà · M. Moretti
Department of Public Health, Experimental and Forensic Medicine, University of Pavia, Pavia, Italy

56.2 Statistical Data About Claims

An interesting study carried out in the USA in 2011 characterized three aspects of malpractice risk among physicians in 25 specialties: the proportion of physicians facing a malpractice claim in a given year, the proportion of physicians making an indemnity payment, and the amount of this payment [3]. Regardless of the different fields of medicine, 7.4% of doctors annually had a claim, whereas 1.6% paid an indemnity. There was significant variation across specialties in the probability of facing a claim, ranging annually from 19.1% in neurosurgery, 18.9% in thoracic–cardiovascular surgery, and 15.3% in general surgery to 5.2% in family medicine, 3.1% in pediatrics, and 2.6% in psychiatry. Interestingly, both emergency medicine and anesthesiology showed results very similar to the general group of physicians, with a rate of claims faced consistently lower than 10% [3]. Another US study published in 2010 reviewed the data on more than 11,500 closed claims made over a 23-year period involving the emergency department [4]. Interestingly, emergency department represented the largest number of claims for an individual specialty. Yet, only a minority of the main defendant were emergency physicians, whereas the great majority of claims were related to physicians of other specialty groups, who either provided direct patient care or consultation for emergency patients. Anesthesiology was associated with the highest average indemnity, followed by neurology and psychiatry. The top ten most common categories of errors were also identified. Errors in diagnosis—including failure to diagnose and diagnosing incorrectly—were identified as the primary misadventure in 37% of all closed claims in the ED. The next highest error category included the improper performance of a procedure (17% of all claims), which was associated with the highest average indemnity payment ($248,422) of all error types. Three of the top ten types of error involved delays in patient care [4]. The most common diagnoses

P. Aseni et al. (eds.), *Operative Techniques and Recent Advances in Acute Care and Emergency Surgery*,
https://doi.org/10.1007/978-3-319-95114-0_56

involved in ED claims were acute myocardial infarction and appendicitis. Bony skeleton fractures appear three times in the top ten diagnoses involved in emergency department closed claims, including forearm fractures, leg fractures, and bony spine fractures (6% altogether) [4]. Claims regarding a patient death represented the 36% of all closed claims arising from the emergency department, 40% of all paid claims. In claims involving a patient death, acute myocardial infarction was the most common diagnosis, followed by chest pain not further defined, aortic aneurysm, symptoms involving the abdomen or pelvis not further defined, and pulmonary embolism. Over a third of closed claims where death occurred were attributed to errors in diagnosis [4].

56.3 Periprocedural Complications in Emergency and Trauma Surgery: The Relevance of Proper Documentation and Disclosure

Even though the diagnostic, therapeutic, and supportive care provided in a department of intensive care or trauma surgery is among the most sophisticated in the whole field of medicine, complications occur, mostly related either to the natural progression of the disease, exposure to nosocomial pathogens, or iatrogenic injury. Sladoz et al. provide a broad and deep framework about legal issues in acute care, pointing out the importance of a philosophy of transparency with respect to complications and iatrogenic injuries, even when related to medical errors [5]. The Center for Medicare and Medicaid Services (CMS), the Joint Commission on the Accreditation of Healthcare Organizations, and many state regulatory agencies advocate that hospitals develop and adhere to disclosure policies and protocols. In the process of disclosure, patients or families are informed early after the recognition that an iatrogenic injury or medical error has occurred. Preliminary studies suggest that full disclosure may decrease litigation. However, the optimal policy and procedure for such disclosure remain somewhat controversial. In fact, the process of disclosure should follow careful deliberation and consideration and should under no circumstances be premature. In general, it is a legal tenet that "anything said or done may be used against the defendant." This is one of the reasons that make the documentation of every event (especially adverse) essential and potentially protective for the doctor in case of a lawsuit.

From a medicolegal standpoint, *the following is a list* of the most important medical records that should be accurately reported.

Medical chart Every medical decision (clinical tests performed) must be documented, and the professional who orders them must be recognized. This is an apparently obvious recommendation, but it is of extreme importance when it comes to the reconstruction of the exact clinical situation and the real medical conduct by a medicolegal expert in case of a liability lawsuit. The clear and thorough explanation of every choice, even though brief, is essential for the doctor to protect himself against wrong evaluations that can lead to hard legal consequences.

Informed consent documents Informed consent is a legal compulsion. Moreover, no doctor can be certain that the "signed consent" can definitely avoid legal liability [6, 7]. Anyway, the signed consent was accurate, and adequate and relevant information were provided truthfully in a form (using nonscientific terms) and language that the patient can understand. The point of the informed consent is for the patient to be capable of picking or rejecting a treatment or a diagnostic procedure [8]. In the field of emergency medicine and surgery, this issue is worthy of a special discussion, which is addressed later in this chapter.

Emergency room assistance sheet or emergency room report This report should include the cause for consultations, the results of any examinations, the anamnesis, the clinical picture, and the diagnosis. If the death of a patient occurs, this emergency room report is fundamental in checking whether it indicates the proper diagnostic tests, whether the results were interpreted correctly, and whether the medical decision was in keeping with the appropriate guidelines of good practice or protocols, where they exist [8].

Nursing documentation Nurses should mention vital signs each time they are measured; the person that gives the drug and medication dose, route, and administration time; requests for care; and any particular decisions made outside the daily working hours. Therefore, it is likely to find very detailed notes in nursing sheets rather than in the medical journal; for this reason, they are more important than generally believed in the reconstruction of the events ex post, for example, in a lawsuit. It is worthy to be underlined that a frank, open, and transparent discussion of iatrogenic injuries and complication among colleagues in a multidisciplinary context is vital both for the reduction of mistakes and even for decreasing the risk of litigation [9]. However, many surgeons still resist open discussion of errors because of a fear of increased malpractice risk. This is exacerbated by the modern malpractice crisis that targets individual physicians, focusing on blame, punishment, and damage reparation. This system encourages secrecy and denial of errors.

56.4 Professional Standards

It is widely shared that any action in the healthcare sector must be performed in accordance with the best practice and professional standards.

This principle is ratified in Article 4 of the Convention on Human Rights and Biomedicine.

> "Article 4—Professional standards Any intervention in the health field, including research, must be carried out in accordance with relevant professional obligations and standards."

Furthermore, the mentioned standards allowing and restricting medical diagnoses and treatments absolutely must be respected for a lot of reasons, and one of them is the constant progress of the medical knowledge and the operative techniques. Moreover, there is a wide range of healthcare quality, from minimal to high-quality standards.

Physicians have an obligation to examine and/or to treat a patient with all the knowledge and the skill that they possess reflecting the best practice according to the current state of the medical science. In determining diagnostic methods and treatments based on the most updated knowledge, there is often a choice of several possible measures which are (a) duty of care in deciding whether to undertake the case, (b) duty of care in deciding what treatment to give, and (c) duty of care in the administration of that treatment. It has to be highlighted that a breach of duty occurs when any of the above duties may give a cause of action for negligence [10].

The adherence to the guidelines, which may consider a medical case (that is not equivalent to the real one encountered in a specific case), is not mandatory [11]. Considering also that they do not cover every clinical situation that a physician can encounter, the guidelines, when available, together with the other scientific resources, are a precious help for the medical doctor, but they are never intended to be followed rigidly or uncritically.

However, even though their use is not compulsory for the clinician, the following scientific resources are of special relevance during trials concerning medical liability, they are often used by experts that take part to lawsuits/trials, and they are also expressly addressed by the members of the Court.

These scientific sources of non-equivalent relevance must also be graduated according to the source hierarchy shown below.

1. Guidelines.
2. Consensus documents.
3. Operational procedures.
4. Evidence-based publications.
5. National literature (medical treatises, etc.)

Though, these documents represent an opportunity for its use or misuse. Moreover, those adhering too strictly to guidelines may be charged with not adopting their best clinical judgment, whereas those deviating from guidelines may be accused of not applying accepted best practices.

In the UK, for instance, guidelines are published not only by scientific associations but also by the Royal College of Physicians, established as a point of reference of prime importance in comparative evaluation between ideal conduct and conduct actually followed by medical and/or healthcare personnel. However, failure to follow a guideline is never, by itself, an evidence of medical mistake. The key step in medical liability litigation is proving that the doctor did not meet the required standard of care, which may be inferred not only from guidelines but also from detailed analysis of all available scientific sources.

The medical literature is sometimes controversial, medications and technologies are in continuous progress, and patients themselves differ. Nonetheless, the Court will assess whether the physician breached his/her duty by doing (or not doing) something that "a reasonably prudent physician would do under similar circumstances."

In addition, the physician should take into account that the legal evaluation of medical responsibility and liability must be made according to the criteria of ex ante evaluation of a doctor's conduct, before the event, i.e., to imagine being in the same space–time circumstances in which the facts under examination took place, bearing in mind the characteristics of the medical and/or healthcare personnel involved (training, age, qualifications, and professional experience) and the technical and instrumental equipment at their disposal [8]. This evaluation is of prime importance in cases of surgical operations (with the intrinsic risk of complications and iatrogenic injuries) and medical treatments of particular technical difficulty. In Italy, the special technical difficulty is expressly mentioned in the civil code as a cause for justification. This circumstance often occurs in an emergency contest, in which the doctor is forced to operate in a critical situation and with unstable patients, and therefore characterized by a high mortality.

A systematic review of the professional adherence to guidelines and protocols in the emergency setting pointed out, interestingly, a higher adherence to diagnostic and organizational recommendations compared to recommendations regarding therapy and treatment [12]. This may indicate that the peculiar clinical context influences adherence to guidelines and protocol recommendations. There are various reasons why, especially in an emergency department, guidelines may not cover all the possible events; moreover, guidelines contain too many recommendations to adhere to, and it is, therefore, difficult to make choices very quickly, as an emergency setting requires. Guidelines for emergency purposes should be translated into more efficient, practical, and feasible protocols, algorithms, and decision trees.

56.5 Informed Consent in Emergency Care

Depending on the respective national legal system, a lot of laws and provisions regulate informed consent in a specific and detailed manner. The right of self-determination results in the right to autonomy with regard to one's own body and health. This consent represents whether, and to what degree, the person concerned allows at that time the medical intervention into his or her body. A patient's consent must be informed to be legally effective; it implies that it must be based on the awareness of the person about the treatment offered and has to be declared before the examination or treatment begins. In general, to give the patient the proper information, the physician must disclose the risks, benefits, and alternatives of the proposed intervention or treatment.

Moreover, to prove an act of true self-determination, the person to be examined must be consciously aware, capable of understanding, and prepared to bear the consequences of his or her decision. Consent also introduces a contract, which requires both disclosure and acceptance. Therefore, consent obtained in the absence of disclosure or from a patient with impaired decision-making capacity is not valid.

Emergency settings imply peculiar situations. The appropriate and valid consent often cannot be obtained, because of the acute clinical conditions of the patient and the necessity to proceed immediately with treatments. As stated in Article 8 of the Convention on Human Rights and Biomedicine (reported below), when because of an emergency situation the appropriate consent cannot be obtained, any medically necessary intervention may be carried out immediately for the benefit of the health of the individual concerned. However, advanced directives and their validity in their respective countries and other previously expressed wishes relating to a medical intervention by the patient also have to be taken into account (Article 9 of the Convention on Human Rights and Biomedicine).

> "Article 8—Emergency situation
> When because of an emergency situation the appropriate consent cannot be obtained, any medically necessary intervention may be carried out immediately for the benefit of the health of the individual concerned.
> Article 9—Previously expressed wishes
> The previously expressed wishes relating to a medical intervention by a patient who is not, at the time of the intervention, in a state to express his or her wishes shall be taken into account."

For emergency medicine specifically, the law acknowledges that uncritically imposing the obligation of informed consent may become deleterious to the patient's health and potentially to the patient's life. Therefore, the largest number of acknowledged exceptions to the doctrine of informed consent derives from the peculiarities in emergency medical circumstances. The general rule is that, in certain emergency medical situations, patient consent is presumed to exist for medical treatment that addresses the emergency [13].

Therefore, when immediate intervention is necessary to prevent death or serious harm to the patient, physicians may treat without having previously obtained the informed consent, when the patient lacks decision-making capacity, and when no one legally authorized to consent on behalf of the patient is available. Usually, relatives (spouse, sons, parents, etc.) are *NOT* authorized to consent on behalf of the patient. They can be informed if the patient agrees, but they never can take decisions about treatments or operations. In Italy, only transplants constitute an exception to this general rule.

The previously mentioned situations are a limited number of exceptions to the duty to obtain informed consent. When the initiation of treatment can be delayed without serious harm, informed consent must be obtained. Even if all the information needed for an informed consent cannot be provided, and the patient is not able to sign the specific form, emergency physicians should, to whatever extent time allows, inform the patient about the treatment they are providing and may not violate the explicit refusal of treatment of a patient with decision-making capacity.

A logical implication of the principles of informed consent is that the patient also has the right not to consent, that is, to refuse treatment. An example could be the refusal to undergo a blood transfusion for religious reasons.

Competent persons are generally permitted to refuse medical treatment, even at the risk of death. Notwithstanding, the essence of the medical profession lies in its fundamental commitment to the preservation of human life and health. Therefore, the right not to consent may represent a conflict for the doctor. Physicians must balance the legal duty of care against the legal and ethical respect for individual autonomy.

In such cases, documentation in the record of determination of capacity, the patient's medical condition, prognosis, and the basis of the no-treatment order is essential.

It is worthy to mention that in the setting of acute care and emergency surgery, the capacity of a patient may be compromised due to the influence of psychotropic medications, sleep deprivation, and depression. Therefore, these conditions have to be considered and documented. Sometimes, a psychiatric consultation can be necessary, to ascertain the presence of psychiatric conditions that can influence the patient's capacity. However, discussing such cases together with colleagues is always a good choice.

Case Scenario

On Saturday, a 73-year-old woman was admitted to the emergency department presenting nausea and dark vomiting going on for several hours. The patient also reported an episode of transient loss of consciousness.

The clinical evaluation did not point out anything remarkable, except abdominal tenderness. Laboratory investigations did not show any pathological results; no chest radiograph or abdominal echography was performed.

Considering the symptoms reported by the woman, a peptic ulcer disease with hematemesis was suspected, and the patient was informed about the need to undergo an esophagogastroduodenoscopy (EGDS). However, the procedure was planned for the following Monday, therefore 2 days after the symptoms begin.

In the next hours, the woman, in the meantime moved to a surgery department, complained of severe abdominal pain, associated with repeated dark vomiting. Details about the patient conditions were not reported on her medical journal, and no medical measures were taken, except for antisecretory drugs therapy and parenteral nutrition.

Suddenly, on Monday morning, the woman had several episodes of jet vomiting and became hemodynamically unstable, with a subsequent cardiorespiratory arrest. The patient could not be revived in spite of all resuscitative measures.

Thus, a forensic autopsy was performed to find out the actual cause of death. The gross examination revealed a wide-neck defect of the left diaphragm with herniation of the fundus of the stomach into the left thoracic cavity, covered by a membranous sheet of tissue (hernia sac). Only mild intrathoracic adhesions were present, and the herniated contents could be easily reduced to the abdomen. The size of the defect was 8 × 6 cm. An atelectasis of the left lung's lower lobe was also observed. The stomach presented an altered shape, without any other pathological finding, neither macroscopic nor microscopic. The gastric content consisted of partially digested food.

Therefore, the cause of death could be identified in a cardiorespiratory arrest due to the compression of the left lung and heart by the large diaphragmatic hernia. Similar cases, though rare, have been reported in literature [14].

Considering the cause of the death, provided by the evidence of the forensic autopsy, a medical mistake was pointed out regarding the diagnosis and treatment of this patient.

Although it is documented that the clinicians firstly addressed their suspects toward a peptic ulcer, focusing their choices entirely on this hypothesis, they failed in following the recommended protocol in case of hematemesis (that specifically suggests an EGDS within 24 h). Therefore, the doctors' behavior has to be considered negligent, as a huge abnormality like an exceptionally oversized diaphragmatic hernia was missed (Figs. 56.1 and 56.2).

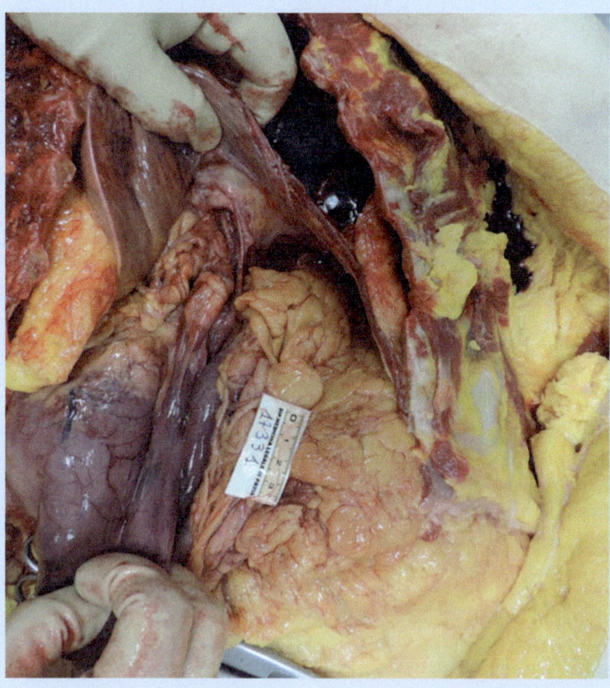

Fig. 56.1 The massive stomach herniation seen from the abdominal cavity during the autopsy

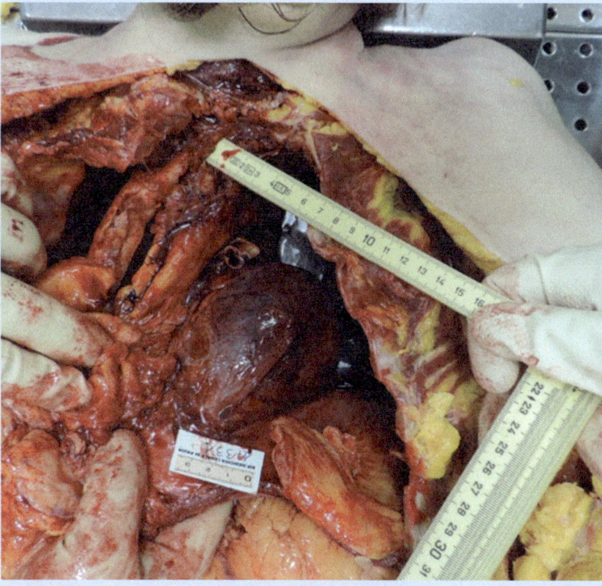

Fig. 56.2 The herniation of the stomach into the thorax through the large diaphragmatic defect observed during the autopsy

The death of the patient was preventable with an accurate physical examination and further diagnostic exams, which would have allowed an early diagnosis and the adequate treatment.

1. Which was the (possible) cause of death?
   A. Respiratory failure due to the impairment of the expansion of the left lung
   B. Hemorrhagic shock
   C. Cardiorespiratory arrest
   D. Cardiogenic shock
2. Which was the cause of the impairment of the expansion of the left lung?
   A. The large diaphragmatic hernia
   B. Respiratory failure
   C. Cardiac arrest
   D. Vomiting
3. Which was the medical mistake in the management of this patient?
   A. Not having followed the best practice and the diagnostic protocol in case of hematemesis.
   B. Lack of attention in the evaluation of the clinical pattern presented by the patient.
   C. Not having performed an accurate objective examination.
   D. All of the previous answers are correct.

Please see Chap. 58 for the correct answer.

References

1. Waxman DA, Greenberg MD, Ridgely MS, Kellermann AL, Heaton P. The effect of malpractice reform on emergency department care. N Engl J Med. 2014;371:1518–25.
2. Massachusetts Medical Society. Investigation of defensive medicine in massachusetts. Informational Report: I-08 – 02. http://www.massmed.org/defensivemedicine/.
3. Jena AB, Seabury S, Lakdawalla D, Chandra A. Malpractice risk according to physician specialty. N Engl J Med. 2011;365:629–36.
4. Brown TW, McCarthy ML, Kelen GD, Levy F. An epidemiologic study of closed emergency department malpractice claims in a national database of physician malpractice insurers. Acad Emerg Med. 2010;17:553–60.
5. Szalados JE. Legal issues in the practice of critical care medicine: a practical approach. Crit Care Med. 2007;35:S44–58.
6. Satyanarayana Rao KH. Informed consent: an ethical obligation or legal compulsion? J Cutan Aesthet Surg. 2008;1:33–5.
7. Dorney MS. Moore v. The Regents of the University of California: balancing the need for biotechnology innovation against the right of informed consent. Berkeley Technol Law J. 1990;5:333.
8. Ferrara SD. Medical malpractice and legal medicine. Int J Legal Med. 2013;127:541–3.
9. Stewart RM, Corneille MG, Johnston J, Geoghegan K, Myers JG, Dent DL, et al. Transparent and open discussion of errors does not increase malpractice risk in trauma patients. Ann Surg. 2006;243:645–9, discussion 649–51.
10. Pandit MS, Pandit S. Medical negligence: coverage of the profession, duties, ethics, case law, and enlightened defense—a legal perspective. Indian J Urol. 2009;25:372–8.
11. Madea B. Handbook of forensic medicine. Hoboken: Wiley; 2014.
12. Ebben RHA, Vloet LCM, Verhofstad MHJ, Meijer S, Mintjes-de Groot JAJ, van Achterberg T. Adherence to guidelines and protocols in the prehospital and emergency care setting: a systematic review. Scand J Trauma Resusc Emerg Med. 2013;21:9.
13. Hartman KM, Liang JDBA. Exceptions to informed consent in emergency medicine. Hosp Physician. 1999. http://www.turner-white.com/pdf/hp_mar99_emergmed.pdf.
14. Testini M, Girardi A, Isernia RM, De Palma A, Catalano G, Pezzolla A, Gurrado A. Emergency surgery due to diaphragmatic hernia: case series and review. World J Emerg Surg. 2017;12:23. https://doi.org/10.1186/s13017-017-0134-5.

Selective Use of Endovascular Techniques in the Damage Control Setting

57

Fabiane Barbosa, Ruggero Vercelli, Marco Solcia, Carmelo Migliorisi, and Antonio Rampoldi

Key Points

- Interventional radiology in damage control setting of the hemodynamically unstable trauma patients is an aggressive and time-restrained algorithm prioritizing saving life of the exsanguinating trauma patient.
- DCIR aims to control hemorrhage by any possible means to save life in an extremely time-conscious, aggressive and minimally invasive manner.
- The hybrid trauma room containing an angiography suite/operating room is a developing program around the world in the attempt to build new facilities to best hemorrhage control of DCIR treatment in severely injured trauma patients.
- The choice of materials, embolic agent, and the operator expertise are critical to the success of DCIR.
- DCIR belongs to a teamwork effort to maintain the patient alive in a very time-conscious procedure, and all decisions should be shared with the trauma team.

57.1 Introduction

The improvement of the acute trauma care workflow performed by a trained multidisciplinary team [1] and the increasing role of interventional radiology (IR) have been changing the management of severely injured patients [2]. Hemorrhage control is time critical, and delaying the operative intervention increases the mortality risks [3]. The hemorrhage control should occur as soon as possible [4], in a time-consciousness protocol to reduce coagulopathies and secondary compartment syndromes' risk [4–6].

Damage control interventional radiology (DCIR) is an aggressive and time-restrained algorithm that prioritizes saving life of the severely traumatized patient with ongoing hemorrhage [1] focusing on hemodynamically unstable patients. Different from DCIR, conventional emergency interventional radiology (CEIR) focuses on hemodynamically stable patients; however, both groups require distinct approaches, methods, and strategies.

The prompt and rapid endovascular strategies in trauma occasions (PRESTO) algorithm addresses and manages the trauma of severe acute hemorrhaging patient from the moment of arrival to the trauma bay until initial completion of hemostasis [1]. This algorithm is based on the motto "Start soon and finish sooner" and aims to shorten the timing of interventional radiology (IR) activation when compared to CEIR. It also relies on the rapid completion of hemostasis in hemodynamically unstable patients, specifically tailoring the damage control. The PRESTO/DCIR algorithm can successfully manage severely injured patients and can increase survival rates [2].

The term "damage control" is derived from the US Navy and describes the capacity of a ship to absorb damage and maintain mission integrity [7]. The concept of "damage control surgery" was developed in the early 1980s to reduce mortality in exsanguinating patients with coagulopathy [8]. In the management of traumatic hemorrhage, the risk of death is increased by a vicious cycle of hypothermia, coagulopathy, and metabolic acidosis known as the triad of death. The "damage control" approach reduces the mortality rate in severely injured patients [9–13]. It is a multistep strategy that aims to restore normal physiology over restoring normal anatomy in hemodynamically unstable patients, controlling but not definitively repairing the injury. Definitive surgery would only occur once all physiological parameters were corrected and normalized [14].

F. Barbosa (✉) · R. Vercelli · M. Solcia · C. Migliorisi
A. Rampoldi
Interventional Radiology, AAST Grande Ospedale metropolitano, Niguarda Hospital, Milan, Italy
e-mail: ruggero.vercelli@ospedaleniguarda.it; MARCO.SOLCIA@OspedaleNiguarda.it; CARMELO.MIGLIORISI@OspedaleNiguarda.it; ANTONIOGAETANO.RAMPOLDI@ospedaleniguarda.it

P. Aseni et al. (eds.), *Operative Techniques and Recent Advances in Acute Care and Emergency Surgery*, https://doi.org/10.1007/978-3-319-95114-0_57

DCIR focuses on hemodynamically unstable patients and aims to control hemorrhage by any possible means to save life in an extremely time-conscious, aggressive, and minimally invasive manner. According to PRESTO/DCIR [1], all procedures from catheterization to the final visual confirmation of embolization are to be completed within a 10-min window for each targeted vessel. The goal of DCIR is not to reach a perfect distal embolization but rather to contain the ongoing bleeding in the fastest way to maintain or re-establish normal hemodynamic values.

The DCIR also develops a crucial role in the presence of arterial hemorrhage after damage control laparotomy. Sometimes the arterial hemorrhage could not be controlled by correction of coagulopathy, and it requires an adjunctive endovascular intervention procedure such as transarterial embolization [15–18].

57.2 Principles, Tools, and Techniques of IR in the Setting of Trauma

It's important to record that DCIR belongs to a teamwork effort to maintain the patient alive in a very time-conscious procedure and all decision should be shared with the trauma team group. As in damage control surgery, the DCIR could be a multistep strategy that aims to maintain the patient alive over restoring normal anatomy, sometimes controlling but not definitively repairing the injury.

The choice of materials, embolic agent, and the operator expertise are critical to ultimate success. Smaller blood vessels typically require femoral access with a 5F sheath, distal catheterization with microcatheters, followed by deployment of microcoils, gel-foam slurry, beads, and glue, based on operator familiarity. In hemodynamically unstable trauma patients, the entity of trauma is usually bigger, and the IR must be more aggressive to save the life of the patient by rapidly controlling exsanguinating hemorrhage. An organ may be sacrificed as life matters most [1], and a balance needs to be struck between precision and suboptimal embolization [19–22]. As the procedure should be done in the shortest time possible, the expertise of IR and the ability with material play a crucial role.

Larger vessels (such as proximal internal iliac and splenic arteries) typically require femoral access with 5F or 6F sheaths followed by deployment of larger coils or Amplatzer plugs [23, 24]. For other arterial injuries, the placement of covered stent grafts is a valid option and usually requires sheath access that can be obtained, depending on the location of the injury, from either the femoral or brachial artery. Usually, femoral access is preferable because stent grafts require sheaths up to 7F or 8F and should be placed over the stiffest wire possible to allow for better support during deployment. The choice of self or balloon-expandible stent grafts depends on the type and the localization of the vascular lesion. Self-expandible stent grafts are more flexible and can be tracked easily through tortuous anatomy; they can conform to different diameters of a single vessel and should be oversized to reach an outward radial force for good vessel wall apposition. They also have higher resistance to crushing or deformation in mobile areas of the body and are produced in a greater range of diameters and lengths; for these reasons, they are more frequently used. Balloon-expandable stent grafts are ideal for immobile and well-protected areas of the body, such as renal, mesenteric, common iliac, and subclavian arteries, as well as ostial lesions. In addition, these stent grafts have higher precision in deployment compared to self-expanding stent grafts [23, 24].

When severely injured patients are hemodynamically unstable, the DCIR suggest abandoning any time-consuming procedure in favor of another for the sake of patient survival. Placing a temporary balloon catheter will maintain sufficient blood flow and pressure, whereby providing the physician enough time to assess and consult with trauma team whether to continue the IR procedure or not. It's important to remember that for an aortic balloon occlusion, it's necessary vascular access with sheaths up to 12Fr. During DCIR procedure, the operator is expected to reassess each maneuver every 5 min. In this setting, failing or time-consuming procedures (>5 min) should be discontinued and replaced by alternative procedures [1].

The use of a hybrid trauma room containing an angiography suite/operating room is the future trend to better DCIR treatment. A time rigorous and specifically designed protocol for hemodynamically unstable patients is crucial to successfully control time and consequently increase survival rates.

Case 1. Mediastinal Hematoma

Male 77 years old hemodynamically unstable with mediastinal hematoma with arterial blushing from the right bronchial artery. The mass effect of the hematoma determined atrial compression and atrial fibrillation (Figs. 57.1 and 57.2).

The right bronchial artery was super-selectively entered, and the embolization was performed with Glubran (Figs. 57.3 and 57.4).

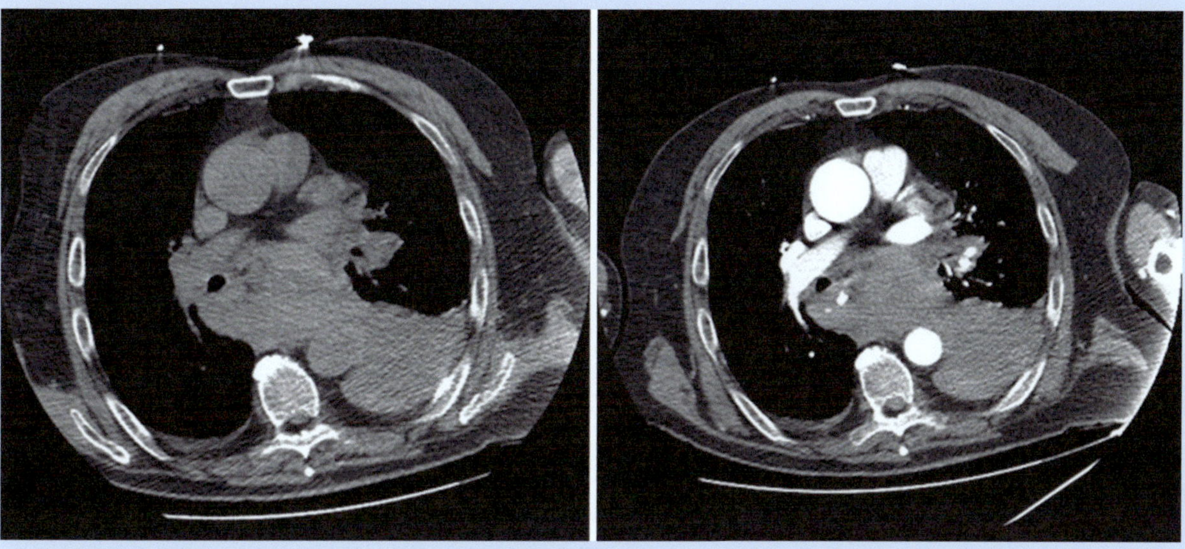

Figs. 57.1 and 57.2 Mediastinal axial CT with and without contrast

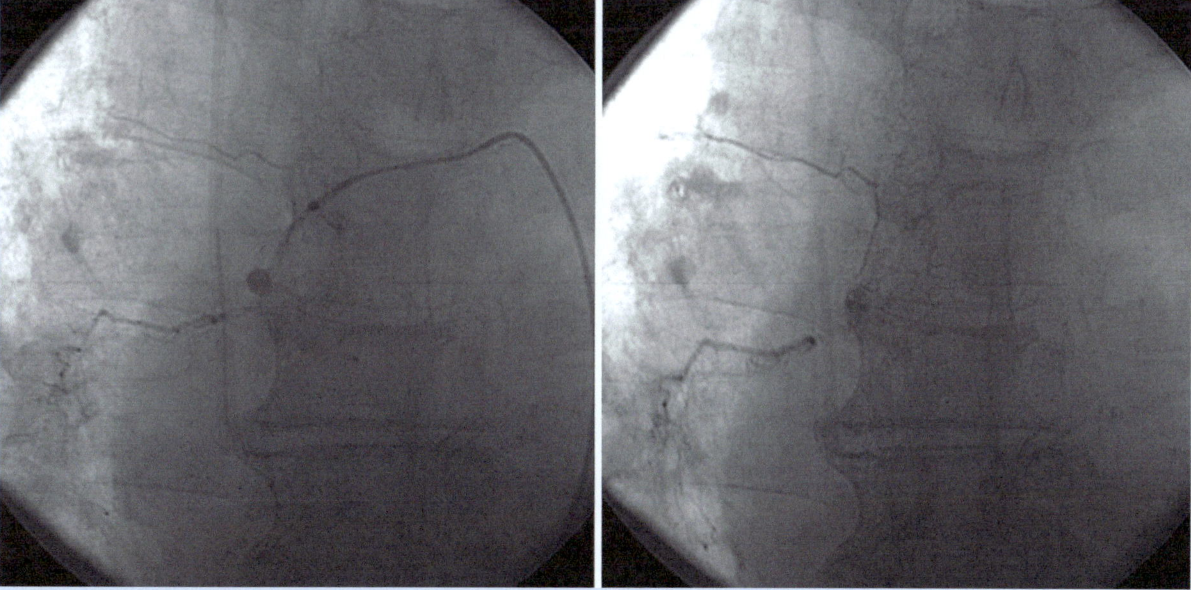

Figs. 57.3 and 57.4 Super-selective entering the right bronchial artery with microcatheter 2.7Fr. After embolization, imaging showing the occluded vessels

Case 2. Axillary Injury

Male 48 years old, hemodynamically unstable trauma with pneumothorax and axillary artery injury.

The angiography confirms the left axillary injury. A cover stent was placed to correct the axillary lesion.

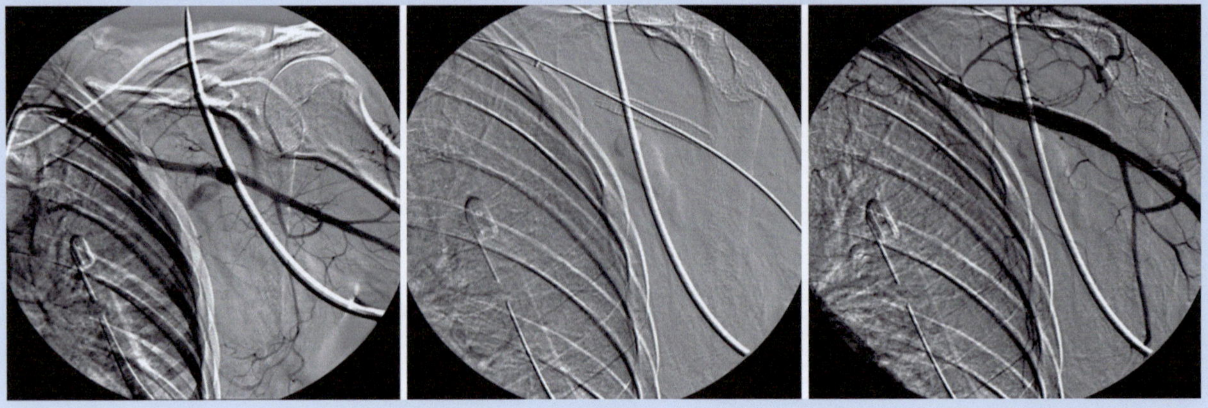

Case 3. Pelvic Fracture with Arterial Bleeding from Left Hypogastric Artery

Female 68 years old with a pelvic and femoral fracture. CT after pelvic packing shows arterial blushing. The angiography confirms blushing from left obturator artery, super-selective catheterization was quickly performed, and the pseudoaneurysm was occluded with Glubran.

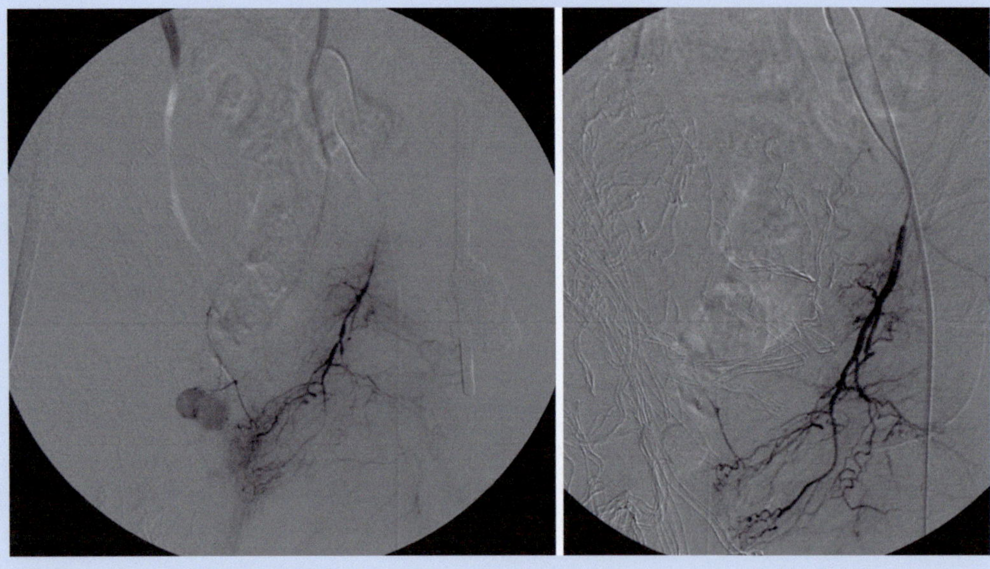

Case 4. Pelvic Fracture with Arterial Bleeding from Hypogastric Artery

Female 38 years old with pelvic fracture. The angiography shows blushing from right obturator artery; quick embolization was performed with Glubran.

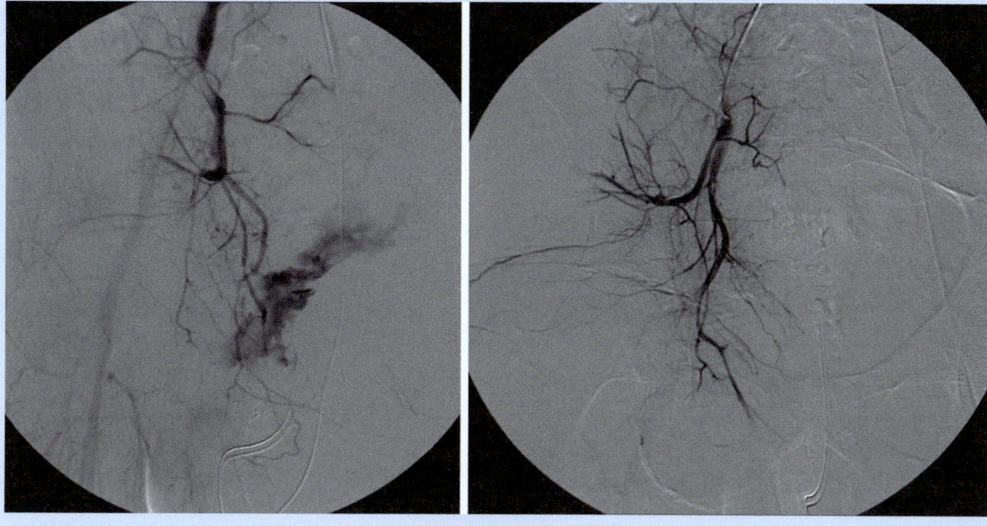

Case 5. Hepatic Injury

Male 50 years old, hemodynamically unstable after motorcycle polytrauma. The axial CT scan shows arterial blushing in the S7 hepatic segment. The angiography confirms the right hepatic blushing. Quick embolization was performed with Glubran. The patient developed a hepatic abscess that was drained; no hepatic dysfunction was observed later.

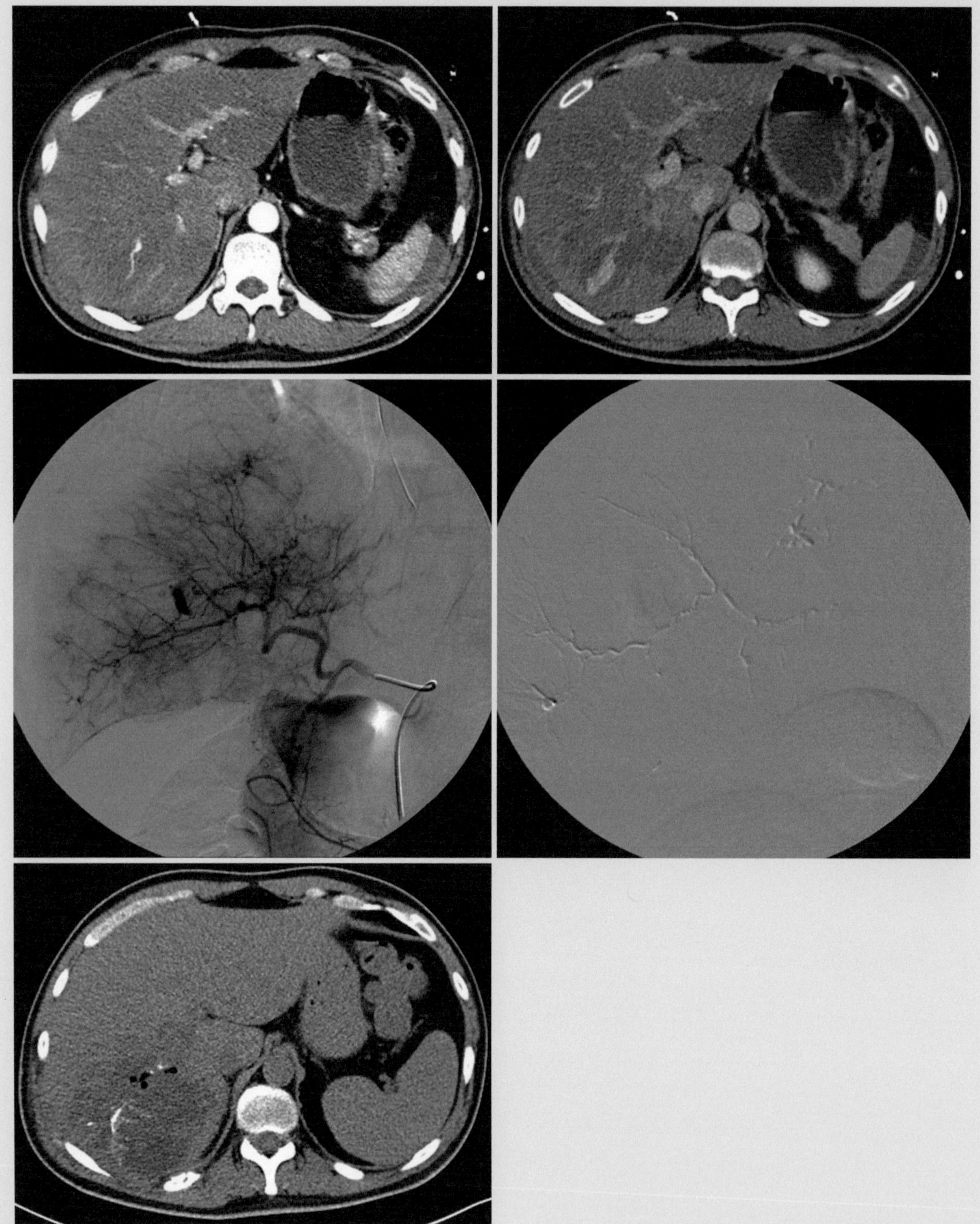

Case 6. Splenic Embolization

Male 66 years old, hemodynamically unstable polytrauma, after falling from the second floor. Axial CT scan shows a grade IV spleen lesion. The angiography confirms CT found. Quick embolization was performed with proximal splenic artery plug.

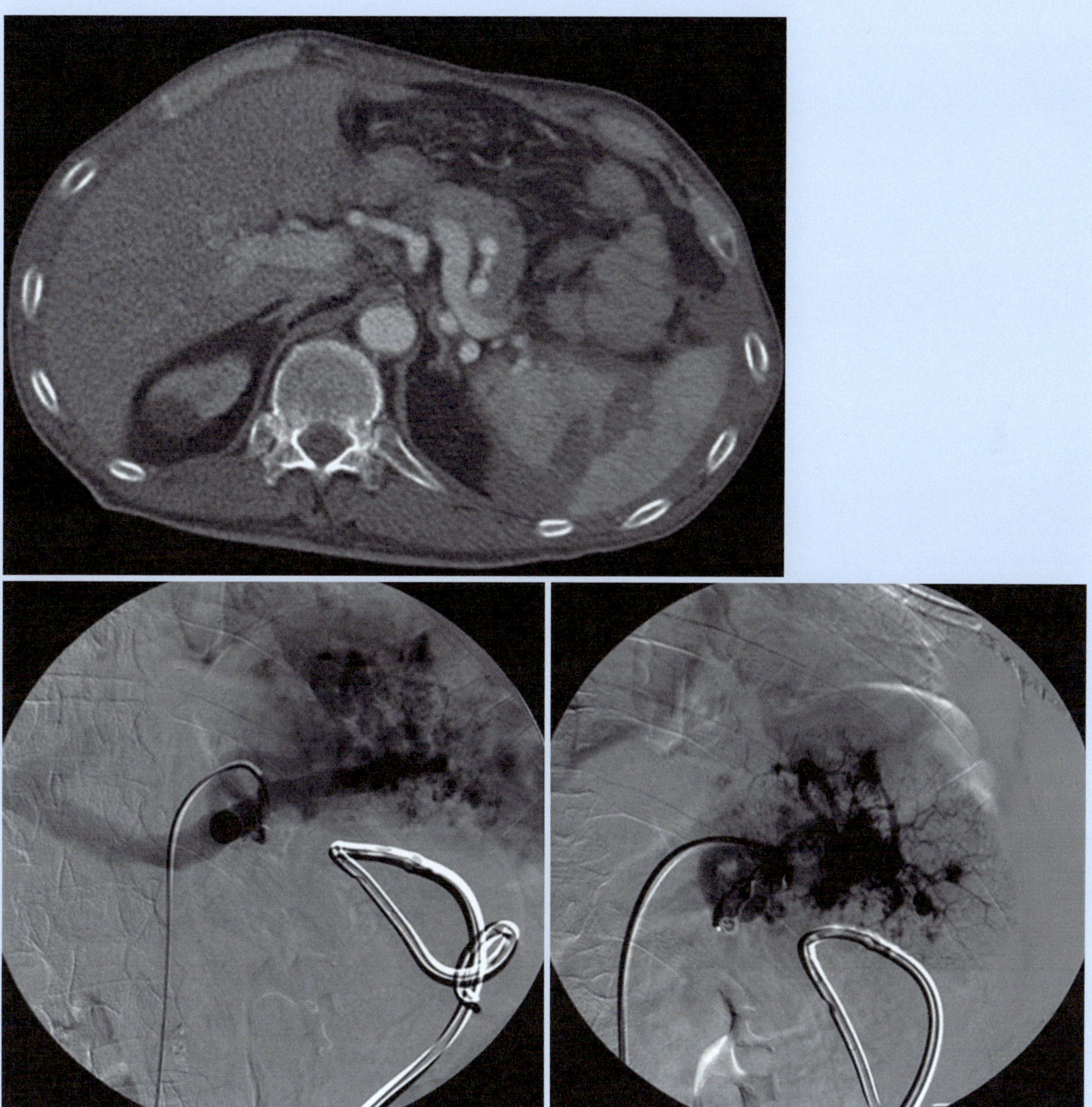

Case 7. Extremity Vascular Injuries

Male 30 years old, hemodynamically unstable polytrauma after a free fall. The angiography confirms the arterial blushing from deep femoral arterial with arteriovenous fistula. The branch was embolized with Glubran. The X-ray shows the Glubran occluding the vessel.

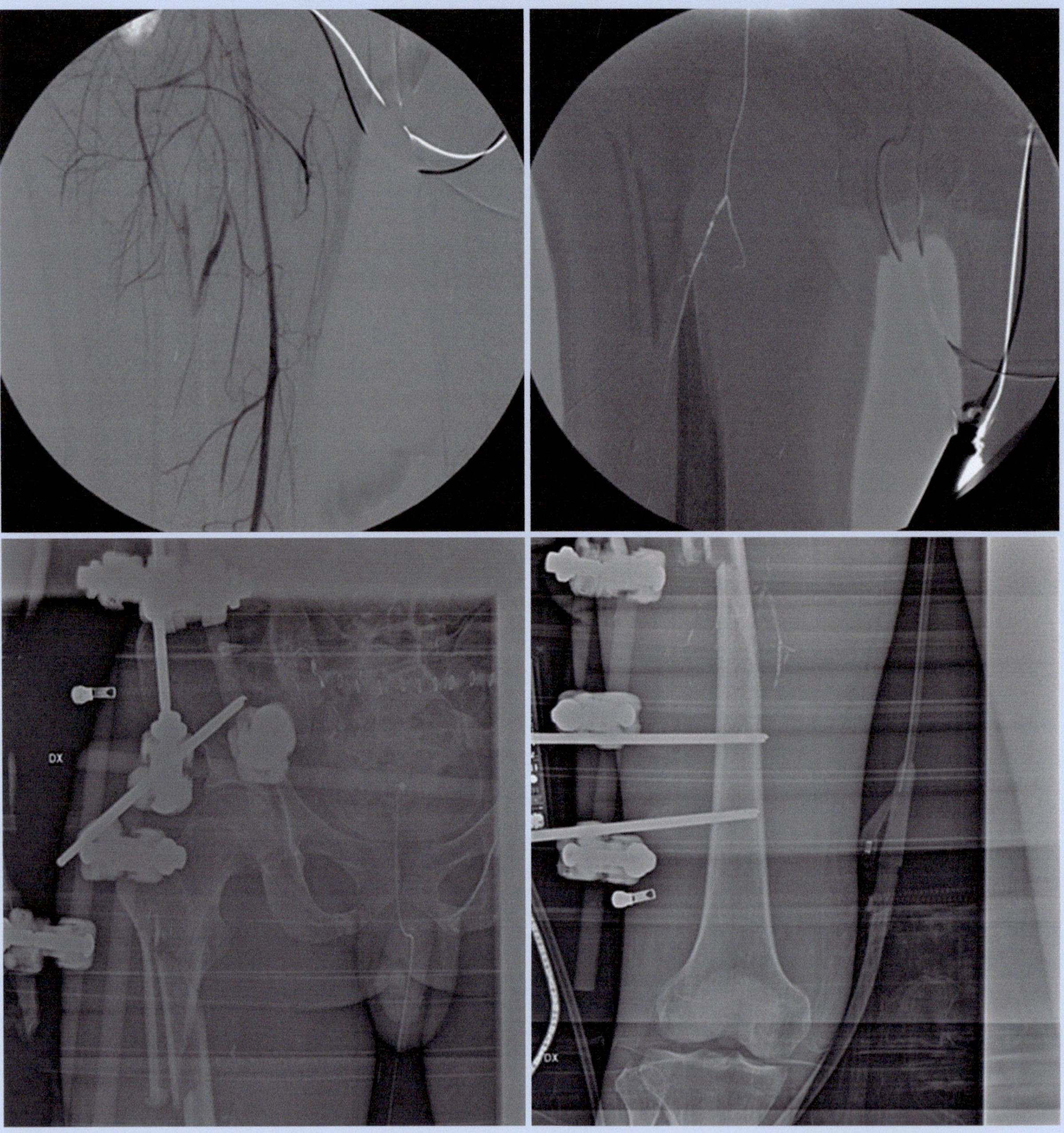

Case 8. Blunt Traumatic Thoracic Aortic Injury

Blunt thoracic aortic injury after a car accident in a hemodynamically unstable patient. Thoracic endovascular aortic repair (TEVAR) was performed.

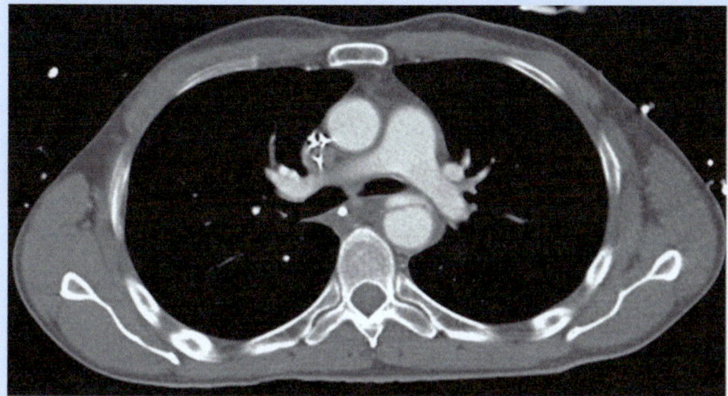

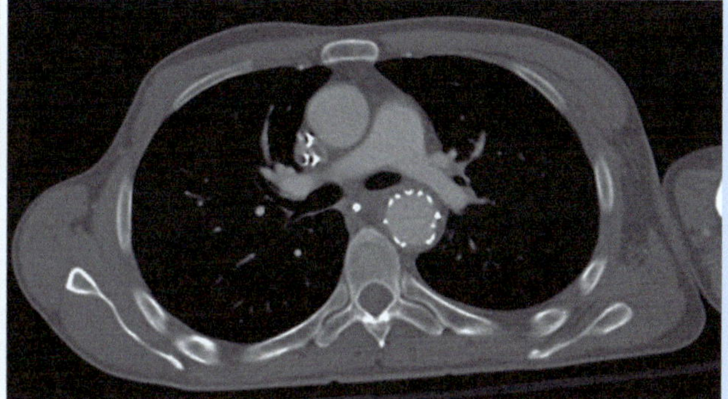

References

1. Matsumoto J, Lohmana BD, Morimotob K, Ichinoseb Y, Hattoric T, Taira Y. Damage control interventional radiology (DCIR) in prompt and rapid endovascular strategies in trauma occasions (PRESTO): a new paradigm. Diagn Interv Imaging. 2015;96:687–91.
2. Kinoshita T, Yamakawa K, Matsuda H, Yoshikawa Y, Wada D, Hamasaki T, Ono K, Nakamori Y, Fujimi S. The survival benefit of a novel trauma workflow that includes immediate whole-body computed tomography, surgery, and interventional radiology, all in one trauma resuscitation room: a retrospective historical control study. Ann Surg. 2017.
3. Clarke JR, Trooskin SZ, Doshi PJ, Greenwald L, Mode CJ. Time to laparotomy for intra-abdominal bleeding from trauma does affect survival for delays up to 90 min. J Trauma. 2002;52:420–5.
4. Kirkpatrick AW, Vis C, Dubé M, Biesbroek S, Ball CG, Laberge J, Shultz J, Rea K, Sadler D, Holcomb JB, Kortbeek J. The evolution of a purpose designed hybrid trauma operating room from the trauma service perspective: the RAPTOR (resuscitation with angiography percutaneous treatments and operative resuscitations). Injury. 2014;45(9):1413–21.
5. Kirkpatrick AW, Balogh Z, Ball CG, Ahmed N, Chun R, McBeth P, et al. The secondary abdominal compartment syndrome: iatrogenic or unavoidable? J Am Coll Surg. 2006;202(4):668–79.
6. Tremblay LN, Feliciano DV, Rozycki GS. Secondary extremity compartment syndrome. J Trauma. 2002;53:833–7.
7. Department of Defense. Surface ship survivability. Washington, DC: US Government Printing Office; 1996. Naval War Publication 3e20.31.
8. Stone HH, Strom PR, Mullins RJ. Management of the major coagulopathy with onset during laparotomy. Ann Surg. 1983;197(5):532–5.
9. Loveland JA, Boffard KA. Damage control in the abdomen and beyond. Br J Surg. 2004;91:1095–101.
10. Moore EE, Burch JM, Franciose RJ, et al. Staged physiologic restoration and damage control surgery. World J Surg. 1998;22:1184–90.
11. Pachter HL, Spencer FC, Hofstetter SR, et al. Significant trends in the treatment of hepatic trauma: experience with 411 injuries. Ann Surg. 1992;215:492–500.
12. Rotondo MF, Schwab CW, McGonigal MD, et al. 'Damage control': an approach for improved survival in exsanguinating penetrating abdominal injury. J Trauma. 1993;35:375–82.
13. Rotondo MF, Zonies DH. The damage control sequence and underlying logic. Surg Clin N Am. 1997;7:761–77.
14. Jaunoo SS, Harji DP. Damage control surgery. Int J Surg. 2009;7(2):110–3.
15. Lin BC, Wong YC, Lim KE, Fang JF, Hsu YP, Kang SC. Management of ongoing arterial haemorrhage after damage control laparotomy: optimal timing and efficacy of transarterial embolization. Injury. 2010;41(1):44–9.
16. Davis KA, Fabian TC, Croce MA, et al. Improved success in nonoperative management of blunt splenic injuries: embolization of splenic artery pseu-doaneurysm. J Trauma. 1998;44:1008–113.
17. Gorich J, Rilinger N, Brado M, et al. Non-operativemanagementof arterialliver hemorrhages. Eur Radiol. 1999;9:60–7.
18. Sclafani SJ, Shaftan GW, Scalea TM, et al. Non-operative salvage of computed tomography-diagnosed splenic injuries: utilization of angiography for triage and embolization for hemostasis. J Trauma. 1995;39:818–25, discussion 826–7.
19. Singh A, Kumar A, Kumar P, Kumar S, Gamanagatti S. "Beyond saving lives": current perspectives of interventional radiology in trauma. World J Radiol. 2017;9(4):155–77.
20. Wallis A, Kelly MD, Jones L. Angiography and embolization for solid abdominal organ injury in adults - a current perspective. World J Emerg Surg. 2010;5:18.
21. Lopera JE. Embolization in trauma: principles and techniques. Semin Intervent Radiol. 2010;27:14–28.
22. Bauer JR, Ray CE. Transcatheter arterial embolization in the trauma patient: a review. Semin Intervent Radiol. 2004;21:11–22.
23. Zhu X, Tam MD, Pierce G, McLennan G, Sands MJ, Wang W. Utility of the Amplatzer Vascular Plug in splenic artery embolization: a comparison study with conventional coil technique. Cardiovasc Intervent Radiol. 2011;34(3):522–31.
24. Kalish J. Selective use of endovascular techniques in the management of vascular trauma. Semin Vasc Surg. 2010;23(4):243–8.

Answers to Quizzes for "Case Scenario"

58

Paolo Aseni

(Q question, N number)

Chapter 2. Q N1: SIRS; Q N2: IL-1 and TNF; Q N3: Infection; Q N4: Balanced pro- and anti-inflammatory cytokines profile (MARS)

Chapter 3. Q N1: Hypovolemic shock; Q N2: Decreased venous return; Q N3: Fluids; Q N4: Dobutamine

Chapter 5. Q N1: 4) We should gather more indexes to assess his volemic status; Q N2: 2 and 4) Thermodilution, vena cava US evaluation; Q N3: 1 and 2) I would have gathered some preoperative information about patient's hemodynamic status; I would have gathered other intraoperative information about patient's hemodynamic status, rather than only diuresis, BP, and CVP; Q N4: 1 and 2) Preload and afterload; heart contractility and heart rate

Comments to the answers Q N1: 4. As mentioned before in this chapter, suggested indexes are not reliable enough in stating patient fluid responsiveness, and other indexes should be gathered. Q N2: 2 and 4: PLR or fluid challenge and lactates are good indexes of hemodynamic status. Vena cava US is not always feasible. This patient underwent colostomy. Therefore, abdominal US is probably not possible due to surgery wound. Even if thermodilution would be an option, in this circumstance, it is probably excessive (low ASA score, uncomplicated surgery). Q N3: 1 and 2) (Preemptive information about hemodynamic status is very important. Recognizing fluid deficit before surgery could have allowed a better preparation of patient and probably would have decreased patient total fluid needs. Intraoperative fluid replacement has been guided only on CVP, BP, and urine output. Other indexes (such as $ScvO_2$, dCO_2, lactates, etc.) should be gathered in order to better manage fluid therapy. As stated in paragraph 3.1 – Crystalloids – above in this chapter, balanced solutions such as Hartman's or Ringer's should be used rather than saline 0.9%.). Q N4: 1 and 2) (Cardiac output determinants are preload, afterload, heart contractility, and rate. Blood pressure, even though it may resemble afterload, should not be considered a direct determinant of cardiac output, while oxygen content is a determinant of tissue perfusion rather than cardiac output.)

Chapter 7. Q N1: B; Q N2: D; Q N3: C; Q N4: D; Q N5: A

Chapter 10. Q N1: C; Q N2: A; Q N3: D; Q N4: D; Q N5: B

Chapter 12. Q N1: Thorax drainage and simultaneous anterior nasal packing positioning; Q N2: Thin slice (1 mm or less) facial CT scan is the gold standard in middle third/orbital/complex facial fractures; its acquisition never significantly increases diagnostic time; Q N3: Performing anterior-posterior nasal packing with silicone dual-lumen devices with separate inflating balloons; Q N4: Facial damage control (manual reduction and temporary stabilization with iron wiring of bone fractures and suture of intra-extraoral wounds) must be done quickly and simultaneously to other maneuvers; Q N5: Diagnostic angiography and superselective embolization with coaxial microcatheter

Chapter 13. Q N1: Yes, but no MR if metallic foreign bodies were suspected; Q N2: Metallosis, due to toxicity of the IOFB, arousing in a few days

Chapter 14. Q N1: A; Q N2: A; Q N3: A

Chapter 15. Q N1: D (While the patient is complaining of difficulty breathing, he has a stable patent airway and normal oxygenation without evidence of impending loss of airway. Plain films of the cervical spine are not sufficient to rule out a cervical spine fracture. The widened mediastinum on chest X-ray is of concern for a vascular injury, and a CTA is the test of choice); Q N2: D (Provided his airway remains patent, he does not require intubation, rather close monitoring. Airway and esophagus should both be evaluated. Some institutions use gastrografin studies to evaluate the esophagus for perforations); Q N3: B (EAST guidelines recommend removal of the c-collar even in obtunded patients which may be safe with a normal CT of the cervical spine. As this is still controversial, it is still prudent to perform an MRI for persistent pain and midline tenderness to rule out

P. Aseni (✉)
Dipartimento di Emergenza Urgenza, ASST Grande Ospedale Metropolitano Niguarda, Milan, Italy

P. Aseni et al. (eds.), *Operative Techniques and Recent Advances in Acute Care and Emergency Surgery*,
https://doi.org/10.1007/978-3-319-95114-0_58

ligamentous injury); Q N4: B (While a large hematoma (D) is evidence of significant bleeding, it does not indicate an absolute indication to consider surgical exploration)

Chapter 16. Q N1: Surgical approach; Q N2: All the above answers are correct

Chapter 22. Q N1: D (FAST (focused assessment sonography for trauma) is mandatory in order to visualize pericardial, pleural, and peritoneal fluid. This diagnostic tool is rapid, easy to use, and accurate; if negative, it may be repeated later especially when cardiac lesions are highly suspected); Q N2: B (The patient is suddenly becoming unstable; immediate surgery is better after a second FAST in order to better localize the injury); Q N3: D (The best approach is considered a left thoracotomy and a transverse sternotomy with control of both internal thoracic arteries: the pericardial sac is opened longitudinally; transverse sternotomy allows better control of cardiac lesions and cardiopulmonary bypass use)

Chapter 23. Q N1: B; Q N2: A; Q N3: C; Q N4: D

Chapter 25. Q N1: B; Q N2: C; Q N3: A; Q N4: A; Q N5: C

Chapter 26. Q N1: A; Q N2: B; Q N3: C

Chapter 27. Q N1: F; Q N2: F; Q N3: E

Chapter 28. Q N1: A; Q N2: C; Q N3: D; Q N4: B and D

Chapter 30. Q N1: A; Q N2: B; Q N3: D

Chapter 31. Q N1: A; Q N2: E; Q N3: D; Q N4: C

Chapter 33. Q N1: A; Q N2: A; Q N3: A; Q N4: A; Q N5: A

Chapter 34. Case scenario N1: Q N1: A; Q N2: D. Case scenario N2: Q N1: B; Q N2: D

Chapter 35. Q N1: D (all the precedent answers are correct); Q N2: D (more than 3); Q N3: B (open **surgery**). **Self-Evaluation Questions**: Q N1: D; Q N2: D; Q N3: D

Chapter 36. Q N1: C; Q N2: D; Q N3: B; Q N4: E; Q N5: B

Chapter 38. (Case scenario N3). Q N1: Correct answers are both B and C. The patient should have good a chance of recovery of its cardiac function for her young age and because of immediate myocardial revascularization; in this case VA-ECMO can be positioned. If cardiac function recovery does not occur, the patient should be transferred to a longer term LVAD implantation and placed on a waiting list for a heart transplant. LVAD has the advantage to avoid patient's exposition to inflammatory effects of extracorporeal circulation; furthermore, LVAD allows a longer period of assistance. Anyway, VA-ECMO has the advantage to support also the right ventricle and the respiratory function. Q N2: Correct answers are A, B, and C, and all present advantages and disadvantages depending on the clinical conditions. In VA-ECMO, cannulation site may include central, right atrium-ascending aorta, or peripheral, femoral artery for blood return to the patient and femoral vein from drainage from inferior vena cava. Central cannulation presents the advantage of using the extracorporeal circulation cannulas, and it is avoided in the upper body hypoxemia and lower limb ischemia (femoral artery injury). In this case it is possible to insert a vent in the left superior pulmonary vein in order to prevent left ventricular distention. Peripheral cannulation has the advantage to close the chest, reducing bleeding and infection problems, and there is no need for chest reopening when the patient is weaned from assistance.

Chapter 39. Q N1: C; Q N2: A

Chapter 40. Q N1: A; Q N2: A

Chapter 41. Q N1: A; Q N2: C; Q N3: B; Q N4: B

Chapter 42. (Case report) Q N1: C; Q N2: D: Q N3: C; Q N4: C; Q N5: C

Chapter 44. Q N1: B; Q N2: A; Q N3: A; Q N4: A; Q N5: C

Chapter 45. Q N1: A; Q N2: B; Q N3: C; Q N4: B; Q N5: D

Chapter 46. Q N1: B; Q N2: D

Chapter 49. Q N1: D; Q N2: A; Q N3: D; Q N4: B; Q N5: B

Chapter 51. Part 1. Q N1: A; Q N2: C; Q N3: B. Part 2. Q N1: A; Q N2: C; Q N3: A

Chapter 52. Q N1: B; Q N2: B; Q N3: A

Chapter 53. Q N1: B; Q N2: B.

Comments to questions N 1 and N 2. Recirculation is the most probable reason for hypoxemia: the oxygenated return cannula is probably positioned in the right atrium near the inferior vena cava where the outflow cannula is draining the venous blood. Typically, in recirculation O_2 saturation in arterial blood is reduced while is high in the drainage line. The O_2 saturation difference between the arterial blood and the drainage line is too low, only 4%, suggesting a recirculation of blood in the right atrium. For this reason cannula position should be checked using transesophageal echocardiography. When there is a recirculation problem, no improvement is obtained by increasing circuit blood flow.

Chapter 54. Q N1: A; Q N2: A; Q N3: D

Chapter 56. Q N1: A; Q N2: A; Q N3: D

Corrections to: Updates in the Management of Anorectal Abscess and Inflammatory or Thrombotic Process

Andreas Ommer, Markus Noll, and Alois Fürst

Correction to:
P. Aseni et al. (eds.), *Operative Techniques and Recent Advances in Acute Care and Emergency Surgery*, https://doi.org/10.1007/978-3-319-95114-0_42

The original version of Chapter 42 was inadvertently published with same figure for figures 42.1 and 42.2. The chapter has been updated. Please find the updated figure 42.1 below, which is published in this version:

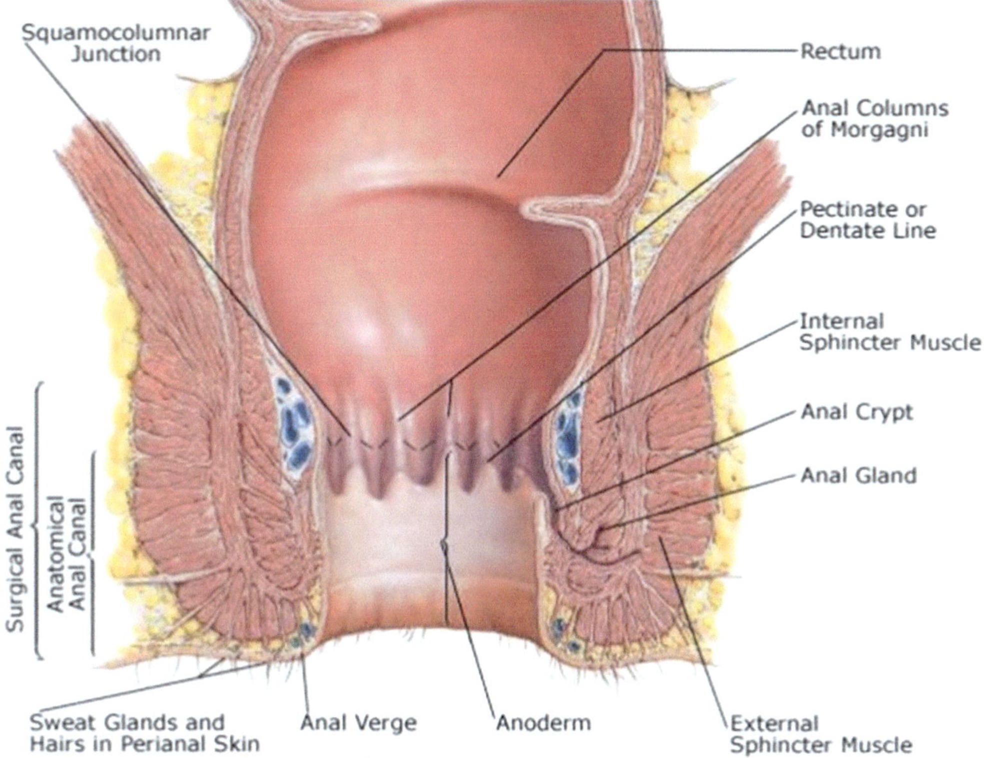

Fig. 42.1 Anatomy of the perianal region

The updated online version for this chapter can be found at https://doi.org/10.1007/978-3-319-95114-0_42

P. Aseni et al. (eds.), *Operative Techniques and Recent Advances in Acute Care and Emergency Surgery*,
https://doi.org/10.1007/978-3-319-95114-0_59

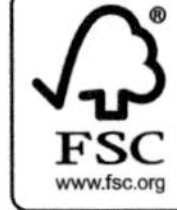

MIX
Papier aus verantwortungsvollen Quellen
Paper from responsible sources
FSC® C105338

If you have any concerns about our products,
you can contact us on
ProductSafety@springernature.com

In case Publisher is established outside the EU,
the EU authorized representative is:
Springer Nature Customer Service Center GmbH
Europaplatz 3, 69115 Heidelberg, Germany

Printed by Libri Plureos GmbH
in Hamburg, Germany